DATE DUE

GAYLORD			PRINTED IN U.S.A.

Cancer in Women

Cancer in Women

Edited by

JOHN J. KAVANAGH, MD
Professor of Medicine
Chief, Section of Gynecologic Medical Oncology
The University of Texas–MD Anderson Cancer Center
Houston, Texas

S. EVA SINGLETARY, MD
Professor of Surgery
Chief, Surgical Breast Section
Department of Surgical Oncology
The University of Texas–MD Anderson Cancer Center
Houston, Texas

NINA EINHORN, MD, PHD
Associate Professor of Gynecologic Oncology
Cancer Foreningen
Radiumhemmet
Karolinska Hospital
Stockholm, Sweden

A. DENNY DePETRILLO, MD, FRCS(C)
Professor, Obstetrics/Gynecology and Surgery
Director, Division of Gynecologic Oncology
Department of Obstetrics and Gynecology
University of Toronto
Toronto, Ontario
Canada

b
**Blackwell
Science**

Editorial Offices:
Commerce Place, 350 Main Street, Malden,
  Massachusetts 02148, USA
Osney Mead, Oxford OX2 0EL, England
25 John Street, London WC1N 2BL, England
23 Ainslie Place, Edinburgh EH3 6AJ, Scotland
54 University Street, Carlton, Victoria 3053, Australia

Other Editorial Offices:
Blackwell Wissenschafts-Verlag GmbH,
  Kurfürstendamm 57, 10707 Berlin, Germany
Blackwell Science KK, MG Kodenmacho Building, 7-
  10 Kodenmacho Nihombashi, Chuo-ku, Tokyo 104,
  Japan

Distributors:

USA
  Blackwell Science, Inc.
  Commerce Place
  350 Main Street
  Malden, Massachusetts 02148
  (Telephone orders: 800-215-1000 or 781-388-8250;
    fax orders: 781-388-8270)

Canada
  Login Brothers Book Company
  324 Saulteaux Crescent
  Winnipeg, Manitoba, R3J 3T2
  (Telephone orders: 204-224-4068)

Australia
  Blackwell Science Pty, Ltd.
  54 University Street
  Carlton, Victoria 3053
  (Telephone orders: 03-9347-0300;
    fax orders: 03-9349-3016)

Outside North America and Australia
  Blackwell Science, Ltd.
  c/o Marston Book Services, Ltd.
  P.O. Box 269
  Abingdon
  Oxon OX14 4YN
  England
  (Telephone orders: 44-01235-465500;
    fax orders: 44-01235-465555)

Acquisitions: Christopher Davis
Production: Irene Herlihy
Manufacturing: Lisa Flanagan
Cover Design: Meral Dabcovich, Visual Perspectives
Typeset by Best-set Typesetter Ltd., Hong Kong
Printed and bound by Braun-Brumfield, Inc.

Printed in the United States of America
98 99 00 01 5 4 3 2 1

Library of Congress Cataloging-in-Publication Data
Cancer in women/edited by John J. Kavanagh . . . [et al.].
     p. cm.
     Includes bibliographical references and index.
     ISBN 0-86542-465-9
     1. Cancer in women. I. Kavanagh, John J.
     [DNLM: 1. Genital Neoplasms, Female. 2. Breast
Neoplasms.   WP 145 C214 1997]
RC281.W65C35   1998
616.99′4′0082—dc21
DNLM/DLC
for Library of Congress   97-43312
                                    CIP

Contents

PART III
Psychosocial and Genetic Aspects

547

List of Contributors

Vera M. Abeler, MD, PhD
Section of Pathology
The Norwegian Radium Hospital
Oslo, Norway

Ingrid Ambus, BA
Research Assistant
Princess Margaret Hospital
Toronto, Ontario
Canada

Sirpa Asko-Seljavaara, MD
Professor and Chief
Department of Plastic Surgery
Helsinki University Central Hospital
Toolo Hospital
Helsinki, Finland

Ahmad Awada, MD
Medical Oncology
Jules Bordet Institute
The University of Brussels
Brussels, Belgium

Richard H. J. Begent, MD, FRCP
Professor of Clinical Oncology
Royal Free Hospital School of Medicine
London, England

John L. Benedet, MD, FRCS(C)
Professor and Head, Department of
    Obstetrics and Gynecology
University of British Columbia;
Head, Division of Gynecologic Oncology
BC Cancer Agency
Vancouver, British Columbia
Canada

**Andrea Bezjak, BMed Sc, MDCM, MSc,
    FRCP(C)**
Assistant Professor
Department of Radiation Oncology
University of Toronto;
Radiation Oncologist
Department of Radiation Oncology
Princess Margaret Hospital/Ontario Cancer
    Institute
Toronto, Ontario
Canada

Diane C. Bodurka, MD
Department of Gynecologic Oncology
The University of Texas–MD Anderson
    Cancer Center
Houston, Texas

Peter Boyle, MD
Division of Gynecology
European Institute of Oncology
Milan, Italy

Molly A. Brewer, DVM, MD
Department of Gynecologic Oncology
The University of Texas–MD Anderson
    Cancer Center
Houston, Texas

Aman U. Buzdar, MD
Internist and Professor of Medicine
Deputy Chairman
Department of Breast and Gynecologic
    Medical Oncology
The University of Texas–MD Anderson
    Cancer Center
Houston, Texas

**David E. C. Cole, MD, PhD, FCCMG,
    FRCP(C)**
Associate Professor
Departments of Laboratory Medicine
    and Pathobiology, Medicine and
    Paediatrics
University of Toronto;
Director, TTH Genetic Repository;
Geneticist, Familial Ovarian Cancer Clinic
The Toronto Hospital
Toronto, Ontario
Canada

**John E. Cullimore, MD, MRCOG,
    FRCSEd**
Consultant Obstetrician and Gynecologist
Princess Margaret Hospital
Swindon, Wiltshire
England

Daniel Dargent, MD
Professor
Hôpital E. Herriot
Lyon, France

Luis Delclos, MD, FACR
Professor of Radiotherapy
Margaret and Ben Love Professorship in
    Clinical Cancer Care in Honor of Dr.
    Charles A. LeMaistre
Department of Radiation Oncology
The University of Texas–MD Anderson
    Cancer Center
Houston, Texas

A. Denny DePetrillo, MD, FRCS(C)
Professor, Obstetrics/Gynecology and
    Surgery
Director, Division of Gynecologic Oncology
Department of Obstetrics and Gynecology
University of Toronto
Toronto, Ontario
Canada

Kapil Dhingra, MD
Assistant Professor of Medicine
Department of Breast Medical Oncology
The University of Texas–MD Anderson
    Cancer Center
Houston, Texas

Eleni Diamandidou, MD
Junior Faculty Associate
Department of Medical Breast Oncology
The University of Texas–MD Anderson
    Cancer Center
Houston, Texas

Brian D. Doan, PhD
Consulting Psychologist
Toronto-Sunnybrook Regional Cancer Centre
North York, Ontario
Canada

Creighton L. Edwards, MD
Professor of Gynecology
Ann Rife Cox Chair
Department of Gynecologic Oncology
The University of Texas–MD Anderson
    Cancer Center
Houston, Texas

Nina Einhorn, MD, PhD
Associate Professor of Gynecologic
    Oncology
Cancer Foreningen
Radiumhemmet
Karolinska Hospital
Stockholm, Sweden

Harold Fox, MD, FRCPath, FRCOG
Emeritus Professor of Reproductive
    Pathology
Department of Pathological Sciences
University of Manchester
Manchester, England

Ralph S. Freedman, MD, PhD
Professor of Gynecologic Oncology
Gynecologist
Department of Gynecologic Oncology
Director of Immunology and Molecular
    Biology Laboratory
The University of Texas–MD Anderson
    Cancer Center
Houston, Texas

Peter T. Grant, MD
Gynecological Cancer Center
Royal Hospital for Women
Randwick, Australia

Neville F. Hacker, MD
Director, Gynecologic Oncology
Gynecological Cancer Center
Royal Hospital for Women
Randwick, Australia

Stacey Hart, PhD
Postdoctoral Fellow
Department of Psychology and Behavioral
    Sciences
Stanford University School of Medicine
Palo Alto, California

A. Peter M. Heintz, MD, PhD
Professor, Department of Obstetrics and
    Gynecology
Gynecological Oncology Center
University of Utrecht
Utrecht, The Netherlands

Frankie Ann Holmes, MD
Adjunct Associate Professor of Medicine
Department of Breast Medical Oncology
The University of Texas–MD Anderson
    Cancer Center;
Texas Oncology, P.A.
Houston, Texas

Lovell A. Jones, PhD
Department of Gynecology
The University of Texas–MD Anderson
    Cancer Center
Houston, Texas

John J. Kavanagh, MD
Professor of Medicine
Chief, Section of Gynecologic Medical
    Oncology
The University of Texas–MD Anderson
    Cancer Center
Houston, Texas

Joseph Kerger, MD
Medical Oncology
Jules Bordet Institute
The University of Brussels
Brussels, Belgium

Kjell E. Kjørstad, MD, PhD
Professor
Department of Gynecology
University of Tromsø
Tromsø, Norway

Stephen S. Kroll, MD
Professor of Plastic Surgery
Department of Plastic Surgery
The University of Texas–MD Anderson
    Cancer Center
Houston, Texas

Andrzej P. Kudelka, MD
Clinical Investigations
Section of Gynecologic Medical Oncology
The University of Texas–MD Anderson
    Cancer Center
Houston, Texas

Lars-Gunnar Larsson, MD
Center of Oncology
University of Umea
Umea, Sweden

Beth Leedham, PhD
Research Associate
Division of Cancer Prevention and Control
    Research
UCLA Jonsson Comprehensive Cancer
    Center
Los Angeles, California

Seymour H. Levitt, MD
Professor and Head
Department of Therapeutic Radiology–Radiation Oncology
University of Minnesota Medical School
Minneapolis, Minnesota

Patrick Maisonneuve, MD
Division of Gynecology
European Institute of Oncology
Milan, Italy

Beth E. Meyerowitz, PhD
Associate Professor
Department of Psychology
University of Southern California
Los Angeles, California

C. Paul Morrow, MD
Charles F. Langmade Professor of Obstetrics and Gynecology
Director of Gynecologic Oncology
University of Southern California School of Medicine
Women's Hospital
Los Angeles, California

Monica Morrow, MD
Professor of Surgery
Northwestern University Medical School;
Director
Lynn Sage Comprehensive Breast Center
Northwestern Memorial Hospital
Chicago, Illinois

K. Joan Murphy, MD
Division of Gynecologic Oncology
Department of Obstetrics and Gynecology
University of Toronto
Toronto, Ontario
Canada

Louise Murphy, BSc
Research Assistant
Princess Margaret Hospital
Toronto, Ontario
Canada

Folke Pettersson, MD, PhD
Gynecologic Oncology
Radiumhemmet
Karolinska Hospital
Stockholm, Sweden

Martine J. Piccart-Gebhart, MD, PhD
Medical Oncology
Head of Chemotherapy Unit
Jules Bordet Institute
The University of Brussels
Brussels, Belgium

Chris D. Platsoucas, PhD
Professor and Chairman
Department of Microbiology and Immunology
Temple University School of Medicine
Philadelphia, Pennsylvania

Jane Poulson, MD, Msc, MDCM, FRCP(C)
Assistant Professor
Department of Medicine
University of Toronto;
Division of General Internal Medicine and Palliative Care
The Toronto Hospital and The Toronto Grace Hospital
Toronto, Ontario
Canada

Ralph M. Richart, MD
Division of Ob/Gyn Pathology
The Sloane Hospital for Women
New York, New York

Barry Rosen, MD
Division of Gynecologic Oncology
Department of Obstetrics and Gynecology
University of Toronto
Toronto, Ontario
Canada

Josée-Anne Roy, MD
Medical Oncology
Jules Bordet Institute
The University of Brussels
Brussels, Belgium

Gordon J. S. Rustin, MD, MSc, FRCP
Director of Medical Oncology
Mount Vernon Hospital
Northwood, Middlesex
England

Eva Rylander, MD, PhD
Professor
Karolinska Institutet;
Division of Obstetrics and Gynaecology
Danderyd Hospital
Stockhom, Sweden

S. Eva Singletary, MD
Professor of Surgery
Chief, Surgical Breast Section
Department of Surgical Oncology
The University of Texas–MD Anderson
   Cancer Center
Houston, Texas

Akira Sugimoto, MD, FRCP(C)
Obstetrics and Gynecology
London Health Science Centre
London, Ontario
Canada

Winston Tam, MD
Department of Obstetrics and Gynecology
University of Toronto
Toronto, Ontario
Canada

Kathryn M. Taylor, PhD
Research Associate Professor
Director of Cancer Risk Information
   Network
York University and Princess Margaret
   Hospital
Toronto, Ontario
Canada

Gillian Thomas, BSc, MD, FRCP(C)
Professor, Department of Radiation Oncol-
   ogy and Obstetrics and Gynecology
University of Toronto;
Head, Division of Radiation Oncology
Toronto-Sunnybrook Regional Cancer Centre
Toronto, Ontario
Canada

Leslee J. Thompson, RN, MScN
Independent Health Care Consultant
Edmonton, Alberta
Canada

Damrong Tresukosol, MD
Department of Obstetrics and Gynecology
Faculty of Medicine
Chulalongkorn University Hospital
Bangkok, Thailand

Apichai Vasuratna, MD
Department of Obstetrics and Gynecology
Faculty of Medicine
Chulalongkorn University Hospital
Bangkok, Thailand

Umberto Veronesi, MD
Scientific Director
European Institute of Oncology
Milan, Italy

Claire F. Verschraegen, MD
Assistant Professor
Section of Gynecologic Medical
   Oncology
The University of Texas–MD Anderson
   Cancer Center
Houston, Texas

Victor G. Vogel, MD, MHS, FACP
Professor of Medicine and Epidemiology
Director, Comprehensive Breast Program
The University of Pittsburgh Cancer
   Institute and The Magee-Womens
   Hospital
Pittsburgh, Pennsylvania

J. Taylor Wharton, MD
Professor of Gynecology
Department of Gynecologic Oncology
Charles B. Baker Chair in Surgery
The University of Texas–MD Anderson
   Cancer Center
Houston, Texas

Preface

Oncologists in all fields now recognize the complexity of their practices. The proliferation of scientific knowledge, particularly molecular biology, has offered new insight into understanding malignancies; however, the conceptualization of such knowledge is often difficult for the practicing physician. In addition, the busy clinician finds it impossible to place the scientific background in a proper perspective owing to the rapidity of translational laboratory developments. Multidisciplinary care is a clear trend that involves meaningful communication among all the major specialists managing the cancer patient. Such communication requires that the specialists acquire a functional amount of knowledge in each other's field. The evolution of women's health care has also necessitated a greater knowledge and understanding on the part of the caregivers to facilitate a more comprehensive approach. The roles of the various specialties in the management of gynecologic and breast malignancies are dynamic, and it is helpful to all individuals, including the patient, if there is a basic understanding of the disease processes and management.

The age of information technology has truly made the practice of medicine an international phenomenon. Clinical expertise and academic accomplishments throughout the world are substantive and worthy of attention. Yet the literature is replete with specialty or regionally dominated publications. The future will undoubtedly be one of international collaboration. Finally, the foundation of all our practices is based on a value structure that evolves in communication with our patients. There is a need for understanding of not only the qualities that make life meaningful, but a sensitivity towards

the end of life. Initially, the text provides a conceptually based scientific framework that is expansive rather than pedantic. The editors urge an understanding of, and an empathy for, the psychosocial and palliative issues that confront all of us in the daily care of our patients. Above all, this textbook is aimed towards providing a functional but sufficiently detailed knowledge for understanding and managing breast and gynecologic cancers.

The book is divided into three major sections: 1) a succinct graphic presentation of the biologic, molecular, and immunologic mechanisms concerned with the diseases; 2) clinically based knowledge for the management of breast and gynecologic malignancies, including special topics, such as the use of laparoscopy; 3) psychosocial-based issues, including palliative care. The text is not meant to be a technical manual for the teaching of radiation therapy or surgical techniques. We feel that these are better addressed in other formats, particularly the classical teacher–student relationship. In addition, tables are used, but to a moderate degree. It is felt that the reference list and other encyclopedic-type texts provide such information. The organization provides a thoughtful and functional knowledge flow for individuals, either in training or in practice, where breast and gynecologic cancer patients are within their scope.

The other major editors (Dr. S. Eva Singletary, Dr. Nina Einhorn, Dr. A. Denny DePetrillo) are recognized authorities in their respective fields. In addition, they represent diverse medical specialty backgrounds. By their nature, these individuals were selected for their in-depth knowledge and basic sense of fairness in dealing with controversial issues. Their task was to ensure that it was not a particular philosophy of care that was expressed, but an equitable presentation of various aspects with adequate references for individual reader deliberation. It is of note that the editors represent a significant body of clinical and academic experience and are known to be excellent practitioners in their field. I express my heartfelt appreciation to the editors for their hard work and thoughtful attention to the textbook.

The editors wish to express their appreciation to all the contributors for the excellent chapters that were provided. In addition, all the authors were very flexible and cooperative in the extensive revision process. I would particularly like to express my thanks and appreciation to Pat Thomas for the organizational aspects of the book. Chris Davis, the executive editor from Blackwell Science, was also very helpful in guiding the project to its completion.

John J. Kavanagh, MD

PART I

Basic Science Principles

CHAPTER 1

Biology of Gynecologic Cancers

CLAIRE F. VERSCHRAEGEN
KAPIL DHINGRA
LOVELL A. JONES

Female gender is determined in utero by estrogenic steroidal influences (Fig. 1-1). Feminization is necessary to develop the complex reproductive apparatus needed for successful pregnancy. The ovary is the reservoir of fertilizable ova and furthermore, regulates the normal menstrual cycle. The uterus provides the milieu for fetal growth and the mammary gland is necessary to sustain the life of the newborn. The reproduction process is only feasible under specific hormonal conditions that modulate the development of the reproductive tract to achieve this goal. We describe the basic endocrinology processes occurring in normal women.

As with any anatomic organs, the reproductive tract and the breasts may potentially be the site of a neoplastic process. Breast cancer is the most frequent cancer of women, affecting one woman in seven (1). Of all pelvic gynecologic cancers, ovarian cancer affects 1 woman in 70 over a lifetime (1). In the United States, 50,000 and 14,000 deaths are attributable each year to breast and ovarian cancers, respectively. How the hormonal environment affects cancer growth is the main subject of this chapter.

During the development of the genital tract, three different types of epithelia come into contact with each other in a small area, and changes occur in the epithelia themselves. Stromal-epithelial interactions are essential for inductive processes and expression of hormonal responses. The müllerian (or paramesonephric) duct develops in a position parallel to each mesonephric duct. The mesonephros and the paramesonephros form the urogenital ridge. In males, the müllerian ducts degenerate in response to the testicular antimüllerian hormones. The most cranial part of the ducts resists degeneration and persists as the appendix testis. The most caudal part participates in the development of the prostatic utricle. In females, the absence of müllerian inhibitory substance allows the paramesonephric ducts to originate the fallopian tubes and the uterus. The cranial portions of the paramesonephric ducts become uterine tubes, with cranial openings into the coelomic cavity persisting as the fimbriated ends. Toward their caudal ends, the paramesonephric ducts approach the midline and cross ventral to the mesonephric ducts. This crossing and ultimate meeting in the midline are caused by the medial migration of the entire urogenital ridge. The region in the midline fusion of the paramesonephric ducts becomes the uterus, and the ridge tissue that is carried along with the paramesonephric ducts forms the broad ligament of the uterus. The blind, caudal ends of the paramesonephric and mesonephric ducts reach the urogenital sinus and form the müllerian (or sinus) tubercle. Morphologic, histochemical, and autoradiographic studies revealed that the development of the vaginal epithelium in mouse and rat is of dual origin. In the human, the fused paramesonephric ducts form the upper part of the vagina, and epithelial tissue from the dorsal wall of the urogenital sinus, close to the müllerian tubercle, hollows out to form the lower part. The development of the vagina is also under hormonal control. Indirect evidence has implicated diethylstilbestrol in the etiology of clear-cell vaginal cancers in the female offspring of pregnant mothers exposed to this drug.

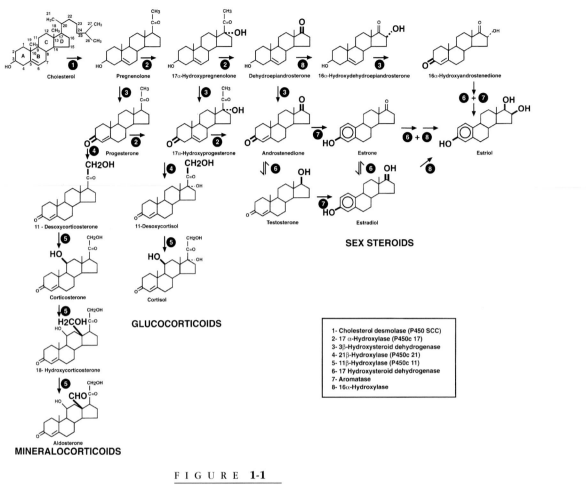

F I G U R E **1-1**

Enzymatic pathways of steroidogenesis.

As the child goes through puberty, the ovaries grow to their adult form. Each month, under the influence of multiple hormones, one dominant follicle matures and releases an ovum ready to be fertilized. Figure 1-2 shows the classic hormonal variations during the menstrual cycle. Figure 1-3 shows the ovarian structure during the different phases of the menstrual cycle. All parts of the ovary except perhaps the surface epithelium are able to secrete the same steroids (progesterone, androstenedione, testosterone, 5α-dihydrotestosterone, estrone, and estradiol) (2). However, the production of these steroids varies with the stage of maturation and the local microenvironment. In vivo the interaction between the three ovarian compartments (theca, follicle, and stroma) directs steroid production. It is accepted that the theca produces the androgen precursors that will be used by the granulosa to make estrogens (3). Because of the presence of a basal membrane between the theca and the granulosa, the follicle receives only steroids produced by the theca (4). In particular, steroids are made from low-density-lipoprotein (LDL) cholesterol brought by the blood supply which cannot cross this barrier. Therefore, steroidogenesis in the granulosa is started from androgen precursors delivered by the theca (5). There is a definite coregulation of gonadotropins and steroids and their respective receptors, which leads to ovulation.

The surface epithelium of the ovary covers the ovary as a continuous sheet. It is disrupted every month by ovulation, which opens this sheet of cells. Repair occurs in 2 to 4 days but leaves a scar. Whether this epithelium is hormonally receptive or productive is not clear (6).

During the menstrual cycle, the cyclical alterations in the hormonal milieu of the breast are associated with profound alterations in the morphology and function of breast epithelium

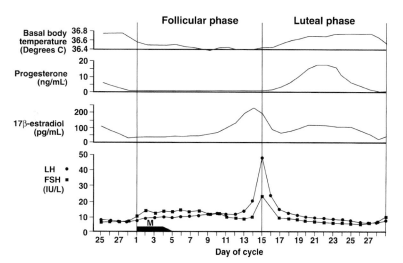

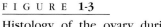

Physiologic variations during the menstrual cycle. LH = luteal phase; FSH = follicle-stimulating hormone.

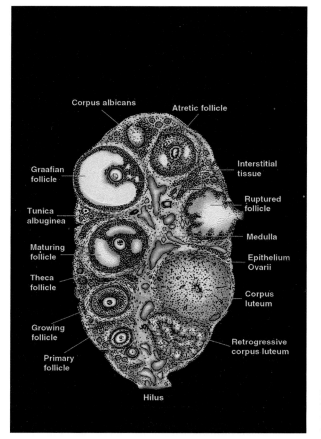

F I G U R E **1-3**

Histology of the ovary during the menstrual cycle.

(7,8). The follicular phase (postmenstrual day 15) of the menstrual cycle is characterized by increasing levels of circulating estrogens secreted by the ovarian follicle (Fig. 1-4). During this phase, the breast lobules are small and composed of few, widely spaced acini, the epithelial cells are small and polygonal with a centrally located nucleus, and mitotic figures are

uncommon. In the luteal phase, under the influence of progesterone, the alveolar cells differentiate into secretory cells and demonstrate the formation of lipid droplets. During this phase, interlobular edema develops and the mammary ducts dilate and may be filled with secretions. The maximum size of lobules and the maximum number of acini are reached between days 20

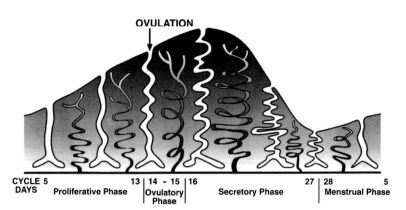

OVULATION

CYCLE 5 DAYS   Proliferative Phase   13 | 14 - 15 | 16   Ovulatory Phase   Secretory Phase   27 | 28   5   Menstrual Phase

F I G U R E **1-4**

Histologic changes of the endometrium during the menstrual cycle.

T A B L E **1-1**

Immunochemistry of Human Endometrium During the Menstrual Cycle

Antigen	Proliferative Phase		Secretory Phase		Presumed Function
	Glands	**Stroma**	**Glands**	**Stroma**	
ER	+	+	+	+	Proliferation
PR	+	+	+	+ (decidua +++)	Secretory differentiation
EGF	+	+	±	+	Proliferation
IGF-I	+	+	±	+	Proliferation
pHER-2/neu	+	−	±	−	Proliferation
Carbohydrate type 3 chains (ABO)					
A	+	−	−	−	—
H	+	−	+	−	Secretory differentiation (glycosylation)
Sialyl T	+	−	+	−	Secretory differentiation (glycosylation)
Relaxin	+	−	+	+ (decidua +++)	Collagenolysis
CD13, CD10	−	+	−	+	Immunomodulators

IGF-I = insulin-like growth factor I; ER = estrogen receptor; PR = progesterone receptor; EGF = epidermal growth factor.

and 26. The peak of mitosis is reached during the second half of the luteal phase and is followed by evidence of programmed cell death, or apoptosis, 3 to 4 days later. Expression of Bcl-2 (a protein that inhibits apoptosis) is observed at a high level during the follicular phase and decreases sharply at the end of the luteal phase, a period that coincides with the morphologic evidence of apoptosis (9). With the onset of menstruation, the secretory activity and tissue edema of the breast decrease, and the epithelial cells degenerate and slough off. The growth and differentiation of mammary epithelium during the menstrual cycle are regulated by a complex interplay between several steroid hormones and their receptors located in the cytosol or the nucleus, and polypeptide growth factors and their receptors located on the cell membrane and the stromal microenvironment.

The uterus is under endocrine control of the hypothalamic-hypopituitary axis (see Fig. 1-4). Responsiveness is mediated by the presence of estrogen and progesterone receptors on epithelial, stromal, and endothelial cells. The vascular supply of the uterus is adapted to the menstrual cycle, and largely influenced by steroid hormones and prostaglandins (10). The endometrial arteries are devoid of subendothelial elastica, allowing rupture during menstruation (11). Subsequent repair occurs by re-epithelialization from the residual glandular epithelium and is probably not under the direct control of steroid hormones.

The concentration of estrogen and progesterone receptors varies with the menstrual cycle, with the highest concentration occurring during the midproliferative cycle. Estrogen promotes receptor formation, and progesterone inhibits receptor formation. Fine hormonal regulation is under autocrine control. Table 1-1 lists some factors that have been implicated in endometrial biology (12). The ultimate function of the uterus is to promote the nidation of the fertilized ovum.

Although the cervix, the vagina, and the vulva are also under hormonal control, the biologically relevant hormonal interactions are less well defined.

Hormones and Growth Factors

Estrogens

Steroidal estrogens are secreted naturally in humans, mainly as 17β-estradiol, estrone, and estriol. These steroids have an 18-carbon structure containing a phenolic A ring with a hydroxyl group at carbon-3, two hexacyclic rings B and C, and a pentacyclic ring D with, in position 17, either a β-hydroxyl group or a ketone (13) (Fig. 1-5). Steroids bind with high affinity to estrogen receptors (ERs) through the phenolic A ring (14). Therefore, any substitutions on the phenolic A ring may impair binding (15). Other nonsteroidal compounds with estrogen-like activity contain a phenolic ring that binds to the ERs. Some have been synthesized and some occur naturally in plants. Diethylstilbestrol is the best example of a synthetic estrogen (16). Naturally occurring estrogen-like substances (phytoestrogens) may be found in flavonoids and coumestan derivatives (17). Steroid estrogens are insoluble in water. They are well absorbed through the skin, the mucus membrane, and the gastrointestinal tract. However, after oral absorption these steroid estrogens are quickly degraded by the liver. There is a conversion to less active products, which are then conjugated with sulfuric and glucuronic acids. A certain proportion of estrogens will be reabsorbed by enterohepatic circulation. The rest is usually excreted by the kidney. In the blood, most steroid estrogens are bound to sex-binding globulin or to albumin.

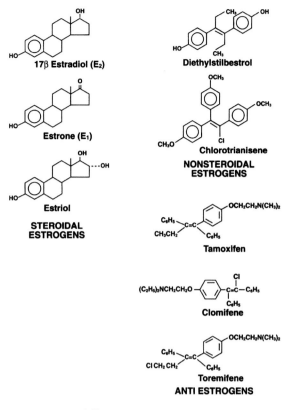

F I G U R E **1-5**

Structure of steroidal estrogens, nonsteroidal estrogens, and antiestrogens.

Some antiestrogens such as tamoxifen and clomifene also contain a phenolic ring that enables the compound to bind to the ER (18). The *cis* or *trans* conformation of the molecule confers an agonist or anti-agonist property, respectively (14).

Because estrogens are obtained by aromatization of androstenedione or testosterone (see Fig. 1-1), inhibitors of the enzymes of steroidogenesis, especially aromatase inhibitors, have been developed for the treatment of breast cancer (Table 1-2).

Progestins

Progestins (Fig. 1-6) are steroid molecules with a delta 4-3-1 A ring structure that binds to the progesterone receptor (PR) (15). This structure can also bind to other steroid receptors such as glucocorticoid, androgen, and mineralocorticoid receptors. Therefore, most progestins also have androgenic capacity. When administrated orally, progesterone is quickly degraded by the liver. The pregnane metabolites are conjugated

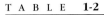

T A B L E   **1-2**

Hormones

Class	Drug	Dose
Estrogens	Diethylstilbestrol	5–15 mg/day orally
	Ethinyl estradiol	0.5–3 mg/day orally
Antiestrogens	Tamoxifen	Up to 40 mg/day orally
	Toremifene	
Progesterones	Megestrol acetate	Up to 160 mg/day orally
	Medroxyprogesterone acetate	Up to 1000 mg/wk IM
Aromatase inhibitors	Anastrazole	1 mg/day orally
Adrenal blocker	Aminoglutethimide	Up to 2 g/day orally
	Trilostane	Up to 480 mg/day orally
	Ketoconazole	Up to 800 mg/day orally
Androgens	Fluoxymesterone	Up to 40 mg/day orally
	Testolactone	Up to 1 g/day orally
GnRH agonists	Leuprolide acetate	7.5-mg depot IM every mo
	Goserelin acetate	3.6-mg depot SC every mo

IM = intramuscularly; SC = subcutaneously.

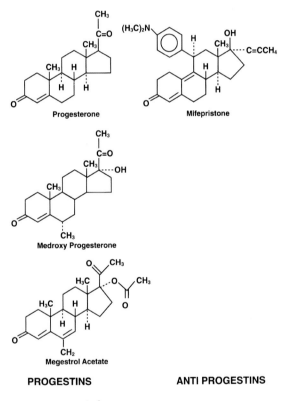

PROGESTINS   **ANTI PROGESTINS**

F I G U R E   **1-6**

Structure of progestins and antiprogestins.

with glucuronic or sulfuric acids and excreted in the urine. Pregnanediol is one of the main metabolites that can be measured in the urine as an index of the endogenous secretion of progesterone. Many analogues of progesterone are less susceptible to degradation by the liver and used orally as contraceptives. Medroxyprogesterone acetate and megestrol acetate are the main progestins used for cancer therapy (19).

The antiprogestin mifepristone (RU 486) acts as a competitive inhibitor of both progesterone and glucocorticoid (20). The 3-one A ring is preserved, allowing receptor binding. However, mifepristone does not bind to receptors for estrogens or mineralocorticoids, and is therefore more specific than other progesterone analogues.

Effects of Estrogen and Progesterone on Breast and Gynecologic Organs

The expression of ER in the mammary epithelium increases during the follicular phase and is downregulated following ovulation, presumably under the influence of progesterone (21,22). The level of PRs does not change very strikingly during the menstrual cycle (22). The synthesis of the PR requires the presence of a functional ER. Estrogens stimulate primarily ductal proliferation while progesterone stimulates lobuloalveolar development. A variety of laboratory, epidemiologic, and clinical evidence suggests a seminal role for steroid hormones in the genesis of breast tumors (23). Breast cancer occurs almost exclusively in women (100:1 female-male ratio). Several reproductive and lifestyle factors whose common effect is an increased cumulative exposure of breast epithelium to female hormones, especially estrogens, are associated with an increased risk of breast cancer. These include early age of menarche, late age of menopause, nulliparity, first pregnancy after age 30, and a first-trimester abortion before the first full-term pregnancy (24). Several investigators observed higher levels of bioavailable estrogens in breast cancer patients as compared to control subjects (25). Some groups reported altered patterns of metabolism of estrogens, that is, a predominance of 16α-hydroxylation and 4-hydroxylation over 2-hydroxylation, as being associated with an increased risk of breast cancer (26). A prominent role for estrogens in the etiology of breast cancer and other cancers such as of the kidney, ovary, and uterus is further supported by animal experiments which showed that estrogen can promote tumor induction by a variety of mammary carcinogens (27). The role of exogenous hormones such as oral contraceptives or postmenopausal hormone replacement therapy in the genesis of breast cancer is controversial. Tamoxifen has been shown to induce a poor-prognosis endometrial carcinoma. The best demonstration of hormonal influence during the embryologic development of the fetus involves the synthetic estrogen diethylstilbestrol, which causes clear-cell carcinoma of the vagina in the offspring of treated mothers (16). The role of estrogens and progestins in the etiology of ovarian and cervical cancers is less clear. However, the use of a contraceptive pill for 5 years is associated with a major reduction in the incidence of ovarian cancer (28).

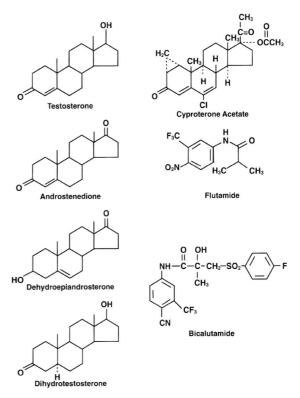

F I G U R E   **1-7**

Structure of androgens (left) and antiandrogens (right).

Androgens

Testosterone (Fig. 1-7) is the principal androgen secreted by the testicle, the ovary, and the adrenal cortex. This steroidal compound is the precursor of estrogen and dihydrotestosterone. Testosterone and analogues bind to its intracellular receptor through the A ring. Binding affinity is increased by reduction at the 5α position (29). The conversion of testosterone to dihydrotestosterone is mediated by the 5α-reductase in the target tissue (30). When administered orally, testosterone is quickly metabolized by the liver. Metabolites include androsterone and androstenedione. They are then conjugated and excreted by the kidney. Alkylation of all steroids in the 17 position retards hepatic metabolism and allows higher serum levels following oral administration (31). The main androgen steroids used in the treatment of cancer are fluorinated compounds such as flu-

oxymesterone, testolactone with a lactone ring in D, and methyltestosterone with an alkyl substitution on 17.

Antiandrogens used in clinics are cyproterone acetate, which is a progesterone analogue with antiandrogen properties (32), and flutamide and bicalutamide, two nonsteroidal antiandrogens (33,34). Flutamide stimulates the production of luteal hormone (LH) and therefore needs to be used in conjunction with gonadotropin-releasing hormone (GnRH) blockage (35). Finasteride is an inhibitor of 5α-reductase that acts directly in the target tissue (36).

Pituitary Peptides

The gonadotropins are secreted in the anterior pituitary by the gonadotropin cells, after stimulation by cyclical release of GnRH. A negative feedback loop controls the secretion of GnRH in the hypothalamus. Gonadotropins include follicle-stimulating hormone (FSH) and LH. Human chorionic gonadotropin (HCG), a gonadotropin analogue, is secreted during pregnancy by the syncytiotrophoblast cells of the fetal placenta as early as 7 days after fertilization. HCG has a luteal function. A closely related glycoprotein is thyrotropin (TSH). Both gonadotropin and thyrotropin share an α-subunit that is encoded by the same gene (37). The biologic specificity is related to the β-subunit, which is encoded by different genes (38). The homology between HCG and LH β-subunits is about 82%, with 150 amino acid residues that are identical. This further contributes to similar biologic actions (39). The α-subunit gene promoter contains regulatory elements called *cyclic adenosine monophosphate (cAMP) regulatory elements* (CREs), which are located in the 5′-flanking region upstream of the transcription initiation site (Fig. 1-8) (40). c-AMP–dependent transcription factors interact with the CRE to promote transcription of the gene. The gene itself is formed of four exons and three introns (41). The introns are spliced during transcription and the messenger RNA (mRNA) is about 800 nucleotides in length. The m-RNA is then translated into a precursor polypeptide containing a 24–amino acid

leader sequence and a 92–amino acid α-subunit sequence. The 24–amino acid leader sequence is rapidly cleaved from the α-subunit (42). Figure 1-9 shows the structure of the α-subunit with two asparagine (Asn) residues that are sites of N-linked attachment of carbohydrate moieties. The carbohydrate groups attached to the subunits are important determinants of biologic activity and metabolic functions of these glycoprotein hormones (43). The β-subunit gene is similarly translated as an amino acid leader sequence followed by the β-subunit polypeptide. The leader sequence is quickly cleaved, allowing the β-subunit to take its final conformation. There is a 12-cysteine motif homology between the β-subunits of these pituitary glycoproteins. The creation of disulfide bonds leads to a β-subunit conformation that is capable of coupling with the α-subunit (44). Each β-subunit is differentially glycosylated with one oligosaccharide group for LH, two for FSH, and six for HCG (45). Each oligosaccharide is branched and has a different composition. The composition of each oligosaccharide

F I G U R E 1-8

Schematic structure of the human α-subunit gene and peptide of the pituitary glycopeptides.

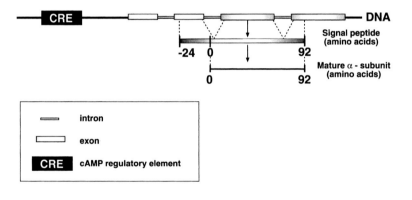

F I G U R E 1-9

Amino acid sequence of the α-subunit peptide of the pituitary glycopeptides.

10
ALA PRO ASP VAL GLN ASP CYS PRO GLU CYS THR LEU GLN GLU ASN PRO
20   30
PHE PHE SER GLN PRO GLY ALA PRO ILE LEU GLN CYS MET GLY CYS CYS
40
PHE SER ARG ALA TYR PRO THR PRO LEU ARG SER LYS LYS THR
50   60
MET LEU VAL GLN LYS ASN VAL THR SER GLU SER THR CYS CYS VAL ALA
70
LYS SER TYR ASN ARG VAL THR VAL MET GLY GLY PHE LYS VAL GLU ASN
80   90
HIS THR ALA CYS HIS CYS SER THR CYS TYR TYR HIS LYS SER-COOH

↓, ASN residues : N-linked attachment sites for carbohydrate moieties.

may play a role in receptor recognition and activation of cellular mechanisms (46). Glycosylation also protects the peptide from degradation in the serum (47). The α-subunit is able to recognize the receptor and induce signal transduction through one of the carbohydrate side chains (46). The role of the β-subunit is less clear. One hypothesis is that when it couples with the α-subunit, it induces a change of conformation in the α-subunit that renders the peptide specific for the target receptor (48). Furthermore, the β-subunit gene contains a 15-bp estrogen-responsive element (ERE), which has been demonstrated for LH (49).

Prolactin is the main hormone regulating lactation (Fig. 1-10). It is part of the somatomammotropic family which also includes growth hormone (GH) and placental lactogen (50). Prolactin and GH are secreted by acidophil cells of the anterior hypophysis. Human placental lactogen is secreted by the placenta. Prolactin is a single polypeptidic chain of 199 amino acids with three disulfide bonds. A tissue-specific transcriptional regulatory protein (PIT-1) binds structurally to the DNA sequences present in two enhancer regions to stimulate gene expression (51). Prolactin gene expression is influenced by calcium and decreased by castration and dopamine agonists such as bromocriptine (42).

Prolactin receptors are present on many breast tumor cells, and in vitro exposure to prolactin can lead to growth stimulation of these cells. The expression of prolactin and estrogen receptors is coordinately regulated in many breast tumor cells. Some recent studies showed the existence of an autocrine growth regulatory loop involving prolactin and its receptors in breast tumors (52,53). Some cervical and uterine tumors secrete prolactin (54).

Transforming Growth Factor-β Family

Transforming growth factor (TGF)-β1 is a ubiquitous polypeptide that exhibits a complex pattern of biologic actions in different systems. Expression of TGF-β2 and TGF-β3 seems to be more limited. The main function of TGF-β involves regulation of cell growth, development, and differentiation, of inflammation, and of immunologic mechanisms (55) (see Chapter 2). TGF-β and related growth factors do have

F I G U R E **1-10**

Amino acid sequence of prolactin.

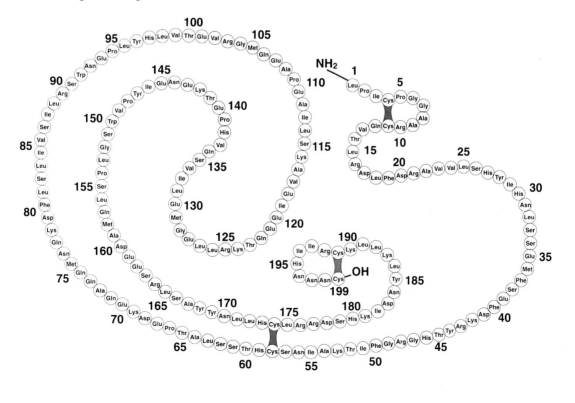

specific receptors that activate a serine/threonine kinase transmembrane pathway (56). Activin and inhibin are members of the TGF-β superfamily, and also signal through similar pathways. There is 40% homology between the β-subunits of inhibin and activin and TGF-β (57).

Inhibin is a heterodimer formed of two polypeptide chains: one α-subunit that has a molecular weight of 18,000 and one β-subunit, either $β_A$ or $β_B$, that is not glycosylated (58). Each β-subunit has a molecular weight of 14,000. Both are secreted as precursor proteins (Fig. 1-11). Inhibin is secreted by the granulosa cells and released in the antral fluid and then in the systemic circulation (59). Inhibin is an inhibitor of FSH secretion (60,61). Heterodimers made of $β_A$ and $β_B$ and homodimers made of either $β_A$-$β_A$ or $β_B$-$β_B$ are called *activins* and stimulate the production of FSH in the pituitary gland (61,62). The β-dimers have a homology with TGF-β, which is also capable of stimulating the production of FSH (63). The actions of inhibin and activin are independent of GnRH (64). However, inhibin modulates the regulation of GnRH receptors in pituitary cells of rats (65). Inhibin exerts its action by inhibiting transcription of the FSH mRNA (66). Inhibin and activin also act as paracrine and autocrine regulators of estrogen and androgen activity (67). In addition, they also have multiple targets and functions outside the reproductive system. The measurement of inhibin serum levels may be used clinically as a marker of the presence of granulosa or Sertoli-Leydig cell tumors.

Insulin-Like Growth Factor Superfamily

Insulin is the most well-known hormone of this family, with two polypeptide chains, A and B, linked by two disulfide bonds. The gene for human insulin is located on chromosome 11. A preproinsulin is produced and metabolized to a proinsulin by microsomal enzymes. This proinsulin is cleaved into equimolar concentrations of insulin and C peptide after transport in the Golgi apparatus of pancreatic B cells (68). However, the most interesting growth factors of this family, which are involved in the hormonal tuning of women, are insulin-like growth factor (IGF)-I, IGF-II, and relaxin. IGFs are also formed from prepropeptides (69). The granulosa cell is the main intraovarian site of IGF-I gene expression in the rats (70); however, in human ovary, IGF-II appears to be more highly

PRECURSORS

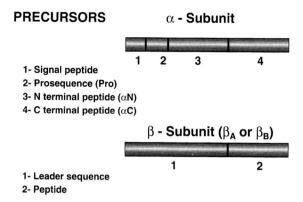

1- Signal peptide
2- Prosequence (Pro)
3- N terminal peptide (αN)
4- C terminal peptide (αC)

1- Leader sequence
2- Peptide

INHIBINS

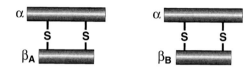

Proteolytic cleavage products with different molecular weight have been identified.

ACTIVINS

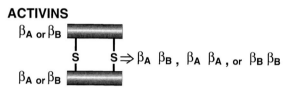

F I G U R E **1-11**

Structure of inhibins and activins.

expressed than IGF-I, suggesting possible species specificity (71). In the ovary, the expression of IGF-I is dependent on the levels of gonadotropin, estradiol, and GH (72). The regulation and action of IGF-I seems to be specific to the organ in which IGF-I is expressed. For example, IGF-I secretion is modulated by GH in opposite directions in the liver (GH increases IGF-I) and the ovary (GH decreases IGF-I) (72). In the hormone-responsive organs, IGF-I seems to act mainly as an autocrine and paracrine hormone. In the ovary, there is a coregulation between the gonadotropins, GnRH, and the IGF system that promotes follicular maturation (73).

Six IGF-binding proteins have been characterized (74). In the plasma, they transport and protect IGF from enzyme degradation. At the organ level, these binding proteins interact with the IGFs to modulate the biologic potency of these growth factors by interfering with receptor recognition (75).

The receptor for IGFs activates a tyrosine kinase transduction pathway (see below). The expression of IGF receptors on the cell membrane might be a determinant of cell growth and transformation. Cells deficient in IGF-I receptors are not susceptible to transformation by the Rous sarcoma virus or bovine papillomavirus (76). Furthermore, malignant cells are not able to maintain their phenotype if they lose the expression of IGF-I receptors (77).

In the breast, IGF-I is expressed in stromal cells, whereas IGF-II is expressed in cancer cells (78). There is a definite coregulation of the IGF system (ligand, binding protein, and receptor) by circulating steroidal hormones such as estrogen, and related drugs such as tamoxifen and retinoids. The former one activates the IGF system whereas the latter two have an inhibitory action (76).

The Fibroblast Growth Factor Family

The fibroblast growth factor (FGF) family includes as least nine distinct proteins encoded by nine different genes (79). The FGFs are mitotic factors for cells of all origins. These growth factors are ubiquitous ones that have been involved in differentiation, angiogenesis, and embryologic development (80). The FGFs are single-chain polypeptides that lack a consensus secretory signal peptide (81). How they are released from their cells of origin is not yet clear. FGFs bind to cellular receptors with high affinity. These receptors are part of the tyrosine kinase receptor family (82). However, FGF can also bind with heparan sulfate chains of heparan-chondroitin sulfate proteoglycan, in a covalent manner (83). This proteoglycan binding may be important to facilitate the binding of FGF to the tyrosine kinase receptors. The exact role of FGF in the ovarian and tumoral microenvironment is not clear. However, many ovarian cancer cell lines bear FGF3 receptors (84). Interactions have been demonstrated between FGF, LH, FSH, and inhibin (85).

The Epidermal Growth Factor Family

The epidermal growth factor (EGF) superfamily contains a subfamily of growth factors that contribute not only to embryonic development but also to tumoral growth. These growth factors are EGF-related peptides that bind to the same family of receptors (86) (Table 1-3). The EGF superfamily also includes other molecules that

Protein	Function
EGF family of proteins	
EGF	Growth factor
Heparin-binding EGF	Growth factor
Transforming growth factor-α	Growth factor
Amphiregulin	Growth factor
Betacellulin	Growth factor
Heregulin α and β	Growth factor
Vaccina virus growth factor	Growth factor
Myxoma virus growth factor	Growth factor
Cripto-1	Growth factor
Other	
Urokinase	Serine protease
Tissue plasminogen activator	Serine protease
Clotting factors (VII, IX, X, XII)	—
LDL receptor	LDL uptake
Laminin B1 chain	Extracellular matrix protein
Thrombospondin	Extracellular matrix protein
EGF receptor family of cell surface tyrosine kinases	
c-erb B/let-23 (EGFR)	p170
c-erb B-2 (HER-2/c-neu)	p185
c-erb B-3 (HER-3)	p160
c-erb B-4 (HER-4)	p180

T A B L E   **1-3**

Epidermal Growth Factor (EGF) and EGF Receptor Families

LDL = low-density lipoprotein.

function as proteases, clotting factors, adhesion and extracellular matrix molecules, and receptors such as the LDL receptor. All these proteins are structurally related through similarities in the last 40 amino acids at their NH$_2$-terminus (87). The presence of three disulfide bonds in this region forms a characteristic three-loop secondary structure. These proteins may be secreted or remain attached to the cell membrane as glycoproteins (87).

The EGF polypeptidic chain consists of 53 amino acids with three internal disulfide bonds (88). The precursor of the EGF chain is a glycoprotein that contains 1217 residues with eight units that do retain a biologic activity similar to that of EGF (89).

Other related peptides are TGF-α, heparin-binding EGF, amphiregulin, betacellulin, and heregulins-α and -β (90). The activity of some of these glycoproteins may be influenced by binding to the extracellular matrix in a way similar to FGF (91). The exact roles of these peptides in normal and tumoral physiology are still unclear.

The receptors for these above-described ligands are part of the EGF receptor (EGFR) family of cell surface tyrosine kinases. All of these peptides, with the exception of heregulins, are able to activate EGFR, a 170-kd protein (92). The receptors c-erb B-3 and c-erb B-4 are the main ones for heregulins. Once heregulin is bound, these receptors can recruit and activate EGFR and c-erb B-2, a 185-kd protein related to EGFR, which was first isolated from human breast carcinoma (93). Receptors for EGFs (see below) are known to be overexpressed in some tumoral cells. The overexpression of the EGFR in breast (94), endometrial (95), and ovarian (96) cancer is a factor of poor prognosis. While the precise role of this growth factor and its receptor in breast cancer is not completely understood, they have been shown to influence the growth and biologic behavior of these cells at physiologically relevant concentrations. Current pilot studies are testing the concept of EGFR expression inhibition for the treatment of breast and ovarian cancers. Different methodologies are being tried, such as transduction in tumor cells overexpressing Her-2/neu of E1A, an adenovirus gene with tumor suppressor activity against HER-2/*neu* oncogene–transformed cells, and vaccination against immunogenic peptides derived from certain intracellular or extracellular domains of HER-2/neu.

Gonadotropin Release Hormones

The GnRH or luteal hormone–releasing hormone (LHRH) is secreted by the hypothalamus as a decapeptide. GnRH affects the secretion of FSH and LH (Fig. 1-12). Receptors to GnRH have been found in a variety of organs including the ovary, the uterus, the placenta, and other hormone-sensitive organs or tumors (97–100). Some ovarian carcinomas are also known to secrete LHRH (101). Two classes of GnRH membrane receptors have been found: one with high affinity/low capacity and one with low affinity/high capacity (102). The respective functions of these receptors are unclear. In primates and rats, LHRH directly regulates the ontogenic development of cellularly and humorally mediated immune responses (103,104). In particular, LHRH stimulates interleukin (IL)-2 receptor expression of rat thymocytes (105).

Clinical studies demonstrated the usefulness of continuous exposure to GnRH agonists in the treatment of breast and other gynecologic

F I G U R E   **1-12**

Schematic view of the hypothalamic-hypopituitary axis. GnRH = gonadotropin-releasing hormone; LH = luteal hormone; FSH = follicle-stimulating hormone.

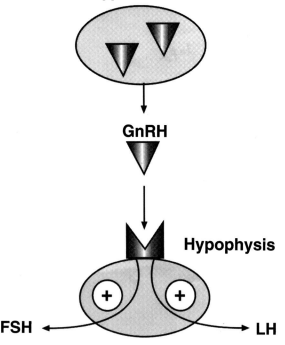

cancers (see Table 1-2). Continuous exposure to GnRH agonists causes a downregulation of LH and FSH receptors in the pituitary, and therefore an inhibition of estrogen formation in the target organs. Furthermore, there could be a direct effect of GnRH on the cancer cells.

The Cytokine Family

The major cytokines include the interferons (106), the ILs (107), the tumor necrosis factors (108), and the colony-stimulating factors (109). mRNAs for these cytokines have been found in tumor cells of gynecologic origin (110). These molecules may influence the hormonal milieu of gynecologic cancers. They are discussed in more detail in Chapter 2.

Receptor Biology

The very existence of multicellular organisms implies that elaborate signaling mechanisms are necessary to communicate with one another. Without intercellular signals, an organism would not be able to coordinate its own metabolism; hence, it would not be able to sustain life. If any of such control fails, it results in embryologic defect, or cancer, which usually kills the multicellular organism.

There are two modes of cell signaling: direct contact between two cells [the best examples are gap junctions and desmosome formations, as well as adhesion mechanisms (111)], or secretion of molecule messengers between two cells. The target cells usually bear receptors that can be intramembranous or intracellular. The receptor becomes activated by binding to the ligand (the signaling molecule). This activation generates a cascade of intracellular signals that alter cell behavior. The signaling molecules may be secreted at a distance from the target cells; this process is called *the endocrine response*. Other signaling molecules may be secreted by various neighboring cells; this process is called *paracrine signaling*. Other

signaling molecules may be secreted by the same cells; this is *autocrine signaling*. These three mechanisms might act together on the same cells, allowing very fine-tuning of the cellular response. Signaling molecules (or ligands) exist in all forms: protein, small peptides, amino acids, nucleotides, steroids, retinoids, fatty acid derivatives, and even some dissolved gases such as nitric oxide and carbon monoxide. Ions and some sugars are also part of the intercellular signaling process.

Intracellular Receptors

Steroid hormones, thyroid hormones, retinoids, and vitamin D are able to diffuse through the cellular membrane and directly bind to intracellular receptor proteins. Each hormone binds to specific receptors. However, all receptors are structurally related (112). Each receptor has a ligand-binding site as well as a DNA-binding site. The DNA-binding site allows receptors to bind to specific DNA sequences, called *response elements*, adjacent to the genes that the ligand regulates. Most steroidal receptors are in the cytosolic fraction, whereas retinoid receptors are usually located in the nucleus.

Retinoid Receptors

The retinoid receptors (Fig. 1-13) are potent regulators of growth and differentiation of both normal and malignant cells. Two classes of retinoid receptors are known: RAR and RXR (113,114). Subtypes of RAR bind specific natural or synthetic retinoid acids (115). RXR forms a heterodimer with RAR before binding to the specific DNA sequences, also called *retinoic acid response elements* (RAREs), which are located in the promoter regions of the genes that the retinoic acid regulates (116). Indirect regulation is also seen with retinoic acids. In this case, there is no direct binding to RAR or RAR/RXR heterodimer to the DNA. The RAR complex binds to a transcription factor, therefore modulating the function of the transcrip-

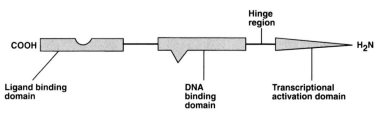

FIGURE 1-13

Schematic view of the retinoid receptor.

tion factor (117). This phenomenon is called *cross-coupling*. There are some hints that the effects of the retinoic acids can also occur at the posttranscriptional level, the translational level, and the posttranslational level. Retinoic acids can modulate the expression of TGF-β, TGF-α, EGF, platelet-derived growth factor (PDGF), FGF, IGFs, as well as cytokines (118). Similarly, retinoic acids can modulate the expression of the PR and the intracellular concentration of progesterone (119). Retinoic acids directly regulate the gene transcription of different enzymes such as alcohol dehydrogenase and phosphoenol pyruvate carboxykinase. The RARE has been identified as a repetitive TGACC motive in the 5′-flanking region of several different genes (120). The same kind of regulation seems very important in the control of the cellular matrix (121). Except for breast cancer cells, the elucidation of the mechanism of action of retinoic acids in gynecologic cancer remains elusive. In breast cancer cell lines, the retinoic acid seems to regulate the expression of estrogen and progesterone receptors as well as the IGF-I receptor (122). Studies of breast cancer prevention with tamoxifen and retinoic acids are ongoing (123,124).

Interestingly, the retinoic acids also are involved in the expression and control of the human papilloma virus (HPV) (125). HPV-16 and -18 as well as some other strains are associated with the development of carcinoma of the cervix or the vulvar area. Infection with HPV leads to cancerization, depending on the differentiation status of the cell (118). Virus formation is not favored when the cell is not very differentiated. Therefore, treatment with retinoids might prevent infection of less differentiated cells. Retinoic acids are also able to repress the transcription of HPV-18/E6-E7 mRNAs in HELA cell lines (126). This might explain why a good response rate was seen with retinoic acid and interferon in the treatment of previously untreated primary cervical cancer (127). Retinoic acids also modulate the expression of transcription factors such as C-Jun and C-Fos (128). The list of transcription factors influenced by retinoic acids is still growing.

Steroidal Receptors

The ER (Fig. 1-14) is a 64-kd protein that shares structural and functional similarities with other members of the steroid receptor superfamily including the progesterone, corticosteroid, thyroid hormone, retinoic acid, and vitamin D receptors (129). Binding of the ligand, estrogen, to the ER results in dimerization of the receptor. This is followed by binding to specific DNA sequences, the EREs, and this interaction leads to the activation of transcription of estrogen-inducible genes that mediate the phenotypic effects of estrogens. The ER has several distinct functional domains (130). The carboxy-terminal domain is the ligand-binding region. This region also contains sequences that participate in receptor dimerization and transcriptional activation (AF-2 domain) following hormone binding. The central region of the ER forms two zinc fingers, which play a role in receptor dimerization and in binding to the ERE. The amino-terminal domain of the ER is responsible for transcriptional activation (AF-1 domain) (see Fig. 1-14). Unlike the carboxy-terminal region, the amino-terminal domain can, in some instances, activate transcription even in the absence of the hormone (131).

FIGURE **1-14**

Schematic view of the estrogen receptor.

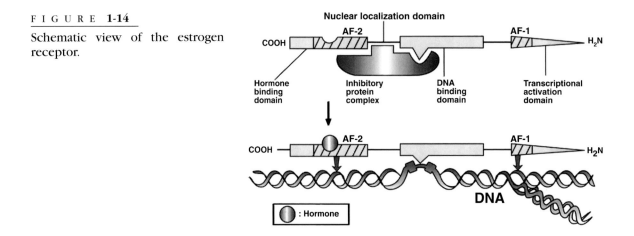

ER-positive breast cancers comprise a heterogeneous group. For example, the clinical response rate to antiestrogens ranges from over 75% for ER-positive, PR-positive tumors to approximately 40% for ER-positive, PR-negative tumors to less than 10% for ER-negative, PR-positive tumors. Therefore, considerable effort has been invested in searching for alterations of the structure and function of steroid receptors in hormone receptor–positive breast tumors. Such variant receptors include those that harbor point mutations, those that are generated by alternative splicing, and those that are generated by posttranslational modifications (132). For example, an exon 5 splice variant is unable to bind the ligand but can activate transcription constitutively and may account for the ER-negative, PR-positive phenotype of some breast tumors. Similarly, variants that lack exon 3 or exon 7 have been described and lead to a nonfunctional ER. Interestingly, the exon 7 splice variant, in addition to being nonfunctional itself, can lead to an inhibition of the action of the wild-type receptor (dominant-negative variant). The ratio of a more commonly occurring variant, clone 4, to the full-length ER transcript may also be relevant to the function of ERs (133).

The mutant ERs provide a logical theoretical explanation for the lack of efficacy of antiestrogen in many ER-positive breast tumors. However, they are not detectable in many breast tumors that are refractory to antiestrogens. Clearly other mechanisms such as alteration of metabolism of antiestrogens (134) or non-ER-related mechanisms of estrogen/antiestrogen action exist in many of these tumors. Similar to ERs, several variants of PRs have also been described recently, but their role in breast cancer is less well understood. Steroid hormone receptors are present in approximately one half to two thirds of all breast tumors. Many breast tumor cell lines can be stimulated to grow by exogenous estrogens and their growth can be inhibited by antiestrogens. Many investigators believe that breast tumor cells that lack hormone receptors have escaped from estrogen dependence and therefore represent a late stage of tumor evolution.

The presence of steroidal receptors on ovarian cancers has not been correlated with hormone responsiveness or prognosis (96,135). In endometrial cancer, the presence of PRs has been correlated with responsiveness to hormones (136) and survival (137).

Transmembranous Receptors

Various types of transmembrane receptors have been described. The best characterized are the ion channel–linked receptors, mainly found at synapses, the G protein–linked receptors, and the enzyme-linked receptors. The ligand activates the receptor by inducing a conformational change. This change allows the phosphorylation and activation of either an intracellular G protein [guanosine triphosphate (GTP) → guanosine diphosphate (GDP)], or an intracellular protein kinase. The G protein–linked receptors are members of a seven-times-across-the-membrane transmembrane protein family. The enzyme-linked receptors are mostly single-pass transmembrane proteins (138) (Fig. 1-15). Here, we only review two types of enzyme-linked receptors: the tyrosine-specific protein kinase and the serine/threonine protein kinase receptors.

F I G U R E **1-15**

Schematic view of the transmembranous receptors. EGF = epidermal growth factor; NGF = nerve growth factor; FGF = fibroblast growth factor; PDGF = platelet-derived growth factor; IGF = insulin-like growth factor; M-CSF = macrophage colony-stimulating factor; VEGF = vascular endothelial growth factor.

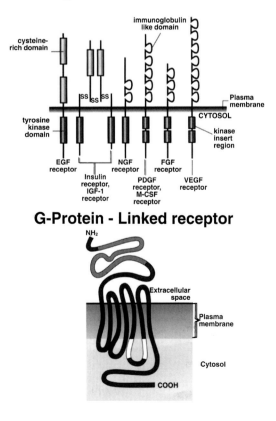

Tyrosine-Specific Protein Kinase Receptors

The tyrosine-specific protein kinase receptors usually consist of a glycosylated extracellular domain and of an intracellular domain, which contains tyrosine kinase activity (Fig. 1-16) (139). When the ligand binds to the extracellular domain, it induces a dimerization of the receptor, which results in activation (140). At this point, the formation of receptor dimers allows a cross-phosphorylation between the numerous tyrosine residues of the tyrosine kinase domains. This is referred to as *autophosphorylation of the receptor dimer*. The signaling cascade is initiated by recruitment of signaling molecules to the autophosphorylation sites. One group of signaling molecules that bind to the autophosphorylation sites share frequently two highly conserved noncatalytic domains, called *SH2* and *SH3* [Src homology regions 2 and 3 (*src* is an oncogene first discovered in the Rous sarcoma virus)], which are essential for the activation of the signaling cascade (Fig. 1-17) (141,142). SH2 domains specifically bind to tyrosine phosphorylated proteins, whereas SH3 domains constitutively bind to proline-rich regions in other signaling molecules. The next proteins to be activated in the signaling cascade are the Ras proteins. The Ras proteins are monomeric GTPases that are active when GTP is bound, and inactive when GDP is bound (143). GTP binding is controlled by a set of activating enzymes that promote the exchange of GDP for GTP and by another set of inhibitory enzymes. The SH3 domains recruited to the receptor complex modulate the activity of these activating and inhibitory enzymes (144). The role of Ras protein is to communicate to the nucleus the message given by the ligand (145). This communication takes place through a serine/threonine phosphorylation cascade that activates kinases such as the mitogen-activating protein (MAP) kinases (146). These kinases are able to induce the production of transcription factors such as Fos (147) or to phosphorylate other transcription factors such as Jun (148). For example, the newly made Fos and the phosphorylated Jun are able to combine together and form an active gene regulatory protein called *AP-1*, which is important in cell differentiation (149).

Any mutations of one of these signaling cascade proteins may be deleterious to the cell. If the signaling cascade becomes activated by hyperactive mutants, cell proliferation is activated and may result in cancer. For example, 30% of human cancers carry a Ras mutation (150). If another mutation inactivates a signaling protein, the cell will stop its development, and may undergo apoptosis. However, inactivation of some proteins in the process of maturation is a normal phenomenon.

Receptors for insulin, IGFs, EGFs, and TGF-α have been identified in a variety of breast tumor cells, ovarian cancer cells, and endometrial cancer cells. Overexpression of some of these receptors is usually a sign of tumor aggressiveness and poor prognosis (94–96). The exact function of these receptors in cancer biology is the basis of active ongoing research. In animal experiments, malignant cell lines can

FIGURE **1-16**

Schematic view of the epidermal growth factor receptor.

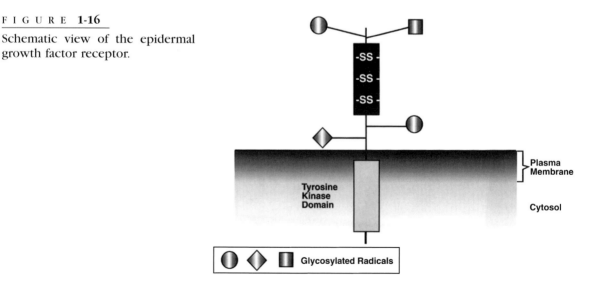

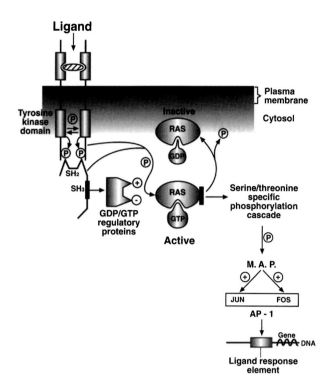

FIGURE **1-17**

Schematic view of the signaling cascade of the tyrosine kinase receptors. MAP = mitogen-activating protein; GTP = guanosine triphosphate; GDP = guanosine diphosphate.

be inhibited by antibodies against the over-expressed receptor, or by transfection with anti-sense oligonucleotides to block the mRNA expression of the receptor. Does inhibition of receptor function lead to cell cycle arrest or differentiation to a more benign pattern? Preclinical studies and phase I trials are using receptor antagonists and kinase inhibitors as anticancer agents to test this hypothesis.

Serine/Threonine Protein Kinase Receptors

In contrast to the serine/threonine-specific protein kinases that are a link to activation of transcription through the tyrosine receptor pathway, the serine/threonine protein kinase receptor is a transmembrane protein that serves as the receptor for TGF-β family members. There are at least five known TGF-β receptors that have been cloned (TGF-β receptor types I, II, III, and V and endoglin) (151). There are probably other binding proteins, but they do not qualify as true receptors (e.g., TGF-β type IV receptor) because they do not play a direct role in signal transduction (152). Type I and II receptors have been studied the most. Their cytoplasmic domain contains a serine/threonine kinase domain that is capable of autophosphorylation (153). The type III receptor is char-

acterized by a very short intracellular domain (41 amino acids), though it has a large extracellular domain. It has been found to exist in a soluble form (154). Endoglin has a structure somewhat similar to the type III receptor; however, TGF-β2 cannot bind to endoglin (155). Type V receptor is less characterized. Signal transduction requires at least intact type I and II receptors. Both receptors form a heterodimer upon recognition and ligation of TGF-β. Type I receptor requires type II receptor to bind the ligand, and type II receptor requires type I receptor to induce signal transduction through cross-phosphorylation of their serine residues (156). The events and molecules implicated in the signaling cascade are not yet well understood. TGF-β causes a reversible G_1 arrest in many different cell types. Therefore, efforts to identify the effects of TGF-β on transcription factors such as Rb and E2F, and on cyclin–cyclin-dependent kinase (cdk) complexes are ongoing (157). TGF-β can induce p21 mRNA transcription. The protein p21 is a cdk inhibitor that inhibits the cyclin E–cdk2 and the cyclin D–cdk4 complexes (158). The end result is an arrest at the G_1 checkpoint, and a decrease in the number of cells that enter into the S-phase (Fig. 1-18). This control of TGF-β on the expression of p21 has been demonstrated in ovarian cancer cell lines (159). However, this is not the

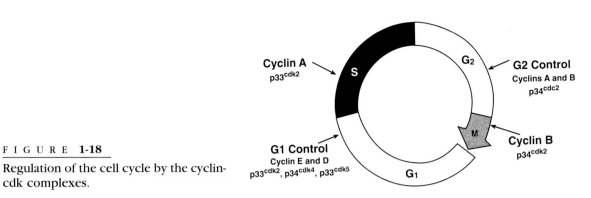

F I G U R E **1-18**

Regulation of the cell cycle by the cyclin-cdk complexes.

only mechanism of action of TGF-β. The TGF-β system (ligands, receptors, and possibly binding proteins) remains very specific for each cell lineage, and induces a very specialized response to the microenvironment. Alteration of the receptor structure may be critical to tumorigenesis. Mutations of the type II receptor have been demonstrated in numerous cancer cell lines. Alterations of the type II receptor prevent the growth inhibitory effects of TGF-β, resulting in uncontrolled cell proliferation (160). Identification of the molecular substrates and effectors that regulate cellular proliferation and differentiation will provide greater insights in our understanding of the TGF-β system.

Conclusions

Many steps are required for a normal cell to be called a cancer cell. What the most relevant step is is not clear and may be different for each cancer. The loss of normal growth pattern, immortalization, metastatic potential, and clonal evolution leading to more and more aberrant genetic material are all characteristics of tumoral cells, yet taken individually, none of them is sufficient to explain the neoplastic phenotype. Some of the mechanisms explaining these biologic behaviors are being thoroughly studied.

Apoptosis or programmed cell death is a normal phenomenon that eliminates cells that are no longer needed by the organism. Programmed cell death is mediated through proapoptotic proteins such as Bax and Bak. Antiapoptotic proteins such as Bcl-2, Bcl-XL, Mcl-1, and A1 undergo heterodimerization with Bax and Bak, hence preventing apoptosis. Inhibitors of the antiapoptotic proteins, Bcl-XS and Bad, indirectly cause apoptosis by binding antiapoptotic proteins and preventing their

dimerization with Bax and Bak (161). Genetic mutations in cancer cells may cause a translocation of antiapoptotic protein genes that leads to increased production of the protein product which may block programmed cell death. Bcl-2 overexpression has been demonstrated in endometrial cancers and in cervical cancers.

Senescence is a normal process of cell life and is mediated at least in part by the telomerase enzymes. Telomeres are located at the end of the chromosomes, and consist of a sequence of six nucleotides (TTAGGG) repeated a hundred to a thousand times. Continuous cell division leads to a shortening of the telomere part of the chromosome. The decreasing length of the chromosome eventually leads to cell death. By a process of reverse transcription, telomerase, a ribonucleoprotein enzyme, makes a DNA copy of its own RNA and fuses it to the 3′ end of the chromosome. Telomerase activity is present in germ cells throughout life. In contrast, somatic cells do not have telomerase activity, and therefore are able to divide only for a limited number of times (40 times for a normal fibroblast) before death. Cancer cells that are immortal usually have acquired telomerase activity. However, telomeres in cancer cells are often smaller than the ones of normal cells. Hence, acquisition of telomerase activity by cancer cells might be a late event in the process of cancerization. Increased telomerase activity has been demonstrated in primary ovarian cancers (162).

Tumor suppressor genes were discovered by A. Knudson, who postulated that two or more mutations were necessary in the process of tumorigenesis (163). Many tumor suppressors have been identified: *p53* (Li-Fraumeni syndrome) and *BRCA1* and *BRCA2* (breast and ovarian cancers) on chromosome 17, *Rb* on chromosome 13 (retinoblastoma), *Wt1* on chromosome 11 (Wilms' tumor), *APC* on chromosome 5 (adenomatous polyposis coli), and others. Normal expression of one of the alleles of these genes is necessary for normal control of the cell cycle. If the expression of both alleles is deficient, either by loss or by mutation, the cell cycle loses its physiologic control, since most of these tumor suppressor molecules control inhibitors of cyclin-cdk complexes (see Fig. 1-18). For example, p21, p27, and p16 are inhibitor proteins that regulate cyclin-cdk expression. In their absence, the cyclin-cdk complexes remain activated, and the cell stays in a mitotic state. p53, and TGF-β and cell-cell contact, are potent stimulators of p21 and p27, respectively, thereby leading to cell cycle arrest in G_1 (164).

Oncogenes are genes that have a positive influence on cell growth. Their normal counterparts, called *proto-oncogenes*, are vital constituents of normal cells and regulate such functions as signal transduction and transcription. Some mutations such as translocation or amplification activate these proto-oncogenes to dominant oncogenes. Alteration of one allele may give rise to a product capable of transforming the cell. The most studied ones are *ras*, *myc*, and *src*, as well as some growth factors (TGF-α, HER-2/*neu*) (165). Other oncogenes are the results of viral infection as observed in cervical cancer. Preclinical experiments are studying antisense oligonucleotides as blocking agents to prevent the translation of the oncogene mRNA (166).

Metastasis is probably a late step of cancerization in most tumors. The metastatic clones must have two essential properties: They must be able to adhere and invade the target organ, and they must be able to grow in the target organ. Metastases are frequently responsible for the death of the patient. Therefore, new therapies, such as inhibitors of matrix-degrading metalloproteinases, a family of at least 11 different enzymes, are targeting some of the metastatic steps (167). The development of metastases in a target organ is probably dependent on a paracrine and autocrine interplay of endogenous and stromal growth factors and their receptors (168). After a critical metastatic mass is obtained, angiogenesis is required for continued growth. Inhibitors of angiogenesis such as the derivative of fumagillin, TNP-470, are presently in phase II studies, and positive results have been observed in controlling cervical cancer (169).

All these steps of carcinogenesis are only possible in a disrupted environment that promotes uncontrolled cellular growth.

We reviewed the current knowledge on hormonal and growth factor interactions in breast and gynecologic physiology, and showed how some mechanisms can be dysregulated and lead to cancerization.

The clinical use of hormones in specific cancer situations is described in the appendix.

Appendix: Hormonal Treatment Options for Gynecologic Cancers

Breast Cancer

The presence or absence of estrogen and progesterone receptors on the primary tumor should be determined.

Premenopausal and Perimenopausal Women

Ovariectomy seems to improve survival (170).

Timing of the mastectomy during the menstrual cycle may influence the prognosis (171).

Hormones may be used if the tumor is receptor positive or receptor status is unknown (see Table 1-2). Hormones are usually given for recurrent cancer (170).

Hormone replacement in patients without evidence of disease is undergoing clinical study (172).

Postmenopausal Women

Hormonal treatment with tamoxifen for a period of 2 to 5 years should be instituted after removal of the primary tumor (170).

Endometrial Adenocarcinoma

For recurrent or metastatic cancer, progestins are used. A 15% to 40% response rate has been reported. The usual dose is 40 mg four times a day for megestrol and 1 g a week for medroxyprogesterone. Other agents that have shown efficacy are tamoxifen and GnRH agonists (173). Low-grade tumors and tumors bearing PRs have a higher likelihood to respond to hormonal manipulations.

Uterine Sarcoma and Mixed Mesodermal Müllerian Tumors

Inoperable low-grade tumor should be treated with a GnRH agonist (174). High-grade lesions have been described anecdotally to respond to hormonal manipulation.

Ovarian Epithelial Tumors

Early studies done in previously untreated patients with ovarian epithelial tumors reported a 50% response rate. Today, there is no consensus of hormonal effectiveness in the treatment of refractory ovarian cancer. Occasional responses and stabilization of disease are observed in 15% of patients with refractory disease (175). The survival rate after hormonal therapy (tamoxifen 20 mg twice a day and leuprolide acetate 7.5 mg every month) is similar to that after second-line chemotherapy (176). No correlation has been established between the presence of steroidal receptors and response to hormonal therapy.

Other Gynecologic Tumors

- Cervical cancer is rarely responsive to hormonal therapy. However, bromocriptine, an inhibitor of prolactin, may be active in rare cases.

- There are no available data on trophoblastic disease.

- Some ovarian stromal cancers can be effectively managed with a GnRH agonist (177).

Acknowledgments

We thank Dr. Gordon Mills for his critical review of this manuscript.

REFERENCES

1. Parker SL, Tong T, Bolden S, Wingo PA. Cancer statistics, 1996. *CA Cancer J Clin* 1996;46:5–27.

2. Hillier SG, Reichert LE, Van Hall EV. Control of preovulatory follicular estrogen biosynthesis in human ovary. *J Clin Endocrinol Metab* 1981; 52:847–856.

3. Tsang BK, Armstrong DT, Whitfield JF. Steroid biosynthesis by isolated human ovarian follicular cells in vitro. *J Clin Endocrinol Metab* 1980;51:1407–1411.

4. McNatty KP, Makris A, DeGrazia C, et al. Steroidogenesis by recombined follicular cells from the human ovary in vitro. *J Clin Endocrinol Metab* 1980;51:1286–1292.

5. Gwynne JI, Strauss JF. The role of lipoproteins in steroidogenesis and cholesterol metabolism in steroidogenic glands. *Endocr Rev* 1982;3:299–329.

6. Clement P. Anatomy and histology of the ovary. In: Kurman R, ed. *Blaustein's pathology of the female genital tract.* New York: Springer, 1994:565.

7. Ferguson DJ, Anderson TJ. Morphological evaluation of cell turnover in relation to the menstrual cycle in the "resting" human breast. *Br J Cancer* 1981;44:177–181.

8. Longacre TA, Bartow SA. A correlative morphologic study of human breast and endometrium in the menstrual cycle. *Am J Surg Pathol* 1986;10:382–393.

9. Sabourin JC, Martin A, Baruch J, et al. *bcl*-2 expression in normal breast tissue during the menstrual cycle. *Int J Cancer* 1994;59:1–6.

10. Fitzpatrick RL, Liggins GC. Effects of prostaglandins on the cervix of pregnant women and sheep. In: Naftolin F, Stubblefield PF, eds. *Dilatation of the uterine cervix.* New York: Raven, 1980:287.

11. Ferenczy A. Studies of the cytodynamics of human endometrial regeneration: II. Transmission electron microscopy and histochemistry. *Am J Gynecol* 1976;124:582–595.

12. Ferenczy A. Anatomy and histology of the uterine corpus. In: Kurman R, ed. *Blaustein's pathology of the female genital tract.* New York: Springer, 1994:327.

13. Murad F, Kuret JA. Estrogens and progestins. In: Goodman Gilman A, Rall TW, Nies AS, Taylor P, eds. *The pharmacological basis of therapeutics.* New York: McGraw Hill, 1993:1384.

14. Jordan VC, Mittal S, Gosden B, et al. Structure-activity relationships of estrogens. *Environ Health Perspect* 1985;61:97–110.

15. Duax WL, Griffin JF, Weeks CM, Wawzark Z. The mechanism of action of steroid antagonists:

insights from crystallographic studies. *J Steroid Biochem* 1988;31:481–492.

16. Giusti RM, Iwamoto K, Hatch EE. Diethyl-stilbestrol revisited: a review of the long term health effects. *Ann Intern Med* 1995;122: 778–788.

17. Makela S, Santti R, McLachlan JA. Phytoestrogens are partial estrogen agonists in the adult male mouse. *Environ Health Perspect* 1995;103 (S7):123–127.

18. Miquel JF, Gilbert J. A chemical classification of nonsteroidal antagonists of sex-steroid hormone action. *J Steroid Biochem* 1988;31:525–544.

19. Wentz AC. Assessment of estrogen and progestin therapy in gynecology and obstetrics. *Clin Obstet Gynecol* 1977;20:461–482.

20. Baulieu EE. Contragestation and other clinical applications of RU 486, an antiprogesterone at the receptor. *Science* 1989;245:1351–1357.

21. Markopoulos C, Berger U, Wilson P, et al. Oestrogen receptor content of normal breast cells and breast carcinomas throughout the menstrual cycle. *BMJ* 1988;296:1349–1351.

22. Battersby S, Robertson BJ, Anderson TJ, et al. Influence of menstrual cycle, parity and oral contraceptive use on steroid hormone receptors in normal breast. *Br J Cancer* 1992;65:601–607.

23. Miller WR. Oestrogens and breast cancer: biological considerations. *Br Med Bull* 1991;47:470–483.

24. Kelsey JL, Gammon MD, John EM. Reproductive factors and breast cancer. *Epidemiol Rev* 1993;15:36–47.

25. el-Aaser AA, el-Merzabani MM, Abu-Bedair FA. Serum estrogen level in Egyptian breast cancer patients. *Tumori* 1985;71:293–295.

26. Osborne MP, Bradlow HL, Wong GY, Telang NT. Upregulation of estradiol C16α-hydroxylation in human breast tissue: a potential biomarker of breast cancer risk. *J Natl Cancer Inst* 1993;85:1917–1920.

27. Guillino PM, Pettigrew HM, Grantham FH. N-Nitrosomethylurea as a mammary gland carcinogen in rats. *J Natl Cancer Inst* 1975;54:401–414.

28. Fathalla MF. Incessant ovulation: a factor in ovarian neoplasia. *Lancet* 1971;2:163.

29. Kovacs WJ, Griffin JE, Weaver DD, et al. A mutation that causes lability of the androgen receptor under conditions that normally promote transformation to the DNA-binding state. *J Clin Invest* 1984;73:1095–1104.

30. Imperato McGinley J, Guerrero L, Gautier T, Peterson RE. Steroid 5-alpha-reductase deficiency in man: an inherited form of male pseudohermaphroditism. *Science* 1974;186: 1213–1215.

31. Wilson JD. Androgens. In: Goodman Gilman A, Rall TW, Nies AS, Taylor P, eds. *The pharmacological basis of therapeutics*. New York: McGraw Hill, 1993:1413.

32. Neri RO. Antiandrogens. *Adv Sex Horm Res* 1976;2:233–262.

33. Marchetti B, Labrie F. Characteristics of flutamide action on prostatic and testicular functions in the rat. *J Steroid Biochem* 1988;29: 691–698.

34. Schellhammer PF, Vogelzang NJ, Sharifi R, et al. Updated results of a randomized, double blind trial in 813 previously untreated metastatic prostate cancer patients comparing the antiandrogens bicalutamide and flutamide in combination with luteinizing hormone releasing hormone analogue therapy. *Proc Am Soc Clin Oncol* 1996;15:245.

35. Geller J, Albert J, Vik A. Advantages of total androgen blockade in the treatment of advanced prostatic cancer. *Semin Oncol* 1988;15:53–61.

36. Gormley GJ, Stoner E, Bruskewitz RC, et al. The effect of finasteride in men with benign prostatic hyperplasia. The finasteride study group. *N Engl J Med* 1992;327:1185.

37. Fiddes JC, Goodman HM. The gene encoding the common alpha subunit of the four human glycoprotein hormones. *J Mol Appl Genet* 1993;1: 3–18.

38. Fiddes JC, Talmadge K. Structure, expression, and evolution of the genes for the human glycoprotein hormones. *Recent Prog Horm Res* 1984;40:43–78.

39. Talmadge K, Boorstein WR, Fiddes JC. The human genome contains seven genes for the β-subunit of chorionic gonadotropin but only one gene for the β-subunit of luteinizing hormone. *DNA* 1983;2:281–289.

40. Akerblom IE, Slater EP, Beato M, et al. Negative regulation by glucocorticoids through interference with a cAMP responsive enhancer. *Science* 1988;241:350–353.

41. Boothby M, Ruddon RW, Anderson C, et al. A single gonadotropin α-subunit gene in normal

tissue and tumor-derived cell lines. *J Biol Chem* 1981;256:5121–5127.

42. Caft KJ, Dufau ML. Gonadotropic hormones: biosynthesis, secretion, receptors, and actions. In: Yen SSC, Jaffe RB, eds. *Reproductive endocrinology*. Philadelphia: WB Saunders, 1991:105.

43. Pierce JG, Parsons TF. Glycoprotein hormones: structure and function. *Annu Rev Biochem* 1981; 50:465–495.

44. Gharib SD, Wierman ME, Shupnik MA, Chin WW. Molecular biology of the pituitary gonadotropins. *Endocr Rev* 1990;11:177–199.

45. Talmadge K, Vamvakopoulos NC, Fiddes JC. Evolution of the genes for the beta subunits of human chorionic gonadotropin and luteinizing hormone. *Nature* 1984;307:37–40.

46. Sairam MR. Role of carbohydrates in glycoprotein hormone signal transduction. *FASEB J* 1989;3:1915–1926.

47. Wilson CA, Leight AJ, Chapman AJ. Gonadotropin glycosylation and function. *J Endocrinol* 1990;125:3–14.

48. Ryan RJ, Charlesworth MC, McCormick DJ, et al. The glycoprotein hormones: recent studies of structure-function relationships. *FASEB J* 1988; 2:2661–2669.

49. Shupnik MA, Weinmann CM, Notides AC, Chin WW. An upstream region of the rat luteinizing hormone β gene binds estrogen receptors and confers estrogen responsiveness. *J Biol Chem* 1989;264:80–86.

50. Niall HD, Hogan ML, Tregear GW, et al. The chemistry of growth hormone and the lactogenic hormones. *Recent Prog Horm Res* 1973;29:387–416.

51. Nelson C, Albert VR, Elsholtz HP, et al. Activation of cell-specific expression of rat growth hormone and prolactin genes by a common transcription factor. *Science* 1988;239:1400–1405.

52. Clevenger CV, Chang WP, Ngo W, et al. Expression of prolactin and prolactin receptor in human breast carcinoma: evidence for an autocrine/paracrine loop. *Am J Pathol* 1995;146: 695–705.

53. Ginsburg E, Vonderhaar BK. Prolactin synthesis and secretion by human breast cancer cells. *Cancer Res* 1995;55:2591–2595.

54. Kazadi BJ, Robledo AMC, Sola GJ, et al. An ovarian sex cord tumor with annular tubules secreting prolactin. *Rev Fr Gynecol Obstet* 1995;90:27.

55. Massague J. The transforming growth factor-β family. *Annu Rev Cell Biol* 1990;6:597–641.

56. Yingling JM, Wang XF, Bassing CH. Signaling by the transforming growth factor-β receptors. *Biochim Biophys Acta* 1995;1242:115–136.

57. Massague J. The TGF-β family of growth and differentiation factors. *Cell* 1987;49:437–438.

58. Vale W, Rivier C, Hsueh A, et al. Chemical and biological characterization of the inhibin family of protein hormones. *Recent Prog Horm Res* 1988;44:1–34.

59. Merchenthaler I, Culler MD, Fetrusz P, Negro-Vilar A. Immunocytochemical localization of inhibin in rat and human reproductive tissues. *Mol Cell Endocrinol* 1987;54:239–243.

60. de Jong FM. Inhibin. *Physiol Rev* 1988;68:555.

61. Carroll RS, Corrigan AZ, Gharib SD, Vale W. Inhibin, activin, and follistatin: regulation of follicle-stimulating hormone messenger ribonucleic acid levels. *Mol Endocrinol* 1989;3:1969–1976.

62. Mason AJ, Berkemeier LM, Schmelzer CH, Schwall RH. Activin B: precursor sequences, genomic structure and in vitro activities. *Mol Endocrinol* 1989;3:1352–1358.

63. Hutchinson LA, Findlay JK, de Vos FL, Robertson DM. Effects of bovine inhibin, transforming growth factor-β and bovine activin-A on granulosa cell differentiation. *Biochem Biophys Res Commun* 1987;146:1405–1412.

64. Vale W, Rivier J, Vaughan J, et al. Purification and characterization of an FSH releasing protein from porcine ovarian follicular fluid. *Nature* 1986;321:776–779.

65. Want OF, Farnworth PG, Findlay JK, Burger HG. Inhibitory effect of pure 31-kilodalton bovine inhibin on gonadotropin-releasing hormone (GnRH)-induced up-regulation of GnRH binding sites in culture rat anterior pituitary cells. *Endocrinology* 1989;124:368.

66. Yen SSC. The human menstrual cycle: neuroendocrine regulation. In: Yen SSC, Jaffe RB, eds. *Reproductive endocrinology*. Philadelphia: WB Saunders, 1991:273.

67. Di Simone N, Crowley WF Jr, Want QF, et al. Characterization of inhibin/activin subunit, follistatin, and activin type II receptors in human ovarian cancer cell lines: a potential role in

autocrine growth regulation. *Endocrinology* 1996;137:486–494.

68. Petersen OH. Control of insulin secretion in pancreatic β-cells. *News Physiol Sci* 1990;5:254.

69. Daughaday WH, Rotwein P. Insulin-like growth factor I and II. Peptide, messenger ribonucleic acid and gene structures, serum and tissue concentrations. *Endocr Rev* 1989;10:68–91.

70. Zhou J, Chin E, Bondy C. Cellular pattern of insulin-like growth factor-I (IGF-I) and IGF-I receptor gene expression in the developing and mature ovarian follicle. *Endocrinology* 1991;129:3281–3288.

71. Hernandez ER, Hurwitz A, Vera A, et al. Expression of the genes encoding insulin-like growth factors and their receptors in the human ovary. *J Clin Endocrinol Metab* 1992;74:419–425.

72. Erickson GF, Nakatani A, Liu XJ, et al. Role of insulin-like growth factors and IGF-binding proteins in folliculogenesis. In: Findlay JK, ed. *Molecular biology of the female reproductive system.* San Diego: Academic, 1994:101–127.

73. Adashi EY, Resnick CE, Brodie AMH, et al. Insulin-like growth factors as intraovarian regulators of granulosa cell growth and function. *Endocr Rev* 1985;6:400–420.

74. Shimasaki S, Ling N. Identification and molecular characterization of insulin-like growth factor binding proteins (IGFBP-1, -2, -3, -4, -5, and -6). *Prog Growth Factor Res* 1991;3:243.

75. Liu XJ, Malkowski M, Guo Y, et al. Development of specific antibodies to rat insulin-like growth factor binding proteins (IGFBP-2 to 6): analysis of IGFBP production by rat granulosa cells. *Endocrinology* 1992;132:1176–1183.

76. LeRoith D, Baserga R, Helman L, Roberts CT Jr. Insulin-like growth factors and cancer. *Ann Intern Med* 1995;122:154–159.

77. Resnicoff M, Sell C, Rubini M, Baserga R. Rat glioblastoma cells expressing an antisense RNA to the insulin-like growth factor-I (IGF-I) receptor are non-tumorigenic and induce regression of wild type tumors. *Cancer Res* 1994;54:2218–2222.

78. Manni A, Badger B, Wei L, et al. Hormonal regulation of insulin-like growth factor II and insulin-like growth factor binding protein expression by breast cancer cells in vivo: evidence for stromal epithelial interactions. *Cancer Res* 1994;54:2934–2942.

79. Tronick SR, Aaronson SA. Growth factors and signal transduction. In: Mendelsohn J, Howley P, Israel MA, Liotta LA, eds. *The molecular basis of cancer.* Philadelphia: WB Saunders, 1995:117–140.

80. Gospodarowicz D. Biological activities of fibroblast growth factors. *Ann NY Acad Sci* 1991;638:1–8.

81. Hearn MT. Structure and function of the heparin-binding (fibroblast) growth factor family. *Baillieres Clin Endocrinol Metab* 1991;5:571–593.

82. Jaye M, Schiessinger J, Dionne CA. Fibroblast growth factor receptor tyrosine kinases: molecular analysis and signal transduction. *Biochim Biophys Acta* 1992;1135:185–199.

83. Klagsbrun M, Baird A. A dual receptor system is required for basic fibroblast growth factor activity. *Cell* 1991;67:229–231.

84. Rosen A, Sevelda P, Klein M, et al. First experience in FGF-(int-2) amplification in women with epithelial ovarian cancer. *Br J Cancer* 1993;67:1122–1125.

85. LaPolt PS, Yamato M, Veljkovic M, et al. Basic fibroblast growth factor induction of granulosa cell tissue-type plaminogen, activator expression and oocyte maturation: potential role as a paracrine ovarian hormone. *Endocrinology* 1990;127:2357–2363.

86. Massague J, Pandiella A. Membrane-anchored growth factors. *Annu Rev Biochem* 1993;62:515–541.

87. Salomon DS, Brandt R, Ciardiello F, Normanno NO. Epidermal growth factor-related peptides and their receptors in human malignancies. *Crit Rev Oncol Hematol* 1995;19:183–232.

88. Carpenter G, Cohen S. Epidermal growth factor and transforming growth factor α. *Baillieres Clin Endocrinol Metab* 1991;5:553.

89. Mroczkowski B, Reich M. Identification of biologically active epidermal growth factor precursor in human fluids and secretions. *Endocrinology* 1993;132:417–425.

90. Campbell I, Bork P. Epidermal growth factor-like molecules. *Curr Opin Struct Biol* 1993;3:385.

91. Ruoslahti E, Yamaguchi Y. Proteoglycans as modulators of growth factor activities. *Cell* 1991;64:867–869.

92. Prigent SA, Lemoine NR. The type 1 (EGFR-related) family of growth factor receptors and their ligands. *Prog Growth Factor Res* 1992;4:1–24.

93. Coussens L, Yang-Feng TL, Liao YC, et al. Tyrosine kinase receptor with extensive homology to

EGF receptor shares chromosomal location with Neu oncogene. *Science* 1985;230:1132–1139.

94. Chrysogelos SA, Dickson RB. EGF receptor expression, regulation, and function in breast cancer. Breast *Cancer Res Treat* 1994;29:29–40.

95. Birmelin G, Zimmer V, Sauerbrei W, et al. Relationship between epidermal growth factor receptor (EGF-R) and various prognostic factors in human endometrial carcinoma. *Int J Gynecol Cancer* 1992;2:66.

96. Scambia G, Benedetti-Panici P, Ferrandina G, et al. Epidermal growth factor, oestrogen and progesterone receptor expression in primary ovarian cancer: correlation with clinical outcome and response to chemotherapy. *Br J Cancer* 1995;72:361–366.

97. Bramley TA, Menzies GS, Baird DT. Specific binding of gonadotrophin-releasing hormone and an agonist to human corpus luteum homogenates characterization, properties, and luteal phase levels. *J Clin Endocrinol Metab* 1985;61:834.

98. Wiznitzer A, Marbach M, Hazum E, et al. Gonadotropin-releasing hormone specific binding sites in uterine leiomyomata. *Biochem Biophys Res Commun* 1988;152:1326–1331.

99. Iwashita M, Evans MI, Catt KJ. Characterization of a gonadotropin-releasing hormone receptor site in term placenta and chorionic villi. *J Clin Endocrinol Metab* 1986;62:127.

100. Emons G, Ortmann O, Becker M, et al. High affinity binding and direct antiproliferative effects of LHRH analogues in human ovarian cancer cell lines. *Cancer Res* 1993;53:5439–5446.

101. Ohno T, Imai A, Furui T, et al. Presence of gonadotropin-releasing hormone and its messenger ribonucleic acid in human ovarian epithelial carcinoma. *Am J Obstet Gynecol* 1993;169:605–610.

102. Emons G, Schally AV. The use of luteinizing hormone releasing hormone agonists and antagonists in gynaecological cancers. *Hum Reprod Update* 1994;9:1364–1379.

103. Marchetti B, Guarcello V, Morale MC, et al. Luteinizing hormone-releasing hormone-binding sites in the rat thymus: characteristics and biological function. *Endocrinology* 1989;125:1025–1036.

104. Mann DR, Ansari AA, Akinbami MA, et al. Neonatal treatment with luteinizing hormone-releasing hormone analogs alters peripheral lymphocyte subsets and cellular and humorally mediated immune responses in juvenile and adult male monkeys. *J Clin Endocrinol Metab* 1994;78:292–298.

105. Batticane N, Morale MC, Gallo F, et al. Luteinizing hormone-releasing hormone signaling at the lymphocyte involves stimulation of interleukin-2 receptor expression. *Endocrinology* 1991;129:277–286.

106. Sen GC, Lengyel P. The interferon system. *J Biol Chem* 1992;267:5017.

107. Bradley EC, Grimm E. Interleukins. In: Holland JF, Frei E, Bast RC, et al, eds. *Cancer medicine.* Philadelphia: Lea & Febiger, 1993:941–948.

108. Spriggs DR. Tumor necrosis factor: basic principles and preclinical studies. In: DeVita VT Jr, Hellman S, Rosenberg SA, eds. *Biologic therapy of cancer.* Philadelphia: JB Lippincott, 1991:354–377.

109. Griffin JD. Clinical applications of colony stimulating factors. *Oncology* 1988;2:15–23.

110. Sancho-Tello M, Perez-Roger I, Imakawa K, et al. Expression of TNFα in the rat ovary. *Endocrinology* 1992;130:1359–1364.

111. Piggot R. *The adhesion molecule facts book.* San Diego: Academic, 1993.

112. Evans RM. The steroid and thyroid hormone receptor superfamily. *Science* 1988;240:889.

113. Giguere V, Ong ES, Segui P, Evans RM. Identification of a receptor for the morphogen retinoic acid. *Nature* 1987;330:624.

114. Mangelsdorf DJ, Ong ES, Dyck JA, Evans RM. Nuclear receptor that identifies a novel retinoic acid-response pathway. *Nature* 1990;345:224.

115. Charpentier B, Bernardon JM, Eustache J, et al. Synthesis, structure-affinity relationships, and biological activities of ligands binding to retinoic acid receptor subtypes. *J Med Chem* 1995;38:4993.

116. Yu VC, Delsert C, Andersen B, et al. RXR-β: a coregulator that enhances binding of retinoic acid, thyroid hormone, and vitamin D receptors to their cognate response elements. *Cell* 1991;67:1251.

117. Schule R, Umesono K, Mangelsdorf DJ, et al. Jun-Fos and receptors for vitamins A and D recognize a common response element in the human osteocalcin gene. *Cell* 1990;61:497.

118. Gudas LJ, Sporn MB, Roberts AB. Cellular biology and biochemistry of the retinoids. In: Sporn MB, Roberts AB, Goodman DS, eds. *The retinoids.* New York: Raven, 1994:443–520.

119. Bagavandoss P, Midgley AR Jr. Lack of difference between retinoic acid and retinol in stimulating progesterone production by luteinizing granulosa cells in vitro. *Endocrinology* 1987; 121:420.

120. Umesono K, Murakami KK, Thompson CC, Evans RM. Direct repeats as selective response elements for the thyroid hormone, retinoic acid, and vitamin D_3 receptors. *Cell* 1991;65:1255–1266.

121. Tsang SS, Li G, Stich HF. Effect of retinoic acid on bovine papillomavirus (BPV) DNA-induced transformation and number of BPV DNA copies. *Int J Cancer* 1988;42:94–98.

122. Clarke CL, Graham J, Roman SD, Sutherland RL. Direct transcriptional regulation of the progesterone receptor by retinoic acid diminishes progestin responsiveness in the breast cancer cell line TA7D. *J Biol Chem* 1991;266:18969–18975.

123. Cobleigh MA, Dowlatshahi K, Deutsch TA, et al. Phase I/II trial of tamoxifen with or without fenretinide, an analog of vitamin A, in women with metastatic breast cancer. *J Clin Oncol* 1993;11:474–477.

124. Harris JR, Lippman ME, Veronesi U, Willet W. Breast cancer (third of 3 parts). *N Engl J Med* 1992;327:473–480.

125. Vasios GW, Gold JD, Petkovich M, et al. A retinoic acid-responsive element is present in the 5′ flanking region of the laminin Bl gene. *Proc Natl Acad Sci USA* 1989;86:9099–9103.

126. Bartsch D, Boye B, Baust C, et al. Retinoic acid-mediated repression of human papillomavirus 18 transcription and different ligand regulation of the retinoic acid receptor β gene in non-tumorigenic and tumorigenic HeLa hybrid cells. *EMBO J* 1992;11:2283–2291.

127. Lippman SM, Kavanagh JJ, Paredes-Espinoza MM, et al. 13-cis retinoic acid plus interferon-alpha 2a in locally advanced squamous cell carcinoma of the cervix. *J Natl Cancer Inst* 1993;85:499–500.

128. Schule R, Rangarajan P, Yang N, et al. Retinoic acid is a negative regulator of AP-1 responsive genes. *Proc Natl Acad Sci USA* 1991;88:6092–6096.

129. Evans RM. The steroid and thyroid hormone receptor superfamily. *Science* 1988;240:889–895.

130. Kumar V, Green S, Stack G, et al. Functional domains of the human estrogen receptor. *Cell* 1987;51:941–951.

131. Tora L, White J, Brou C. The human estrogen receptor has two independent nonacidic transcriptional activation functions. *Cell* 1989; 54:477–487.

132. McGuire WL, Chamness GC, Fuqua SAW. The importance of normal and abnormal oestrogen receptor in breast cancer. *Cancer Surv* 1992; 14:31–40.

133. Murphy LC, Dotzlaw H, Hamerton J, Schwarz J. Investigation of the origin of variant, truncated estrogen receptor-like mRNAs identified in some human breast cancer biopsy samples. *Breast Cancer Res Treat* 1993;26:149–161.

134. Osborne CK, Coronado E, Allred DC, et al. Acquired tamoxifen resistance: correlation with reduced breast tumor levels of tamoxifen and isomerization of trans-4-hydroxytamoxifen. *J Natl Cancer Inst* 1991;83:1477–1482.

135. Kieback DG, McCamant SK, Press MF, et al. Improved prediction of survival in advanced adenocarcinoma of the ovary by immunocytochemical analysis of the composition adjusted receptor level of the estrogen receptor. *Cancer Res* 1993;53:5188–5192.

136. Kauppila A. Progestin therapy of endometrial, breast and ovarian carcinoma. *Acta Obstet Gynecol Scand* 1984;63:441–450.

137. Ingram SS, Rosenman J, Heath R, et al. The predictive value of progesterone receptor levels in endometrial cancer. *Int J Radiat Oncol Biol Phys* 1989;17:21–27.

138. Berridge MJ, Bourne H, Hafen E, et al. Cell signaling. In: Alberts B, Bray D, Lewis J, et al, eds. *Molecular biology of the cell*. New York: Garland, 1994:721.

139. Carpenter G. Receptors for epidermal growth factor and other polypeptide mitogens. *Annu Rev Biochem* 1987;56:881.

140. Fantl WJ, Johnson DE, Williams LT. Signalling by receptor tyrosine kinases. *Annu Rev Biochem* 1993;62:453–481.

141. Mayer BJ, Baltimore D. Signalling through SH2 and SH3 domains. *Trends Cell Biol* 1993;3:8.

142. Pawson T, Gish G. SH2 and SH3 domains: from structure to function. *Cell* 1992;71:359–362.

143. Bollag G, McCormick F. Putting back the GTP. *Curr Biol* 1992;2:329.

144. Pawson T, Schlessinger J. SH2 and SH3 domains. *Curr Biol* 1993;3:434.

145. Lowy DR, Willumsen BM. Function and regulation of Ras. *Annu Rev Biochem* 1993;62: 851–891.

146. Nishida E, Gotoh Y. The MAP kinase cascade is essential for diverse signal transduction pathways. *Trends Biochem Sci* 1993;18:128–131.

147. Franza BR, Rauscher FJ, Josephs SF, Curran T. The Fos complex and Fos-related antigens recognize sequence elements that contain AP-1 binding sites. *Science* 1988;239:1150–1153.

148. Nakabeppu Y, Ryder K, Nathans D. DNA binding activities of three murine jun proteins: stimulation by Fos. *Cell* 1988;55:907–915.

149. Varmus HE. Oncogenes and transcriptional control. *Science* 1987;238:1337–1339.

150. Berridge MJ, Bourne H, Hafen E, et al. Cell signaling, In: Alberts B, Bray D, Lewis J, et al, eds. *Molecular biology of the cell.* New York: Garland, 1994:763–766.

151. Lin HY, Lodish HF. Receptors for the TGF-β superfamily: multiple polypeptides and serine/threonine kinases. *Trends Cell Biol* 1993;3:14.

152. Moustakas A, Takumi T, Lin HY, Lodish HF. GH3 pituitary tumor cells contain heteromeric type I and type II receptor complexes for transforming growth factor beta and activin-A. *J Biol Chem* 1995;270:765.

153. Bassing CH, Yingling JM, Howe DJ, et al. A transforming growth factor beta type I receptor that signals to activate gene expression. *Science* 1994;263:87–89.

154. Lopez-Casillas F, Cheifetz S, Doody J, et al. Structure and expression of the membrane proteoglycan betaglycan, a component of the TGF-beta receptor system. *Cell* 1991;67:785–795.

155. Cheifetz S, Bellon T, Cales C, et al. Endoglin is a component of the transforming growth factor beta receptor system in human endothelial cells. *J Biol Chem* 1992;267:19027–19030.

156. Wrana JL, Attisano L, Wieser R, et al. Mechanism of activation of the TGF-beta receptor. *Nature* 1994;370:341–347.

157. Laiho M, DeCaprio JA, Ludlow JW, et al. Growth inhibition by TGF-beta linked to suppression of retinoblastoma protein phosphorylation. *Cell* 1990;62:175–185.

158. Datto MB, Li Y, Panus JF, et al. Transforming growth factor beta induces the cyclin-dependent kinase inhibitor p21 through a p53-independent mechanism. *Proc Natl Acad Sci USA* 1995;92: 5545.

159. Elbendary A, Berchuck A, Davis P, et al. Transforming growth factor beta 1 can induce CIP1/WAF1 expression independent of the p53 pathway in ovarian cancer cells. *Cell Growth Differ* 1994;5:1301–1307.

160. Park K, Kim SJ, Bang YJ, et al. Genetic changes in the transforming growth factor beta type II receptor gene in human gastric cancer cells: correlation with sensitivity to growth inhibition by TGF-beta. *Proc Natl Acad Sci USA* 1994;91: 8772–8776.

161. Mikulski S. Pathogenesis of cancer in view of mutually opposing apoptotic and anti-apoptotic growth signal. *Int J Oncol* 1994;4:1257.

162. Counter C, Hirte H, Bacchetti S, Harley C. Telomerase activity in human ovarian carcinoma. *Proc Natl Acad Sci USA* 1994;91:2900–2904.

163. Knudson A, Strong L. Mutation and cancer: a model for Wilms' tumor of the kidney. *J Natl Cancer Inst* 1972;48:313–324.

164. Polyak K, Kato J, Solomon M, et al. p27kip1, a cyclin-cdk inhibitor, links transforming growth factor-β and contact inhibition to cell cycle arrest. *Genes Dev* 1994;8:9–22.

165. Krontiris T. Oncogenes. *N Engl J Med* 1995;333: 303–306.

166. Askari F, McDonnell WM. Antisense-oligonucleotide therapy. *N Engl J Med* 1996;334:316–318.

167. Sato H, Takino T, Okada Y, et al. A matrix metalloproteinase expressed on the surface of invasive tumor cells. *Nature* 1994;370:61–65.

168. Verschraegen C, Giovanella B, Mendoza J, Stehlin J. Specific organ metastases of human melanoma cells injected in the arterial circulation of nude mice. *Anticancer Res* 1991;11:529–535.

169. Levy T, Kudelka A, Verschraegen C, et al. A phase I study of TNP-470 administered to patients with advanced squamous cell carcinoma of the cervix. *Proc Am Assoc Cancer Res* 1996;37: 166.

170. Early Breast Cancer Trialists' Collaborative Group. Systemic treatment of early breast cancer by hormonal, cytotoxic, or immune therapy: 133 randomised trials involving 31,000 recurrences and 24,000 deaths among 75,000 women. *Lancet* 1992;339:1, 71.

171. Senie RT, Rosen PP, Rhodes P, Lesser ML. Timing of breast cancer excision during the menstrual cycle influences duration of disease-free survival. *Ann Intern Med* 1991;115:337–342.

172. Theriault RL, Sellin RV. A clinical dilemma: estrogen replacement therapy in post-menopausal women with a background of primary breast cancer. *Ann Oncol* 1991;2:709–717.

173. Moore TD, Phillips PH, Nerenstone SR, Cheson BD. Systemic treatment of advanced and recurrent endometrial carcinoma: current status and future directions. *J Clin Oncol* 1991;9: 1071–1088.

174. Bremen T, Waibel S, Bender G, et al. Partial tumor remission in recurrent low malignant stromal endometriosis following GnRH agonist treatment. *Cancer Hum Reprod GnRH analogues* 1990;3:189.

175. Kavanagh JJ, Kudelka AP, Verschraegen CF. Role of hormonal therapy in management of ovarian cancer. In: Gerschenson D, McGuire W, eds. *Controversies in management.* New York: Churchill Livingstone, in press.

176. Lopez A, Tessadrelli A, Kudelka AP, et al. Combination therapy with leuprolide acetate and tamoxifen in refractory ovarian cancer. *Int J Gynecol Cancer* 1996;6:15.

177. Fishman A, Kudelka AP, Tresukosol D. Leuprolide acetate in the treatment of refractory or persistent ovarian granulosa cell tumor. *J Reprod Med* 1996;41:393–396.

CHAPTER 2

Progress Toward Tumor-Specific Immunity in Carcinomas of the Ovary and Breast

RALPH S. FREEDMAN
ANDRZEJ P. KUDELKA
CLAIRE F. VERSCHRAEGEN
CHRIS D. PLATSOUCAS

New Technologies in Immunology

Phenomenal breakthroughs in human tumor immunology and the production of novel therapeutic products, also called *biologic response modifiers* (BRMs), have led to the development of effective immunotherapy strategies for cancer patients. From a historical perspective, the first BRMs were developed in the 1960s, 1970s, and 1980s. They had a complex composition with multiple biologic actions or pleiotropic effects that were difficult to resolve in vivo. These early BRMs, which included *Corynebacterium parvum*, bacille Calmette-Guérin (BCG), leukocyte interferon (IFN), and viral oncolysates, produced some significant clinical responses, although the precise mechanisms of action of these agents were difficult to resolve. The clinical results obtained with this first generation of BRMs for the treatment of gynecologic malignancies are reviewed elsewhere (1).

Clinical and laboratory applications of the hybridoma and recombinant DNA technologies have fostered the field of clinical immunology and have led to the identification and isolation of a number of human cytokines and antibodies with therapeutic potential. Cytokines can be produced either by normal or by malignant cells. They may exert their actions either on cells that produce these molecules (autocrine effect) or on other cells in close proximity to the producer cells (paracrine effect) (2). Cytokines have to be distinguished from hormones, which typically act on cells at a distance from the producer cells (endocrine effect). A number of cytokines have been genetically engineered by recombinant DNA technology, and may be almost identical to the naturally occurring molecules. Differences in structure are usually limited to the type and amount of glycosylation. Recombinant interleukin-2 (rIL-2), recombinant interferon-α (rIFN-α), recombinant interferon-γ (rIFN-γ), and recombinant granulocyte colony-stimulating factor (rG-CSF) are examples of recombinant cytokines that have established roles in the therapeutic armamentarium of cancer (3–5). The production and the secretion of cytokines by various human tissues can be measured with accuracy (at the picogram level or lower) by using sensitive standardized immunoassays, available in kit form. Reverse transcriptase–polymerase chain reaction is used to detect and quantitate RNA transcripts of cytokines produced in tissues and in cell populations of interest (Fig. 2-1).

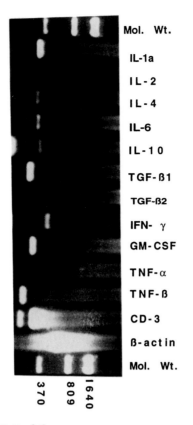

FIGURE **2-1**

Cytokine-specific transcripts identified in an RNA extract of a CD8⁺ ovarian tumor-infiltrating lymphocyte (TIL)–derived T-cell line by reverse transcriptase–polymerase chain reaction. RNA was extracted from the CD8⁺ T-cell line with guanidine thiocyanate/phenol, and complementary DNA (cDNA) was made using murine reverse transcriptase (Gibco BRL). The cDNA was amplified with Taq polymerase (Perkin-Elmer) using primers for the indicated cytokines. Controls included transcription of endogenous CD3 and β-actin messenger RNA (mRNA). The amplified DNA products were displayed on a 1.5% agarose/TBE gel containing 0.5 mg of EtBr per milliliter and photographed under ultraviolet light. Molecular weight markers are shown in nucleotide base pairs. Transcripts are shown for interleukin (IL)-1α, IL-4, IL-6, IL-10, transforming growth factor (TGF)-β1, interferon (IFN)-γ, granulocyte-macrophage colony-stimulating factor (GM-CSF), and tumor necrosis factor (TNF)-β. Transcripts not detected included IL-2, TGF-β2, and TNF-α. (Experiment by M. Nash, PhD.)

Hybridoma technology has led to the production of different monoclonal antibodies (mAbs) that have been used to identify and clone a number of cytokines produced by the hemopoietic system or by tumor cells (6,7). Certain of these molecules play important roles

in the induction or modulation of tumor immunity. The use of mAbs that recognize lymphocyte cell surface antigens by automated fluorescence procedures, such as fluorescence-activated cell sorter (FACS) analysis (8), has made it possible to 1) identify and isolate subsets of mononuclear leukocytes that are involved in tumor immunity, and 2) to monitor the activation of these cells in vivo before and after treatment with agents that modulate tumor immunity. FACS methods that can measure functional properties of cells such as in vitro cytotoxicity (9) and cytokine production (10) have also been developed. Other mAbs also recognize tumor-associated antigens. Detection of the CA-125 antigen with the OC-125 mAb is now well established as an indicator of response to therapy in patients with ovarian cancer. The mAbs with cell surface reactivity have also been conjugated to radioisotopes (radioimmunoconjugates), or to plant or bacterial toxins (immunotoxins). Clinical trials with these products are in progress. The recent development of immunoconjugates of human mAbs, including two developed by our group, that recognize tumor-associated antigens (11–13) has opened up new opportunities for in vivo diagnosis and immunotherapy.

This chapter focuses on the development and application of new strategies to enhance specific or adaptive (new terminology) immunity in the treatment of ovarian and breast cancers. New concepts of tumor vaccinology and of gene transfer methods to enhance tumor-specific immunity are also discussed.

Cancer and Specific Immunity

Tumors may be infiltrated by large numbers of lymphocytes referred to as *tumor-infiltrating lymphocytes* (TILs) or as *tumor-associated lymphocytes* when the cells are derived from malignant effusions. These cells may be responsible for an active immune response of the host specifically directed against the tumor (14,15). TILs have been detected in high numbers in tumors of certain patients with a more favorable prognosis and an increased pattern of survival (16–18). Some investigators (18–23) found significant correlations between T-cell infiltrates and clinical stage or prognosis of breast cancer, but others (23,24) did not.

Cell populations of hemopoietic origin can be distinguished from one another by utilizing mAbs that recognize specific molecules designated by the prefix *CD* (cluster of differentiation) (6). The CD-labeled molecules may be either ligands or receptors (Table 2-1). Fresh TILs from most human solid tumors, including carcinomas of the ovary and breast, are primarily derived from T lymphocytes that express the CD3⁺CD8⁺TCRαβ⁺ or CD3⁺CD8⁺TCRαβ⁺ phenotype. Specific cytotoxicity activity has been attributed to a subset of CD8⁺ T cells. In contrast, T- and B-cell helper functions are an important function of CD4⁺ T-cell subsets. These cells are easily identified by FACS (Fig. 2-2) or by immunohistochemistry using lymphocyte surface antigen–specific mAbs. CD4⁺ T cells can be further subdivided into helper T cells that are type 1 (Th1) or type 2 (Th2). Th1 cells mainly synthesize IFN-γ, granulocyte-macrophage colony-stimulating factor (GM-CSF), and interleukin (IL)-2; Th2 cells secrete IL-4, IL-5, IL-6, and IL-10. Other mononuclear leukocytes are present in smaller numbers and include CD3⁺TCRγδ⁺ cells, non-T lymphocytes such as B cells (CD19⁺ or CD20⁺), natural killer (NK) cells (CD16⁺), and lymphokine-activated killer cells (LAK) which have the CD3⁻CD56⁺ phenotype (i.e., non-T cells), as well as cells of the macrophage-monocyte lineage (CD14⁺ or CD68⁺) and dendritic cells (lineage negative).

There are two types of T-cell receptors (TCRs), the αβTCR and the γδTCR, which are also recognized with mAbs. The αβTCR, which is the most common type expressed by T cells, is made of disulfide-linked polypeptide chains and together with the CD3 complex is responsible for the specific activation of T cells.

A number of activation markers expressed on TILs, including HLA-DR, CD69, CD43, and CD38, are present on a high proportion of breast TILs, suggesting that numerous T cells may be activated in these tumors (25–28).

Fresh TILs from patients with malignant melanoma (29–31) or ovarian carcinomas contain substantial proportions of identical α- and β-chain TCR transcripts, suggesting that they are composed primarily of oligoclonal T cells (32–36). Breast TILs also contain significant proportions of oligoclonal T cells that preferentially utilize the Vβ3.1 and Vβ14 TCR gene segments (32–37) (Heckel MD, Klonowski KD, Schwarting R, Platsoucas CD, unpublished results, 1996). The oligoclonality of the T cells suggests that TILs have undergone specific, albeit unknown antigen-driven proliferation and clonal expansion in vivo at the site of the tumor.

Adaptive immunity is the result of a number of ligand-receptor interactions culminating in the activation of several signaling pathways, as shown schematically in Figure 2-3. The tumor cell might sometimes behave as an antigen-presenting cell. Peptide derived from protein within the cell is presented by the major histo-

TABLE 2-1

Examples of Commonly Used Clusters of Differentiation (CD)

CD Marker	Marker Description	Main Expressing Cells
CD3	Monomorphic complex	T cells
CD4	Coactivation molecule	T cell, monocytes, dendritic cells
CD8	Coactivation molecule	T cells
CD16	Fc receptor	NK cells, monocytes
CD20	EBV receptor	B cells
TCRαβ	Receptor for binding peptide—MHC ligand	T cells
TCRγδ	Receptor on T cells with NK-like function	T cells
CD56	Activation molecule	T cells or LAK cells
CD68	Differentiation antigen	Monocytes
CD69	Activation molecule	T cells
CD38	Activation molecule	T cells
CD43	Activation molecule	T cells
CD28	Receptor for costimulatory molecule	T cells
CD80	Costimulatory molecule	Dendritic cells, monocytes
CD86	Costimulatory molecule	Dendritic cells, monocytes

EBV = Epstein-Barr virus; MHC = major histocompatibility complex; NK = natural killer; LAK = lymphokine-activated killer.

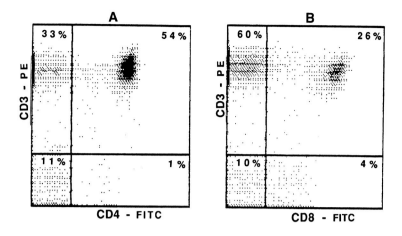

F I G U R E **2-2**

Immunofluorescence analysis of peritoneal exudate cells from a patient with epithelial ovarian cancer, after removal of the granulocyte fraction. Fifty-four percent of the leukocytes were dual positive with anti-CD3 and anti-CD4 monoclonal antibodies (mAbs) (*A*), and 26% were dual positive with anti-CD3 and anti-CD8 mAbs (*B*). To identify the percentage of dual-positive cells, mAbs labeled with two different fluoresceins, phycoerythrin (PE) and fluorescein isothiocyanate (FITC), were used. A live scatter "gate" was used to identify the cell population of interest. Control readings (not shown) were first obtained with a labeled mAb that has the same isotype as the anti-CD mAb, but that is nonreactive with human cells.

F I G U R E **2-3**

Simplified schema showing activation of a T cell through the T-cell receptor complex (TCR-CD3) by a peptide presented in association with the major histocompatibility complex (MHC) as a competent antigen-presenting cell. This represents the first signal. Second signaling results from ligand-receptor interaction of the costimulatory molecules. Also shown are the main signaling pathways leading to activation of the interleukin (IL)-2 cytokine gene.

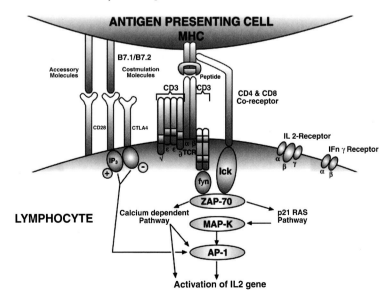

compatibility complex (MHC) protein, on the cell surface, for binding by the TCR. Other molecules such as B7.1 (CD80) and B7.2 (CD86) provide costimulatory signals through another group of receptors on the T cell, CD28 and CTLA-4. Yet other molecules referred to as *adhesion molecules* may result in additional signals to enhance the effect that either may direct cytotoxic action against the target tumor cells or may result in the production and secretion of cytokines that facilitate tumor destruction or growth inhibition. The initial signal is provided through the TCR-CD3 protein complex, assisted by the CD4 and CD8 cofactors (see Fig. 2-3). Secondary signals are provided through costimulation. Optimum activation of T-cell functions can only occur when the correct peptide binds to the TCR with an exact matching motif and when proper signaling is permitted to occur through the intracellular portions of the CD3 molecule and the costimulatory molecules. Malfunction or anergy may result when the first or second signals are interrupted or when improper peptide presentation occurs. Figure 2-3 summarizes the molecular interactions leading to specific or MHC-restricted activation of T lymphocytes, and includes some of the main signaling pathways. Essentially, these interactions involve phosphorylation of kinases (or phosphatase activity) and a cascade of reactions that result in the activation of genes that encode for cytotoxic and other specific functions of these cells (38–40).

Recovery and Characterization of TIL-Derived T Cells in Cancers of the Ovary and Breast

Ovarian Cancer

Ovarian tumor cells and ovarian TILs are easily recovered often in large numbers from abdominal ascites (41). They can also be recovered from biopsy specimens of metastases on the peritoneum or serosa obtained at the time of tumor-reductive laparotomy. On average 200×10^6 mononuclear leukocytes can be harvested from a liter of malignant ascites, or 20×10^6 mononuclear leukocytes from a gram of solid tumor tissue (41). A number of investigators developed T-cell lines from ascites or from solid tumors of patients with ovarian cancer in high concentrations of rIL-2. Most of these T-cell

lines only exhibited MHC unrestricted cytotoxicity, i.e., the T-cell lines exhibit killing against allogeneic (MHC unrelated) as well as against autologous (from the same patient) tumor cells (42–44).

T-cell lines have also been developed from ascites or from solid tumors of ovarian cancer in low concentrations of rIL-2 (41,45–47). These T-cell lines are either $CD3^+CD8^+CD4^-TCR\alpha\beta^+$ or $CD3^+CD8^-CD4^+TCR\alpha\beta^+$. Certain T-cell lines of the $CD3^+CD8^+CD4^-$ phenotype exhibit cytotoxicity primarily against autologous ovarian tumor cells, and do not lyse ovarian tumor cells from other patients or K562 cells (45–47). Blocking experiments using appropriate mAbs demonstrated that the TCR-CD3 complex on the T cells and MHC class I antigens on the tumor cells are involved in the cytolytic process (46). $CD3^+CD8^-CD4^+$, rIL-2–dependent T-cell lines exhibit mainly MHC-unrestricted cytotoxicity and lyse both autologous and allogeneic targets. TILs from certain patients with malignant melanoma and ovarian carcinomas demonstrate many of the characteristic features of a T-cell immune response, such as oligoclonality (29–31), surface expression of activation markers (14), and proliferation in response to low concentrations of rIL-2 (41,45,46,48–56). The production and secretion of cytokines with tumor inhibitory properties comprise a further mechanism whereby T cells might produce a therapeutic response. $CD4^+TCR\alpha\beta^+$ and $CD8^+TCR\alpha\beta^+$ TILs produce and secrete large amounts of IFN-γ and tumor necrosis factor (TNF)-α both in vitro and in vivo. In the presence of low concentrations of rIL-2 (20 IU) in vitro, IFN-γ and TNF-α are detected either in an antigen-dependent (in the presence of autologous tumor) and in an antigen-independent manner (in the presence of allogeneic or HLA-mismatched tumor) (48,57). IFN-γ may exhibit cytostatic effects against tumor cells either directly or by inducing the production of amino acid metabolites that inhibit the proliferation of tumor cells.

Breast Cancer

Studies on T-cell immune responses in breast carcinoma are not as extensive or conclusive as those of melanoma and ovarian carcinoma. A number of investigators (49–65) developed T-cell lines derived from TILs or from draining lymph nodes of patients with breast carcinoma. Certain of these T-cell lines are $CD4^+$ and produce cytokines in response only to autologous tumor cells, that is, autologous tumor specificity (50,51). Other T-cell lines exhibit MHC-unrestricted cytotoxicity against breast tumor cells, which is mediated through their αβTCR. These T cells recognize a protein epitope of the ductal epithelial mucin produced by breast or pancreatic adenocarcinomas (62,63,66,67). In addition, cytotoxic T-cell lines from patients with breast or pancreatic adenocarcinomas recognize Epstein-Barr virus (EBV)–immortalized B cells transfected with epithelial mucin complementary DNA (cDNA) (66,67). This recognition of mucin by MHC-unrestricted T cells may be done in a superantigen-like manner where the repetitive motif binds directly to a TCR site other than that responsible for antigen/MHC recognition. Furthermore, a nonapeptide from the tandem repeat domain of mucin is recognized by MHC-restricted T cells in association with HLA-A11. These T cells were derived from the lymph nodes of an HLA-A11$^+$ patient with breast cancer or from peripheral blood of normal donors by in vitro stimulation with the P9-17 peptide (68). Fresh (not cultured) TILs from patients with breast carcinoma and other cancers respond poorly to TCR/CD3 ligation and produce significantly reduced amounts of IL-2, IFN-γ, and TNF in comparison to peripheral blood mononuclear cells (25,69–75), although TILs from malignant melanoma and ovarian carcinoma demonstrate many characteristic features of a T-cell immune response, such as oligoclonality (29,31–33), surface expression of activation markers [reviewed in (14)], and the ability to proliferate in response to low concentrations of rIL-2 (41–43,48–56). Limiting dilution studies demonstrated that breast carcinoma TILs contained significantly decreased frequencies of proliferating T-lymphocyte precursors (PTL-P) (68,70, 74). However, despite impaired proliferative responses, TILs exhibit relatively high frequencies of potential cytotoxic T-lymphocyte (CTL) precursors (CTL-P) against unknown antigens (determined in a lectin-dependent cytotoxicity assay) (70,71,73). These results suggest that the activation and proliferation potential of TILs is impaired and this may play an important role in the inability of TILs to contain the tumor. This impaired activation and proliferation of breast and other TILs is poorly understood. Although suppressor cells may be responsible for this impaired activation and proliferation, different mechanisms may contribute

(see Inhibitory Effects of Cytokines on Tumor Immunity).

Tumor Antigen Expression and Active Immunity in Ovarian and Breast Cancers

The potentiation of an autologous tumor-specific response requires the presence of T cells that have been specifically activated by antigens expressed by the tumor cell. In contrast to previously held views, these antigens are situated initially inside the cell. Certain antigens such as those associated with mucins or superantigens are exceptions to this general rule. Polypeptides or proteins are digested by enzymes into short-chain peptides, 8 to 10 amino acids long. These peptides are transferred under the influence of the *transporter associated with antigen processing genes* (*TAP*) (76) to the tumor cell surface in association with MHC antigens. Activation of the T cells by these antigens requires that the MHC allele and its motif-matching peptide be recognizable by specific binding regions of the TCR.

Intensive research efforts are ongoing to characterize the structures that are recognized by cytotoxic lymphocytes on tumor cells. T-cell lines with autologous tumor-specific cytotoxicity against melanoma lysed equally well certain allogeneic melanoma cells that shared HLA-A2 or other class I HLA antigens, but did not lyse autologous normal lymphocytes (77,78). Experiments that were conducted with anti-HLA class I–specific antibodies demonstrated significant but not total inhibition of the lysis of melanoma (50) and ovarian targets (45,46). Therefore, other structures in addition to the MHC are involved in the activity of cytotoxic T cells. Through their TCR, both CD4$^+$ and CD8$^+$ T cells recognize peptides presented in association with MHC (45,46,79–82). Most of the current information that is available on human tumor antigens recognized by T cells is from studies of malignant melanoma (81–85). These antigens include MAGE-1 (81–85), tyrosinase (82), gp100 (83), MART-1 (84), and melanin A (85). Peptides derived from these antigens are recognized in association with certain HLA allotypes (e.g., HLA-A1 with MAGE-1 peptides). MAGE-3 (86) is one of 12 members of the MAGE family of tumor antigens. Different MAGE-3 peptides are recognized by cytotoxic T cells on autologous and heterologous melanoma tumor cells in association with HLA-Al (86) and HLA-A2, respectively. MAGE-1 and MAGE-3 transcripts have also been found in 12% of breast carcinomas (87). Two other tumor antigens designated *BAGE* (88) and *GAGE* (89) have been isolated from malignant melanoma. T cells recognize the peptides derived from these antigens on melanoma tumor cells, in association with HLA-Cw*1601 (88) and HLA-Cw*0601 (89), respectively. BAGE and GAGE transcripts have been identified in about 10% of breast carcinomas (88,89). *MAGE*, *BAGE*, and *GAGE* genes are also expressed in fresh epithelial ovarian carcinomas (90).

MAGE-1 (81,91), MAGE-3 (86), BAGE (88), and GAGE (89) are not expressed in normal tissues with the exception of the testis. They may be tumor-specific antigens in female patients and tumor-associated antigens in male patients. Tyrosinase (82,92), MART-1/melan (84,85), gp100 (83), and gp75 (93) do not appear to be expressed in breast carcinoma. These antigens are mostly of the tumorassociated type rather than the tumor-specific type because they are also expressed on normal cells. Tumor-specific antigens usually result from point mutations. Information on structures recognized by breast and by ovarian T cells is scarce (94,95).

Overexpression of HER-2/*neu* proto-oncogene has been detected in 20% to 40% of patients with breast cancer and ovarian cancer, and may correlate with poor prognosis (96–98). Although this is a normal protein, its overexpression may induce cytotoxic T cells (99). Two HER-2/neu peptides that bind to HLA-A2 induce T-cell growth from peripheral mononuclear cells of normal donors (99). A HER-2/neu peptide (designated *GP2*) is recognized in association with HLA-A2 tumor-specific T cells of patients with breast or ovarian carcinoma (92,94,95,100). HLA-2 is expressed in approximately 50% of the white population (101), and HLA-A1 in approximately 10% to 20%.

Wild-type and mutated forms of the tumor suppressor gene, *p53*, are overexpressed in approximately 50% of patients with breast carcinoma (102). The presence of point mutations in *p53* has been associated with substantially increased tumorigenicity and metastatic potential in breast cancer (103–105). Three codons of the *p53* gene have a high frequency of mutations but point mutations have been demonstrated in many codons. No particular mutations predominate in breast cancer. Peripheral mononuclear cells of patients that exhibit in vivo anti-p53 antibody responses to breast carcinoma and whose tumors overexpress *p53* are induced to proliferate in vitro in the presence of wild-type *p53* (106). Cytotoxic lymphocytes from normal donors (106–109) or experimental animals (110,111) can be induced against peptides derived from wild-type or mutant *p53*. Mutated as well as wild-type *p53* peptides demonstrated strong affinity for HLA-A2 and certain other HLA class I molecules (112–114). However, there is no information that particular mutations predominate in breast cancer.

Carcinoembryonic antigen (CEA), an oncofetal antigen, is expressed in a number of cancers, including breast cancer for which CEA expression has been demonstrated in approximately 50% of patients (115). Immunization of mice with a recombinant vaccinia vector expressing the *CEA* gene (*rV-CEA*) partially protected the animals from a syngeneic murine colon adenocarcinoma transduced with the human *CEA* gene (116). Immunization of mice with *rV-CEA* and recombinant vaccinia murine B7-1 (costimulatory molecule) resulted in complete protection and in the generation of specific anti-CEA T-cell responses (117). MHC-restricted cytotoxic T-cell lines recognizing CEA peptides were developed from peripheral mononuclear cells of patients immunized with rV-CEA (115,118). These MHC-restricted T cells were able to lyse autologous EBV-transformed B-cell lines transduced with the CEA gene as well as CEA-expressing carcinoma cells (115). Human anti-CEA T cells can thus be developed by immunizing patients with rV-CEA.

It is probable that T cells infiltrating breast or ovarian carcinomas recognize peptides on the tumor cells in association with MHC molecules. These peptides may be derived from tumor antigens, oncogene proteins, tumor suppressor genes, or oncofetal antigens. New recombinant or peptide-based vaccines can then be designed as specific immunotherapy for the treatment of patients with breast or ovarian carcinomas. Since peptide-based tumor vaccines may be too restricted for many human tumors, other approaches may be needed that incorporate multiple epitopes (119).

HLA Expression and Tumor Immunity

Defective assembly or expression of the MHC class I and class II molecules by cancer cells may contribute to the lack of in vivo activation of T lymphocytes. Certain tumors lose selectively A2 expression. Downregulation of MHC alleles is not always restricted to particular alleles, for example, HLA-A2, and other alleles are frequently involved as well (120–122). Restoration of an effective MHC expression may increase susceptibility to T cells as seen in a human melanoma cell line transduced with HLA-A2, which exhibited increased susceptibility to an HLA-restricted CD8$^+$ cytotoxic T-cell clone (123). MHC and its allelic expression can also be upregulated to normal levels in some but not all specimens after the tumor cells are exposed to IFN-γ or IFN-γ plus TNF-α (122). Upregulation of MHC class I antigens may be required for T cell–mediated immunity (124).

Several studies examined the expression of MHC antigens on ovarian carcinoma cell lines or tumor tissues (120,121,125–127). Previous immunohistochemical studies of tissue sections obtained from patients with ovarian carcinoma revealed a variable degree of expression of HLA class I antigens on ovarian tumor cells (121). MHC class I expression was found in over 95% of ovarian carcinomas, although downregulation of certain MHC class I alleles, including HLA-A2, was observed in a number of tumor specimens. We found that HLA class I and class II expression varied extensively among ovarian carcinoma cells and higher expression of HLA class I molecules correlated with larger numbers of infiltrating T lymphocytes in ovarian tissues (127). Moreover, TIL-derived T-cell lines are easier to develop from tumors expressing a high level of HLA class I (127). Assessment of the surface density expression of HLA and allelic antigens on tumor cells might be helpful in identifying patients who might benefit from active specific immunotherapy strategies. Incorporation of cytokines such as the IFNs in immunotherapeutic strategies may also help to upregulate tumor MHC expression so that these tumors become better targets for tumor-specific immunotherapy (124).

Costimulation and Dendritic Cells

The costimulatory molecules B7.1 (CD80) and B7.2 (CD86) are cell ligands primarily found on antigen-presenting cells such as cells of the macrophage-monocyte lineage, B cells, and dendritic cells (128,129). The B7.1 or B7.2 costimulatory molecules may bind to specific receptors on the T cell (CD28 or CTLA-4) and

provide the second signal that is required for activation of the TCR-CD3 complex. CTLA-4 may have a significantly higher affinity for B7.1 and B7.2 than CD28 has. Activation of CTLA-4 by B7.1 or B7.2 may in fact shut down the activation of the T cell or induce apoptosis (130). Less than 5% of mononuclear leukocytes in the peritoneal cavity of ovarian cancer patients are dendritic cells (131). These cells can be cultured in a medium containing GM-CSF and TNF-α (Fig. 2-4). Dendritic cells were identified by FACS as lineage-negative (lack specific surface markers for T cells, B cells, monocytes, and NK cells), DR-positive cells. These cells are recognized by FACS as being CD4$^+$ and CD86$^+$ and have the features of mature dendritic cells. CD80 antigen (B7.1) was virtually absent. Dendritic cells may present antigenic peptide to CD8$^+$TCRαβ$^+$ or CD4$^+$TCRαβ$^+$ cells through their MHC molecules. The costimulatory molecules of antigen-presenting cells may, however, be downregulated by cytokines produced in the

F I G U R E **2-4**

Microphotograph of dendritic cells in culture showing cytoplasmic processes. (By B. Melichar.)

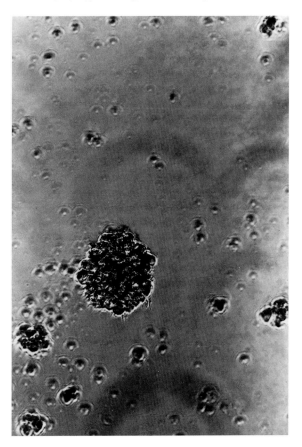

tumor microenvironment. This could be one of the mechanisms by which a tumor may block the activation of cytotoxic or tumor inhibitory cytokine-producing T cells. Other surface molecules such as intercellular adhesion molecule (ICAM)-1 may also function as accessory signaling factors (132). Antigen-presenting cells can present peptides from processed tumor-associated antigens to activate CD8$^+$ and CD4$^+$ T lymphocytes. Alternatively, peptides associated with MHC molecules of adjacent tumor cells might be passively transferred onto the MHC of antigen-presenting cells. Specific activation of lymphocytes could result in proliferation of the activated lymphocytes, cytotoxic activity, or production of specific cytokines in vivo. To investigate the role of costimulation in vivo, we have designed a pilot clinical trial that will employ a canary pox vector, ALVAC B7.1, to express the CD80 (B7.1) gene product into autologous ovarian tumor cells ex vivo. Irradiated intact ovarian tumor cells will be used as an intraperitoneal autologous tumor vaccine in the treatment of ovarian cancer patients who have failed standard chemotherapy.

Inhibitory Effects of Cytokines on Tumor Immunity

A tumor may produce or secrete into the microenvironment immunosuppressant factors that can downregulate or block immunologic effects directed against itself (133). The observed impaired responses may be caused by defects in the signal transduction mechanisms leading to T-cell activation, or downregulation of the MHC or of the costimulatory molecules directly affecting the TCR sites. Subsets of CD8$^+$ cells or CD4$^+$ cells also secrete cytokines such as IFN-γ, TNF-α, and GM-CSF that activate cell-mediated immunity, whereas other lymphocytes produce cytokines (IL-4, IL-5, and IL-6), that drive the differentiation of B cells.

The mechanisms responsible for reduced expression of MHC on tumor cells are largely unknown. However, both transforming growth factor (TGF)-β and IL-10 decreased the expression of HLA molecules on tumoral or normal cells in in vitro studies (134–136). Moreover, both TGF-β (137–140) and IL-10 (141) may suppress the production of cytokines and the lytic functions of T cells and monocytes.

TGF-β is a large family of growth-modifying proteins and is produced by many cells includ-ing platelets, activated macrophages, monocytes, activated T lymphocytes, B cells, and osteoblasts. One isotype, TGF-β1, was detected in the plasma of patients with breast cancer, whereas TGF-β2 was not (140,142). TGF-β2 has been found in malignant melanoma cells (137,138), a finding that appears to correlate with more aggressive behavior of the tumor (139). Three independent studies showed that expression of the TGF-β protein on breast cancer cells in vivo also correlates with a more aggressive disease pattern (140,143,144). TGF-β molecules have a variety of inhibitory effects on the immune system including arrest of T-cell proliferation (145), inhibition of proliferative and lytic activity of cytotoxic LAK precursor cells (136) and of T cells (146), and inhibition of IL-2–induced cytotoxic activity of monocytes in the absence of IFN-γ (147–149). TGF-β also decreased the expression of the IL-2 receptor (γ type) on monocytes (148), induced apoptosis of activated T cells (150), and inhibited the expression of HLA class I and class II antigens on normal tissues (151) and of HLA class II antigens on certain tumor cell lines (152). Although most experiments attributed immunosuppressive properties to TGF-β, others showed that TGF-β can induce CD4$^+$ memory cells in vitro to secrete IL-2 and IFN-γ (153). In contrast to these studies, other studies showed TGF-β1 in vitro to have costimulatory functions on T cells (153–155). A recent study showed that tumor cells from epithelial ovarian cancer express all three isotypes of TGF-β (β1, β2, and β3), although quantitation of protein expression was not performed (156). In the ascitic fluid of ovarian cancer patients, a 25-kd fragment of TGF-β suppressed LAK activity (157). We recently showed that RNA extracts of ovarian tumor tissues and of peritoneal exudates from patients with ovarian cancer express messenger RNA (mRNA) transcripts of TGF-β1 and TGF-β2 (158). In contrast, RNA extracts from ovarian TILs express mRNA transcripts of TGF-β1 but not TGF-β2. Since TGF-β has both autocrine and paracrine effects, and is associated with more aggressive behavior in certain tumors, a decrease in the production of TGF-β by these tumors could possibly change their phenotype to a less aggressive form. A reduction of the inhibitory influence of TGF-β on immunocompetent cells might also result in improved responsiveness of patients to active immunotherapy strategies. A decrease in the production of TGF-β can be accomplished by surgical debulking or by chemotherapeutic means (133). Other cytokines or antisense TGF-β have been used to reduce TGF-β production by tumor cells in vivo (159). Intraperitoneal priming injections of rIFN-γ and rIL-2 in patients with ovarian cancer resulted in an increased expression of HLA class I and class II antigens on the tumor cells of the peritoneal cavity (160). Intraperitoneal rIFN-γ was also associated with a reduction of TGF-β2 expression in peritoneal tumor cells in certain patients. These preliminary findings suggest that the local presence of IFN-γ could trigger opposing effects on HLA and TGF-β2 expression in patients with ovarian cancer. Critical studies are needed to understand the functions of TGF-β in malignancy, their interactions with receptors on both normal and malignant cells at the tumor site, and ways of modulating endogenous production.

IL-10 is a homodimer that has a molecular mass of 39 kd. IL-10 is produced by monocytes and certain IL-2–stimulated CD4$^+$ and CD8$^+$ T cells. IL-10 is an inhibitor of cell-mediated immunity that, with other autoregulatory molecules, modulates the mechanisms of apoptosis of activated T cells and hence may prevent uncontrolled lymphoproliferative disorders, although there is also some evidence for a stimulatory role on adaptive immunity (161–163). IL-10 causes significant reduction in CD3$^+$, CD2$^+$, CD4$^+$, and CD8$^+$ T lymphocytes in the blood of human subjects (164). IL-10 inhibits the expression of HLA class II antigens on monocytes in vitro (135) and of HLA class I antigens on tumor cells (134). Moreover, IL-10 inhibits the production of IL-2 and IFN-γ by activated T cells (137). IL-10 mRNA has been detected in certain tumors, for example, basal and squamous cell carcinomas of the skin (165), bronchial carcinoma (166), melanoma (167), renal cell carcinoma (168), and ovarian cancer (169–171). However, ovarian tumor cell lines do not produce IL-10. IL-10 mRNA has also been detected on certain CD4$^+$ TILs (the type 2 helper T cell) and less frequently on CD8$^+$ TILs. Further studies are needed to determine 1) the immunobiologic role of IL-10 in ovarian cancer, 2) which cells within these tumors produce IL-10, and 3) how IL-10 production can be controlled.

Biotherapy of Cancer

In vivo murine models show that therapy with the cytokine IL-2 alone can result in significant tumor regression (172,173). Potential mechanisms involved in this antitumor effect include the activation of LAK cells, the generation of CTLs against the tumor, and the secondary induction of other cytokines such as TNF-α or IFN-γ.

In murine models with metastatic tumors, IL-2–expanded TILs had potent antitumor activity when treated with high-dose cyclophosphamide and rIL-2 (172,173). TIL-derived T cells were many times more effective than LAK cells on a per cell basis in causing the rejection of pulmonary metastases. These TILs were also antigen specific and MHC restricted. Based on these experiments, Rosenberg et al (174,175) developed an adoptive immunotherapy strategy in which patients with various solid tumors (primarily melanoma) received their own in vitro rIL-2–expanded TILs and high doses of intravenous rIL-2. Clinical responses were observed in patients from whom TILs could be expanded to at least 10^{10} cells. Certain patients who had failed to respond to rIL-2 alone responded to TILs. An overall response rate of 34% was observed among 86 patients with melanoma. Responding patients exhibited higher levels of in vitro cytotoxicity (≥10%) against autologous melanoma cells, and their TILs also secreted GM-CSF and often IFN-γ and TNF-α (176). TILs from responding patients expanded more rapidly in culture and tended to be derived from subcutaneous lesions rather than lymph node metastases.

Biotherapy of Ovarian Cancer

Since ovarian cancer primarily involves structures in the abdominal cavity, intraperitoneal therapy applications are very appealing. There are pharmacologic and potential therapeutic advantages to intraperitoneal administration of cytokines. Trials with *C. parvum* (177), rIFN-α (178,179), rIFN-γ (180,181), rIL-2 (182–185), and rIL-2 plus LAK (186,187) produced surgically documented responses. The results of these studies are summarized in Tables 2-2 to 2-4. Intraperitoneal rIFN-α with or without chemotherapy resulted in surgically confirmed responses in the range of 30% to 40% (179,188). Intraperitoneal IFN-γ given twice weekly produced a complete surgical response rate of 23% with a 62% projected 3-year survival in the responding patients (180). Intraperitoneal rIL-2 was administered to small numbers of patients

T A B L E   **2-2**

Toxicity and Clinical Activity from Intraperitoneal Recombinant Interferon-α (rIFN-α) ± Cisplatin (CDDP) in Patients with Ovarian Carcinoma

Study	Year	No. of Patients (MRD)		Dosing	Schedule	Toxicity (Frequency)	Response
Berek	1985	14 (7)	rIFN-α[a]	5–50 × 10⁶ U	Wkly ×8 cycles	Fever >39° (18%) Emesis (37%) Abdominal pain (22%)	CR—4 PR—1
Willemse	1990	20 (11)	rIFN-α[a]	50 × 10⁶ U	Wkly ×8 cycles	Fever >39° (43%)	CR—5, PR—4 (PFI 6–13+ mo)
Nardi	1990	14 (11)	rIFN-α[a]	50 × 10⁶ U	Biwkly ×4—repeat at 14–17 wk	Catheter infection (3)	CR—7 (6/7 cyto+)
			CDDP	90 mg/m²	wk 7, 10, 20, 23	Adhesions and chemical peritonitis (−9)	7 patients survive >22 mo
Berek	1991	24 (9)	rIFN-α[a] CDDP	10–50 × 10⁶ U 45–75 mg/m²	q 2–3 wk × 6	Renal (12%) ↑ Malaise, fever, diarrhea, emesis (30%) (above 25/60 dose)	CPR—2–15 mo, 19 mo PR—3, mean survival 18 mo
Markman	1992	43 (15)	rIFN-α[a] CDDP	25 × 10⁶ U 60 mg/m²	q 3 wk × 6	Adhesions Neurotoxicity (14%)	PR—1/18 evaluable patients
Frasci	1993	41 (18)	rIFN-α[a] Mitoxantrone CDDP	30 × 10⁶ IU/m² 20 mg/m² 75 mg/m²	q 3 wk × 4	Severe abdominal pain (37%)	CR—23/37 4 year DFS = 50% (CRs)
Frasci	1994	21 (11)	rIFN-α[b] Carboplatin	30 × 10⁶ IU/m² 150 mg/m²	q wk × 12	Grade 3–4 Myelosuppression (30%)	10/11 CR had < 5 mm residual 4/9 CR had > 5 mm residual

MRD = mimimum residual disease, usually individual tumors ≤5 mm in diameter; CR = complete response; PR = partial response; CPR = complete pathologic response.

[a] Schering.
[b] First line treatment.

T A B L E   **2-3**

Toxicity and Clinical Activity after Intraperitoneal Recombinant Interferon-γ in Patients with Advanced Ovarian Cancer

Study	Year	No. of Patients (MRD)	Dose	Schedule	Duration	Toxicity	Response
Allavena	1990	7	0.5 mg[a]	3× wkly	9 wk	Fever, malaise (no fibrosis)	0
D'Aquisto	1988	27 (5)	0.05–8 × 10⁶ U/m²[b]	Wkly		None severe	0 (1 NED 12 mo)
Colombo	1992	8 (8)	2 × 10⁶ U/m²[c]	2× wkly	3 mo	Abdominal discomfort (no fibrosis)	CR (1) 28 mo PR (2) 20, 11 mo
Pujade	1996	108 (33)	2 × 10⁶ U/m²[c]	2× wkly	3 mo	Fever, malaise, abdominal pain, perforation, leukopenia, LFT↑	23% surgical CR; 62% PFI
Greiner	1992	6	0.1–0.5–100 × 10⁶ U[a]	Wkly Wkly	2 wk 8 wk	Catheter infection	0

NED = no incidence of disease; MRD = minimal residual disease; LFT = liver function test; CR = complete response; PR = partial response.

[a] Biogen, 1 mg = 2 × 10⁷ U.
[b] Schering, 1 mg = 2.6 × 10⁶ U.
[c] Roussel.

T A B L E **2-4**

Toxicity and Clinical Activity from Intraperitoneal Recombinant Inter-
leukin-2 (rIL-2) Alone or with Lymphokine-Activated Killer Cells
(LAK) in Patients with Advanced Ovarian Cancer

Study	No. of Patiens (MRD)	Dosing (Not Corrected for International Units)	Schedule	Local Toxicity	Systemic Toxicity				Response
					N&V/D	↑ Wt	↓ Plat	Other	
Intraperitoneal rIL-2 Alone									
Lotze (88)	7* (1)	10^4 to 3×10^5 U/kg[a]	tid/7 days	Adhesions	+/+	—	—	↑ Cr, ↑ bili	0
Chapman (88)	7 (5)	10^5 to 10^7 U/m^{2a}	3 days/wk	Sepsis	+	+	—	↑ Cr, ↑ glucose	CA-125 ↓
Beller (89)	8 (2)	2×10^3 U to 2×10^4 U[a]	5 days/wk	—	—	—	—	Neuropathy	CA-125 ↓
Melioli (89)	6*	3.4×10^5 U to 1×10^6 U[b]	14 days	Peritonitis	—	+	+	Dyspnea	0
Edwards (95)	42 (19)	10^4–5×10^6 U	A. 24°/wk B. 7 days alternate wks	Perforation	—	—	—	Hypotension	CR 7, PR 2
Intraperitoneal IP rIL-2 + LAK									
Stewart (90)	10 (3)	(i) IL-2 (IV)[c] 5×10^5 U 2×10^6 U 8×10^6 U (ii) Leukapheresis (iii) LAK + IL-2 (IP)	× 6 doses (Days 1–12) Days 15–18 Days 19–21	Hematemesis Adhesions Infections Ascites	+/+	+	+	—	PR 1
Steiss (90)	10/20* (10)	(i) IL-2 10^6 IU/kg (IV)[a] (ii) Leukapheresis (iii) LAK + IL-2 (IP) IL-2 2.5×10^3 U/kg (tid)	tid/3 days 5 days 5 days	Abdominal pain, fibrosis, perforation	+	+	+	—	PR 2

MRD = minimum residual disease; nd = no data; N&V/D = nausea vomiting/diarrhea; Wt = weight; Plat = platelets; IP = intraperitoneal; Cr = creatinine; bili = bilirubin; CR = complete response; PR = partial response.

*Included nonovarian causes of carcinomatosis.

[a] Chiron-Cetus (×6 IU).

[b] Glaxo.

[c] Roche.

at different dosages and schedules (182–184). In a study of intraperitoneal rIL-2, nine responses (including seven complete responses) were reported for patients who had received either of two low-dose schedules of rIL-2 (184). An important aspect of the studies with intraperitoneal administration of cytokines is that responses were most frequent in patients who had minimal residual tumor, usually 5 mm or less, and that tumors with larger diameters responded less frequently. Initial trials with rIFN-α or IL-2 explored high doses of cytokines. Dose-limiting toxicities included abdominal pain, adhesions, sepsis, and neurotoxicity in up to 14% of patients who received chemotherapy with cisplatin and IFN-α (188–190). Prior cisplatin exposure may have contributed to the occurrence of neurotoxicity after IP therapy. Intraperitoneal injection of interleukin at lower doses had fewer systemic side effects compared with the intravenous or subcutaneous routes. Moreover, responses were observed at doses well below the maximum tolerated doses for these agents. The extended half-life characteristics of intraperitoneal cytokines may favor biologically active lower dosing schedules. We showed that daily bolus injections of rIL-2 (0.6 × 10^6 IU/m^2) administered each day for 4 days produced no significant local or systemic toxicities. IL-2 was detected in the peritoneal cavity (20–30 ng/mL) over a 12- to 24-hour period following the intraperitoneal injection (185). The concentration of rIL-2 during the beta phase (20–30 ng/mL) is similar to the concen-

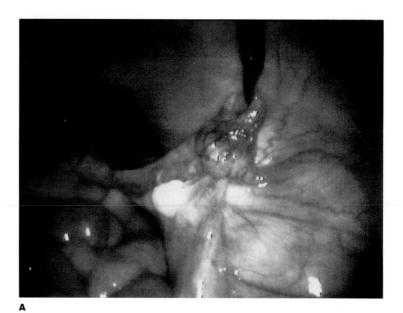

A

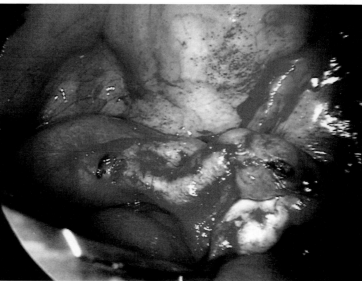

B

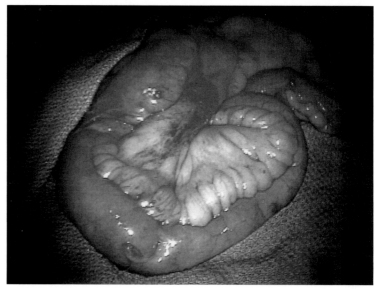

C

tration of rIL-2 used in vitro (600 IU/mL) to expand ovarian TILs. This rIL-2 dose ($0-6 \times 10^6$ IU/m²) did not produce detectable serum levels of IL-2 or detectable TNF-α in the peritoneal cavity. These findings could account for the absence of significant systemic or local toxicity with this dose and schedule of intraperitoneal rIL-2. A phase II study is currently underway to evaluate a similar dose of rIL-2 administered at weekly intervals.

Peritoneal exudate lymphocytes (obtained after intraperitoneal rIL-2 treatments) exhibit substantial in vitro cytotoxicity against ovarian and nonovarian tumor cell targets, when comparison is made with pretreatment lymphocytic cytotoxicity levels. Intraperitoneal treatment with rIL-2 also results in the production of endogenous IFN-γ in the peritoneal cavity (185). This finding suggests that T cells might be activated in vivo by intraperitoneal rIL-2, although other cells such as NK cells might also produce IFN-γ. We also detected an increase in IL-10 concentrations after intraperitoneal rIL-2. IL-10 levels in peritoneal cavity fluids can be lowered if needed by reducing the rIL-2 dose approximately sixfold and by delivering this dose over 6 hours instead of by bolus (Freedman RS, unpublished data, 1997).

Few trials have been conducted in ovarian cancer patients utilizing cytokine-activated lymphocytes. Initial studies (186,187) were conducted with lymphocytes obtained from peripheral blood after intravenous or intraperitoneal priming with IL-2 (see Table 2-4). LAK cells were obtained by leukapheresis, which frequently resulted in clinically significant thrombocytopenia. Two partial responses were observed in ovarian patients in whom prior chemotherapy had failed. We recently described a method for expanding large numbers (up to 10^{11}) of TILs in a low concentration of rIL-2 (Chiron-Cetus, Emeryville, CA) (41). Ovarian TILs expanded from ascites or from solid tumor were administered with low-dose IL-2 (0.6×10^6 IU/m²) intraperitoneally to patients with advanced ovarian carcinoma in whom standard chemotherapy had failed. Side effects were manageable and minor responses were observed in four patients. This was a pilot study and all of the patients had tumors that were suboptimal for an intraperitoneal approach.

To explore the role of CD8[+] or CD4[+] T-cell populations in vivo, we developed a procedure for expanding purified TILs (either CD8[+]TCR$\alpha\beta$[+] or CD4[+]TCR$\alpha\beta$[+]) in sufficient numbers (41). One patient with fallopian tube metastases was treated with intraperitoneal purified CD8[+] TILs plus low-dose rIL-2 (0.03 mg/m²) or 600,000 IU/m², and had surgically confirmed control of her peritoneal cavity disease at subsequent laparoscopy (Fig. 2-5). The CA-125 values, which were elevated prior to the treatment, remained quite stable during this period. At a subsequent laparotomy, 14 months after the start of therapy, the previously involved tube and the ovary were removed, and were found to be pathologically normal. However, tumor metastases developed at extraperitoneal sites. This finding suggests that other routes of administration might be needed in certain cases to control tumor growth at sites outside of the peritoneal cavity. A second patient who was treated with intraperitoneal purified CD4[+] TILs plus intraperitoneal rIFN-γ plus rIL-2 had stable disease for 5 months, as determined by computed tomography. Serum CA-125 values decreased by more than 50% following the intraperitoneal treatment. These clinical trials of intraperitoneal administration of TILs and low-dose rIL-2 established the feasibility of this technique in patients exposed to extensive prior chemotherapy. Toxicity is manageable, and most patients can be treated in an outpatient setting. We also found that temporary vascular-type catheters (5Fr) inserted intraperitoneally by interventional radiologists can be utilized over prolonged periods for intraperitoneal therapy. Future efforts aimed at improving the proportion of patients from whom TILs can be expanded ex vivo may include costimulation and other cytokines such as IL-12. In another intraperitoneal approach, T lymphocytes retargeted with a bispecific antibody directed to the CD3 molecule on T lymphocytes and the folate receptor on ovarian carcinoma cells were utilized, and complete responses were reported in 3 of 26 patients (191).

Chemoimmunotherapy of Ovarian Cancer

The combination of cytokines with chemotherapy may have synergistic activity as observed in in vitro and in vivo animal studies (192–195). In vitro experiments showed that the combination of cisplatin and rIL-2 increases the antitumor effect of macrophages. Chemotherapy agents have been incorporated into chemoimmunotherapy regimens with rIL-2, rIFN-α, and other cytokines for malignant melanoma, renal cell carcinoma, and other tumors (196). The mechanisms responsible for the additive or synergistic effects of biologic agents on chemotherapy are presently unknown. Chemotherapy agents may alter the membrane physiology of tumor cells and render these cells more susceptible to lysis by effector lymphocytes that have been activated by cytokines (197). Chemotherapy may also potentiate the induction of active immunity against tumor cells in vivo (194,195,198), reducing the numbers of tumor cells that secrete cytokines that are inhibitory to the growth of tumor cells (192).

A limited number of chemoimmunotherapy trials have been performed on patients with ovarian cancer (188,190,195,199,200). Alberts et al (197) reported negative results from a randomized trial conducted in patients with ovarian cancer who received platinum or doxorubicin-based chemotherapy either with or without BCG. IFN-α was administered intraperitoneally in combination with cisplatin, with variable results with evidence of clinical responses (see Table 2-2) (188–190). These results suggest that 60 mg of cisplatin can be administered in the same cycle together with 25×10^6 U rIFNα2b (188). Alternatively, carboplatin, which is less neurotoxic and renotoxic, can be given at a dose of 150 mg/m^2 in the same cycle as 30×10^6 U/m^2 rIFNα2b (200). In a recent analysis of a Gynecologic Oncology Group trial with *cis*-diamminedichloroplatinum (CDDP) and rIFN-α, Markman (190) found only one response in 18 evaluable patients. However, this trial may have included a larger number of patients whose tumors were progressing after chemotherapy or who had more extensive metastases, and entry of some patients was delayed up to 12 weeks after surgery. In a recent Japanese trial (201), 13 patients with ovarian cancer received rIL-2–expanded TILs derived from chemotherapy-naive tumors. TILs were reinfused without rIL-2 in patients who responded to chemotherapy and disease-free survival was compared with that in a similar group of patients who received no additional treatment after completing their planned courses of chemotherapy. The control group included patients whose TILs could not be expanded. The disease-free survival rate for the TIL-treated patients was significantly different: 82.1% versus 54.5% for the control group at 3 years ($p < 0.05$). Patients received less than 10^{10} TILs and surprisingly no rIL-2 was administered. This trial did not use randomization and the observation that ovarian cancer patients had a longer survival following therapy with TILs needs further confirmation.

Conclusions

Trials of intraperitoneal administration of certain cytokines such as rIFN-α and rIFN-γ, and preliminary studies with rIL-2 showed promising activity in patients with ovarian carcinoma, especially those patients who had small residual tumor burdens after prior surgery and chemotherapy. In contrast, systemic administration routes will be required for most patients with breast cancer. It is clear that carefully planned sequences and dosing schedules of cytokines used alone or in combinations will be needed to obtain the maximum effectiveness. Such studies have not yet been done. Intraperitoneal injections of new cytokines such as rIL-12, which is a high-molecular-weight heterodimer, offer the possibility that adaptive immunity can be enhanced through upregulation of Th1-type lymphocyte functions. This drug is interesting because it has the potential for effective combinations with other cytokines such as rIL2 or with tumor vaccines and with novel approaches that utilize costimulation. A number of interesting tumor vaccine approaches are also about to enter clinical trials. Such studies include the use of intact tumor cells modified through gene transfer techniques to express molecules involved with costimulation as well as cytokines such as IFN-γ and IL-2. Highly effective bioimmunotherapeutic approaches for malignancies such as ovarian cancer and breast cancer are now within our grasp. This is made possible by the advances in molecular immunology, development of novel recombinant cytokines and gene transfer approaches, and carefully designed, scientifically based clinical trials.

Acknowledgments

We thank Ms. Barbara Wilson for typing the manuscript. This work was supported in part by grant EDT-56 from the American Cancer Society; grants RO1-CA64943, MO1-RR02558, and UO1-CA97-001 from the National Institutes of Health; and Core Grant 16672 to The University of Texas M. D. Anderson Cancer Center.

REFERENCES

1. Freedman RS. Recent immunologic advances affecting the management of ovarian cancer. *Clin Obstet Gynecol* 1985;28:849–867.

2. Vilcek J, Junming L. Immunology of cytokines: an introduction. In: Thompson A, ed. *The cytokine handbook.* San Diego: Academic, 1994:1–19.

3. Borden EC, Sondel PM. Lymphokines and cytokines as cancer treatment. *Cancer* 1991;65: 800–814.

4. Witt PL, Lindner DJ, D'Cunha D, Borden EC. Pharmacology of interferons: induced proteins, cell activation, and antitumor activity. Chabner B, Longo D, eds. In: *Cancer chemotherapy and biotherapy: principles and practice.* 2nd ed. Philadelphia: Lippincott-Raven, 1991:585–607.

5. Petros WP, Peters WP. Colony-stimulating factors. Chabner B, Longo D, eds. In: *Cancer chemotherapy and biotherapy.* Philadelphia: Lippincott-Raven, 1996:639–654.

6. Nomenclature Committee of the 4th International Workshop on Human Leukocyte Differentiation Antigens. Workshop antigen designation. *J Immunol* 1989;143:758–759.

7. Cantor H, Boyse EA. Functional subclasses of T lymphocytes bearing different Ly antigens I: the generation of functionally distinct T cell subclasses is a differentiative process independent of antigen. *J Exp Med* 1975;141:1376–1389.

8. Zagursky RJ, Sharp D, Solomon KA, Schwartz A. Quantitation of cellular receptors by a new immunocytochemical flow cytometry technique. *Biotechniques* 1995;18:504–509.

9. Papadopoulos NG, Dedoussis GVG, Spanakos G. An improved fluorescence assay for the determination of lymphocyte-mediated cytotoxicity using flow cytometry. *J Immunol Methods* 1994; 177:101–111.

10. Picker LJ, Singh MK, Zdraveski Z. Direct demonstration of cytokine synthesis heterogeneity among human memory/effector T cells by flow cytometry. *Blood* 1995;86:1408–1419.

11. Freedman RS, Ioannides CF, Mathioudakis G, Platsoucas CD. Novel immunologic strategies for the treatment of ovarian carcinoma based on cell surface recognition. *Am J Obstet Gynecol* 1992; 167:1470–1478.

12. Freedman RS, Ioannides CG, Tomasovic B. Development of a cell surface reacting human monoclonal antibody agent in ovarian carcinoma. *Hybridoma* 1991;10:21–33.

13. Vriesendorp HM, Quadri SM, Jaeckle KA, et al. Proposal for translational analysis and development of clinical radiolabeled immunoglobulin therapy. *Radiother Oncol* 1996;41:151–161.

14. Platsoucas CD. Autologous tumor-specific T cells in malignant melanoma. *Cancer Metastasis Rev* 1991;10:151–176.

15. Kreider JK, Bartlett GL, Butkiewiz BL. Relationship of tumor leucocytic infiltration to host defense mechanisms and prognosis. *Cancer Metastasis Rev* 1984;3:53–74.

16. Mihm MC, Clark WJ, From L. The clinical diagnosis, classification and histogenetic concepts of the early stages of cutaneous malignant melanomas. *N Engl J Med* 1971;184:1078–1083.

17. Cochran AJ. Histology and prognosis in malignant melanoma. *J Pathol* 1969;97:459–468.

18. Aaltomaa S, Lipponen P, Eskelinen M, et al. Lymphocyte infiltrates as a prognostic variable in female breast cancer. *Eur J Cancer* 1992;28: 859–864.

19. Black MM, Barclay TH, Hankey BF. Prognosis in breast cancer utilizing histologic characteristics of the primary tumor. *Cancer* 1975;36: 2048–2055.

20. Berg JW. Morphologic evidence for immune response to breast cancer: a historical review. *Cancer* 1971;28:1453–1456.

21. Hamlin IM. Possible host resistance in carcinoma of the breast. *Br J Cancer* 1968;22:381–401.

22. Shimokawara I, Imamura M, Yamanaka N, et al. Identification of lymphocyte subpopulations in human breast cancer tissue and its significance: an immunoperoxidase study with anti-human T- and B-cell sera. *Cancer* 1982;49:1456–1464.

23. Bishop HM, Blamey RW, Elston CW, et al. Relationship of estrogen-receptor status to survival in breast cancer. *Lancet* 1979;2:283–284.

24. Dawson PJ, Karrison T, Ferguson DJ. Histologic features associated with longterm survival in breast cancer. *Hum Pathol* 1986;17:1015–1021.

25. Hurlimann J, Saraga P. Mononuclear cells infiltrating human mammary carcinomas: immunohistochemical analysis with monoclonal antibodies. *Int J Cancer* 1985;35:753–762.

26. Whitwell HL, Hughes HPA, Moore M, Ahmed A. Expression of major histocompatibility antigens and leucocyte infiltration in benign and malignant human breast disease. *Br J Cancer* 1984;49:161–172.

27. Whitford P, Mallon EA, George WD, Campbell AM. Flow cytometric analysis of tumour infiltrating lymphocytes in breast cancer. *Br J Cancer* 1990;62:971–975.

28. Rubbert A, Manger B, Lang N, et al. Functional characterization of tumor-infiltrating lymphocytes, lymph-node lymphocytes and peripheral-blood lymphocytes from patients with breast cancer. *Int J Cancer* 1991;49:25–31.

29. Chen PF, Li YD, Pollock R, et al. Fresh tumor-infiltrating lymphocytes from certain patients with malignant melanoma are comprised of oligoclonal T-cells: sequence analysis of the αβ T-cell receptor cDNAs. *Proc Am Assoc Cancer Res* 1992;A1843.

30. Lin WL, Chen PF, Freedman RS, Platsoucas CD. Fresh (uncultured) tumor-infiltrating lymphocytes (TIL) from patients with malignant melanoma or ovarian carcinoma are comprised of oligoclonal T cells. *J Immunol* 1993;150:A176.

31. Isabelle P, Even J, Pannetier C, et al. Oligoclonality of tumor-infiltrating lymphocytes from human melanoma. *J Immunol* 1994;153:2807–2818.

32. Mackensen A, Ferradini L, Carcelain G, et al. Evidence for in situ amplification of cytotoxic T lymphocytes with antitumor activity in a human regression melanoma. *Cancer Res* 1993;53:3569–3573.

33. Weidmann E, Elder EM, Trucco M, et al. Usage of T-cell receptor V beta chain genes in fresh and cultured tumor-infiltrating lymphocytes from human melanoma. *Int J Cancer* 1993;54:383–390.

34. Ferradini L, Mackenson A, Genevee C, et al. Analysis of T-cell receptor variability in tumor-infiltrating lymphocytes from a human regressive melanoma. Evidence for situ T cell clonal expansion. *J Clin Invest* 1993;91:1183–1190.

35. Mackenson A, Carcelain G, Viel S, et al. Direct evidence to support the immunosurveillance concept in a human regressive melanoma. *J Clin Invest* 1994;93:1397–1402.

36. Straten PT, Scholler J, Hou-Jensen K, Zeuthen J. Preferential usage of T-cell receptor alpha beta variable regions among tumor-infiltrating lymphocytes in primary human malignant melanomas. *Int J Cancer* 1994;56:78–86.

37. Klonowski KD, Heckel MD, Schwarting R, et al. Characterization of tumor-infiltrating lymphocytes (TIL) in human breast carcinoma: evidence of an oligoclonal T-cell infiltrate. *FASEB J* 1996;10:A1471.

38. Paul WE, Seder RA. Lymphocyte responses and cytokines. *Cell* 1994;76:241–251.

39. Weiss A, Littman DR. Signal transduction by lymphocyte antigen receptors. *Cell* 1994;76:263–274.

40. Taniguchi T. Cytokine signaling through non-receptor protein tyrosine kinases. *Science* 1995;268:251–255.

41. Freedman RS, Tomasovic B, Templin S, et al. Large-scale expansion in interleukin-2 of tumor-infiltrating lymphocytes from patients with ovarian carcinoma for adoptive immunotherapy. *J Immunol Methods* 1994;167:145–160.

42. Allavena P, Zanaboni F, Rossini S, et al. Lymphokine activated killer activity of tumor associated and peripheral blood lymphocytes isolated from patients with ascites ovarian tumors. *J Natl Cancer Inst* 1986;77:8863–8868.

43. Wang YL, Li WY, Lushing S. Lymphocytes infiltrating human ovarian tumors: synergy between tumor necrosis factor alpha and interleukin-2 in the generation of CD8$^+$ effector from tumor-infiltrating lymphocytes. *Cancer Res* 1989;49:5979–5985.

44. Ferrini S, Biassoni R, Moretta A, et al. Clonal analysis of T lymphocytes isolated from ovarian carcinoma ascitic fluid. Phenotype and functional characterization of T-cell clones capable of lysing autologous carcinoma cells. *Int J Cancer* 1985;36:337–343.

45. Ioannides CG, Platsoucas CD, Rashed S, et al. Tumor cytolysis by lymphocytes infiltrating ovarian malignant ascites. *Cancer Res* 1991;51:4257–4265.

46. Ioannides CG, Freedman RS, Platsoucas CD, Kim Y-P. Cytotoxic T cell clones isolated from ovarian tumor-infiltrating lymphocytes recognize multiple antigenic epitopes on autologous tumor cells. *J Immunol* 1991;146:1700–1707.

47. Peoples GE, Goedegebuure PS, Andrews JVR, et al. HLA-A2 presents shared tumor-associated antigens derived from endogenous proteins in ovarian cancer. *J Immunol* 1993;151:5481–5491.

48. Kooi S, Freedman RS, Rodriquez-Villanueva J, Platsoucas CD. Cytokine production by T-cell lines derived from tumor-infiltrating lymphocytes (TIL) from patients with ovarian carcinoma: tumor-specific immune responses and inhibition of antigen-independent cytokine production by ovarian tumor cells. *Lymphokine Cytokine Res* 1993;12:429–437.

49. Balch CM, Riley LB, Bae YJ, et al. Patterns of human tumor-infiltrating lymphocytes in 120 cancers. *Arch Surg* 1990;125:200–205.

50. Itoh K, Platsoucas CD, Balch CM. Autologous tumor-specific cytotoxic T lymphocytes in the infiltrate of human metastatic melanomas. *J Exp Med* 1984;168:1419–1441.

51. Nanno M, Seki H, Mathioudakis G, et al. γδ T cell antigen receptors expressed on tumor infiltrating lymphocytes from patients with solid tumors. *Eur J Immunol* 1992;22:679–687.

52. Salmeron MA, Morita T, Seki H, et al. Lymphokine production by human melanoma tumor-infiltrating lymphocytes. *Cancer Immunol Immunother* 1992;35:211–217.

53. Yagita M, Itoh K, Owen-Schaub LB, et al. Involvement of both TAC and non-TAC IL-2 binding peptides in the interleukin-2-dependent proliferation of human tumor infiltrating lymphocytes. *Cancer Res* 1989;49:1154–1159.

54. Ioannides CG, Freedman RS, Platsoucas CD. OKT4 monoclonal antibody-induced activation of an autoreactive T cell clone. *Cell Immunol* 1989;123:244–252.

55. Freedman RS, Edwards CL, Kavanagh JJ, et al. Intraperitoneal adoptive immunotherapy of ovarian carcinoma with tumor-infiltrating lymphocytes and low dose recombinant interleukin-2: a pilot trial. *J Immunother* 1994;16:198–210.

56. Freedman RS. Immunotherapy for peritoneal ovarian carcinoma metastasis using ex vivo expanded tumor infiltrating lymphocytes. In: Sugarbaker PH, ed. *Peritoneal carcinomatosis: principles of management.* Boston: Kluwer Academic, 1996:115–146.

57. Schwartzentruber DJ, Topalian SL, Mancini M, Rosenberg SA. Specific release of granulocyte macrophage colony stimulating factor, tumor necrosis factor alpha, and IFN-gamma by human tumor infiltrating lymphocytes after autologous tumor stimulation. *J Immunol* 1991;146:3674–3681.

58. Schwartzentruber DJ, Solomon D, Rosenberg SA, Topalian SL. Characterization of lymphocytes infiltrating human breast cancer: specific immune reactivity detected by measuring cytokine secretion. *J Immunother* 1992;12:1–12.

59. Skornick Y, Topalian SL, Rosenberg SA. Comparative studies of the long-term growth of lymphocytes from tumor infiltrates, tumor-draining lymph nodes, and peripheral blood by repeated in vitro simulation with autologous tumor. *J Biol Response Modifier* 1990;9:431–438.

60. Okubo M, Sato N, Wada Y, et al. Identification by monoclonal antibody of the tumor antigen of a human autologous breast cancer cell that is involved in cytotoxicity by a cytotoxic T-cell clone. *Cancer Res* 1989;49:3950–3954.

61. Kaieda T, Imawari M, Yamasaki Z, et al. Identification of a tumor-associated target antigen, ATM-1, for a human T-cell clone with activated killer activity and its existence in sera of cancer patients. *Cancer Res* 1988;48:4848–4854.

62. Jerome KR, Barnd DL, Bendt KM, Boyer CM. Cytotoxic T-lymphocytes derived from patients with breast adenocarcinoma recognized an epitope present on the protein core of mucin molecule preferentially expressed by malignant cells. *Cancer Res* 1991;51:2908–2916.

63. Barnd DL, Lan MS, Metzgar RS, Finn OJ. Specific MHC-unrestricted recognition of tumor-associated mucins by human cytotoxic T cells. *Proc Natl Acad Sci USA* 1989;86:7159–7163.

64. Hoover SK, Frank JL, Mc Crady C, et al. Activation and in vitro expansion of tumor-reactive T lymphocytes from lymph nodes draining human primary breast cancer. *J Surg Oncol* 1991;46:117–124.

65. Baxevanis CN, Dedoussis GVZ, Papadopoulos NG, et al. Tumor specific cytolysis by tumor infiltrating lymphocytes in breast cancer. *Cancer* 1994;74:1275–1282.

66. Jerome KR, Bu D, Finn OJ. Expression of tumor-associated epitopes on Epstein-Barr virus-immortalized B-cells and Burkitt's lymphomas transfected with epithelial mucin complementary DNA. *Cancer Res* 1992;52:5985–5990.

67. Jerome KR, Domenech N, Finn OJ. Tumor-specific cytotoxic T cell clones from patients with breast and pancreatic adenocarcinoma recognize EBV-immortalized B cells transfected with polymorphic epithelial mucin complementary DNA. *J Immunol* 1993;151:1654–1662.

68. Domenech N, Henderson RA, Finn OJ. Identification of an HLA-A11-restricted epitope from the tandem repeat domain of the epithelial tumor antigen mucin. *J Immunol* 1995;155:4766–4774.

69. Miescher S, Whiteside TL, Carrel S, Von Vliedner V. Functional properties of tumor-infiltrating and blood lymphocytes in patients with solid tumors: effects of tumor cells and their supernatants on proliferative responses of lymphocytes. *J Immunol* 1986;136:1899–1907.

70. Miescher S, Whiteside TL, Moretta L, Von Fliedner V. Clonal and frequency analyses of tumor-infiltrating lymphocytes from human solid tumors. *J Immunol* 1987;138:4001–4004.

71. Miescher S, Stoeck M, Qiao L, et al. Proliferative and cytolytic potentials of purified human tumor-infiltrating T lymphocytes: impaired response to mitogen-driven stimulation despite T-cell receptor expression. *Int J Cancer* 1988;42: 659–666.

72. Whiteside TL, Miescher S, Hurlimann J, et al. Separation, phenotyping and limiting dilution analysis of T-lymphocytes infiltrating human solid tumors. *Int J Cancer* 1986;37:803–811.

73. Stoeck M, Miescher S, Qiao L, et al. Stimulation of FACS-analyzed CD4$^+$ and CD9$^+$ human tumor-infiltrating lymphocytes with ionomycin + phorbol-12,13-dibutyrate does not overcome their proliferative deficit. *Clin Exp Immunother* 1990;79:105–108.

74. Whiteside TL, Miescher S, Hurlimann J, et al. Clonal analysis and in situ characterization of lymphocytes infiltrating human breast carcinomas. *Cancer Immunol Immunother* 1986;23: 169–178.

75. Vitolo D, Zerbe T, Kanbour A, et al. Expression of mRNA for cytokines in tumor-infiltrating mononuclear cells in ovarian adenocarcinoma and invasive breast cancer. *Int J Cancer* 1992;51: 573–580.

76. Germain RN. MHC-associated antigen processing, presentation, and recognition. *Immunologist* 1995;3:185–190.

77. Wolfel T, Klehman E, Muller C, et al. Lysis of human melanoma cells by autologous cytolytic T cell clones. Identification of human histocompatibility leukocyte antigen A2 as a restriction element for three different antigens. *J Exp Med* 1989;170:797–810.

78. Darrow T, Slingluff CL Jr, Seigler JF. The role of HLA class I antigens in recognition of melanoma cells by tumor specific cytotoxic T lymphocytes. *J Immunol* 1989;142:3329–3335.

79. Allen PM, Strydom DJ, Unanue ER. Processing of lysozyme by macrophages: identification of the determinant recognized by two T-cell hybridomas. *Proc Natl Acad Sci USA* 1984;81: 2489–2493.

80. Nixon DF, Townsend AR, Elvin JG, et al. HIV-1 gag-specific CTL defined with recombinant vaccinia virus and synthetic peptides. *Nature* 1988;336:484–487.

81. Van der Bruggen P, Traversari C, Chomez P, et al. A gene encoding an antigen recognized by cytolytic T cells on a human melanoma. *Science* 1991;254:1643–1647.

82. Brichard V, Van Pel A, Wolfel T, et al. The tyrosinase gene codes for an antigen recognized by autologous cytolytic T lymphocytes on HLA-A2 melanomas. *J Exp Med* 1993;178:489–495.

83. Bakker ABH, Schreurs MWJ, de Boer AJ, et al. Melanocyte lineage-specific antigen gp100 is recognized by melanoma-derived tumor infiltrating lymphocytes. *J Exp Med* 1994;179:1005–1009.

84. Kawakami Y, Eliyahu S, Sakaguchi K, et al. Identification of the immunodominant peptides of the MART-1 human melanoma antigen recognized by the majority of HLA-A2-restricted tumor infiltrating lymphocytes. *J Exp Med* 1994; 180:347–352.

85. Coulie PG, Brichard V, Van Pel A, et al. A new gene coding for a differentiation antigen recognized by autologous cytolytic T lymphocytes on HLA-A2 melanomas. *J Exp Med* 1994;180:35–42.

86. Gaugler B, Van den Eynde B, Van der Bruggen P, et al. Human gene MAGE-3 codes for an antigen recognized on a melanoma by autologous cytolytic T lymphocytes. *J Exp Med* 1994; 179:921–930.

87. Van der Bruggen P, Bastin J, Gajewski T, et al. A peptide encoded by human gene MAGE-3 and presented by HLA-A2 induces cytolytic T lymphocytes that recognize tumor cells expressing MAGE-3. *Eur J Immunol* 1994;24:3038–3043.

88. Boel P, Wildmann C, Sensi ML, et al. BAGE: a new gene encoding an antigen recognized on human melanoma cytolytic T lymphocytes. *Immunity* 1995;2:167–175.

89. Van den Eynde B, Peeters O, De Backer O, et al. A new family of genes coding for an antigen recognized by autologous cytolytic T lymphocytes on a human melanoma. *J Exp Med* 1995;182:689–698.

90. Ruzzo V, Dalerba P, Ricci A, et al. MAGE, BAGE and GAGE gene expression in fresh epithelial ovarian carcinomas. *Int J Cancer* 1996;67: 457–460.

91. Brasseur F, Marchand M, Vanwijk R, et al. A human gene MAGE-1, which codes for a tumor-rejection antigen, is expressed by some breast tumors. *Int J Cancer* 1992;52:839–841.

92. Wolfel T, Van Pel A, Brichard V, et al. Two tyrosine nonapeptides recognized on HLA-A2 melanomas by autologous cytolytic T lymphocytes. *Eur J Immunol* 1994;24:759–764.

93. Wang RF, Robbins PF, Kawakami Y, et al. Identification of a gene encoding a melanoma tumor antigen recognized by HLA-A31 restricted tumor-

infiltrating lymphocytes. *J Exp Med* 1995;181: 799–804.

94. Fisk B, Blevins TL, Wharton JT, Ioannides CG. Identification of an immunodominant peptide of the HER-2/neu protooncogene recognized by ovarian tumor-specific cytotoxic T lymphocyte lines. *J Exp Med* 1995;181:2100–2117.

95. Peoples GE, Goedegebuure PS, Smith R, et al. Breast and ovarian cancer-specific cytotoxic T lymphocytes recognize the same HER2/neu-derived peptide. *Proc Natl Acad Sci USA* 1995; 92:432–436.

96. Tandon AK, Clark GM, Chamness GC, et al. HER-2/neu oncogene protein and prognosis in breast cancer. *J Clin Oncol* 1989;7:1120–1128.

97. Allred DC, Clark GM, Gandon AK, et al. HER-2/neu in node-negative breast cancer: prognostic significance of overexpression influenced by the presence of in situ carcinoma. *J Clin Oncol* 1992;10:599–605.

98. Slamon DJ, Godolphin W, Jones LA, et al. Studies of the HER-2/neu proto-oncogene in human breast and ovarian cancer. *Science* 1989; 244:707–712.

99. Disis ML, Smith JW, Murphy AE, et al. In vitro generation of human cytolytic T-cells specific for peptides derived from the HER-2/neu proto-oncogene protein. *Cancer Res* 1994;53:1071–1076.

100. Linehan DC, Goedegebuure PS, Peoples GE, et al. Tumor-specific and HLA-A2-restricted cytolysis by tumor-associated lymphocytes in human metastatic breast cancer. *J Immunol* 1995;155: 4486–4491.

101. Imanishi T, Akaza T, Kimura A, et al. Allele and haplotype frequencies for HLA and complement loci in various ethnic groups. In: *The Eleventh International Histocompatibility Workshop and Conference, Yokohamashi, Japan, 1991.* 1065–1120.

102. Callahan R, Cropp CS, Merlo GR, et al. Somatic mutations and human breast cancer. A status report. *Cancer* 1992;69:1582–1588.

103. Sawan A, Randall B, Angus B, et al. Retinoblastoma and p53 gene expression related to relapse and survival in human breast cancer: an immunohistochemical study. *J Pathol* 1992;168: 23–28.

104. Vogelstein B. A deadly inheritance. *Nature* 1990;348:681–682.

105. Wang NP, To H, Lee WH, Lee EY. Tumor suppressor activity of rb and p53 genes in human

breast carcinoma cells. *Oncogene* 1993;8:279–288.

106. Tilkin AF, Lubin R, Soussi T, et al. Primary proliferative T cell response to wild-type p53 protein in patients with breast cancer. *Eur J Immunol* 1995;25:1765–1769.

107. Houbiers JG, Nijam HW, Van der Burg SH, et al. In vitro induction of human cytotoxic T lymphocyte responses against peptides of mutant and wild-type p53. *Eur J Immunol* 1992;23: 2072–2077.

108. Nijman HW, Van der Burg SH, Vierboom MP, et al. p53, a potential target for tumor-directed T cells. *Immunol Lett* 1994;40:171–178.

109. Roepke M, Regener M, Claesson MH. T cell-mediated cytotoxicity against p53-protein derived peptides in bulk and limiting dilution cultures of healthy donors. *Scand J Immunol* 1995;42:98–103.

110. Yanuck M, Carbone DP, Pendleton CD, et al. A mutant p53 tumor suppressor protein is a target for peptide-induced $CD8^+$ cytotoxic T-cells. *Cancer Res* 1993;53:3257–3261.

111. Ciernik IF, Berzofsky J, Carbone DP. Mutant oncopeptide immunization induces CTL specifically lysing tumor cells endogenously expressing the corresponding intact mutant p53. *Hybridoma* 1995;14:139–142.

112. Stuber G, Leder GH, Storkus WT, et al. Identification of wild-type and mutant p53 peptides binding to HLA-A2 assessed by a peptide loading-deficient cell line assay and a novel major histocompatibility complex class I peptide binding assay. *Eur J Immunol* 1994;24:765–768.

113. Zeh HJ, Leder GH, Lotze MT, et al. Flow-cytometric determination of peptide-class I complex formation. Identification of p53 peptides that bind to HLA-A2. *Hum Immunol* 1994; 39:79–86.

114. Gnjatic S, Bressac-de Paillerets B, Guillet JG, Choppin J. Mapping and ranking of potential cytotoxic T epitopes in the p53 protein: effect of mutations and polymorphism on peptide binding to purified and refolded HLA molecules. *Eur J Immunol* 1995;25:1638–1642.

115. Schlom J, Kantor J, Abrams S, et al. Strategies for the development of recombinant vaccines for the immunotherapy of breast cancer. *Breast Cancer Res Treat* 1996;38:27–39.

116. Kaufman H, Schlom J, Kantor J. A recombinant vaccinia virus expressing human carcinoembry-

onic antigen (CEA). *Int J Cancer* 1991;48:900–907.

117. Hodge JW, McLaughlin JP, Abrams SI, et al. Admixture of a recombinant vaccinia virus containing the gene for the costimulatory molecule B7 and a recombinant vaccinia virus containing a tumor-associated antigen gene results in enhanced specific T-cell responses and anti tumor immunity. *Cancer Res* 1995;55:3598–3602.

118. Tsang KY, Zaremba S, Nieroda CA, et al. Generation of human cytotoxic T cells specific for human carcinoembryonic antigen epitopes from patients immunized with recombinant vaccinia-CEA vaccine. *J Natl Cancer Inst* 1995;87:982–990.

119. Melief CJM, Offringa R, Toes REM, Kast WM. Peptide-based cancer vaccines. *Cancer* 1996;8:651–657.

120. Wang P, Vánky F, Klein E. Assembly of MHC class I restricted auto tumor specific CD4+CD8− T-cell clones established from autologous mixed lymphocyte tumor cell culture (MLTC). *Int J Cancer* 1992;51:962–967.

121. Végh Z, Wang P, Vánky F, Klein E. Selective downregulated expression of major histocompatibility complex class I alleles in human solid tumors. *Cancer Res* 1993;53:2416–2420.

122. Vánky F, Hising C, Sjöwall K., et al. Interferon-γ and tumor necrosis factor-α treatment of *ex vivo* human carcinoma cells potentiates their interaction with allogeneic lymphocytes. *J Interferon Cytokine Res* 1996;16:201–207.

123. Rivoltini L, Barrachini KC, Viggiano V, et al. Quantitative correlation between HLA class I allele expression and recognition of melanoma cells by antigen-specific cytotoxic T lymphocytes. *Cancer Res* 1995;55:3249–3257.

124. Yang Y, Nunes FA, Brencsi K, et al. Cellular immunity to viral antigens limits E1-deleted adenoviruses for gene therapy. *Proc Natl Acad Sci USA* 1994;91:4407–4411.

125. Festenstein H, Bridges J, Navarrete C. MHC expression on tumour cells. In: Sharp F, Mason WP, Leake RE, eds. *Ovarian cancer: biological and therapeutic challenges*. New York: Chapman and Hall, 1990:97–109.

126. Kabawat SW, Bast RC Jr, Welch WR, et al. Expression of major histocompatibility antigens and nature of inflammatory cellular infiltrate in ovarian neoplasms. *Int J Cancer* 1983;32:547–554.

127. Kooi S, Zhang H-Z, Patenia R, et al. HLA class I expression on human ovarian carcinoma cells correlates with T-cell infiltration *in vivo* and T-cell expansion *in vitro* in low concentrations of recombinant interleukin-2. *Cell Immunol* 1996;174:116–128.

128. Townsend SE, Allison JP. Tumor rejection after direct costimulation of CD8+ T cells by B7-transfected melanoma cells. *Science* 1993;259:368–370.

129. Schwartz RH. Advances in immunoregulation and immunotherapy. *Immunologist* 1995;3:244–246.

130. Krummel MF, Allison JP. CD28 and CTLA-4 have opposing effects on the response of T cells to stimulation. *J Exp Med* 1995;182:459–465.

131. Melichar B, Savary CA, Kudelka AP, et al. Dendritic cells in ascites associated with peritoneal carcinomatosis (Poster Discussion). *Proc Am Assoc Cancer Res* 1997:A234.

132. Cavallo F, Martin-Fontecha A, Bellone M, et al. Co-expression of B7-1 and ICAM-1 on tumors is required for rejection and the establishment of a memory response. *Eur J Immunol* 1995;25:1154–1162.

133. Greenburg PD. Adoptive T cell therapy of tumors: mechanisms operative in the recognition and elimination of tumor cells. *Adv Immunol* 1991;49:281–355.

134. Matsuda M, Salazar F, Petersson M. Interleukin-10 pretreatment protects target cells from tumor- and allo-specific cytotoxic T cells and downregulates HLA class I expression. *J Exp Med* 1994;180:2371–2376.

135. de Waal MR, Haanen J, Spits H. Interleukin-10 (IL-10) and viral IL-10 strongly reduce antigen-specific human T cell proliferation by diminishing the antigen-presenting capacity of monocytes via downregulation of class II major histocompatibility complex expression. *J Exp Med* 1991;174:915–924.

136. Kasid A, Bell GI, Director EP. Effects of transforming growth factor-β on human lymphokine activated killer cell procedures. *J Immunol* 1988;141:690–698.

137. Albino AP, Davis BM, Nanus DM. Induction of growth factor RNA expression in human malignant melanoma: markers of transformation. *Cancer Res* 1991;51:4815–4820.

138. Samid D, Shack S, Myers CE. Selective growth arrest and phenotypic reversion of prostate cancer cells in vitro by nontoxic pharmacological concentrations of phenylacetate. *J Clin Invest* 1993;91:2288–2295.

139. Reed JA, McNutt NS, Prieto VG, Albino AP. Expression of transforming growth factor-β2 in malignant melanoma correlates with the depth of tumor invasion. *Am J Pathol* 1994;45:97–104.

140. Walker RA, Dearing SJ. Transforming growth factor-β1 in ductal carcinoma *in situ* and invasive carcinomas of the breast. *Eur J Cancer* 1992;28:641–644.

141. Bost KL, Biegligk SC, Jaffe BM. Lymphokine mRNA expression by transplantable murine B lymphocytic malignancies: tumor-derived IL-10 as a possible mechanism for modulating the antitumor response. *J Immunol* 1995;154:718–729.

142. Wakefield LM, Letterio JL, Chen T. Transforming growth factor-β1 circulates in normal human plasma and is unchanged in advanced metastatic breast cancer. *Clin Cancer Res* 1995;1: 129–136.

143. Gorsch SM, Memoli VA, Stukel TA, et al. Immunohistochemical staining for transforming growth factor-β1 associates with disease progression in human breast cancer. *Cancer Res* 1992;52:6949–6952.

144. Dalal BI, Kewon PA, Greenburg AH. Immunocytochemical localization of secreted transforming growth factor-β1 to the advancing edges of primary tumors and to lymph node metastases of human mammary carcinoma. *Am J Pathol* 1993;143:381–389.

145. Kehrl JH, Wakefield LM, Roberts AB. Production of transforming growth factor beta by human T lymphocytes and its potential role in the regulation for T cell growth. *J Exp Med* 1986;163:1037–1050.

146. Mule JJ, Schwarz AB, Roberts AB, et al. Transforming growth factor-beta inhibits the in vivo generation of lymphokine-activated killer cells and cytotoxic T cells. *Cancer Immunol Immunother* 1988;26:95–100.

147. Tsunawaki S, Sporn M, Ding A, Nathan C. Deactivation of macrophages by transforming growth factor-β. *Nature* 1988;334:260–264.

148. Bosco MC, Espinoza-Delgado I, Schwabe M. The gamma subunit of the interleukin-2 receptor is expressed in human monocytes and modulated by interleukin-2, interferon-γ, and transforming growth factor-β1. *Blood* 1994;83: 3462–3467.

149. Espinoza-Delgado I, Bosco MC, Musso T. Inhibitory cytokine circuits involving transforming growth factor-β, interferon-α, and interleukin-2 in human monocyte activation. *Blood* 1994;83:3332–3338.

150. Weller M, Constam DB, Malipiero U, Fontana A. Transforming growth factor-β2 induces apoptosis of murine T cell clones without downregulating bcl-2 mRNA expression. *Eur J Immunol* 1994;24:1293–1300.

151. Donnet-Hughes A, Schriffin EJ, Huggett AC. Expression of MHC antigens by intestinal epithelial cells. Effect of transforming growth factor-beta-2 (TGF-β2). *Clin Exp Immunol* 1995;99: 240–244.

152. Czarniecki CW, Chiu HH, Wong GHW, et al. Transforming growth factor-β1 modulates the expression of class II histocompatibility antigens on human cells. *J Immunol* 1988;140:4217–4223.

153. Swain SL, Huston G, Tonkonogy S, Weinberg A. Transforming growth factor-β and IL-4 cause helper T cell precursors to develop into distinct effector helper cells that differ in lymphokine secretion pattern and cell surface phenotype. *J Immunol* 1991;147:2991–3000.

154. Lee HM, Rich S. Differential activation of CD8+ T cells by transforming growth factor-β1. *J Immunol* 1993;151:668–677.

155. Cerwenka A, Bevec D, Majkic O, et al. TGF-β1 is a potent inducer of human effector T cells. *J Immunol* 1994;153:4367–4377.

156. Henriksen R, Gobl A, Wilander E, et al. Expression and prognostic significance of TGF-beta isotypes, latent TGF-beta 1 binding protein, TGF-beta type I and type II receptors, and endoglin in normal ovary and ovarian neoplasms. *Lab Invest* 1995;73:213–220.

157. Hirte H, Clark DA. Generation of lymphokine-activated killer cells in human ovarian carcinoma ascitic fluid: identification of transforming growth factor-β as a suppressive factor. *Cancer Immunol Immunother* 1991;32:296–302.

158. Nash MA, Edwards CL, Kavanagh JJ, et al. Differential expression of cytokine transcripts in human epithelial ovarian carcinoma by solid tumor specimens, peritoneal exudate cells containing tumor, TIL-derived T-cell lines and established tumor cell lines (submitted).

159. Fakhrai H, Dorigo O, Shawler DL, et al. Eradication of established intracranial rat gliomas by transforming growth factor β antisense gene therapy. *Proc Natl Acad Sci USA* 1996;93: 2909–2914.

160. Freedman RS, Nash MA, Zhang HZ, et al. Intraperitoneal (IP) injection of rIFN-γ and rIL-2 modulate expression of HLA class I and II and TGFβ2 on tumor cells from epithelial ovarian

carcinoma (EOC) patients (pts). *Proc Am Assoc Cancer Res 1996*:A3334.

161. Cohen SBA, Katsikis PD, Feldmann M, Londei M. IL-10 enhances expression of the IL-2 receptor α chain on T cells. *Immunology* 1994;83: 329–332.

162. Schwartz MA, Hamilton LD, Tardelli L, et al. Stimulation of cytolytic activity by interleukin-10. *J Immunother* 1994;16:95–104.

163. Spagnoli GC, Juretic A, Schultz-Thater E. On the relative roles of interleukin-2 and interleukin-10 in the generation of lymphokine-activated killer cell activity. *Cell Immunol* 1993;146:391–405.

164. Chernoff AE, Granowitz EV, Shapior L, et al. A randomized, controlled trial of IL-10 in humans. *J Immunol* 1995;154:5492–5499.

165. Kim J, Modlin RL, Moy RL, et al. IL-10 production in cutaneous basal and squamous cell carcinomas. A mechanism for evading the local T cell immune response. *J Immunol* 1995;155: 2240–2247.

166. Smith DR, Kunkel SL, Burdick MD, et al. Production of interleukin-10 by human bronchogenic carcinoma. *Am J Pathol* 1994;145:18–25.

167. Chen Q, Daniel V, Maher DW, Hersey P. Production of IL-10 by melanoma cells: examination of its role in immunosuppression mediated by melanoma. *Int J Cancer* 1994;56:755–760.

168. Nakagomi H, Pisa P, Pisa EK, et al. Lack of interleukin-2 (IL-2) expression and selective expression of IL-10 mRNA in human renal cell carcinoma. *Int J Cancer* 1995;673:366–371.

169. Pisa P, Halapi E, Pisa EK, et al. Selective expression of interleukin 10, interferon γ, and granulocyte-macrophage colony stimulating factor in ovarian cancer biopsies. *Proc Natl Acad Sci USA* 1992;89:7708–7712.

170. Gotlieb WH, Abrams JW, Watson JM, et al. Presence of interleukin 10 (IL-10) in the ascites of patients with ovarian and other intra-abdominal cancers. *Cytokine* 1992;4:385–390.

171. Freedman R, Nash M, Edwards C, et al. Cytokine transcripts of peritoneal exudate cells (PEC) and TIL-derived T-cell lines from patients with epithelial ovarian carcinoma (EOC) and established EOC tumor cell lines. In: *9th International Congress of Immunology 1995.* 1995: A3974.

172. Rosenberg SA, Spiess P, Lafreniere R. A new approach to the adoptive immunotherapy of cancer with tumor infiltrating lymphocytes. *Science* 1986;233:1318–1321.

173. Spiess PJ, Yan JC, Rosenberg S. Tumor infiltrating lymphocytes expanded in recombinant interleukin-2 mediate potent anti-tumor activity in vivo. *Cancer Res* 1988;48:206–212.

174. Rosenberg SA, Packard BS, Aebersold PM. Use of tumor-infiltrating lymphocytes and interleukin-2 in the immunotherapy of patients with metastatic melanoma. A preliminary report. *N Engl J Med* 1988;319:1676–1680.

175. Rosenberg SA, Yang JC, Topalian SL, et al. Treatment of 283 consecutive patients with metastatic melanoma or renal cell cancer using high-dose bolus interleukin-2. *JAMA* 1994;271: 907–913.

176. Schwartzentruber DJ, Ham SS, Dadmarz R, et al. In vitro predictors of therapeutic response in melanoma patients receiving tumor-infiltrating lymphocytes and interleukin-2. *J Clin Oncol* 1994;12:1475–1483.

177. Bast RC Jr, Berek JS, Obrist R. Intraperitoneal immunotherapy of human ovarian carcinoma with *Corynebacterium parvum. Cancer Res* 1983;43:1395–1401.

178. Berek JS, Hacker NF, Lichtenstein A, et al. Intraperitoneal recombinant alpha-interferon for 'salvage' immunotherapy in stage III epithelial ovarian cancer: a Gynecologic Oncology Group Study. *Cancer Res* 1985;45:4447–4453.

179. Willemse PHB, De Vries EGE, Mulder NH, et al. Intraperitoneal human recombinant interferon alpha-2b in minimum residual ovarian cancer. *Eur J Cancer* 1990;26:353–358.

180. Pujade-Lauraine E, Guastella JP, Colombo N, et al. Intraperitoneal recombinant interferon-gamma in ovarian cancer patients with residual disease at second-look laparotomy. *J Clin Oncol* 1996;14:343–350.

181. Greiner JW, Guadagni F, Goldstein D, et al. Intraperitoneal administration of interferon-gamma to carcinoma patients enhances expression of tumor associated glycoprotein-72 and carcinoembryonic antigen on malignant ascites cells. *J Clin Oncol* 1992;10:735–746.

182. Chapman PB, Kolitz JE, Hakes TB, et al. A phase I trial of intraperitoneal recombinant interleukin-2 in patients with ovarian carcinoma. *Invest New Drugs* 1988;6:179–188.

183. Panici PB, Scambia G, Greggi S, et al. Recombinant interleukin-2 continuous infusion in ovarian cancer patients with minimal residual

disease at second look. *Cancer Treat Rep* 1989; 16:123–127.

184. Edwards RP, Lembersky BC, Kunschner AJ, et al. Intraperitoneal interleukin-2 produces durable responses for refractory ovarian cancer. *Proc Am Soc Clin Oncol* 1995:A997.

185. Freedman RS, Gibbons JA, Giedlin M, et al. Immunopharmacology and cytokine production of a low dose schedule of intraperitoneal administered human recombinant interleukin-2 in patients with advanced epithelial ovarian carcinoma. *J Immunother* 1977;19:443–451.

186. Urba WJ, Clark JW, Steis RG. Intraperitoneal lymphokine-activated killer cell/interleukin-2 therapy in patients with intra-abdominal cancer: immunologic considerations. *J Natl Cancer Inst* 1989;81:602–611.

187. Stewart JA, Belinson JL, Moore AL, et al. Phase I trial of intraperitoneal recombinant interleukin-2/lymphokine-activated killer cells in patients with ovarian cancer. *Cancer Res* 1990;50:6302–6310.

188. Berek JS, Welander C, Schink JC, et al. A phase I-II trial of intraperitoneal cisplatin and α-interferon in patients with persistent epithelial ovarian cancer. *Gynecol Oncol* 1991;40:237–243.

189. Nardi M, Cognetti F, Pollera CF. Intraperitoneal recombinant alpha-2-interferon alternating with cisplatin as salvage therapy for minimal residual-disease ovarian cancer. A phase II study. *J Clin Oncol* 1990;8:1036–1041.

190. Markman M, Berek JS, Blessing JA, et al. Characteristics of patients with small-volume residual ovarian cancer unresponsive to cisplatin-based ip chemotherapy: lessons learned from a gynecologic oncology group phase II trial of ip cisplatin and recombinant α-interferon. *Gynecol Oncol* 1992;45:3–8.

191. Canevari S, Stoter G, Arienti F, et al. Regression of advanced ovarian carcinoma by intraperitoneal treatment with autologous T lymphocytes retargeted by a bispecific monoclonal antibody. *J Natl Cancer Inst* 1995;87:1463–1469.

192. Mitchell MS. Combining chemotherapy with biological response modifiers in treatment of cancer. *J Natl Cancer Inst* 1988;80:1445–1450.

193. Sznol M, Longo DL. Chemotherapy drug interactions with biological agents. *Semin Oncol* 1993;20:80–93.

194. Papa MZ, Yang, JC, Vetto JT, et al. Combined effects of chemotherapy and interleukin-2 in the therapy of mice with advanced pulmonary tumors. *Cancer Res* 1988;48:122–129.

195. Eggermont AMM, Sugarbaker PH. Efficacy of intracavitary administration of cyclophosphamide, interleukin-2 and lymphokine activated killer cells against established intra-peritoneal tumor. *Acta Med Austriaca* 1989;16:47–51.

196. Legha SS, Buzaid AC. Role of recombinant interleukin-2 in combination with interferon-alpha and chemotherapy in the treatment of advanced melanoma. *Semin Oncol* 1993;20:27–32.

197. Alberts DS, Mason-Liddil N, O'Toole RV, et al. Randomized phase III trial of chemoimmunotherapy in patients with previously untreated stages III and IV suboptimal disease ovarian cancer: a Southwest Oncology Group study. *Gynecol Oncol* 1989;32:8–15.

198. Formelli F, Rossi C, Sensi ML, Parmiani G. Potentiation of adoptive immunotherapy by *cis*-diamminedichloroplatinum (II), but not by doxorubicin, on a disseminated mouse lymphoma and its association with reduction of tumor burden. *Int J Cancer* 1988;42:952–957.

199. Frasci G, Tortoriello A, Facchini G, et al. Intraperitoneal (IP) cisplatin-mitoxantrone-interferon-alpha 2b in ovarian cancer patients with minimal residual disease. *Gyn Oncol* 1993; 50:60–67.

200. Frasci G, Tortoriello A, Facchini G, et al. Carboplatin and alpha-2b interferon intraperitoneal combination as first-line treatment of minimal residual ovarian cancer. A pilot study. *Eur J Cancer* 1994;30:946–950.

201. Fujita K, Ikarashi H, Takakuwa K. Prolonged disease-free period in patients with advanced epithelial ovarian cancer after adoptive transfer of tumor-infiltrating lymphocytes. *Clin Cancer Res* 1995;1:501–507.

$\mathscr{P}$ART II

Clinical Applications

SECTION 1

Breast

CHAPTER *3*

Breast Cancer Risk Factors and Preventive Approaches to Breast Cancer

VICTOR G. VOGEL

*P*ublic attention and awareness about breast cancer have been heightened by the diagnosis of the disease in prominent political and social figures and by national campaigns that present breast cancer as a public health problem. Programs that promote the benefits of screening mammography also focus attention on breast cancer, as does media coverage of research reports about the genetic basis of the disease. For these and perhaps other reasons, the public is anxious about breast cancer, and many women perceive their risk of dying of breast cancer to be very high in the short term (1). Although for most women the actual risk is significantly lower than the perceived risk, women consult physicians regularly to obtain information to control their risk for breast cancer. Available data suggest that a balanced presentation by health-care professionals about the risk factors for breast cancer and the strategies to lower the risk may reduce anxiety regardless of whether a woman actively adopts measures to reduce her risk.

For clinicians, an understanding of the factors that affect a woman's risk for breast cancer results in better comprehension of the biologic processes that lead to the disease and allows the clinician to give informed, objective responses to patients' questions. This, in turn, reduces patients' anxiety and improves clinical management of the woman at risk. It also facilitates the design and adoption of improved preventive strategies for breast cancer. In this chapter, I review the factors that lead to an increased or decreased risk for breast cancer, examine models that allow clinicians to quantify a woman's risk of developing breast cancer, define techniques for counseling women to decrease their risk, and briefly review clinical methods currently being evaluated for the primary prevention of breast cancer.

Factors That Increase Risk

Clinicians and epidemiologists evaluate risk to identify those women who require special management and to increase understanding of the biologic processes that lead to breast cancer. *Risk* is a relative term derived by comparing the incidence of a disease in a group having a particular risk factor or trait with the incidence of the same disease in a comparison group of individuals who do not carry the risk factor but who are in every other way the same. If risk calculations are derived from retrospective data, risk is expressed as the odds ratio, or the ratio of the odds of having the disease in those with the trait of interest compared with the odds of having the disease in those without the trait. If a trait is evaluated in a prospective study, the risk of disease can be expressed as the ratio of the incidence of the disease in those with the trait divided by the incidence of the disease in those without the trait. This ratio is known as the *relative risk* and can be viewed as the level of increased risk of developing the disease associated with the risk factor. For example, a relative risk (or an odds ratio) of 1.8 means that a person with a given trait or characteristic is 1.8 times more likely to develop the disease than is someone without the trait. A trait associated with a relative risk of this magnitude can also be described as being associated with an 80% increase in risk.

It is important to recognize that the presence of a risk factor does not guarantee the development of a disease just as the absence of a risk factor does not confer absolute protection against the disease. The relationship between a risk factor and the proportion of cases of a disease that it may cause is known as the *attributable risk*. Calculation of attributable risk requires knowledge of the prevalence of a particular risk factor in the population of interest and the relative risk associated with

that risk factor (2). For example, a risk factor that is present in 20% of the population and that has an associated relative risk of 1.5 has an attributable risk of 0.09 or 9%, meaning that the presence of this risk factor explains 9% of the incidence of the disease in the population. Common breast cancer risk factors (3) and their associated relative risks, population prevalence, and attributable risks are shown in Table 3-1.

Few breast cancer risk factors have a population prevalence greater than 10% to 15%, although some are associated with very large relative risks (e.g., mutated genes, cellular atypia), making them important to consider in the clinical management of breast cancer risk (4). Traits associated with large relative risks are rare; common risk factors are associated with relative risks less than 2.0 so that the attributable risk for any particular risk factor is small, as shown in Table 3-1. In addition, because many women possess multiple risk factors for breast cancer and because of the epidemiologic confounding that may occur in evaluating both relative and attributable risks, it may not be pos-

T A B L E   3-1

Risk Factors for Breast Cancer, Their Relative Risks, and the Associated Population Attributable Risk

Risk Factor (3)	Comparison Category	Risk Category	Relative Risk	Prevalence (4)	Population Attributable Risk*
Age at menarche	16 yr	Younger than 12 yr	1.3	16%	0.05
Age at menopause	45–54 yr	After 55 yr	1.5	6%	0.03
Age at first live birth	Before 20 yr	Nulliparous or older than 30 yr	1.9	21%	0.16
Benign breast disease	No biopsy or fine-needle aspiration	Any benign disease	1.5	15%	0.07
		Proliferative disease	2.0	4%	0.04
		Atypical hyperplasia	4.0	1%	0.03
Family history of breast cancer	No first-degree relative affected	Mother affected	1.7	8%	0.05
		Two first-degree relatives affected	5.0	4%	0.14
Obesity	10th percentile	90th percentile	1.2	18%	0.03
Alcohol use	Nondrinker	Moderate drinker	1.7	12%	0.08
Estrogen replacement therapy	Never used	Current use ages 50–59 yr	1.5	18%	0.08

*As defined by Lilienfeld and Lilienfeld (2); population attributable risk = (prevalence × relative risk)/[(prevalence × relative risk − 1) + 1].

sible to sum the attributable risks in Table 3-1 to obtain a summary attributable risk. If the risk factors were independent and there were no interactions among them affecting the respective levels of risk associated with them, then the complement of the summary attributable risk (i.e., 1 − attributable risk) would be the product of the complements of the individual attributable risks (5). If this assumption holds, then the summary attributable risk for the risk factors listed in Table 3-1 is 47%. Previously published estimates of the summary population attributable risk for breast cancer range from 21% in premenopausal women to 29% in postmenopausal women (6) to 55% in women in the Breast Cancer Detection and Demonstration Project (BCDDP) (5). Attributable risk does not establish causality, and it is clear that nearly half the attributable risk for breast cancer remains unexplained (7). Nevertheless, it is instructive to examine what is known regarding established risk factors for breast cancer.

Age

All women are at risk for breast cancer, and the most important single risk factor is age. The risk of breast cancer increases throughout a woman's lifetime (4): The annual incidence of breast cancer in U.S. women 80 to 85 years old is 15 times higher than the incidence among women 30 to 35 years old (412 cases/100,000 women/yr at age 80 compared with 27.9 cases/100,000 women/yr at age 30). It is not yet known whether these observed differences are explained by the accumulation of a number of events that occur throughout a woman's lifetime or by a single event that is triggered with greater frequency in older than in younger women.

Race and ethnicity modify the effect of age on the risk of breast cancer. For example, African-American women younger than 50 have a higher age-specific incidence of breast cancer than do their white American counterparts, but older African-Americans have a lower age-specific incidence than do older white Americans (4). There is not yet an adequate explanation for these differences. Furthermore, the breast cancer incidence for Hispanic women living in North America is only 40% to 50% as great as the incidence among non-Hispanic white women. Asian women born in Asia have an extremely low lifetime risk of breast cancer, but their daughters born in North America have the same lifetime risk of breast cancer as do

American white women (8). No explanation, including dietary factors, yet accounts for these observed differences.

Gynecologic Events

The extensive epidemiologic literature about the risk factors for breast cancer is derived from both case-control and cohort studies. Most breast cancer risk factors relate to gynecologic or endocrinologic events in a woman's life (3,9–12). Age at menarche is related to a woman's chance of developing breast cancer: Compared with women who experience menarche at age 16, girls who experience menarche 2 to 5 years earlier have a 10% to 30% greater risk of developing breast cancer later in life. A similar observation has been made for the timing of events at the other end of the reproductive spectrum, the age at menopause. The average age at menopause in the United States is slightly older than 51 years. If women who experience menopause between the ages of 45 and 55 years are used as the referent group, women who experience menopause at age 55 or older have a 50% higher risk of subsequently developing breast cancer, and women who cease menstruating at age 45 or earlier have a 30% lower risk of subsequently developing breast cancer. These data, along with the observations about the age at menarche, indicate that one way of expressing the risk of breast cancer in relation to gynecologic events is simply to count the number of ovulatory menstrual cycles that a woman experiences in her lifetime. Early menarche and late menopause lead to an increased total lifetime number of menstrual cycles and a corresponding 30% to 50% increase in breast cancer risk. Conversely, late menarche and early menopause lead to a reduction in breast cancer risk of similar magnitude. Consistent with this observation is the fact that oophorectomy before the age of menopause (especially before the age of 40) lowers the risk of breast cancer by approximately two thirds (9).

It is tempting to say that the explanation for these observations is the level of circulating estrogen to which a woman is exposed in her lifetime. In an adult woman, the predominant circulating estrogen is estradiol, and most of this is bound to sex hormone–binding globulin (SHBG). A smaller proportion is bound to albumin. Between menarche and menopause, a woman is exposed to higher static levels of circulating estradiol (bound to either SHBG or albumin as well as freely circulating). Cell proliferation is low during the follicular phase of the menstrual cycle and does not increase with the preovulatory peak in estradiol (13). Following ovulation, progesterone stimulates cell proliferation to three times the follicular rates. If fertilization and pregnancy do not occur, progesterone levels fall, breast cell division decreases, and apoptosis follows (14). During pregnancy, circulating levels of both estrogen and progesterone remain elevated. In animal models, progesterone is a potent mitogen to breast cells, possibly making them more susceptible to the effects of breast carcinogens (13). During the second half of pregnancy, however, cell differentiation occurs in the breast, and proliferation decreases.

Pregnancy at a young age, especially before the age of 20, markedly reduces the incidence of subsequent breast cancer (9). Conversely, both nulliparity and age older than 30 at the time of the first live birth are associated with nearly a doubling of the risk of subsequent breast cancer (12). Pregnancies not ending in the birth of a viable fetus do not confer a reduction in the risk of breast cancer (15). For obvious technical, practical, and ethical reasons, there are no data from women that provide a histologic explanation for the protection from breast cancer brought about by early pregnancy.

Benign Breast Disease

Symptomatic changes in the breast are quite common in clinical practice. Various published studies reported that as many as two thirds of women have symptoms and signs variously described as pain, lumps, tenderness, nodularity, or thickening of the breasts (16). Some studies showed a correlation between risk factors for breast cancer and those for benign breast disease (17), while others did not (18). The latter studies raised the possibility that benign breast disease is not a precursor of breast cancer. Few benign lesions show amplification of the HER-2/*neu* oncogene or mutation of the *TP53* tumor suppressor gene (19). The significance of these findings remains to be determined. Although there is some correlation between the presence of nodularity on physical examination and the appearance of the mammogram, benign disease of the breast is not more common in women with other risk factors

for breast cancer such as a family history of the disease. The signs and symptoms of benign breast disease often resolve without treatment and usually do not require breast biopsy for definitive diagnosis; fewer than 20% of women in North America have undergone a biopsy for benign breast disease by age 50 (20). Benign breast disease that results in biopsy does increase the risk of subsequently developing breast cancer (21).

The clinical lexicon is replete with creative, if not accurately descriptive terms for benign breast disease: chronic cystic mastitis, fibroadenoma, fibrocystic disease, and so on. Among women undergoing biopsy for benign breast disease, the risk of subsequent breast cancer is not uniform. The most informative classification schema is based on histopathology: It divides benign disease into proliferative and nonproliferative categories (22). The important subclassifications of proliferative disease are listed in Table 3-2 with their associated relative risks. Proliferative disease accounts for between one fourth and one third of all biopsies for benign disease, and 5% to 10% of the proliferative lesions show cellular atypia, the histologic change associated with the highest risk (22–26). The atypical features are similar to some found in carcinoma in situ. Increasing use of mammographic screening has led to increased identification of women with proliferative lesions of the breast (27).

Cystic disease also increases risk. While early benign disease classification schemes did not include sclerosing adenosis among the lesions that increase risk, recent data indicate that sclerosing adenosis increases the risk of breast cancer by approximately 70%, which justifies its inclusion among proliferative disease without atypia (28). A family history of breast cancer in first-degree relatives has an additive effect on the subsequent risk of breast cancer (22,25,26). While fewer than 5% of women with a biopsy showing no proliferative changes develop breast cancer over the subsequent 25 years, nearly 40% of women with a family history of breast cancer and atypical hyperplasia subsequently develop breast cancer. Biopsy before the age of 50 to 55 years may be associated with a fivefold to sixfold increase in the risk of breast cancer, while biopsy at older ages is associated with only half this risk (21).

Familial breast cancers show an increased prevalence of medullary histology, and it is well established that in younger women invasive

T A B L E   **3-2**

Classification of Benign Breast Disease and the Risk for Subsequent
Development of Breast Cancer (22–26)*

Benign Lesion	Description	Associated Relative Risk for Breast Cancer	
		With Family History of Breast Cancer	**Without Family History of Breast Cancer**
Proliferative disease without atypia	—	2.4–2.7	1.7–1.9
Moderate and florid ductal hyperplasia of the usual type	Most common type of hyperplasia; cells do not have the cytologic appearance of lobular or apocrine-like lesions; florid lesions have a proliferation of cells that fill more than 70% of the involved space	—	—
Additional lesions	Intraductal papilloma, radial scar, sclerosing adenosis, apocrine metaplasia	—	—
Atypical hyperplasia		11.0	4.2–4.3
Atypical ductal hyperplasia	Has features similar to ductal carcinoma in situ but lacks the complete criteria for that diagnosis		
Atypical lobular hyperplasia	Defined by changes that are similar to lobular carcinoma in situ but lack the complete criteria for that diagnosis	—	—
Nonproliferative	Normal glandular histology, cysts, duct ectasia, mild hyperplasia, fibroadenoma	1.2–2.6	0.9–1.0

*Relative risks represent the range of values reported in the published literature.

breast cancer is of higher grade, is more proliferative, has an increased thymidine labeling index and S-phase fraction, and has increased expression of proliferation-associated proteins (29). Early-onset breast cancers also have an excess of invasive ductal carcinoma with a predominant intraductal component, although familial breast cancers do not.

One emerging use of benign breast pathology is in the clinical evaluation of women with a familial predisposition to breast cancer. Among women with normal findings on clinical examination, bilateral fine-needle aspiration of all four breast quadrants yields cytologic evidence of proliferative breast disease in 30% to 40% of patients who have two or more first-degree relatives with breast cancer, compared with only 13% of women without a family history of breast cancer (30,31). The subsequent appearance of breast cancer in some women with these abnormalities suggests that cytohistologic changes may precede the development of breast cancer in women with predisposing risk factors. These changes may also serve as intermediate biologic end points in clinical prevention trials that enroll these women as subjects. Other studies showed an increasing proportion of overexpression of breast cancer–associated biologic markers in fine-needle breast aspirates from women with risk factors for breast cancer (32). More aspirates from women with atypia than from women with proliferative changes only had elevations in epidermal growth factor receptor (EGFR), p53, and aneuploidy. The incorporation of cyto-histologic changes into routine clinical risk assessment awaits the completion of confirmatory studies. Use of these changes in clinical decision making (e.g., the decision to undergo prophylactic mastectomy) has not been evaluated.

It is an extremely interesting observation that estrogen replacement therapy lowers the risk of breast cancer in women with proliferative benign breast disease with or without atypia (33). A history of proliferative benign

T A B L E   3-3

Indications for Breast Cancer Risk Counseling

1 More than two first-degree relatives with breast, ovarian, or other cancers
2 Two or more generations affected
3 First-degree relatives with bilateral breast cancer
4 Multiple primary tumors, breast or other
5 Early-onset cancer (younger than 45 years)
6 Sarcomas, adrenocortical carcinomas, or other rare cancers in relatives
7 Ataxia telangiectasia in relatives
8 Premalignant histology on breast biopsy
9 Relative with a known mutation in a susceptibility gene
10 Women considering prophylactic mastectomy or oophorectomy

Source: Reproduced by permission from Peters J. Breast cancer genetics: relevance to oncology practice. *Cancer Control* 1995;2:195–208.

breast disease is not, therefore, a contraindication to estrogen replacement therapy.

Family History of Breast Cancer

Genetic factors contribute to approximately 5% of all breast cancers but to 25% of those diagnosed before age 30 (34). Early-onset breast cancer is that which occurs before age 50, when there is a flattening in the rate of increase in the age-specific incidence rates. A number of factors can indicate a need to explore more fully the history of breast cancer in a family. These factors are listed in Table 3-3 (35). Risk can be quantified rapidly and simply by assessing the number and degree of a woman's relatives affected with breast cancer and their ages at diagnosis. This is illustrated in Table 3-4 (36). Having more relatives diagnosed with breast cancer before the age of 50 increases the cumulative lifetime risk of developing the disease to near 50%, indicating the autosomal dominant behavior of some syndromes of genetically predisposed breast cancer.

Mutation of one gene, *BRCA1*, appears to account for 45% of families with a significantly high incidence of breast cancer and at least 80% of families with an increased incidence of both early-onset breast cancer and ovarian cancer (37,38). *BRCA1* is located on chromosome 17q and appears to encode a tumor suppressor protein that acts as a negative regulator of tumor

Affected Relative	Age of Affected Relative (yr)	Cumulative Breast Cancer Risk by Age 80 (%)
One first degree	<50	13–21
	50	9–11
One second degree	<50	10–14
	50	8–9
Two first degree	Both <50	35–48
	Both ≥50	11–24
Two second degree[b]	Both <50	21–26
	Both ≥50	9–16

T A B L E   3-4

Breast Cancer Risk Estimates for Members of Moderate-Risk Families[a]

[a] Risk estimates are derived by including age extremes from the risk tables calculated by Claus et al (34) as modified by Hoskins et al (36). For example, for affected relatives younger than 50 years, the lower limit is the calculated risk if the affected relative is in the 40- to 49-year age group and the upper limit is the calculated risk for a relative in the 20- to 29-year age group. Thus, these figures represent the range of risk based on age and are not confidence intervals.

[b] Both paternal or both maternal.

Source: Reproduced by permission from Hoskins KF, Stopfer JE, Calzone KA, et al. Assessment and counseling for women with a family history of breast cancer—a guide for clinicians. *JAMA* 1995;273:577–585.

growth (39,40). It is a large gene containing 5592 nucleotides spread over 100,000 bases of genomic DNA (41). It is composed of 22 coding exons that produce a protein containing 1863 amino acids. At the amino-terminal end of the protein there is a region that is thought to interact with other amino acids or to form protein complexes, suggesting a role for *BRCA1* in regulating DNA transcription. Mutations in *BRCA1* may also play a role in the progression of sporadic breast cancer (40,42). Family studies showed that predisposition to cancer is inherited as a dominant genetic trait, but the associated allele behaves in a recessive way in somatic cells. An inherited copy of the mutant allele causes familial predisposition to cancer, and mutation of the other, paired allele begins the progression toward malignancy.

Reported mutations to the *BRCA1* gene are of several types: frameshift (insertion or deletion of two or more nucleotides resulting in altered translation of the protein), nonsense (nucleotide substitution producing a stop codon and termination of protein translation), missense (change of a single amino acid), and splice-site (which also causes production of an aberrant protein) (41). Mutations result in a truncated protein in 86% of the patients tested to date. All of these mutations appear to be rare in the general population, occurring in somewhere between 1 in 200 and 1 in 500 persons. One particular mutation (185delAG), however, appears to occur in as many as 1% of Ashkenazi-Jewish individuals (43). Confirmatory studies of these preliminary findings are necessary, as are precautions to guard against the unethical or inappropriate use of testing in narrowly targeted populations (44).

The presence of a mutated *BRCA1* gene with a resultant truncated protein has important clinical consequences, as shown in Table 3-5

(45). The relative risk of breast cancer associated with a *BRCA1* mutation is greater than 200 before the age of 40 but drops to 15 in the seventh decade of life (45). The penetrance of the phenotype in carriers of mutated genes is estimated to be 87% for breast cancer and 44% for ovarian cancer by age 70. There is also evidence of allelic heterogeneity, with 29% of *BRCA1* mutations conferring a high risk of ovarian cancer and 71% conferring a moderate risk. If these observations hold true, the average lifetime risk of ovarian cancer in *BRCA1* mutation carriers will be approximately 40%.

Young women with a diagnosis of breast cancer who have multiple affected relatives have a higher likelihood of being mutation carriers. Approximately 45% of families with increased susceptibility to breast cancer carry mutations of *BRCA1* (37). Hoskins et al (36) divided these women into two groups. The first group, those from moderate-risk families, are characterized by a "less striking" family history, an absence of ovarian cancer, and an older average age at diagnosis. High-risk families are generally characterized by the occurrence of breast cancer in at least three close relatives that follows an autosomal dominant pattern. Available data show that 26% of families with three affected members diagnosed before age 60 and 60% of families with four or more members show *BRCA1* mutations (37). The presence of even one case of ovarian cancer in the family makes a *BRCA1* mutation more likely, and a case of male breast cancer makes a *BRCA1* mutation less likely (46). Breast cancer is often diagnosed at an early age (<45 years), and there may be cases of ovarian cancer as well. A description of the evaluation of moderate-risk families is beyond the scope of this chapter; the reader is referred to the appropriate quantitative models (47,48) and review articles (36) for guidance.

T A B L E **3-5**				
Estimated Cumulative Risks of Breast and Ovarian Cancer in *BRCA1* Gene Carriers		**Cumulative Risk**		
	Age (yr)	**Breast Cancer**	**Ovarian Cancer**	**Either Cancer**
	30	0.032	0.0017	0.034
	40	0.191	0.0061	0.195
	50	0.508	0.227	0.619
	60	0.542	0.298	0.678
	70	0.850	0.633	0.945

Source: Reproduced by permission from Easton DF, Ford BP, Bishop DT, the Breast Cancer Linkage Consortium. Breast and ovarian cancer incidence in BRCA1-mutation carriers. *Am J Hum Genet* 1995;56:265–271.

Current technology permits sequencing of the entire *BRCA1* gene in individuals with an increased likelihood of carrying a mutated gene, particularly in women with breast cancer. Once a woman with a diagnosis of breast cancer is identified by DNA sequencing methodology as having a mutated *BRCA1* allele, additional women at risk in her family may be screened using allele-specific oligonucleotides that efficiently screen for the known mutation (41). Families can also be screened with assays that evaluate the presence of a truncated *BRCA1* protein (49), but these assays are investigational, and precise estimates of test-related sensitivity and specificity are not yet available. Furthermore, the predictive value of a positive test result will depend significantly on the prior probability of carrying a mutation in the individual being tested. A negative test result is only informative in a woman from a family where a known *BRCA1* mutation exists. Her risk of breast cancer would then be equal to that of a woman in the general population. In a family undergoing genetic testing where no *BRCA1* mutation is found, risk should be calculated using quantitative models just referenced and described elsewhere in this chapter.

Because *BRCA1* is an autosomal gene, it can be carried and transmitted by men in the affected families. Although the risk of breast cancer in the male carriers appears to be negligible, there is a threefold risk of prostate cancer and a fourfold risk of colon cancer in male mutation carriers. A second breast cancer gene, *BRCA2*, which localizes to chromosome 13, confers risks for breast and ovarian cancer in women similar to those conferred by *BRCA1* and is associated with an increased risk of breast cancer in male carriers (36,50). Several other genetic syndromes (e.g., the Li-Fraumeni syndrome, caused by mutations in the *TP53* gene) predispose carriers to an increased risk of developing breast cancer, but they are rare and beyond the scope of this chapter. The reader is referred to a comprehensive review of familial cancer risk for details and management recommendations (51).

Women without a diagnosis of breast cancer with increased pretest probabilities of carrying a *BRCA1* mutation can be identified on the basis of the number of their relatives diagnosed with breast cancer and their ages at diagnosis (36,47,48,52). Not all women who are at risk for breast cancer because of a family history of the disease will elect to undergo genetic testing, however. Women who have regular breast examinations by a physician, who believe that mammography effectively detects early breast cancer, and who believe that breast cancer is curable report that they would accept genetic susceptibility testing for breast cancer (53). The proportion of women who actually choose to have testing following counseling is the focus of several ongoing research studies. Guidelines for the responsible use of genetic testing are outlined in Table 3-6 (54–58). All subjects who

T A B L E   **3-6**

Responsible Use of Presymptomatic Genetic Testing for Cancer Susceptibility (54-58)

Cancer susceptibility testing is currently investigational and not routine.
Testing should be voluntary and free from professional and family pressure to participate.
Persons have the right to know the results of their testing.
Persons have the right *not* to know their genetic predispositions.
Participation in genetic testing should be based on understanding and should require fully informed consent.
Testing can have long-lasting and profound psychosocial consequences.
Cancer risk counseling is a prerequisite for testing.
Predisposition testing is most appropriate for diseases that are preventable or treatable.
Results of genetic testing must be private and confidential.
Regulation may be necessary to avoid employment and insurance discrimination.
Vulnerable populations such as minors and incompetent adults need extra protections.
Resources and access to testing should be equitably distributed.
Additional research is needed on specific criteria for test sensitivity, specificity, and effectiveness.
Research into clinical and psychological implications of susceptibility testing is needed.
Ethical consultation and supervision of testing programs are helpful at the current stage of test development.
Quality assurance should include standards for laboratories and professional personnel.

undergo genetic susceptibility testing should undergo counseling. Counseling is necessary to educate the subject about risk, to explain the process and limitations of genetic testing, to assess and manage anxiety and other psychopathology, and to review clinical management options. There are also important legal and ethical complexities that must be considered. The counseling process is complex, and the reader is referred to appropriate reviews (35,36,55,56,59). Patients should be referred to trained and experienced genetics counselors whenever possible.

Management options for women who carry *BRCA1* mutations include mammographic screening, prophylactic mastectomy, and participation in investigational chemoprevention trials, all discussed later in this chapter. The effect of either oral contraceptives or estrogen replacement therapy on the risk of breast cancer in carriers of *BRCA1* mutations is unknown. Ovarian cancer screening with CA-125 antigen and transvaginal ultrasound remains investigational.

Mammographic Parenchymal Pattern

In 1976, Wolfe (60) proposed a classification system for mammograms based solely on the radiographic appearance of the breast parenchyma. Four parenchymal patterns (N1, P1, P2, DY) were associated with a stepwise increase in breast cancer risk. Meta-analysis of multiple published studies revealed a fivefold increase in risk for high-risk parenchymal patterns in prospective cohort studies and a twofold increase in risk in retrospective case-control studies (61). High-risk patterns are more prevalent in countries with an increased incidence of breast cancer than in countries with a lower incidence (62). Women showing the P1 pattern (mostly fat with <25% prominent duct pattern) or the DY pattern (sheet-like areas of increased density) are more likely to have a finding of lobular carcinoma in situ in breast biopsy specimens (63).

Because Wolfe's original classification scheme was somewhat subjective, other investigators sought to assess breast density more quantitatively. Using a compensating polar planimeter, Saftlas et al (64) measured breast densities in mammograms taken prior to a diagnosis of breast cancer. There was a linear increase in the risk of breast cancer with increasing breast density. Using a referent group in whom less than 5% of the mammogram area was dense, they calculated the odds ratio for subsequent development of breast cancer to be 4.3 for women in whom more than 65% of the breast area was dense. In a recent follow-up study of participants in the BCDDP, mammographic densities were evaluated using a computerized planimeter prior to the development of breast cancer in 1880 women who subsequently developed breast cancer (65). High densities with either the P2 (prominent linear and nodular ductal densities that occupy 25%–100% of the breast area) or the DY pattern of Wolfe were associated with odds ratios of 3.2 and 2.9, respectively, of developing breast cancer. Women who had a quantitative breast density of 75% or greater by planimetry had a fivefold increased risk of breast cancer. In the BCDDP, 28% of the incident breast cancer cases were associated with a breast density of 50% or greater. This technique appears to be an independent measure of breast cancer risk although it has not gained wide acceptance in clinical practice.

A mechanistic explanation for the differences in radiographic breast density may lie in plasma lipid levels. In one study, mammographic density was associated with plasma levels of high-density lipoprotein (HDL) cholesterol, low-density lipoprotein (LDL) cholesterol, triglycerides, and apoprotein B, and urinary excretion of the mutagen malondialdehyde (66). The relationship of these observations to breast cancer risk remains to be defined.

Few correlations between mammographic appearance and histopathology have been published. One autopsy study that allowed comparison of breast histopathology with whole breast mammograms of formalin-fixed mastectomy specimens showed that in most women the mammographic parenchymal pattern is confounded by obesity, the normal aging process, and genetic factors (67). Correspondingly, the correlation of the mammographic pattern with the amount of breast parenchyma and the presence of fibrocystic changes was poor. Mammographic lucency was closely associated with age, obesity, and large breast size. These observations suggest that parenchymal pattern may not, in fact, be an independent predictor of the risk of breast cancer.

Risk Factors of Uncertain Significance

Body Size and Obesity

Although body weight and measures of body size are positively associated with the risk of developing breast cancer in postmenopausal women, a negative association between weight and breast cancer risk has been found in premenopausal women (11,68–71). On the other hand, data about height as an independent risk factor are conflicting, and no plausible mechanism has been proposed that would explain the interactive effect of body size and menopausal status on the risk of breast cancer. Some studies reported either that a weight gain in adulthood is associated with increased risk of breast cancer or that the ratio of central to peripheral fat distribution affects risk (68,70). Whether this is related to endogenous estrogen production by adipose tissue remains speculative. The effect of obesity on other risk factors for breast cancer is not well studied, with the exception of the association of obesity or large body size with early age at menarche. It is not clear whether significant weight reduction has a substantial protective effect on breast cancer risk.

Exercise

That physical exercise may be biologically linked to breast cancer risk is plausible because strenuous physical activity is associated with an increase in luteal-phase defects, anovulation, and depressed serum estradiol levels (72). Exercise may also influence the prevalence of obesity, but large body mass has actually been associated with reductions in the risk of premenopausal breast cancer, as noted earlier. Both the timing of weight change in adulthood and body fat distribution may be important determinants of risk, but additional studies are needed to clarify the hormonal consequences of physical activity and obesity.

Studies showing that moderate physical activity can have a protective effect against the development of breast cancer (73) have been difficult to confirm (74,75). Various studies of different designs showed nonsignificant protection afforded by physical activity, or an unexpected increased risk among the most physically active women, either premenopausal (76) or postmenopausal (72). Studies of women with nonsedentary occupations suggested that physical activity at work may lower the risk of dying of breast cancer by approximately 15% (77), but results have been inconsistent (78).

Some of these earlier studies may have been handicapped by an inability to control for other breast cancer risk factors, to accurately measure physical activity, or to account for changes in activity over time. More recent research done with greater methodologic rigor did show that the average number of hours spent in physical exercise activities per week from menarche to early middle age is a significant predictor of reduced breast cancer risk. In one study, women who spent 1 to 3 hours per week in physical activity reduced their risk of breast cancer by 30% relative to inactive women, and those who exercised at least 4 hours per week reduced the risk by 50%. The effect was greatest for women who had at least one child, and the effect was not lost among obese women (79). The interaction of physical activity with other breast cancer risk factors is not yet clear, and more information is required. It is not known, for example, whether physical activity can reduce the risk associated with genetic predisposition or proliferative benign breast disease. Women with these conditions should be counseled that there is uncertainty about the protective effect of physical exercise in the setting of their risk factor profiles.

Diet

Fat consumption in the diet was thought to influence the risk of breast cancer, largely on the basis of the observation that the age-adjusted incidence rates for breast cancer are highest in countries with the highest levels of dietary fat consumption (80). Case-control and prospective cohort studies, however, showed either weak or nonexistent associations between dietary fat and the risk of breast cancer (3). For example, the Nurses' Health Study, a prospective evaluation of more than 90,000 registered nurses in the United States, found equal risks for breast cancer across all levels of dietary fat and fiber consumption for both premenopausal and postmenopausal women (81). The explanation for these apparently conflicting observations may lie in the micronutrient components of the diets consumed rather than in the levels of total fat or calories.

Supporting the view that dietary subcomponents may affect cancer risk more than fat or total calories consumed is the fact that some polyunsaturated fatty acids can serve as substrates for prostaglandin synthesis and are implicated in tumorigenesis (82). Other polyunsaturated fatty acids have a double bond between the third and fourth carbon atoms (so-called omega-3 fatty acids) and are competitive inhibitors of prostaglandin endoperoxidase synthetase. It is possible, therefore, that the omega-3 fatty acids (such as eicosapentaenoic or docosahexaenoic acids) may act as dietary inhibitors of carcinogenesis. This protective effect is suggested by the lower age-standardized breast cancer incidence rates from countries around the world where the consumption of fish oil (a rich source of omega-3 fatty acids) is high (83,84). These data suggest a protective effect from fish oils, but additional studies in women are needed before dietary modification or supplementation can be recommended as a proven breast cancer prevention strategy.

Similar suggestive but unconfirmed data exist for populations with increased dietary consumption of soybeans. Increased soy protein consumption is significantly correlated with a reduction in the risk of breast cancer (85). Asians, for example, eat diets rich in soybean products and have breast cancer death rates one third to one half those of women in the West (86). Foods made from soybeans contain large quantities of isoflavones, which are phytoestrogens with weak estrogen agonist activity and may interfere with the breast cancer–promoting effects of physiologic estrogen (87). These promising compounds merit additional clinical investigations. Until these studies are completed, it is not yet appropriate to suggest to women that they can significantly lower their risk of breast cancer by increasing their consumption of soybean products.

Vitamins

The antioxidant vitamins A, C, and E have potential preventive properties because endogenous production of hydrogen peroxide has been associated with tumor cell proliferation, may confer a growth advantage to tumor cell populations, and may contribute to the malignant phenotype (88). Antioxidant vitamins may reduce the risk of cancer through their functions as free radical scavengers and as blockers

of nitrosation reactions (89). Despite these plausible hypotheses, the epidemiologic evidence demonstrating a significant relationship between either serum levels or dietary intake of vitamins C and E and reduced risk of breast cancer is limited and inconsistent (89,90). The epidemiologic and prospective cohort data for vitamin A intake suggest a modest protective effect against breast cancer among women in is highest intake quartiles (91,92), but it is not yet known whether supplemental vitamin A will reduce the risk of breast cancer for women with average dietary intakes of vitamin A. While clinical studies are in progress to address that question, women should be cautioned not to exceed the recommended daily doses of vitamins—particularly the fat-soluble vitamins A and E—that have known and potentially serious toxicities at higher doses.

Alcohol

There are several mechanisms through which ethanol may increase the risk of breast cancer. It may 1) induce increased levels of circulating estrogen, 2) stimulate hepatic metabolism of carcinogens such as acetaldehyde, 3) facilitate transport of carcinogens into breast tissue, 4) stimulate pituitary production of prolactin, 5) modulate cell membrane integrity with an effect on carcinogenesis, 6) aid production of cytotoxic protein products, 7) impair immune surveillance, 8) interfere with DNA repair, 9) promote production of toxic congeners, 10) increase exposure to toxic oxidants, or 11) reduce intake and bioavailability of protective nutrients (93–95). Few of these mechanisms have been studied, however, either in experimental animals or in humans, with the exception of the effect of alcohol consumption on plasma and urinary hormone concentrations in premenopausal women. When female volunteers aged 21 to 40 years were given a controlled diet that included 30 g of alcohol daily (equivalent to about two drinks) through three menstrual cycles, significant increases were seen in periovulatory plasma levels of dehydroepiandrosterone sulfate, estrone, and estradiol. Luteal-phase increases in levels of urinary estrone, estradiol, and estriol were also recorded (96). Although no changes were found in the percentage of bioavailable estradiol, the increased total estradiol levels in the periovulatory phase suggest elevated absolute amounts of bioavailable estradiol. These results imply that there are major effects of alcohol on both estrogen production and metabolism. It is not clear whether increased levels of bioavailable estradiol increase either the risk of breast cancer or the chance that a breast cancer will contain measurable estrogen receptors, but it is clear that alcohol may play some role.

Individual studies of the effect of alcohol intake on breast cancer risk showed no increase in risk for daily ethanol intakes of less than 6 g, with the risk increasing linearly to an odds ratio of 2.4 for intakes between 33 and 45 g/day (97). Studies also showed little effect on risk from alcohol consumption in early adult life, and a relative risk of approximately 1.2 for consumption of each 13 g/day in later adult life (98).

Meta-analysis of the published literature relating alcohol consumption and breast cancer revealed strong evidence of a dose-response relationship with a very modest slope (99). The relative risks of breast cancer associated with consumption of one, two, or three drinks per day are 1.11, 1.24, and 1.38, respectively. Although nearly all studies in the meta-analysis were adjusted for known breast cancer risk factors and socioeconomic factors, the individual studies remain confounded by a number of biases (95). The data do not support a recommendation that women should abstain from alcohol to reduce their breast cancer risk. Furthermore, the beneficial effects of light to moderate alcohol consumption on overall mortality must be taken into consideration before abstinence can be recommended as a breast cancer control strategy (100,101). Nevertheless, women who are at increased risk for breast cancer and at low risk of heart disease may wish to consider limiting their alcohol consumption.

Oral Contraceptives

The relationship between oral contraceptive use and breast cancer risk has been the subject of numerous epidemiologic investigations over the past several decades (102–107). Earlier studies (102,103) showed little relationship between oral contraceptive use and breast cancer, but recent studies (106) demonstrated an increased risk among certain subsets of users, especially among women diagnosed with breast cancer before age 35 or who have used oral contraceptives for 10 years or longer. Relative risks are as high as threefold for women who began oral contraceptive use before age 18 and continued usage for more than 10 years. Increased risk is

also observed for women who used oral contraceptives within 5 years of their cancer diagnosis or who had cancers diagnosed at advanced stages. Oral contraceptive use in the reported case-control studies appears to increase the risk of premenopausal, bilateral breast cancer (108). It is not clear whether the reported increased risk in younger women is due to patterns of use or to specific disease characteristics of the breast cancers such as hormone receptor status or proliferative activity.

With data from eight population-based case-control studies of oral contraceptive use and breast cancer risk among women younger than 45 years, it is possible to estimate that there is a 3.1% increase in breast cancer risk per year of oral contraceptive use (107). This risk increases to 3.8% per year of oral contraceptive use before a first birth. Nevertheless, the absolute risk of breast cancer among younger women in the general population is small, and oral contraceptive use might add one or two additional cases for every 100,000 women in this age group.

Among older women, some studies showed a decreasing risk with either increasing intervals since first or last use of oral contraceptives. This may indicate that oral contraceptives merely advance the presentation of disease rather than acting as a true causal factor (109). Taken together, these studies showed inconsistent patterns of use among those women with excess risk. Because the relative risks in these studies were usually twofold or less, there is the possibility that the positive findings might have been influenced by the selective use of screening among the users with the introduction of both detection and lead-time biases. This possibility is supported by multiple studies showing that oral contraceptive users tend to have tumors that are smaller and less often of late stage than do nonusers (110–112).

In summary, the risk of breast cancer associated with oral contraceptive use is small and is greatest among younger women who use oral contraceptives for prolonged periods of time. There is little evidence to indicate that elimination of oral contraceptive use would have an important effect on breast cancer incidence rates.

Estrogen Replacement Therapy

It is generally accepted that endogenous estrogens play some role in the causation of breast cancer (10,11), but the risk of breast cancer among women using estrogen replacement therapy after menopause is the subject of controversy and conflicting data in the medical literature (113). Although steroid hormones are not known to act as tumor-initiating agents, in postmenopausal women obesity is positively associated both with elevated concentrations of endogenous estrogens (114) and with moderate elevations in the risk of breast cancer. Obesity is characterized by increased peripheral aromatization of precursor androgens to estrogens (115), which is the main source of estrogens in postmenopausal women (116). Intake of replacement hormones in doses adequate for relief of postmenopausal symptoms usually produces serum estradiol levels equivalent to those of the midfollicular phase of the normal menstrual cycle in a premenopausal woman (117) and plasma estradiol levels up to five times higher than those in an untreated postmenopausal woman. Although direct epidemiologic evidence linking endogenous estrogen levels to breast cancer is limited, serum levels of estrogen appear to be related to the risk of developing breast cancer after adjusting for body mass. The odds ratio for the highest quartile of estradiol serum levels is 1.8 when compared with the lowest quartile, and the odds ratios for the highest quartile of estrone are threefold higher (118). Both free estradiol and that bound to albumin appear to increase risk, while estradiol bound to SHBG does not, possibly because it is less biologically active. These observations indicate that factors that either increase the endogenous production of estrogen or reduce the binding of estradiol to SHBG may increase a woman's risk of developing breast cancer.

Our understanding of the effect of progestational agents on the breast is incomplete. Animal studies indicated that the administration of progestagens before a chemical carcinogen inhibits tumor production, while treatment with progestagens after the initiating agent has the opposite effect (119). Human breast epithelial cells proliferate in response to estrogens, and the presence of progesterone further increases cell division (120). Despite these laboratory observations, combined estrogen and progestin hormone replacement therapy in middle-aged women did not increase the risk of breast cancer in some studies (121), but increased it slightly in others (122). The epidemiologic data related to this association are limited, however,

because addition of progestins to hormone replacement regimens is a relatively recent practice and the observation times for women taking progestins are short. It is reassuring that depot medroxyprogesterone acetate, a potent, long-acting injectable progestagen contraceptive, does not increase the risk of breast cancer overall, although the remote possibility exists that it might accelerate the growth of occult cancers (123). More human observational data are required before the effect of combined estrogen and progestin therapy on the breast can be completely understood.

Most studies that evaluated estrogen replacement therapy following menopause and its possible role in the development of breast cancer found no overall increase in risk (33,124–129), though several studies demonstrated a modest overall increase (130,131). Such studies may be confounded, however, by a bias in treatment selection that denies hormone replacement therapy to women with a family history of breast cancer (132). If physicians are less likely to prescribe estrogen for women with a family history of breast cancer, a lack of association or a spurious inverse relationship between estrogen use and breast cancer risk may appear.

Despite methodologic rigor and careful selection of subjects, individual reports about the effect of estrogen replacement therapy on breast cancer risk provide conflicting results. Because individual studies may be subject to serious limitations owing to small numbers of subjects and short observation times, meta-analyses have been done to combine available data and to increase the power of the analyses. Meta-analysis is a systematic and quantitative statistical method of combining data across studies to increase statistical power and to generalize results. Meta-analyses of the effect of estrogen replacement therapy on the risk of breast cancer have yielded mixed results.

At least three meta-analyses to determine the effect of noncontraceptive estrogen replacement therapy on breast cancer risk have been published (133–135). None of the studies found a positive association between estrogen replacement therapy and risk of breast cancer when women who had ever used estrogen were compared with women who had never used it. One study (135) was unable to conclude whether there was an effect of duration of use on the risk of breast cancer, and one study found no effect (134). In a third meta-analysis that used studies published in the English-language literature between 1966 and 1989, Steinberg et al (133) found that the risk of breast cancer did not increase for women who experienced any type of menopause until after at least 5 years of estrogen use. After 15 years of use, the risk of breast cancer increased 30% (relative risk = 1.3), but the increase in risk was largely due to studies that included premenopausal women or women using estradiol with or without progestin, for whom the relative risk was 2.2 after 15 years. Of greatest concern was the finding that the relative risk was 3.4 among women with a family history of breast cancer (at least one first-degree relative) who had used estrogen replacement therapy compared with 1.5 for women with a family history who had not used estrogen replacement therapy. However, the increased risk among women with a family history may be due to the difference in preparations of estrogen used in the United States and Europe.

These results do not provide definitive evidence that hormone replacement therapy with low-dose conjugated estrogens, including therapy in high-risk women, increases the risk of breast cancer. The possibility remains, however, that the risk may be moderately increased with long durations of use (>5 years), with higher doses, and with unconjugated estrogens (e.g., estradiol). Because the data were derived from analyses of retrospectively constructed subsets, the risk of estrogen replacement therapy for women with a family history of breast cancer is unclear.

Unlike the studies of replacement hormones given after menopause, most studies of oral contraceptive use, as noted earlier in this chapter, showed no associated increase in the risk of breast cancer (136–138), and one study suggested a reduced risk in oral contraceptive users (139).

The morbidity and mortality associated with estrogen deficiency in postmenopausal women are substantial. Estrogen deficiency causes hot flashes, mood swings, and genital atrophy with resultant dyspareunia. These symptoms are relieved by estrogen replacement therapy. More importantly, the risk of death from cardiovascular disease increases 18-fold after menopause (140), and elevated levels of total cholesterol and LDL cholesterol have been causally related to an increased risk of coronary vascular disease. Cohort studies indicated reductions in total mortality, coronary heart disease mortality,

and hip fracture incidence among current users of estrogen replacement therapy (141). Increased incidences of breast and endometrial cancers appear to be offset by reduced risks of other neoplasms.

The use of estrogen replacement therapy after menopause has a favorable influence on HDL cholesterol, LDL cholesterol, and total cholesterol levels. Estrogen supplementation reduces the risk for coronary heart disease (142), and estrogen replacement therapy has a vascular protective effect (143). In addition, numerous studies demonstrated that all-cause mortality and mortality from coronary heart disease and cerebrovascular disease are reduced in women who have used estrogen replacement therapy (144). Estrogen supplementation can also reduce or prevent trabecular bone loss and the development of osteoporosis (145,146), another cause of significant postmenopausal morbidity.

Contrary to these arguments for the use of estrogen replacement therapy, there are data showing that breast cancer risk is lower among women who experience menarche at a later age, who have fewer ovulatory menstrual cycles during their lifetime, or who are younger at menopause, whether the menopause is natural or surgically induced (147,148). Despite these observations, the lower risk of breast cancer among women who have lower endogenous estrogen levels does not necessarily imply an increased risk of breast cancer in women who receive estrogen replacement therapy at menopause.

In light of the published benefits of estrogen replacement therapy with regard to quality of life, reduction of cardiovascular morbidity and mortality, and reduction of morbidity and mortality attributable to osteoporosis, estrogen replacement therapy must be considered in postmenopausal women. It is unreasonable to reject such therapy as inappropriate for women at increased risk (149–151). One useful strategy is to assist a woman in weighing the risks and benefits of estrogen replacement therapy in her personal clinical situation. For example, postmenopausal women taking hormone replacement therapy can expect a 35% reduction in the risk of coronary heart disease and a 25% reduction in the lifetime risk of hip fracture (144). The change in life expectancy associated with taking hormone replacement therapy is related to the underlying risks of heart disease, osteoporosis, and breast cancer in each individual and varies from 8 months to more than 2 years. Net benefit may be derived from hormone replacement therapy even if it is associated with a small increase in the risk of breast cancer. Published evaluations of individual risks and benefits are available (144) and should be consulted to assist in clinical decision making. Discussion of the effect of hormone replacement therapy on overall quality of life should be included in the clinical discussion. Estrogen replacement therapy should then be offered to women who accept the potential risks and known benefits (144,152).

Environment (Radiation)

Few environmental exposures have been definitely associated with increased risk of breast cancer, but exposure to ionizing radiation is known to increase the risk. Exposure to atomic bomb irradiation, chest fluoroscopy for tuberculosis, treatment of postpartum mastitis, diagnostic roentgenography for scoliosis, and therapeutic irradiation for breast cancer are all associated with an increased risk of subsequent breast cancer (153). Relative risks vary from 1.2 to 2.4 and are related to both total dose and age at exposure, with younger women being at greater risk than older women (153,154).

Of particular concern are individuals who are heterozygotes for the ataxia telangiectasia (*ATM*) gene, who make up about 1% of the general population. Female AT heterozygotes who are exposed to ionizing radiation have nearly a sixfold increased risk of developing breast cancer compared with nonexposed control subjects (155). This observation raises concerns about the safety of mammographic screening in women who are AT heterozygotes, but there are no current public health recommendations regarding screening of these women. Recent cloning of the gene (156) makes it likely that AT heterozygotes can be identified, but a strategy to systematically identify and counsel these women remains to be defined.

Quantitative Risk Assessment

Women who are at increased risk for breast cancer can be identified using individual risk factors one at a time (see Table 3-1). This approach does not permit combining risk factors, however, nor does it lend itself readily to calculating a woman's lifetime probability of developing breast cancer. Multivariate risk models allow determination of composite relative risk for breast cancer along with a cumulative lifetime risk adjusted both for all risk factors taken together and for competing causes of mortality, expressed as the percentage chance that a woman will ever develop breast cancer. Published data are derived largely from studies of white women, and the generalizability of the data to other racial and ethnic groups is uncertain.

The model developed by Gail et al (21) is a widely used method of quantifying a woman's risk of developing breast cancer. It is being used for risk evaluation in the Breast Cancer Prevention Trial, a clinical study to determine the worth of tamoxifen in preventing breast cancer in women who are at increased risk (157). The model allows estimation of the likelihood that a woman of a given age with certain risk factors will develop breast cancer over a specified interval. The model was derived using 4496 matched pairs of subjects from the BCDDP, a mammography screening project carried out between 1973 and 1980 involving more than 280,000 women. Each pair of subjects included a woman with breast cancer and a matched control subject. Using logistic regression techniques, Gail et al examined a number of possible risk factors for breast cancer including the use of various medications, including hormones; cigarette smoking and alcohol consumption; height; gynecologic history, including a woman's age at menarche and at first childbirth; history of breast biopsy; and family history of breast cancer in first-degree relatives (i.e., mother, sisters, or daughters). The risk factors were adjusted simultaneously for the presence of the other risk factors, and only five factors were shown to be significant predictors of the lifetime risk of breast cancer:

Current age

Age at menarche

Number of breast biopsies

Age at first live birth

Family history of breast cancer in first-degree relatives

Each risk factor is grouped into categories as shown in Table 3-7. The procedure to determine a woman's risk is straightforward. Age at menarche is considered alone, and its associated relative risk is referenced in the table. Next, a woman's age and the number of breast biopsies (incisional, excisional, or fine-needle aspirations but not cyst aspirations) performed for benign breast disease are then considered together, and a second relative risk is derived from Table 3-7. A breast biopsy showing atypical hyperplasia doubles the risk estimate shown in the table. To obtain the final relative risk for the model, a woman's age at the time of first live birth is considered together with the number of first-degree relatives with breast cancer.

Consider, for example, a 45-year-old woman who reports menarche at age 12, one breast biopsy, no children, and a sister with breast cancer. Table 3-7 shows that the relative risk associated with menarche at age 12 is 1.099. For a woman younger than 50 having one biopsy, the associated relative risk is 1.698. Finally, a nulliparous woman with one affected first-degree relative with breast cancer has an asso-

ciated relative risk of 2.756. These three relative risks are then multiplied together to obtain a summary relative risk: $1.099 \times 1.698 \times 2.756 = 5.14$, or 5.0 for practical purposes.

This number, 5.0, represents this woman's lifetime relative risk of developing breast cancer when compared with a woman of the same age without any of the identified risk factors. A relative risk is not very useful, however, for providing information about an individual's risk of breast cancer. Recognizing this, Gail et al calculated lifetime probabilities of developing breast cancer with a given relative risk and adjusting for competing causes of death (a woman cannot develop breast cancer if she first dies of another disease). These data are shown in Table 3-8, which contains estimates of developing breast cancer during 10, 20, or 30 years of follow-up. The table shows an "initial rela-

T A B L E   **3-7**

Gail's Risk Model and Associated Relative Risks (21)*

Risk Factor (Code No.)		Associated Relative Risk	No. of Cases (n = 2852)	No. of Controls (n = 3146)
Age at menarche (yr)				
≥14 (0)		1.000	790	926
12–13 (1)		1.099	1554	1735
<12 (2)		1.207	508	485
No. of biopsies				
Age <50 yr				
0 (0)		1.000	635	794
1 (1)		1.698	113	93
≥2 (2)		2.882	66	24
Age ≥50 yr				
0 (0)		1.000	1551	1817
1 (1)		1.273	312	300
≥2 (2)		1.620	175	118
Age at first live birth (yr)	No. of relatives			
<20 (0)	0 (0)	1.000	167	285
	1 (1)	2.607	44	40
	2 (2)	6.798	8	0
20–24 (1)	0 (0)	1.244	708	1042
	1 (1)	2.681	208	123
	2 (2)	5.775	25	5
25–29 or nulliparous (2)	0 (0)	1.548	968	1106
	1 (1)	2.756	247	178
	2 (2)	4.907	46	20
≥30 (3)	0 (0)	1.927	307	291
	1 (1)	2.834	87	50
	2 (2)	4.169	19	6

*Relative risk compared with that of an individual of the same age without any risk factors is estimated by locating the person's associated relative risk for age at menarche, number of biopsies, and the combination of age at first live birth and number of relatives and multiplying these three numbers together.

Source: Gail MH, Brinton LA, Byar DP, et al. Projecting individualized probabilities of developing breast cancer for white females who are being examined annually. *J Natl Cancer Inst* 1989;81:1879–1886.

T A B L E **3-8**

Projected Probability (%) of Developing Breast Cancer within 10, 20, or 30 Years of Follow-Up (21)

Initial Age (yr)	Years of Follow-Up	Later Relative Risk[a]	Initial Relative Risk[a,b]					
			1.0	2.0	5.0	10.0	20.0	30.0
20	10	—	0.0	0.1	0.2	0.5	1.0	1.4
	20	—	0.5	1.0	2.5	4.9	9.5	14.0
	30	—	1.7	3.4	8.3	15.9	29.3	40.5
30	10	—	0.5	0.9	2.3	4.4	8.7	12.8
	20	—	1.7	3.3	8.1	15.6	28.8	39.9
	30	1.0	3.2	4.8	9.5	16.9	29.9	40.8
		2.0	4.7	6.3	10.9	18.2	30.9	41.7
		5.0	8.9	10.4	14.9	21.8	34.0	44.3
		10.0	15.6	17.1	21.2	27.6	38.8	48.3
		20.0	27.6	28.8	32.3	37.8	47.4	55.5
		30.0	37.7	38.7	41.8	46.4	54.7	61.7
40	10	—	1.2	2.5	6.1	11.8	22.2	31.3
	20	1.0	2.8	4.0	7.5	13.1	23.4	32.4
		2.0	4.3	5.5	8.9	14.5	24.5	33.4
		5.0	8.6	9.7	13.1	18.3	28.0	36.4
		10.0	15.4	16.4	19.5	24.4	33.3	41.1
		20.0	27.4	28.4	30.9	35.2	42.7	49.5
		30.0	37.7	38.5	40.7	44.3	50.8	56.6
	30	1.0	4.4	5.6	9.1	14.6	24.6	33.5
		2.0	7.4	8.6	11.9	17.3	27.0	35.6
		5.0	15.9	17.0	20.0	24.9	33.7	41.5
		10.0	28.3	29.2	31.8	35.9	43.4	50.0
		20.0	47.5	48.1	50.0	53.1	58.5	63.4
		30.0	61.2	61.6	63.1	65.3	69.3	72.8
50	10	—	1.6	3.1	7.6	14.6	27.1	37.7
	20	—	3.2	6.4	15.1	27.9	47.8	61.9
	30	—	4.4	8.5	19.9	35.5	57.8	71.7
60	10	—	1.8	3.6	8.6	16.5	30.1	41.5
	20	—	3.0	5.9	14.0	25.9	44.6	58.2
70	10	—	1.4	2.7	6.7	12.9	24.1	33.7

[a] The initial relative risk corresponds to the initial age. If the initial age is <50 and if the initial age plus the follow-up specified is >50, then a later relative risk at age 50 should also be specified. If the initial age is ≥50, only the initial relative risk is required. If the initial age is <50 and if the initial age plus the years of follow-up does not exceed 50, then only an initial relative risk is required.

[b] Values in columns are projected probabilities expressed as percentages.

Source: Gail MH, Brinton LA, Byar DP, et al. Projecting individualized probabilities of developing breast cancer for white females who are being examined annually. *J Natl Cancer Inst* 1989;81:1879–1886.

tive risk" and a "later relative risk." As explained in the footnote to Table 3-8, the initial relative risk corresponds to the subject's initial age (i.e., her age at evaluation). If the initial age is less than 50 and the woman will be older than 50 at the end of the specified follow-up period, then a later relative risk should be specified using the age term in Table 3-7. For the woman illustrated above, her initial relative risk is 5.0, but she becomes older than 50 during the first follow-up interval of 10 years, indicating that a later relative risk must be calculated. In Table 3-7, we see that the associated relative risk for a woman older than 50 with one biopsy is

1.273. The later relative risk then becomes: 1.099 × 1.273 × 2.756 = 3.85.

The probabilities in Table 3-8 are approximations, at best. For our 45-year-old patient, we begin in the initial relative risk column labeled 5.0. Looking down the column to the line that corresponds to an initial age of 40 years and 10 years of follow-up, we find a 10-year probability of developing breast cancer of 6.1%. For 20 years of follow-up, we calculated a later relative risk of 3.85, which is between 2.0 and 5.0. The 20-year probability of breast cancer with an initial relative risk of 5.0 and a later relative risk of 2.0 is 8.9%; for an initial relative risk of 5.0 and a later relative risk of 3.8 the 20-year probability is 13.1%. Therefore, this woman's 20-year probability of developing breast cancer is approximately 12%. Finally, her 30-year probability is between 11.9% and 20%, or about 17%.

There are limitations to the use of the Gail model. Investigators who have attempted to validate the model found that it overpredicted absolute breast cancer risk by 33% among women aged 25 to 61 years who did not receive annual screening (158). Most of the overprediction is confined to premenopausal women who do not adhere to guidelines for annual mammographic screening (159) and to women with extensive family histories of breast cancer in whom other risk models may be more appropriate. I consider one of those models later in this chapter. Critics of the Gail model also suggest that there are ethical questions regarding the value of individual breast cancer risk prediction in the absence of safe and effective preventive regimens. Conversely, it may be unethical not to offer counseling to women who overestimate their risk and live with inappropriate anxiety or elect unnecessary procedures such as prophylactic mastectomy.

Alternatives to the Gail model are available. These models offer the advantage of counting the number of first- or second-degree relatives affected with breast cancer and considering their ages at diagnosis (36,48,52). Both of these factors are known to affect the risk of developing breast cancer and are not considered in the Gail model. A practical modification of one of these models is shown in Table 3-4. More complete risk assessment tables are available in the literature (36,48,52), and all permit calculation of a lifetime probability of developing breast cancer.

Any valid estimate of a woman's lifetime probability of developing breast cancer can be used for counseling purposes and for making decisions about clinical management of risk. The clinician should be positive in his or her recommendations and deliver clear messages regarding risk management, emphasizing that risk calculations should be used only to estimate the probability of developing the disease and not the risk of dying of breast cancer (36). Previous research suggests that counseling about risk may have unwanted psychological effects (160), so counseling should include an assessment of risk perception. Women younger than 50 who are at increased risk for breast cancer tend to overestimate their risk, even as much as 20-fold (1). A substantial proportion of women who have abnormal-appearing mammograms but not cancer report significant impairments in mood and daily functioning (161,162), and more than one fourth of high-risk women may have clinically elevated levels of psychological distress (163). Psychological distress may, in turn, interfere with adherence to recommended breast screening (162–166) or other preventive behaviors. While the preliminary studies showed a greater likelihood of having prior mammograms among women with higher self-perceived risks of breast cancer (167), more research is needed to define at what level risk perception becomes inhibitory rather than motivating. Because of these recognized concerns about psychological issues, it is important to explore a woman's fears about breast cancer, and the clinician should ask each patient if her worries about breast cancer impede her daily functioning. If simple reassurance and encouragement do not relieve anxiety or the patient cannot participate in making clinical decisions because of her anxiety, psychological consultation is warranted.

Management of Women at Increased Risk

Optimal preventive strategies for breast cancer have not yet been identified, although a great deal of research is being conducted in this area. In this section, I highlight current information about mammographic screening prescriptions, prophylactic mastectomy, and primary prevention that will guide clinicians in selecting interventions for women who are at increased risk. Clinicians are referred to several excellent reviews that cover clinical management strategies in greater detail (168–170).

Mammographic Screening Prescriptions

Annual mammographic screening in women 50 years and older reduces mortality by 25% to 30% (171), and there is little debate that screening should be employed in postmenopausal women. There is also growing evidence that screening offers benefit in women between the ages of 40 and 49 years (172), but uncertainty about the magnitude of the benefit remains (173). Only one prospective, randomized comparison of mammographic screening in women younger than 50 years has been published (174), but technical limitations prevent acceptance of the trial's negative findings as definitive (175).

The performance profile of any screening test is related not only to the clinical characteristics of the test (e.g., the sensitivity and specificity of the test), but also to the prevalence of the disease in the population being screened (176). In a population of women younger than 50 years who are at increased risk of breast cancer, the prevalence of the disease is increased, and therefore the performance outcomes of screening mammography should not differ from the outcomes of mammographic screening in older populations who have the same breast cancer prevalence (177). In fact, imaging breast cancers appears to be as efficient in very young women as in older women (178). These observations support annual mammographic screening for women 40 to 49 years old who are at average risk for breast cancer, but the data do not address the question of screening women younger than 40 years who are at increased risk. I review that question next. ·

Mammographic screening offers several benefits as well as potential risks. The benefits include a demonstrated decrease in mortality for women older than 50 years, the ability to use conservative surgery for smaller, less advanced breast cancers, and the psychological reassurance gained by a woman after negative mammography findings (161). The drawbacks of screening include physical discomfort from compression techniques and the fact that screening increases the likelihood of women having to undergo additional investigations including breast ultrasound, fine-needle aspiration, needle biopsy, or open biopsy. In addition, there is the possibility of overtreating lesions that are actually benign clinically and that would not have come to clinical attention in the absence of screening (179). Unnecessary surgery and radiation therapy may be used to treat these lesions that impose no true threat to health. Screening mammography has inherent limitations in its sensitivity: As many as 15% of negative mammography results may be false negative (180). The false reassurance that follows a negative mammography result may lead to decreased compliance with attendance at future scheduled screenings, and this issue has not been investigated in women who are at increased risk. There is also some psychologi-

cal morbidity associated with undergoing mammographic screening (161,162).

There are more than 20 million women between the ages of 30 and 39 in the United States, and as many as 20% of these women may be at increased risk for breast cancer (173). Anecdotal reports indicated that mammography visualizes 90% of breast cancers occurring in younger women (178). Although there are no data about the outcome of mammographic screening in women younger than 40, these anxious patients often demand that clinicians do something to help them manage their risk. This is a challenge in the absence of a proven benefit from any specific screening regimen. To do no screening until age 40 in women who are at increased risk may miss an opportunity to prevent mortality from breast cancer, yet it is also possible that screening women before age 40 will incur expense without offering benefit. Clinicians must discuss these uncertainties with patients who request screening before age 40, and they must also inform patients that their health insurance carrier may not cover the cost of their screening mammograms even though mammograms in older women are paid for.

If a clinician decides that screening should begin at age 30, the initial consideration is whether the younger woman is attempting to become pregnant, is pregnant, or is lactating. Although the radiation dose to a fetus from a screening mammogram is minimal, the exposure must be avoided. Equally important, the benign nodular densities that appear in the breasts of lactating and pregnant women generate an increased number of false-positive mammographic readings that must also be avoided. Pregnant and lactating women who are at increased risk of breast cancer must delay initiation of screening mammography until they are no longer attempting to conceive children. Equally important, any symptomatic breast lesion in a pregnant woman must be evaluated aggressively to rule out the possibility of malignancy.

If a woman age 30 or older is not pregnant and there is evidence of genetic predisposition or familial clustering of breast cancer or an increased risk profile for breast cancer, annual mammographic screening may begin. In a woman without a genetic predisposition to breast cancer but who has had a breast biopsy showing either lobular carcinoma in situ or proliferative disease with or without atypia, initiation of annual mammographic screening is warranted after the biopsy that establishes the diagnosis. In women with none of these findings but who have Gail model risk scores of 5 or higher, initiation of annual mammographic screening at age 30 is advised, on the basis of the disease prevalence considerations explained previously. Most of the women with elevated Gail model risk scores will have multiple affected first-degree relatives with breast cancer or a history of breast biopsy or both (21).

Because adequate mammographic visualization can be difficult in young women with dense breasts (178), ultrasonography should accompany screening mammography to distinguish the frequent cystic lesions that occur in these young women from the solid lesions that require biopsy for diagnosis. This strategy will minimize the number of biopsies performed in young women who receive regular screening.

Prophylactic Mastectomy

There are several possible reasons why prophylactic mastectomy might appear to be a desirable clinical strategy for the control of breast cancer. These include elimination of the risk of developing breast cancer, removal of occult carcinomas, and improvement of psychological distress related to unreasonable fears about the risk of developing breast cancer. Indications for prophylactic mastectomy may include genetic risk, proliferative benign breast disease with or without atypia, and lobular carcinoma in situ. A prophylactic mastectomy is an operation that removes the total breast, tail of Spence, lower axillary lymph nodes, areola, and nipple (181,182). It is typically followed by a reconstructive procedure for cosmetic reasons.

Experimental studies of prophylactic mastectomy in rats given chemical carcinogens showed that tumors occur despite total mastectomy (183), and similar observations have been made in mice that develop spontaneous breast malignancies without mammary carcinogens (184). Pathologic examination of the chest wall and axilla in women undergoing mastectomy for breast cancer shows extension of breast tissue well into the axilla and pectoral fascia (185), indicating that total extirpation of the breast requires even more extensive surgery than a total mastectomy. Less extensive subcutaneous mastectomies are known to be followed by invasive carcinomas in up to 1% of patients (186–188). Although as many as 5% of prophylactic mastectomy specimens contain

occult carcinomas (187), there are no data comparing the outcomes of patients managed with prophylactic mastectomy with a similar group of women at increased risk who are followed with close surveillance including mammographic screening and timely biopsy when clinically indicated. Nonrandomized, prospective data do show, however, that prophylactic mastectomy does reduce the subsequent incidence of invasive breast cancer to less than 1% of patients (189). Because of these facts, prophylactic mastectomy for women at increased risk of breast cancer must still be recommended with caution.

Available data also indicate that rather than relieving anxiety, prophylactic mastectomy may increase it and cause other adverse psychological consequences. After prophylactic mastectomy and reconstruction, 20% of women believe their breasts are either too small or in the wrong position, 100% lose erogenous sensitivity in the nipple-areola complex, and 60% report markedly negative changes in their sexual lives (190). Based on these observations, it is difficult to argue in favor of prophylactic mastectomy as an effective preventive procedure with satisfactory clinical and psychological outcomes.

Even though the decision to undergo prophylactic mastectomy may have profound physical and psychological implications for the woman at increased risk, it may be appropriate in a small subset of patients. There are published recommended criteria for third-party payer coverage of prophylactic mastectomy. These include lobular or ductal carcinoma in situ; severe dysplasia; personal history of breast cancer or personal history of breast cancer in the opposite breast; one first-degree relative with bilateral, premenopausal breast cancer; desmoid tumor of the breast or giant fibroadenoma; cystosarcoma phyllodes; significant virginal hypertrophy; or postinjection silicone mastopathy (191). These criteria may be overly aggressive, and not all clinicians would recommend prophylactic surgery for these conditions. Slightly more conservative considerations leading to a decision for prophylactic mastectomy are reviewed in Table 3-9. The presence of lobular carcinoma in situ or atypical lobular or ductal hyperplasia in the setting of a history of breast cancer in first-degree relatives increases the risk of breast cancer significantly (21,192). In these patients, the physician may initiate discussion of the possibility of prophylactic mastectomy with the understanding that one half or more of the patients with these predisposing histologic lesions will never develop breast cancer, making the procedure unnecessary for them. There are currently no validated clinical markers available to determine which patients with these predisposing conditions will develop malignancy.

Women who carry genes that increase the risk of breast cancer (e.g., *BRCA1*, *BRCA2*,

TP53, *ATM*, etc.) have more than a 60% chance of developing breast cancer by age 50 and may want to consider prophylactic mastectomy (38,55). In women whose risk profiles show them to be at increased risk of breast cancer but who have negative results on genetic testing, a history of repeated breast biopsies in the presence of dense breast parenchyma, a history of proliferative benign breast disease on biopsy, or manifestations of extreme anxiety about developing breast cancer should lead the clinician to discuss prophylactic mastectomy with the patient. The physician should never force the decision on the patient and should carefully explore the relative advantages and disadvantages of the procedure, including the lack of certainty that the patient will develop breast cancer and the rare chance that a prophylactic procedure will not prevent breast cancer from occurring (56). For some patients at increased risk, careful consideration of these risks and benefits will lead to a decision to have prophylactic mastectomy and will reduce anxiety.

T A B L E **3-9**

Considerations in the Decision for Prophylactic Mastectomy

Carriers of *BRCA1*, *BRCA2*, *p53*, ataxia-telangiectasia, or other predisposing genes
In the absence of genetic testing, a family history that makes a genetic syndrome likely (e.g., bilateral, premenopausal breast cancer in one or more first-degree relatives or multiple affected relatives in several generations)
Women with a multivariate relative risk score >10 or a lifetime probability of breast cancer >20%
Family history of breast cancer in first-degree relative(s) *plus* a breast biopsy showing atypical hyperplasia
Lobular carcinoma in situ *plus* a family history of breast cancer in first-degree relatives
Increased objective risk *plus* repeated breast biopsies with significant scarring resulting in a difficult physical examination and/or multiple nodular densities on the mammogram
Psychological disability due to extreme fear of cancer

Primary Prevention

The optimal strategy to control breast cancer is to prevent it from ever occurring, but there are no proven strategies for the primary prevention of breast cancer. Table 3-10 lists the approaches that are currently under investigation for the prevention of breast cancer. Several strategies

T A B L E **3-10**

Strategies for Detection and Prevention of Breast Cancer

Method	Example	Limitation
Initiation of screening at an early age	Begin annual mammography at age 30	No demonstrated benefit
Prophylactic mastectomy	In a woman with family history, atypical hyperplasia, etc.	Psychological, physical implications; questionable effectiveness
Antiestrogens	Tamoxifen	Investigational; endometrial carcinoma, thrombosis, menopausal symptoms
Retinoids	Fenretinide	Investigational; night blindness, hepatic toxicity
Gonadotropin-releasing hormone agonists	Leuprolide	Investigational; limited human data
Progestogen antagonists	RU 486	Investigational; limited experience with long-term administration
Phytoestrogens	Soy products	Unknown bioavailability; no controlled observations

that may eventually be employed to prevent breast cancer are reviewed later in the chapter. All of these pharmacologic approaches remain investigational, however, and should not be used for the clinical management of women at increased risk of breast cancer until ongoing investigations of the agents are completed.

Tamoxifen

Prevention of Contralateral Breast Cancer
Detailed information on the incidence of second primary breast cancers is available from a comprehensive overview of the world's literature on the use of tamoxifen as adjuvant therapy for breast cancer (193). An unexpected observation from these trials was the reduction in the incidence of contralateral breast cancers in patients receiving tamoxifen. The overview presents data from more than 18,000 women enrolled in 42 separate randomized, placebo-controlled trials for whom information is available about second primary breast cancers occurring as long as 10 years after the initial diagnosis. There were 184 women (2.0%) with second primary breast cancers among 9135 women treated with placebo versus 122 with second primary breast cancers (1.3%) among 9128 women who received 10 to 40 mg of tamoxifen for a median of 2 years (193). A dose-response relationship was observed for the duration of tamoxifen therapy: For women who received therapy for less than 2 years, the reduction in the actuarial odds of a second primary breast cancer was only 26%, compared with a 37% reduction for women with therapy for exactly 2 years and a 56% reduction for women who received adjuvant tamoxifen for more than 2 years. Other studies demonstrated that tamoxifen adjuvant therapy for short durations (e.g., 48 weeks) may not be sufficient to provide protection against the development of second primary breast cancers (194).

Tamoxifen is an antiestrogen that binds to the estrogen receptor, resulting in altered RNA transcription, decreased cell proliferation, and partial estrogen agonist activity. Tamoxifen may also cause apoptosis of potentially malignant cells; modulation of production of transforming growth factors; decreases in circulating insulin-like growth factor I; increases in circulating levels of SHBG that may decrease the availability of free estrogen, removing a stimulus for tumor cell growth; and increases in levels of circulating natural killer cells (195).

Cardiovascular Effects In addition to these observed reductions in the odds of developing a second primary breast cancer, the overview data demonstrate a 12% reduction in nonbreast cancer deaths, a 25% reduction in deaths from vascular disease, and a 9% reduction in other causes of death. A major proportion of the reduction in noncancer deaths is due to a reduction in cardiovascular disease mortality (196,197), and these results are due, in part, to decreases in LDL cholesterol observed as early as 2 months after the initiation of tamoxifen therapy. These reductions are followed at 6 months by either no change or an increase in HDL cholesterol, a fall in LDL cholesterol, and an increase in triglyceride levels (198,199). Tamoxifen's estrogenic effect on the liver may lead to increased synthesis of very-low-density-lipoprotein cholesterol and increased triglyceride levels, decreased levels of apolipoprotein B synthesis, and increased levels of apolipoprotein A-I synthesis, with resultant increased levels of HDL cholesterol (200,201). Longitudinal observations of women at risk for heart disease are limited, but available data indicate that a 15% to 20% decrease in LDL cholesterol may result in a 6% to 20% decrease in coronary heart disease (202,203).

The effect of tamoxifen on the development of atherosclerotic cardiovascular disease may also relate to its antithrombotic properties. Postmenopausal women taking tamoxifen show an average drop of only 10% in antithrombin III levels during therapy, while fibrinogen levels decline 16% or more (204). Population studies demonstrated a relationship between fibrinogen levels, myocardial infarction, and stroke, with lower fibrinogen levels associated with lower cardiovascular risk (205,206). Concerns about the durability of these effects arise from studies of former users of tamoxifen that show reversal of the increases in HDL cholesterol at the cessation of tamoxifen therapy (207). A final assessment of the effect of tamoxifen on the risk of morbidity and mortality from cardiovascular disease in healthy women awaits completion of ongoing studies.

Effects on Bone Bone loss in postmenopausal women is caused primarily by loss of estrogen production by the ovaries. Decreased concentrations of circulating estrogen lead to increased bone resorption, decreased bone density, and osteoporosis with fractures, a major cause of morbidity in women older than 55 (208).

Tamoxifen decreases rates of resorption of trabecular bone in experimental animals, with a resultant net preservation of bone density (209–212). In rats that have undergone oophorectomy, tamoxifen also blocks both bone loss (209) and an increase in osteoclast number and activity (211).

Tamoxifen appears to preserve bone mineral density in postmenopausal women (213,214), presumably because of its estrogenic effect on osteoclasts, which slows bone resorption. Experimental data in vitro showing that tamoxifen blocks bone resorption induced by parathyroid hormone, prostaglandin E_2, and 1,25-dihydroxyvitamin D_3 support these clinical observations of benefit (215). Of some concern is the observation that tamoxifen may reduce bone mineral density in premenopausal women by 1.9% annually while increasing bone density in postmenopausal women by 1.8% (216). Prospective, randomized studies of women taking tamoxifen for the primary prevention of breast cancer will clarify this issue.

Toxicity Associated with Tamoxifen Tamoxifen therapy is associated with a variety of symptomatic toxicities including gynecologic symptoms (particularly hot flashes and vaginal discharge in perimenopausal women) (157). Early reports of an increased risk of thrombotic events were not confirmed in subsequent prospective trials with prolonged periods of observation (197), and no hepatic neoplasms have been reported in women taking the usually prescribed 20 mg daily despite preliminary reports of hepatic neoplasms in women taking 40 mg daily (217). Isolated reports of an increased incidence of gastrointestinal neoplasms occurring in women exposed to tamoxifen (218) were not confirmed in the overview analysis that showed a reduction in all second primary malignancies except endometrial cancer among women taking tamoxifen for the adjuvant treatment of breast cancer (193). Similar negative conclusions were also reached when early reports of ocular toxicity associated with tamoxifen were investigated with properly conducted prospective studies.

A well-established consequence of tamoxifen therapy is an increased incidence of endometrial carcinoma. In a randomized trial from Sweden that used 40 mg of tamoxifen daily, the incidence of uterine tumors (both endometrial carcinomas and uterine sarcomas) was 6.5-fold higher in the women who received

tamoxifen than in those who received placebo, and the cumulative frequency of uterine tumors was 0.4% in the control group, 0.9% in women who received tamoxifen for 2 years, and 5.5% in women treated with tamoxifen for 5 years (217,219). In another trial using tamoxifen, 30 mg daily for 48 weeks, the incidence ratio for endometrial carcinomas was 1.9, with cumulative incidences after 10 years of 0.3% and 1.0% in the patients receiving placebo and tamoxifen, respectively (194,220).

Additional data are available from the National Surgical Adjuvant Breast and Bowel Project trial B-14 that included 1419 women randomly assigned to receive tamoxifen, 1220 who entered the study after randomization had been performed but who were taking tamoxifen, and 1424 women randomly assigned to receive placebo (control patients). After an average time of study between 5 and 8 years, 2 patients in the placebo group and 24 in the tamoxifen group developed endometrial carcinoma (221). A number of women in both groups had used estrogen replacement therapy for various periods of time, and the relative contribution of the estrogen therapy to the risk of endometrial carcinoma in these women is unknown. The hazard rate in the placebo group was 0.2 per 1000 women compared with 1.6 per 1000 women in the tamoxifen group (relative risk = 7.5). Occurrences of endometrial carcinoma in the placebo group subsequent to the initial publication of the study have lowered the estimated relative risk to approximately 4.0. Endometrial sampling and abdominal or vaginal ultrasound examination of the endometrium before and during tamoxifen therapy are currently being investigated for their ability to detect early malignancy and to lower the chance of dying of endometrial cancer after exposure to tamoxifen.

Breast cancer patients enrolled in clinical trials may be different in many ways from healthy women in the population who might use tamoxifen for the primary prevention of breast cancer. Population-based studies of breast cancer patients who have used tamoxifen for less than 2 years showed a 50% reduction in the risk of contralateral breast cancer and no increase in the risk of either ovarian or endometrial cancer (222). Such studies also showed a twofold risk of endometrial cancer with cumulative tamoxifen doses higher than 15 g (i.e., 2 years of 20 mg daily) (223). The effect of prolonged administration of tamoxifen to healthy women can only be addressed in a clinical trial.

Retinoids

Retinyl acetate and the synthetic retinoid N-(4-hydroxyphenyl)-retinamide (4-HPR, fenretinide) are effective inhibitors of chemically induced breast cancer in rats (224). Fenretinide reduces the incidence and time to appearance of these tumors, and doses up to 200 mg daily with a 3-day drug holiday monthly can be administered chronically to humans, without significant toxicity. The effect of fenretinide is enhanced in rats by oophorectomy, but the drug does not affect circulating levels of estradiol, testosterone, dehydroepiandrosterone sulfate, prolactin, luteinizing hormone, follicle-stimulating hormone, or SHBG.

Retinoids induce the synthesis of transforming growth factor-α, a growth factor that negatively modulates cancer growth, and they lower the levels of insulin-like growth factor I, a potent mitogen for transformed breast epithelium, in both breast cancer cell lines and breast cancer patients (225).

Gonadotropin-Releasing Hormone Agonists

Many risk factors for breast cancer (e.g., age at menarche, age at menopause, age at first live birth) are biologic events mediated by estrogen and progesterone. Both hormones induce growth of the breast epithelium, and this sex steroid–driven breast epithelial proliferation may increase the risk of carcinogenesis by accelerating the occurrence of somatic genetic errors (13,226). Although breast cell proliferation increases in early pregnancy, cell proliferation decreases during the second half of pregnancy when cell differentiation occurs (227). This may account for the small protective effect conferred by pregnancy and delivery that occur at an early age. Some investigators hypothesized that any genetic damage acquired by breast cells during the premenopausal period is not lost following menopause and that this is reflected in the rising breast cancer incidence rates that are observed with advancing age (13), but this hypothesis has not been confirmed.

If one accepts this hypothesis, then suppression of ovarian steroidogenesis should have a favorable effect on breast cancer risk. Opti-

mally, this suppression should occur after the first full-term pregnancy and before age 40. The potentially adverse long-term consequences of such suppression are not yet known. If this were to be done for durations as long as 15 years, the theoretical predicted reduction in the lifetime risks of cancer of the breast, ovary, and endometrium are 70%, 45%, and 84%, respectively, based on a published model (228).

Other Agents

Epidemiologic observations show that breast cancer incidence rates are significantly lower in Asia than in the West (229). These differences may be related to high intakes of polyunsaturated fatty acids, β-carotene, or soy protein, or a combination of these. Breast cancer incidence rates are 40% to 50% lower among Asian women with the highest levels of consumption of soy proteins than among Western women (230). This may be related to the presence of naturally occurring phytoestrogens found in soy products. Phytoestrogens may suppress either the production or the activity of endogenous estrogens and may, thereby, function as inhibitors of hormone-dependent carcinogenesis. No controlled investigations for the prevention of breast cancer with these agents are being conducted yet.

Clinical Trials in Chemoprevention of Breast Cancer

Chemoprevention is the use of specific natural or synthetic chemical agents to reverse, suppress, or prevent carcinogenic progression to invasive cancer (231,232). The ability of tamoxifen to prevent breast cancer, lower cardiovascular mortality, and prevent bone fractures is being evaluated in the Breast Cancer Prevention Trial, a randomized, prospective clinical trial comparing tamoxifen with placebo in women at increased risk of breast cancer (157). The trial began in 1992 and will follow 13,000 women during 5 years of drug administration and 2 additional years of observation. The trial is conducted by the National Surgical Adjuvant Breast and Bowel Project with support from the National Cancer Institute and other government agencies. Eligible women include all those age 60 or older and women between the ages of 35 and 59 who are at increased risk of breast cancer as determined by the Gail model. Participants may not take oral contraceptives or replacement hormones during the trial, but non-hormonal medications are permitted for the management of elevated blood lipid levels or prevention of osteoporosis. The study will evaluate the effect of tamoxifen on both lipids and bone mineral density. The utility of endometrial screening is also being investigated. Results from the Breast Cancer Prevention Trial will not be available for several years, and until the studies in progress are completed and demonstrate a definite benefit from the active agent compared with placebo along with an acceptable toxicity profile, it is inappropriate to prescribe tamoxifen or any other agent with potential for the chemoprevention of breast cancer.

Several investigators conducted a pilot trial of ovarian steroid suppression using leuprolide acetate depot as the gonadotropin-releasing hormone agonist along with replacement doses of conjugated estrogen and medroxyprogesterone acetate to eliminate the hypoestrogenic side effects of the gonadotropin-releasing hormone agonist (226). Symptoms with this regimen are tolerable, but loss of bone density in the lumbar region of the spine necessitates addition of an androgen to the regimen. Favorable changes in mammographic density have been reported with this regimen, but it is not known whether this approach will result in the predicted lowering of the risk of breast cancer. It is certainly too early to apply this prevention strategy outside the context of a clinical trial.

A prospective clinical trial is being conducted in Italy to investigate the ability of 4-HPR to reduce the incidence of second primary breast cancers in women with a first breast cancer (233). Eligible women are 35 to 65 years old with T1 or T2 primary breast cancers, axillary lymph nodes negative for cancer, and no evidence of distant disease who did not receive either adjuvant endocrine therapy or chemotherapy. The results of that study will be important for many obvious reasons, as is the observation in rats that tamoxifen and 4-HPR result in enhanced inhibition of mammary carcinogenesis and reduction in tumor-related mortality (234). If both retinoids and tamoxifen are shown individually to prevent breast cancer in women, additional clinical trials of combination therapy will be warranted.

Finally, a very large clinical trial is being conducted in the United States to evaluate the effect of several interventions on chronic diseases in women. The Women's Health Initiative is both a prospective, randomized trial and an observational study that will evaluate the effect of diet on the risks of breast cancer, colon cancer, and cardiovascular disease; the effect of estrogen replacement therapy on the risk of cardiovascular disease, osteoporosis, and breast cancer; and the effect of calcium supplementation and vitamin D on osteoporosis and other risk factors (235). The trial, which began in 1994, will ultimately enroll more than 100,000 participants and will continue as long as 15 years or until significant end points are achieved.

Conclusions

The ultimate goal when studying breast cancer epidemiology is to identify effective strategies for primary prevention. Potentially effective interventions that may significantly reduce the incidence of breast cancer in the near future are being evaluated. Interim management options can be employed until effective primary prevention is available.

REFERENCES

1. Black WC, Nease RF Jr, Tosteson ANA. Perceptions of breast cancer risk and screening effectiveness in women younger than 50 years of age. *J Natl Cancer Inst* 1995;87:720–731.

2. Lilienfeld AM, Lilienfeld DE. *Foundations of epidemiology.* New York: Oxford University Press, 1980:217, 346–347.

3. Harris JR, Lippman ME, Veronesi U, et al. Breast cancer. *N Engl J Med* 1992;327:319–328.

4. Dawson DA, Thompson GB. Breast cancer risk factors and screening: United States, 1987. National Center for Health Statistics. *Vital Health Stat* 10 1989;172:1–60.

5. Bruzzi P, Green SB, Byar DP, et al. Estimating the population attributable risk for multiple risk factors using case-control data. *Am J Epidemiol* 1985;122:904–914.

6. Seidman H, Stellman SD, Mushinski MH. A different perspective on breast cancer risk factors: some implications of the nonattributable risk. *CA Cancer J Clin* 1982;32:301–313.

7. Madigan MP, Ziegler RG, Benichou J, et al. Proportion of breast cancer cases in the United States explained by well-established risk factors. *J Natl Cancer Inst* 1995;87:1681–1685.

8. Buell P. Changing incidence of breast cancer in Japanese-American women. *J Natl Cancer Inst* 1973;51:1479–1483.

9. Kelsey JL. A review of the epidemiology of human breast cancer. *Epidemiol Rev* 1979;1:74–109.

10. Kelsey JL, Berkowitz GS. Breast cancer epidemiology. *Cancer Res* 1988;48:5615–5623.

11. Kelsey JL, Gammon MD. Epidemiology of breast cancer. *Epidemiol Rev* 1990;12:228–240.

12. Kelsey JL, Gammon MD, John EM. Reproductive factors and breast cancer. *Epidemiol Rev* 1993;15:36–47.

13. Spicer DV, Krecker EA, Pike MC. The endocrine prevention of breast cancer. *Cancer Invest* 1995;13:495–504.

14. Anderson TJ, Ferguson DJP, Raab GM. Cell turnover in the "resting" human breast: influence of parity, contraceptive pill, age, and laterality. *Br J Cancer* 1982;46:376–382.

15. Daling JR, Malone KE, Voigt LF, et al. Risk of breast cancer among young women: relationship to induced abortion. *J Natl Cancer Inst* 1994;86:1584–1592.

16. Ernster VL. The epidemiology of benign breast disease. *Epidemiol Rev* 1981;3:184–202.

17. Black MM, Modan B, Lubin F, et al. A nationwide study of breast disease. *Cancer* 1988;61:2547–2551.

18. Yu H, Rohan TE, Howe GR, et al. Risk factors for fibroadenoma: a case-control study in Australia. *Am J Epidemiol* 1992;135:247–258.

19. Millikan R, Hulka B, Thor A, et al. p53 mutations in benign breast tissue. *J Clin Oncol* 1995;13:2293–2300.

20. Vogel VG. High-risk populations as targets for breast cancer prevention trials. *Prevent Med* 1991;20:86–100.

21. Gail MH, Brinton LA, Byar DP, et al. Projecting individualized probabilities of developing breast cancer for white females who are being examined annually. *J Natl Cancer Inst* 1989;81:1879–1886.

22. Dupont WD, Page DL. Risk factors for breast cancer in women with proliferative breast disease. *N Engl J Med* 1985;312:146–151.

23. Page DL, Dupont WD, Rogers LW, et al. Atypical hyperplastic lesions of the female breast: a long-term follow-up study. *Cancer* 1985;55:2698–2708.

24. Carter CL, Corle DK, Micozzi MS, et al. A prospective study of the development of breast cancer in 16,692 women with benign breast disease. *Am J Epidemiol* 1988;128:467–477.

25. London SJ, Connolly JL, Schnitt SJ, et al. A prospective study of benign breast disease and the risk of breast cancer. *JAMA* 1992;267:941–944.

26. Dupont WD, Parl FF, Hartman WH, et al. Breast cancer risk associated with proliferative disease and atypical hyperplasia. *Cancer* 1993;71:1258–1265.

27. Rubin E, Visscher DW, Alexander RW, et al. Proliferative disease and atypia in biopsies performed for nonpalpable lesions detected mammographically. *Cancer* 1988;61:2077–2082.

28. Jensen RA, Page DL, Dupont WD, et al. Invasive breast cancer risk in women with sclerosing adenosis. *Cancer* 1989;64:1977–1983.

29. Marcus JN, Watson P, Page DL, et al. Pathology and heredity of breast cancer in younger women. *Monogr Natl Cancer Inst* 1994;16:23–34.

30. Skolnick MH, Cannon-Albright LA, Goldgar DE, et al. Inheritance of proliferative breast disease in breast cancer kindreds. *Science* 1990;250:1715–1720.

31. Ward JH, Marshall CJ, Schumann GB, et al. Detection of proliferative breast disease by four-quadrant fine-needle aspiration. *J Natl Cancer Inst* 1990;82:964–966.

32. Fabian CJ, Kamel S, Kimler BF, et al. Potential use of biomarkers in breast cancer risk assessment and chemoprevention trials. *Breast J* 1995;1:236–242.

33. Dupont WD, Page DL, Rogers LW, et al. Influence of exogenous estrogens, proliferative breast disease, and other variables on breast cancer risk. *Cancer* 1989;63:948–957.

34. Claus EB, Risch N, Thompson WD. Genetic analysis of breast cancer in the Cancer and Steroid Hormone Study. *Am J Hum Genet* 1991;48:232–242.

35. Peters J. Breast cancer genetics: relevance to oncology practice. *Cancer Control* 1995;2:195–208.

36. Hoskins KF, Stopfer JE, Calzone KA, et al. Assessment and counseling for women with a family history of breast cancer. A guide for clinicians. *JAMA* 1995;273:577–585.

37. Easton DF, Bishop DT, Ford D, Crockford GP, the Breast Cancer Linkage Consortium. Genetic linkage analysis in familial breast and ovarian

cancer: results for 214 families. *Am J Hum Genet* 1993;52:678–701.

38. Miki Y, Swensen J, Shattuck-Eidens D, et al. A strong candidate for the breast and ovarian cancer susceptibility gene BRCA1. *Science* 1994;266:66–71.

39. Merajver SD, Pham TM, Caduff RF, et al. Somatic mutations in the BRCA1 gene in sporadic ovarian tumors. *Nat Genet* 1995;9:439–443.

40. Thompson ME, Jensen RA, Obermiller PS, et al. Decreased expression of BRCA1 accelerates growth and is often present during sporadic breast cancer progression. *Nat Genet* 1995;9:444–450.

41. Shattuck-Eidens D, Mclure M, Semerd J, et al. A collaborative survey of 80 mutations in the BRCA1 breast and ovarian cancer susceptibility gene. Implications for presymptomatic testing and screening. *JAMA* 1995;273:535–541.

42. Chen Y, Chen C-F, Riley DJ, et al. Aberrant subcellular localization of BRCA1 in breast cancer. *Science* 1995;270:789–791.

43. Struewing JP, Abeliovich D, Peretz T, et al. The carrier frequency of the BRCA1 185delAG mutation is approximately 1 percent in Ashkenazi Jewish individuals. *Nat Genet* 1995;11:190–200.

44. Goldgar DF, Reilly PR. A common BRCA1 mutation in the Ashkenazim. *Nat Genet* 1995;11:113–114.

45. Easton DF, Ford BP, Bishop DT, the Breast Cancer Linkage Consortium. Breast and ovarian cancer incidence in BRCA1-mutation carriers. *Am J Hum Genet* 1995;56:265–271.

46. Stratton M, Ford DF, Bishop DT, et al. Familial male breast cancer is not linked to the BRCA1 locus on chromosome 17q. *Nat Genet* 1994;7:103–107.

47. Slattery ML, Kerber RA. A comprehensive evaluation of family history and breast cancer risk—the Utah population database. *JAMA* 1993;270:1563–1568.

48. Claus EB, Risch N, Thompson WD. Autosomal dominant inheritance of early-onset breast cancer: implications for risk prediction. *Cancer* 1994;73:643–651.

49. Hogervorst FBL, Cornelius RS, Bout M, et al. Rapid detection of BRCA1 mutations by the protein truncation test. *Nat Genet* 1995;10:208–212.

50. Wooster R, Neuhausen SL, Mangion J. Localization of a breast cancer susceptibility gene BRCA2 to chromosome 13q12-13. *Science* 1994;265:2088–2090.

51. Offit K, Brown K. Quantitation of familial cancer risk: a resource for clinical oncologists. *J Clin Oncol* 1994;12:1724–1736.

52. Anderson DE, Badzioch MD. Risk of familial breast cancer. *Cancer* 1985;56:383–387.

53. Chaliki H, Loader S, Levenkron JC, et al. Women's receptivity to testing for a genetic susceptibility to breast cancer. *Am J Public Health* 1995;85:1133–1135.

54. Li FP, Garber JE, Friend SH, et al. Recommendations on predictive testing for germ line p53 mutations among cancer-prone individuals. *J Natl Cancer Inst* 1992;84:1156–1160.

55. Biesecker BB, Boehnke M, Calzone K, et al. Genetic counseling for families with inherited susceptibility to breast and ovarian cancer. *JAMA* 1993;269:1970–1974.

56. King M-C, Rowell S, Love SM. Inherited breast and ovarian cancer: What are the risks? What are the choices? *JAMA* 1993;269:1975–1980.

57. Statement of the American Society of Human Genetics on genetic testing for breast and ovarian cancer predisposition. *Am J Hum Genet* 1994;55:i–iv.

58. National Advisory Council for Human Genome Research. Statement on the use of DNA testing for presymptomatic identification of cancer risk. *JAMA* 1994;271:785.

59. Vogel VG. Counseling the high-risk woman. In: Stoll BA, ed. *Reducing breast cancer risk in women.* Boston: Kluwer Academic, 1995:69–80.

60. Wolfe JN. Risk for breast cancer development determined by mammographic parenchymal pattern. *Cancer* 1976;37:2486–2492.

61. Warner E, Lockwood G, Tritchler D, Boyd NF. The risk of breast cancer associated with mammographic parenchymal patterns: a meta-analysis of the published literature to examine the effect of method of classification. *Cancer Detect Prev* 1992;16:67–72.

62. Gravelle IH, Bulbrook RD, Wang DY, et al. A comparison of mammographic parenchymal patterns in premenopausal Japanese and British women. *Breast Cancer Res Treat* 1991;18(suppl 1):S93–S95.

63. Beute BJ, Kalisker L, Hutter RVP. Lobular carcinoma in situ of the breast: clinical, pathological, and mammographic features. *AJR Am J Roentgenol* 1991;157:257–265.

64. Saftlas AF, Hoover RN, Brinton LA, et al. Mammographic densities and risk of breast cancer. *Cancer* 1991;67:2833–2838.

65. Byrne C, Schairer C, Wolfe J, et al. Mammographic features and breast cancer risk: effects with time, age, and menopause status. *J Natl Cancer Inst* 1995;87:1622–1629.

66. Boyd NF, Connelly P, Byng J, et al. Plasma lipids, lipoproteins, and mammographic densities. *Cancer Epidemiol Biomarkers Prev* 1995;4: 727–733.

67. Bartow SA, Pathak DR, Mettler FA, et al. Breast mammographic pattern: a concatenation of confounding and breast cancer risk factors. *Am J Epidemiol* 1995;142:813–819.

68. Tretli S. Height and weight in relation to breast cancer morbidity and mortality: a prospective study of 570,000 women in Norway. *Int J Cancer* 1989;44:23–30.

69. London S, Willett WC. Diet, body size and breast cancer risk. *Rev Endocr Related Cancer* 1988;31:19–25.

70. Willett WC, Browne ML, Bain C, et al. Relative weight and risk of breast cancer among premenopausal women. *Am J Epidemiol* 1985; 122:731–740.

71. Brinton LA. Ways that women may possibly reduce their risk of breast cancer. *J Natl Cancer Inst* 1994;86:1371–1372. Editorial.

72. Dorgan JF, Brown C, Barrett M, et al. Physical activity and risk of breast cancer in the Framingham Heart Study. *Am J Epidemiol* 1994; 139:662–669.

73. Frisch RE, Wyshak G, Albright NL, et al. Lower prevalence of breast cancer and cancers of the reproductive system among former college athletes compared to non-athletes. *Br J Cancer* 1985;52:885–891.

74. Paffenbarger RS Jr, Hyde RT, Wing AL. Physical activity and incidence of cancer in diverse populations: a preliminary report. *Am J Clin Nutr* 1987;45:312–317.

75. Paffenbarger RS Jr, Lee I-M, Wing AL. The influence of physical activity on the incidence of site-specific cancers in college alumni. *Adv Exp Med Biol* 1992;322:7–15.

76. Albanes D, Blair A, Taylor PR. Physical activity and risk of cancer in the NHANES I population. *Am J Public Health* 1989;79:744–750.

77. Vena JE, Graham S, Zielezny M, et al. Occupational exercise and risk of cancer. *Am J Clin Nutr* 1987;45:318–327.

78. Pukkala E, Poskiparta M, Apter D, Vihko V. Life-long physical activity and cancer among Finnish female teachers. *Eur J Cancer Prev* 1993; 2:369–376.

79. Bernstein L, Henderson BE, Hanisch R, et al. Physical exercise and reduced risk of breast cancer in young women. *J Natl Cancer Inst* 1994;86:1403–1408.

80. Prentice RL, Sheppard L. Dietary fat and cancer: consistency of the epidemiologic data, and disease prevention that may follow from a practical reduction in fat consumption. *Cancer Causes Control* 1990;1:81–97.

81. Willett WC, Hunter DJ, Stampfer MJ, et al. Dietary fat and fiber in relation to the risk of breast cancer: an eight-year follow-up. *JAMA* 1992;268:2037–2044.

82. Jurkowski JJ, Cave WT Jr. Dietary effects of menhaden oil on the growth and membrane lipid composition of rat mammary tumors. *J Natl Cancer Inst* 1984;74:1145–1150.

83. Kaizer L, Boyd NF, Kriukov V, et al. Fish consumption and breast cancer risk: an ecological study. *Nutr Cancer* 1989;12:61–68.

84. Hursting SD, Thornquist M, Henderson MM. Types of dietary fat and the incidence of cancer at five sites. *Prev Med* 1990;19:242–253.

85. Lee HP, Gourley L, Duffy SW, et al. Dietary effects on breast cancer risk in Singapore. *Lancet* 1991;337:1197–2000.

86. Shimizu H, Ross RK, Bernstein L, et al. Cancer of the prostate and breast among Japanese and white immigrants in Los Angeles County. *Br J Cancer* 1991;63:963–966.

87. Barnes S, Peterson G, Grubbs C, et al. Potential role of dietary isoflavones in the prevention of cancer. *Adv Exp Med Biol* 1994;354:135–147.

88. Djuric Z, Evertt CK, Luongo DA. Toxicity, single-strand breaks, and 5 hydroxymethyl-2'-deoxyuridine formation in human breast epithelial cells treated with hydrogen peroxide. *Free Radic Biol Med* 1993;14:541–547.

89. Knekt P. Vitamin E and cancer: epidemiology. *Ann NY Acad Sci* 1992;669:269–279.

90. Garland M, Willett WC, Manson JE, et al. Antioxidant micronutrients and breast cancer. *J Am Coll Nutr* 1993;12:400–411.

91. Hunter DJ, Manson JE, Colditz GA, et al. A prospective study of the intake of vitamins C, E, and A and the risk of breast cancer. *N Engl J Med* 1993;329:234–240.

92. Willett WC, Hunter DJ. Vitamin A and cancers of the breast, large bowel, and prostate: epidemiologic evidence. *Nutr Rev* 1994;52:S53–S59.

93. Schatzkin A, Longnecker MP. Alcohol and breast cancer: where are we now and where do we go from here? *Cancer* 1994;74:1101–1110.

94. Blot WJ. Alcohol and cancer. *Cancer Res* 1992;52:2119s–2123s.

95. Rosenberg L, Metzger LS, Palmer JR. Alcohol consumption and risk of breast cancer: a review of the epidemiologic evidence. *Am J Epidemiol* 1993;15:133–144.

96. Reichman ME, Judd JT, Longscope C, et al. Effects of alcohol consumption on plasma and urinary hormone concentrations in premenopausal women. *J Natl Cancer Inst* 1993;85:722–727.

97. Longnecker MP, Paganini-Hill A, Ross RK. Lifetime alcohol consumption and breast cancer risk among postmenopausal women in Los Angeles. *Cancer Epidemiol Biomarkers Prev* 1995; 5:721–725.

98. Longnecker MP, Newcombe PA, Mittendorf R, et al. Risk of breast cancer in relation to lifetime alcohol consumption. *J Natl Cancer Inst* 1995;87:923–929.

99. Longnecker MP. Alcoholic beverage consumption in relation to risk of breast cancer: meta-analysis and review. *Cancer Causes Control* 1994;5:73–82.

100. Friedman LA, Kimball AW. Coronary heart disease mortality and alcohol consumption in Framingham. *Am J Epidemiol* 1986;124:481–489.

101. Klatsky AL, Friedman GD, Siegelaub AB. Alcohol and mortality. A ten-year Kaiser-Permanente experience. *Ann Intern Med* 1981;95:139–145.

102. Vessey MP, Doll R, Jones K, et al. An epidemiological study of oral contraceptives and breast cancer. *BMJ* 1979;1:1755–1758.

103. Pike MC, Henderson BE, Krailo MD, et al. Breast cancer in young women and use of oral contraceptives: possible modifying effects of formulation and age at use. *Lancet* 1983;2:926–930.

104. McPherson K, Vessey MP, Neil A, et al. Early oral contraceptive use and premenopausal breast cancer in Sweden and Norway: possible effects of different pattern of use. *Int J Epidemiol* 1989;18:527–532.

105. Kay CR, Hannaford PC. Breast cancer and the pill—a further report from the Royal College of General Practitioners' oral contraception study. *Br J Cancer* 1988;58:675–680.

106. Brinton LA, Daling JR, Liff JM, et al. Oral contraceptives and breast cancer risk among younger women. *J Natl Cancer Inst* 1995; 87:827–835.

107. Henderson BE, Bernstein L. Endogenous and exogenous hormonal factors. In: Harris JR, Lippman ME, Morrow M, Hellman S, eds. *Diseases of the Breast.* Philadelphia: Lippincott-Raven, 1996:185–200.

108. Ursin G, Aragaki CC, Paganini-Hill A, et al. Oral contraceptives and premenopausal bilateral breast cancer: a case-control study. *Epidemiology* 1992;3:414–419.

109. Wingo PA, Lee NC, Ory HW, et al. Age-specific differences in the relationship between oral contraceptive use and breast cancer. *Cancer* 1993;71:1506–1517.

110. Rookus MA, van Leeuwen FE. Oral contraceptives and risk of breast cancer in women aged 20–54 years. The Netherlands Oral Contraceptives and Breast Cancer Study Group. *Lancet* 1994;344:844–851.

111. WHO Collaborative Study of Neoplasia and Steroid Contraceptives. Breast cancer and combined oral contraceptives: results from a multinational study. *Br J Cancer* 1990;61:110–119.

112. Schesselman JJ, Stadel BV, Korper M, et al. Breast cancer detection in relation to oral contraception. *J Clin Epidemiol* 1992;45:449–459.

113. Hulka BS. Hormone-replacement therapy and the risk of breast cancer. *CA Cancer J Clin* 1990;40:289–296.

114. Cauley JA, Gutai JP, Kuller LH, et al. The epidemiology of serum sex hormones in postmenopausal women. *Am J Epidemiol* 1989; 129:1120–1131.

115. Hershcopf RJ, Bradlow HL. Obesity, diet, endogenous estrogens, and the risk of hormone-sensitive cancer. *Am J Clin Nutr* 1987;45: 283–289.

116. Grodin JM, Siiteri PK, MacDonald PC. Source of estrogen production in postmenopausal women. *J Clin Endocrinol Metab* 1973;36:207–214.

117. Adami H-O, Persson I. Hormone replacement and breast cancer a remaining controversy? *JAMA* 1995;274:178–179. Editorial.

118. Toniolo PO, Levitz M, Zeleniuch-Jacquotte A, et al. A prospective study of endogenous estrogens and breast cancer in postmenopausal women. *J Natl Cancer Inst* 1995;87:190–197.

119. Russo J, Tay LK, Russo IH. Differentiation of the mammary gland and susceptibility to carcinogenesis. *Breast Cancer Res Treat* 1982;2:5–73.

120. Key TJ, Pike MC. The role of oestrogens and progestagens in the epidemiology and prevention of breast cancer. *Eur J Cancer Clin Oncol* 1988;24:29–43.

121. Stanford JL, Weiss NS, Voigt LF, et al. Combined estrogen and progestin hormone replacement therapy in relation to risk of breast cancer in middle-aged women. *JAMA* 1995;274:137–142.

122. Colditz GA, Hankison SE, Hunter DJ, et al. The use of estrogens and progestins and the risk of breast cancer in postmenopausal women. *N Engl J Med* 1995;332:1589–1593.

123. Skegg DCG, Noonan EA, Paul C, et al. Depot medroxyprogesterone and breast cancer—a pooled analysis of the World Health Organization and New Zealand Studies. *JAMA* 1995; 273:799–804.

124. Gambrell RD Jr, Maier RC, Sanders BI. Decreased incidence of breast cancer in post-menopausal estrogen-progestogen users. *Obstet Gynecol* 1983;62:435–443.

125. Brinton LA, Hoover R, Fraumeni JF Jr. Menopausal estrogens and breast cancer risk: an expanded case-control study. *Br J Cancer* 1986;54:825–832.

126. Lippman ME, Swain SM. Endocrine-responsive cancers of humans. In: Wilson JD, Foster DW, eds. *Williams textbook of endocrinology.* 8th ed. Philadelphia: WB Saunders, 1992:1577–1597.

127. Bergkvist L, Adami H-O, Person I, et al. The risk of breast cancer after estrogen and estrogen-progestin replacement. *N Engl J Med* 1989;321: 293–297.

128. Kaufman DW, Palmer JR, de Mouzon J, et al. Estrogen replacement therapy and the risk of breast cancer: results from the case-control surveillance study. *Am J Epidemiol* 1991;134: 1375–1385.

129. Newcomb PA, Longnecker MP, Storer BE, et al. Long-term hormone replacement therapy and risk of breast cancer in postmenopausal women. *Am J Epidemiol* 1995;142:788–795.

130. Mills PK, Beeson WL, Phillips RL, Fraser GE. Prospective study of exogenous hormone use and breast cancer in Seventh-Day Adventists. *Cancer* 1987;64:591–597.

131. Hunt K, Vessey M. Long-term effects of post-menopausal hormone therapy. *Br J Hosp Med* 1987;38:450–453, 456–460.

132. Barrett-Connor E. Postmenopausal estrogen replacement and breast cancer. *N Engl J Med* 1989;321:319–320. Editorial.

133. Steinberg KK, Thacker SB, Smith SJ, et al. A meta-analysis of the effect of estrogen replacement therapy on the risk of breast cancer. *JAMA* 1991;265:1985–1990.

134. Armstrong BK. Oestrogen therapy after the menopause—boon or bane? *Med J Aust* 1988;143:213–214.

135. Dupont WD, Page DL. Menopausal estrogen replacement therapy and breast cancer. *Arch Intern Med* 1991;151:67–72.

136. Schlesselman JJ, Stadel BV, Murray P, Lai S. Breast cancer in relation to early use of oral contraceptives—no evidence of a latent effect. *JAMA* 1988;259:1828–1833.

137. Lipnick RJ, Buring JE, Hennekens CH, et al. Oral contraceptives and breast cancer—a prospective cohort study. *JAMA* 1986;255:58–61.

138. Sattin RW, Rubin GL, Wingo PA, et al. Oral-contraceptive use and the risk of breast cancer. *N Engl J Med* 1986;315:405–411.

139. The Centers for Disease and Control Cancer and Steroid Hormone Study: long-term oral contraceptive use and the risk of breast cancer. *JAMA* 1983;249:1591–1595.

140. Carr BR. Disorders of the ovary and female reproductive tract. In: Wilson JD, Foster DW, eds. *Williams textbook of endocrinology.* 8th ed. Philadelphia: WB Saunders, 1992:733–798.

141. Folsom AR, Mink PJ, Sellers TA, et al. Hormonal replacement therapy and morbidity and mortality in a prospective study of postmenopausal women. *Am J Public Health* 1995;85:1128–1132.

142. Barrett-Connor E, Bush TJ. Estrogen and coronary heart disease in women. *JAMA* 1991;265: 1861–1867.

143. Paganini-Hill A, Ross RK, Henderson BE. Post-menopausal oestrogen treatment and stroke: a prospective study. *BMJ* 1988;297:519–522.

144. Grady D, Rubin SM, Petitti DB, et al. Hormone therapy to prevent disease and prolong life in postmenopausal women. *Ann Intern Med* 1992;117:1016–1037.

145. Ettinger B, Genant HK, Conn CE. Post-menopausal bone loss is prevented by treatment with low-dose estrogen with calcium. *Ann Intern Med* 1987;106:40–45.

146. Kiel DP, Felson DT, Anderson JJ, et al. Hip fracture and the use of estrogens in postmenopausal women. *N Engl J Med* 1987;317:1169–1174.

147. Henderson BE, Ross R, Bernstein L. Estrogens as a cause of human cancer: the Richard and Hinda Rosenthal Foundation Award Lecture. *Cancer Res* 1988;48:246–253.

148. Bernstein L, Ross RK, Henderson BE. Prospects for the primary prevention of breast cancer. *Am J Epidemiol* 1992;135:142–152.

149. Stoll BA. Hormone replacement therapy in women treated for breast cancer. *Eur J Cancer Clin Oncol* 1989;25:1909–1913.

150. Theriault RL, Sellin RV. A clinical dilemma: estrogen replacement therapy in postmenopausal women with a background of primary breast cancer. *Ann Oncol* 1991;2:709–717.

151. Cobleigh MA, Berris RF, Bush T, et al. Estrogen replacement therapy in breast cancer survivors—a time for change. *JAMA* 1994;272: 540–545.

152. American College of Physicians. Guidelines for counseling postmenopausal women about preventive hormone therapy. *Ann Intern Med* 1992;117:1038–1041.

153. Boice JD, Harvey EB, Blettner M, et al. Cancer in the contralateral breast after radiotherapy for breast cancer. *N Engl J Med* 1992;326:781–785.

154. Hoffman DA, Lonstein JE, Norin MM, et al. Breast cancer in women with scoliosis exposed to multiple diagnostic x-rays. *J Natl Cancer Inst* 1989; 81:1307–1312.

155. Swift M, Morrell D, Massey RB, Chase CL. Incidence of cancer in 161 families affected by ataxia telangiectasia. *N Engl J Med* 1991;325:1831–1836.

156. Savitsky K, Bar-Shira A, Gilad S, et al. A single ataxia telangiectasia gene with a product similar to PI-3 kinase. *Science* 1995;268:1749–1753.

157. Nayfield SG, Karp JE, Ford LG, et al. Potential role of tamoxifen in prevention of breast cancer. *J Natl Cancer Inst* 1991;83:1450–1459.

158. Spiegelman D, Colditz GA, Hunter D, Hertzmark E. Validation of the Gail et al model predicting individual breast cancer risk. *J Natl Cancer Inst* 1994;86:600–607.

159. Bondy ML, Spitz MR, Halabi S, et al. Low incidence of familial breast cancer among Hispanic women. *Cancer Causes Control* 1992;3:377–382.

160. Lerman C, Rimer BK, Engstrom PF. Cancer risk notification: psychological and ethical implications. *J Clin Oncol* 1991;9:1275–1282.

161. Lerman C, Rimer B, Trock B, et al. Psychological and behavioral implications of abnormal mammograms. *Ann Intern Med* 1991;114:657–661.

162. Lerman C, Trock B, Rimer B, et al. Psychological side-effects of breast cancer screening. *Health Psychol* 1991;10:259–267.

163. Kash JM, Holland JC, Halper MS, et al. Psychological distress and surveillance behaviors of women with a family history of breast cancer. *J Natl Cancer Inst* 1992;84:24–30.

164. Lerman C, Schwartz M. Adherence and psychological adjustment among women at high risk for breast cancer. *Breast Cancer Res Treat* 1993; 28:145–155.

165. Alagna SW, Morokoff PJ, Bevett JM, et al. Performance of breast self-examination by women at high risk for breast cancer. *Women Health* 1987;12:29–46.

166. Lerman C, Rimer B, Trock B, et al. Factors associated with repeat adherence to breast cancer screening. *Prev Med* 1990;19:279–290.

167. Vogel VG, Graves DS, Vernon SW, et al. Mammographic screening of women with increased risk of breast cancer. *Cancer* 1990;66:1613–1620.

168. Vogel VG, Yeomans A, Higginbotham E. Clinical management of women at increased risk for breast cancer. *Breast Cancer Res Treat* 1993; 28:195–210.

169. Morrow M. Identification and management of women at increased risk for breast cancer development. *Breast Cancer Res Treat* 1994;31:53–60.

170. Bilimoria M, Morrow M. The woman at increased risk for breast cancer: evaluation and management strategies. *CA Cancer J Clin* 1995;45:263–278.

171. Hurley SF, Kaldor JM. The benefits and risk of mammographic screening for breast cancer. *Epidemiol Rev* 1992;14:101–130.

172. Smart CR, Hendrick RE, Rutledge JH, et al. Benefit of mammography screening in women ages 40 to 49 years—current evidence from randomized controlled trials. *Cancer* 1995;75: 1619–1626.

173. Vogel VG. Screening younger women at risk for breast cancer. *Monogr Natl Cancer Inst* 1994; 16:55–60.

174. Miller AB, Baines CJ, To T, et al. Canadian National Breast Screening Study. I. Breast cancer and death rates among women aged 40 to 49 years. *Can Med Assoc J* 1992;147:1459–1476.

175. Sickles EA, Kopans DB. Deficiencies in the analysis of breast screening data. *J Natl Cancer Inst* 1993;85:1621–1624.

176. Sackett DL, Haynes RB, Guyatt GH, Tugwell P. *Clinical epidemiology—a basic science for clinical medicine.* Boston: Little, Brown, 1991:69–152.

177. Mettlin C. Breast cancer risk factors—contributions to planning breast cancer control. *Cancer* 1992;69:1904–1910.

178. Meyer JE, Kopans DB, Oot R. Breast cancer visualized by mammography in patients under 35. *Radiology* 1983;147:93–94.

179. Lantz PM, Remington PL, Newcomb PA. Mammography screening and increased incidence of breast cancer in Wisconsin. *J Natl Cancer Inst* 1991;83:1540–1546.

180. Svane G, Potchen EJ, Siena A, Azavedo E. How to interpret a mammogram. In: *Screening mammography—breast cancer diagnosis in asymptomatic women.* St. Louis: CV Mosby, 1993:148.

181. Bland KI, O'Neal B, Weiner LJ, et al. One-stage simple mastectomy with immediate reconstruction for high-risk patients. *Arch Surg* 1986; 121:221–225.

182. Rubin LR. Prophylactic mastectomy with immediate reconstruction for the high-risk woman. *Clin Plast Surg* 1984;11:369–381.

183. Wong JH, Jackson CF, Swanson JS, et al. Analysis of the risk reduction of prophylactic partial mastectomy in Sprague-Dawley rats with 7,12-dimethylbenzathracene-induced breast cancer. *Surgery* 1986;99:67–71.

184. Nelson H, Miller SH, Buck D, et al. Effectiveness of prophylactic mastectomy in the prevention of breast tumors in C3H mice. *Plast Reconstr Surg* 1989;83:662–669.

185. Temple WJ, Lindsay RL, Magi E, et al. Technical considerations for prophylactic mastectomy in patients at high risk for breast cancer. *Am J Surg* 1991;161:413–415.

186. Goodnight JE Jr, Quagliana JM, Mortoan DL. Failure of subcutaneous mastectomy to prevent the development of breast cancer. *J Surg Oncol* 1984;26:198–201.

187. Pennisi VR, Capozzi A. Subcutaneous mastectomy data: a final statistical analysis of 1500 patients. *Aesthetic Plast Surg* 1989;13:15–21.

188. Ziegler LD, Kroll SS. Primary breast cancer after prophylactic mastectomy. *Am J Clin Oncol* 1991;14:451–454.

189. Hartmann L, Jenkins R, Schaid D, et al. Prophylactic mastectomy: preliminary retrospective cohort analysis. Proc Am Assoc Cancer Res 1997;38:A168.

190. Wapnir IL, Rabinowitz B, Greco RS. A reappraisal of prophylactic mastectomy. *Surg Gynecol Obstet* 1990;171:171–184.

191. American Society of Plastic and Reconstructive Surgeons. *Position paper on prophylactic mastectomy.* Arlington Heights, IL: American Society of Plastic and Reconstructive Surgeons, 1989.

192. Claus EB, Risch N, Thompson WD, et al. Relationship between breast histopathology and family history of breast cancer. *Cancer* 1993;71:147–153.

193. Early Breast Cancer Trialists' Collaborative Group. Systemic treatment of early breast cancer hormonal, cytotoxic, or immune therapy. *Lancet* 1992;339:1–15.

194. Andersson M, Storm HH, Mouridsen HT. Carcinogenic effects of adjuvant tamoxifen treatment and radiotherapy for early breast cancer. *Acta Oncol* 1992;31:259–263.

195. Vogel VG. Tamoxifen for the prevention of breast cancer. In: De Vita VT Jr, Helman S, Rosenberg SA, eds. *Important advances in oncology—1995.* Philadelphia: JB Lippincott, 1995:187–200.

196. McDonald CC. Fatal myocardial infarction in the Scottish adjuvant tamoxifen trial. *BMJ* 1991; 303:435–437.

197. Rutqvist LE, Mattson A. Cardiac and thromboembolic morbidity among postmenopausal women with early-stage breast cancer in a randomized trial of adjuvant tamoxifen. *J Natl Cancer Inst* 1993;85:1398–1406.

198. Bruning PF, Bonfrer JMG, Hart AAM, et al. Tamoxifen, serum lipoproteins and cardiovascular risk. *Br J Cancer* 1988;58:497–499.

199. Love RR, Newcomb PA, Wiebe DA, et al. Effects of tamoxifen therapy on lipid and lipoprotein levels in postmenopausal patients with node-negative breast cancer. *J Natl Cancer Inst* 1990;82:1327–1332.

200. Windler E, Kovanen PT, Chao YS, et al. The estradiol stimulated lipoprotein receptor of rat liver: a binding site that mediates uptake of rat lipoproteins containing apoproteins B and E. *J Biol Chem* 1980;255:10464–10471.

201. Stacls B, Anwer J, Chan L, et al. Influence of development, estrogens, and food intake on apolipoproteins A-I, A-III, and E in RNA in rat liver and intestine. *J Lipid Res* 1989;30: 1137–1147.

202. Bush T, Fried LP, Barrett-Connor E. Cholesterol, lipoprotein and coronary heart disease in women. *Clin Chem* 1988;34:60–70.

203. Yusuf SA, Wittes J, Friedman L. Overview of results of randomized clinical trials in heart disease. II: unstable angina, heart failure, primary prevention with aspirin and risk factor modification. *JAMA* 1988;260:2259–2263.

204. Love RR, Wiebe DA, Newcomb PA, et al. Effects of tamoxifen on cardiovascular risk factors in postmenopausal women. *Ann Intern Med* 1991;115:860–864.

205. Kannel WB, Wolf PA, Castelli WP, et al. Fibrinogen and risk of cardiovascular disease. *JAMA* 1987;258:1183–1186.

206. Hoffman CJ, Miller RH, Lawson WE, et al. Elevation of factor VII activity and mass in young adults at risk of ischemic heart disease. *J Am Coll Cardiol* 1989;14:941–946.

207. Cuzick J, Allen D, Baum M, et al. Long-term effects of tamoxifen—Biological Effects of Tamoxifen Working Party. *Eur J Cancer* 1993;29:15–21.

208. Barrett-Connor E. Postmenopausal estrogen, cancer and other considerations. *Women Health* 1986;11:179–195.

209. Jordan VC, Phelps E, Lingren JU. Effect of anti-estrogens on bone in castrated and intact female rats. *Breast Cancer Res Treat* 1987;10:31–35.

210. Turner RT, Wakley GK, Hannon KS, et al. Tamoxifen prevents the skeletal effects of ovarian hormone deficiency in rats. *J Bone Miner Res* 1987;2:449–456.

211. Turner RT, Wakley GK, Hannon KS, et al. Tamoxifen inhibits osteoclast-mediated resorption of trabecular bone in ovarian hormone deficient rats. *Endocrinology* 1988;122:1146–1150.

212. Wakley GK, Hannon KS, Bell NA, et al. The effects of tamoxifen on the osteopenia induced by sciatic neurotomy in the rat: histomorphometric study. *Calcif Tissue Int* 1988;43:383–388.

213. Love RR, Mazess RB, Borden HS, et al. Effects of tamoxifen on bone mineral density in postmenopausal women with breast cancer. *N Engl J Med* 1992;326:852–856.

214. Kristensen B, Ejlertsen B, Dalgaard P, et al. Tamoxifen and bone metabolism in postmenopausal low-risk breast cancer patients: a randomized study. *J Clin Oncol* 1994;12:992–997.

215. Stewart PJ, Stern PH. Effects of the antiestrogens tamoxifen and clomiphene on bone resorption in vitro. *Endocrinology* 1986;118:125–131.

216. Powles TJ, Hickish TF, Kanis JA, Ashley S. Tamoxifen preserves bone mineral density in post-menopausal women but causes loss of bone density in premenopausal women. *Proc Am Soc Clin Oncol* 1995;14:A165.

217. Fornander T, Rutvqvist LE, Cedermark B, et al. Adjuvant tamoxifen in early breast cancer: occurrence of new primary cancers. *Lancet* 1989;1:117–120.

218. Rutqvist LE, Johansson H, Signomklao T, et al. Adjuvant tamoxifen therapy for early stage breast cancer and second primary malignancy. *J Natl Cancer Inst* 1995;87:645–651.

219. Fornander T, Hellstrom A-C, Moberger B. Descriptive clinicopathological study of 17 patients with endometrial cancer during or after adjuvant tamoxifen in early breast cancer. *J Natl Cancer Inst* 1993;85:1850–1855.

220. Andersson M, Storm HH, Mouridsen HT. Incidence of new primary cancers after adjuvant tamoxifen therapy and radiotherapy for early breast cancer. *J Natl Cancer Inst* 1991;83:1013–1017.

221. Fisher B, Costantino JP, Redmond CK, et al. Endometrial cancer in tamoxifen-treated breast cancer patients: findings from the National Surgical Adjuvant Breast and Bowel Project (NSABP) B-14. *J Natl Cancer Inst* 1994;86:527–537.

222. Cook LS, Weiss NS, Schwartz SM, et al. Population-based study of tamoxifen therapy and subsequent ovarian, endometrial, and breast cancers. *J Natl Cancer Inst* 1995;87:1359–1364.

223. van Leeuwen FE, Benraadt J, Coebergh JW, et al. Risk of endometrial cancer after tamoxifen treatment of breast cancer. *Lancet* 1994;343:448–452.

224. Vogel VG, Lippman SM, Boyd N. Is breast cancer preventable? *Can J Oncol* 1991;1:28–37.

225. Torrisi R, Pensa F, Orengo, MA, et al. The synthetic retinoid fenretinide lowers plasma insulin-like growth factor I levels in breast cancer patients. *Cancer Res* 1993;53:4769–4771.

226. Spicer DV, Pike MC. Breast cancer prevention through modulation of endogenous hormones. *Breast Cancer Res Treat* 1993;28:179–193.

227. Battersby A, Anderson TJ. Proliferative and secretory activity in the pregnant and lactating human breast. *Virchows Arch A Pathol Anat Histopathol* 1988;413:189–196.

228. Pike MC. Age-related factors in cancers of the breast, ovary, and endometrium. *J Chronic Dis* 1987;40(suppl):59s–69s.

229. Vogel VG. Early detection, epidemiology, and prevention of breast cancer. *Curr Opin Oncol* 1992;4:1017–1026.

230. Lee HP, Gaurley L, Duffy SW, et al. Dietary effects on breast cancer risks in Singapore. *Lancet* 1991;337:1197–1200.

231. Sporn MB. Carcinogenesis and cancer: different perspectives on the same disease. *Cancer Res* 1991;51:6215–6218.

232. Lippman SM, Benner SE, Hong WK. Cancer chemoprevention. *J Clin Oncol* 1994;12:851–873.

233. Costa A, Formelli F, Chiesa F, et al. Prospects of chemoprevention of human cancers with the synthetic retinoid fenretinide. *Cancer Res* 1994;54:2032s–2037s.

234. Ratco TA, Detrisac CJ, Dinger NM, et al. Chemopreventive efficacy of combined retinoid and tamoxifen treatment following surgical excision of a primary cancer in female rats. *Cancer Res* 1989;49:4472–4476.

235. Rossouw J, Finnegan L, Pottern L, et al. The evolution of the Women's Health Initiative: perspectives from the NIH. *J Am Med Wom Assoc* 1995;150:50–55.

CHAPTER 4

Controversies in Breast Cancer Screening Guidelines

LARS-GUNNAR LARSSON

*I*n parts of the world with a Western lifestyle, such as the United States, Canada, Europe, Australia, and New Zealand, breast cancer is very common and constitutes 20% to 30% of all incident cancers in women. In these regions, breast cancer is usually also the most frequent cause of cancer death among women. In the United States, where lung cancer during recent years has replaced breast cancer as the leading cause of cancer-related death, breast cancer is still—because of its age distribution—the malignancy that causes the most lost woman-years of life. In the regions mentioned above, about 1 woman in 10 will develop breast cancer during her lifetime, and the disease is sufficiently common to be felt as a real threat by most women.

Many risk factors for the development of breast cancer are known but none of them has a character that at present makes general, primary preventive measures possible. Therefore, much interest during the past decades has focused on methods for early detection and treatment, with the aim of preventing metastatic, lethal cancer. This chapter discusses the three methods of mass breast cancer screening in widespread use at this time: breast self-examination (BSE), clinical breast examination (CBE), and mammography. Other available detection methods either are not sensitive or specific enough (e.g., thermography, diaphanoscopy, and ultrasonography) or are too complicated and expensive (e.g., computed tomography and magnetic resonance imaging) to be used for mass breast cancer screening,

even if they may have some potential as supplemental diagnostic tools in clinical situations.

Breast Self-Examination

In the absence of screening, more than 90% of breast cancers are detected by women themselves through the incidental finding of a lump or irregularity in the breast parenchyma. It is natural to assume that increased awareness among women may lead to earlier diagnosis and increased curability of breast cancer. Programs promoting BSE have been developed in many countries. The information on BSE is disseminated by cancer societies and health authorities. Written information is usually in the form of pamphlets. BSE campaigns will probably be most efficient if this written information is supplemented by practical training in BSE given during visits to physicians' offices, through courses at places of work, and so on.

Many studies on BSE have been reported (1). Most concern compliance rates in relation to mode of instruction, age, education, social and economic factors, and other variables. Even after intensive education, the general rate of compliance with regular monthly BSE seems to be rather low and is seldom higher than 50%.

Two studies deserve special comment as they tried to show whether screening with BSE really reduces the breast cancer mortality rate. The UK Trial of Early Detection of Breast Cancer, which was set up in 1979, used a semi-experimental approach by comparing breast cancer mortality in three regions: one where women were invited to undergo annual CBE and biannual mammography, one where women received intensive education in BSE, and one control region without a screening program. After a follow-up of about 10 years, no difference in the breast cancer mortality rate was found between the BSE and the control regions (2). In Finland, a very ambitious BSE education program was conducted between 1973 and 1975 (3). A cohort study was performed some years later of women who had returned self-administered calendars recording their practice of BSE over a 2-year period. Compared with the general Finnish population, the cohort had a 25% lower breast cancer mortality rate (3). However, because of possible selection bias (only women who returned calendars were included in the cohort), no definite conclusions could be drawn from this observation.

Even though there is at present no scientifically solid evidence that BSE reduces the breast cancer mortality rate, it seems very likely that BSE in some women prevents lethal disease. BSE is an inexpensive measure, and it can be repeated at short intervals; these are good reasons to promote the general use of BSE in women older than 40 years.

Clinical Breast Examination

Breast cancer is only rarely an incidental finding at routine clinical examination. Nevertheless, all clinicians should be well acquainted with the technique of CBE, and CBE should be included in routine physical examinations, especially of women older than 40. Including CBE in the physical examination also gives the physician an opportunity to instruct the patient in BSE.

During the 1950s and 1960s, some screening trials with CBE were performed. However, CBE is a very inefficient screening instrument. Even though the cumulative incidence of breast cancer over an extended period of time is quite high, the prevalence of palpable cancer at a given time is very low. In the middle of the 1960s, a population-based study of screening with CBE was performed in Malmö, Sweden (4). The results were disappointing. In women 40 to 70 years old, breast cancer was detected in only 2.1 per 1000 women at the first screening and 1.2 per 1000 women at rescreening

17 months later. The rate of benign lesions detected was more than 10 times as high, and a large number of diagnostic biopsies had to be performed. The conclusion was that screening with CBE was inefficient and would create huge practical problems.

In many screening programs, a combination of mammography and CBE is used as the primary screening instrument. This is discussed further in the next section on mammography. Neither BSE nor CBE can replace mammography in screening for breast cancer, but both can serve as supplements to mammography.

Mammography

The superiority of mammography among breast cancer screening methods lies in its ability to detect nonpalpable early cancer and precancerous lesions (cancer in situ). Mammography uses low-voltage x-rays, which in combination with compression of the breast makes it possible to image the soft tissues in great detail. Although mammography was developed already during the 1930s, it was not until the beginning of the 1960s that mammography's capacity to detect subclinical cancers—and thereby its potential for screening—was recognized (5). Once these benefits were recognized, some centers in the United States and Europe began to use mammography for screening. A large number of more or less systematic studies of screening mammography have been reported to date. Most interesting of these are the randomized trials that try to elucidate the effect of screening on breast cancer mortality rates. Both randomized and nonrandomized studies of mammography have also greatly contributed to the knowledge of the biology of early breast cancer.

To judge from the Swedish experience, the first screening (the "prevalence screening") of an unselected group of previously unscreened women aged 40 to 69, usually reveals four to six invasive cancers and one to two cancers in situ per 1000 women examined. About half of the cancers are subclinical, and the distribution of pathologic stages is clearly shifted toward more early stages compared with the stage distribution for spontaneously detected cancers (6). The cancer detection rate increases with age from about 1.5 per 10,000 women screened in the age group 40 to 44 years to about 10 per 10,000 women screened in the age group 65 to

69 years. At rescreening of the same population 2 years later, the breast cancer detection rate is usually about the same as at the prevalence screening; the majority of detected cancers are now subclinical, and the shift in the stage distribution toward early pathologic stages is even more pronounced than at the prevalence screening. A small number of cancers will always appear between screening rounds. These so-called interval cancers tend to have a stage distribution rather similar to that for spontaneously detected cancers.

Randomized Trials

Early cancers detected by screening seem to have a good prognosis, to judge from survival curves. However, this is not sufficient proof of a benefit from screening. One reason is *lead-time bias*, which refers to the fact that if detection by screening is pushed back in time, then measurement of survival can spuriously suggest a benefit. A second reason is *length-biased sampling*, which concerns the fact that screening preferably selects less malignant, slowly growing tumors that have a long preclinical stage.

To study whether screening really reduces breast cancer mortality rates, the Health Insurance Plan of Greater New York trial was started in 1963 (the "HIP trial"). From the insurance register, 31,000 women aged 40 to 64 were randomly selected and invited to undergo screening with mammography and CBE, repeated yearly for 4 consecutive years. This group was compared with a control group of similar size and composition. Only 65% of invited women participated. After 9 years of observation, the breast cancer mortality rate was about 30% lower in the invited group than in the control group, a statistically significant difference (7). The effect was confined to women 50 years or older; there was no benefit for women aged 40 to 49 years. However, results after 18 years of follow-up indicated a similar reduction in the breast cancer mortality rate of about 25% for women younger than as well as older than 50 (8).

In Europe, the development of screening mammography was influenced by studies conducted in Sweden during the 1970s. In 1977, after two pilot studies (9,10) had shown that mammography alone with one oblique projection could be used as an effective and inexpensive primary screening instrument,

Sweden's National Board of Health and Welfare initiated a population-based randomized study (the "two-county trial") of screening mammography. Women aged 40 or older were invited to undergo periodic screening with one-projection mammography repeated at 2- to 2.5-year intervals. After an observation time of 7 years, a significant reduction of about 30% in the breast cancer mortality rate was observed among women who were 40 to 74 years old at the time of randomization (11). Similar to the reports of the HIP trial, the early reports found no benefit in women aged 40 to 49 at the time of invitation, but prolonged observation revealed a small but not statistically significant mortality benefit in this age group (12). In addition to the two-county trial, three more randomized trials of screening mammography were started in Sweden between 1976 and 1981 in Malmö (13), Stockholm (14), and Gothenburg.

As the four Swedish randomized trials had a rather similar design, pooled analyses of these trials have been performed to obtain more precise risk estimates and allow statistically more meaningful stratification into age groups. These analyses included about 157,000 women in the invited group and about 126,000 in the control group, with attendance rates varying between 74% and 89% in the different trials. The first published results of this overview (15,16,17) showed that after an observation period of 6 to 12 years, among women in the invited group, there was a statistically significant reduction of approximately 30% in the breast cancer mortality rate in the 50 to 69 age group while the reduction in the breast cancer mortality rate in the 40 to 49 age group was small and statistically not significant. A further analysis after 4 more years of observation, however, showed an almost statistically significant reduction of approximately 20% in the breast cancer mortality rate in women who were 40 to 49 years old at the time of invitation (18,19).

Randomized trials of screening mammography have also been performed in the United Kingdom (Edinburgh) and Canada. The Edinburgh trial, started in 1978, recruited women 45 to 65 years old and included annual CBE plus biannual mammography. After 10 years of observation, a 14% to 21% statistically nonsignificant reduction in the breast cancer mortality rate was found independent of age at the time of invitation (20).

The Canadian National Breast Screening Study (NBSS) recruited participants between

1980 and 1985. It included two separate randomized studies. In one study, NBSS 1, women aged 40 to 49 were randomly assigned to undergo either annual mammography plus CBE or only initial CBE. In the other trial, NBSS 2, annual mammography plus CBE was compared with annual CBE alone in women aged 50 to 59. After an observation period of about 7 years, none of these trials showed a difference in breast cancer mortality between the two compared groups (21,22). For the 40- to 49-year age group, this result is not surprising as no trial so far had shown a clear benefit of screening after such a short follow-up. More puzzling is the result in the 50- to 59-year age group, in which one would expect an obvious benefit of mammography after 7 years. The selection caused by the design of the studies—actually only a minority of the invited women participated in the trials—may also have reduced the possibility of positive result (23–25). Results after longer follow-up will, however, be interesting to follow.

With regard to the collective evidence, there is little doubt at present that screening with mammography or mammography plus CBE in women aged 50 to 69 reduces the breast cancer mortality rate by about 30% within the first 7–10 years of observation (26). The results reported in the randomized trials are dominated by the prevalence screening and the first few rescreenings; the effect of periodic screening over a long time has been impossible to study. In the HIP trial, the systematic screening in the study group was limited to the first 4 years, and in the Swedish trials, the control groups were invited to undergo screening some years after the time of randomization. It seems likely, however, that the real, long-term reduction in the breast cancer mortality rate in women who start screening at age 50 is at least on the order of 30%.

Some Nonrandomized Studies

The largest systematic but not randomized study of screening mammography is the Breast Cancer Detection Demonstration Project (BCDDP) in the United States, which started in 1973 and recruited more than a quarter of a million women aged 35 to 74 years. The participants were screened on an annual basis using a combination of medical history, CBE, mammography, and until 1977, thermography. The participants were also taught BSE and advised to perform it monthly. Several reports from this project gave information on cancer detection rates in women according to age, mode of detection, stage distribution of detected cancers, and survival according to stage (27,28). Survival curves from this study strongly support the concept that breast cancer detected early by screening mammography really is a curable disease even if the possibility of lead-time bias and length-biased sampling means that the studies cannot prove that screening really causes a reduction in breast cancer mortality.

Several nonrandomized, population-based studies have been reported from Europe. The most well known are the DOM (Diagnostisch Onderzoek Mammacarcinoom) and Nijmegen projects in the Netherlands (29,30) and the Florence project in Italy (31), which provided valuable information on interval cancers and early indicators of screening efficacy (32–34). The DOM and Florence projects also conducted case-control studies within the invited populations. These studies seemed to show that screening reduced the risk of dying of breast cancer by 50% to 70% (31,35). However, it has later been shown that this type of analysis has a serious bias, as women not complying with screening ("refusers") a priori represent a high-risk group.

Questions Related to Screening Mammography

In the following sections, some special questions related to screening mammography are discussed.

Mammography in Women Aged 40 to 49 Years

The great controversy at present concerns the age group 40 to 49. Early results from the randomized trials failed to show a reduction in the breast cancer mortality rate in this group. However, prolonged follow-up of the pooled data from the Swedish trials suggested a benefit on the order of 20%. Similar results were obtained by a meta-analysis of all randomized controlled trials of screening mammography (36). The present knowledge is summarized in Table 4-1. Some of the reported benefits have no doubt been caused by continued screening after age 50, but the magnitude of this influence is at present unknown (37–39).

None of the trials reported so far were specifically designed to answer the question of whether it is more beneficial to start screening

T A B L E   **4-1**

Relative Risks of Dying of Breast Cancer (Invited Group Versus Control Group) in the Age Group 40 to 49: Results of Randomized Trials

Trial	Relative Risk	95% Confidence Interval
Health Insurance Plan	0.77	0.55–1.11
Malmö	0.67	0.35–1.27
Kopparberg*	0.67	0.37–1.22
Ostergötland*	1.02	0.59–1.77
Stockholm	1.08	0.54–2.17
Gothenburg	0.59	0.33–1.06
Edinburgh	0.73	0.43–1.25
Canadian National Breast Screening Study (NBSS) 1	1.10	0.79–1.54
Pooled Swedish rials	0.77	0.59–1.01
Meta-analysis, all trials	0.85	0.71–1.01
Meta-analysis, all trials (except NBSS 1)	0.76	0.62–0.93

† Kopparberg and Ostergötland are the two counties in the "two-county trial."

Sources: Falun meeting on breast cancer screening with mammography in women aged 40–49 years: report of the organizing committee and collaborators. Int J Cancer 1996;64:693–699. Smart CR, Hendrick RE, Rutledge JH, Smith RA. Benefit of mammography screening in women aged 40–49 years—current evidence from randomized controlled trials. *Cancer* 1995;75:1619–26.

around age 40 than at age 50. Some years ago, a trial was started in the United Kingdom to compare women invited to undergo annual mammography screening at ages 40 to 41 with a control group not invited until age 50. Under the auspices of the International Union Against Cancer and with the support of the National Cancer Institute of the United States, an extended inter-European trial with similar design ["Eurotrial 40" (40)] is planned at present. If this trial is realized, the combined United Kingdom and European trials will contain 150,000 women in the invited group and 300,000 in the control group, and the first mortality analyses will be possible around the year 2010.

In Sweden, a huge amount of information on screening mammography has accumulated since the middle of the 1980s. At present, all Swedish counties actively invite women to periodic screening with mammography, and the compliance rate is high. As about half of the counties use 40 years as the lower age limit and the other half use 50 years, and as the counties started screening at different times, there are opportunities for retrospective comparative cohort studies that may elucidate the effect of different starting ages. Such studies are planned at present.

However, the problem with the age group 40 to 49 goes beyond demonstrating a significant reduction in breast cancer mortality rates. The low prevalence of mammographically detectable cancer in this age group makes the mortality gain in absolute terms small even if a relative benefit can be demonstrated. Mammography seems also to detect breast cancer less efficiently in the age group 40 to 49 than in older women. One would expect the ratio between the detection rate and the annual incidence rate registered in the region before screening began to be more or less constant regardless of age. However, this is not the case. At prevalence screenings in Sweden, this ratio has as a rule been 1 to 2 in the age group 40 to 49 compared with 3 or more in the older age groups. One reason for this trend is certainly that the dense parenchyma in the premenopausal breast makes the cancers less easy to detect. Another cause could be that breast cancers in women aged 40 to 49 on average grow more rapidly and therefore are more difficult to detect early by screening (41,42).

Another area of concern in the age group 40 to 49 is that the rate of mammographically uncertain findings requiring supplementary examinations and biopsies is rather high in relation to the cancer detection rate (6,43). In the Stockholm trial (43), which invited women aged 40 to 65, it was calculated that false-positive findings in the first screening round resulted in a cost of around $1 million per 100,000 women screened and that about 40% of this cost was associated with examinations performed in women younger than 50. Even more important is, of course, the anxiety caused among the women concerned, especially as it often took considerable time before cancer could be regarded as excluded. At present, many believe that screening before age 50 does more harm than good.

Mammography Alone Versus Mammography Plus Clinical Breast Examination

In the United States and Canada, screening consists of mammography plus CBE, while in Sweden and some other European countries, mammography alone is used as the primary screening instrument. An argument for CBE is that some palpable cancers (~5%) are not detected by mammography. This is especially common for lobular carcinomas. The advantages of using mammography alone as the primary screening instrument are the considerably lower costs and the sharp demarcation obtained between the screening procedure and the clinical situation. The results can be illustrated by a screening program in a Swedish county (6) of women aged 40 to 69. The attendance rate was 87% at the first screening and 78% at the second screening. Of 1000 women at the first screening, 46 were recalled for supplementary mammography; only 9 of these were referred for clinical examination and biopsy. Five of these women had cancer as demonstrated by histologic examination. The figures found at rescreening 2 years later were very similar.

Active Invitation Versus General Recommendations

In many countries, including the United States, the impetus for screening comes mainly from general recommendations issued by health authorities, cancer societies, and specialist organizations; women are not actively invited to undergo mammography. Whether a woman undergoes screening then becomes largely dependent on her own initiative and responsibility. The problem with this approach is the generally low attendance rate, usually below 50%, and the great dependence on factors such as education, social class, income, and geographic location. Active invitation of women in concerned age groups is much more effective, producing attendance rates usually on the order of 70% to 90%.

Interval Between Screening Rounds

All screening is based on periodic examinations; this is necessary for a quantitative effect. The optimal interval between consecutive screenings is not known but ongoing randomized studies in the United Kingdom and Finland are comparing different screening intervals. Current recommendations are mainly based on the experience with so-called interval cancers. There is general agreement that the interval between consecutive screening rounds should not be shorter than 1 year and not longer than 3 years. Indications that breast cancers in younger women (40–49 years) may grow more rapidly (41,42) speak in favor of annual screening in this age group.

Type of Mammography

Since the 1960s, when the HIP trial was started, considerable technical developments in mammography have led to reductions in the radiation dose and improvements in the quality of the image. This progress has been made possible by the development of special machines that generate optimal low-energy x-rays, special devices for compression of the breast, more sensitive films, and intensifying screens and grids. The importance of mammography quality assurance programs has been recognized in all countries with screening programs, and in addition to monitoring the quality of mammography equipment, countries can monitor medical parameters such as cancer detection rates and rates of recall for supplementary mammography, CBE, or biopsy to determine the efficacy of screening programs. Mammography has essentially become a subspecialty of radiology, and radiologists who practice mammography are usually required to complete special training programs and courses.

Unlike clinical mammography, which is done using three projections (mediolateral, craniocaudal, and mediolateral oblique), screening mammography uses one projection (mediolateral oblique) or two projections (mediolateral oblique and craniocaudal). There seem to be negligible differences between one- and two-projection screening mammography with regard to the cancer detection rate, but two-projection mammography reduces the rate of recall for supplementary mammography (44) and is therefore now generally preferred, especially in younger women. Independent reading of the mammograms by two radiologists has often been recommended and in one systematic study increased the cancer detection rate by 15% (45).

Radiation Risks

The radiation risks of mammography have been much discussed. That ionizing radiation can cause breast cancer is well known from epidemiologic analyses of atomic bomb survivors and cohorts of women exposed to ionizing radiation for medical reasons (46). As a rule, the doses that have induced breast cancer have been higher than 0.5 Gy, but theoretical risks of lower doses can be calculated by linear extrapolation. During the 1960s, when mammography was first used for screening, the doses were relatively high (50 mGy or more) and even though the theoretical risk of breast cancer induction was low, this theoretical risk caused concern about mass screening with mammography and frightened many women away from participation in screening programs. Owing to technical developments, radiation doses have decreased dramatically and at present are ideally about 4 mGy for two-projection mammography. In practice, a dose of 5 to 10 mGy per screening seems more realistic as the conditions are not always ideal and as some women are recalled for supplementary mammography. The theoretical risk of radiation-induced breast cancer after such low doses is very low in absolute terms. However, because mammography is an intervention performed in a population without known disease, the risk must be weighed against the assumed benefit. The benefit-risk ratio can be expressed as "years of life saved by screening detection of breast cancer"/"years of life lost because of radiation-induced breast cancer." Estimates of this ratio are complicated by the fact that different epidemiologic materials lead to rather different risk assumptions. Other complications for the theoretical risk calculations are the accumulation of the radiation dose over time and the latency time for radiation-induced cancer. Even with the most pessimistic risk assumptions it is, however, obvious that the benefit to risk ratio is very high for women who start screening at age 50 or later. Due to the still somewhat uncertain benefit of screening in women between 40 and 50 the radiation risk may still be an argument, but probably not a very strong one, against mammography screening in this age group.

Specific High-Risk Groups

Some groups of women have an exceptionally high risk of breast cancer. One group is, of course, women operated on for breast cancer. Such women have a high risk of developing a new cancer in the contralateral breast and, after breast-conserving treatment, a new cancer or recurrence in the ipsilateral breast. Another group consists of women operated on for benign breast lesions with proliferative, atypical epithelial changes or cancer in situ. The mentioned groups are usually followed with CBE two to three times per year and mammography annually regardless of age.

Women with a genetic predisposition to breast cancer constitute another high-risk group. During recent years, mutations in specific genes (*BRCA1*, *BRCA2*, and others) were found in women with hereditary breast cancer and also in healthy women from families with high rates of breast cancer (47). The latter women have an exceptionally high risk of developing breast cancer, often at a remarkably young age. If bilateral mastectomy is not performed, these women may require close surveillance with mammography, CBE, and other screening methods such as ultrasonography and magnetic resonance imaging. However, little is known at present about the effectiveness of such surveillance.

Older Women

Mammographic screening in women older than 70 is so far insufficiently studied. Of the randomized studies to date, only the two-county trial had no upper age limit for invited women and because of a low compliance rate among the oldest women, only the age group 70 to 74 has been included in the mortality analyses. The reduction in the breast cancer mortality rate in this age group seemed to be insignificant, but these results have little relevance because the group was small and screening in women older than 70 was terminated after the second screening round (15). In a separate report from the two-county trial (48), a significant reduction in the breast cancer mortality rate of 32% was found in women who were 65 to 74 years old at the time of randomization. However, it is not known to what degree this benefit derived from women older than 70. Several studies have shown that the cancer detection rate is high and the rate of false-positive findings is low in old women; the fatty, unstructured breast in these women seems to be an ideal object for mammography (6,10,48).

Some have argued against screening in older women, citing the opinion that breast cancer is not as lethal in older women as in younger women and also referring to the relatively short normal life expectancy in the elderly. The first assumption does not seem to be true: Several studies showed that the relative survival for elderly breast cancer patients is worse than that for younger ones (49,50). Concerning the second argument, women between 70 and 80 years old without breast cancer now have an expected survival of 15 to 10 years. There are certainly good reasons to focus more interest on screening in elderly women—perhaps especially those between 70 and 75 years old.

Cost-Benefit Considerations

Several cost-benefit calculations have been reported on the basis of experience from the randomized trials. For the age group 50 to 69, the cost per year of life saved has been calculated to be $3000 to $5000 in Europe (51); similar calculations in the United States (52) revealed costs on the order of $15,000 to $30,000. The higher calculated costs in the United States are due to annual instead of biannual screening, more expensive mammography, compulsory CBE, and a higher biopsy rate. For the age group 40 to 49, all calculations are very uncertain because the reduction in the mortality rate is still unclear. Assuming, however, a reduction in the breast cancer mortality rate of 20%, the cost in the United States has been calculated to be $40,000 to $50,000 per year of life saved (53).

On the whole, the cost-benefit analyses suggest that the costs of breast cancer screening are reasonable compared with costs of other life-saving measures such as kidney and heart transplantations and some radical treatment for symptomatic cancer.

Screening Guidelines in Different Countries

Most developed countries with a high incidence of breast cancer have issued more or less official guidelines on screening for breast cancer. In 1983, the American Cancer Society (ACS) in cooperation with the National Cancer Institute (NCI) presented such guidelines. They recommended monthly BSE for all women older than 20, CBE every 3 years between ages 20 and 40, annual CBE after age 40, and mammography every 1 to 2 years between ages 40 and 50 and annually after age 50. In 1993, after an international workshop (54), NCI omitted the recommendations for screening with CBE and mammography in women younger than 50. However, as a result of a new conference in January 1997 (55) both NCI and ACS now recommend annual mammography starting at age 40.

In Sweden, the National Board of Health and Welfare in 1986 issued recommendations to the county councils (which are responsible for the health service) on active invitation to screening mammography. The Board recommended that counties use a lower age limit not below 40 and not over 50 and an upper age limit of 75. For women younger than 55, screening every 18 months was recommended; for women older than 55, biannual screening was recommended. In 1989, the Board recommended that in case of scarce resources, women aged 50 to 69 should be given priority. As a result, the whole country is at present covered by screening programs with 40 as the lower age limit in about half of the counties. At present, a revision of the 1986 guidelines is being prepared within the National Board of Health and Welfare.

Systems similar to the Swedish one, which is based on active invitation, have been introduced in the United Kingdom, Finland, the Netherlands, and Iceland, but with 50 years as the lower age limit. In the cancer control program of the European Union, mammographic screening is given high priority and strongly recommended for all women aged 50 to 69.

Some Concluding Remarks

At present, there is almost universal consensus concerning the value of mammographic screening in women aged 50 to 69. Besides reducing the breast cancer mortality rate, screening also increases the possibility of breast-conserving treatment and reduces the need for adjuvant endocrine or cytotoxic treatment.

Screening in women younger than 50 is still controversial, even if there are some indications that screening in the age group 40 to 49 reduces the relative breast cancer mortality rate. The evidence, however, is not too convincing, especially as some part of the registered benefit certainly derives from continued screening after age 50. On the debit side is a high rate of uncertain findings in relation to the rate of detected cancers. More knowledge of the effect of screening on breast cancer mortality rates in this age group can probably be obtained by retrospective epidemiologic analyses of the large body of data from the Swedish service screening. The ongoing UK trial and the planned Eurotrial (40) may ultimately answer the question of whether it is beneficial to start screening at age 40 instead of age 50, but answers will not be available until around the year 2010.

A reasonable compromise at present could be to start screening at age 45. The prevalence of detectable cancer before this age is very low, and the benefit, if any, of screening in age 40–44 must be marginal and can hardly outweigh the negative side effects. More attention should be focused on women older than 70, especially those aged 70 to 74, in whom considerable benefit can be expected. In countries without active invitation to screening, much could be gained by efforts to increase the compliance rate in screening programs, which at present is low among some categories of women.

A woman attending screening usually regards it as a means of either excluding breast cancer or detecting a cancer that can be easily cured but that if not detected by screening might have killed her. This is of course a great simplification of the reality. All women who participate in screening should be informed about some simple principles of the procedure. They should thus know that an essential benefit can be obtained only by repeated screenings at regular intervals. They should also know that screening can never detect all breast cancers and, of course, not prevent the development of cancer later on. Finally, they should be aware of the considerable probability of uncertain results, which may cause anxiety and inconvenience in the form of supplemental examinations and biopsies.

In a way, screening for early detection of breast cancer is a medical anomaly that converts many perfectly healthy women into patients. However, until acceptable primary preventive methods are found, screening will probably continue to be the most effective way to reduce the consequences of breast cancer.

REFERENCES

1. Baines CJ. Breast self-examination. *Cancer* 1992;69(suppl 7):1942–1946.
2. UK Trial of Early Detection of Breast Cancer Group. Breast cancer mortality after 10 years in the UK trial of early detection of breast cancer. *Breast* 1993;2:13–20.
3. Gastrin G, Miller AB, To T, et al. Incidence and mortality from breast cancer in the Mama program for breast screening in Finland, 1973–1986. *Cancer* 1994;73:2168–2174.
4. Langeland P. Population screening for female breast tumours. A clinical investigation. *Acta Radiol Suppl* 297;1970.
5. Egan RL. Experience with mammography in a tumor institution. Evaluation of 1000 studies. *Radiology* 1960;75:894–900.
6. Thurfjell EL, Lindgren JA. Population-based mammography screening in Swedish clinical practice: prevalence and incidence screening in Uppsala county. *Radiology* 1994;193:351–357.
7. Shapiro S. Evidence on screening for breast cancer from a randomized trial. *Cancer* 1977;39:2772–2782.
8. Shapiro S. Determining the efficacy of breast cancer screening. In: Fortner JG, Rhoads JE, eds. *Accomplishments in cancer research.* Philadelphia: JB Lippincott, 1989:61–74.
9. Jakobsson S, Lundgren B, Melander O, Norin T. Mass-screening of a female population for detection of early carcinoma of the breast. *Acta Radiol* 1975;14:424–432.
10. Lundgren B, Jakobsson S. Single view mammography. A simple and efficient approach to breast cancer screening. *Cancer* 1976;38:1124–1129.
11. Tabar L, Fagerberg CJG, Gad A, et al. Reduction in mortality from breast cancer after mass screening with mammography. *Lancet* 1985;1:829–832.
12. Tabar L, Fagerbert G, Chen HH, et al. Screening for breast cancer in women aged under 50: mode of detection, incidence, fatality and histology. *J Med Screen* 1995;2:94–98.
13. Andersson J, Aspegren K, Janzon L, et al. Mammographic screening and mortality from

breast cancer: the Malmö mammographic screening trial. *BMJ* 1988;297:943–948.

14. Frisell J, Lidbrink E, Hellström L, Rutqvist LE. Follow-up after 11 years. Update of mortality results in the Stockholm mammographic screening trial. In: Lidbrink E. Mammographic screening for breast cancer. Aspects on benefit and risks (dissertation). Stockholm: Karolinska Institute, 1995.

15. Nyström L, Rutqvist LE, Wall S, et al. Breast cancer screening with mammography: overview of Swedish randomised trials. *Lancet* 1993;341: 973–978.

16. Nyström L, Larsson LG, Rutqvist LE, et al. Determination of cause of death among breast cancer cases in the Swedish randomized mammography screening trials. A comparison between official statistics and validation by an endpoint committee. *Acta Oncol* 1995;34:145–152.

17. Larsson LG, Nyström L, Wall S, et al. The Swedish randomised mammography screening trials: analysis of their effect on the breast cancer related excess mortality. *J Med Screen* 1996;3: 129–132.

18. Falun meeting on breast cancer screening with mammography in women aged 40–49 years: report of the organising committee and collaborators. *Int J Cancer* 1996;64:693–699.

19. Larsson LG, Andersson I, Bjurstam N, et al. Updated overview of the Swedish randomized trials on breast cancer screening with mammography: age group 40–49 at randomization. *JNCI* 1997; monograph No. 22:57–61.

20. Alexander FE, Anderson TJ, Brown HK, et al. The Edinburgh randomised trial of breast cancer screening: results of 10 years of follow-up. *Br J Cancer* 1994;70:542–548.

21. Miller AB, Baines CJ, To T, Wall C. Canadian National Breast Screening Study #1. Breast cancer detection and death rates among women aged 40 to 49 years. *Can Med Assoc J* 1992;147: 1459–1476.

22. Miller AB, Baines CJ, To T, Wall C. Canadian National Breast Screening Study #2. Breast cancer detection and death rates among women aged 50 to 59 years. *Can Med Assoc J* 1992; 147:1477–1488.

23. Boyd NF, Jong RA, Yaffe MJ, et al. A critical appraisal of the Canadian National Breast Cancer Screening Study. *Radiology* 1993;189:661–663.

24. Tarone RE. The excess of patients with advanced breast cancer in young women screened with mammography in the Canadian National Breast Screening Study. *Cancer* 1995;75:997–1003.

25. Baines CJ. The Canadian National Breast Screening Study. *Ann Intern Med* 1994;120: 326–334.

26. Shapiro S. Screening: assessment of current studies. *Cancer* 1994;74:231–238.

27. Baker LH. Breast Cancer Detection Demonstration Project: five-year summary report. *CA Cancer J Clin* 1982;32:194–225.

28. Smart CR, Hartmann WH, Beahrs OH, Garfinkel L. Insights into breast cancer screening of younger women. *Cancer* 1993;72:1449–1456.

29. de Waard F, Collette HJA, Romback JJ, et al. The DOM project for the early detection of breast cancer, Utrecht, the Netherlands. *J Chronic Dis* 1984;37:1–44.

30. Peeters PHM, Verbeek ALM, Hendriks JHCL, van Bon MJH. Screening for breast cancer in Nijmegen. Report of 6 screening rounds, 1975–1986. *Int J Cancer* 1989;43:226–230.

31. Palli D, Del Turco MR, Buitti E, et al. A case-control study of the efficacy of a non-randomized breast cancer screening program in Florence (Italy). *Int J Cancer* 1986;38:501–504.

32. Peeters PHM, Verbeek ALM, Hendriks JHCL, et al. The occurrence of interval cancers in the Nijmegen screening programme. *Br J Cancer* 1989;59:929–932.

33. Paci E, Ciatto S, Buiatti E, et al. Early indicators of efficacy of breast cancer screening programmes. Results of the Florence district programme. *Int J Cancer* 1990;46:198–202.

34. Peer P, Holland R, Hendriks J, et al. Age-specific effectiveness of the Nijmegen population-based breast cancer-screening program: assessment of early indicators of screening effectiveness. *J Natl Cancer Inst* 1994;86:436–441.

35. Collette HJA, Day NE, Rombach JJ, de Waard F. Evaluation of screening for breast cancer in a non-randomised study (the DOM project) by means of a case-control study. *Lancet* 1984;1 2:1224–1226.

36. Smart CR, Hendrick RE, Rutledge JH, Smith RA. Benefit of mammography screening in women aged 40–49 years—current evidence from randomized controlled trials. *Cancer* 1995;75:1619–1626.

37. Shapiro S, Venet W, Strax P, et al. Ten- to fourteen-year effect of screening on breast cancer mortality. *J Natl Cancer Inst* 1982;60:349–355.

38. de Koning HJ, Boer R, Warmerdam PG, et al. Quantitative interpretation of age-specific mortality reductions from the Swedish breast cancer-screening trials. *J Natl Cancer Inst* 1995;87:1217–1223.

39. Tabar L, Duffy SW, Chen HH. Re: Quantitative interpretation of age-specific mortality reductions from the Swedish breast cancer-screening trials. *J Natl Cancer Inst* 1996;88:52–53.

40. *Eurotrial 40. A randomized population-based trial on the efficacy of screening mammography in women under 50. Study protocol.* Geneva, International Union Against Cancer, September 1995.

41. Peer P, van Dijck J, Hendriks J, et al. Age-dependent growth rate of primary breast cancer. *Cancer* 1993;71:3547–3551.

42. Tabar L, Fagerberg G, Chen HH, et al. Tumour development, histology and grade of breast cancers: prognosis and progression. *Int J Cancer* 1996;66:413–419.

43. Lidbrink E, Elfving J, Frisell J, Jonsson E. Neglected aspects of false positive findings of mammography in breast cancer screening: analyses of false positive cases from the Stockholm trial. *BMJ* 1996;312:273–312.

44. Thurfjell E, Taube A, Tabar L. One- versus two-view mammography screening. A prospective population-based study. *Acta Radiol* 1994;35:340–344.

45. Thurfjell E, Lernevall A, Taube A. Benefit of independent double reading in a population-based mammography screening program. *Radiology* 1994;191:241–244.

46. United Nations Scientific Committee on the Effects of Atomic Radiation. *1994 Report.* New York: United Nations, 1994.

47. Olsson H, Borg Å. Genetic pre-disposition to breast cancer. *Acta Oncol* 1996;35:1–8.

48. Chen HH, Tabar L, Fagerberg G, Duffy SW. Effect of breast cancer screening after age 65. *J Med Screen* 1995;2:10–14.

49. Adami HC, Malker B, Holmberg L, et al. The relationship between survival and age at diagnosis in breast cancer. *N Engl J Med* 1986;14:559–563.

50. Constanza ME. Breast cancer screening in older women. Synopsis of a forum. *Cancer* 1992;69 (suppl):1925–1931.

51. de Koning H, van Ineveld M, van Oortmarssen G, et al. Breast cancer screening and cost-effectiveness: policy alternatives, quality of life considerations and the possible impact of uncertain factors. *Int J Cancer* 1991;49:531–537.

52. Elixhauser A. Costs of breast cancer and the cost-effectiveness of breast cancer screening. *Int J Techol Assess Health Care* 1991;7:604–615.

53. Rosenquist CJ, Lindfors KK. Screening mammography in women aged 40–49 years: analysis of cost-effectiveness. *Radiology* 1994;191:647–650.

54. Fletcher SW, Black W, Harris R, et al. Report of the International Workshop on Screening for Breast Cancer. *J Natl Cancer Inst* 1993;85:1644–1656.

55. NIH consensus development conference on breast cancer screening for women ages 40–49. Jan 21–23, 1997. Program and abstracts. National Inst. Health, 1997.

CHAPTER 5

Indications and Techniques for Breast Biopsy

MONICA MORROW

*T*he most common clinical indications for breast biopsy are a dominant breast mass, pathologic nipple discharge, or an abnormal-appearing mammogram. The determination of what constitutes a dominant mass is frequently difficult, particularly in the premenopausal woman. The normal glandular tissue of the breast is nodular, and this nodularity is usually most pronounced in the upper outer quadrant of the breast and the inframammary ridge area. Such nodularity, particularly when it waxes and wanes during the menstrual cycle, is a physiologic process and is not an indication for breast biopsy. Breast nodularity is often accompanied by breast pain. Breast pain is an uncommon presenting symptom of breast carcinoma; fewer than 10% of patients with cancer have pain as an associated symptom. In the absence of clinical or mammographic evidence of a breast mass, breast pain should be managed nonoperatively. This is true even when the pain appears to be localized, because surgery, including radical surgical approaches such as mastectomy, is rarely successful in eradicating breast pain.

Dominant Masses

Dominant masses are characterized by their persistence throughout the menstrual cycle. They may be discrete or poorly defined, but differ in character from the surrounding breast tissue and the corresponding area in the contralateral breast. The differential diagnosis of dominant breast masses includes macrocysts, fibroadenoma, prominent areas of fibrocystic change, fat necrosis, and carcinoma. A dominant breast mass palpated in a premenopausal woman should be aspirated to determine if it is a cyst. Cysts are usually well demarcated from the surrounding breast tissue, and are somewhat mobile and firm. Cysts that are very full are often quite hard, and may be difficult to distinguish from solid masses by physical examination. Cysts require biopsy only if the aspirated fluid is bloody, the palpable abnormality does not resolve completely after the aspiration of fluid, or the same cyst recurs multiple times in a short time interval. The routine cytologic examination of cyst fluid is not indicated because of the low likelihood of carcinoma in the absence of the clinical findings just noted. In addition, the cytologic identification of atypical cells in cyst fluid is not uncommon, resulting in the clinical dilemma of a patient whose cyst resolves with aspiration, whose mammogram appears normal, and who has a cytology indicating the need for a biopsy. Ciatto et al (1) performed cytology on 6782 cyst fluid aspirates. Atypical cells were identified in 1677 and no cancers were identified. Five intracystic papillomas were found, but bloody fluid was present in all of these aspirates.

Cysts can occur at any age, but are particularly common in women in their 40s and those who are perimenopausal. In postmenopausal women who are not taking exogenous estrogen, cysts are uncommon and should be regarded with a higher degree of suspicion than in the premenopausal years. Aspiration is still an

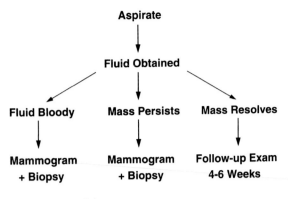

F I G U R E **5-1**

Algorithm for the evaluation and management of breast cysts.

appropriate first step, but a repeat examination 4 to 6 weeks after aspiration to check for recurrence of the cyst is essential. The algorithm for cyst management is summarized in Figure 5-1.

Noncystic masses in premenopausal women that are clearly different from the surrounding breast tissue should be evaluated by biopsy using one of the techniques described later in the chapter. Observation for one or two menstrual cycles is only appropriate for vague asymmetry or nodularity, when it is unclear that a dominant mass is present. A dominant breast mass should not be dismissed as a cyst unless the diagnosis is documented by sonography or aspiration.

In postmenopausal women, clinical examination of the breasts is frequently easier owing to atrophy of the nodular glandular elements. Benign breast problems causing palpable masses are less frequent in this age group, and carcinoma is more common; therefore, small areas of nodularity that might be observed in a premenopausal woman should be considered for prompt biopsy in a postmenopausal woman.

Nipple Discharge

Nipple discharge is a common complaint, but an uncommon sign of breast carcinoma. Three percent to 11% of women with carcinoma have an associated nipple discharge. The likelihood of a nipple discharge being secondary to malignancy increases with age. In one study, 32% of women over age 60 presenting with nipple discharge and no mass had carcinoma, compared

to 7% of women under age 60 with the same presentation (2). The initial step in the evaluation of nipple discharge is to determine whether it is physiologic or pathologic. Discharges are classified as pathologic if they are spontaneous, and localized to one duct. Pathologic discharges may be bloody or serous, and are almost always unilateral. In contrast, physiologic discharges occur only with nipple compression, frequently originate from multiple ducts, and are often bilateral. The clinical evaluation of a pathologic discharge should include testing the fluid for occult blood and identifying the quadrant of the breast from which the discharge originates. Although 70% to 85% of the discharges due to carcinoma contain blood (3), a nonbloody discharge that meets the other criteria of a pathologic discharge is an indication for a breast biopsy. Cytology is not usually useful in the evaluation of nipple discharge because the absence of malignant cells does not reliably exclude carcinoma, and positive cytologic findings will not differentiate between intraductal and invasive carcinoma.

As part of the evaluation of a pathologic discharge, a mammogram should be obtained to look for nonpalpable masses, calcifications, or dilated ducts. When a discharge occurs in association with a mass, the mass should be evaluated by biopsy. In the absence of a mass, a terminal duct excision should be performed. The role of galactography in the management of nipple discharge is controversial. Tabar et al (4) studied 116 women undergoing galactography for pathologic discharge. Ductal lesions were visualized in all women, but how this altered the surgical approach or avoided surgery is not clear. Galactography may be useful in identifying lesions in the periphery of the breast that would not be removed with a standard terminal duct excision, or in minimizing the amount of the ductal system that is removed in women of childbearing age. However, galactography does not provide a definitive diagnosis for intraductal lesions and does not obviate the need for histologic sampling in women with pathologic discharges.

Mammographic Abnormalities

In many surgical practices, a mammographic abnormality is one of the most frequent indications for breast biopsy. The initial clinical step in the evaluation of a mammographic abnormality is a careful physical examination. If there is any question about whether a palpable finding corresponds to a mammographically identified mass, a radiopaque marker should be placed on the abnormality and repeat mammographic views obtained. If the clinical and mammographic lesions correspond, the lesion can be approached as a palpable abnormality. If there is any doubt about this correspondence, a needle localization biopsy is the most prudent course.

The classic mammographic signs of clinically occult malignancy are clustered microcalcifications and small masses. A review of 5500 mammographically generated biopsies identified microcalcifications as the indication for biopsy in 45% of patients, masses in 43%, masses containing microcalcifications in 6%, and asymmetric density in 5% (5). The positive predictive value of most mammographic findings is low and cancer is identified in only 20% to 35% of biopsy specimens in most series (6–9). Special mammographic views are frequently helpful in the evaluation of equivocal findings on two-view mammography, and these views should be obtained prior to making a final determination of the need for biopsy. Morrow et al (9) studied 267 consecutive patients referred to a surgeon because of an abnormal-appearing mammogram. Sixty-seven percent of the group had an incomplete radiologic workup, and spot compression and magnification views were obtained before the need for biopsy was determined. After the additional evaluation, only 150 of the 267 abnormalities were found to be suspicious enough to warrant biopsy. Even when biopsy is clearly indicated on the basis of the initial mammogram, magnification views are useful in delineating the extent of the lesion.

Techniques of Breast Biopsy

Palpable Masses

Palpable breast masses can be diagnosed with fine-needle aspiration (FNA) biopsy, core cutting needle biopsy, excisional biopsy, or incisional biopsy. The accuracy, techniques, and advantages of each of these approaches are discussed.

Fine-Needle Aspiration

FNA is becoming increasingly popular for the diagnosis of dominant breast masses. Accuracy rates for FNA are high. A review of seven published reports of 4943 FNA procedures noted a sensitivity of 87%, and the incidence of insufficient specimens varied from 4% to 13% (10). Kline et al (11) reviewed 3545 breast aspirates and reported a 9.6% rate of false-negative results. In half of the false-negative cases the needle tract did not extend into the tumor. Other factors reported to be associated with false-negative aspirates include small tumor size, fibrotic tumors, and infiltrating lobular, tubular, and cribriform histologies (11–13). False-positive aspirates are extremely uncommon, being reported in fewer than 1% of cases in most large series (10–14).

FNA has the advantage of being quick, relatively painless, and inexpensive to perform. Results are available within 24 hours, and immediate interpretation of smears is often feasible. Since the diagnosis of malignancy by FNA is quite reliable, treatment options can be discussed with the patient and definitive surgery performed without the need for a biopsy. This approach avoids the problem of incorporating the biopsy incision in the definitive surgical resection. Aspirates that are interpreted as suspicious or atypical are an indication for a surgical biopsy. Insufficient specimens provide no useful information and are an indication for a repeat FNA or another type of biopsy. In one series (14), physician experience was the factor that correlated best with a low rate of insufficient specimens.

The major drawback to the use of FNA in many institutions is the lack of an experienced cytopathologist. In addition, FNA will not reliably distinguish invasive from intraductal carcinoma, potentially leading to the overtreatment of gross ductal carcinoma in situ, and FNA provides no histologic detail such as the presence of an extensive intraductal component associated with the invasive cancer, which might influence the extent of a lumpectomy.

The major controversy surrounding the use of FNA is the management of the dominant mass with a benign aspirate. The so-called triple test uses physical examination, mammography, and FNA in an attempt to avoid surgical biopsy of benign breast lesions. When all three of these modalities indicate benign disease, the chance of carcinoma being present is 0.6% according to one review (15). However, Bell et al (16) noted a 3.4% incidence of carcinoma in 285 women for whom the results of the triple test were negative. When one considers observation of a dominant mass in the setting of negative triple test results, all elements of the triple test must be evaluable. The extremely low incidence of malignancy cited above does not apply in patients in whom the mass is not visible on the mammogram, or those with an insufficient cytologic aspirate. In addition, the accuracy of a clinical or mammographic diagnosis of a benign lesion is lowest in young women, the group in whom biopsy is most likely to be omitted. If a dominant mass is to be observed, a defined follow-up plan must be established to allow for the early detection of missed cancers. The use of FNA in the evaluation of solid masses is summarized in Figure 5-2.

Technique The breast mass is fixed in the operator's nondominant hand and the skin is cleansed with antiseptic. A small amount of 1% lidocaine is used to anesthetize the skin at the puncture site. Needles varying in size from 21 to 27 gauge have been used for FNA. The use of a syringe holder, which aids in creating a vacuum for aspiration, is preferred although a standard syringe can also be used. The needle is inserted into the mass, and when firm tissue is encountered, suction is applied from the syringe. The needle is moved back and forth within the tumor to facilitate dislodging cells. When aspirated material is visible in the hub of the needle, a satisfactory specimen has usually been obtained. In order to minimize the number of insufficient specimens, a second aspirate is

obtained through the same skin puncture site. Depending on the preference of the cytologist, the aspirated material is smeared onto microscope slides or placed into a fixative for cell block preparation.

There are no real contraindications to aspiration cytology. The procedure may be done in anticoagulated patients as long as firm pressure is applied to the site at the completion of the aspiration. Mammography done within 2 weeks of an FNA may result in false-positive readings due to hematoma obscuring the regular contours of benign breast masses (17). The most common complication of FNA is bruising. Pneumothorax has been reported after the procedure, but is very rare. This complication can be prevented by avoiding a direct perpendicular approach to lesions deep within the breast.

Core Cutting Needle Biopsy

Core cutting needle biopsies have many of the advantages of FNA, but because a core of tissue is obtained for histologic examination, more details of tumor structure are available and ductal carcinoma in situ can be identified. The adequacy of the specimen can be evaluated at the time of the biopsy, allowing additional tissue to be removed when the specimen appears to be nothing but fat, and the material is suitable for interpretation by any pathologist. Fentiman et al (18) performed core biopsy on 135 patients with breast cancer and 107 (79%) were successfully diagnosed. In a similar study of 150 core biopsies, Minkowitz et al (19) determined an 89% sensitivity and a 100% specificity for the core technique. In both series, a higher incidence of false-negative results was reported

F I G U R E **5-2**

Algorithm for the management of solid breast masses using fine-needle aspiration (FNA) cytology. The decision to follow a solid mass on the basis of benign findings by physical examination, mammography, and FNA should be made after a consideration of the patient's age and other recognized breast cancer risk factors.

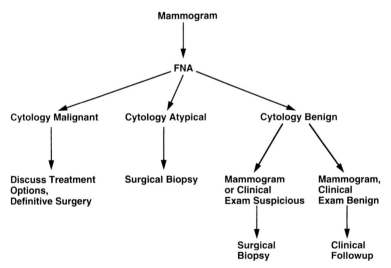

for small tumors. Shabot et al (20) prospectively compared the diagnostic accuracy of aspiration cytology and core needle biopsy in 81 patients with breast masses. Aspiration cytology was diagnostic in 95% of patients, compared to a 70% diagnostic rate for core biopsy ($p = 0.008$). False-positive diagnoses are rare with the core biopsy technique, but could occur with lesions such as radial scars. False-negative results may occur with extremely hard tumors, because the sampling needle is deflected into the surrounding fat. The choice between core biopsy and FNA is often dependent on the availability of a cytopathologist.

Technique Core needle biopsies can be performed with Tru-Cut needles or the spring-loaded Bioptycut device. The Bioptycut needle has a higher diagnostic sensitivity than the Tru-Cut needle (21), but it is also more expensive. Seeding of core needle tracts with tumor cells has been reported, so it is prudent to place the biopsy tract so that it will be excised during definitive therapy. This is probably a theoretical concern in patients undergoing breast-conserving surgery who will receive irradiation, but in patients undergoing mastectomy, excision of the puncture site is desirable. Complications of core biopsy are uncommon and include hematoma, infection, and pneumothorax.

Excisional Biopsy

Excisional biopsy is the complete removal of a breast abnormality. When the excisional biopsy of a cancer includes a margin of normal breast tissue, it will often serve as the definitive lumpectomy. Excisional biopsy is an outpatient procedure that can almost always be performed using local anesthesia supplemented with intravenous sedation as necessary. In the past, patients undergoing a breast biopsy were often admitted to the hospital and given general anesthesia, with a plan to proceed directly to a mastectomy if a frozen section revealed carcinoma. There is little rationale for such an approach today. Data from retrospective and prospective trials demonstrate no survival advantage for patients undergoing biopsy followed immediately by definitive surgery when compared to patients undergoing two separate operative procedures (22,23). The performance of a separate biopsy (two-step procedure) allows the clinician to review the pathology of the entire malignancy before discussing treatment options, and

allows the patient to seek consultation with a radiation oncologist or a reconstructive surgeon prior to making a treatment choice. For many women, the time for consultation with other members of the breast cancer care team and the option of a second opinion are critical to the decision-making process. Delays of up to 1 month from the time of diagnosis to definitive therapy have not been shown to alter prognosis (22,23), so performing definitive surgery is not an emergency.

Prior to an excisional biopsy, high-quality diagnostic mammography that includes magnification views of the site of the palpable abnormality should be performed. The purpose of this is to assess the extent of the palpable mass and any associated nonpalpable component, and to ensure that no nonpalpable abnormali-

F I G U R E **5-3**

A mammogram obtained following a breast biopsy that demonstrated a 1-cm carcinoma. The large postbiopsy hematoma affects the surrounding breast parenchyma, and limits the assessment of the patient's suitability for breast-conserving therapy.

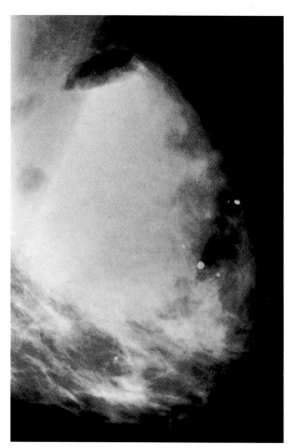

ties are present elsewhere in either breast. This information is essential to evaluate the patient's suitability for breast-conserving therapy if a diagnosis of cancer is made. Adequate mammograms in the immediate postbiopsy period are often difficult to obtain, owing to pain on compressing the breast or hematoma and post-biopsy inflammation obscuring the breast parenchyma (Fig. 5-3). Using information obtained from magnification mammography of the primary tumor site, Kearney and Morrow (24) obtained histologically negative margins with a single conservative diagnostic biopsy in 227 (95%) of 239 patients. Magnification mammography also readily identifies patients requiring wider excisions for complete tumor removal (25).

Technique Cosmetic outcome and the possible need for definitive cancer surgery must be balanced when one considers the site of incision. Incisions in Langer's lines usually produce the best cosmetic result for lesions in the upper half of the breast. In the lower half of the breast the choice between a radial incision and an incision in Langer's lines will depend on the contour of the breast and the amount of tissue to be excised (Fig. 5-4).

When malignancy is suspected, the incision should be placed over the mass to allow its removal as a single specimen, and to provide adequate visualization to achieve hemostasis. This approach will also facilitate re-excision of

the cavity when necessary to obtain cancer-negative margins. Tunneling for small distances to improve cosmesis is appropriate, but the use of circumareolar incisions to remove lesions in the periphery of the breast should be avoided.

Skin removal is neither necessary nor desirable unless the lesion is adherent to the dermis. An important step in avoiding visible depressions in the breast contour is preservation of the subcutaneous fat. Once the skin is incised, the breast tissue should be divided to a point 0.5 to 1.0 cm superficial to the breast mass and then excision is carried out (Fig. 5-5). Lesions that appear to be fibroadenomas can be shelled out at the level of the capsule as long as care is taken to remove the entire lesion. Other masses should be removed with a small margin (5–10 mm) of normal breast tissue. Electrocautery should be used with care until the lesion has been removed, because thermal injury makes evaluation of margins difficult and may interfere with the histologic diagnosis of small tumors.

Proper specimen management is critical to the success of an excisional biopsy. If a margin of normal tissue has been removed as part of the biopsy, orienting sutures should be placed. The use of two sutures will allow orientation of the specimen by the pathologist. The intact specimen should be examined to confirm that the lesion in question has been removed. When there is suspicion of malignancy, the adequacy of the margins can be grossly assessed. The

FIGURE **5-4**

Incision placement for breast biopsy. The dotted lines indicate Langer's lines and solid lines illustrate the site of incision placement in different parts of the breast.

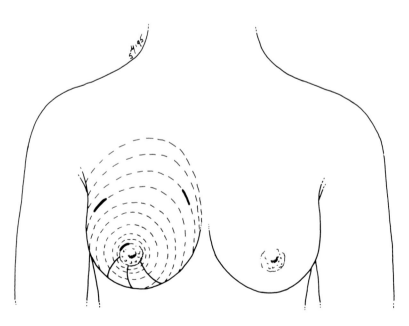

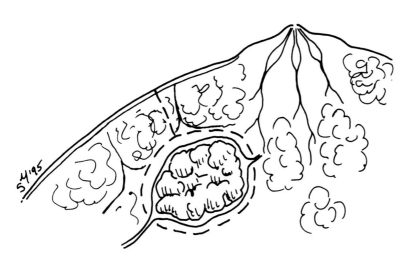

FIGURE **5-5**

Approach to lesions within the substance of the breast by incising the subcutaneous tissue and overlying parenchyma (dotted line) to a point approximately 1 cm superficial to the lesion.

specimen is sent fresh to pathology and margins are inked to allow identification of patients who require re-excision.

Prior to closure, careful palpation of the biopsy site should be carried out to confirm removal of the lesion in its entirety. Meticulous hemostasis is important, and use of drains should be avoided. Reapproximation of the breast parenchyma should also be avoided because this often distorts the contour of the breast and worsens the cosmetic result. This distortion is often not evident when the patient is supine with her arms relaxed. The deep dermis is reapproximated with several interrupted sutures and a subcuticular skin closure is utilized. Complications of excisional biopsy are uncommon and include infection, hematoma, and failure to remove the palpable mass.

Incisional Biopsy

The use of incisional biopsy is reserved for masses too large to be excised as a diagnostic procedure, most commonly locally advanced breast cancer. Today there are few indications for incisional biopsy. Diagnostic material can be obtained using FNA or core needle biopsy with lower morbidity and lower cost, and immuno-histochemical techniques allow the determination of hormone receptor status and the study of tumor markers from small specimens. Incisional biopsy is appropriate when it becomes apparent intraoperatively that what appeared to be a dominant mass is a diffuse process within the breast. This situation usually occurs with benign fibrocystic changes, and rather than remove an entire quadrant of the breast, an inci-

sional biopsy of the clinical abnormality should be performed.

Nipple Discharge

Terminal Duct Excision

The standard method for the diagnosis of pathologic nipple discharge is a terminal duct excision. Terminal duct excision, like other excisional breast biopsies, is an outpatient procedure that is readily performed under local anesthesia, usually with supplemental sedation. Patients should be advised preoperatively that there may be some permanent numbness of the nipple-areolar complex following the biopsy, and women of childbearing age will be unable to lactate. In the patient who has had preoperative galactography demonstrating a localized ductal abnormality, a needle localization of the abnormality may be performed. This approach may be advantageous in the young patient who wishes to maintain the ability to lactate in the future.

Technique A circumareolar incision is placed over the quadrant of the breast where the discharge originates (Fig. 5-6A). The incision may involve up to one half of the circumference of the areola if necessary for exposure. Incisions of more than half of the areolar circumference risk devascularization of the nipple-areolar complex. With the knife, the nipple is dissected free from the underlying breast tissue as a full-thickness dermal flap (Fig. 5-6B). Dissection deep to the level of the dermis runs the risk that the ductal pathology, which is usually proximal

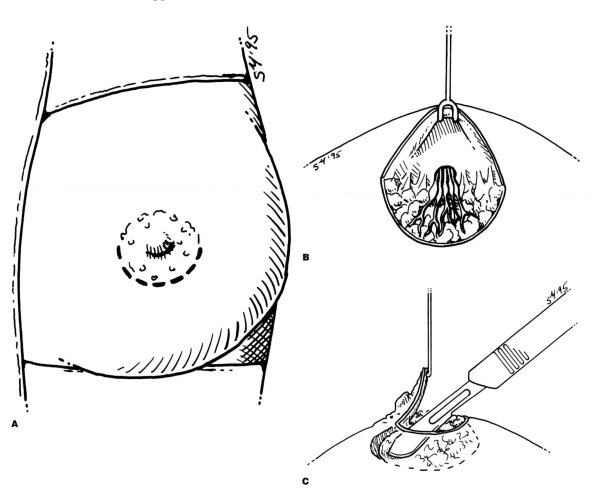

FIGURE **5-6**

A. A circumareolar incision centered over the discharging duct is used for terminal duct excision. B. The nipple-areolar complex is dissected free from the underlying breast tissue as a full-thickness dermal flap. C. If a single abnormal duct is not identified intraoperatively, the entire central core of ductal tissue is excised.

in the duct, will not be removed. As the nipple is dissected free and the proximal ducts are divided, the abnormal duct can usually be identified visually or by the presence of discharge. Some surgeons prefer to cannulate the discharging duct with a fine probe prior to making the incision. If a single abnormal duct is identified, it is followed distally in the breast for a distance of 2 to 3 cm and then transected. The point of transection should be observed for discharge, which would indicate that the pathology was more peripheral in the duct. Ligation of the transected duct is unnecessary. If an abnormal duct is not identified intraoperatively, the entire central core of ductal tissue is excised to a depth of 2 to 3 cm (Fig. 5-6C). Attempts

to reapproximate the breast tissue should be avoided. An excellent cosmetic result is obtained with careful approximation of the dermis and subcuticular closure of the skin.

Mammographic Abnormalities

Needle Localization Biopsy

The most important factors in the success of a needle localization biopsy are accurate placement of the guide, a thorough understanding by the surgeon of the relationship between the guide and the mammographic abnormality, and communication between the surgeon and the radiologist. Gallagher et al (26) reviewed 100 consecutive needle localization biopsies performed by a single surgeon in a 1-year period. In 96 procedures the wire was within 5 mm of the abnormality. The median specimen volume was 6.0 cm³, and one patient required a second biopsy because of failure to excise the lesion. Other series reported that 59% to 78% of localizations are within 1 cm of the target (27–29). Whether a guidewire, dye, or a combination of the two is used appears to be primarily a matter of preference. Failure rates of needle localization biopsy vary widely, ranging from less than 1% to 18% (30,31), but most modern series reported failure to excise the mammographic lesion in 1% to 2% (32–34) of patients.

The majority of needle localization biopsies can be done under local anesthesia, with supplemental sedation as necessary. As discussed previously, most mammographically identified breast abnormalities are benign, and the routine removal of very large amounts of breast tissue should be avoided.

Technique Prior to beginning the procedure, the surgeon must carefully review the mammograms to understand the relationship between the localizing wire and the mammographic abnormality. Marking the point where the wire enters the skin with a radiopaque marker makes it easy to determine how much of the wire is within the breast. The ideal localization is one in which the wire passes through the abnormality. Wire placement more than 1 cm from the target is not particularly helpful to the surgeon, and repositioning should be considered. Measurements of the distance from the localizing wire to the lesion, taken with the patient erect and the breast compressed, are of little use to the surgeon in the operating room.

Incision placement is critical to the success of needle localization biopsy. The incision should be placed at the point of entry of the wire into the breast only when the wire has a short course within the breast. When the wire traverses a large amount of the breast, the incision should be made just proximal to the area of the pathology and the wire identified within the breast parenchyma (Fig. 5-7). The appropriate location for the incision can be determined by noting the relationship between the nipple, the entry point of the wire in the skin, and the lesion on both mammographic views. Incision over the area of the pathology allows the use of a smaller incision, facilitates hemostasis, and allows the removal of a single specimen. In addition, if a carcinoma requiring re-excision lumpectomy is identified, the re-excision is readily accomplished.

After the breast tissue is entered, the localizing wire is identified within the breast parenchyma. When this is accomplished, the distal portion of the wire is stabilized with a clamp and the remainder of the wire is brought into the incision. Caution should be used when dividing breast tissue with the cautery prior to the identification of the wire, because the wire can be readily transected with the cautery. Care should be taken at all times to avoid pulling on the wire, grasping it with clamps, or moving it to determine its course within the breast. These maneuvers, particularly in women with fatty breasts, run the risk of dislodging the wire from the area of the target.

The breast tissue over the proximal portion of the wire is incised until the area of the pathology is approached. This approach is facilitated by the use of a guidewire with a thickened distal segment, with the thickened segment positioned in the lesion. When the

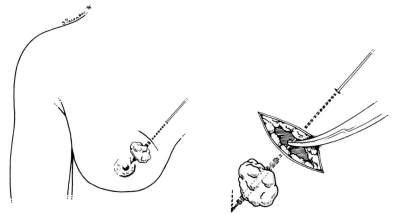

F I G U R E **5-7**

Incisions for needle localization breast biopsy should be placed adjacent to the area of pathology, not at the entry point of the wire into the breast. The wire is then identified in the breast parenchyma and brought into the wound.

change in the caliber of the wire is identified, the dissection is moved away from the wire to allow removal of the entire lesion with a small margin of normal breast tissue. Cautery should be avoided in the area of the lesion, because cautery artifact can make both the diagnosis of small lesions and an assessment of margin status difficult.

Specimen radiography is a mandatory part of needle localization biopsy. It is the only way to determine whether calcifications have been removed, and although many mammographically identified masses are palpable intraoperatively, a specimen radiograph ensures that the palpable abnormality corresponds to the mammographic lesion being sought, and serves as a record that the lesion has been removed. The specimen is marked with orienting sutures and the pathologist is provided with a copy of the specimen radiograph. As with other breast biopsies, inking of the specimen to determine margin status should be routine. Frozen section has little role in the management of nonpalpable abnormalities. Sacchini et al (35) reported a 12% discordance rate between frozen section and permanent section results in a series of 403 nonpalpable abnormalities. Problems were primarily due to the inability to reliably distinguish atypical hyperplasia from intraductal carcinoma, and difficulties in identifying a small area of invasion in large areas of intraductal carcinoma. Frozen section of small lesions runs the risk of distorting all of the available diagnostic material with frozen section artifact. The widespread availability of immunohistochemical hormone receptor determination, and the fact that a diagnostic needle localization is rarely undertaken with a plan to proceed to definitive surgery, make frozen section unnecessary in the management of nonpalpable abnormalities.

When the specimen radiograph fails to confirm the presence of the lesion, both the surgeon and the radiologist should review the localization films to determine whether the lesion was truly localized. If, in retrospect, the lesion was not localized, further excision of breast tissue at the site of the wire is of little merit and the procedure should be terminated. Failure to localize the lesion is a relatively uncommon cause of failure to excise a mammographic abnormality. More commonly, limited exposure from a poorly placed incision and traction on the localizing wire are the causes of failure. If the localization appears to be on target, the removal of additional breast tissue from the distal portion of the biopsy cavity will usually result in excision of the mammographic abnormality. If the lesion is not visualized in the second specimen, the procedure should be terminated. When the patient can comfortably tolerate compression, a mammogram should be obtained to confirm persistence of the lesion and a repeat biopsy undertaken.

In addition to failure to remove the mammographic abnormality, complications of needle localization biopsy include retention of a portion of the wire in the breast, infection, and hematoma.

Image-Guided Core Needle Biopsy

An alternative to excisional biopsy in the management of mammographic abnormalities is stereotactic core needle biopsy. Nonpalpable masses can also be sampled using ultrasound guidance. The potential advantages of a core biopsy include less pain, the absence of surgical scars, and lower cost compared to open surgical biopsy. A review of seven series comparing stereotactic core biopsies to surgical excision demonstrated sensitivities ranging from 71% to 100% for core biopsy when the technique was used in selected patients (36). The sensitivity of the procedure varies with the type of lesion being targeted, and is lower for microcalcifications than mass lesions (36,37). The routine use of specimen radiography with core biopsies done for calcifications will allow a determination that the appropriate area has been sampled. As experience has been gained with the core biopsy technique, a number of core diagnoses that are indications for surgical biopsy have been identified. The most frequently encountered of these is atypical ductal hyperplasia, which is associated with carcinoma in 30% to 50% of cases (38,39). A core diagnosis of radial scar is also an indication for a surgical biopsy to exclude coexistent carcinoma. Another indication for a repeat biopsy is lack of concordance between the core biopsy findings and the appearance of the mammographic target. Prior to core biopsy, a differential diagnosis for the mammographic abnormality should be developed. Lack of concordance between the histologic diagnosis and the mammographic diagnosis suggests that the lesion may not have been sampled, and is an indication for a repeat biopsy. Dershaw et al (38) observed this problem in 15 of 314 women undergoing core biopsy. A diagnosis of lobular carcinoma in situ should not be accepted as a cause for a mammographic abnormality, and is an indication for repeat biopsy.

One limitation of core biopsy is that it does not always provide the accurate characterization of an entire malignant lesion, which is essential for treatment planning. Jackman et al (39) observed that of 43 lesions diagnosed by core biopsy as intraductal carcinoma, 8 (19%) contained invasive carcinoma. Similar results were reported by Parker et al (37) in their large multi-institutional series. The clinical implications of an incomplete diagnosis are reflected in the series of Evans (40), in which 12% of patients diagnosed with carcinoma by core biopsy required more than one surgical procedure.

Contraindications to core biopsy include very-low-suspicion mammographic abnormalities that can be safely followed, patients with lesions that cannot be accurately targeted such as lesions immediately beneath the skin or those that are diffuse, and patients who are unable to cooperate with the procedure. Breast implants and extremely small lesions that would be completely removed with the procedure are also contraindications. The cost-effectiveness of core biopsy varies with the degree of suspicion of the lesion being sampled and the type of local therapy selected after cancer is diagnosed (36,40).

REFERENCES

1. Ciatto S, Cariaggi P, Bulgaresi P. The value of routine cytologic examination of cyst fluids. *Acta Cytol* 1987;31:301–304.

2. Seltzer M, Perloff L, Kellye R, Fitts W. The significance of age in patients with nipple discharge. *Surg Gynecol Obstet* 1979;131:519–522.

3. Murad T, Contesso G, Mouriesse H. Nipple discharge from the breast. *Ann Surg* 1989;195:250–264.

4. Tabar L, Dean PB, Pentek Z. Galactography: the diagnostic procedure of choice for nipple discharge. *Radiology* 1983;149:31–38.

5. Talamonti M, Morrow M. The abnormal mammogram. In: Harris JR, Lippman M, Morrow M, Hellman S, eds. *Diseases of the breast*. New York: Lippincott-Raven, 1996:114–121.

6. Silverstein M, Gamagami P, Colburn W, et al. Nonpalpable breast lesions: diagnosis with slightly overpenetrated screen-film mammogra-

7. phy and hook wire directed biopsy in 1014 cases. *Radiology* 1989;171:633–638.

7. Wilhelm MC, Edge S, Cole D, et al. Nonpalpable invasive breast cancer. *Ann Surg* 1991;213:600–605.

8. Knutzen A, Gisvold J. Likelihood of malignant disease for various categories of mammographically detected, nonpalpable breast lesions. *Mayo Clin Proc* 1993;68:454–460.

9. Morrow M, Schmidt R, Cregger B, et al. Preoperative evaluation of abnormal mammographic findings to avoid unnecessary breast biopsies. *Arch Surg* 1994;129:1090–1096.

10. Hamond S, Keyhani-Rafagha S, O'Toole RV. Statistical analysis of fine needle aspiration of the breast. A review of 678 cases plus 4265 cases from the literature. *Acta Cytol* 1987;31:276–280.

11. Kline TS, Joshi LP, Neal HS. Fine needle aspiration of the breasts: diagnoses and pitfalls. *Cancer* 1979;44:1458–1464.

12. Lamb J, Anderson TJ. Influence of cancer histology on the success of fine needle aspiration of the breast. *J Clin Pathol* 1989;42:733–735.

13. Patel JJ, Gartell PC, Smallwood JA, et al. Fine needle aspiration cytology of breast masses; an evaluation of its accuracy and reasons for diagnostic failure. *Ann R Coll Surg Engl* 1987;69:156–159.

14. Barrows GH, Anderson TJ, Lamb JL, Dixon JM. Fine needle aspiration of breast cancer. Relationship of clinical factors to cytology results in 689 primary malignancies. *Cancer* 1986;58:1493–1498.

15. Donegan WL. Evaluation of a palpable breast mass. *N Engl J Med* 1992;327:937–942.

16. Bell DA, Hajdu SI, Urban JA, Gaston JP. Role of aspiration cytology in the diagnosis and management of mammary lesions in office practice. *Cancer* 1983;51:1182–1189.

17. Sickles EA, Klein DL, Goodson WH, Hunt TIC. Mammography after needle aspiration of palpable breast masses. *Am J Surg* 1983;145:395–397.

18. Fentiman IS, Millis RR, Hayward JL. Value of needle biopsy in the outpatient diagnosis of breast cancer. *Arch Surg* 1989;115:652–654.

19. Minkowitz S, Moskowitz R, Khafuf R, Alderete MN. Tru-Cut needle biopsy of the breast. An analysis of its specificity and sensitivity. *Cancer* 1985;57:320–323.

20. Shabot MM, Goldberg IM, Schick P, et al. Aspiration cytology is superior to TruCutR needle biopsy in establishing the diagnosis of clinically

suspicious breast masses. *Ann Surg* 1982; 196:122–126.

21. McMahon AJ, Lutfy AM, Matthew A, et al. Needle core biopsy of the breast with a spring-loaded device. *Br J Surg* 1992;79:1042–1045.

22. Fisher ER, Sass R, Fisher B. Biologic considerations regarding the one and two step procedures in the management of patients with invasive carcinoma of the breast. *Surg Gynecol Obstet* 1985;161:245–249.

23. Bertario L, Reduzzi D, Piromalli D, et al. Outpatient biopsy of breast cancer: influence on survival. *Ann Surg* 1985;201:64–67.

24. Kearney T, Morrow M. Effect of re-excision on the success of breast conserving surgery. *Ann Surg Oncol* 1995;2:303–307.

25. Morrow M, Schmidt R, Hassett C. Patient selection for breast conservation therapy with magnification mammography. *Surgery* 1995;118:621–626.

26. Gallagher WJ, Cardenosa G, Rubens JR, et al. Minimal-volume excision of nonpalpable breast lesions. *Am J Radiol* 1989;153:957–961.

27. Gisvold JJ, Martin JK. Pre-biopsy localization of nonpalpable breast masses. *Am J Radiol* 1984;143:477–481.

28. Tinnemans JGM, Wobbes TH, Hendricks KJC, et al. Localization and excision of nonpalpable breast lesions: a surgical evaluation of three methods. *Arch Surg* 1987;122:802–806.

29. Bigelow R, Smith R, Goodman PA, Wilson GS. Needle localization of nonpalpable breast masses. *Arch Surg* 1985;129:565–569.

30. Roses DF, Mitnick J, Harris MN, et al. The risk of carcinoma in wire localization biopsies for mammographically detected clustered calcifications. *Surgery* 1991;110:877–886.

31. Norton LW, Zeligman BE, Pearlman NW. Accuracy and cost of needle localization breast biopsy. *Arch Surg* 1988;123:947–950.

32. Meyer JE, Eberlein TJ, Stomper PC, Sonnenfeld MR. Biopsy of occult breast lesions. Analysis of 1261 abnormalities. *JAMA* 1990;263:2341–2343.

33. Thompson WR, Bowen JR, Dorman BA, et al. Mammographic localization and biopsy of nonpalpable breast lesions. *Arch Surg* 1991; 126:730–734.

34. Alexander HR, Candela FC, Dershaw DD, Kinne DW. Needle localized mammographic lesions. Results and evolving treatment strategy. *Arch Surg* 1990;125:1441–1444.

35. Sacchini V, Luini A, Agristi R, et al. Nonpalpable breast lesions. Analysis of 952 operated cases. *Breast Cancer Res Treat* 1995;36:32–59.

36. Morrow M. When can stereotactic core biopsy replace excisional biopsy? A clinical perspective. *Breast Cancer Res Treat* 1995;36:1–9.

37. Parker SH, Burbank F, Jackman RJ, et al. Percutaneous large core breast biopsy: a multi-institutional study. *Radiology* 1994;193:359–364.

38. Dershaw DD, Liberman L, Abramson AF. Non-diagnostic stereotaxic core breast biopsy: results of re-biopsy. *Radiology* 1996;198:323–325.

39. Jackman RJ, Nowels KW, Shepard MJ, et al. Stereotaxic large-core needle biopsy of 450 nonpalpable breast lesions with surgical correlation in lesions with cancer or atypical hyperplasia. *Radiology* 1994;193:91–95.

40. Evans WP. Stereotactic core biopsy. In: Harris JR, Lippman ME, Morrow M, Hellman S, eds. *Diseases of the breast*. Philadelphia: Lippincott-Raven, 1996:144–152.

CHAPTER 6

Breast-Conserving Therapy for Early-Stage Breast Cancer

UMBERTO VERONESI

History of Breast-Conserving Therapy

The treatment of breast cancer remained substantially unchanged for some 80 years after the publication by Halsted in 1892 of the first report of radical mastectomy. Some variations in surgical technique were introduced during the first half of this century, either to reduce the extent of surgical ablation (for instance, conservation of the pectoralis major muscle) or to enlarge the extent of the tissues removed (for instance, removal of the internal mammary nodes). The need for extirpation of the entire breast was, however, never put under discussion. A handful of pioneers challenged the necessity of radical mastectomy, but they never received attention or recognition. Among them, one should mention the German gynecologist Hirsch (1), the French radiotherapist Baclesse (2), the English surgeon Keynes (3), and the American surgeon Crile (4).

Some 30 years ago, the issue of breast conservation was introduced with force in many cancer centers, for the following reasons: 1) All controlled studies comparing highly aggressive local-regional treatments with less aggressive ones showed no differences in survival. 2) The new concept of the natural history of breast cancer included the principle that prognosis depended chiefly on the presence or absence of occult metastatic foci in distant organs. 3) The introduction of mammography made it possible to identify nonpalpable, clinically silent lesions. All these events, which occurred in the 1960s, laid the groundwork for a more scientific approach to breast preservation.

Unfortunately, the first randomized trial comparing breast-conserving therapy with mastectomy (5), conducted in the 1960s at Guy's Hospital in London, showed a worrying increase in mortality rates among women treated with a breast-conserving procedure. It is now recognized that the failure of the London trial was due to the inadequate radiotherapeutic and surgical approaches (axillary dissection was not performed in node-positive patients, and insufficient doses of radiotherapy were delivered to the breast and axilla). However, the results from the Guy's Hospital study, published in 1972 (5), made it ethically difficult for institutional review boards to accept further proposals for randomized trials comparing radical mastectomy with less radical surgical procedures. Fortunately, in 1969, at a meeting of breast cancer experts called by the World Health Organization in Geneva (6), a proposal for such a trial presented by the Milan Cancer Institute won approval despite considerable opposition. The Milan trial was designed to compare the Halsted mastectomy with extensive breast resection and complete axillary dissection followed by radiotherapy to the ipsilateral breast with a dose of 50 Gy plus a boost dose to the scar of an additional 10 Gy. This trial was completed by the end of the 1970s, and the results were published in 1981 (7). The results showed similar rates of local recurrence and identical long-term survival rates with both treatments, indicating that appropriate breast-conserving therapy is as safe as the Halsted mastectomy. The results of the Milan trial were confirmed by subsequent trials in various countries.

Results of Randomized Trials

Only the most important randomized trials with at least 300 patients are considered in this review.

Trials Comparing Conservative Treatment with Mastectomy

As previously mentioned, the first trial comparing conservative treatment with mastectomy was conducted at Guy's Hospital in London (5). The study was conducted between 1961 and 1970 and involved a total of 370 patients. The patients were randomly assigned to one of two groups. The first group was treated with radical mastectomy plus radiotherapy to the axilla, supraclavicular triangle, and internal mammary chain (25–27 Gy). The second group was treated with breast resection plus radiotherapy to the breast (35–38 Gy) and regional nodes (25–27 Gy) similar to the mastectomy group. The early results of this trial, published in 1972 (5), showed that among stage II patients treated conservatively, there was a significant increase in the local-regional recurrent rate and a reduced survival rate. A more recent report of this trial showed that even in stage I patients, mastectomy was superior to conservative treatment (8).

The Milan trial conducted between 1973 and 1980 was the first to show that breast-conserving therapy is a safe method of treatment in patients with small cancers of the breast. This trial randomly assigned 701 patients with T1N0 breast carcinoma to undergo either Halsted mastectomy or quadrantectomy, axillary dissection, and radiotherapy of 60 Gy to the breast only (QUART). Early data were published in 1977 (9,10), and more complete results were published in 1981 (7). The results showed identical disease-free and overall survival rates in both groups. The results were confirmed in more recent publications (11) after 16 years of follow-up.

Data from the National Surgical Adjuvant Breast and Bowel Project (NSABP) B-06 trial were first published in 1985 (12) and were updated in 1989 (13) and 1995 (14). This trial was started in 1976 and accrued a total of 1855 patients who were randomly assigned to undergo total mastectomy, lumpectomy, or lumpectomy plus radiotherapy (50 Gy). In addition, all patients were treated with a subtotal axillary dissection. Patient accrual into this trial stopped in 1984. Although the survival rates did not differ between the three groups, patients treated conservatively had a considerably higher rate of local recurrence (39% for patients treated with lumpectomy and 10% for patients treated with lumpectomy plus radiotherapy) than did patients treated with mastectomy. In the lumpectomy-plus-radiotherapy group, patients who had positive lymph nodes and were treated with adjuvant chemotherapy had a reduced rate of local recurrence, while in the lumpectomy-only group, the use of adjuvant chemotherapy did not affect the local recurrence rate.

Between 1980 and 1986, the European Organization for Research and Treatment of Cancer (EORTC) carried out an extensive trial in Europe (15). A total of 903 patients with stage I or II disease were randomly assigned to undergo breast resection, axillary dissection, and radiotherapy to the breast (50 Gy plus 25 Gy with an iridium implant) or modified radical mastectomy. The interesting aspect of the EORTC trial was the inclusion of patients with large tumors (≤5 cm). The data obtained from the trial helped to confirm previous results. The survival curves of the two groups were superimposable even though the rate of local recurrence was higher in the group treated with breast conservation (15).

Between 1983 and 1989, the Danish Breast Cooperative Group conducted a randomized trial comparing breast-conserving therapy with mastectomy in 905 patients. Breast-conserving therapy consisted of wide breast resection plus axillary dissection and radiotherapy to the ipsilateral breast (50 Gy plus 10–25 Gy). A total of 450 patients were assigned to receive breast-conserving therapy, whereas 455 were assigned to undergo mastectomy. The survival and local-regional recurrence rates were equal in the two groups (16).

Trials Comparing Two Different Conservative Procedures

As previously mentioned, the NSABP B-06 trial (14) compared two different conservative treatments (lumpectomy and lumpectomy plus radiotherapy) and showed similar survival rates with both treatments but a fourfold increase

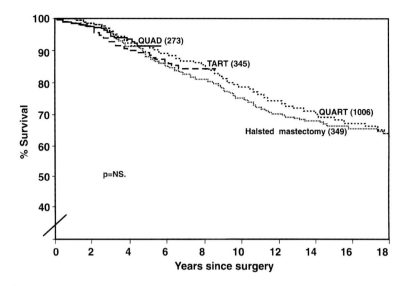

Cumulative incidence of local recurrence according to treatment in the first, second, and third Milan trials. NS = not significant; QUAD = quadrantectomy plus axillary dissection; QUART = quadrantectomy and axillary dissection plus radiotherapy; TART = lumpectomy and axillary dissection plus radiotherapy. (Reproduced by permission from Veronesi U, Salvadori B, Luini A, et al. Breast conservation is a safe method in patients with small cancer of the breast. Long-term results of three randomized trials on 1,973 patients. *Eur J Cancer* 1995;31: 1574-1579.)

Overall survival according to treatment in the first, second, and third Milan trials. NS = not significant; QUAD = quadrantectomy plus axillary dissection; QUART = quadrantectomy and axillary dissection plus radiotherapy; TART = lumpectomy and axillary dissection plus radiotherapy. (Reproduced by permission from Veronesi U, Salvadori B, Luini A, et al. Breast conservation is a safe method in patients with small cancer of the breast. Long-term results of three randomized trials on 1,973 patients. *Eur J Cancer* 1995;31:1574-1579.)

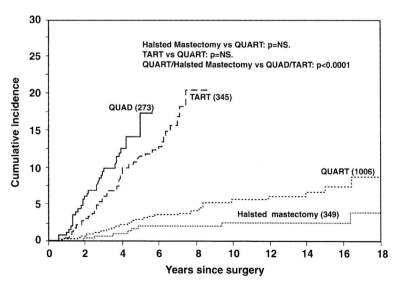

in local recurrences in patients not receiving radiotherapy.

Between 1981 and 1988, the Uppsala-Orebro Breast Cancer Study Group randomly assigned 381 patients to receive either sector resection plus axillary dissection (194 patients) or sector resection plus axillary dissection followed by radiotherapy (54 Gy; 187 patients) (17). Local recurrences were two times more frequent in patients treated with resection without radiotherapy than they were in patients who received resection plus radiotherapy. Survival curves were similar in the two groups (17,18).

In the second Milan trial, conducted between 1985 and 1987, a total of 705 patients were randomly assigned to undergo either QUART (50 plus 10 Gy) or lumpectomy and axillary dissection plus radiotherapy (45 plus 15 Gy by interstitial radioactive iridium). The results showed similar survival curves but a threefold increase in local recurrences in the lumpectomy group (19).

A third clinical trial was conducted in Milan between 1988 and 1989. A total of 567 women with early breast cancer (tumor diameter <2.5 cm) were randomly assigned to undergo QUART or quadrantectomy and axillary dissection but no radiotherapy (QUAD). The local recurrence rate was considerably higher in patients treated with QUAD than it was in patients treated with QUART (20). The annual rate of recurrence was 3.3% in the QUAD group and 0.46% in the QUART group. However, in women older than 55 years, the recurrence rate was low even in the QUAD group (annual rate of 1.5%) (Figs. 6-1 and 6-2).

Issues in Breast-Conserving Therapy

The introduction of breast-conserving therapy raised a series of issues, some of which have not yet been resolved. These issues are discussed in this section. In the case of controversial issues, the available data are reviewed, and recommendations for treatment are given.

Significance of Size of Primary Tumor

One of the most important issues in breast-conserving therapy is the indication for breast-conserving therapy in relation to the size of the primary carcinoma. The first Milan trial accrued

patients with tumors less than 2 cm in maximum diameter (7). The two major subsequent trials of the NSABP (14) and EORTC (15) explored the possibility of expanding the indications for breast-conserving therapy to include treatment of tumors up to 4 cm (NSABP) or 5 cm (EORTC) in diameter.

The results of these trials showed that size of the primary carcinoma is not a limiting factor for breast conservation. In addition, the long-term results of the NSABP and EORTC studies showed no survival differences when breast-conserving therapy was compared with mastectomy. However, the size of the tumor is an important factor in breast conservation from the standpoint of quality of results. If the size of the breast is small, breast conservation is unsatisfactory even for small tumors and is impractical for large tumors.

Another important issue in breast-conserving therapy is the presence of tumor cells at the resection margins. In the NSABP trial (12,13), margin positivity was a criterion for exclusion from the breast conservation group and assignment to treatment with mastectomy. Other studies provided evidence that even when margins are positive, a re-resection will, in the majority of patients, result in clear margins and maintain the patient as a candidate for breast conservation (21). In this context, the NSABP trial clearly showed that margin negativity does not indicate the absence of residual cancer cells: In some 40% of patients with negative margins treated with lumpectomy, a local relapse occurred, showing that in spite of margin negativity, cancer cells were in fact present in the residual mammary tissue (13). These data have strongly called in question the reliability of the status of resection margins as a predictor of local recurrence. It must be added that in the second Milan trial, in the lumpectomy-plus-radiotherapy group, patients with positive resection margins had a limited increase in local recurrences compared with patients with negative margins (19,22). In the Milan trials, the status of the resection margins of the quadrantectomy specimen was not considered important because with this quadrantectomy, positive margins are exceptionally rare.

Proper Extent of Local Excision

The proper extent of local resection is one of the crucial problems of breast conservation. How large must the resection margins be to avoid an excess risk of local recurrence? The final answer should result from the judgment of the surgeon once he or she has discussed with the patient the various options and the cosmetic expectations. What is certain is that the wider the excision, the lower the risk for local recurrences; the survival duration is not affected by the extent of resection. What should be avoided is the sharp and sometimes brutal request of the surgeon that a woman choose between "lumpectomy" (with a high risk of local relapses) and "mastectomy." The surgeon must inform the patient that many intermediate options, among them wide tylectomy, sector resection, and quadrantectomy, are also available and result in very low rates of local recurrence and acceptable cosmetic outcomes. Otherwise, under the pressure of their anxiety, most patients will choose mastectomy, which can be avoided in most patients. This rudimental way of approaching the patient with incomplete information has most likely resulted in increased rates of unnecessarily mutilated women in many countries.

On the other hand, the surgeon must know that a wide excision of normal breast tissue around the primary carcinoma will create a large defect in the breast that will require remodeling of the breast shape.

With the techniques available today, it is possible to achieve better aesthetic results than were previously possible with breast-conserving therapy. Even when the cosmetic result of the treated breast is good, this breast is often smaller than the opposite breast. If the difference is minimal, surgical correction of the contralateral breast is not needed, and the edema resulting from subsequent radiotherapy to the treated breast will help to restore the symmetry between the two sides. If the difference is considerable, the opposite breast should be remodeled as well.

Role of Axillary Dissection

The need for axillary dissection as part of breast-conserving therapy is a subject of debate. Axillary dissection has been a constant component of breast cancer surgery since the first Halsted mastectomy. Axillary dissection was originally considered an important therapeutic procedure because gross axillary involvement was very common in patients treated during the first half of the century. However, the role of this procedure has slowly changed over the past

20 years. Axillary dissection has become an "informational" procedure in women with a clinically uninvolved axilla, with the aim of discovering occult lymph node metastases.

In the case of axillary involvement, an indicator of poor prognosis, adjuvant systemic treatment needs to be considered. In very small early breast carcinomas (<1 cm), the risk of occult axillary involvement is on the order of 5% to 10%. The morbidity associated with dissecting axillary nodes, which are normal in 90% to 95% of these women with tumors smaller than 1 cm, is a heavy price to pay for obtaining, in only a minority of women, information that may be helpful in the planning of subsequent therapeutic programs. Moreover, many recent studies showed that useful prognostic information can be obtained with accurate pathologic, biologic, and molecular biologic examination of the primary carcinoma (23,24). It appears, therefore, that axillary dissection in patients with small carcinomas of the breast and with clinically negative nodes may represent overtreatment (25). In women with carcinomas smaller than 1 cm, axillary dissection will probably soon be abandoned. In exceptional cases where a tumor of such small size shows unfavorable prognostic characteristics (histopathologic grade 3, high proliferative index, absence of estrogen receptors, etc), adjuvant treatment may be applied. An alternative treatment of the clinically negative axilla may be the administration of radiotherapy, which if strictly limited to the axillary field should not create any risk of damage to the brachial plexus. A trial designed to evaluate the ability of radiotherapy to destroy occult cancer foci in clinically negative patients is in progress in Milan. A new solution to the problem of the axillary dissections in axillary negative patients is the "sentinel node" technique, recently proposed. With this method, which employs either a blue dye or a radioactive colloid albumin, the first axillary node draining the mammary lymph from the area where the tumor is located is isolated, removed, and histologically examined. If negative, the remaining nodes will be negative, with an accuracy around 95%, and axillary dissection may be avoided (26).

Role of Radiotherapy

The importance of radiotherapy in breast-conserving therapy is well established. There is no doubt that the administration of radiotherapy after surgical treatment for breast carcinoma considerably reduces the risk of local recurrence.

In the NSABP experience, among women treated with lumpectomy with free resection margins, the risk of local recurrences was 40% without the use of adjuvant radiotherapy but only 10% with the use of radiotherapy. Similar results were observed in two other clinical trials of lumpectomy with or without radiotherapy: the Uppsala trial (18) and the Milan 3 trial (20).

Nonetheless, some aspects of the role of radiotherapy need further discussion. The first is the fact that although radiotherapy reduces the risk of local recurrence, it does not influence the overall survival of the patient. Therefore, the patient must be aware that choosing not to undergo radiotherapy will increase the risk of local relapse (which may be quantified) but will not increase the risk of dying of breast cancer.

The second aspect is the effectiveness of radiotherapy in different age groups. According to the Milan experience, radiotherapy is essential in young women and important in middle-aged women but considerably less important in women older than 55. Among patients who undergo adequate local treatment such as quadrantectomy but who do not receive radiotherapy, the annual rate of local recurrence is 1.53% among women older than 55 years, compared with 2.99% in women between 45 and 55 years old and 6.93% in women younger than 45 (11). Women older than 55, when informed about the low annual rate of local relapse with surgery alone, may decide not to undergo radiotherapy.

Biologic Significance of Local Recurrence

The biologic significance of locally recurrent disease after breast-conserving therapy is an area of controversy. Two recent articles (27,28) were devoted to clarifying whether local recurrences represent the expression of a particularly aggressive tumor type or simply reflect the result of incomplete removal of the primary carcinoma.

Several studies were conducted to identify risk factors for the development of local recurrences. Among these risk factors are the histologic type, pathologic grade, proliferative rate, the presence of an extensive intraductal component (EIC), resection margin status, peritu-

moral lymphatic spread, and other biologic and biomolecular markers (29–32). It would be useful to be able to distinguish markers for increased risk of local recurrence from markers that may also indicate an increased risk for the development of distant disease.

With this objective, an extensive study was recently conducted in Milan. A review of 2233 patients treated with quadrantectomy and radiotherapy showed that a number of biologic and pathologic factors influence the local spread of disease, the development of distant metastases, or both.

Patient age and peritumoral vascular invasion were found to be predictors of both local and distant recurrences, while tumor size and axillary lymph node involvement appeared to be associated only with an increased risk of distant disease. The presence of an EIC appeared to be an important predictor of local recurrence but not distant metastases. This specific risk appears to be inversely proportional to the extent of resection of normal breast tissue around the primary carcinoma: In patients treated with quadrantectomy, the presence of an EIC has limited prognostic value for local recurrences, while in patients treated with lumpectomy, the presence of an EIC has much greater prognostic significance (11).

The data from the Milan study showed a probability of recurrence, starting from the second year after surgery, of about 1% per year. In patients who had a local recurrence, the potential for distant metastases varied greatly according to the time elapsed between the surgical removal of the primary tumor and the appearance of the local recurrence. The risk of developing a distant metastasis was more than six times greater in patients who had a local recurrence in the first year after primary surgery than it was in patients who had a local recurrence more than 3 years after the primary procedure. The relative risk decreased to 2.2 in patients with a local recurrence in the second year after surgery and to 1.2 in patients with a local recurrence in the third year. The 5-year survival rate for patients who experienced local recurrences was approximately 70% (28).

How, then, should local relapse be managed in terms of both local and systemic treatment? If the local recurrence is a small (<1 cm) single mass and is strictly limited to the scar of the previous resection, a re-resection of the breast may be indicated. If the recurrences are multiple, of large size, or not strictly limited to the site of the previously resected primary carcinoma, a mastectomy should be performed. For local recurrences occurring during the first 2 years after surgery, in young patients (<35 years old), or in patients with evidence of peritumoral lymphatic invasion, systemic therapy should be recommended. On the other hand, for local relapses occurring more than 2 years after surgery, in patients whose primary carcinoma contained an EIC, or in patients who were treated with inadequate surgery, additional systemic therapy may be avoided.

Role of Plastic Surgery in Breast-Conserving Therapy

The cosmetic requirements of breast surgery create a role for the plastic surgeon in the treatment of primary breast cancer. As the surgical reshaping of the contralateral breast to achieve a symmetric result becomes increasingly common, the role of the plastic surgeon in breast-conserving therapy is becoming more important. A team that includes the leading breast surgeon, the plastic surgeon, and a pathologist and a radiologist (for intraoperative pathologic and radiologic verifications) appears to provide the ideal cooperative approach to effectively treating primary breast carcinoma. We are facing a period during which, owing to extensive detection campaigns, most breast carcinomas are discovered at a very early phase of development, when the disease is local and the risk of dissemination is very low. Under these conditions, the greatest efforts must be concentrated on appropriate local-regional treatment to maximize local control of the disease and to minimize cosmetic defects.

Preoperative Chemotherapy To Enable Breast-Conserving Therapy

Many patients with medium or large tumors (>3 cm) who, because of the dimensions of their tumors, are not candidates for conservative surgery may be treated with breast-conserving therapy after the administration of preoperative chemotherapy for a short period. Generally, three or four courses of combination chemotherapy can reduce the size of the tumor enough to allow a conservative breast resection. In a significant percentage of patients, the mass will disappear clinically, while the complete pathologic disappearance of the carcinoma is a rare event (33,34). In one of the main studies of preoperative chemotherapy (33), no significant differences were seen in the response rates of primary carcinomas to the various combinations of chemotherapeutic agents utilized (Table 6-1).

Recommendations for the surgical approach after preoperative chemotherapy were recently set forth. First, the extent of tumor regression must be evaluated not only by careful and frequent physical examination, but also by strict mammographic monitoring. Tumor measurements should be recorded after each physical examination. Second, when choosing the type of operation, the surgeon should consider not only the size of the tumor but also the volume of the breast and the possible cosmetic

Drug Regimen (No. of Cycles)	N	Positive Nodes (%)	LR	DR	Negative Nodes (%)	LR	DR
CMF (3)	32	23 (71.9)	3	9	9 (28.1)	2	—
CMF (4)	33	19 (57.6)	2	6	14 (42.4)	—	2
FAC (3)	30	19 (63.3)	1	6	11 (36.7)	1	—
FAC (4)	32	11 (34.3)	1	1	21 (65.6)	1	2
FEC (3)	33	24 (72.7)	1	10	9 (27.3)	—	2
FNC (3)	33	15 (45.5)	—	4	8 (54.5)	—	3
ADM (3)	33	25 (75.8)	4	4	8 (24.2)	1	1
Total	226	136 (60.1)	12	45	90 (39.9)	5	10

T A B L E **6-1**

Local (LR) and Distant Recurrences (DR) as First Event According to Axillary Nodal Status and Type of Chemotherapy (Milan Study)

CMF = cyclophosphamide, methotrexate, fluorouracil; FAC = fluorouracil, doxorubicin, cyclophosphamide; FEC = fluorouracil, etoposide, cisplatin; FNC = fluorouracil hitoxantrone cyclophosphamide; ADM = doxorubicin.

Source: Veronesi U, Bonadonna G, Zurrida S. Conservation surgery after primary chemotherapy in large carcinomas of the breast. *Ann Surg* 1995; 222:612–618.

outcome. Third, while at the operating table, the surgeon must be assisted by an experienced pathologist who will carefully examine the specimen and perform multiple biopsies to obtain samples for frozen-section evaluation when necessary to quantify the extent of tumor regression. Fourth, microcalcifications must always be considered carefully, because they are unlikely to disappear after chemotherapy, and the re-excised specimen must contain all of them. Fifth, the placement of tattoo marks on the skin to guide the surgeon must be done prior to the institution of chemotherapy. Sixth, when breast remodeling is performed hastily or without sufficient care, the poor cosmetic result abrogates the raison d'être of the whole approach.

The main problem associated with pre-operative chemotherapy is patients' fear of such treatment. Very often women are frightened by the idea of starting treatment with chemotherapy instead of surgery. Because chemotherapy is considered by many patients to be a sign of utmost gravity of disease, serious depression may ensue. Moreover, unpleasant side effects, particularly alopecia, are a deterrent to this approach. Therefore, the task of future research should be the identification of a combination of drugs that will minimize side effects but maintain good efficacy in the control of the primary carcinoma.

Conclusions

Breast-conserving therapy is becoming increasingly common in breast cancer treatment. Further improvements in the early diagnosis of breast cancer will emphasize this trend in the future. Survival rates after conservative surgery are equal to those obtained with radical mastectomy. However, excessively conservative surgery or the withholding of radiotherapy will increase the risk of local recurrence, leading to a high rate of salvage mastectomies. Finally, the possibility of saving the breast when a tumor is discovered while still small is an important motivation for the participation of women in screening and early detection programs.

REFERENCES

1. Hirsch J. Radiumchirurgia des brust Krebses. *Dtsch Med Wochenschr* 1927;43:1419–1421.

2. Baclesse F. Roentgen therapy as the sole method of treatment of cancer of the breast. *Am J Roent Radium Ther Nucl Med* 1949;62:311–313.

3. Keynes G. Conservative treatment of cancer of the breast. *BMJ* 1937;2:643–647.

4. Crile G Jr. Results of simplified treatment of breast cancer. *Surg Gynecol Obstet* 1964;118:517–523.

5. Atkins H, Hayward JL, Klugman DJ, Wayte AB. Treatment of early breast cancer: a report after 10 years of clinical trial. *BMJ* 1972;2:423–429.

6. *Meeting of investigators for evaluation of methods and diagnosis and treatment of breast cancer. Final report.* World Health Organization, Geneva, December 8–12, 1969.

7. Veronesi U, Saccozzi R, Del Vecchio M, et al. Comparing radical mastectomy with quadrantectomy, axillary dissection, and radiotherapy in patients with small cancers of the breast. *N Engl J Med* 1981;305:6–11.

8. Hayward JL. The Guy's trial of treatment of early breast cancer. *World J Surg* 1988;1:314–316.

9. Veronesi U. New trends in the treatment of breast cancer at the Cancer Institute of Milan. *AJR Am J Roentgenol* 1977;128:287–289.

10. Veronesi U, Banfi A, Saccozzi R, et al. Conservative treatment of breast cancer. *Cancer* 1977;39:2822–2826.

11. Veronesi U, Salvadori B, Luini A, et al. Breast conservation is a safe method in patients with small cancer of the breast. Long-term results of three randomized trials on 1,973 patients. *Eur J Cancer* 1995;31:1574–1579.

12. Fisher B, Bauer M, Margolese R, et al. Five-year results of a randomized clinical trial comparing total mastectomy and segmental mastectomy with or without radiation in the treatment of breast cancer. *N Engl J Med* 1985;312:665–673.

13. Fisher B, Redmond C, Poisson R, et al. Eight-year results of a randomized clinical trial comparing total mastectomy and lumpectomy with or without irradiation in the treatment of breast cancer. *N Engl J Med* 1989;320:822–828.

14. Fisher B, Anderson S, Redmond CK, et al. Reanalysis and results after 12 years of follow-up in a randomized clinical trial comparing total mastectomy with lumpectomy with or without irradiation in the treatment of breast cancer. *N Engl J Med* 1995;333:1496–1498.

15. van Dongen JA, Bartelink H, Fentiman IS. Randomized clinical trial to assess the value of breast-conserving therapy in stage I and II breast

cancer, EORTC 10801 Trial. National Institutes of Health Consensus Development Conference on the Treatment of Early-Stage Breast Cancer. *Monogr Natl Cancer Inst* 1992;11:15–18.

16. Blichert-Toft M, Rose C, Andersen JA, et al. Danish randomized trial comparing breast conservation therapy with mastectomy: six years of life-table analysis. National Institutes of Health Consensus Development Conference on the Treatment of Early-Stage Breast Cancer. *Monogr Natl Cancer Inst* 1992;11:19–25.

17. The Uppsala-Orebro Breast Cancer Study Group. Sector resection with or without postoperative radiotherapy for stage I breast cancer: a randomized trial. *J Natl Cancer Inst* 1990;31:277–280.

18. Liljegren G, Holmberg L, Adami HO, et al. Sector resection with or without postoperative radiotherapy for stage I breast cancer: five-year results of a randomized trial. Uppsala-Orebro Breast Cancer Study Group. *J Natl Cancer Inst* 1994;86:652–654.

19. Veronesi U, Volterrani F, Luini A, et al. Quadrantectomy versus lumpectomy for small size breast cancer. *Eur J Cancer* 1990;26:671–673.

20. Veronesi U, Luini A, Del Vecchio M, et al. Radiotherapy after breast-preserving surgery in women with localized cancer of the breast. *N Engl J Med* 1993;328:1587–1591.

21. Schmitt SY, Abner A, Gelman R, et al. The relationship between microscopic margins of resection and the risk of local recurrence in patients treated with breast conserving surgery and radiation therapy. *Cancer* 1994;74:1746–1751.

22. Veronesi U, Andreola S, Agresti R, et al. The examination of resection margins with conservative surgery: what is the value? In: Wise L, Johnson H Jr, eds. *Controversies in management.* New York: Futura, 1994:165–168.

23. Silvestrini R, Daidone MG, Luisi A, et al. Biologic and clinicopathologic factors as indicators of specific relapse types in node-negative breast cancer. *J Clin Oncol* 1995;13:697–704.

24. Silvestrini R, Daidone MG, Benini E. Validation of p53 accumulation as a predictor of distant

metastasis at 10 years of follow-up in 1400 node-negative breast cancers. *Clin Cancer Res* 1996;2: 2007–2013.

25. Greco M, Agresti R, Raselli R, et al. Axillary dissection can be avoided in selected breast cancer patients: analysis of 401 cases. *Anticancer Res* 1996;16:3913–3918.

26. Veronesi U, Paganelli G, Galimberti V, et al. Sentinel-node biopsy to avoid axillary dissection in breast cancer with clinically negative lymphnodes. *Lancet* 1997;349:1864–1867.

27. Fisher B, Anderson S, Fisher ER, et al. Significance of ipsilateral breast tumor recurrent after lumpectomy. *Lancet* 1991;338:327–331.

28. Veronesi U, Marubini E, Del Vecchio M, et al. Local recurrences and distant metastases after conservative breast cancer treatment: partly independent events. *J Natl Cancer Inst* 1995;87: 19–27.

29. Schnitt SJ, Connolly JL, Harris JR, et al. Pathologic predictors of early local recurrence in stage I and II breast cancer treated by primary radiation therapy. *Cancer* 1984;53:1049–1057.

30. Stotter AT, McNeese MD, Ames FC, et al. Predicting the rate and extent of locoregional failure after breast cancer. *Cancer* 1989;64:2217–2225.

31. Recht A, Schnitt SJ, Connolly JL, et al. Prognosis following local or regional recurrence after conservative surgery and radiotherapy for early stage breast carcinoma. *Int J Radiat Oncol Biol Phys* 1989;16:3–9.

32. Holland R, Veling SH, Mravunac M, et al. Histologic multifocality of Tis, T1–2 breast carcinomas. Implications for clinical trials of breast conserving surgery. *Cancer* 1985;56:979–990.

33. Bonadonna G, Veronesi U, Brambilla C, et al. Primary chemotherapy to avoid mastectomy in tumors with diameters of three centimeters or more. *J Natl Cancer Inst* 1990;82:1539–1545.

34. Veronesi U, Bonadonna G, Zurrida S. Conservation surgery after primary chemotherapy in large carcinomas of the breast. *Ann Surg* 1995; 222:612–618.

CHAPTER 7

Overview of Breast Reconstruction

STEPHEN S. KROLL
SIRPA ASKO-SELJAVAARA

Growing Interest in Breast Reconstruction

Twenty-five years ago, postmastectomy breast reconstruction was rare, even in the United States. The results were inconsistent and, more often than not, unsatisfying. Today breast reconstruction is common, particularly in cancer centers in the United States but also increasingly in medical centers throughout the world (1–4). At the University of Texas M. D. Anderson Cancer Center in Houston, Texas, for example, breast reconstruction is now the most commonly performed major reconstructive operation. The reasons for this increase include better reconstructive techniques with improved results, increasing awareness on the part of women about the availability of breast reconstruction, an improved climate of cooperation between oncologic and reconstructive surgeons, and increased availability of plastic surgeons capable of performing breast reconstruction. These changes have resulted in fewer limitations, lowered psychological stress, and a more complete rehabilitation for breast cancer patients.

Rationale for Breast Reconstruction

Mastectomy, in the eyes of a woman who is compelled to submit to it for treatment of breast cancer, is often considered a deforming operation. Some women are able to cope with the deformity with ease, but many (if not most) others are not (5). Especially in the woman with large breasts, unilateral mastectomy causes an asymmetry that must be corrected by wearing an external breast prosthesis. Although the prosthesis is concealed by clothing, many women complain that it is uncomfortable, limits the type of clothing that they can wear, and can become dislodged during strenuous activities like swimming and dancing. Moreover, each morning when the prosthesis is applied, the patient is reminded of her deformity. Breast reconstruction serves to correct many of these problems, allowing women who are psychologically or physically uncomfortable with their deformity to regard themselves once again as completely feminine, attractive, and normal.

The goal of breast reconstruction is to restore symmetry and a normal female contour so that the patient will appear normal in her clothing without having to wear a prosthesis. Patients should be warned not to expect the breasts to look normal in the unclothed state. A normal clothed appearance, however, is a realistic goal that can almost always be met so that the patient's expectations will rarely be disappointed. The surgeon may well strive to accomplish something better and not infrequently may achieve a result that does appear nearly normal without clothing (Fig. 7-1). Nevertheless, it is unwise to promise that quality of result to a patient. It is better to promise less than can be delivered, because the vagaries of blood supply and scar behavior make the results of even the best surgeons' work impossible to predict accurately. Patients are never unhappy when the results exceed their expectations.

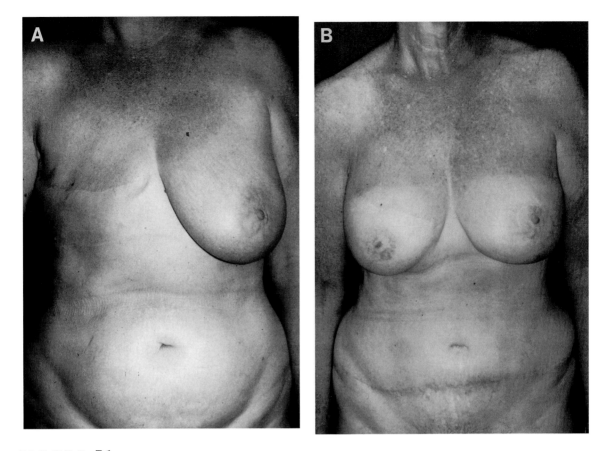

F I G U R E **7-1**

A. A 49-year-old woman after right modified radical mastectomy. [Reproduced by permission from Kroll SS. Breast reconstruction with the transverse rectus abdominis myocutaneous (TRAM) flap. In: Kroll SS, ed. *Reconstructive plastic surgery for cancer.* Philadelphia: Mosby, 1996:276–285.] *B*. The patient 6 years after right TRAM flap breast reconstruction and left mastopexy. (Reproduced by permission from Kroll SS, Miller MJ, Schusterman MA, et al. Rationale for elective contralateral mastectomy with immediate bilateral reconstruction. *Ann Surg Oncol* 1994;1:457–461.)

Available Methods

Reconstructive surgeons and their patients have a wide variety of methods of breast reconstruction available to them. These methods can be divided into two general categories: those based on implants and those based on autogenous tissues. Implant-based methods include simple implant insertion (6–8), tissue expansion with subsequent implant placement (9,10), and the latissimus dorsi myocutaneous flap used over an implant (11,12). Autogenous tissue methods involve the use of flaps including the transverse rectus abdominis myocutaneous (TRAM) flap (13–15), the gluteal free flaps (16–19), and other less commonly used free flaps such as the

lateral thigh flap (20) and the extended latissimus dorsi flap (21). All the autogenous methods create a breast mound without using an alloplastic implant. As such, they tend to be more complex than those methods that utilize an implant but generally lead to better and more consistently successful results.

Implant-Based Reconstructions

The simplest method of breast mound reconstruction is just to replace the breast tissue with an implant and then cover it with locally available skin. This is most often possible when the original breast is very ptotic and when much of the breast skin has been preserved in the mas-

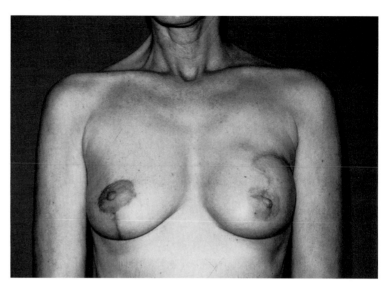

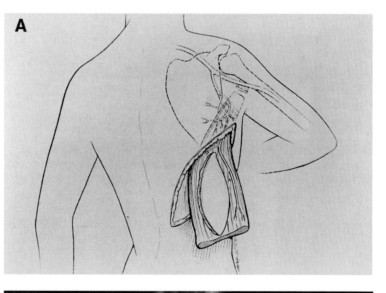

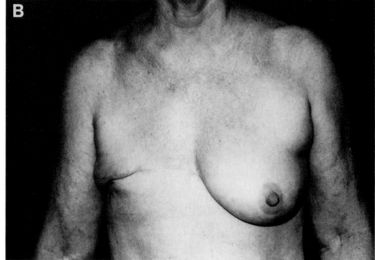

FIGURE 7-2

A 48-year-old woman 1 year after left breast reconstruction with a silicone gel implant and right mastopexy.

FIGURE 7-3

A. The latissimus dorsi flap plan. (Reproduced by permission from Singletary SE, Hortobagyi GN, Kroll SS. Surgical and medical management of local-regional treatment failures in advanced primary breast CA. *Surg Oncol Clin North Am* 1995;4:671–684.) *B.* A 60-year-old woman after right modified radical mastectomy. *C.* The result of reconstruction with a latissimus dorsi flap overlying a silicone gel implant. *D.* The donor site.

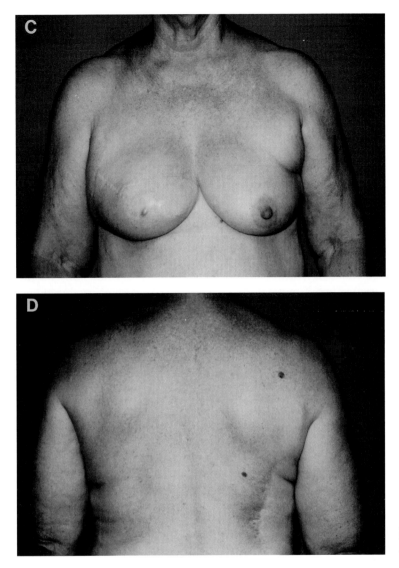

FIGURE **7-3**
Continued

tectomy. Generally the preference is to place the implant beneath the pectoralis major muscle, at least in the upper pole of the breast, to reduce the risk of capsular contracture (22). Combined with an opposite mastopexy to provide symmetry, simple implant insertion in this situation can lead to a very acceptable result with a minimum of additional surgery.

If there is insufficient local skin to provide coverage of the implant and permit adequate breast ptosis, tissue expansion can be used to overcome the skin deficiency and allow successful breast mound reconstruction without importing distant skin and creating additional scarring (Fig. 7-2). The textured expanders have been more successful than the smooth-walled ones (23–25); the former allow more rapid expansion with less capsular contracture. Expansion should begin within 2 weeks after

surgery, before a rigid scar capsule has had a chance to form. The expander should ultimately be overfilled so that the reconstructed breast is larger than the opposite normal one. This overexpanded state should be maintained for at least 4 months so that the skin expansion becomes relatively permanent. The device is then replaced by a permanent implant of the proper size to match the opposite breast.

Tissue expansion and simple implant placement appeal to many women because these techniques do not require extensive surgery and no visible scars are created other than those required by the mastectomy. Unfortunately, the long-term results with implant-based methods have not equaled those obtained with autogenous tissue. Capsular contracture (26) occurs in virtually all patients with implants, and in breast reconstruction, unlike breast augmentation, the prosthesis is close to the skin so the contracture is readily apparent. We found that within 5 years, two thirds of our patients who had breast reconstruction with smooth-walled silicone gel implants developed a noticeable capsular contracture, and at least one third required a surgical correction (27). Although capsular contracture rates using polyurethane foam–covered implants were lower, those devices are no longer available. Newer textured saline implants are advertised as having a lower contracture rate than the smooth-walled implants, but it is unclear whether this is really true. The M. D. Anderson experience to date suggests that the risk of capsular contracture using the newest textured implants probably is lower than that with smooth-walled implants, but the risk, along with that of deflation, infection, and rippling, is still significant enough to make implant-based reconstruction unpredictable.

The use of the latissimus dorsi myocutaneous flap over an implant is a time-tested technique that is capable of achieving quite good results (Fig. 7-3). By bringing new skin from the back to replace the skin removed in the mastectomy, the vagaries of tissue expansion are avoided, and re-establishment of breast shape and ptosis is predictably achieved. Unfortunately, capsular contracture is not prevented. For this reason, we have become less enthusiastic about the standard latissimus dorsi flap (used with an implant) than we were in years past.

Implant-based reconstruction has several other risks in addition to capsular contracture. Periprosthetic infection occurs in approximately 1% of patients, and requires removal of the implant. Implant shell failure with leakage of the contents is common in implants that have been in place for many years, and requires implant replacement. Some patients have had to have their implants removed because of chronic unexplained pain, even when capsular contracture was absent. If the patient gains weight, the normal breast gets larger while the implant-based one does not. Finally, there are questions about silicone's relationship with autoimmune diseases (28–32). We are not convinced, at the time of this writing, that a causative relationship exists. Nevertheless, we cannot dismiss the possibility entirely. Moreover, even if there is no causative relationship, the anxiety about the risks of silicone implants has been a serious problem for women with implant-based reconstruction and for their surgeons. For all these reasons, the alternative of reconstruction with only autogenous tissue has become increasingly popular.

Autogenous Tissue Reconstruction

Autogenous tissue breast reconstruction is more complex than reconstruction with implants, but it confers many long-term advantages. First, all the risks and anxieties associated with silicone implants are eliminated. Second, because the mature normal breast is largely composed of fat, reconstruction with subcutaneous fatty tissues creates a breast mound that looks and feels much like a real breast. The reconstructed breast also physically mimics a real breast, exhibiting ptosis and falling off to the side naturally when the patient is supine. Third, if the patient gains weight, the reconstructed breast (containing fatty tissues) will get larger just like a real breast. Finally, because the breast mound is entirely autogenous tissue, severed nerve endings can grow into it, and some degree of normal sensation is usually restored.

TRAM Flap

The most commonly used technique for autogenous tissue breast reconstruction, both in our institution and elsewhere, is that involving the TRAM flap (13–15,33). The TRAM flap combines the transfer of enough tissue to easily reconstruct one breast (and often two breasts) with a donor site that is easily hidden by clothing (Fig. 7-4). In some patients, the removal of redundant tissue on the lower abdomen improves the appearance of the donor site, although this does not invariably occur. The TRAM flap procedure is technically not overly difficult, and failures in experienced hands (although not necessarily in inexperienced ones) are uncommon. For these reasons, use of the TRAM flap has become the most popular and commonly used method of breast reconstruction in our institution.

There are several variations of the TRAM flap, but they can be divided into two categories: the conventional TRAM flap and the free TRAM flap (3,33–35). The conventional TRAM flap gets its blood supply from the superior epigastric vessels (36,37) via the full length of the rectus abdominis muscle between the xiphoid and the lower edge of the flap (Fig. 7-5). In healthy nonsmoking patients, the blood supply from one muscle alone is usually adequate; in patients who smoke and in others at higher risk of complications, the use of two pedicles is

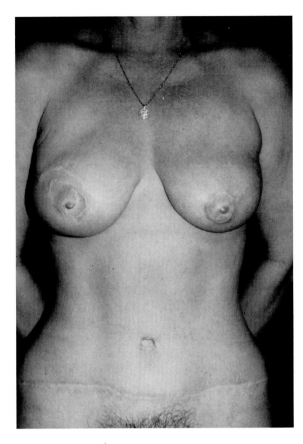

F I G U R E **7-4**

A 43-year-old woman 2 years after bilateral immediate free TRAM flap breast reconstruction. (Reproduced by permission from Kroll SS, Miller MJ,
Schusterman MA, et al. Rationale for elective contralateral mastectomy with immediate bilateral
reconstruction. *Ann Surg Oncol* 1994;1:457–461.)

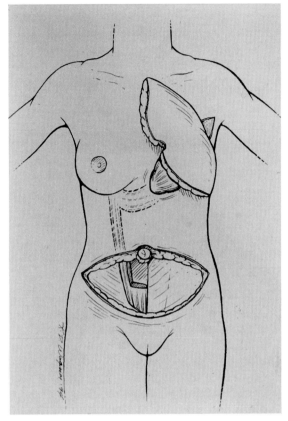

F I G U R E **7-5**

The conventional TRAM flap. The flap is left
attached to the muscle pedicle and transferred
through a subcutaneous tunnel to the chest wall.
(Reproduced by permission from Singletary SE,
Hortobagyi GN, Kroll SS. Surgical and medical management of local-regional treatment failures in
advanced primary breast CA. *Surg Oncol Clin
North Am* 1995;4:671–684.)

T A B L E **7-1**

Incidence of Ischemic Necrosis
in 331 TRAM Flaps

		Percentage of Flaps			
TRAM Type	n	Total Loss	Major Loss	Minor Loss	Fat Necrosis
Free	136	0.7	0.7	2.9	11.0
Conventional	195	0.0	2.1	21.0	25.6

TRAM = transverse rectus abdominis myocutaneous.

better and will reduce the incidence of flap
necrosis. The conventional TRAM flap is
capable of achieving excellent results (Fig. 7-6).
It has the advantage of not requiring microvascular equipment or expertise, but it has two disadvantages compared to the free TRAM flap: It
requires the sacrifice of more muscle and has a
less robust blood supply.

The free TRAM flap is more technically
complex in that it requires specialized equipment and surgeons who are trained in microvascular free tissue transfer. It does, however, have
several important advantages. First, the blood
supply to the flap is more direct and therefore
more effective (Table 7-1) (37). Partial flap loss
is much less common in patients who have

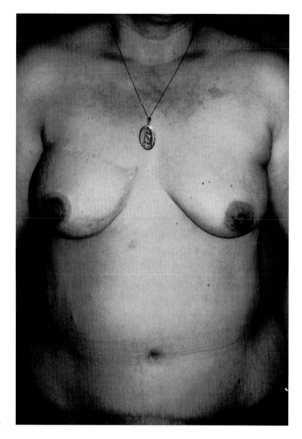

FIGURE **7-6**

A 43-year-old woman 8 years after reconstruction of the right breast with a conventional TRAM flap.

reconstruction with the free TRAM flap, and when it does occur, it tends to be minor in degree (38). In addition, because of the more robust blood supply, the surgeon has more freedom to bend and twist the flap into whatever shape is required to create an aesthetically successful breast. For these reasons, the average aesthetic results of free TRAM flap reconstruction tend to be slightly better than those achieved with conventional flaps (38).

Second, the amount of muscle sacrificed in performing a free TRAM flap is much less than that required using a conventional flap. This leads to a stronger postoperative abdominal wall, at least as measured by the ability to perform sit-ups (39). Moreover, the upper part of the abdominal wall is not disturbed at all. This is especially important because the epigastric region can be a frequent source of prolonged pain in conventional TRAM flap patients, especially in older women. With the free flap, epigastric abdominal wall disruption is completely eliminated. Consequently, the free

TRAM flap patients have less postoperative pain and a faster recovery.

The most significant long-term risk of any type of TRAM flap breast reconstruction is development of a postoperative abdominal bulge or hernia. When severe, this complication can be devastating and must be prevented at all cost. We found that if the abdominal wall is securely repaired by approximating the internal oblique fascia to the midline fascia deep to the linea alba with heavy suture material (such as No. 1 Prolene or Novafil), postoperative bulges and hernias are extremely rare (40). The weak fascia of the anterior rectus sheath lateral to the midline should not be relied on. On rare occasions, if the closure is unusually tight or if the fascia is of poor quality and does not hold the suture well, synthetic mesh is used to reinforce the abdominal wall further. In most cases, however, even after bilateral reconstruction, mesh is not necessary.

Gluteal Flaps

The superior and inferior gluteal free flaps are good autogenous tissue sources that can be used as an alternative to the TRAM flap or in patients in whom a TRAM flap cannot be used because of a previous abdominoplasty or other surgery. The gluteal flap reconstruction is technically more difficult to perform than the TRAM flap procedure, however, often requiring a vein graft and more time to perform. They also cause donor site changes that can be visible even through clothing when the patient is wearing pants. Consequently, they have not become as popular as the TRAM flap for general breast reconstruction. Both flaps are useful, however, in patients who have had a previous unilateral TRAM flap reconstruction and who subsequently develop a new contralateral breast cancer. In such patients, a gluteal free flap can be a good alternative capable of matching the existing TRAM flap reconstruction fairly well.

Extended Latissimus Dorsi Flap

The second most commonly used autogenous tissue breast reconstruction technique in our institution, after the TRAM flap procedure, is the extended latissimus dorsi flap method (21). This is a technically simple method that has a high success rate and is capable of achieving excellent results (Fig. 7-7). The method is identical to the standard latissimus dorsi flap procedure except that additional subcutaneous fat and skin are transferred with the flap so that an implant is not required. Operative time is less than that for any of the other autogenous tissue techniques. Failure is rare, unless the thoracodorsal vessels have previously been injured. Shaping of the breast is somewhat more difficult than with the TRAM flap, but the ultimate result is usually similar. The main disadvantage of the extended latissimus dorsi flap is the donor site scarring (Fig. 7-8). Many women do not seem to mind these scars, possibly in part because they do not usually look at them. The donor deformity is noticeable and can be visible when the patient is wearing a bathing suit. In spite of this, however, the method has become quite popular.

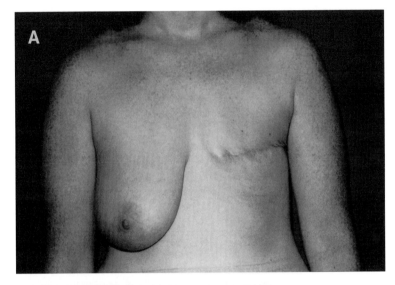

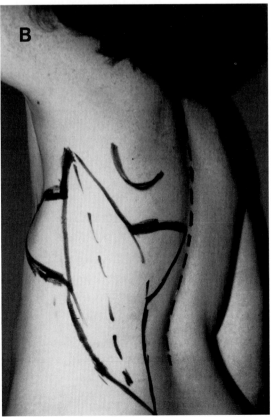

FIGURE 7-7

A. A 31-year-old woman after a left modified radical mastectomy. *B.* A "fleur-de-lis" pattern for an extended latissimus dorsi flap. *C.* The patient 2 years after reconstruction.

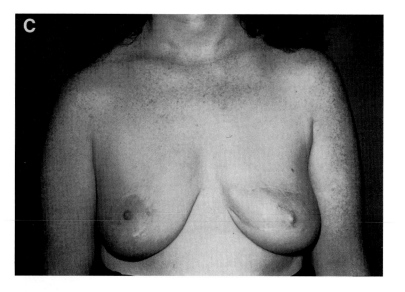

FIGURE 7-7

Continued

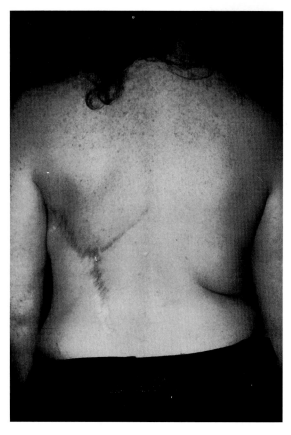

FIGURE 7-8

The donor site scarring from the "fleur-de-lis" type of extended latissimus dorsi flap.

"Ruben's Fat Pad" Flap

"Ruben's fat pad" flap technique (41) uses fatty tissue in the flank overlying the iliac crest. This free flap procedure is more technically difficult than the TRAM flap one, but has a relatively well-hidden donor site scar and the advantage of being available for use even for the patient who has had a previous TRAM flap or abdominoplasty. Usage of Ruben's flap is relatively new, and not enough of these procedures have been done to fairly assess its reliability or place in breast reconstruction. Nevertheless, this promising method is being used increasingly when a TRAM flap is not possible, and it deserves further study.

Immediate Versus Delayed Breast Reconstruction

Delayed breast reconstruction, performed months or years after the mastectomy, has stood the test of time and has several advantages. Women who have lived with their mastectomy scars for some time are usually sure of their motivations and tend to be satisfied with the results, even when less than perfect. Any required adjuvant chemotherapy or radiation will have been completed and will not interfere with the reconstruction. If they have survived many years without cancer, these women are usually oncologically stable and not likely to develop unexpected tumor recurrence. Nevertheless, immediate reconstruction has grown in popularity and is the preferred approach for most patients with early breast cancer (1,2,42,43).

Immediate reconstruction has a number of significant advantages. It is more convenient for patients, accomplishing most of their reconstructive needs simultaneously with the removal of their malignancy. Immediate reconstruction is psychologically easier because the patient is not confronted with the deformity of mastectomy. It is also less expensive than delayed reconstruction because one less hospitalization is required (44). With one less anesthetic induction, the patient is exposed to less anesthesia risk. Finally, the aesthetic results of immediate reconstruction tend to be better than those of delayed reconstruction because of the ability to preserve and use uninvolved breast skin (38).

Immediate reconstruction is especially advantageous to patients undergoing breast reconstruction with a free flap. After axillary dissection, the thoracodorsal artery and vein are usually exposed and available for use as recipient vessels. This recipient vessel exposure shortens the operating time for the reconstructive surgeon and eliminates the possibility of vascular injury when the vessels have to be dissected out of scar tissue in a delayed reconstruction.

Immediate reconstruction, especially when combined with a skin-preserving mastectomy, requires teamwork and coordination between the plastic and general surgical teams. The quality of the result depends not only on the work of the reconstructive surgeon but also on that of the general surgeon. He or she must be capable of working with limited skin incisions and yet maintaining sufficient blood supply to the mastectomy flaps that they remain viable. If use of a free flap is planned, the thoracodorsal vessels must be properly exposed and uninjured. The general surgeon is therefore an important member of the team.

Immediate breast reconstruction does not increase the likelihood of cancer recurrence, either locally or systemically (2,45). At the University of Texas M. D. Anderson Cancer Center,

immediate reconstruction has been combined with skin-preserving mastectomy in more than 550 patients. Although local recurrences have occurred, the incidence of such events is similar to that found in patients in other comparable series treated without either immediate reconstruction or skin-preserving mastectomy (Table 7-2). We therefore see no reason why this reconstructive option should be denied to patients with early (T1 and T2) breast cancer who desire it. For patients with more advanced (T3) malignancies, immediate reconstruction is more controversial. Some surgeons prefer to avoid immediate reconstruction for such patients because they will often require urgent postoperative adjuvant radiotherapy or chemotherapy, or both, and the surgeon does not want to subject the flap to radiotherapy or run the risk that a surgical complication of the reconstruction might delay adjuvant treatment. Our own opinion at this time is that immediate reconstruction can be indicated for selected patients with T3 tumors but that because postoperative radiotherapy is more difficult after reconstruction, the radiation therapist should be consulted and the situation discussed prior to the surgery.

Role of Nipple and Areolar Reconstruction

Nipple reconstruction is technically simple and can generally be accomplished in an office or clinic setting using local anesthesia. Not all patients request reconstruction of the nipple, but for those who accept it, nipple reconstruction can add a significant degree of realism to the reconstructed breast. Because nipple reconstruction adds so much to breast reconstruction with so little risk, we believe that surgeons should encourage their patients to undergo it

		Percentage of Patients		
	n	Recurrence	Metastasis	Death
All patients	545	2.6	5.1	2.2
Length (yr) of follow-up				
>1	394	3.6	6.9	3.0
>2	278	4.0	7.9	3.6
>3	176	5.1	9.7	4.0
>4	95	4.2	6.3	1.1
>5	39	7.8	10.3	2.6

T A B L E **7-2**

Local Tumor Recurrence, Metastasis, and Mortality in Patients with T1 and T2 Breast Cancer Undergoing Skin-Preserving Mastectomy with Immediate Reconstruction

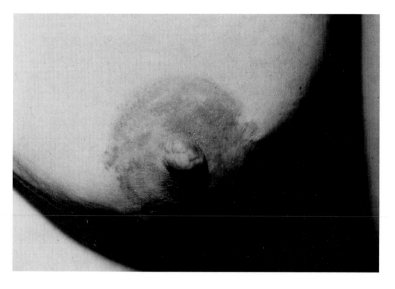

FIGURE 7-9

A reconstructed nipple-areolar complex. The use of medical-grade tattooing to simulate an areola not only is relatively painless, but also provides color to the nipple, reconstructed with small local flaps, as well. (Reproduced by permission from Kroll SS. Nipple and areolar reconstruction. In: Kroll SS, ed. *Reconstructive plastic surgery for cancer.* Philadelphia: Mosby, 1996: 314–318.)

by making it as painless, convenient, and inexpensive as possible. This is facilitated by reconstructing the areola with tattooing rather than a skin graft (46,47), because tattooing can be performed in the office or clinic with minimal anesthesia. It is possible to perform the areolar tattooing immediately following the nipple reconstruction, but the results seem to be better if the tattooing is delayed for a few weeks. Tattooing also permits coloration of the nipple itself, something a skin graft cannot accomplish (Fig. 7-9). For these reasons, nipple reconstruction methods that require skin grafting are best avoided.

Complications

Complications of implant-based reconstruction include capsular contracture, periprosthetic infection, leakage, and breast asymmetry, as discussed earlier. Infection requires that the implant be removed and not replaced (except by autogenous tissue). Leaking or deflated implants, and those that are rendered severely asymmetric by changes in the patient's weight, are ordinarily replaced with new ones in a relatively simple surgical procedure. Treatment of capsular contracture, if it causes severe disfigurement or pain, is more difficult. Release of the capsule relieves the symptoms, but the problem usually recurs quickly unless the implant is replaced with something different (such as autogenous tissue). Capsular contracture is especially likely in patients treated with radiotherapy (48), so implants should be avoided if irradiation is planned (49). Should a patient

with an implant subsequently need radiotherapy, however, the implant is not ordinarily removed until the capsular contracture becomes symptomatic.

Complications are not rare after autogenous tissue reconstruction, but they are usually self-limited and do not lead to failure of the reconstruction. Most of them, in fact, will resolve without further surgery. Partial loss of a TRAM flap may require early surgical revision (50). Extensive flap loss may require augmentation or replacement with another flap (51). If such additional surgery is necessary, we prefer to do it early so that delays in the administration of adjuvant treatment are minimized.

Hernias and abdominal bulges occur in between 1% and 4% of TRAM flap patients and usually appear a few months after the reconstruction. Most such abdominal wall problems can be repaired successfully, and virtually all of them can be if the TRAM flap was unilateral (52). Synthetic mesh may be necessary to reinforce the abdominal wall in this situation. Because an abdominal bulge or hernia does not interfere with adjuvant treatment, its repair is generally deferred until all such treatment is completed.

Integration of Multimodality Therapy

Immediate reconstruction does not hinder administration of postoperative adjuvant chemotherapy or irradiation unless healing of the reconstructed breast is significantly delayed. Such delays in wound healing are usually caused by flap ischemia and partial necrosis, especially if the necrosis is not corrected by early debridement and surgical revision. Partial flap necrosis is much less common after reconstruction with free TRAM flaps than with conventional TRAM flaps (53); this is one reason why we prefer free TRAM flaps and use them regularly.

Similarly, the late appearance of fat necrosis (which can cause one or more firm nodules of scar tissue in the periphery of the reconstructed breast) is related to flap blood supply and is much less common with free TRAM flaps than conventional ones. Fat necrosis can be confused with tumor recurrence and for this reason often causes concern in the patient and oncologist. If the mass suspected of being fat necrosis is in a typical location (usually the point in the reconstructed breast most distant from its blood supply) and if it appears to be softening and decreasing in size with time, it can probably be treated with observation and benign neglect. If there is doubt about the diagnosis, needle biopsy can be used for confirmation. If the mass is getting larger, however, biopsy should be performed immediately. If the nodule is attached to the skin, it is probably not fat necrosis and biopsy is required.

Conclusions

Breast reconstruction is of great assistance to women who have difficulty coping with the deformity caused by mastectomy. Many methods of breast reconstruction are available, and all have advantages and devotees. Our own preference, for patients who are suitable candidates, is to use only autologous tissues. Our first choice for most patients is the free TRAM flap. We find this technique, especially when combined with a skin-preserving mastectomy and used for immediate reconstruction, to be exceedingly reliable and effective. Other effective but less frequently used methods of breast reconstruction are the extended latissimus dorsi flap, the gluteal free flaps, and the "Ruben's fat pad" flap techniques. For patients who are not appropriate candidates for autologous tissue reconstruction, or for those who for their own reasons prefer the use of breast implants, implant-based reconstruction can also be effective. Provided that patients have reasonable expectations, breast reconstruction usually succeeds in achieving its goals, and most patients are highly satisfied with the outcome.

REFERENCES

1. Noone RB, Murphy JB, Spear SL, Little JW. A 6-year experience with immediate reconstruction after mastectomy for cancer. *Plast Reconstr Surg* 1985;76:258–269.

2. Noone RB, Frazier TG, Noone GC, et al. Recurrence of breast carcinoma following immediate reconstruction: a 13-year review. *Plast Reconstr Surg* 1994;93:96–106.

3. Suominen E, Asko-Seljavaara S, Tuominen H, Tukainen E. Free microvascular TRAM flaps for breast reconstruction: the first 50 patients. *Eur J Plast Surg* 1995;18:1–6.

4. DeMay M, Lejour M, Declety A, Meythiaz A. Late results and current indications of latissimus dorsi breast reconstructions. *Br J Plast Surg* 1991;44:1–4.

5. Schain WS, Wellisch DK, Pasnau RO. The sooner the better: a study of psychological factors in women undergoing immediate versus delayed breast reconstruction. *Am J Psychiatry* 1985;142:40–46.

6. Little JW, Golembe EV, Fisher JB. The "living bra" in immediate and delayed reconstruction of the breast following mastectomy for malignant and nonmalignant disease. *Plast Reconstr Surg* 1981;68:392.

7. Woods JE. Breast reconstruction: current state of the art. *Mayo Clin Proc* 1986;61:579–585.

8. Jarrett JR, Cutler RG, Teal DF. Subcutaneous mastectomy in small, large, or ptotic breasts with immediate placement of implants. *Plast Reconstr Surg* 1978;62:702.

9. Gibney J. Use of a permanent tissue expander for breast reconstruction. *Plast Reconstr Surg* 1989;84:607–617.

10. Becker H. Breast reconstruction using an inflatable breast implant with detachable reservoir. *Plast Reconstr Surg* 1984;73:678–683.

11. Bostwick J, Vasconez LO, Jurkiewicz MJ. Breast reconstruction after a radical mastectomy. *Plast Reconstr Surg* 1978;61:682.

12. Biggs TM, Cronin ED. Technical aspects of the latissimus dorsi myocutaneous flap in breast reconstruction. *Ann Plast Surg* 1981;6:381.

13. Hartrampf CR Jr, Scheflan M, Black PW. Breast reconstruction with a transverse abdominal island flap. *Plast Reconstr Surg* 1982;69:216–224.

14. Hartrampf CR Jr, Bennett GK. Autogenous tissue reconstruction in the mastectomy patient:

a critical review of 300 patients. *Ann Surg* 1987;205:508–518.

15. Elliott LF, Hartrampf CR Jr. Tailoring of the new breast using the transverse abdominal island flap. *Plast Reconstr Surg* 1983;72:887–893.

16. Shaw WW. Breast reconstruction by superior gluteal microvascular free flaps without silicone implants. *Plast Reconstr Surg* 1983;72:490–499.

17. Nahai F. Inferior gluteus maximus musculocutaneous flap for breast reconstruction. *Perspect Plast Surg* 1992;6:65.

18. Codner MA, Nahai F. The gluteal free flap breast reconstruction: making it work. *Clin Plast Surg* 1994;21:289–296.

19. Shaw WW. Microvascular free flaps: the first decade. *Clin Plast Surg* 1983;10:3–20.

20. Elliott LF, Beegle PH, Hartrampf CR Jr. The lateral transverse thigh free flap: an alternative for autogenous-tissue breast reconstruction. *Plast Reconstr Surg* 1990;85:169–181.

21. McCraw JB, Papp C, Edwards A, McMellin A. The autogenous latissimus breast reconstruction. *Clin Plast Surg* 1994;21:279–288.

22. Woods JE, Irons GB, Arnold PG. The case for submuscular implantation of prostheses in reconstructive surgery. *Ann Plast Surg* 1980;5: 115.

23. Spear SL, Stefan MM, Travaglino-Parda R. Breast reconstruction with expanders and implants. In: Kroll SS, ed. *Oncologic plastic surgery: reconstructive surgery for cancer patients.* Philadelphia: Mosby, 1996:305–313.

24. Ohlsen HL. A clinical comparison of the tendency to capsular contracture between smooth and textured gel-filled silicone mammary implants. *Plast Reconstr Surg* 1992;90:247–254.

25. Pollack H. Breast capsular contracture: a retrospective study of textured versus smooth silicone implants. *Plast Reconstr Surg* 1993;91: 404–407.

26. McCraw JB, Maxwell GP. Early and late capsular "deformation" as a cause of unsatisfactory results in the latissimus dorsi breast reconstruction. *Clin Plast Surg* 1988;15:717–726.

27. Kroll SS, Baldwin BJ. A comparison of outcomes using three different methods of breast reconstruction. *Plast Reconstr Surg* 1992;90:455–462.

28. Heggers JP, Kossovsky N, Parsons RW, et al. Biocompatibility of silicone implants. *Ann Plast Surg* 1983;11:38–45.

29. McGrath MH, Burkhardt BR. The safety and efficacy of breast implants for augmentation mammaplasty. *Plast Reconstr Surg* 1984;74:550–560.

30. Kossovsky N, Heggers JP, Robson MC. The bioreactivity of silicone. In: Williams DF, ed. *CRC critical reviews in biocompatibility.* Boca Raton: CRC Press, 1987:53–85.

31. Brody GS, Conway DP, Deapen DM, et al. Consensus statement on the relationship of breast implants to connective-tissue disorders. *Plast Reconstr Surg* 1992;90:1102–1105.

32. Fisher JC. The silicone controversy—when will science prevail? *N Engl J Med* 1992;326:1696–1698.

33. Schusterman MA, Kroll SS, Miller MJ, et al. The free TRAM flap for breast reconstruction: a single center's experience with 211 consecutive cases. *Ann Plast Surg* 1994;32:234–242.

34. Holmstrom H. The free abdominoplasty flap and its use in breast reconstruction. *Scand J Plast Reconstr Surg* 1979;13:423.

35. Grotting JC, Urist MM, Maddox WA, Vasconez LO. Conventional TRAM flap versus free microsurgical TRAM flap for immediate breast reconstruction. *Plast Reconstr Surg* 1989;83:842–844.

36. Moon HK, Taylor GI. The vascular anatomy of rectus abdominis musculocutaneous flaps based on the deep superior epigastric system. *Plast Reconstr Surg* 1988;82:815–829.

37. Boyd JB, Taylor GI, Corlett R. The vascular territories of the superior epigastric and the deep inferior epigastric systems. *Plast Reconstr Surg* 1984;73:1–14.

38. Kroll SS, Coffey JA Jr, Winn RJ, Schusterman MA. A comparison of factors affecting aesthetic outcomes of TRAM flap breast reconstruction. *Plast Reconstr Surg* 1995;96:860–864.

39. Kroll SS, Schusterman MA, Reece GP, et al. Abdominal wall strength, bulging, and hernia after TRAM flap breast reconstruction. *Plast Reconstr Surg* 1995;96:616–619.

40. Kroll SS, Marchi M. Comparison of strategies for preventing abdominal-wall weakness after TRAM flap breast reconstruction. *Plast Reconstr Surg* 1992;89:1045–1053.

41. Hartrampf CR Jr, Noel RT, Drazan L, et al. Ruben's fat pad for breast reconstruction: a periiliac soft-tissue free flap. *Plast Reconstr Surg* 1994;93:402–407.

42. Beasley ME. The pedicled TRAM as preference for immediate autogenous tissue breast reconstruction. *Clin Plast Surg* 1994;21:191–205.

43. Vinton AL, Traverso LW, Zehring RD. Immediate breast reconstruction following mastectomy is as safe as mastectomy alone. *Arch Surg* 1990; 125:1303–1308.

44. Elkowitz A, Colen S, Slavin S, et al. Various methods of breast reconstruction after mastectomy: an economic comparison. *Plast Reconstr Surg* 1993;92:77–83.

45. Kroll SS, Ames F, Singletary SE, Schusterman MA. The oncologic risks of skin preservation at mastectomy with immediate breast reconstruction. *Surg Gynecol Obstet* 1991;172:17–20.

46. Spear SL, Convit R, Little JW. Intradermal tattoo as an adjunct to nipple-areolar reconstruction. *Plast Reconstr Surg* 1989;83:907–911.

47. Kroll SS. Nipple and areolar reconstruction. In: Kroll SS, ed. *Oncologic plastic surgery: reconstructive surgery for cancer patients.* Philadelphia: Mosby, 1996:314–318.

48. Schuster RH, Kuske RR, Young VL, Fineberg B. Breast reconstruction in women treated with radiation therapy for breast cancer: cosmesis, complications, and tumor control. *Plast Reconstr Surg* 1992;90:445–454.

49. Kroll SS, Schusterman MA, Reece GP, et al. Breast reconstruction with myocutaneous flaps in previously irradiated patients. *Plast Reconstr Surg* 1994;93:460–469.

50. Kroll SS. The early management of flap necrosis in breast reconstruction. *Plast Reconstr Surg* 1991;87:893–901.

51. Kroll SS, Freeman P. Striving for excellence in breast reconstruction: the salvage of poor results. *Ann Plast Surg* 1989;22:58–64.

52. Kroll SS, Schusterman MA, Mistry D. The internal oblique repair of abdominal bulges secondary to TRAM flap breast reconstruction. *Plast Reconstr Surg* 1995;96:100–104.

53. Schusterman MA, Kroll SS, Weldon ME. Immediate breast reconstruction: why the free TRAM over the conventional TRAM flap? *Plast Reconstr Surg* 1992;90:255–262.

CHAPTER 8

Adjuvant Therapy for Breast Cancer

AHMAD AWADA

JOSEPH KERGER

JOSÉE-ANNE ROY

MARTINE J. PICCART-GEBHART

*B*reast cancer, once it has recurred at distant sites, is a lethal disease. This rule, which has very few exceptions, highlights the crucial role of adjuvant therapy in the treatment of early breast cancer. The major end point of adjuvant therapy is cure for a larger and larger proportion of patients.

Slow but constant progress is being made in the identification of effective adjuvant therapy regimens; however, there is increasing awareness that these treatments may not be devoid of serious side effects in the long run. This chapter summarizes the current knowledge in the changing field of adjuvant therapy as well as the most promising new approaches in the early stages of clinical development.

Adjuvant Therapy for Node-Positive Breast Cancer

Hormonal Therapy

Hormonal manipulation has been used for the treatment of breast cancer for a century (1). However, the effectiveness of hormonal agents as adjuvant therapy was not widely appreciated until the publication in 1988 of an overview of randomized trials (2), the first update of which was published in 1992 (3). The roles of tamoxifen and ovarian ablation as adjuvant therapy for breast cancer were closely examined in these reports.

Tamoxifen

In the 1992 overview (3), data on 30,000 women enrolled in randomized trials of adjuvant tamoxifen were analyzed. These trials included not only trials of tamoxifen versus no tamoxifen but also trials of tamoxifen plus chemotherapy versus the same chemotherapy alone (Table 8-1). Data on recurrence and mortality at 10 years were analyzed for the entire cohort and for particular subsets, such as node-negative and node-positive patients.

Tamoxifen was found to produce a significant reduction in the annual odds of recurrence and death. Indirect comparisons strongly suggested that women 50 years or older, those with estrogen receptor–positive tumors, and those who took tamoxifen for at least 2 years had a greater benefit with therapy. However, the reductions in the annual odds of mortality for tamoxifen given for an average of 2 years or for an average of more than 2 years were comparable, with overlapping confidence intervals, leaving uncertainty about the optimal duration of treatment. Results recently issued by three cooperative groups shed light on this important question (4–6). More than 3500 post-menopausal patients with operable node-positive or node-negative invasive breast cancer were randomized in the Swedish trial to receive tamoxifen for 2 or 5 years (4). At a median follow-up of 5½ years, there was a significant improvement in event-free survival and overall survival rates for the patients receiving tamoxifen for 5 years.

138

T A B L E   **8-1**

Overview of Findings from Early Breast Cancer Trialists' Collaborative
Group 1992[a]

Treatment	Reduction in Annual Odds of		Absolute Difference at 10 Years in	
	Recurrence (%)	Mortality (%)	Recurrence-Free Survival (%)	Survival (%)
Ovarian ablation in patients <50 yr old	26 ± 6	25 ± 7	10.2 ± 2.7	10.6 ± 2.7
Tamoxifen[b]	25 ± 2	17 ± 2	6.6 ± 0.9	6.2 ± 0.9
Node-negative patients	28 ± 4	17 ± 5	5.1 ± 1.4	3.5 ± 1.4
Node-positive patients	33 ± 2	18 ± 2	8.8 ± 1.1	8.2 ± 1.1
Polychemotherapy[b]	28 ± 3	16 ± 3	8.4 ± 1.3	6.3 ± 1.4
Node-negative patients	26 ± 7	18 ± 8	7.1 ± 2.7	4.0 ± 2.8
Node-positive patients	30 ± 3	18 ± 3	8.7 ± 1.5	6.8 ± 1.6

[a] Based on 133 randomized trials conducted between 1957 and 1985 involving 75,000 women (3).
[b] Overall analysis.

In the National Surgical Adjuvant Breast and Bowel Project (NSABP) trial B-14 (5), 1172 breast cancer patients with node-negative and estrogen receptor–positive tumors were randomized to stop tamoxifen treatment after 5 years or to pursue the drug for an additional 5 years. Preliminary results indicate no further benefit from use of tamoxifen for more than 5 years.

The results of a small Scottish trial were similar: No additional benefit was observed in patients randomized to continue tamoxifen indefinitely as compared to patients receiving treatment for 5 years, and there was a suggestion that treatment for longer than 5 years may increase the risk of endometrial carcinoma (6).

While we wait for the results of other important clinical trials addressing the issue of the optimal duration of tamoxifen therapy, it seems reasonable to adopt 5-year tamoxifen therapy in daily clinical practice.

In addition to a significant reduction in the annual odds of recurrence and death, adjuvant tamoxifen confers additional advantages, such as a reduction in the incidence of contralateral breast cancer and potential protection from cardiovascular events and physiologic bone loss.

A reduction in the incidence of contralateral breast cancer in patients receiving adjuvant tamoxifen was observed in several trials (7,8). Similarly, the 1992 overview (3) reported that contralateral breast cancer developed in 2% (184/9135) of the control patients, in contrast with 1.3% (122/9128) of the tamoxifen-treated patients (3).

Both the Stockholm trial (9) and the Scottish trial (10) showed a decreased number of cardiac events in women receiving adjuvant tamoxifen. In the 1992 overview analysis (3), tamoxifen was associated with a reduction of 12% [standard deviation (SD) = 6, $p = 0.05$] in non-breast-cancer deaths in general and a 25% (SD = 13, $p = 0.06$) reduction in death from vascular causes. This trend in decreased cardiac events may be explained by favorable changes in the lipid profile observed after adjuvant tamoxifen therapy for 2 and 5 years (11).

Tamoxifen given to postmenopausal women for 5 years also may preserve bone mineral density in the lumbar region of the spine (12). This effect on bone may eventually translate into a reduction in lumbar spine fractures in women taking tamoxifen for long periods.

Ovarian Ablation

The role of ovarian ablation as an effective form of adjuvant therapy in premenopausal women with breast cancer was a major finding of the 1992 overview (3) and was nicely reviewed by Davidson (13). The 1992 overview found that women younger than 50 years who had an ovarian ablation had a recurrence-free survival rate of 58.5% at 10 years compared with 48.3% in the control group (see Table 8-1).

The overview also examined the effectiveness of chemotherapy plus ovariectomy in women younger than 50 years. By indirect comparison, chemotherapy plus ovariectomy did not seem to yield better results than did ovariectomy alone. Data on the effectiveness of adjuvant ovariectomy with respect to hormone receptor levels were not available in the overview, mainly because these trials were conducted before the era of hormone receptor determination.

Permanent ovarian ablation may be detrimental for younger women. Severe menopausal symptoms such as hot flashes, dysuria, and dyspareunia may develop with the rapid decrease in plasma levels of sex hormones and may be very difficult to alleviate with nonhormonal therapy. Furthermore, suppression of ovarian function for long periods can lead to an increased risk of osteoporosis (14) and ischemic heart disease (15).

Strategies to suppress ovarian function temporarily rather than permanently have been developed recently, with the hope of reducing the incidence and severity of the aforementioned complications. Several ongoing trials are assessing the value of luteinizing hormone –releasing hormone (LHRH) agonists given for 2 to 5 years in premenopausal women with early breast cancer. It is hoped that these trials will help to define the effectiveness of LHRH agonists alone or in combination with chemotherapy. The effectiveness of total estrogen blockade, in which an LHRH agonist is combined with an antiestrogen compound, will also be assessed in some of these trials.

Chemotherapy

According to the 1992 overview (3), polychemotherapy is an effective form of adjuvant therapy for node-positive breast cancer, reducing the annual odds of recurrence and mortality by 30% and 18%, respectively (see Table 8-1). This effect was more pronounced in younger women than in patients older than 50 years and persisted when patients with involvement of four or more axillary nodes were included in the analysis.

The overview clearly indicated that combination chemotherapy is superior to single-agent cytotoxic therapy. Of note, most of the trials of combination chemotherapy included in the overview used cyclophosphamide, methotrexate, and fluorouracil (CMF) (16) or CMF-like regimens.

Role of Anthracyclines

Doxorubicin (17) and its analogue epirubicin (18) are considered the most active cytotoxic drugs against advanced or metastatic breast cancer. When given as single agents at full doses as primary chemotherapy, they prove to be nearly as effective as several standard combinations. In two major trials conducted in patients with metastatic breast cancer, the combination of fluorouracil, doxorubicin, and cyclophosphamide (FAC) was superior to CMF regimens with regard to objective response rate, complete responses, time to progression, and even survival, and fluorouracil, epirubicin, and cyclophosphamide (FEC) produced results comparable to those produced by FAC (19,20).

Anthracyclines were introduced into the adjuvant treatment of node-positive breast cancer more than 20 years ago. However, no firm or definitive conclusions can be drawn today regarding the efficacy of these drugs in the adjuvant setting. This is mainly due to methodologic problems with the design of the published randomized trials, as explained here.

Data from a number of randomized trials comparing anthracycline- with non-anthracycline-containing regimens are presented in Table 8-2 (21–35). Unfortunately, the nonoptimal design of most of these studies has precluded true assessment of the independent value of the anthracyclines as an adjuvant. Since CMF represents the best-studied and most commonly used adjuvant chemotherapy regimen, the utility of anthracyclines would best have been defined by a randomized trial comparing CMF with CAF or CEF; however, no such study has been extensively published so far. Instead, anthracycline-containing regimens have generally been compared with non-anthracycline-containing combinations other than CMF.

The NSABP trials B-11 and B-12 (21) compared a three-drug regimen [melphalan, doxorubicin, and fluorouracil (PAF)] with a two-drug regimen [melphalan and fluorouracil (PF)]. At 6 years of follow-up, PAF was superior to PF in patients younger than 48 years and in patients aged 50 to 59 with negative progesterone receptor status. In women older than 60 years and women aged 50 to 59 with positive progesterone receptor status, PF and PAF

T A B L E   **8-2**

Randomized Trials of Anthracycline-Containing Versus Non-Anthracycline-Containing
Regimens in Node-Positive Breast Cancer

Design/Group (Reference)	Regimens	No. of Patients	Median Follow-up Time (yr)	Disease-Free Survival Rate (%)			Overall Survival Rate (%)		
				+Aa	−Aa	P	+Aa	−Aa	P
3-Drug vs 2-drug regimen									
National Surgical Adjuvant Breast and Bowel Project (NSABP) B-11 (21)	PAF vs PF	707	5	51	44	0.007	65	59	NS
NSABP B-12 (21)	PAFT vs PFT	1106	5	64	63	NS	77	78	NS
Dissimilar regimens									
Oncofrance (22)	AVCF vs CMF	249	10	54	43	0.04	67	61	0.01
Bordeaux (23)	3 MThVn/3 EVM vs CMF	228	5	78	67	0.05	—	—	NS
NSABP B-15 (24)	4 AC VS 6 CMF	2194	3	62	63	NS	83	82	NS
Sequential vs alternating regimens									
Eastern Cooperative Oncology Group (ECOG) (25)	CMFPT/VAThHT vs CMFPT	533	5	70	63	0.04	77	79	NS
Milan Istituto Nazionale per lo Studio e la Cura dei Tumori (1–3 N+) (26)	8 CMF + 4A vs 12 CMF	486	5	72	74	NS	86	89	NS
Milan Istituto Nazionale per lo Studio e la Cura dei Tumori (≥4 N+) (27,28)	4 A + 8 CMF vs (2 CMF/1A) × 4	403	10	42	28	0.002	58	44	0.002
Similar regimens									
Southeastern Cancer Study Group (SECSG) (29,30)	CAF vs CMF	527	5	—	—	—	74	68	NS
International Cancer Cooperative Group (ICCG) (31,32)	Various FEC vs CMF	760	5	61	58	NS	79	76	NS
National Cancer Institute of Canada (NCI-C) (33)	CEF vs CMF	710	3	73	65	0.03	84	81	NS
Different dose and/or dose intensity									
Cancer and Leukemia Group (CALG) B-8541 (34)	High-dose CAF	513	3.4	74	—	—	92	—	—
	Moderate-dose CAF	507	—	70	—	—	90	—	—
	Lose-dose CAF	509	—	63	—	<0.001	84	—	0.004
NSABP B-22 (35)	Standard-dose AC	746	3	73	—	—	89	—	—
	High-dose AC	737	—	70	—	NS	89	—	NS
	High-dose intensity AC	755	—	74	—	—	87	—	—

+Aa = anthracycline-containing; −Aa = non-anthracycline-containing; A = doxorubicin; C = cyclophosphamide; E = epirubicin; F = fluorouracil; H = fluoxymesterone; M = methotrexate; P = prednisone; T = tamoxifen; Th = thiotepa; V = vincristine; Vn = vindesine;
NS = not significant.

plus tamoxifen produced equivalent long-term results. The lack of difference in the latter patient subset could be explained by a negative interaction between tamoxifen and certain antineoplastic agents or by reduced effectiveness of anthracycline against well-differentiated steroid receptor–positive tumors.

The Oncofrance trial (22) randomly assigned women to receive either CMF or doxorubicin, vincristine, cyclophosphamide, and fluorouracil (AVCF). With 10-year follow-up, the disease-free and overall survival rates were superior in the subset of premenopausal patients treated with AVCF, but in view of schedule and drug differences and an imbalance in nodal involvement between the two study groups, it is not clear how much of the improvement can be attributed to the use of doxorubicin.

Another French group (23) conducted a trial that randomly assigned women to receive either six courses of CMF intravenously or three courses of mitomycin C, thiotepa, and vindesine followed by three courses of epirubicin, vincristine, and methotrexate. This trial enrolled 228 node-positive, receptor-negative premenopausal patients. Five-year results showed a slightly better relapse-free survival rate in the epirubicin-containing treatment group, but the overall survival rate was similar. The epirubicin-containing regimen was more toxic.

The NSABP trial B-15 (24) examined both the role of doxorubicin in adjuvant therapy and the duration of adjuvant therapy. More than 2000 node-positive breast cancer patients were randomly assigned to receive four courses of doxorubicin and cyclophosphamide (AC) given over 3 months; CMF for 6 months; or four courses of AC given over 3 months followed by reinduction with CMF 6 months later. There were no statistically significant differences in relapse-free or overall survival rates at a median follow-up of 3 years. Given this similar efficacy, short-course AC might be preferable to conventional CMF: AC is better tolerated, so compliance is higher, and AC is also more convenient, as it is given over 3 instead of 6 months. It must be stressed that the shorter duration of AC might have precluded the detection of a difference in treatment outcome in favor of the anthracycline-containing regimen.

The Milan group compared 12 courses of intravenous CMF with eight cycles of CMF followed by four courses of doxorubicin in breast cancer patients with one to three positive nodes and could not detect any significant difference in outcome after a median follow-up of 5 years (26). The same investigators also tested the Norton-Simon hypothesis of sequential administration of potentially non-cross-resistant chemotherapy regimens in a higher-risk group of patients—those with more than three involved axillary nodes. The investigators observed better relapse-free and overall survival rates with sequential chemotherapy (four courses of doxorubicin followed by eight cycles of CMF) than with alternating chemotherapy (two cycles of CMF followed by one cycle of doxorubicin for a total of 12 courses) (27,28). The promising results with this sequential program warrant confirmatory trials, which are presently under way.

Few randomized trials directly compared the classic CMF regimen with similar cyclophosphamide, doxorubicin, and fluorouracil (CAF) or FEC combinations. At 3 and 5 years of follow-up, the results of the Southeastern Cancer Study Group (29,30), which used "equitoxic" regimens of CMF (cyclophosphamide 600 mg/m^2, methotrexate 60 mg/m^2, and fluorouracil 600 mg/m^2) and CAF (cyclophosphamide 450 mg/m^2, doxorubicin 45 mg/m^2, and fluorouracil 450 mg/m^2), with a lower dose intensity for the CAF regimen, and of the International Cancer Cooperative Group (31,32), which compared various schedules of CMF and FEC, did not clearly show a benefit for anthracycline-containing combinations. However, with a median follow-up of 3 years, the National Cancer Institute of Canada (NCI-C) study of CMF versus CEF, which enrolled premenopausal patients only and used a relatively intensive CEF regimen, demonstrated a significant advantage in relapse-free survival with CEF (33). These results need to be confirmed with a longer follow-up. Meanwhile, the results of another FEC-versus-CMF trial launched by the Danish Breast Cancer Group are eagerly awaited.

The relationship between dose and long-term results remains controversial. With regard to the anthracyclines, only two studies prospectively addressed this question. The results of the Cancer and Leukemia Group B-8541 trial (34) suggested either a dose-response effect or a threshold effect: Inferior results were seen in the low-dose treatment group (cyclophosphamide 300 mg/m^2, doxorubicin 30 mg/m^2, fluorouracil 300 mg/m^2 for four cycles), but similar results were observed so far for the high-dose (cyclophosphamide 600 mg/m^2, doxorubicin 60 mg/m^2, fluorouracil 600 mg/m^2 for four cycles) and moderate-dose (cyclophosphamide 400 mg/m^2, doxorubicin 40 mg/m^2, fluorouracil 400 mg/m^2 for six cycles) regimens. In fact, the so-called high-dose CAF regimen could be viewed as a standard-dose regimen, whereas the dose and dose intensity of the low-dose treatment group could be viewed as insufficient or inadequate. This potential threshold effect was not detected after a similar follow-up period in the NSABP B-22 protocol (35), which investigated a fixed dose of doxorubicin in combination with more dose-intense or higher-dose cyclophosphamide.

In summary, in spite of 20 years of randomized clinical trials, the role of anthracyclines in adjuvant therapy for node-positive breast cancer remains controversial. Additional randomized trials, longer follow-up of some of the more recent studies, or a meta-analysis of all existing trials will be needed to clarify this important issue. It must be stressed, however, that anthracycline-based regimens have never produced therapeutic results inferior to those produced by CMF regimens. The higher toxicity associated with anthracyclines (discussed later in this chapter) and the remaining uncertainty regarding the long-term survival advantage in the adjuvant setting should raise caution about their widespread use in unselected patients outside the context of randomized clinical trials.

Duration of Adjuvant Chemotherapy

Several prospective, randomized trials addressed the optimal duration of adjuvant chemotherapy (24,36–38). In general, prolonged, relatively low-dose combination regimens for longer than 6 months do not produce better long-term results, and one single perioperative chemotherapy cycle seems to be inadequate (39).

Timing of Adjuvant Chemotherapy

Preclinical models suggest that early initiation of adjuvant chemotherapy may be important to obtain optimal therapeutic results. One study even suggested that perioperative chemotherapy may be a way to prevent accelerated tumor proliferation after surgery (40). Retrospective analyses of the time variable in clinical trials of adjuvant chemotherapy produced conflicting results. In most published studies, adjuvant chemotherapy was required to start within 30 days after surgery. In the prospective trial conducted by the Ludwig Breast Cancer Study Group, the addition of one perioperative course of CMF plus prednisone to six classic CMF-prednisone cycles started 3 to 4 weeks after the surgical procedure did not produce any additional benefit (39).

Primary Chemotherapy

There is clearly renewed interest in primary or "neoadjuvant" chemotherapy following the growing popularity of breast-conserving surgery in the management of breast cancer (41). Numerous trials of primary chemotherapy, most of them nonrandomized, were conducted during the past decade, first in patients with locally advanced but more recently also in patients with operable breast cancer (Table 8-3). Impressive objective response rates and even complete responses were observed in most of these studies, allowing for breast-conserving strategies (42–51). Evaluation of the long-term impact of primary chemotherapy in operable breast cancer, however, must await maturation of ongoing or recently closed randomized clinical trials.

In the meantime, locally advanced breast cancer is the optimal model in which to compare various chemotherapeutic regimens for their potential to induce marked, or even complete, tumor regressions. The European Organization for Research and Treatment of Cancer Breast Cancer Cooperative Group, in collaboration with the NCI-C and the Schweizerische Arbeitsgemeinschaft für Klinische Krebsforschung, has recently closed for accrual a large clinical trial in which patients with locally advanced breast cancer are randomly assigned to receive either a short, "accelerated," and intensive neoadjuvant epirubicin-cyclophosphamide regimen given with granulocyte colony-stimulating factor support or six 1-month cycles of the Canadian "CEF" regimen given without granulocyte colony-stimulating factor. Taxoids are obviously strong candidates for becoming the most widely used drugs in the neoadjuvant chemotherapy setting for these high-risk patients (52).

Sequencing of Chemotherapy and Radiation Therapy

In spite of two decades of clinical trials, the optimal sequence for administering adjuvant

T A B L E   **8-3**

Studies of Primary Chemotherapy in Surgically Resectable Breast Cancer

Group (Reference)	No. of Patients	Type of Elective Locoregional Therapy	Chemotherapeutic Regimen	Response Rate (%)		
				Complete and Partial	Complete	Pathologic Complete
Jacquillat (42)	250	RT	Vinblastine, thiotepa, methotrexate, 5-fluorouracil, ± doxorubicin, ± tamoxifen	75	30	—
Forrest (43)	27	Surgery	Cyclophosphamide, doxorubicin, vincristine, and prednisone	72	NR	NR
Smith (44)	50	Surgery → RT	5-fluorouracil by CI, epirubicin, and cisplatin	98	66	27
Smith (45)	64	RT → Surgery	CMF or MMM	69	17	—
Mauriac (46)	134	RT in patients w/CR	EVM × 3 + MTV × 3	63	33	—
Scholl (47)	153	RT	FAC	82	30	—
Bonadonna (48)	227	Surgery	Doxorubicin or CMF or FAC	78	21	4
Bonadonna (49)	210	Surgery	Doxorubicin	74	12	1.5
Fisher (50)	549	Surgery	Doxorubicin and cyclophosphamide	80	37	NR
Powles (51)	101	Surgery → RT*	Methotrexate, mitoxantrone, and tamoxifen ± mitomycin C	85	19	10

NR = not reported; CR = complete response; RT = radiation therapy; CMF = cyclophosphamide, methotrexate, and 5-fluorouracil; MMM = methotrexate, mitoxantrone, and mitomycin C; EVM = epirubicin, vincristine, and methotrexate; MTV = mitomycin C, thiotepa, and vindesine; FAC = fluorouracil, doxorubicin, and cyclophosphamide; CI = continuous infusion.

Source: Adapted from Bonadonna G, Valagussa P, Zucorli R, Salvadori B. Primary chemotherapy in surgically resectable breast cancer. *CA Cancer J Clin* 1995;45:227–243.

*Two patients did not receive radiotherapy.

chemotherapy and radiation therapy has not yet been determined. Possible sequence options are chemotherapy followed by radiation therapy, concomitant treatment, sandwich radiation therapy, and radiation therapy followed by chemotherapy (53).

Retrospective data are conflicting. Delaying radiation therapy may result in increased local recurrence rates, and the safety of postponing radiation therapy until the end of chemotherapy in patients who have had lumpectomy or partial mastectomy has not been formally demonstrated. On the other hand, in node-positive breast cancer patients with a high risk of systemic recurrence, early initiation of adjuvant chemotherapy and full-dose chemotherapy may be important, especially in view of the fact that local radiation therapy is unlikely to have a sig-

nificant impact on long-term survival. Several prospective trials were initiated with the hope of clarifying this important sequencing issue.

Results of the first randomized trial assessing the sequence of chemotherapy and radiation therapy after conservative surgery for early breast cancer are now available (54). Two hundred forty-four patients with stage I or II breast cancer, considered to be at substantial risk for systemic metastases, were randomized to receive a 12-week course of chemotherapy either before or after radiation therapy. The 5-year actuarial rates of cancer recurrence at any site and of distant metastases in the radiotherapy-first group and the chemotherapy-first group were 38% and 31% ($p = 0.17$) and 36% and 25% ($p = 0.05$), respectively. The overall survival rates were 73% and 81%

(p = 0.11), respectively. Of interest, a lower chemotherapy dose intensity was delivered to the radiotherapy-first group.

As the authors concluded, the results of this study suggest that it is preferable to give a 12-week course of chemotherapy followed by radiation therapy rather than the opposite sequence. Whether these results can be extrapolated to longer chemotherapy regimens is unknown.

Adjuvant Chemoendocrine Therapy

Several prospective, randomized trials compared the simultaneous administration of adjuvant chemotherapy and hormonal therapy with adjuvant chemotherapy alone or adjuvant hormonal therapy alone. Unfortunately, many of these trials were initiated before determination of tumor hormone receptor status became routine.

In premenopausal women, even when the benefits of ovarian ablation seem to be similar in magnitude to those of chemotherapy, this does not mean that chemotherapy and ovarian ablation are equivalent (3). In the Scottish Cancer Trials Breast Group trial (55), which slowly accrued 332 premenopausal women with node-positive breast cancer and compared ovarian ablation with CMF given for six to eight cycles, there was no statistically significant difference in relapse-free or overall survival rates

T A B L E   **8-4**

Randomized Trials of Chemoendocrine Therapy in Postmenopausal Women with Node-Positive Breast Cancer

Group/Trial (Reference)	Regimen	No. of Patients	Median Follow-up Time (yr)	Relapse-free Survival Rate (%)	p	Overall Survival Rate (%)	p
HT vs CHT							
IBCSG (56)	Control	156	7	24	—	47	—
	PT	153	—	36	0.003	51	NS
	CMFP + T	154	—	51	—	57	—
DBCG 82-C (57)	T	458	4	49	—	68	—
	CMF + T	432	—	56	—	66	—
	T + RT	457	—	60	0.03	71	NS
Case Western (58)	T	48	4.6	53	—	78	—
	CMFVP + T	46	—	78	0.04	79	NS
NSABP B-16 (59)	T	376	3	67	—	85	—
	AC + T	377	—	84	0.0004	93	0.04
	T	298	3	66	—	84	—
	MelAF + T	—	—	83	0.0002	84	NS
NCI-C (60)	T	705	7.5	—	—	—	—
	CMF + T	—	—	—	NS	—	NS
CT vs CHT							
NSABP B-09 (61)	MelF	941	5	47	—	67	—
	MelF + T	950	—	52	0.002	67	NS
Crowe (62)	CMF	99	10	36	—	42	—
	CMF + T (+ BCG)	212	—	47	0.02	57	NR
CT vs HT vs CHT							
Southwest Oncology Group (SWOG) (63)	CMFVP	894	4.3	—	—	78	—
	T	—	—	—	NS	77	NS
	CMFVP + T	—	—	—	—	73	—
GROCTA (64,65)	CMF/E	84	3.3	—	—	—	—
	T	89	—	—	0.000	—	0.002
	CMF/E + T	94	—	—	—	—	—

A = doxorubicin; BCG = bacille Calmette-Guérin; C = cyclophosphamide; CHT = combined chemoendocrine therapy; CT = chemotherapy; E = epirubicin; F = fluorouracil; HT = hormonal therapy; Mel = melphalan; M = methotrexate; N/R = not reported; NS = not significant; P = prednisone; RT = radiation therapy; T = tamoxifen; IBCSG = International Breast Cancer Study Group; DBCG = Danish Breast Cancer Group; GROCTA = Breast Cancer Adjuvant Chemo-hormone Therapy Cooperative Group (ITALY).

at 8 years between the two groups. However, ovarian ablation was associated with improved survival in patients with estrogen receptor–rich tumors, and CMF was associated with improved survival in patients with estrogen receptor–poor or –negative tumors.

A number of trials comparing adjuvant chemotherapy and castration (accomplished by surgical ovarian ablation or use of LHRH analogues) either alone or in combination are currently in progress and should help to refine adjuvant therapy for premenopausal patients in the near future. The role of tamoxifen given after chemotherapy is also being explored by the European Organization for Research and Treatment of Cancer Breast Cancer Cooperative Group and by the NCI-C in two parallel ongoing trials.

In postmenopausal women, the addition of chemotherapy to tamoxifen produced conflicting results (Table 8-4). Some of these trials showed that chemoendocrine therapy improves relapse-free survival, but the impact on overall survival is less apparent (56–65). It will be interesting to see whether the next overview of adjuvant therapy trials will confirm the trend in improved relapse-free survival and overall survival for combined chemoendocrine therapy in postmenopausal women that was suggested by the 1992 overview (3). Also, the magnitude of this benefit in relation to hormone receptor status needs to be elucidated.

In any event, many questions related to chemoendocrine therapy remain unanswered: Which patients are most likely to benefit from combined treatment? What is the optimal chemotherapy regimen? Which is more effective—simultaneous or sequential administration of tamoxifen? (Do antagonisms exist between tamoxifen and some cytotoxic drugs?) What is the optimal duration of hormonal therapy?

Until these questions are resolved, a reasonable treatment approach to node-positive breast cancer patients is that recently outlined by an international panel (66).

Adjuvant Therapy for Node-Negative Breast Cancer

About half of all patients newly diagnosed as having breast cancer are node negative, and this proportion is increasing with more aggressive screening (67). Although node-negative patients clearly have a more favorable outlook than node-positive breast cancer patients, 20% to 30% of node-negative patients will die of their disease.

A well-validated and easily obtainable prognostic factor is the pathologic tumor size. The 5-year survival rate for patients with invasive tumors less than 1 cm in diameter is as high as 98% (68), and such patients have a projected relapse-free survival rate of 88% at 20 years (69). On the other hand, for patients with tumors larger than 2 cm in diameter, the risk of developing distant metastasis is greatly increased (70,71). For tumors between 1 and 2 cm, hormone receptor status, tumor grade, and presence or absence of vascular invasion are currently used to select patients most suitable for adjuvant therapy, but these selection criteria remain unsatisfactory.

There is a crucial need to identify and validate new, powerful prognostic factors and to determine the optimal adjuvant treatment in relation to them. New prognostic factors currently under study are reviewed later in this chapter.

Although the 1992 overview of adjuvant therapy trials (3) showed a statistically significant reduction in relapse-free survival and mortality at 10 years for node-negative patients who received either tamoxifen or polychemotherapy, it should be kept in mind that the majority of patients selected for these trials were those who had tumors larger than 3 cm in diameter or estrogen receptor–negative tumors measuring 1 to 3 cm in diameter.

Future trials for node-negative breast cancer should focus on patients with intermediate-sized tumors (1–2 cm) and the presence of one or more adverse prognostic factors.

Adjuvant Therapy in Older Women with Breast Cancer

The management of breast cancer in older women is becoming a major challenge as the general population ages. Two randomized trials specifically addressed the effectiveness of adjuvant tamoxifen in 170 and 320 women 65 years or older with node-positive breast cancer (72,73). In both trials, patients treated with tamoxifen had a significant improvement in recurrence-free survival but not in overall survival. The lack of significant improvement in overall survival in these two trials is probably due to the small numbers of patients studied.

Indeed, the 1992 overview (3) indicated that the use of tamoxifen improves relapse-free and overall survival rates for postmenopausal women, including those older than 70 years (3). As expected, tamoxifen therapy is of greatest benefit in patients whose primary tumors are estrogen and progesterone receptor positive.

In contrast, adjuvant chemotherapy in older women has been studied only minimally, and therefore the 1992 overview (3) is of little help. In one adjuvant chemotherapy trial in which patients with node-positive breast cancer received a doxorubicin-containing chemotherapy regimen, patients older than 65 years had disease-free and overall survival rates similar to those of their younger counterparts at a median follow-up of 7.3 years (74). Severe leukopenia was the only toxicity found to be more common in older patients (74).

A cost-effectiveness analysis examining total and active life expectancy outcomes in elderly patients receiving chemotherapy for node-negative breast cancer was recently published (75). The authors concluded that a small survival benefit for adjuvant chemotherapy in elderly patients is likely, but the cost associated with this benefit is high.

In summary, there is a clear need to conduct clinical trials of adjuvant chemotherapy for elderly patients, who represent an increasing proportion of breast cancer patients and for whom the benefits and risks of adjuvant therapy have not been properly assessed so far.

Long-Term Side Effects of Adjuvant Therapy

Over the past 5 years, the oncology community has become increasingly aware of possible long-term side effects of adjuvant therapies given to breast cancer patients.

Side Effects of Tamoxifen

Several investigators (8,76,77) reported the occurrence of endometrial cancer in patients taking adjuvant tamoxifen, in the context of several prospective randomized clinical trials (Table 8-5).

A retrospective analysis done on 53 patients with endometrial carcinoma revealed that 15 of these patients had taken tamoxifen for breast carcinoma and that several of these 15 patients presented with high-grade endometrial cancers that had a poor prognosis (78). This aggressive biologic behavior was not observed in patients who developed secondary endometrial cancer within the NSABP B-14 trial (76). A case-control study done in the Netherlands (79) supported the hypothesis that tamoxifen increases the risk of endometrial cancer: A relative risk of 1.3 [95% confidence interval (CI), 0.7–2.4] was found for women using tamoxifen. Furthermore, women who had used tamoxifen for more than 2 years had a relative risk of 2.3 (95% CI, 0.9–5.9) compared with never users. In this study, there was a significant trend for increased endometrial cancer risk with longer tamoxifen use and also with a higher cumulative tamoxifen dose.

Surprisingly, an excess risk of gastrointestinal cancers has also been found in tamoxifen-treated patients (relative risk, 1.9; 95% CI, 1.2–2.9) (77). These data on second cancers obviously need confirmation since they may represent an artifact: Women taking tamoxifen have a prolonged survival and may therefore be at increased risk of developing other neoplasias.

Two other side effects of tamoxifen are worth mentioning: the increased risk of devel-

T A B L E   **8-5**

Cases of Endometrial Cancer Reported in Randomized Trials of Tamoxifen

Trial (Reference)	No. of Patients	Median Follow-up Time (yr)	Cases of Endometrial Cancer		Relative Risk (95% CI)
			Tamoxifen	Control	
Stockholm Trial (8)[a]	1846	9.5	14	2	6.4 (1.4–28.0)
NSABP B-14 (76)[b]	2843	8	15	0	7.5 (1.7–32.7)
Scandinavian Trials (77)[c]	4914	9	34	8	4.1 (1.9–8.9)

[a] Tamoxifen, 40 mg daily for 2 or 5 yr.

[b] Tamoxifen, 20 mg daily for at least 5 yr.

[c] Tamoxifen, 30 or 40 mg daily for 1 or 2 yr.

oping venous thromboses and tamoxifen-related retinopathy. In the NSABP B-14 trial, 2843 node-negative women were randomly assigned to receive tamoxifen, 20 mg daily, or a placebo (76). Phlebitis was documented in only two patients in the placebo group but in 12 patients receiving tamoxifen, including one patient who died of a pulmonary embolism.

To investigate the incidence and course of ocular toxicity in patients receiving tamoxifen, 20 mg daily, a prospective study (80) was conducted in 63 patients. Retinopathy or keratopathy or both developed in four patients after a median duration of 25 months. In another study, screening of 135 asymptomatic tamoxifen-treated women revealed that two patients had changes consistent with tamoxifen-induced retinopathy (81). The authors of this study concluded that routine ophthalmologic screening was not necessary in tamoxifen-treated patients.

Side Effects of Chemotherapy

In addition to a number of acute side effects such as gastrointestinal distress, hair loss, and myelosuppression, chemotherapy can induce permanent ovarian dysfunction in premenopausal patients, causing menopausal symptoms and resulting in the potential increased risk of developing ischemic heart disease or osteoporosis. Administration of chemotherapy has also been implicated in the development of venous thromboses (82).

Recently, the Milan group reported on the occurrence of second malignancies following their adjuvant treatment program, in which CMF was given to women with resectable breast cancer (83). At 15 years, the cumulative actuarial risk of second malignancies was 6.7% ± 0.8% for the total series. The cumulative risk was 6.4% ± 0.9% in women who had received CMF adjuvant therapy, while it was 8.4% ± 2.9% after local-regional treatment alone, suggesting the lack of an increased risk of second malignancies following CMF chemotherapy. Of note, three cases of acute nonlymphoblastic leukemia developed, all in the chemotherapy group, for a cumulative risk of 0.23% ± 0.15%.

The picture may be somewhat different for patients receiving anthracycline-based chemotherapy. Indeed, several worrisome reports (84–88) of acute myeloid leukemia following anthracycline-based chemotherapy have now been published (Table 8-6). Some of these leukemias showed the typical 11q23 translocation observed with leukemia secondary to topoisomerase II inhibitors. Of note, some cases of acute myeloid leukemia occurring after anthracycline-based therapy for advanced breast cancer have also been reported (89). A synergistic effect in leukemogenesis between anthracyclines and alkylating agents has been proposed but remains hypothetical.

The use of anthracyclines may also be hampered by their potential long-term, drug-related cardiotoxicity—mainly chronic cardiomyopathy,

T A B L E **8-6**

Cases of Acute Myeloid Leukemia (AML) Reported in Breast Cancer Adjuvant Studies

Group (Reference)	Type of Study	Regimen (Dose of Anthracycline in mg/m²)	No. of Patients Receiving Anthracycline	No. of Cases of AML (Previous RT)	Presence of 11q23	Months Between Study Entry and AML (Median)
Buzdar (84)	Retrospective study	FAC	736	8 (7)	—	68
Riggi (85)	Randomized trials	EC (60 × 2) vs CMF	577	2 (—)	—	22
		FEC (50) vs FEC (75)	621	1 (1)	—	48
Shepherd (86)	Randomized trial	CEF (60 × 2) vs CMF	351	3 (2)[a]	1	18
DeCillis (87)	Randomized trial	AC (60)[b]	2548	6 (2)	3	14
Linassier (88)	Retrospective study	CN (12) F[c]	—	5 (5)[d]	3	16

[a] One case of acute lymphocytic leukemia was also described.

[b] This trial compares different doses of C, i.e., 1200 mg/m² × 4 or 2400 mg/m² × 2 or 2400 mg/m² × 4.

[c] Two patients also received vinblastine.

[d] Four patients received adjuvant chemotherapy, while one received anthracycline for metastatic disease.

RT = radiation therapy; F = fluorouracil; A = doxorubicin; C = cyclophosphamide; E = epirubicin × 2 given on days 1 and 8; M = methotrexate; N = mitoxantrone.

ischemic heart disease, and congestive heart failure. Clear data on anthracycline-induced cardiomyopathy in the adjuvant setting are relatively sparse, and in most of the adjuvant trials performed so far, the incidence of cardiomyopathy was not prospectively or extensively evaluated. With a total cumulative dose of 400 mg/m^2 or less of doxorubicin or 720 mg/m^2 or less of epirubicin, the incidence of congestive heart failure was estimated to be about 1%; the incidence was somewhat higher (2%) after both doxorubicin and radiation therapy to the left breast (90). However, additional factors such as the schedule of drug administration (for example, high-dose bolus) and concomitant use of anthracyclines and newer chemotherapy agents, such as the taxoids, could further increase the risk of developing cardiac events. Therefore, monitoring of anthracycline cardiotoxicity will need to be reinforced in the coming years (91).

Future Directions

The latest developments in the field of adjuvant therapy for early breast cancer and some of the highest priorities for future clinical research are discussed.

New Prognostic Factors in Early Breast Cancer

For two decades, clinicians have used information about the number of involved axillary nodes, tumor size, hormone receptor status, and tumor histology as the best but still suboptimal way to predict outcome in patients with early breast cancer. More recently, a rapidly growing number of biologic markers have been proposed as new prognostic factors, but none of them has yet been incorporated into general clinical practice. In addition to problems of quality control in the evaluation of these markers, there are problems in the design of the studies published to date: The new markers were examined individually rather than by multivariate analysis, retrospectively rather than prospectively, and in small trials with a short follow-up period. These important methodologic and statistical problems were extensively discussed by McGuire (92), Gasparini et al (93), and Knoop et al (94).

At present, these new "prognostic factors" should be considered investigational. They include markers related to tumor proliferation (Ki 67, S-phase fraction, thymidine labeling index, and cyclin D1), tumor growth (epidermal growth factor receptor, c-erb B-2 or Neu, insulin-like growth factor, and the H-*ras* oncogene product), growth suppression or metastasis (*p53*, *RB*, and *nm23*), invasion (cathepsin D, urokinase plasminogen activator/plasminogen activator inhibitor 1, and collagenase type IV), adhesion (laminin receptor), and angiogenesis. Table 8-7 summarizes our current knowledge in this developing field.

New Predictive Factors in Early Breast Cancer

A *predictive factor* is defined as a factor allowing the selection of patients most likely to respond to a specific form of therapy. The prototypical predictive factor in breast cancer, known for 20 years, is tumor estrogen receptor content, which correlates with the probability of response to endocrine therapy.

It is only in the past 5 years that other gene products known to play an important role in tumor biology have been investigated as potential predictors of response to hormonal or chemotherapeutic agents. Tumors with pS2 expression were found to be more likely than tumors without pS2 expression to respond to hormonal treatment (95), while tumors expressing c-erb B-2 (96,97), epidermal growth factor receptor (98), or urokinase-type plasminogen activator (99) were poorly responsive to endocrine therapy. P-glycoprotein overexpression was associated with resistance to anthracyclines (100). Of note, all the studies mentioned above were performed in patients with metastatic disease. As far as adjuvant treatment is concerned, Muss et al (101) showed recently that overexpression of c-erb B-2 may identify the subset of patients who are most likely to benefit from higher doses of adjuvant FAC chemotherapy. This elegant study needs additional follow-up and the findings need to be confirmed by other groups (102).

Finally, a number of in vitro studies showed interesting correlations between overexpression of heat shock proteins (103) or mutant-type p53 (104) and decreased sensitivity to chemotherapy.

More studies of this kind in the adjuvant setting are clearly needed: They may spare thousands of patients toxic and costly treatment, and may allow for targeting of specific thera-

T A B L E **8-7**

Examples of Investigational Prognostic Markers in Breast Cancer

Marker	No. of Studies (Median No. of Patients)	Proposed Function	Expression in Breast Tumors, % (Range)	Correlation with Prognosis in Multivariate Analysis (No. of Studies)		Comments
				Yes	No	
erb B-1	13 (212)	Gene product = EGF-R = growth factor receptor	EGF-R: 45 (22–91)	4	4	Conflicting results
erb B-2	38 (380)	Gene product = 185-kd protein p185 = growth factor receptor	erb-B2 gene overexpression: 20–25 p185 positivity: 19 (9–33)	13	13	Conflicting results, poor prognosis in node-positive patients; inverse correlation with ER and PgR; positive correlation with tumor grade, size, and mitotic activity
uPA/PAI1	14 (223)	Local invasiveness marker	High uPA: 42 (29–58)	12	2	High contents of uPA or PAI1 = poor prognosis
p53 (Mutant)	12 (260)	Gene product = 53 kd = suppression of cell proliferation and malignant transformation	p53 positivity: 28 (13–52)	11	0	p53 overexpression = poor prognosis; inverse correlation with ER and PgR; positive correlation with tumor grade
nm23	4 (range; 24–130)	Antimetastatic gene	NR	NR	2	Decreased level of nm23 RNA and nm23 protein = poor prognosis
CD-31 antibody, factor VIII related antigen	14 (73)	Tumor angiogenesis	NR	8	2	Intense neovascularization = poor prognosis

EGF-R = epidermal growth factor receptor; ER = estrogen receptor; NR = not reported; PAI1 = plasminogen activator inhibitor; PgR = progesterone receptor; uPA = urokinase plasminogen activator.

Source: Adapted from Knoop AS, Laenkholm AV, Mirza MR, et al. Prognostic and predictive factors in early breast cancer. ESMO Educational Book, 1994:9–18.

pies to subsets of patients likely to derive the greatest benefit.

New Directions in Adjuvant Endocrine Treatment

In spite of one trial that found that amino-glutethimide as adjuvant endocrine therapy for postmenopausal women was not effective (105), it is likely that the newest aromatase inhibitors, with their increased therapeutic ratio in advanced breast cancer (106), will soon be tested in the adjuvant setting, alone or in combination with tamoxifen.

New antiestrogen products such as toremifene and the pure antiestrogen ICI 182780 may also have a role in the treatment of early breast cancer in view of their well-documented activity in advanced disease (107,108).

Fenretinide, a synthetic retinoid, definitely deserves investigation in the adjuvant setting. Preclinical data demonstrate a decreased incidence of carcinogen-induced mammary tumors with the use of fenretinide and enhanced inhibition of breast carcinogenesis when the drug is combined with ovariectomy (109). Furthermore, fenretinide significantly enhanced the efficacy of tamoxifen against breast cancer growth. A large, placebo-controlled phase III trial, recently closed, will determine the role of fenretinide, if any, in preventing contralateral primary breast cancer (110). The trial enrolled 3000 women with a previous diagnosis of localized breast cancer (110). In the adjuvant setting, trials comparing tamoxifen with tamoxifen plus fenretinide are ready to begin on both sides of the Atlantic Ocean. It is hoped that the combination regimen will increase disease-free and overall survival rates.

New Chemotherapeutic Agents and New Combination Regimens

The past 10 years has witnessed the clinical development of a number of new cytotoxic drugs with innovative mechanisms of action.

Vinorelbine, the taxoids (paclitaxel and docetaxel), thymidylate synthase inhibitors (e.g., tomudex), gemcitabine, and camptothecin analogues (topotecan and irinotecan) have demonstrated interesting activity in advanced breast cancer (52,111,112). One of these compounds, docetaxel, induces unusually high response rates in liver metastases (113). This activity may be of interest in the adjuvant setting: Goldhirsch et al (114) recently showed that adjuvant treatments in current use improve patient outcome mainly by reducing the incidence of first local, regional, or distant soft tissue relapses, while first recurrences in bone or viscera appear to be much less influenced.

Combination regimens that include new, active compounds are now under active investigation against metastatic disease in phase I/II trials. High objective response rates and sometimes high complete remission rates have been reported (115–119). However, these dose-finding studies included very small numbers of patients, and further studies specifically addressing the antitumor activity of these drugs are needed. The role of these new combinations in the management of primary breast cancer should be assessed

through properly designed randomized clinical trials.

Renewed Interest in Drug Sequencing

The effects of some chemotherapy regimens are sequence dependent—that is, the effects of the regimens differ depending on the timing of administration of the drugs in the same cycle. When anthracyclines and taxoids are given in combination according to prolonged schedules of drug administration, the observed side effects appear to be dependent on drug sequencing; it is less clear whether the antitumor activity of this combination is sequence dependent. Interestingly, pharmacokinetic studies do not always explain sequence-dependent differences, which suggests that other mechanisms may be operative at the cellular level (120).

Bonadonna et al (28) showed the superiority of sequential versus alternating schedules of doxorubicin and CMF in the adjuvant setting.

Encouraged by this observation, by the feasibility of sequential administration of doxorubicin and high-dose cyclophosphamide, and by the partial non-cross-resistance between paclitaxel and doxorubicin, Memorial Sloan-Kettering Cancer Center launched a study of rapid sequential administration of maximum tolerated doses of doxorubicin, paclitaxel, and cyclophosphamide with granulocyte colony-stimulating factor support in patients with four or more positive nodes (121). This innovative regimen might be a candidate for future prospective randomized clinical trials in the adjuvant setting.

Dose-Intensive Adjuvant Therapy for "High-Risk" Early Breast Cancer

Results of preclinical experiments conducted in mammary tumor models and retrospective analyses of a number of clinical trials in breast cancer patients suggest a possible role for dose-intensive therapies in the treatment of this disease.

While suboptimal doses of adjuvant chemotherapy are associated with inferior results (34,122), the role of high-dose chemotherapy remains controversial (123).

In the past years the results of many small phase I and II trials using high-dose chemotherapy given as single agents or combinations have been published (124,125). The results are promising in comparison with results of historical studies. However, this comparison is seriously hampered by the strict patient selection process for these toxic programs (123,126). Fortunately, randomized clinical trials in patients with stage II disease (five or more positive nodes), stage III disease, and inflammatory breast cancer are currently under way (127). The first results are expected toward the end of this century. Table 8-8 summarizes some important randomized clinical trials in progress.

New Modulating Agents

The former generation of "modulating" agents such as leucovorin, pentoxifylline, toremifene, and cyclosporine has been used in combination with anticancer drugs with the hope of avoiding or overcoming chemotherapy resistance. So far, none of these approaches has been tested in the adjuvant setting, as a clear-cut advantage over conventional treatment could not be shown in advanced disease.

More recently, monoclonal antibodies have been used against the HER-2/neu protein with encouraging preliminary results. Pietras et al (128) showed that a monoclonal antibody to the HER-2/neu receptor can block DNA repair following cisplatin exposure in human breast and ovarian cancer cells. Moreover, this antibody enhanced the cytotoxicity of cisplatin (129), carboplatin (130), and doxorubicin (130) against human breast tumor cells. Paclitaxel was combined with anti–growth factor receptor monoclonal antibodies (anti–epidermal growth factor

T A B L E **8-8**

Ongoing Randomized Phase III Trials of High-Dose Adjuvant Chemotherapy with Hematopoietic Stem Cell Support

Country (Group)	No. of Involved Axillary Nodes	Induction Regimen	Randomization Arms
USA (CALGB)	>10	CAF × 4	C, B, P* (high dose) vs C, B, P (conventional dose)
USA (ECOG)	>10	CAF × 4	C, T* vs no further therapy
The Netherlands	>10	FEC × 4	C, T, Cb* vs FEC × 1
France (PEGASE 01)	>8	FEC × 4	C, M, Mx* vs no further therapy
Sweden	>5	FEC	C, T, Cb* vs FEC increasing dose + GCSF

*Peripheral stem cell support.

A = doxorubicin; B = carmustine; C = cyclophosphamide; Cb = carboplatin; E = epirubicin; F = fluorouracil; GCSF = granulocyte colony-stimulating factor; M = melphalan; Mx = mitoxantrone; P = cisplatin; T = thiotepa.

T A B L E **8-9**

Antiangiogenic and Antimetastatic Drugs in Early Clinical Development

Drug	Mechanism of Action	Clinical Experience	
		Mode of Administration	Toxicity
AGM-1470	Inhibition of endothelial cell proliferation	IV	Asymptomatic retinal hemorrhages
r Platelet factor 4	Inhibition of endothelial cell proliferation	Intratumoral or IV	Local pain
Pentosan polysulfate	Inhibition of endothelial cell proliferation	IV or orally	Reversible anticoagulant effects
Razoxane	Antimetastatic	Orally	Neutropenia
BB-2516	Metalloproteinase inhibitor	Orally	Too early to tell

IV = intravenously.

Source: Adapted from Gasparini G, Harris AL. Clinical importance of the determination of tumor angiogenesis in breast carcinoma: much more than a new prognostic tool. *J Clin Oncol* 1995;13:765–782.

receptor ARMA 528, anti–HER 2 ARMA 4 D5) in breast cancer xenografts, with interesting results (131).

A monoclonal antibody against HER-2/neu is presently being investigated in a phase III trial in association with front-line chemotherapy for metastatic breast cancer patients whose tumors overexpress the Neu protein. If this study leads to a prolongation of progression-free survival, it will undoubtedly stimulate the evaluation of this monoclonal antibody in the adjuvant setting.

Differentiating, Antiangiogenic, and Antimetastatic Drugs

Results of several preclinical studies suggest the possible efficacy of novel treatment approaches, including the use of differentiating agents, such as retinoic acid derivatives, and agents interfering with metastasis and angiogenesis (40). Table 8-9 summarizes the early clinical experience with some of the antiangiogenic and antimetastatic drugs (132).

These new agents are not expected to show activity in the presence of bulky disease but may delay tumor progression following response to cytotoxic drugs. The demonstration of such an effect in metastatic disease, if achieved without significant toxicity, would encourage the design of prospective adjuvant clinical trials with these agents.

Conclusions

Systemic adjuvant treatment for early breast cancer is a therapeutic field in constant evolution.

The most important message of this chapter is that "optimal" adjuvant therapy for patients with early-stage breast cancer is adjuvant therapy within the framework of a prospective clinical trial. Too many uncertainties remain about the risk-benefit ratio of the therapies in current use for patients to be treated outside of clinical trials.

The future of adjuvant therapy for breast cancer is promising: A number of innovative treatment approaches based on new cellular targets will soon enter the clinical arena. With improved knowledge of clinical trial methodology, let us hope that these new strategies will benefit from an adequate evaluation early on.

Acknowledgments

The authors want to thank M. Delval and P. Adam for their excellent secretarial work and the Fonds JC Heuson de Recherche en Cancérologie Mammaire and the Fonds National de la Recherche Scientifique (Belgium) for supporting the clinical research fellowships of J. A. Roy, MD, and A. Awada, MD, respectively.

REFERENCES

1. Beatson GT. On the treatment of inoperable cases of carcinoma of the mamma: suggestions for a new method of treatment. *Lancet* 1896;2:104–107, 162–165.

2. Early Breast Cancer Trialists' Collaborative Group. The effects of adjuvant tamoxifen and of cytotoxic therapy on mortality in early breast cancer: an overview of 61 randomised trials among 28,896 women. *N Engl J Med* 1988; 319:1681–1692.

3. Early Breast Cancer Trialists' Collaborative Group. Systemic treatment of early breast cancer by hormonal, cytotoxic or immune therapy. 133 randomized trials involving 31,000 recurrences and 24,000 deaths among 75,000 women. *Lancet* 1992;339:1–15, 71–85.

4. Swedish Breast Cancer Cooperative Group. Randomized trial of 2 versus 5 years of adjuvant tamoxifen in postmenopausal early-stage breast cancer. *Proc Am Soc Clin Oncol* 1996;15:126. Abstract 171.

5. Fisher B, Dignam J, Wieand S, et al. Duration of tamoxifen (TAM) therapy for primary breast cancer: 5 versus 10 years (NSABP B-14). *Proc Am Soc Clin Oncol* 1996;15:113. Abstract 118.

6. Stewart HJ, Forrest AP, Everington D, et al. Randomised comparison of 5 years of adjuvant tamoxifen with continuous therapy for operable breast cancer. *Br J Cancer* 1996;74: 297–299.

7. Fisher B, Costantino J, Redmond C, et al. A randomized clinical trial evaluating tamoxifen in the treatment of patients with node-negative breast cancer who have estrogen-receptor-positive tumors. *N Engl J Med* 1989;320: 479–484.

8. Fornander T, Rutqvist LE, Cedermark B, et al. Adjuvant tamoxifen in early breast cancer: occurrence of new primary cancers. *Lancet* 1989;1:117–120.

9. Rutqvist LE, Matson A, for the Stockholm Breast Cancer Study Group. Cardiac and thromboembolic morbidity among postmenopausal women with early stage breast cancer in a randomized trial of adjuvant tamoxifen. *J Natl Cancer Inst* 1993;85:1398–1406.

10. McDonald CC, Stewart HJ. Fatal myocardial infarction in the Scottish adjuvant tamoxifen trial. The Scottish Breast Cancer Committee. *BMJ* 1991;303:435–437.

11. Love RR, Wiebe DA, Feyzi JM, et al. Effects of tamoxifen on cardiovascular risk factors in postmenopausal women after 5 years of treatment. *J Natl Cancer Inst* 1994;86:1534–1539.

12. Love RR, Barden HS, Mazess RB, et al. Effect of tamoxifen on lumbar spine bone mineral density in postmenopausal women after 5 years. *Arch Intern Med* 1994;154:2585–2588.

13. Davidson NE. Ovarian ablation as treatment for young women with breast cancer. *Monogr Natl Cancer Inst* 1994;16:95–99.

14. Cauley JA, Seeley DG, Ensrud K, et al, for the Study of Osteoporotic Fractures Research Group. Estrogen replacement therapy and fractures in older women. *Ann Intern Med* 1995; 122:9–16.

15. Barrett-Connor E, Bush TL. Estrogen and coronary heart disease in women. *JAMA* 1991;265: 1861–1867.

16. Bonadonna G, Valagussa P, Moliterni A, et al. Adjuvant cyclophosphamide, methotrexate and fluorouracil in node-positive breast cancer. The results of 20 years of follow-up. *N Engl J Med* 1995;332:901–906.

17. Bonadonna G, Valagussa P, Brambilla C, et al. Adjuvant and neoadjuvant treatment of breast cancer with chemotherapy and/or endocrine therapy. *Semin Oncol* 1991;18:515–524.

18. Bonadonna G, Gianni L, Santoro A, et al. Drugs ten years later: epirubicin. *Ann Oncol* 1993; 4:359–369.

19. French Epirubicin Study Group. A prospective randomized phase III trial comparing combination chemotherapy with cyclophosphamide, fluorouracil, and either doxorubicin or epirubicin. *J Clin Oncol* 1988;6:679–688.

20. French Epirubicin Study Group. A prospective randomized trial comparing epirubicin monochemotherapy to two fluorouracil, cyclophosphamide, and epirubicin regimens differing in epirubicin dose in advanced breast cancer patients. *J Clin Oncol* 1991;9:305–312.

21. Fisher B, Redmond C, Wickerham DL, et al. Doxorubicin-containing regimens for the treatment of stage II breast cancer: the National Surgical Adjuvant Breast and Bowel Project Experience. *J Clin Oncol* 1989;7:572–582.

22. Misset JL, Gil-Delgado M, Chollet P, et al. Ten years results of the French trial comparing Adriamycin, vincristine, 5-fluorouracil and cyclophosphamide to standard CMF as adjuvant therapy for node-positive breast cancer. *Proc Am Soc Clin Oncol* 1992;11:54. Abstract 41.

23. Mauriac L, Durand M, Chauvergne J, et al. Randomized trial of adjuvant chemotherapy for operable breast cancer comparing i.v. CMF to an epirubicin-containing regimen. *Ann Oncol* 1992;3:439–443.

24. Fisher B, Brown AM, Dimitrov NV, et al. Two months of doxorubicin-cyclophosphamide with and without interval reinduction therapy compared with 6 months of CMF in positive-node breast cancer patients with tamoxifen-nonresponsive tumors: results from the National Surgical Adjuvant Breast and Bowel Project B-15. *J Clin Oncol* 1990;8:1483–1496.

25. Tormey DC, Gray R, Abeloff MD, et al. Adjuvant therapy with a doxorubicin regimen and long term tamoxifen in premenopausal breast cancer patients: an Eastern Cooperative Oncology Group trial. *J Clin Oncol* 1992;10: 1848–1856.

26. Moliterni A, Bonadonna G, Valagussa P, et al. CMF with or without doxorubicin in the adjuvant treatment of resectable breast cancer with one to three positive axillary nodes. *J Clin Oncol* 1991;9:1124–1130.

27. Buzzoni R, Bonadonna G, Valagussa P, Zambetti M. Adjuvant chemotherapy with doxorubicin plus cyclophosphamide, methotrexate and fluorouracil in the treatment of resectable breast cancer with more than three positive axillary nodes. *J Clin Oncol* 1991;9:2134–2140.

28. Bonnadonna G, Zambetti M, Valagussa P. Sequential or alternating doxorubicin and CMF regimens in breast cancer with more than three positive nodes: ten-year results. *JAMA* 1995; 273:542–547.

29. Carpenter JT, Velez-Garcia E, Aron BS, et al. Prospective randomized comparison of cyclophosphamide, Adriamycin, and fluorouracil (CAF) vs CMF for breast cancer with positive axillary nodes: a Southeastern Cancer Group study. *Proc Am Soc Clin Oncol* 1991;10:45. Abstract 54.

30. Carpenter JT, Velez-Garcia E, Aron BS, et al. Five-year results of a randomized comparison of CAF versus CMF for node positive breast cancer. *Proc Am Soc Clin Oncol* 1994;13:66. Abstract 68.

31. Coombes RC, Bliss JM, Marty M, et al. A randomized trial comparing adjuvant FEC with CMF in premenopausal patients with node positive resectable breast cancer. *Proc Am Soc Clin Oncol* 1991;10:41. Abstract 37.

32. Marty M, Bliss JM, Coombes RC, et al. CMF versus FEC chemotherapy in premenopausal women with node positive breast cancer: results of a randomized trial. *Proc Am Soc Clin Oncol* 1994;13:62. Abstract 50.

33. Levine M, Bramwell V, Bowman D, et al. A clinical trial of intensive CEF versus CMF in premenopausal women with node positive breast cancer. *Proc Am Soc Clin Oncol* 1995;14:103. Abstract 112.

34. Wood WC, Budman DR, Korzun AH, et al. Dose and dose intensity of adjuvant chemotherapy for stage II, node-positive breast carcinoma. *N Engl J Med* 1994;330:1253–1259.

35. Dimitrov N, Anderson S, Fisher B, et al. Dose intensification and increased total dose of adjuvant chemotherapy for breast cancer: findings from NSABP B-22. *Proc Am Soc Clin Oncol* 1994;13:64. Abstract 58.

36. Bonadonna G. Conceptual and practical advances in the management of breast cancer. Karnofsky Memorial Lecture. *J Clin Oncol* 1989;7:1380–1397.

37. Levine MN, Gent M, Hryniuk WM, et al. A randomized trial comparing 12 weeks versus 36 weeks of adjuvant chemotherapy in stage II breast cancer. *J Clin Oncol* 1990;8:1217–1225.

38. Rivkin SE, Green S, Metch B, et al. One versus 2 years of CMVFP adjuvant chemotherapy in axillary node-positive and estrogen receptor-negative patients: a Southwest Oncology Group study. *J Clin Oncol* 1993;11:1710–1716.

39. Ludwig Breast Cancer Study Group. Combination adjuvant chemotherapy for node-positive breast cancer. Inadequacy of a single perioperative cycle. *N Engl J Med* 1988;319:677–683.

40. Folkman J. Angiogenesis in cancer, vascular, rheumatoid and other disease. *Nat Med* 1995;1:27–31.

41. Bonadonna G, Valagussa P, Zucorli R, Salvadori B. Primary chemotherapy in surgically resectable breast cancer. *CA Cancer J Clin* 1995;45:227–243.

42. Jacquillat C, Weil M, Baillet F, et al. Results of neoadjuvant chemotherapy and radiation therapy in the breast conserving treatment of 250 patients with all stages of infiltrative breast cancer. *Cancer* 1990;66:119–129.

43. Forrest AP, Chatty U, Miller WR, et al. A human tumor model. *Lancet* 1986;2:840–842.

44. Smith IE, Jones AL, O'Brien ME, et al. Primary medical (neoadjuvant) chemotherapy for operable breast cancer. *Eur J Cancer* 1993;29A:1796–1799.

45. Smith IE, Walsh G, Jones A, et al. High complete remission rates with primary neoadjuvant infusional chemotherapy for large early breast cancer. *J Clin Oncol* 1995;13:424–429.

46. Mauriac L, Durand M, Avril A, Dilhuydy JM. Effects of primary chemotherapy in conservative treatment of breast cancer patients with operable tumors larger than 3 cm: results of a randomized trial in a single centre. *Ann Oncol* 1991;2:347–354.

47. Scholl SM, Fourquet A, Asselain B, et al. Neoadjuvant versus adjuvant chemotherapy in premenopausal patients with tumors considered too large for breast conserving surgery. Preliminary results of a randomized trial: S6. *Eur J Cancer* 1994;30A:645–652.

48. Bonadonna G. Evolving concepts in the systemic adjuvant treatment of breast cancer. *Cancer Res* 1992;52:2127–2137.

49. Bonadonna G, Valagussa P, Brambilla C, et al. Response to primary chemotherapy increases rates of breast preservation and correlates with prognosis. *Proc Am Soc Clin Oncol* 1994;13:107. Abstract 230.

50. Fisher B, Rockette H, Robidoux A, et al. Effect of preoperative therapy for breast cancer on local-regional disease: first report of NSABP B-18. *Proc Am Soc Clin Oncol* 1994;13:64. Abstract 57.

51. Powles TJ, Hickish TF, Makris A, et al. Randomized trial of chemoendocrine therapy started before or after surgery for treatment of primary breast cancer. *J Clin Oncol* 1995;13:547–552.

52. Piccart MJ. Taxoid compounds in breast cancer: current status and future prospects. In: Muggia FM, ed. *Concepts, mechanisms and new targets for chemotherapy.* Boston: Kluwer Academic, 1995:185–208.

53. Recht A. The integration of radiation and chemotherapy for patients treated with breast

cancer conserving surgery. In: ASCO Educational Book. Philadelphia: American Society of Clinical Oncology, Spring 1994:11–14.

54. Recht A, Come SE, Henderson IG, et al. The sequencing of chemotherapy and radiation therapy after conservative surgery for early-stage breast cancer. *N Engl J Med* 1996;334:1356–1361.

55. Scottish Cancer Trials Breast Group and ICRF Breast Unit, Guy's Hospital, London. Adjuvant ovarian ablation versus CMF chemotherapy in premenopausal women with pathological stage II breast carcinoma: the Scottish trial. *Lancet* 1993;341:1293–1298.

56. Goldhirsch A, Gelber RD. Adjuvant chemoendocrine therapy alone for postmenopausal patients: Ludwig studies III and IV. *Recent Results Cancer Res* 1989;115:153–162.

57. Mouridsen HT, Rose C, Overgaard M, et al. Adjuvant treatment of postmenopausal patients with high risk primary breast cancer. Results from the Danish adjuvant trials DBCG 77C and DBCG 82C. *Acta Oncol* 1988;27:699–705.

58. Pearson OH, Hubay CA, Gordon NH, et al. Endocrine versus endocrine plus five-drug chemotherapy in postmenopausal women with stage II estrogen receptor-positive breast cancer. *Cancer* 1989;64:1819–1823.

59. Fisher B, Redmond C, Legault-Poisson S, et al. Postoperative chemotherapy and tamoxifen compared with tamoxifen alone in the treatment of positive-node breast cancer patients aged 50 years and older with tumors responsive to tamoxifen: results from the National Surgical Adjuvant Breast and Bowel Project B-16. *J Clin Oncol* 1990;8:1005–1018.

60. Pritchard K, Zee B, Paul N, et al. CMF added to tamoxifen as adjuvant therapy in postmenopausal women with node-positive estrogen and/or progesterone receptor positive breast cancer: negative results from a randomized clinical trial. *Proc Am Soc Clin Oncol* 1994;13:65. Abstract 61.

61. Fisher B, Redmond C, Brown A, et al. Adjuvant chemotherapy with and without tamoxifen in the treatment of primary breast cancer: 5-year results from the National Surgical Adjuvant Breast and Bowel Project Trial. *J Clin Oncol* 1986;4:459–471.

62. Crowe JP, Gordon NH, Shenk RR, et al. Short-term tamoxifen plus chemotherapy: superior results in node-positive breast cancer. *Surgery* 1990;108:619–628.

63. Rivkin SE, Green S, Metch B, et al. Adjuvant CMFVP versus tamoxifen versus concurrent CMFVP and tamoxifen for postmenopausal, node-positive, and estrogen receptor-positive breast cancer patients: a Southwest Oncology Group Study. *J Clin Oncol* 1994;12:2078–2085.

64. Boccardo F, Rubagotti A, Bruzzi P, et al. Chemotherapy versus tamoxifen versus chemotherapy plus tamoxifen in node-positive, estrogen receptor-positive breast cancer patients: results of a multicentric Italian study. *J Clin Oncol* 1990;8:1310–1320.

65. Boccardo F, Rubagotti A, Amoroso D, et al. (GROCTA) Chemotherapy versus tamoxifen versus chemotherapy plus tamoxifen in node-positive estrogen-receptor positive breast cancer patients. *Eur J Cancer* 1992;28:673–680.

66. Goldhirsch A, Wood WC, Senn HJ, et al. Meeting highlights: international consensus panel on the treatment of primary breast cancer. *J Natl Cancer Inst* 1995;87:1441–1445.

67. Devesa SS, Blot WJ, Stone BJ, et al. Recent cancer trends in the United States. *J Natl Cancer Inst* 1995;87:175–182.

68. Carter CL, Allen C, Henson DE. Relation of tumor size, lymph node status, and survival in 24,740 breast cancer cases. *Cancer* 1989;63:181–187.

69. Rosen PP, Groshen S, Saigo PE, et al. Pathological prognostic factors in stage I (T1N0M0) and stage II (T1N1M0) breast carcinoma: a study of 644 patients with a median follow-up of 18 years. *J Clin Oncol* 1989;7:1239–1251.

70. Silvestrini R, Daidone MG, Luisi A, et al. Biologic and clinicopathologic factors as indicators of specific relapse types in node-negative breast cancer. *J Clin Oncol* 1995;13:697–704.

71. Quiet CA, Ferguson DJ, Weichelbaum RR, Hellman S. Natural history of node-negative breast cancer: a study of 826 patients with long-term follow-up. *J Clin Oncol* 1995;13:1144–1151.

72. Cummings FJ, Gray R, Davis T, et al. Adjuvant tamoxifen treatment of elderly women with stage II breast cancer. *Ann Intern Med* 1985;103:324–329.

73. Castiglione M, Gelber RD, Goldhirsch A. Adjuvant systemic therapy for breast cancer in the elderly: competing causes of mortality. *J Clin Oncol* 1990;8:519–526.

74. Muss H, Cooper MR, Hoen H, et al. Adjuvant chemotherapy in older women with node posi-

tive breast cancer: the Piedmont Oncology Association experience. *Proc Am Soc Clin Oncol* 1992;11:147. Abstract 408.

75. Desch CE, Hillner BE, Smith TJ, Retchin SM. Should the elderly receive chemotherapy for node-negative breast cancer? A cost-effectiveness analysis examining total and active life-expectancy outcomes. *J Clin Oncol* 1993;11:777–782.

76. Fisher B, Costantino JP, Redmond CK, et al. Endometrial cancer in tamoxifen-treated breast cancer patients: findings from the National Surgical Adjuvant Breast and Bowel Project (NSABP) B-14. *J Natl Cancer Inst* 1994; 86:527–537.

77. Rutqvist LE, Johansson H, Signomklao T, et al. Adjuvant tamoxifen therapy for early stage breast cancer and second primary malignancies. *J Natl Cancer Inst* 1995;87:645–651.

78. Magriples U, Naftolin F, Schwartz PE, Carcangiu ML. High-grade endometrial carcinoma in tamoxifen-treated breast cancer patients. *J Clin Oncol* 1993;11:485–490.

79. Van Leeuwen FE, Benraadt J, Coebergh JW, et al. Risk of endometrial cancer after tamoxifen treatment of breast cancer. *Lancet* 1994; 343:448–452.

80. Pavlidis NA, Petris C, Briassoulis E, et al. Clear evidence that long-term, low-dose tamoxifen treatment can induce ocular toxicity. A prospective study of 63 patients. *Cancer* 1992; 69:2961–2964.

81. Heier JS, Dragoo RA, Enzenauer RW. Screening for ocular toxicity in asymptomatic patients treated with tamoxifen. *Am J Ophthalmol* 1994;117:772–775.

82. Levine MN, Gent M, Hirsh J, et al. The thrombogenic effect of anti-cancer drug therapy in women with stage II breast cancer. *N Engl J Med* 1988;318:404–407.

83. Valagussa P, Moliterni A, Terenziani M, et al. Second malignancies following CMF-based adjuvant chemotherapy in resectable breast cancer. *Ann Oncol* 1994;5:803–808.

84. Buzdar A, Iwaniec J, Kau S, et al. Secondary leukemia following adjuvant doxorubicin-containing chemotherapy for (stage II or III) breast cancer. *Proc Am Soc Clin Oncol* 1991;10:59. Abstract 112.

85. Riggi M, Riva A. Therapy-related leukemia: what is the role of 4-epi-doxorubicin? *J Clin Oncol* 1993;11:1430–1431.

86. Shepherd L, Ottaway J, Myles J, Levine M. Therapy-related leukemia associated with high dose 4-epi-doxorubicin and cyclophosphamide used as adjuvant chemotherapy for breast cancer. *J Clin Oncol* 1994;12:2514–2515.

87. DeCillis A, Anderson S, Wickerham DL, et al. Acute myeloid leukemia in NSABP B-25. *Proc Am Soc Clin Oncol* 1995;14:98. Abstract 92.

88. Linassier C, Barin C, Brémond JL, et al. Leucémies aiguïs myéloblastiques induites par mitoxantrone dans le cadre d'un traitement pour cancer du sein. *Bull Cancer (Paris)* 1995;82:240. Abstract.

89. Pedersen-Bjergaard J, Sigsgaard TC, Nielsen D, et al. Acute monocytic or myelomonocytic leukemia with balanced chromosome translocations to band 11q23 after therapy with 4-epidoxorubicin and cisplatin or cyclophosphamide for breast cancer. *J Clin Oncol* 1992; 10:1444–1451.

90. Valagussa P, Zambetti H, Biasi S, et al. Cardiac effects following adjuvant chemotherapy and breast irradiation in operable breast cancer. *Ann Oncol* 1994;5:209–216.

91. Shapiro CL, Henderson IC. Late cardiac effects of adjuvant therapy: too soon to tell? *Ann Oncol* 1994;5:196–198. Editorial.

92. McGuire WL. Breast cancer prognostic factors: evaluation guidelines. *J Natl Cancer Inst* 1991; 83:154–155.

93. Gasparini G, Pozza F, Harris AL. Evaluating the potential usefulness of new prognostic and predictive indicators in node-negative breast cancer patients. *J Natl Cancer Inst* 1993; 85:1206–1219.

94. Knoop AS, Laenkholm AV, Mirza MR, et al. Prognostic and predictive factors in early breast cancer. ESMO European Society for Medical Oncology, Lugano (Switzerland) 1994: 9–18.

95. Schwartz LH, Koerner FC, Edgerton SM, et al. pS2 expression and response to hormonal therapy in patients with advanced breast cancer. *Cancer Res* 1991;51:624–628.

96. Leitzel K, Teramoto Y, Konrad K, et al. Elevated serum c-erbB-2 antigen levels and decreased response to hormone therapy of breast cancer. *J Clin Oncol* 1995;13:1129–1135.

97. Gusterson BA, Gelber RD, Goldhirsch A, et al. Prognostic importance of c-erbB-2 expression in breast cancer. *J Clin Oncol* 1992;10:1049–1056.

98. Nicholson S, Sainsburg JRC, Halcrow P, et al. Expression of epidermal growth factor receptors associated with lack of response to endocrine therapy in recurrent breast cancer. *Lancet* 1989;1:182–185.

99. Foekens JA, Look MP, Peters HA, et al. Urokinase-type plasminogen activator and its inhibitor PAI-1: predictors of poor response to tamoxifen therapy in recurrent breast cancer. *J Natl Cancer Inst* 1995;87:751–756.

100. Gasparini G, Bevilacqua P, Pozza F, et al. P-Glycoprotein expression predicts response to chemotherapy in previously untreated advanced breast cancer. *Breast* 1993;2:27–32.

101. Muss HB, Thor AD, Berry DA, et al. c-ErbB-2 expression and response to adjuvant therapy in women with node-positive early breast cancer. *N Engl J Med* 1994;330:1260–1266.

102. Goldhirsch A, Gelber R. Understanding adjuvant chemotherapy for breast cancer. *N Engl J Med* 1994;330:1308–1309.

103. Giocca DR, Fuqua SAW, Lock-Lim S, et al. Response of human breast cancer cells to heat shock and chemotherapeutic drugs. *Cancer Res* 1992;52:3648–3654.

104. Lowe SW, Ruley HE, Jacks T, Housman DE. p53-dependent apoptosis modulates the cytotoxicity of anticancer agents. *Cell* 1993;74:957–967.

105. Jones AL, Powles TJ, Law M, et al. Adjuvant aminoglutethimide for postmenopausal patients with primary breast cancer: analysis at 8 years. *J Clin Oncol* 1992;10:1547–1552.

106. Goss PE, Gwyn KMEH. Current perspectives on aromatase inhibitors in breast cancer. *J Clin Oncol* 1994;12:2460–2470.

107. Vogel CL, Shemano I, Schoenfelder J, et al. Multicenter phase II efficacy trial of toremifene in tamoxifen-refractory patients with advanced breast cancer. *J Clin Oncol* 1993;11:345–350.

108. Howell A, DeFriend D, Robertson J, et al. Response to a specific antiestrogen (ICI 182780) in tamoxifen-resistant breast cancer. *Lancet* 1995;345:29–30.

109. McCormick DL, Mehta RG, Thompson CA, et al. Enhanced inhibition of mammary carcinogenesis by combined treatment with N-(4-hydroxyphenyl) retinamide and ovariectomy. *Cancer Res* 1982;42:508–512.

110. Costa A, Formelli F, Chiesa F, et al. Prospects of chemoprevention of human cancers with the synthetic retinoid fenretinide. *Cancer Res* 1994;54(suppl 7):2032s–2037s.

111. Hortobagyi GN. Future directions for vinorelbine (Navelbine). *Semin Oncol* 1995;22(suppl 5):80–87.

112. Piccart M. Docetaxel. A new defence in the management of breast cancer. *Anticancer Drugs* 1995;6(suppl 4):7–11.

113. Awada A, Cvitovic E, Piccart MJ. Cancer du sein et métastases hépatiques: nouveaux espoirs? *Bull Cancer (Paris)* 1995;82:478. Abstract.

114. Goldhirsch A, Gelber RD, Price KN, et al. Effect of systemic adjuvant treatment on first sites of breast cancer relapse. *Lancet* 1994;343:377–381.

115. Gianni L. Use of paclitaxel with other anticancer agents. *Proc EORTC Early Drug Development Meeting* 1995:54-55.

116. Tolcher AW, Gelmon KA. Interim results of a phase I/II study of biweekly paclitaxel and cisplatin in patients with metastatic breast cancer. *Semin Oncol* 1995;22(suppl 8):28–32.

117. Dieras V, Gruia G, Pouillart P, et al. Phase I study of the combination of docetaxel (D) and doxorubicin (DX) in 1st line CT treatment of metastatic breast cancer (MBC). *Eur J Cancer* 1995;31A(suppl 5):s194. Abstract 935.

118. Fumoleau P, Delecroix V, Gentin M, et al. Docetaxel in combination with vinorelbine as 1st line chemotherapy in patients with MBC: phase I dose finding study. *Eur J Cancer* 1995;31A(suppl 5):s195. Abstract 938.

119. Friedman MA. New directions for breast cancer therapeutic research. *Hematol Oncol Clin North Am* 1994;8:113–119.

120. Roy JA, Awada A, Kusenda Z, Piccart MJ. Sequence dependent effect (SDE) of chemotherapy (CT agents): a review. Presented at the 19th International Congress of Chemotherapy, Montreal, July 1995.

121. Seidman AD, Hudis CA, Norton L. Memorial Sloan-Kettering Cancer Center experience with paclitaxel in the treatment of breast cancer: from advanced disease to adjuvant therapy. *Semin Oncol* 1995;22(suppl 8):3–8.

122. Henderson IC, Hayes DF, Gelman R. Dose response with treatment of breast cancer: a critical review. *J Clin Oncol* 1988;6:1501–1515.

123. Hortobagyi GN. High-dose chemotherapy is not an established treatment for breast cancer. ASCO Educational Book, Springer 1995:341–346.

124. Antman KH, Souhami RL. High-dose chemotherapy in solid tumours. *Ann Oncol* 1993;4(suppl 1):529–544.

125. Antman KH. Dose intensive adjuvant therapy in breast cancer. ASCO Educational Book, 1994: 80–83.

126. Crump M, Pruice M, Goss PE. Outcome of extensive evaluation of women with ≥10 positive axillary lymph nodes prior to adjuvant therapy for breast cancer. *Proc Am Soc Clin Oncol* 1995;13:102. Abstract 107.

127. Smigel K. Phase III ABMT studies under way. *J Natl Cancer Inst* 1995;87:952–955.

128. Pietras RJ, Fendly BM, Chazin VR, et al. Antibody to HER-2/neu receptor blocks DNA repair after cisplatin in human breast and ovarian cancer cells. *Oncogene* 1994;9:1829–1838.

129. Hancock MC, Langton BC, Chan T, et al. A monoclonal antibody against the c-erbB-2 protein enhances the cytotoxicity of cis-diamminedichloroplatinum against human breast and ovarian tumor cell lines. *Cancer Res* 1991;51: 4575–4580.

130. Pegram MD, Pietras RJ, Slamon DJ. Monoclonal antibody to HER-2/neu gene product potentiates cytotoxicity of carboplatin and doxorubicin in human breast tumor cells. *Proc Am Assoc Cancer Res* 1992;23:442. Abstract 2639.

131. Baselga J, Norton L, Coplan K, et al. Antitumor activity of paclitaxel in combination with anti-growth factor receptor monoclonal antibodies in breast cancer xenografts. *Proc Am Assoc Cancer Res* 1994;35:380. Abstract 2262.

132. Gasparini G, Harris AL. Clinical importance of the determination of tumor angiogenesis in breast carcinoma: much more than a new prognostic tool. *J Clin Oncol* 1995;13:765–782.

CHAPTER 9

Radiotherapy for Breast Cancer

SEYMOUR H. LEVITT

*R*adiotherapy has been an integral part of the management of breast cancer since the discovery of the therapeutic benefits of radiation in the late 1800s. The evolution of the use of radiotherapy for breast cancer treatment since that time has been well described (1). The early use of radiotherapy, either alone or in conjunction with radical mastectomy, was based on the premise that breast cancer spreads in an orderly fashion from the primary tumor through the lymph nodes. This halstedian paradigm, named after the surgeon who initially described this view of the disease, suggested that some early disease is curable if adequate local treatment is given. Based on this view, several modifications to mastectomy have been tried, including extended radical mastectomy and the incorporation of postmastectomy radiotherapy, to better ensure local disease control. Several randomized clinical trials clearly proved, and long-term results confirmed, that the addition of radiotherapy after mastectomy significantly improves local control (2–5). However, whether the addition of radiotherapy produces a survival benefit is less clear, and this fact continues to generate questions about the importance of controlling local disease.

In the 1970s, several developments in breast cancer research had a strong impact on the role of radiotherapy in the treatment of breast cancer. Studies by Stjernsward and Cuzick (6–8) suggested that postmastectomy radiotherapy may actually decrease survival, studies on the use of chemotherapy showed survival benefits (9,10), and a new paradigm was introduced that viewed breast cancer as a systemic disease (11). All of these changes converged to call into question the importance of controlling local disease in curing disease and to call into question the role of radiotherapy.

Throughout these years, retrospective studies (12) and critical assessments of the Stjernsward and Cuzick studies (13) argued for a positive effect of local control on survival. Recent long-term follow-up of some of these trials (2,14), along with emerging biologic data on breast tumors (15), gave rise to the most recent paradigm, which maintains that some early disease is curable if adequate local treatment is given. This paradigm, newly named the *sequential view* of the disease (16), resurrects the importance of local disease control and therefore the importance of adequate radiotherapy in curing some disease.

Regardless of the continual debate over the impact of local control on survival, reducing the risk of or delaying local recurrence is generally supported as an essential goal of patient care because of the psychological trauma of disease recurrence.

Because the successful treatment of breast cancer depends on the integration of different treatment modalities, improved dialogue between surgeons, radiation oncologists, and medical oncologists is needed, beginning at the time of diagnosis. This seems common sense, yet all too often radiation oncologists are not included in the diagnostic evaluation of a patient and see a patient only after surgery and after systemic therapies have been initiated. One implicit purpose of this chapter is to show that the essential role of radiotherapy in the treatment of breast cancer mandates the inclusion of radiation oncologists in the initial treatment planning for breast cancer patients.

Treatment by Stage of Disease

Ductal Carcinoma In Situ

Increased diagnosis of ductal carcinoma in situ (DCIS) in recent years has led to increased focus on the best treatment for this type of breast carcinoma. Although mastectomy is the traditional treatment, excision alone or with radiotherapy has become more widely used because of the good results obtained with conservative surgery for early invasive disease. Results of retrospective and randomized studies suggest that the addition of radiotherapy improves local disease control. The average local failure rate is about 20% in studies of excision alone versus 10% in studies of excision with irradiation (17). The National Surgical Adjuvant Breast and Bowel Project (NSABP) trial B-17, a large randomized trial comparing these two treatments (18), as well as a meta-analysis of 12 trials comparing wide excision alone versus wide excision with radiotherapy versus mastectomy (19), found similar results. Recently published long-term findings of a collaborative international study from nine institutions of 259 patients with DCIS treated with conservative surgery and irradiation revealed an actuarial rate of local failure of 19% and an actuarial cause-specific survival rate of 96% at 15 years (20) (Table 9-1). Studies currently under way will help better determine the role of radiotherapy in the treatment of DCIS (17).

Although conservative surgery and irradiation is becoming more widely accepted and is used for the majority of women with DCIS, certain features may indicate the need for mastectomy. These features include diffuse or high-grade lesions and young patient age (17). For women in whom conservative surgery is indicated, several pathologic and histologic features of the tumor are used to determine whether radiotherapy is needed. Of the histologic subtypes—micropapillary, papillary, solid, cribriform, and comedo—the comedo type suggests the most aggressive disease and a higher probability of recurrence and malignant changes. Margin status and lesion size are important pathologic indicators of the risk of recurrence (17). The role of radiotherapy as determined by these prognostic factors is shown in Figure 9-1, which outlines a fairly standard current approach to treating DCIS. Although a standard prognostic classification system for DCIS has yet to be identified, attempts have been made to classify patients according to whether they are candidates for mastectomy, excision with radiation, or excision alone (21).

Early Disease: Stages I and II

Conservative surgery (lumpectomy) followed by radiotherapy is now considered standard treatment for many women with early breast cancer. Long-term results of randomized studies showing comparable survival between patients treated with mastectomy and patients treated with conservative surgery plus irradiation (Table 9-2) (22–28) led in 1990 to the following statement by the National Cancer Institute: "Breast conservation treatment is an appropriate

TABLE **9-1**

Actuarial Outcome Data at 5, 10, and 15 Years for Patients with Ductal Carcinoma In Situ Treated with Conservative Surgery and Radiotherapy

	At 5 Years		At 10 Years		At 15 Years	
Outcome	**%**	**95% CI**	**%**	**95% CI**	**%**	**95% CI**
Overall survival	98	97–100	94	91–97	87	81–93
Cause-specific survival	99	98–100	97	95–99	96	93–99
Freedom from distant metastases	99	98–100	97	95–99	96	94–99
Local failure	7	4–10	16	11–21	19	13–25
Contralateral breast cancer	2	0–4	6	3–9	9	4–13

CI = confidence interval.

Source: Reproduced by permission from Solin LJ, Kurz J, Fourquet A, et al. Fifteen year results of breast conserving surgery and definitive breast irradiation for the treatment of ductal carcinoma in situ (intraductal carcinoma) of the breast. *J Clin Oncol* 1996;14:757.

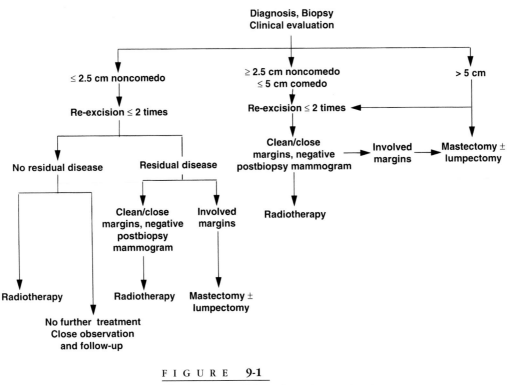

FIGURE 9-1

Management of ductal carcinoma in situ.

method of primary therapy for the majority of women with stage I-II breast cancer and is preferable because it provides survival rates equivalent to those of total mastectomy and axillary dissection while preserving the breast" (29).

Although the majority of stage I and II breast cancer patients are eligible for breast-conserving surgery, the potential increased risk of local failure for some patients requires careful patient selection. A report on standards of care for breast-conserving therapy issued in 1992 by a joint committee of the American College of Surgeons, the American College of Radiology, the College of American Pathologists, and the Society of Surgical Oncology outlines both absolute and relative contraindications for breast-conserving therapy (30). Absolute contraindications include two or more gross tumors in separate quadrants of the breast, diffuse indeterminate or malignant-appearing microcalcifications, and previous irradiation of the region. Breast-conserving therapy is also contraindicated in women in the first or second trimester of pregnancy. Relative contraindications include a large tumor-to-breast ratio, large breast size, tumor located beneath the nipple, and a history

of connective tissue disease. Several of these relative contraindications—for example, large breasts and nipple involvement—are predictors of poorer cosmetic results. The variation between women in expectations and wishes regarding cosmetic outcome makes these contraindications truly relative (31).

Other controversial contraindications potentially associated with increased risk of recurrence are young age, family history of breast cancer, and certain pathologic features of the tumor (32). Two important pathologic features are margin status and the presence of extensive intraductal component (EIC). Figure 9-2 shows a fairly standard approach to the treatment of patients with early disease. Patients with clear margins and those with close margins without EIC are candidates for radiotherapy. Patients with involved margins are generally treated with mastectomy with or without reconstruction, with additional postmastectomy chest wall irradiation given to patients at high risk for recurrence (33). Whether involved margins and the presence of EIC are associated with increased local failure rates remains open to debate, however. A clear and uniform classification

T A B L E   **9-2**

Randomized Trials of Mastectomy Versus Conservative Surgery and Radiotherapy

Trial (Years) (No. of Patients)	Local Recurrence Rate		Survival Rate		Length of Follow-up (Survival)
	M	CS + RT	M	CS + RT	
Gustave-Roussy (22) (1972–1979) (n = 179)	14%*	9%*	65%	73%	15 y
NCI Milan (23,24) (1973–1980) (n = 701)	2%	4%	69%	71%	13 y
NSABP B-06 (25) (1976–1984) (n = 1843)	8%	10%	71%	76%	8 y
NCI (26) (1979–1987) (n = 237)	6%	20%	85%	89%	5 y
EORTC (27) (1980–1986) (n = 903)	9%	13%	75%	75%	7 y
Danish Breast Cancer Group (1983–1987) (n = 905)	4%	3%	82%	79%	6 y

*First cause of failure.

CS = conservative surgery; EORTC = European Organization for Research and Treatment of Cancer; M = mastectomy; NCI = National Cancer Institute; NSABP = National Surgical Adjuvant Breast and Bowel Project; RT = radiotherapy.

Source: Reproduced by permission from Harris JR, Morrow M. Treatment of early-stage breast cancer. In: Harris JR, Morrow M, Hellman S, eds. *Diseases of the breast*. Philadelphia: Lippincott-Raven, 1996:492–493.

system for margin status is still lacking among treatment centers (32), and while the results of several studies indicate that EIC is associated with increased local failure rates (34,35), other findings do not (36).

Regardless of the extent of excision (mastectomy or lumpectomy), the addition of radiotherapy significantly improves local disease control and results in a demonstrated survival benefit. This is confirmed by long-term results from the Stockholm trial of postmastectomy irradiation (4) (Table 9-3) and by the more recent studies on conservative surgery (24,37–39). In addition, the extent to which radiotherapy is needed to achieve local control is reflected in data from the NSABP B-06 trial, which showed a significantly higher rate of mastectomies among node-negative patients initially treated with lumpectomy alone than among patients treated with lumpectomy and irradiation (84% versus 66%, p = 0.006) (40). Maintenance of

local control is clearly important because it spares patients the physical and psychological hardships associated with a recurrence. The effect of local control on survival, although highly controversial, appears to grow over time, and recent findings strongly suggest a small but clinically important survival benefit with radiation (41,42) (Tables 9-3 and 9-4).

Of current interest is the definition of subgroups of patients with early breast cancer in whom radiotherapy may not be needed. Since systemic adjuvant therapies are now a standard part of treatment for patients with breast disease of all stages, even node-negative disease, it is important to be able to identify patients in whom further adjuvant treatment is unnecessary to avoid the unnecessary psychological, economic, and physical costs of extra treatment. To date, subgroups of patients in whom radiotherapy can safely be withheld have not been identified (43).

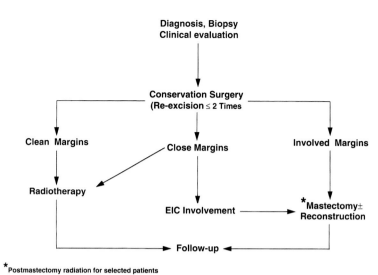

F I G U R E   **9-2**

Management of early breast cancer.   *Postmastectomy radiation for selected patients

T A B L E   **9-3**

Stockholm Trial of Postoperative Radiotherapy

Event	Postoperative Radiotherapy		Surgery Alone		Rate Ratio (95% Confidence Interval)	p Value (Log-Rank)
	Patients	Events (%)	Patients	Events (%)		
Pathologically negative nodes	204		197			
Treatment failure*		74 (36%)		99 (50%)	0.65 (0.48–0.88)	<0.01
Local-regional recurrence		10 (5%)		45 (23%)	0.25 (0.15–0.42)	<0.001
Distant metastases		52 (26%)		49 (25%)	1.02 (0.69–1.50)	0.94
Death		66 (33%)		74 (38%)	0.87 (0.63–1.21)	0.40
Breast cancer death		47 (23%)		43 (22%)	1.05 (0.70–1.59)	0.80
Pathologically positive nodes	118		120			
Treatment failure*		76 (64%)		94 (78%)	0.64 (0.47–0.87)	<0.01
Local-regional recurrence		18 (15%)		58 (48%)	0.29 (0.18–0.45)	<0.001
Distant metastases		61 (52%)		83 (69%)	0.66 (0.48–0.92)	0.02
Death		72 (61%)		84 (70%)	0.82 (0.60–1.12)	0.21
Breast cancer death		59 (50%)		81 (68%)	0.70 (0.50–0.98)	0.04

*Treatment failure defined as local-regional recurrence, distant metastases, or death without recurrence.

Source: Reproduced by permission from Harris JR, Morrow M. Treatment of early-stage breast cancer. In: Harris JR, Morrow M, Hellman S, eds. *Diseases of the breast*. Philadelphia: Lippincott-Raven Publishers, 1996:514. Data from Ruqvist L, Pettersson D, Johansson M. Adjuvant radiation therapy versus surgery alone in operable breast cancer: long-term follow-up in a randomized clinical trial. *Radiat Oncol* 1993;26:104.

Locally Advanced Disease

The current standard treatment for locally advanced disease favors a multimodal approach that combines primary chemotherapy, adjuvant radiotherapy, and either mastectomy or lumpectomy. Several studies indicate the increased benefit to locoregional control and survival with multimodality therapy. A study by Klefstrom et al of 120 stage III breast cancer patients randomized into three different treatment schemes, surgery plus chemotherapy, surgery plus radiotherapy, and surgery plus radiotherapy plus chemotherapy, reported a 5-year disease-free survival of 30%, 22%, and 67%, respectively (44). Another study by Perez et al, which examined three different treatment schemes of combined mastectomy and radiotherapy with or

T A B L E   **9-4**

Five-Year Survival Benefit with the Addition of Radiotherapy to Lumpectomy in Node-Negative Breast Cancer Patients: Combined Results of Uppsala-Orebro, Canadian, and NSABP B-06 Trials*

Treatment	Overall Survival	Difference in Survival	Probability of a Positive Treatment Effect	Annual Mortality Rate	Relative Reduction in Annual Mortality Rate (SE)
Lumpectomy	87.5%	—	—	2.7%	—
Lumpectomy + RT	88.7%	1.27%	79%	2.4%	9.6% (±13.7%)

RT = radiotherapy; SE = standard error.

*Based on bayesian analysis.

Source: Reproduced by permission from Levitt SL, Aeppli DM, Nierengarten ME. The impact of radiation on early breast carcinoma survival: a bayesian analysis. *Cancer* 1996;78:1038.

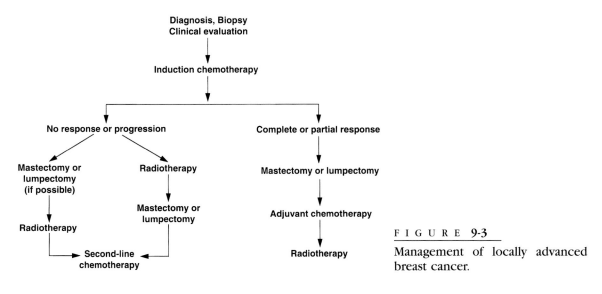

F I G U R E   **9-3**

Management of locally advanced breast cancer.

without chemotherapy in locally advanced non-inflammatory breast cancer patients, reported locoregional tumor control at 5 years of 91% for combined chemotherapy, radiotherapy, and mastectomy, 80% for irradiation and mastectomy, 54% for irradiation and chemotherapy, and 31% for irradiation alone. Corresponding actuarial 10-year disease-free survival rates were 36%, 19%, 10%, and 11% (45). The benefit of treating patients with adjuvant irradiation in combination with systemic therapy and surgery is further highlighted in a recent study by Fisher et al that examined the significance of extra-capsular nodal extension (ECE) on locoregional failure and survival in 82 stage II or III breast cancer patients treated by systemic chemotherapy or hormonal therapy without locoregional radiation (46). Based on the patterns of failure of these patients, the authors recommended breast/chest wall and supraclavicular radiation for all patients with pathological evidence of ECE who have had a level I and II axillary dis-

section regardless of the number of positive axillary nodes.

The use of induction chemotherapy followed by surgery and radiation is another approach to treating locally advanced patients. The use of primary chemotherapy developed after trials of radiation alone failed to provide optimal treatment because of increased complications stemming from the need for higher radiation dose to control gross disease (47–49). Good tumor shrinkage with the use of induction chemotherapy resulted in trials that examined whether adjuvant radiotherapy or mastectomy offered better local control. Two randomized trials failed to show any significant difference in relapse rates or survival between the two treatments when they were combined with chemotherapy (50,51).

The sequencing of mastectomy and radiation after primary chemotherapy for advanced disease is uncertain. Many centers perform surgery first after chemotherapy and reserve

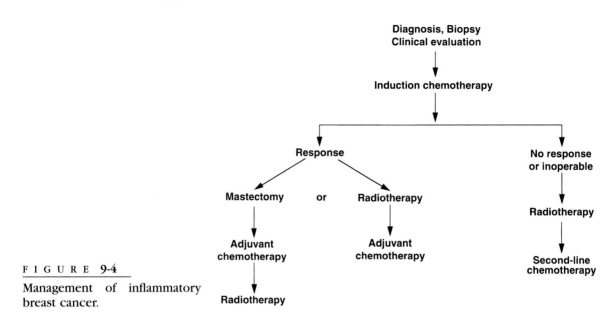

FIGURE 9-4

Management of inflammatory breast cancer.

radiotherapy to the chest wall and nodal areas until the completion of chemotherapy (52). Results from the National Cancer Institute of Italy and the University of Texas M. D. Anderson Cancer Center suggest the inclusion of maintenance chemotherapy after this regimen to improve outcomes (53,54). A fairly standard approach to treating locally advanced disease is shown in Figure 9-3. A similar combined-modality approach is used for patients with inflammatory disease and is shown in Figure 9-4.

Other approaches under investigation for the treatment of advanced disease also suggest an important role for radiotherapy. Breast-conserving therapy followed by radiation is one approach that has produced favorable results in carefully selected patients. Studies from the M. D. Anderson Cancer Center demonstrated local recurrence rates of less than 10% in carefully selected patients who respond well to systemic chemotherapy (55–58). In these studies, patient selection for breast-conserving therapy after neoadjuvant chemotherapy was based on tumor size (solitary primary tumor of 4 cm or less or two primary tumors within a sphere of 4 cm); the absence of skin involvement or tumor fixation to the chest wall; a tumor-to-breast ratio favorable for cosmetic outcomes; the absence of palpable or small, low, mobile axillary lymph nodes; the absence of collagen vascular disease; and the absence of extensive lymphatic involvement in the breast (58). Total excision of the gross tumor in these patients allowed for a reduced radiation dose to avoid cosmetic complications. Other studies also indicate breast-

conserving therapy for some patients with locally advanced disease (59), although recommendations for standard care in these patients must await long-term results.

The combined use of radiotherapy and autologous bone marrow transplantation after conventional or high-dose chemotherapy is another treatment under investigation for advanced disease. Early results from a pilot study by the Cancer and Leukemia Group B of stage II and III patients with 10 or more positive nodes treated with mastectomy followed by conventional-dose plus high-dose chemotherapy with autologous bone marrow transplantation and radiotherapy indicate that the addition of radiotherapy helps to lower the frequency of chest wall and regional lymph node recurrence (60,61). The pilot study concluded that radiotherapy is an important component of this treatment regimen. Later analysis demonstrated that the high frequency of hematologic toxicity found with the addition of radiotherapy in this study was primarily due to the lower blood cell counts of patients prior to radiotherapy (62).

Specific Issues in Radiotherapy for Breast Cancer

Node-Negative Patients

Studies are examining whether breast-conserving surgery without radiotherapy is indicated in certain subsets of node-negative patients. Results so far do not indicate a group of patients in whom adjuvant radiotherapy can be omitted without compromise of optimal local disease control (43).

Pregnant Patients

Radiotherapy is contraindicated in pregnant patients because it is not possible to shield the fetus from internal radiation scatter. Lumpectomy and axillary dissection during the third trimester followed by radiotherapy after delivery is possible (52).

Older Women

Different treatment for older women based on age has not yet been indicated. For early-stage disease, conservative surgery with radiotherapy is a viable option, as it is in younger patients. Because disease is often more indolent in women older than 65, studies are under way to determine whether less aggressive treatment is adequate for these women. The Cancer and Leukemia Group B is conducting a study to assess whether radiotherapy can be omitted in some of these women with early-stage T1-2 disease (63).

Radiotherapy after Local Recurrence

For most women treated initially with mastectomy, the treatment of a local recurrence with radiotherapy results in complete disease regression. However, a large number of women still have a further locoregional recurrence, which may be due to delayed radiotherapy or inade-

quate technique (4,64,65). One good argument for the use of prophylactic irradiation after mastectomy is the difficulty of controlling locoregional disease once it recurs. The 16-year follow-up of the Stockholm study of adjuvant radiotherapy versus surgery alone found that the overall proportion of patients with locoregional disease at death or last follow-up was significantly higher among patients treated with surgery alone than it was among patients treated with adjuvant radiotherapy (16% versus 6%, $p < 0.01$) (4).

The importance of adequate technique is highlighted by a series of patients treated with radiotherapy for recurrence at the Mallinckrodt Institute of Radiology. The 5-year failure rate was 25% when adequate chest wall irradiation was given but 64% when only small fields were treated. An adequate radiation technique significantly reduced the risk of further recurrence in the supraclavicular nodes from 16% in untreated patients to 6% in irradiated patients (64). This study showed that achievement of long-term local control is highly dependent on the volume of disease remaining at the time of irradiation (Table 9-5). For gross disease that precludes excision, a proper radiation dose is necessary to achieve local control. A detailed discussion of the appropriate radiation technique for achieving long-term control after recurrence can be found elsewhere (66).

Studies on the use of radiotherapy to treat recurrences in patients treated initially with mastectomy and irradiation are few and small, although the results do indicate some palliative benefit from limited doses of radiation. Similarly, there is little information on the use of

TABLE 9-5

Chances of In-field Tumor Recurrence According to Radiation Dose and Extent of Surgery*

Dose (Gy)	Complete Excision	Residual Tumor ≤ 3 cm	Tumor > 3 cm or Diffuse or Multiple Tumors
≤49.99	1/9 (11%)	2/7 (29%)	7/8 (88%)
50–54.99	1/26 (4%)	1/5 (20%)	7/15 (47%)
55–59.99	1/21 (5%)	2/9 (22%)	2/11 (18%)
60–64.99	4/22 (18%)	0/9 (0%)	10/20 (50%)
≥65	0/2 (0%)	0/6 (0%)	7/15 (47%)

*Patients treated to small fields excluded.

Source: Reproduced by permission from Recht A, Hayes DF, Eberkin TJ, Sadowsky NL. Local-regional recurrence after mastectomy or breast conserving therapy. In: Harris JR, Lippman ME, Morrow M, Hellman S, eds. *Diseases of the breast.* Philadelphia: Lippincott-Raven, 1996:653. Data from Halvorson KJ, Perez CA, Kuske RR, et al. Isolated local-regional recurrence of breast cancer following mastectomy: radiotherapeutic management. *Int J Radiat Oncol Biol Phys* 1990;19:851.

radiotherapy to treat recurrences after breast-conserving surgery either alone or with irradiation, with several small studies reporting inconclusive results (66). Five recent randomized trials of the combined use of radiotherapy and hyperthermia to treat recurrent breast cancer revealed promising results for control of local disease (67).

Complications

Many of the acute complications of modern radiotherapy, such as erythema, edema, and mild tiredness, are short-term conditions that become neither chronic nor life-threatening. Chronic, more serious conditions such as arm edema, decreased arm mobility, soft tissue necrosis, rib fractures, radiation pneumonitis, and brachial plexopathy are possible but occur very infrequently when an appropriate radiation technique is used (31). Improved radiation techniques have also minimized radiation-induced cardiac morbidity and carcinogenesis, which were major complications prior to modern radiotherapy. Cause-specific mortality data from the updated Cuzick meta-analysis show that cardiac deaths accounted for increased mortality in the older trials that used orthovoltage techniques (2). The updated Cuzick meta-analysis and a combined analysis of the Stockholm and Oslo trials (14) showed that increased cardiac morbidity and mortality were not evident with the use of modern megavoltage techniques. A further study from Stockholm showed that patients who received the highest volume of irradiation had the most increased risk of cardiac mortality (68).

The risk of radiation-induced cancers, including sarcomas, leukemia, and lung cancer, has substantially decreased with the current technique of treating only the tangential breast fields. Among breast cancer patients currently treated with radiotherapy, the excess risk of death due to radiation-induced cardiac mortality or secondary cancers is estimated to be less than 1%. Patients younger than 45 at the time of diagnosis and treatment have a higher risk of radiation-related contralateral breast cancer, whereas patients older than 45 have little if any risk (69,70).

A fairly new concern is the development of breast cancer after chest irradiation for Hodgkin's disease. A recent study indicated a high risk for women treated with radiotherapy for childhood Hodgkin's disease (71). Women who were 16 years or younger at the time of treatment had the highest risk of developing breast cancer.

Radiotherapy and Systemic Therapies

For both early and advanced breast cancer, study results indicate improved local control and survival with the combined use of adjuvant radiotherapy and chemotherapy after breast-conserving surgery or mastectomy. This is especially true for patients with four or more positive nodes. Studies reported a locoregional recurrence rate of 10% in patients with one to three positive nodes treated with chemotherapy alone compared with 20% to 30% in patients with four or more positive nodes or primary tumors 5 cm or larger (72–75). For these women at high risk, the combination of chemotherapy and radiotherapy produces better locoregional control and disease-free survival rates than either adjuvant modality alone does (76,77).

The proper sequencing of radiotherapy and chemotherapy after surgery remains an important and controversial aspect of treatment. A recently published trial by the Joint Center for Radiation Therapy examined this question in a subgroup of patients considered at increased risk for systemic metastases (i.e., nearly all the patients had positive nodes). In that trial, 244 stage I and II patients treated with breast-conserving surgery were randomly assigned to receive a 12-week course of chemotherapy either before or after radiotherapy (78). At a median follow-up in surviving patients of 58 months, the authors found an increased risk of local recurrence in the group who received chemotherapy first (14% versus 5%) and an increased risk of distant recurrence in the group who received radiotherapy first (32% versus 20%). These results suggest that a 12-week course of chemotherapy before radiotherapy may result in a better outcome for patients at increased risk for systemic metastases. Although the possible detrimental effects of delaying radiotherapy were not addressed in this study, an earlier study by the same authors found that delaying radiotherapy for more than 16 weeks after surgery resulted in a 5-year actuarial local control rate of 28% versus 5% in patients treated within 16 weeks (79). Similarly, another study reported a significant increase in the relapse rate at 5 years for women in whom radiotherapy was not delivered until at least 120 days after surgery (80). Other studies, however, found no difference in local control rates based on the timing of radiation delivery (81,82).

Quality of Life

Survival remains the primary goal of breast cancer treatment, but it is not the only goal. This fact is emphasized by the shift from radical mastectomy to breast-conserving therapy for many women with early breast cancer. Many women who opt for breast-conserving therapy rather than mastectomy have a better body image and sexual functioning without an increased fear of recurrence (83). However, in some women the fear of recurrence associated with breast-conserving surgery outweighs the possible benefit of improved cosmesis (84). Addressing the different expectations and desires of each woman in her treatment choice is integral to incorporating quality-of-life considerations into the decision-making process. In addition, good communication between physician and patient is important to help manage the anxiety and depression that frequently accompany the diagnosis and treatment of this disease and that diminish the quality of life. A pilot study that assessed the main treatment factors affecting quality of life in breast cancer patients found that patient-centered care (tailoring treatment choice to fit the particular needs and wishes of each patient), good communication between physician and patient, psychological support from the physician, the availability of additional services to help provide emotional support, and continuity of care affected quality of life during treatment (85). A compendium of different tests to measure quality of life in breast cancer patients was recently published (86).

Conclusions

Radiotherapy is an integral part of breast cancer management. Radiotherapy after mastectomy or conservative surgery significantly improves local control rates and has a demonstrated ability to improve survival. Appropriate radiotherapy technique is critical for optimal disease control and improved survival, as reflected in the better outcomes of trials that employed modern radiotherapy techniques. Essential to a good radiation oncology center is a state-of-the-art team of radiation oncologists, medical physicists, and technicians, as well as state-of-the-art equipment, including linear accelerators, simulators, and treatment-planning computers. With improved treatment planning and delivery, radiotherapy is becoming increasingly effective in delivering optimal doses to the tumor while minimizing doses to normal tissue. In breast cancer management, the incidence of complications following chest wall irradiation has been drastically reduced, as has the incidence of radiation-induced malignancies.

Acknolwedgments

I wish to thank Mary Beth Nierengarten for editorial assistance.

REFERENCES

1. Mansfield CM. *Early breast cancer: its history and results of treatment. Experimental biology and medicine: monographs on interdisciplinary topics*, vol. 5. Basel: S. Karger, 1976.

2. Cuzick J, Stewart H, Rutqvist L, et al. Cause-specific mortality in long-term survivors of breast cancer who participated in trials of radiotherapy. *J Clin Oncol* 1994;12:447–453.

3. Host H, Brennhovd IO. The effect of post-operative radiation therapy in breast cancer. *Int J Radiat Oncol Biol Phys* 1977;2:1061–1067.

4. Rutqvist LE, Pettersson D, Johansson H. Adjuvant radiation therapy versus surgery alone in operable breast cancer: long-term follow-up of a randomized clinical trial. *Radiother Oncol* 1993;26:104–110.

5. Uematsu M, Boarnstein BA, Recht A, et al. Long-term results of post-operative radiation therapy following mastectomy with or without chemotherapy in stage I-III breast cancer. *Int J Radiat Oncol Biol Phys* 1993;25:765–779.

6. Cuzick J, Stewart H, Peto R, et al. Overview of randomized trials comparing radical mastectomy without radiotherapy against simple mastectomy with radiotherapy in breast cancer. *Cancer Treat Rep* 1987;71:7–14.

7. Cuzick J, Stewart H, Peto R, et al. Overview of randomized trials of postoperative adjuvant radiotherapy in breast cancer. *Cancer Treat Rep* 1987;71:15–25.

8. Stjernsward J. Can survival be decreased by postoperative irradiation? *Int J Radiat Oncol Biol Phys* 1977;2:1171–1175.

9. Bonadonna G, Brusamolino E, Valagussa P, et al. Combination chemotherapy as an adjuvant treatment in operable breast cancer. *N Engl J Med* 1976;294:405–410.

10. Fisher B, Redmond C, Elias EG, et al. Adjuvant chemotherapy for breast cancer: an overview of NSABP findings. *Int Adv Surg Oncol* 1982;5: 65–90.

11. Fisher B. Laboratory and clinical research in breast cancer—a personal adventure: the David A. Karnofsky Memorial Lecture. *Cancer Res* 1980;40:3863–3874.

12. Fletcher GH, McNeese MD, Owald MJ. Long-range results for breast cancer patients treated by radical mastectomy and postoperative radiation without adjuvant chemotherapy: an update. *Int J Radiat Oncol Biol Phys* 1989;17:11–14.

13. Levitt SH. Is there a role for post-operative adjuvant radiation in breast cancer? Beautiful hypothesis versus ugly facts. 1987 Gilbert H. Fletcher Lecture. *Int J Radiat Oncol Biol Phys* 1988;14: 787–796.

14. Auquier A, Rutqvist LE, Host H, et al. Postmastectomy megavoltage radiotherapy: the Oslo and Stockholm trials. *Eur J Cancer* 1992;28:433–437.

15. Tubiana M. Postoperative radiotherapy and the pattern of distant spread in breast cancer. In: Fletcher GH, Levitt SH, eds. *Non-disseminated breast cancer: controversial issues in management.* Berlin: Springer, 1993:11–26.

16. Hellman S. Karnofsky Memorial Lecture. Natural history of small breast cancers. *J Clin Oncol* 1994;12:2229–2234.

17. Wood WC. Management of lobular carcinoma in situ and ductal carcinoma in situ of the breast. *Semin Oncol* 1996;23:446–452.

18. Fisher ER, Constantino J, Fisher B, et al. Pathologic findings from the National Surgical Adjuvant Breast Project (NSABP) protocol B-17. *Cancer* 1995;75:1310–1319.

19. Bradley SJ, Weaver DW, Bouwman DL. Alternatives in the surgical management of in situ breast cancer. A meta-analysis of outcome. *Am Surg* 1990;56:428–432.

20. Solin LJ, Kurz J, Fourquet A, et al. Fifteen year results of breast conserving surgery and definitive breast irradiation for the treatment of ductal carcinoma in situ (intraductal carcinoma of the breast). *J Clin Oncol* 1996;14:754–763.

21. Silverstein MJ, Poller DN, Waisman JR, et al. Prognostic classification of breast ductal carcinoma-in-situ. *Lancet* 1995;345:1154–1157.

22. Arriagada R, Le MG, Rochard F, Contesso G. Conservative treatment versus mastectomy in early breast cancer: patterns of failure with 15 years of follow-up results. *J Clin Oncol* 1996; 14:1558–1564.

23. Veronesi U, Banfi A, Salvadori B, et al. Breast conservation is the treatment of choice in small breast cancer: long-term results of a randomized clinical trial. *Eur J Cancer* 1990;26:668–670.

24. Veronesi U, Luini A, Galimberti V, Zurrida S. Conservation approaches for the management of stage I/II carcinoma of the breast: Milan Cancer Institute trials. *World J Surg* 1994;18:70–75.

25. Fisher B, Redmond C, Poisson R, et al. Eight-year results of a randomized clinical trial comparing total mastectomy and lumpectomy with or without irradiation in the treatment of breast cancer. *N Engl J Med* 1989;320:822–828.

26. Lichter A, Lippman M, Danforth D, et al. Mastectomy versus breast conserving therapy in the treatment of stage I and II carcinoma of the breast: a randomized trial at the National Cancer Institute. *J Clin Oncol* 1992;10:976–983.

27. van Dongen JA, Bartelink H, Fentiman IS, et al. Randomized clinical trial to assess the value of breast-conserving therapy in stage I and II breast cancer: EORTC 10801 trial. *Monogr Natl Cancer Inst* 1992;11:15–18.

28. Blichert-Toft M, Rose C, Andersen J, et al. Danish randomized trial comparing breast conservation therapy with mastectomy: six years of life-table analysis. *Monogr Natl Cancer Inst* 1992;11:19–25.

29. NIH Consensus Conference. Treatment of early-stage breast cancer. *JAMA* 1991;265:391–395.

30. Winchester D, Cox J. Standards for breast conservation treatment. *CA Cancer J Clin* 1992;42: 134–162.

31. Harris JR, Morrow M. Local management of invasive breast cancer. In: Harris JR, Lippman ME, Morrow M, Hellman S, eds. *Diseases of the breast.* Philadelphia: Lippincott-Raven, 1996: 487–547.

32. Recht A. Selection of patients with early stage invasive breast cancer for treatment with conservative surgery and radiation therapy. *Semin Oncol* 1996;23:19–30.

33. Love S, Parker B, Ames M, et al. Practice guidelines for breast cancer. *Cancer J Sci Am* 1996;2(suppl 3A):S7–S21.

34. Paterson DA, Anderson TJ, Jack WJL, et al. Pathological features predictive of local recur-

rence after management by conservation of invasive breast cancer: importance of noninvasive carcinoma. *Radiother Oncol* 1992;25:176–180.

35. Vicini FA, Recht A, Abner A, et al. Recurrence in the breast following conservative surgery and radiation therapy for early-stage breast cancer. *Monogr Natl Cancer Inst* 1992;11:33–39.

36. Solin LJ, Fowble BL, Schultz DJ, Goodman RL. The significance of the pathology margins of the tumor excision on the outcome of patients treated with definitive irradiation for early stage breast cancer. *Int J Radiat Oncol Biol Phys* 1991;21:279–287.

37. Fisher B, Anderson S, Redmond CK, et al. Reanalysis and results after 12 years of follow-up in a randomized clinical trial comparing total mastectomy with lumpectomy with or without irradiation in the treatment of breast cancer. *N Engl J Med* 1995;333:1456–1461.

38. Liljegren G, Holmberg L, Adami HO, et al. Sector resection with or without postoperative radiotherapy for stage I breast cancer: five-year results of a randomized trial. Uppsala-Orebro Breast Cancer Study Group. *J Natl Cancer Inst* 1994;86:717–722.

39. Whelan T, Clark R, Roberts R, et al. Ipsilateral breast tumor recurrence postlumpectomy is predictive of subsequent mortality: results from a randomized trial. Investigators of the Ontario Clinical Oncology Group. *Int J Radiat Oncol Biol Phys* 1994;30:11–16.

40. Kemperman H, Borger J, Hart A, et al. Prognostic factors for survival after breast conserving therapy for stage I and II breast cancer. The role of local recurrence. *Eur J Cancer* 1995;31A: 690–698.

41. Levitt SH, Aeppli DM, Nierengarten ME. The impact of radiation on early breast carcinoma survival: a bayesian analysis. *Cancer* 1996;78: 1035–1042.

42. National Cancer Institute. Reanalysis of the NSABP protocol B06, Emmes Corporation. CancerNet, National Cancer Institute, April 11, 1994.

43. Morrow M, Harris JR, Schnitt SJ. Local control following breast-conserving surgery for invasive cancer: results of clinical trials. *J Natl Cancer Inst* 1995;87:125–129.

44. Klefstrom P, Grohn P, Heinonen E, et al. Adjuvant postoperative radiotherapy, chemotherapy, and immunotherapy in stage III breast cancer. II. 5-year results and influence of levamisole. *Cancer* 1987;60:936–942.

45. Perez CA, Graham ML, Taylor ME, et al. Management of locally advanced carcinoma of the breast. I. Non-inflammatory. *Cancer* 1994;74: 453–465.

46. Fisher BJ, Perera FE, Cooke AL, et al. Extracapsular axillary extension in patients receiving adjuvant systemic therapy: an indication for radiotherapy. *Int J Radiat Oncol Biol Phys* 1982; 8:31–36.

47. Bedwinek J, Rao D, Perez C. Stage III and localized stage IV breast cancer: irradiation alone vs. irradiation plus surgery. *Int J Radiat Oncol Biol Phys* 1982;8:31–36.

48. Sheldon T, Hayes DF, Cady B, et al. Primary radiation for locally advanced breast cancer. *Cancer* 1987;60:1219–1225.

49. Spanos W, Montague E, Fletcher G. Late complications of radiation only for advanced breast cancer. *Int J Radiat Oncol Biol Phys* 1980;6: 1473–1476.

50. DeLena M, Varini M, Zucali R. Multimodal treatment for locally advanced breast cancer. *Cancer Clin Trials* 1981;4:229–236.

51. Perloff M, Lesnick G, Korzun A. Combination chemotherapy with mastectomy or radiotherapy for stage III breast carcinoma: a Cancer and Leukemia Group B study. *J Clin Oncol* 1988; 6:261–269.

52. Harris JR, Morrow M, Bonadonna G. Cancer of the breast. In: De Vita VT, Hellman S, Rosenberg SA, eds. *Cancer: principles and practices of oncology.* 4th ed. Philadelphia: JB Lippincott, 1993:1264–1332.

53. Hortobagyi GN. Comprehensive management of locally advanced breast cancer. *Cancer* 1990; 66:1367–1391.

54. Valagussa P, Zambetti M, Bonadonna G. Prognostic factors in locally advanced noninflammatory breast cancer. Long-term results following primary chemotherapy. *Breast Cancer Res Treat* 1990;15:137–147.

55. Feldman LD, Hortobagyi GN, Buzdar AU, et al. Pathological assessment of response to induction chemotherapy in breast cancer. *Cancer Res* 1986;46:2578–2581.

56. Hortobagyi GN, Blumenschein GR, Spanos W, et al. Multimodal treatment of locoregionally advanced breast cancer. *Cancer* 1983;51: 763–768.

57. Segel MC, Paulus DD, Hortobagyi GH. Advanced primary breast cancer: assessment at

mammography of response to induction chemotherapy. *Radiology* 1988;169:49–54.

58. Singletary SE, McNeese MD, Hortobagyi GN. Feasibility of breast-conservation surgery after induction chemotherapy for locally advanced breast carcinoma. *Cancer* 1992;69:2849–2852.

59. Kuske RR, Farr GH, Harris K, et al. Is breast preservation possible in women with large, locally advanced breast cancers? *J La State Med Soc* 1993;145:165–167.

60. Marks LB, Halperin EC, Prosnitz LR, et al. Post-mastectomy radiotherapy following adjuvant chemotherapy and autologous bone marrow transplantation for breast cancer patients with ≤10 positive axillary lymph nodes. *Int J Radiat Oncol Biol Phys* 1992;23:1021–1026.

61. Peters WP, Ross M, Vredenburgh JJ, et al. High-dose chemotherapy and autologous bone marrow support as consolidation after standard-dose adjuvant therapy for high-risk primary breast cancer. *J Clin Oncol* 1993;11:1132–1143.

62. Marks LB, Rosner GL, Prosnitz LR, et al. The impact of conventional plus high dose chemotherapy with autologous bone marrow transplantation on hematologic toxicity during subsequent local-regional radiotherapy for breast cancer. *Cancer* 1994;74:2964–2971.

63. Shank B. Ageism or acumen—the treatment of older women with breast cancer. *Int J Radiat Oncol Biol Phys* 1996;34:753–754.

64. Halverson KJ, Perez CA, Kuske RR, et al. Isolated local-regional recurrence of breast cancer following mastectomy: radiotherapeutic management. *Int J Radiat Oncol Biol Phys* 1990;19:851–858.

65. Kenda R, Lozza L, Zucali R. Results of irradiation in the treatment of chest wall recurrent breast cancer. *Radiother Oncol* 1992;24:S41. Abstract.

66. Recht A, Hayes DF, Eberlein TJ, Sadowsky NL. Local-regional recurrence after mastectomy or breast-conserving therapy. In: Harris JR, Lippman ME, Morrow M., Hellman S, eds. *Diseases of the breast.* Philadelphia: Lippincott-Raven, 1996:649–667.

67. Vernon CC, Hand JW, Field SB, et al. Radiotherapy with or without hyperthermia in the treatment of superficial localized breast cancer: results from five randomized controlled trials. *Int J Radiat Oncol Biol Phys* 1996;35:731–744.

68. Rutqvist LE, Lax I, Fornander T, Johansson H. Cardiovascular mortality in a randomized trial of adjuvant radiation versus surgery alone in primary breast cancer. *Int J Radiat Oncol Biol Phys* 1992;22:887–896.

69. Boice JD Jr, Harvey EB, Blettner M, et al. Cancer in the contralateral breast after radiotherapy for breast cancer. *N Engl J Med* 1992;326:781–785.

70. Shapiro CL, Recht A. Late effects of adjuvant therapy for breast cancer. *Monogr Natl Cancer Inst* 1994;16:101–112.

71. Bhatia S, Robison LL, Oberlin O, et al. Breast cancer and other second neoplasms after childhood Hodgkin's disease. *N Engl J Med* 1996;334:745–751.

72. Fowble B. The role of postmastectomy adjuvant radiotherapy for operable breast cancer. In: Fowble B, Goodman RL, Glick JH, Rosato EF, eds. *Breast cancer treatment: a comprehensive guide to management.* St. Louis: Mosby-Year Book, 1991:289–309.

73. Griem KL, Henderson IC, Gelman R, et al. The 5-year results of a randomized trial of adjuvant radiation therapy after chemotherapy in breast cancer patients treated with mastectomy. *J Clin Oncol* 1987;5:1546–1555.

74. Stefanik D, Goldberg R, Byrne P, et al. Local-regional failure in patients treated with adjuvant chemotherapy for breast cancer. *J Clin Oncol* 1985;3:660–665.

75. Sykes HF, Sim DA, Wong CJ, et al. Local-regional recurrence in breast cancer after mastectomy and Adriamycin-based adjuvant chemotherapy: evaluation of the role of postoperative radiotherapy. *Int J Radiat Oncol Biol Phys* 1989;16:641–647.

76. Overgaard M, Christensen JJ, Johansen H, et al. Evaluation of radiotherapy in high-risk breast cancer patients: report from the Danish Breast Cancer Cooperative Group (DBCG 82) trial. *Int J Radiat Oncol Biol Phys* 1990;19:1121–1124.

77. Ragaz J, Jackson SM, Plenderleith IH, et al. Can adjuvant radiotherapy improve the overall survival of breast cancer patients in the presence of adjuvant chemotherapy? 10 year analysis of the British Columbia randomized trial. *Proc Am Soc Clin Oncol* 1993;12:10. Abstract.

78. Recht A, Come SE, Henderson IC, et al. The sequencing of chemotherapy and radiation therapy after conservative surgery for early-stage breast cancer. *N Engl J Med* 1996;334:1356–1361.

79. Recht A, Harris JR, Come SE. Sequencing of irradiation and chemotherapy for early-stage breast cancer. *Oncology* 1994;8:19–28.

80. Hartsell WF, Recine DC, Griem KL, Murthy AK. Delaying the initiation of intact breast irradiation for patients with lymph node positive breast cancer increases the risk of local recurrence. *Cancer* 1995;76:2497–2503.

81. McCormick B, Norton L, Yao TJ, et al. The impact of the sequence of radiation and chemotherapy on local control after breast-conserving surgery. *Cancer J Sci Am* 1996;2:39–45.

82. Wallgren A, Bernier J, Gelber RD, et al. Timing of radiotherapy and chemotherapy following breast-conserving surgery for patients with node-positive breast cancer. *Int J Radiat Oncol Biol Phys* 1996;35:649–659.

83. Hietanen PS. Measurement and practical aspects of quality of life in breast cancer. *Acta Oncol* 1996;35:39–42.

84. Fallowfield LJ, Baum M, Maguire GP. Effects of breast conservation on psychological morbidity associated with diagnosis and treatment of early breast cancer. *BMJ* 1986;293:1331–1334.

85. Hietanen P, ed. Finnish Hospital League. *The quality of life in a breast cancer patient.* Jyvaskyla, Finland: Gummelius Press, 1990.

86. Fallowfield LJ. Assessment of quality of life in breast cancer. *Acta Oncol* 1995;34:689–694.

CHAPTER *10*

Advanced Breast Carcinoma, Locoregional Recurrences, and Distant Metastases

S. EVA SINGLETARY
AMAN U. BUZDAR
ELENI DIAMANDIDOU

Although the frequency of locally advanced breast cancer has decreased to less than 5% of breast cancers detected in mammographically screened populations, it represents 30% to 50% of newly diagnosed breast cancer cases in medically underserved areas of the United States and in many other countries (1,2). Because the greatest risk for patients with locally advanced breast cancer is the development of distant metastases and subsequent death, the goals of surgery are maximal locoregional control with minimal disfigurement and accurate staging to determine prognosis and thus the need for postoperative adjuvant therapy. Close cooperation between the medical and surgical oncologists and the reconstructive surgeon is required to determine the feasibility of breast preservation and to assess the advisability of major resections of either persistent advanced primary disease or locoregional recurrences. If life expectancy is very short, as with patients who have bulky visceral disease or metastases nonrespondent to multiple chemotherapy regimens, the true benefit of a complex but technically feasible operation should be evaluated carefully. However, in selected patients, surgery may achieve quality palliation of the local symptoms of pain, hemorrhage, and malodorous ulceration.

Locally Advanced Disease

Evolution of Standard Treatment

In 1943, on the basis of the outcomes of 1135 breast cancer patients treated with radical mastectomy from 1915 to 1942, Haagensen and Stout (3) defined the clinical features of locally advanced breast cancer that predicted a 50% or higher chance of local recurrence and a 0% five-year survival rate: extensive edema involving more than two thirds of the breast, satellite skin nodules, "inflammatory" carcinoma, and edema of the arm. Patients with less extensive skin edema (one third of the breast), skin ulcerations, a tumor fixed to the chest wall, or fixed axillary lymph nodes had a local recurrence rate of 40%, with a long-term survival rate of less than 5%. Because surgery alone for locally advanced breast cancer produced such poor results, high-dose radiotherapy subsequently replaced surgery as the local therapy of choice, producing an overall 5-year survival rate of 21% in combined series (4–6). Unfortunately, high-dose radiotherapy was often associated with severe side effects such as fibrosis and skin ulceration, brachial plexopathy, and lymphedema of the arm. During the 1960s and early 1970s, procedures designed to lower the total dose of radiation—preoperative radiotherapy followed by radical mastectomy or, conversely, a debulking extended simple mastectomy followed within 2 to 3 weeks by irradiation—became the standard treatment for patients with locally advanced breast cancer treated at major institutions in this country (7).

In the early 1970s, the paradigm that survival from breast cancer depends on the eradication of occult micrometastases was introduced. This concept led to the integration of systemic chemotherapy into a combined-modality approach with local therapy. Today, with the increasing use of induction (preoperative) chemotherapy, the extent of surgery, if any, that is necessary after downstaging of the tumor remains unclear.

Role of Surgery Following Induction Chemotherapy

In a Cancer and Leukemia Group B study (8), 87 patients with locally advanced breast cancer were randomly assigned to receive radiotherapy or mastectomy after downstaging with a doxorubicin-based induction chemotherapy regimen. Locoregional relapse rates and duration of disease control were not significantly different between the mastectomy and radiotherapy groups (19% and 29 months versus 27% and 24 months, respectively). Survival was equivalent regardless of the modality of local therapy used. In the Milan study (9) with a follow-up of 10 years, for patients who had a complete remission with preoperative doxorubicin-based combination chemotherapy, the locoregional recurrence rate was 40% in 65 patients treated with surgery alone and 51% in 95 patients treated with radiotherapy alone.

A recent update of the National Cancer Institute's pilot trial (10), in which 43% of patients had inflammatory breast cancer, revealed a 16% local failure rate in 31 patients treated with radiotherapy but no surgery who had complete responses with induction chemotherapy as confirmed by needle biopsies. The actuarial 5-year rate of local recurrence as the first sign of relapse was 23%. Similarly, Jacquillat et al (11) reported a locoregional recurrence rate of 13% [subsequently updated to 18% (12)] for 98 patients with stage III disease treated with doxorubicin-based induction chemotherapy and both external and interstitial radiotherapy but no surgery. Eighty percent of patients were described as having an excellent or good cosmetic result. However, the late complications of radiation alone as treatment for advanced breast cancer may create considerable long-term morbidity in patients who have chemosensitive tumors and survive for a long time (13).

For the past 20 years, patients with primary breast cancers larger than 5 cm in diameter (T3), with skin or chest wall involvement (T4), or with matted or fixed axillary lymph nodes (N2) have been treated at The University of Texas M. D. Anderson Cancer Center with a multimodal approach comprising induction chemotherapy followed by surgery or irradiation or both.

In the first M. D. Anderson clinical trial of this multimodal approach, induction combination chemotherapy was administered to 174 evaluable patients (191 registered) with noninflammatory stage III breast cancer. Seventeen percent of the patients had a complete remission and 71% had a partial remission after three cycles of 5-fluorouracil, doxorubicin, and cyclophosphamide (FAC) therapy (14). Radiation alone was then given to the chest wall and regional lymph nodes of patients with an excellent tumor response and minimal residual disease. A combination of irradiation and complete mastectomy with limited axillary lymph node dissection was used for patients who had residual tumor of substantial volume. After completion of locoregional therapy, FAC was reinitiated and continued until the total dose of 450 mg/m² of doxorubicin was reached, at which time treatment with cyclophosphamide, methotrexate, and 5-fluorouracil (CMF) was instituted for a total treatment period of 2 years. The induction chemotherapy was well tolerated, and the surgical procedures were completed without an increased rate of infection or delayed wound healing (15).

A histologically confirmed response in the mastectomy specimen after induction chemotherapy was an excellent prognostic factor for survival (16,17). The number of positive axillary nodes after induction chemotherapy was also an excellent prognostic factor for survival, with actuarial 5-year survival rates of 70% for patients with negative lymph nodes, 62% for patients with 1 to 3 positive lymph nodes, 47% for patients with 4 to 10 positive lymph nodes, and 21% for patients with more than 10 positive lymph nodes (Fig. 10-1) (17). The 5-year disease-free survival rates were 72%, 46%, 35%, and 6%, respectively. When subsets of patients with four or more positive lymph nodes were combined, the overall survival rate at 5 years was 38%, and the disease-free survival rate was only 20%. Of the subset of 22 patients whose tumors showed a minor or no clinical response to induction chemotherapy in this protocol,

Actuarial survival of patients with locally advanced breast cancer by the number of axillary lymph nodes still positive for metastatic disease after induction chemotherapy. (Reproduced by permission from McCready DR, Hortobagyi GN, Kau SW, et al. The prognostic significance of lymph node metastases after preoperative chemotherapy for locally advanced breast cancer. *Arch Surg* 1989; 124:21–25.).

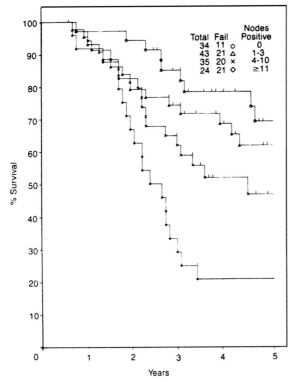

only 7 were alive at 5 years, for a disease-free survival rate of 16% (18). This dismal survival rate associated with macroscopic residual disease after induction chemotherapy parallels M. D. Anderson results obtained with mastectomy and postoperative irradiation but no systemic therapy for locally advanced breast carcinoma (19). An alternative treatment option for patients with four or more positive lymph nodes after induction chemotherapy is enrollment in a randomized trial of standard chemotherapy (e.g., FAC) with or without consolidation therapy with high-dose chemotherapy regimens (e.g., cisplatin, etoposide, and cyclophosphamide) or a crossover chemotherapy regimen of promising new agents such as paclitaxel (20,21).

The next M. D. Anderson clinical trial (1985–1989) was designed to determine whether the extent of residual disease in the mastectomy specimen after induction chemotherapy could be used as a guide to plan postoperative adjuvant treatment. Three cycles of vincristine, doxorubicin, cyclophosphamide, and prednisone (VACP) were administered at 21-day intervals, and then a modified radical mastectomy (complete removal of all breast tissue including the nipple-areolar complex, and axillary lymph node dissection) was performed. Patients with histologically confirmed complete remission and those with less than $1\,cm^3$ of residual tumor received five additional cycles of VACP; those with no response to induction chemotherapy were crossed over to receive five cycles of methotrexate, 5-fluorouracil, and vinblastine (MFVb). Patients with partial responses were randomly assigned to receive five additional cycles of either VACP or MFVb. All patients received radiation to the chest wall and regional lymph nodes. Eight patients whose tumors remained inoperable after initial induction chemotherapy underwent irradiation before mastectomy and MFVb. The irradiation had a minimal effect on wound healing as long as wound tension and thin skin flaps were avoided. If mastectomy resulted in a large defect, flap coverage consisting of healthy autogenous tissue was preferred to the use of skin grafts.

Of 193 evaluable patients in this trial (200 registered), 161 had a partial or greater clinical response to the three cycles of induction chemotherapy. No statistically significant difference ($p = 0.64$) was detected in the 4-year survival rates for the MFVb and VACP groups (75% and 58%, respectively) (22). Of the 32 patients in this study whose tumors showed a minor or no response to induction chemotherapy, only 16 remain alive (8 are disease free) at the time of writing. The lack of impact on survival of the crossover regimen was probably due to the absence of effective second-line therapy in this study. However, the downstaging observed—17 mastectomy specimens had no evidence of residual tumor, and 54 mastectomy specimens had less than $1\,cm^3$ of tumor—led us to consider the possibility of performing breast preservation surgery for locally advanced disease.

Breast Preservation Surgery

To assess the feasibility of breast preservation surgery after tumor downstaging, we performed a retrospective review that correlated the clinical and mammographic responses with the histologic findings in the mastectomy specimen and with subsequent locoregional relapse (23). Of the 161 patients with chemoresponsive tumors, 18 were excluded either because they refused total mastectomy (n = 8) or because their tumor response could not be fully analyzed (n = 10). The tumors of the remaining 143 patients who had either a complete response (16%) or a partial response (84%) were then staged according to the 1988 American Joint Committee on Cancer staging system (24): 17% were stage IIB (T3, N0), 36% were stage IIIA (T1-3, N2), 41% were stage IIIB (T4, N0-3), and 6% were stage IV (positive supraclavicular lymph nodes). According to strict eligibility criteria for breast preservation (Table 10-1), 33 (23%) of the 143 patients who responded to induction chemotherapy could

have had a segmental mastectomy (wide local excision) and axillary node dissection rather than a modified radical mastectomy. None of the total mastectomy specimens from these 33 patients were found to have tumor in other quadrants of the breast, and at a median follow-up of 34 months, none of the patients had experienced a chest wall recurrence. In contrast, of 110 patients who were not considered to be good candidates for breast preservation surgery, 55 (50%) had tumor in other quadrants: 22 (40%) involving two quadrants, 9 (16%) involving three quadrants, and 24 (44%) involving the entire breast.

The factors most commonly associated with multiple-quadrant involvement were persistent skin edema (65%), residual tumor size larger than 4 cm (56%), extensive intramammary lymphatic invasion (20%), and known mammographic evidence of multicentric disease (16%). Of the 110 patients who were not candidates for breast preservation, 17 (15%) had recurrence in the chest wall after radiotherapy. Of these 17 patients, 13 (76%) had persistent skin edema before mastectomy, 2 (12%) had known extensive intramammary lymphatic invasion, and 2 (12%) had extensive multicentric disease. These findings led to the objective of the third M. D. Anderson clinical trial (1989–1992): to determine prospectively what fraction of patients with locally advanced breast cancer become eligible for breast preservation surgery after tumor downstaging with induction chemotherapy and choose that alternative. Of 203 evaluable patients with stage IIA through stage IV breast cancer who completed four cycles of induction chemotherapy (FAC) from 1989 to 1991, 51 (25%) elected breast preservation and the procedure was performed (Fig. 10-2). The breast preservation rate for patients with ulcerative lesions or dermal lymphatic involvement (stage IIIB) was only 6%. With a median follow-up time of longer than 43 months (range, 29–61 months), only 4 patients had relapses in the breast, and at the time of this report 2 of these patients remained disease free after mastectomy.

Schwartz et al (25) reported that 39% of stage II and III patients who received induction chemotherapy until maximum clinical response was achieved underwent breast preservation surgery. With a median follow-up time of 29 months, only one patient had developed recurrent disease in the breast. Since 1990, these

T A B L E   **10-1**

Criteria for Breast Preservation Surgery after Induction Chemotherapy for Locally Advanced Breast Cancer

Complete resolution of skin edema (peau
  d'orange)
Residual tumor size <5 cm
Absence of extensive intramammary lymphatic
  invasion
Absence of extensive suspicious microcalcifications
No known evidence of multicentricity
Patient's desire for breast preservation

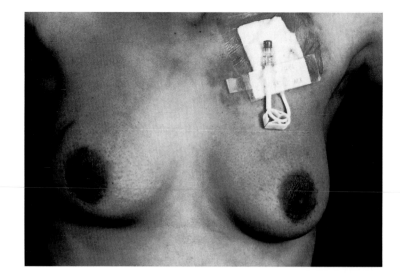

F I G U R E **10-2**

A 39-year-old woman with T2, N2, M0 carcinoma of the right breast who underwent segmental mastectomy and axillary lymph node dissection after four cycles of induction chemotherapy with 5-fluorouracil, doxorubicin, and cyclophosphamide (FAC). No residual tumor was found in the breast or axillary nodes. Postoperatively, she completed five additional cycles of FAC followed by radiation to the breast and peripheral lymphatics. She was free of disease at her 5-year follow-up.

investigators have performed breast preservation in approximately three fourths of their patients who responded to induction chemotherapy.

To determine whether induction chemotherapy yields higher survival and breast preservation rates than does postoperative adjuvant chemotherapy in patients with large primary breast tumors, Scholl et al (26) randomly assigned 390 premenopausal patients with T2-3, N0-1, M0 breast cancer to receive either four cycles of induction chemotherapy with FAC followed by irradiation, surgical excision of any persistent tumor, and an axillary node dissection (n = 200), or irradiation with or without surgery followed by four cycles of adjuvant chemotherapy with FAC (n = 190). Of the 153 patients in the induction chemotherapy arm who were evaluable after four cycles of FAC, 82% experienced tumor regression of greater than 50%. Sixty-one percent of patients with residual disease after four cycles of FAC achieved a complete response with irradiation. Thirty percent of the patients in this treatment arm underwent limited excision, and 18% of these patients underwent mastectomy, for a breast preservation rate of 82%. Of the 143

evaluable patients in the postoperative adjuvant treatment arm, 85% experienced tumor regression of greater than 50% with irradiation. Thirty percent of the patients then underwent limited excision, and 23% underwent mastectomy, for a breast preservation rate of 77%. At a median follow-up time of 54 months, the 5-year survival probability was higher in patients who received induction chemotherapy than in those who received postoperative adjuvant therapy (86% versus 78%, $p = 0.039$). However, no differences in disease-free intervals or local recurrence rates were detected between the induction chemotherapy and adjuvant chemotherapy groups.

Recently, this approach of induction chemotherapy has been used even in patients with smaller primary tumors (2–5 cm). In the pilot study of Bonadonna et al (27) of 227 women with primary tumors at least 3 cm in largest diameter without skin or chest wall involvement, patients whose tumors were downstaged by induction chemotherapy to less than 3 cm at the time of surgery underwent quadrantectomy (minimum margin of 2 cm) and irradiation (5 fractions per week for a total dose of 60 Gy in 6 weeks). One of five different drug regimens was used for three to four cycles preoperatively, with additional postoperative chemotherapy (two to three cycles) given to patients with positive nodes or with negative nodes but estrogen receptor–negative tumors. Clinical response was determined by palpation prior to surgery. Of 200 evaluable patients, 21% had complete responses, 57% had partial responses, 15% had objective improvement, and 3% had progressive disease. Response rates were unrelated to the drug regimen used. Breast preservation was possible in 91% of patients with an initial tumor size of 3 to 5 cm (n = 183) and in 73% of patients with an initial tumor size larger than 5 cm (n = 37). At a median follow-up time from completion of induction chemotherapy of 30 months, the local recurrence rate was 2%, and the overall survival rate was 93%. These encouraging preliminary results suggest that breast preservation may be an appropriate treatment option for selected patients with locally advanced breast cancer.

If breast preservation surgery is performed, radiopaque hemoclips should be placed at the base of the excision defect in the breast to guide the radiotherapist in planning the radiation fields (28).

Currently, regardless of whether the breast is preserved or removed, a level I and II axillary lymph node dissection (removal of lymph nodes lateral and posterior to the pectoralis minor muscle) is included for histologic assessment of tumor response to the induction chemotherapy and for identification of patients who may qualify for dose-intensive chemotherapy programs (i.e., patients with four or more positive nodes after induction chemotherapy). The necessity of axillary lymph node dissection and its future role in treatment are being addressed in clinical trials. For example, in the current clinical trial at M. D. Anderson, patients with T2-3, N0-1 breast cancer are initially randomized to receive either paclitaxel or standard FAC preoperatively. After the completion of induction chemotherapy, patients who have become candidates for breast preservation and who have clinically negative axilla are further randomly assigned to undergo either observation of the axilla or a standard level I and II axillary lymph node dissection (Fig. 10-3). This is then followed by completion of systemic therapy and breast irradiation that includes the lower axilla and the supraclavicular fossa in patients with a nondissected axilla.

Treatment Options for Unresectable Tumors

Patients whose tumors remain unresectable after doxorubicin-based induction combination chemotherapy and preoperative irradiation should be offered systemic therapy. The optimal regimen is determined by patient and tumor characteristics. Patients with strongly positive estrogen or progesterone receptor status and especially those with a long tumor history or well-differentiated tumor histology should be given a course of hormonal therapy. In this

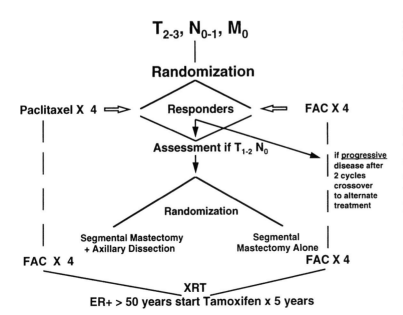

T_{2-3}, N_{0-1}, M_0

Randomization

Paclitaxel X 4 ⟹   Responders   ⟸ FAC X 4

Assessment if T_{1-2} N_0

if **progressive** disease after 2 cycles crossover to alternate treatment

Randomization

Segmental Mastectomy + Axillary Dissection   Segmental Mastectomy Alone

FAC X 4   FAC X 4

XRT
ER+ > 50 years start Tamoxifen x 5 years

F I G U R E   **10-3**

Treatment schema for T2-3, N0-1 breast carcinoma comparing 5-fluorouracil, doxorubicin, and cyclophosphamide (FAC) with paclitaxel. Patients who become candidates for breast preservation surgery after induction chemotherapy are randomly assigned to segmental mastectomy either with or without axillary node dissection. ER+ = estrogen receptor positive; XRT = radiation therapy.

setting, tamoxifen (29,30) would be the initial choice for both postmenopausal and premenopausal patients, although surgical oophorectomy (31) or administration of a luteinizing hormone–releasing hormone analogue (32) might be an acceptable substitute in the latter patients. All other patients should be offered second-line cytotoxic therapy or participation in clinical trials of investigational agents (33–35). Paclitaxel has become the de facto second-line regimen in the United States as there is no cross-resistance of this agent with doxorubicin. The probability of response with paclitaxel is 20% to 30% in patients previously treated with doxorubicin (19,20,36,37). Other agents with potential usefulness in this situation include the vinca alkaloids [vinblastine and vinorelbine (Navelbine)] used as single agents or in combination with other drugs, such as methotrexate, mitomycin, and 5-fluorouracil with folinic acid (33,35). When used as second-line therapy for metastatic breast cancer, these regimens result in response rates of 30% to 40%, but their activity in patients with anthracycline-resistant and radioresistant tumors remains to be defined. Another option to be considered is the use of intra-arterial chemotherapy. Investigators (38,39) reported a high response rate and very rapid responses after intra-arterial administration of chemotherapy, even in patients with recurrent breast cancer or tumors refractory to standard chemotherapy. Mitoxantrone, fluoropyrimidines, and mitomycin are agents frequently used for intra-arterial therapy. However, intra-arterial therapy requires a team with extensive experience in this type of treatment because of the toxicities and complications related to this procedure.

Several novel therapies are being explored for the treatment of breast cancer. Among new cytotoxic agents, docetaxel (Taxotere), vinorelbine, the anthrapyrazoles (losoxantrone and others), and new folate antagonists (edatrexate) have demonstrated activity against breast cancer, while many others are in phase I/II trials (33,34). Monoclonal antibodies, radioimmunoconjugates, immunotoxins, and several forms of gene therapy are proceeding through early clinical development (40–42). Patients with unresectable tumors after induction chemotherapy and radiotherapy are encouraged to participate in these clinical trials when possible.

If the tumor becomes operable after second-line systemic therapy, completion of locoregional therapy with surgical resection is advisable for optimal local and systemic control.

High-dose chemotherapy is being investigated in patients with high-risk primary breast cancer, including those with locally advanced breast cancer (43). However, one of the lessons learned from the high-dose chemotherapy protocols for metastatic breast cancer was that patients with previously demonstrated resistance to chemotherapy do not benefit from this procedure (44). Therefore, patients with no response or progression of disease after induction chemotherapy are not advised at this time to participate in high-dose chemotherapy programs outside of clinical trials.

Reconstructive Surgery

In some patients with locally advanced breast cancer who need or elect to have standard mastectomy, breast reconstructive surgery for cosmesis is often delayed until completion of both adjuvant chemotherapy and irradiation. As most locoregional recurrences are in the skin or subcutaneous tissue of the chest wall (45,46), a flat postmastectomy chest wall often makes irradiation technically easier than does a reconstructed breast mound.

Because of loss of skin elasticity and fibrosis of underlying tissues after irradiation, tissue expansion for implant reconstruction in an irradiated field has had disappointing results, with a high complication rate as well as patient discomfort and dissatisfaction (47,48). In contrast, the use of a myocutaneous flap for breast reconstruction, either before or after irradiation, has not interfered with the resumption of chemotherapy or the ability to detect locoregional recurrence (49–51). Irradiation of the reconstructed breast mound flap has not impaired the flap's blood supply or significantly affected the cosmetic result (52). Thus, in selected patients with an excellent response to chemotherapy or when palliative debulking surgical procedures are needed, the preference is to use an autogenous flap to create a breast mound or to provide skin coverage of the operative defect without the use of skin grafts. The two most frequently used tissue flaps are the myocutaneous flaps based on the latissimus dorsi and rectus abdominis muscles and their blood supplies.

The latissimus dorsi myocutaneous flap consists of an elliptical island of skin carried on the latissimus dorsi muscle (28). This muscle has a single dominant vascular pedicle from the thoracodorsal artery at its insertion and, at its origin, multiple segmental pedicles originating from some of the lumbar and lower six intercostal arteries. The advantages of the latissimus dorsi flap include its reliable blood supply and the relative rarity of donor-site morbidity. It also is a relatively thin flap, so it matches the thickness of the native chest wall skin fairly closely and is therefore excellent for providing coverage of a soft tissue defect (Fig. 10-4). The chief disadvantage of the latissimus dorsi flap is its limited size; an implant is usually required if the patient desires a reconstructed breast mound. The amount of available surplus skin varies from patient to patient, but in general, the latissimus dorsi flap is never more than 10 cm wide or 20 cm long.

The rectus abdominis myocutaneous flap (53,54) is an abdominal skin island flap based on the rectus abdominis muscle, whose blood supply is normally provided by the superior epigastric vessels at the junction of the costal margin and the xiphoid process. However, if a free flap is used, the inferior epigastric vessels are usually anastomosed to the thoracodorsal vascular bundle in the axilla. Rectus abdominis flaps can be quite large and are therefore most useful for defects too large to repair with a latissimus dorsi flap. Their chief disadvantage is that they tend to be bulky, so they do not match the thickness of the native chest wall skin well. This thickness, however, can occasionally become an advantage if the defect is located directly over a missing breast (Fig. 10-5). In such a case, the surgeon can simultaneously cover the wound and use the excess flap bulk to reconstruct a breast.

There are two main types of rectus abdominis flaps: the transverse rectus abdominis myocutaneous (TRAM) flap and the vertical rectus abdominis myocutaneous (VRAM) flap. The TRAM flap has a greater arc of rotation and a more symmetric and easily concealed donor site. The VRAM flap leaves a more noticeable donor scar but is technically easier to construct and has a more reliable blood supply. In general, the TRAM flap is used most often when cosmetic considerations are important or when

FIGURE **10-4**

A 42-year-old patient presented with an 8 × 10-cm carcinoma of the left breast that involved the overlying skin (*A, B*). The patient refused induction chemotherapy or radiation therapy. To provide coverage of the skin defect after a modified radical mastectomy (*C*), an island of skin carried on the latissimus dorsi muscle was used as a myocutaneous flap (*D*). The patient had excellent range of motion 10 days after surgery (*E*). (Reproduced by permission from Singletary SE. Breast surgery. In: Roh MS, Ames FC, eds. *Atlas of advanced oncologic surgery*. New York: Gower Medical, 1993:14.1–14.9.).

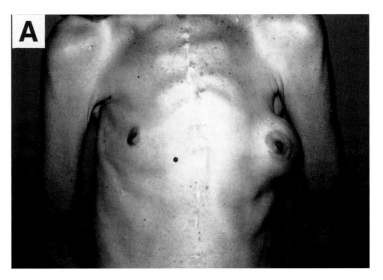

F I G U R E **10-4**

Continued

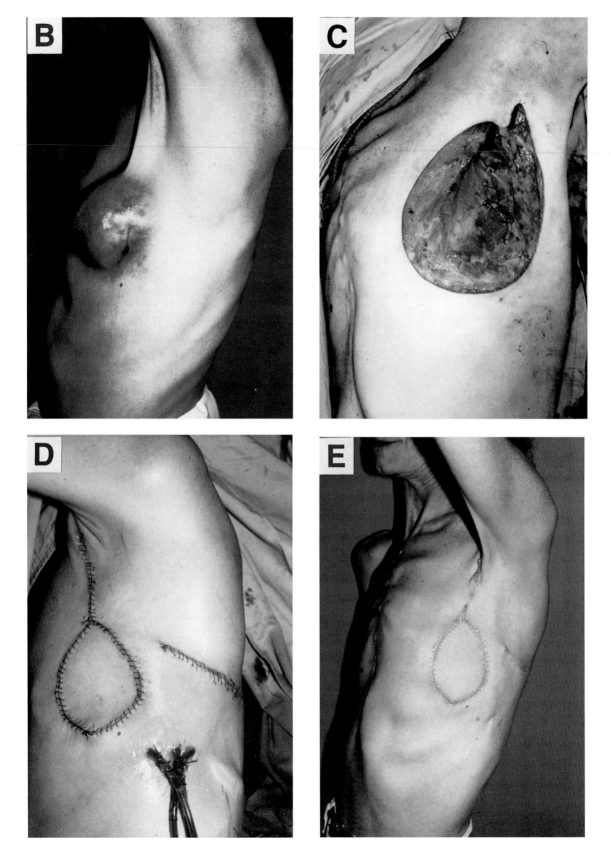

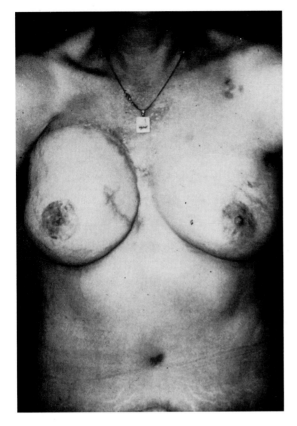

F I G U R E   **10-5**

Soft tissue and skin coverage provided by a transverse rectus abdominis myocutaneous flap after a debulking mastectomy for locally advanced carcinoma of the right breast. Nipple reconstruction was performed 6 weeks later by tattooing.

the surgeon is trying to reconstruct a breast. Use of the VRAM flap is more common when cosmesis is unimportant and wound coverage is the only goal.

When patients have a history of heavy smoking, lower abdominal scarring, or diabetes or require a larger lateral flap, the skin island flap should be placed more cephalad on the abdominal wall to improve the flap's blood supply; alternatively, a double-pedicled or microsurgically augmented flap should be considered.

Chest Wall Resections

The availability of tissue flaps carrying their own blood supply has improved surgeon's ability to perform complex chest wall resections for persistent advanced primary disease or locoregional recurrences. The indications for full-thickness chest wall resection are control of

local symptoms, removal of a site of sepsis, and osteoradionecrosis (55). The defect must be covered with a well-vascularized flap of nonirradiated tissue, but the blood supply to the flap itself may have been irradiated before flap transfer (52). In the M. D. Anderson series (56) of 61 patients with locally recurrent breast cancer or radionecrosis infection of the chest wall, prior irradiation of the internal mammary artery, the nutrient vessel to the rectus abdominis flap, or the thoracodorsal artery, which provides blood to the latissimus dorsi flap, did not compromise the viability of any of the flaps used for wound coverage. It is best to cover the wound with the largest flap that can be raised without creating excessive tension when the donor site is closed. In patients with radionecrosis, the surgical defect to be covered is often 50% to 75% larger than the actual size of the resected area, owing to retraction of the edges of the surgical wound as the irradiation-induced contracture or scarring is released. Moreover, it is often advisable to resect additional damaged but viable tissue at the margin of the radionecrosis provided that the size of the flap is sufficient to cover the resulting wound. This reduces the incidence of wound complications and prevents further progression of the radionecrosis.

The rectus abdominis flap is capable of covering a wide area from the clavicle to the costal margin and from the sternum to the midaxillary line. The bulkiness of this flap provides enough chest wall stability that up to five ribs or the entire sternum can be resected without the need for prosthetic mesh. When there is a defect of three or more ribs, however, it may be advisable to stabilize the defect with mesh anyway. Although the mesh is not necessary for survival, its use improves chest wall mechanics and reduces the duration of ventilator dependence and hospital stay. Provided that the mesh is covered by well-vascularized tissue, the risk of infection and extrusion is relatively small (57). Marlex, a nonabsorbable durable mesh, can be used for flat surfaces of the chest wall. For larger defects, a "sandwich" of Marlex mesh and methyl methacrylate can be formed to create a more anatomically normal contour (58).

Other alternatives to the latissimus dorsi and rectus abdominis flaps include the pectoralis major myocutaneous flap (59) and the omental flap (60). These flaps are rarely used today because they require split-thickness skin grafts, they give a less satisfactory cosmetic result, and they lack inherent strength.

Locoregional Recurrences

Local recurrence after mastectomy is defined as the recurrence of breast cancer on the chest wall at the site of a previous mastectomy, either in the skin flaps or along the surgical scar. *Regional recurrence* after primary treatment is defined as recurrence of breast cancer in the regional lymphatics in the axilla or in the internal mammary nodal chain. Tumor involvement of the supraclavicular nodal basin is now categorized as distant disease (M1) by the American Joint Committee on Cancer (24).

Risk factors for locoregional recurrence are four or more positive axillary nodes, primary tumor size larger than 5 cm, macroscopic extranodal disease in the axilla, and extensive dermal lymphatic invasion (61–63). The type of mastectomy (radical, modified radical, or extended simple) has not been shown to affect the locoregional recurrence rate (45). Although systemic chemotherapy may lower the incidence of locoregional recurrence as compared with surgery alone, adding radiotherapy to chemotherapy after mastectomy for patients with operable stage III disease lowered the locoregional recurrence rate from 18% to only 8% (45). Similarly, radiation decreased the rate of locoregional relapse following mastectomy and FAC adjuvant therapy from 14% to 5% in patients with 4 to 10 positive nodes and from 21% to 8% in patients with more than 10 positive nodes (45).

Of 367 evaluable patients registered (n = 391) in M. D. Anderson protocols (21) for locally advanced breast cancer (1974–1989) in which a doxorubicin-based induction combination chemotherapy regimen plus local surgery or irradiation, or both, was used, only 57 (16%) patients developed a locoregional recurrence as a first site of relapse (chest wall, 72%; regional nodal basins including the supraclavicular area, 21%; or both, 7%). The initial tumor stage was T2 in 2% of patients, T3 in 17%, and T4 in 81%. Matted axillary nodes (N2) had been present in 37%. Eleven of the 57 patients had shown resistance to prior induction chemotherapy. Surgery (usually a total mastectomy with level I and/or II axillary node dissection) had been performed in 51 patients, and consolidation therapy with irradiation had been performed in 29 patients.

Five patients had received irradiation only without mastectomy.

Unfortunately, 17 of these patients with locoregional recurrences also had synchronous distant metastasis; their median survival time from the first recurrence (regional or distant) was 5 months. The median survival time from recurrence for the 40 patients whose first relapse was locoregional only was 16 months (range, 1–109 months); only 1 patient was still alive without disease at the time of this writing (21).

Although locoregional recurrence has historically been considered a harbinger of distant metastases and subsequent death, selected patients experience a long disease-free interval and occasionally long-term survival (64–66). A multifactorial analysis (67) of prognostic variables for survival following locoregional recurrence of operable breast cancer demonstrated 5-year actuarial overall survival rates of 44% to 49% for patients with isolated chest wall or nodal disease as compared with 21% to 24% for patients with multiple or concomitant locoregional recurrences. In a subset of patients whose chest wall recurrences were excised or were less than 3 cm and who had a disease-free interval of at least 2 years from primary treatment, the 5-year disease-free and overall survival rates were 54% and 67%, respectively. Other investigators also observed that solitary recurrences of tumor of limited volume with a long interval between primary treatment and relapse may identify a subset of patients with a favorable prognosis (68–70).

Thus, for selected patients, surgical attempts to render the patient free of disease may influence the course of the disease. For the majority of patients with locoregional recurrences, however, improvement in survival will require the development of more effective systemic approaches.

Systemic treatment for patients with locoregional recurrence depends on several factors. Patients who develop recurrent disease while receiving induction or postoperative adjuvant chemotherapy or within 6 months of the last chemotherapy treatment are considered to have a tumor that is resistant to front-line therapy. Consequently, their best option would be second-line chemotherapy or, in patients with estrogen receptor–positive tumors, hormonal therapy.

Patients who have relapses more than 6 months after the last dose of front-line chemotherapy may still benefit from the same regimen used for reinduction chemotherapy. In fact, the longer the interval between the last dose of adjuvant chemotherapy and relapse, the higher the probability of response to reinduction with the same regimen. Maintenance of optimal dose intensity appears to be important during adjuvant chemotherapy and probably during induction and reinduction therapy too. Hematopoietic growth factors (granulocyte colony-stimulating factor and granulocyte-macrophage colony-stimulating factor) are excellent aids in the maintenance of dose intensity, even in patients with prior exposure to chemotherapy and radiotherapy (71).

For patients who respond well to reinduction therapy, consolidation therapy with high-dose chemotherapy [with autologous bone marrow (ABM) or peripheral blood stem cell (PBSC) support] represents an exciting investigational option (72). However, to date, no definite survival benefit has been demonstrated for this procedure. The observation that high tumor grade and c-*erb* B-2 overexpression may help predict which patients are more likely to respond to high-dose chemotherapy still needs to be confirmed (73,74).

No conclusive data are available to show that radiotherapy alters survival duration; instead, radiotherapy may only reduce the frequency of local failure as the first site of relapse. However, many studies showed that irradiation can effectively control local recurrences in only 50% to 60% of patients not treated by primary radiation (75,76). To avoid symptomatic local recurrence and its emotional sequelae, irradiation should be considered for patients at high risk for recurrent disease.

Systemic Therapy for Metastatic Disease

The incidence of breast cancer has risen steadily over the past decades. Approximately 100,000 women die each year in Western Europe and North America as a result of breast cancer; in the United States alone, 46,000 women died of breast cancer in 1995 (77).

While early disease is frequently curable with combined-modality therapy, the prognosis of patients with recurrent disease is not as favorable. With currently available therapy, a high fraction of patients with recurrent disease have objective tumor shrinkage but only a small frac-

tion of patients who have complete remission remain in remission (78–80).

In patients with metastatic breast cancer, the optimal selection of therapy for individual patients is guided by several factors: the extent of disease, the pattern and aggressiveness of the recurrence, estrogen and progesterone receptor status, and the patient's menstrual status. For patients with rapidly progressive disease, chemotherapy can often produce objective responses more quickly than other treatment modalities can. For less aggressive disease and for patients with no vital organ involvement and positive estrogen and progesterone receptor status, endocrine therapies should be considered.

Combinations of hormonal agents with chemotherapy (81), rotation of chemotherapeutic regimens (82), and more recently, high-dose chemotherapy with or without the support of ABM transplantation or PBSC transplantation (43,44,83–85) may result in higher objective response rates, but it is still unclear whether these treatments result in improved long-term survival rates.

Patients who have a relapse after a disease-free interval of longer than 2 years with the dominant site of the metastasis in bones or soft tissue and whose tumor is estrogen or progesterone receptor positive have much longer median survival times (83 months) than do patients with the same characteristics but with the site of relapse in a visceral organ (56 months). The median survival of patients who either have a relapse in less than 2 years or have a tumor that is estrogen or progesterone receptor negative is much worse (15–29 months), particularly if the site of the metastases is visceral (86).

Prior adjuvant chemotherapy and response to anthracycline-based regimens play an important role in subsequent responses to secondary chemotherapies and overall survival. Most first-line chemotherapy regimens for metastatic disease include CMF or FAC combinations (87,88). These regimens produce response rates in untreated patients in the range of 50% to 80%, with a median survival time of 2 years (89,90).

Anthracycline-containing combinations are considered the most active agents presently available for advanced breast cancer, with response rates ranging from 20% to 75% (the higher response rates are observed in patients who have not received prior anthracycline chemotherapy or have chemoresponsive tumors) (91–93). Evidence for a dose-response relationship for anthracyclines has also been described (94–96). Patients previously treated with anthracycline-based chemotherapy whose tumors did not respond or recurred soon after completion of chemotherapy usually have lower response rates (20%–27%) to second-line chemotherapy (97). Patients with anthracycline-resistant tumors represent a particularly difficult clinical situation with limited therapeutic options and poor prognosis (98,99).

Vinorelbine (Navelbine), a new vinca alkaloid, is one of the chemotherapeutic drugs shown to produce acceptable response rates (16%–40%) when used as a second-line regimen even in anthracycline-resistant tumors (100–104).

Several other drugs have been used alone or in combination in the setting of salvage therapy, including mitomycin C, vinblastine, 5-fluorouracil (weekly, continuous infusion, or bolus every 3 weeks), methotrexate, and mitoxantrone (105–112). Response rates with these agents have ranged from 7% to 40% (105–112).

Taxanes

Taxanes (paclitaxel and docetaxel) recently became available for the treatment of patients resistant to first-line therapy, and both drugs have significant antitumor activity in this patient population. These drugs have a novel and unique mechanism of action.

For patients with metastatic disease who have received prior adjuvant treatment, paclitaxel is often used as a first-line treatment. Multiple schedules of administration were tested in phase I trials, but in most of the current regimens, the drug is administered over 3, 24, or 96 hours. Response rates in patients who have not previously received anthracycline-based chemotherapy but whose tumors responded to prior therapy range from 32% to 62%. The drug doses evaluated have ranged from 135 to 250 mg/m^2 given over 3 to 24 hours (21,113,114). In patients with anthracycline-resistant tumors, response rates have ranged from 15% to 48% (17,115–117).

Docetaxel, a semisynthetic taxoid, promotes the polymerization of tubulin into stable microtubules. Docetaxel given by 1-hour infusion in patients with metastatic breast cancer and with three or fewer previous chemotherapy regimens produced response rates between 31% and 70% (118,119).

Combinations of paclitaxel or docetaxel with anthracyclines, cyclophosphamide, cisplatin, vinorelbine, 5-fluorouracil, and other agents are under investigation, and some triple-drug regimens have also been studied. Recently, the results of a study using combinations of paclitaxel and doxorubicin were published (120). Reported response rates were as high as 90%, but there was associated higher cardiotoxicity (120).

Other New Cytotoxic Drugs

Several new chemotherapeutic drugs have been developed over the past 5 to 10 years and are presently being evaluated for the treatment of metastatic breast cancer.

Camptothecin, a plant alkaloid with broad-spectrum activity, was isolated from *Camptotheca acuminata* more than two decades ago. More recently, several novel semisynthetic and synthetic analogues designed to be less toxic and to overcome the problems associated with pharmaceutical formulations of natural products have appeared. These analogues inhibit both DNA and RNA synthesis by topoisomerase I–mediated effects (121). Topotecan and irinotecan (CPT-11) were given to patients with metastatic breast cancer who had received minimal or no prior chemotherapy and produced response rates (mainly partial remissions) of 23% to 36% (122,123). There are no sufficient data for duration of response.

Gemcitabine is a pyrimidine antimetabolite. It inhibits DNA synthesis and has a long accumulation phase. Gemcitabine was given to patients with minimally treated metastatic breast cancer and produced response rates of 29% (all partial remissions) (124).

High-Dose Chemotherapy

Breast cancer is now the most common disease for which high-dose chemotherapy with ABM or PBSC support is performed in the United States.

In 1984, Hryniuk and Bush (125) introduced the concept of dose intensity (drug dose administered expressed as mg/m^2/wk) to quantify dose-response effects using breast cancer as a model. They hypothesized that dose intensity correlates with response, which in turns correlates with survival. However, for some drugs, there may be little or no advantage to dose escalation. For example, for vinblastine, the dose-response curve for antitumor activity plateaus after a small dose escalation, but its sensitivity and toxicity to normal tissues continue to increase with further dose escalations (126). On the other hand, for alkylating agents at a dose level within the intrinsic tumor resistance range, dose escalations will not be effective. However, once the resistance level is exceeded, dose escalation may prove to be much more effective in killing tumor cells. This concept led to the initiation of high-dose chemotherapy regimens for patients with breast cancer.

Even prior to initiation of high-dose chemotherapy with ABM or PBSC support, Bonadonna and Valagussa (127) showed that patients who received adjuvant chemotherapy at higher doses had significantly better disease-free and overall survival rates. Later, studies using high-dose combination alkylating agents with ABM/PBSC support demonstrated a high frequency of objective responses, especially complete responses, even in very heavily pretreated patients with refractory metastatic disease (128). The encouraging early results prompted Peters et al (129) to conduct a trial of high-dose combination alkylating agents with ABM support as consolidation for patients with metastatic breast cancer who experienced a complete remission after intensive doxorubicin-based induction therapy. Patients had documented metastatic disease and estrogen and progesterone receptor–negative tumors. Approximately half of these patients were premenopausal, and half of them had not received prior adjuvant chemotherapy. The performance status of all patients was excellent (Zubrod scale score of 0–1). The results of this study were updated at the 1996 American Society of Clinical Oncology meeting (130). The reported overall survival rate for all randomized patients with complete tumor responses was 25% at 5 years. Patients randomly assigned to undergo observation followed by transplantation at the time of relapse had a superior overall survival time compared with patients who received transplants immediately (3.2 years versus 1.9 years, $p = 0.04$).

The drawback for the ABM/PBSC trials is the lack of an appropriate control group of patients who received standard chemotherapy for metastatic breast cancer. One of the most controversial points is the selection criteria for patients entering the ABM/PBSC studies. In the high-dose trials, most patients were chemosensitive during induction therapy. This is not always the case in patients treated with standard chemotherapy. In addition, patients in the high-dose trials usually had more limited disease, good performance status, and minimal comorbidity, all of which are features predicting superior survival.

Interestingly, the results of a 10-year follow-up study of premenopausal women with metastatic breast cancer treated with standard doxorubicin-based chemotherapy showed an overall median survival time of 35 months (131). Subgroup analysis showed that estrogen receptor–negative patients had a shorter overall median survival time than did estrogen receptor–positive patients (30 months compared to 42 months). These results indicate that premenopausal women with metastatic breast cancer treated with standard chemotherapy have a survival time comparable to that in most recently reported ABM/PBSC-treated groups (130). In addition, patients treated with standard chemotherapy have significantly fewer side effects from chemotherapy, better quality of life, and owing to the lower cumulative cyclophosphamide dose, a lower risk of treatment-related leukemias (132).

Endocrine Therapy

Endocrine therapy is an option for the treatment of estrogen or progesterone receptor–positive advanced disease. Hormonal therapy has been shown to be effective in 25% to 30% of unselected patients; in patients with receptor-positive status, the response rate is approximately 50%.

The goal of endocrine therapy for breast cancer is to decrease or stop the growth of estrogen-dependent tumors by reducing estrogen levels or blocking the interaction of estrogen with its receptor (133). Prediction of response to endocrine therapy is based on the presence of hormone receptors in the tumor. For patients with both estrogen and progesterone receptor positivity, response rates can be as high as 70%, compared with 30% in patients whose tumor is positive for either receptor and 11% in patients whose tumor is negative for both receptors (134). Previous response to endocrine therapy is a useful indication that the tumor is hormone dependent and that the likelihood of response to a second-line hormonal therapy is therefore high. Hormonal receptors are also more likely to be present in tumors of postmenopausal women (approximately 63%) than in tumors of premenopausal women (approximately 45%).

Currently, the most commonly applied endocrine manipulations include surgical oophorectomy or radiation castration (in premenopausal women), antiestrogens, progestins, luteinizing hormone–releasing hormone agonists (in premenopausal women), and aromatase inhibitors.

Tamoxifen

Tamoxifen is now the most prescribed hormonal treatment for patients with primary and metastatic breast cancer. Tamoxifen has been the standard first-line therapy for metastatic breast cancer in postmenopausal women since the late 1970s.

Tamoxifen has also been used in premenopausal women with receptor-positive metastatic disease. Tamoxifen was compared to oophorectomy in two trials (135,136). The difference in median survival between patients treated with tamoxifen and those treated with oophorectomy did not reach statistical significance. However, in both studies, hormone receptor status was not available for all of the patients.

Progestins

Progestins have been used for the treatment of metastatic breast cancer for more than three decades (137,138). The response rates appear to be similar to those seen with other endocrine therapies. An overall response rate of 25% was reported for megestrol acetate as second-line therapy in advanced disease (139).

Luteinizing Hormone-Releasing Hormone Agonists

Luteinizing hormone–releasing hormone agonists have most commonly been used in premenopausal women with metastatic breast cancer. In large studies, the reported response rates ranged from 33% (hormone receptor–negative patients) to 49% (hormone receptor–positive patients) (140,141).

Aromatase Inhibitors

Selective aromatase inhibitors, including anastrozole, letrozole, formestane, and trilostane,

have been developed over the years in an attempt to reduce associated side effects, eliminate the need for concomitant steroid supplementation, and increase the specificity while retaining clinical efficacy.

Anastrozole is a competitive and highly selective nonsteroidal inhibitor of aromatase. It has no activity against desmolase or other enzymes involved in steroid biosynthesis. The recommended dose of 1 mg/day is based on the results of two large randomized trials (142,143). The doses tested were 1 mg/day (which completely suppresses estradiol but not estrone) and 10 mg/day (which suppresses both estradiol and estrone). These two doses were compared with 40 mg of megestrol acetate four times a day. There was no statistically significant difference in median time to objective progression among the three treatment groups or between the two dose levels. Given the similar efficacy and favorable safety profile, oral nonsteroidal aromatase inhibitors such as anastrozole should be considered in patients who are candidates for further hormonal therapy after tamoxifen treatment.

REFERENCES

1. Seidman H, Gell SK, Silverberg E, et al. Survival experience in the Breast Cancer Detection Demonstration Project. *CA Cancer J Clin* 1987; 37:258–290.

2. Zeichner GI, Mohar BA, Ramirez UMT. Epidemiologia del cancer de mama en el Instituto Nacional de Cancerologia (1989–1990). *Cancerologia* 1993;39:1825–1830.

3. Haagensen CD, Stout AP. Carcinoma of the breast. II. Criteria of operability. *Ann Surg* 1943; 118:859–870, 1032–1051.

4. Baclesse F. Roentgen therapy alone as the method of treatment of cancer of the breast. *AJR Am J Roentgenol* 1949;62:311–319.

5. Fletcher GH, Montague ED. Radical irradiation of advanced breast cancer. *AJR Am J Roentgenol* 1965;93:573–584.

6. Harris JR, Sawicka J, Gelman R, Hellman S. Management of locally advanced carcinoma of the breast by primary radiation therapy. *Int J Radiat Oncol Biol Phys* 1983;9:345–349.

7. Rodger A, Montague ED, Fletcher G. Preoperative or postoperative irradiation as adjunctive treatment with radical mastectomy in breast cancer. *Cancer* 1983;51:388–392.

8. Perloff M, Lesnick GJ, Korzun A, et al. Combination chemotherapy with mastectomy or radiotherapy for stage III breast carcinoma: a Cancer and Leukemia Group B study. *J Clin Oncol* 1988;6:261–269.

9. Valagussa P, Zambetti M, Bonadonna G, et al. Prognostic factors in locally advanced noninflammatory breast cancer: long-term results following primary chemotherapy. *Breast Cancer Res Treat* 1990;15:137–147.

10. Pierce LJ, Lippman M, Ben-Baruch N, et al. The effect of systemic therapy on local-regional control in locally advanced breast cancer. *Int J Radiat Oncol Biol Phys* 1992;23:949–960.

11. Jacquillat CL, Baillet F, Weil M, et al. Results of a conservative treatment combining induction (neoadjuvant) and consolidation chemotherapy, hormonotherapy, and external and interstitial irradiation in 98 patients with locally advanced breast cancer (IIIA–IIIB). *Cancer* 1988;61:1977–1982.

12. Baillet F, Housset M, Weil M, et al. Study of 58 local-regional failures after conservative treatment involving neoadjuvant chemotherapy and exclusive radiotherapy in 304 breast cancer patients. In: *Fourth International Congress on Anti-Cancer Chemotherapy. Paris, France* 1993; 23:63.

13. Spanos WJ Jr, Montague ED, Fletcher GH. Late complications of radiation only for advanced breast cancer. *Int J Radiat Oncol Biol Phys* 1980;6:1473–1476.

14. Hortobagyi GN, Ames FC, Buzdar AU, et al. Management of stage III primary breast cancer with primary chemotherapy, surgery, and radiation therapy. *Cancer* 1988;62:2507–2516.

15. Broadwater JR, Edwards MJ, Kuglen C, et al. Mastectomy following preoperative chemotherapy. *Ann Surg* 1991;213:126–129.

16. Feldman LD, Hortobagyi GN, Buzdar AU, et al. Pathological assessment of response to induction chemotherapy in breast cancer. *Cancer Res* 1986;46:2578–2581.

17. McCready DR, Hortobagyi GN, Kau SW, et al. The prognostic significance of lymph node metastases after preoperative chemotherapy for locally advanced breast cancer. *Arch Surg* 1989;124:21–25.

18. Singletary SE, Hortobagyi GN, Kroll SS. Surgical and medical management of local-regional treatment failures in advanced primary breast cancer. *Surg Oncol Clin N Am* 1995;4:671–684.

19. Strom EA, McNeese MD, Fletcher GH, et al. Results of mastectomy and postoperative irradiation in the management of locoregionally advanced carcinoma of the breast. *Int J Radiat Oncol Biol Phys* 1991;21:319–323.

20. Rowinsky EK, Casenave LA, Donehower RC. Taxol: a novel investigational antimicrotubule agent. *J Natl Cancer Inst* 1990;82:1247–1259.

21. Holmes FA, Walters RS, Theriault RL, et al. Phase II trial of taxol, an active drug in the treatment of metastatic breast cancer. *J Natl Cancer Inst* 1991;83:1797–1805.

22. Hortobagyi GN, Singletary SE, Buzdar AU, et al. Primary chemotherapy for breast cancer: M. D. Anderson experience. In: Banzet P, ed. *Proceedings of the 3rd international congress on neo-adjuvant chemotherapy.* New York: Springer, 1991:145–148.

23. Singletary SE, McNeese MD, Hortobagyi GN. Feasibility of breast conservation surgery after induction chemotherapy for locally advanced carcinoma. *Cancer* 1992;69:2849–2852.

24. American Joint Committee on Cancer. *Manual for staging of cancer.* 3rd ed. Philadelphia: JB Lippincott, 1988:145–150.

25. Schwartz GF, Birchansky CA, Komarnicky LT, et al. Induction chemotherapy followed by breast conservation for locally advanced carcinoma of the breast. *Cancer* 1994;73:362–369.

26. Scholl SM, Fourquet A, Asselain B, et al. Neoadjuvant versus adjuvant chemotherapy in premenopausal patients with tumours considered too large for breast conserving surgery: preliminary results of randomised trial: S6. *Eur J Cancer* 1994;30A:645–652.

27. Bonadonna G, Veronesi U, Brambilla C, et al. Primary chemotherapy for resectable breast cancer. *Recent Results Cancer Res* 1993;127:113–117.

28. Singletary SE. Breast surgery. In: Roh MS, Ames FC, eds. *Atlas of advanced oncologic surgery.* New York: Gower Medical, 1993:14.1–14.9.

29. Kiang DT, Kennedy BJ. Tamoxifen (antiestrogen) therapy in advanced breast cancer. *Ann Intern Med* 1977;87:687–690.

30. Jaiyesimi IA, Buzdar AU, Decker DA, Hortobagyi GN. Use of tamoxifen for breast cancer: twenty-eight years later. *J Clin Oncol* 1995;13:513–529.

31. Kennedy BJ, Fortuny IE. Therapeutic castration in the treatment of advanced breast cancer. *Cancer* 1964;17:1197–1202.

32. Manni A, Santen R, Harvey H, et al. Treatment of breast cancer with gonadotrophin-releasing hormone. *Endocr Rev* 1986;7:89–94.

33. Hortobagyi GN. Overview of new treatments for breast cancer. *Breast Cancer Res Treat* 1992;21:3–13.

34. Chevallier B, Fumoleau P, Kerbrat P, et al. Docetaxel is a major cytotoxic drug for the treatment of advanced breast cancer: a phase II trial of the clinical screening cooperative group of the European Organization for Research and Treatment of Cancer. *J Clin Oncol* 1995;13:314–322.

35. Toussaint C, Izzo J, Spielmann S, et al. Phase I/II trial of continuous infusion vinorelbine for advanced breast cancer. *J Clin Oncol* 1994; 12:2102–2112.

36. Pazdur R, Kudelka AP, Kavanagh JJ, et al. The taxoids: paclitaxel (Taxol) and docetaxel (Taxotere). *Cancer Treat Rev* 1993;19:351–386.

37. Seidman AD, Reichman BS, Crown JPA, et al. Paclitaxel as second and subsequent therapy for metastatic breast cancer: activity independent of prior anthracycline response. *J Clin Oncol* 1995; 13:1152–1159.

38. Smith IE, Walsh G, Jones A, et al. High complete remission rates with primary neoadjuvant infusional chemotherapy for large early breast cancer. *J Clin Oncol* 1995;13:424–429.

39. Schneebaum S, Walker MJ, Young D, et al. The regional treatment of liver metastases from breast cancer. *J Surg Oncol* 1994;55:26–32.

40. Goodman GE, Hellstrom I, Brodzinsky L, et al. Phase I trial of murine monoclonal antibody L6 in breast, colon, ovarian and lung cancer. *J Clin Oncol* 1990;8:1083–1092.

41. Baselga J, Norton L, Masui H, et al. Antitumor effects of doxorubicin in combination with anti-epidermal growth factor receptor monoclonal antibodies. *J Natl Cancer Inst* 1993;85:1327–1333.

42. Trail PA, Willner SJ, Lasch AJ, et al. Cure of xenografted human carcinomas by BR96-doxorubicin immunoconjugates. *Science* 1993; 261:212–215.

43. Peters WP, Ross M, Vredenburgh JJ, et al. High-dose chemotherapy and autologous bone marrow support as consolidation after standard-dose adjuvant therapy for high-risk primary breast cancer. *J Clin Oncol* 1993;11:1132–1143.

44. Dunphy FR, Spitzer G, Buzdar AU, et al. Treatment of estrogen receptor negative or hormonally refractory breast cancer with double high-dose chemotherapy intensification and bone marrow support. *J Clin Oncol* 1990; 8:1207–1216.

45. Buzdar AU, McNeese MD, Hortobagyi GN, et al. Is chemotherapy effective in reducing the local failure rate in patients with operable breast cancer? *Cancer* 1990;65:394–399.

46. Ung O, Langlands AO, Barraclough B, Boyages J. Combined chemotherapy and radiotherapy for patients with breast cancer and extensive nodal involvement. *J Clin Oncol* 1995;13:435–443.

47. Halpern J, McNeese MD, Kroll SS, Ellerbrock N. Irradiation of prosthetically augmented breasts: a retrospective study on toxicity and cosmetic results. *Int J Radiat Oncol Biol Phys* 1990;18:189–191.

48. Rosato RM, Dowden RV. Radiation therapy as a cause of capsular contracture. *Ann Plast Surg* 1994;32:342–345.

49. Kroll SS, Ames FC, Singletary SE, Schusterman MA. The oncologic risks of skin preservation at mastectomy when combined with immediate reconstruction of the breast. *Surg Gynecol Obstet* 1991;172:17–20.

50. Schusterman MA, Kroll SS, Miller MJ, et al. The free transverse rectus abdominis musculocutaneous flap for breast reconstruction: one center's experience with 211 consecutive cases. *Ann Plast Surg* 1994;32:234–242.

51. Slavin SH, Love SM, Goldwyn RM. Recurrent breast cancer following immediate reconstruction with myocutaneous flaps. *Plast Reconstr Surg* 1994;93:1191–1204.

52. Kroll SS, Schusterman MA, Reece GP, et al. Breast reconstruction with myocutaneous flaps in previously irradiated patients. *Plast Reconstr Surg* 1994;93:460–469.

53. Hartrampf CR, Scheflan M, Black PW. Breast reconstruction with a transverse abdominal island flap. *Plast Reconstr Surg* 1982;69:216–224.

54. Ishii CH, Bostwick J, Raine TJ, et al. Double-pedicled transverse abdominis myocutaneous flap for unilateral breast and chest wall reconstruction. *Plast Reconstr Surg* 1985;76:901–907.

55. McKenna RJ, McMurtrey MJ, Larson DL, Mountain CF. A perspective on chest wall resection in patients with breast cancer. *Ann Thorac Surg* 1984;38:482–486.

56. McKenna RJ, Mountain CF, McMurtrey MJ, et al. Current techniques for chest wall reconstruction: expanded possibilities for treatment. *Ann Thorac Surg* 1988;46:508–512.

57. Kroll SS, Walsh G, Ryan B, King RC. Risks and benefits of using Marlex mesh in chest wall reconstruction. *Ann Plast Surg* 1993;31:303–306.

58. McCormack PM, Bains MS, Burt ME, et al. Local recurrent mammary carcinoma failing multimodality therapy. *Arch Surg* 1989;124:158–161.

59. Starzynski TE, Snyderman RK, Beattie EJ Jr. Problems of major chest wall reconstruction. *Plast Reconstr Surg* 1969;44:525–535.

60. Jurkiewicz MJ, Arnold PG. The omentum: an account of its use in the reconstruction of the chest wall. *Ann Surg* 1977;185:548–554.

61. Fowble B, Gray R, Gilchrist K, et al. Identification of a subgroup of patients with breast cancer and histologically positive axillary nodes receiving adjuvant chemotherapy who may benefit from postoperative radiotherapy. *J Clin Oncol* 1988;6:1107–1117.

62. Valagussa P, Bonadonna G, Veronesi U. Patterns of relapse and survival following radical mastectomy. *Cancer* 1978;41:1170–1178.

63. Aberizk WJ, Silver B, Henderson IC, et al. The use of radiotherapy for treatment of isolated regional recurrence of breast cancer after mastectomy. *Cancer* 1986;58:1214–1218.

64. Bedwinek JM, Lee J, Fineberg B, Ocwieza M. Prognostic indicators in patients with isolated local-regional recurrence of breast cancer. *Cancer* 1981;47:2232–2235.

65. Griem KL, Henderson IC, Gelman R, et al. The 5-year results of a randomized trial of adjuvant radiation therapy after chemotherapy in breast cancer patients treated with mastectomy. *J Clin Oncol* 1987;5:1546–1555.

66. Holmes FA, Buzdar AU, Kau S-W, et al. Combined-modality approach for patients with isolated recurrences of breast cancer (IV-NED). The M. D. Anderson experience. *Breast Dis* 1994; 7:7–20.

67. Halverson KJ, Perez CA, Kuske RR, et al. Survival following locoregional recurrence of breast cancer: univariate and multivariate analysis. *Int J Radiat Oncol Biol Phys* 1992;23:285–291.

68. Crowe JP Jr, Gordon NH, Antunez AR, et al. Local-regional breast cancer recurrence following mastectomy. *Arch Surg* 1991;126:429–432.

69. Janjan NA, McNeese MD, Buzdar AU, et al. Management of locoregional recurrent breast cancer. *Cancer* 1986;58:1552–1556.

70. Probstfeld MR, O'Connell TX. Treatment of locally recurrent breast carcinoma. *Arch Surg* 1989;124:1127–1130.

71. Neidhart JA. Dose-intensive treatment of breast cancer supported by granulocyte-macrophage colony-stimulating factor. *Breast Cancer Res Treat* 1991;20(suppl):S15–S23.

72. Neidhart JA, Morris DM, Herman TS. Dose-intensification chemotherapy for patients with advanced breast cancer. *Semin Radiat Oncol* 1994;4:236–241.

73. Muss HB, Thor AD, Berry DA, et al. c-erb B-2 expression and response to adjuvant therapy in women with node-positive early breast cancer. *N Engl J Med* 1994;330:1260–1266.

74. Resnick JM, Sneige N, Kemp BL, et al. p53 and c-erb B-2 expression and response to preoperative chemotherapy in locally advanced breast cancer. *Breast Dis* 1995;8:149–158.

75. Pierce LJ, Lichter AS, Archer P. Indications, integration, and technical aspects of local-regional irradiation in the management of advanced breast cancer. *Semin Radiat Oncol* 1994;4: 242–253.

76. Singletary SE. Surgical management of locally advanced breast cancer. *Semin Radiat Oncol* 1994;4:254–259.

77. Wingo PA, Tong T, Bolden S. Cancer statistics. *CA Cancer J Clin* 1995;45:8–30.

78. Garber JE, Henderson IC. The use of chemotherapy in metastatic breast cancer. *Hematol Oncol Clin North Am* 1989;3:807–821.

79. Greengerg PAC, Hortobagyi GNH, Smith T, et al. Long-term follow-up of patients with complete remission following combination chemotherapy for metastatic breast cancer. *J Clin Oncol* 1996;14:2197–2205.

80. Sledge GW Jr, Antman KH. Progress in chemotherapy for metastatic breast cancer. *Semin Oncol* 1992;19:317–332.

81. Paridaens R, Heuson JC, Julien JC, et al. Assessment of estrogenic recruitment before chemotherapy in advanced breast cancer: preliminary results of a double-blind randomized study of the EORTC Breast Cancer Cooperative Group. *J Steroid Biochem Mol Biol* 1990;6:1109–1113.

82. Paridaens R, Van Zijl J, Van der Merwe J, et al. Comparison between the alternating and the sequential administration of three different chemotherapy regimens in advanced breast cancer. A randomized study of the EORTC Breast Cancer Cooperative Group. Communication at the 5th EORTC Breast Cancer Working Conference, Leuven, Belgium, September 3–6, 1991.

83. Jones RB, Shpall EJ, Shogan J, et al. The Duke AFM program. Intensive induction chemotherapy for metastatic breast cancer. *Cancer* 1990; 66:431–436.

84. Antman K, Gale RP. Advanced breast cancer, high-dose chemotherapy and bone marrow autotransplants. *Ann Intern Med* 1988;108: 570–574.

85. Wallerstein R Jr, Spitzer G, Dunphy F, et al. A phase II study of mitoxantrone, etoposide, and thiotepa with autologous bone marrow support for patients with relapsed breast cancer. *J Clin Oncol* 1990;8:1782–1788.

86. Vogel CL, Azevedo S, Hilsenbeck S, et al. Survival after first recurrence of breast cancer: the Miami experience. *Cancer* 1992;70:129–135.

87. Hayes DF, Henderson IC, Shapiro CL. Treatment of metastatic breast cancer: present and future prospects. *Semin Oncol* 1995;22:5–21.

88. Henderson IC, Harris JR, Kinne DW, et al. Cancer of the breast. In: De Vita VT Jr, Hellman S, Rosenberg SA, eds. *Cancer: principles and practice of oncology.* 3rd ed. Philadelphia: JB Lippincott, 1989:1197–1258.

89. Henderson IC. Chemotherapy for metastatic disease. In: Harris JR, Hellman S, Henderson IC, Kinne DW, eds. *Breast diseases.* 2nd ed. Philadelphia: JB Lippincott, 1991:604–665.

90. Mouridsen HT. Systemic therapy of advanced breast cancer. *Drugs* 1992;44:17–28.

91. Neidhart JA, Gochnour D, Roach R, et al. A comparison of mitoxantrone and doxorubicin in breast cancer. *J Clin Oncol* 1986;4:672–677.

92. Henderson IC, Allegra JC, Woodcock T, et al. Randomized clinical trial comparing mitoxantrone with doxorubicin in previously treated patients with metastatic breast cancer. *J Clin Oncol* 1989;17:560–571.

93. Jain KK, Casper ES, Geller NL, et al. A prospective randomized comparison of epirubicin and doxorubicin in patients with advanced breast cancer. *J Clin Oncol* 1985;3:818–826.

94. Hortobagyi GN, Bodey GP, Buzdar AU, et al. Evaluation of high-dose versus standard FAC chemotherapy for advanced breast cancer in protected environment units, a prospective randomized study. *J Clin Oncol* 1987;5:254–364.

95. Habeshaw T, Paul J, Jones R, et al. Epirubicin at two dose levels with prednisolone as treatment for advanced breast cancer, the results of a randomized trial. *J Clin Oncol* 1991;9:295–304.

96. Piccart M, van der Schueren E, Bruningx P, et al. High-dose-intensity (DI) chemotherapy (CT) with epiadriamycin (E), cyclophosphamide (C) and r-metHuG-CSF (AMGEN) in breast cancer (BC) patients. *Eur J Cancer* 1991;27:S56.

97. Porkka K, Blomquvist C, Rissanen P, et al. Salvage therapies in women who fail to respond to first-line treatment with fluorouracil, epirubicin, and cyclophosphamide for advanced breast cancer. *J Clin Oncol* 1994;12:1639–1647.

98. Buzdar AU. Chemotherapeutic approaches to advanced breast cancer. *Semin Oncol* 1988; 15:65–70.

99. Buzdar AU, Legha SS, Hortobagyi GN, et al. Management of breast cancer patients failing adjuvant chemotherapy with Adriamycin-containing regimens. *Cancer* 1981;47:1798–2802.

100. Weber B, Vogel C, Jones S, et al. A U.S. multicenter phase II trial of Navelbine in advanced breast cancer. *Proc Am Soc Clin Oncol* 1993; 12:61. Abstract.

101. Agostara B, Gebbia V, Testa A, et al. Mitomycin-C and vinorelbine as second line chemotherapy for metastatic breast carcinoma. *Tumori* 1994; 80:33–36.

102. Jones S, Winer E, Vogel C. A randomized comparison of vinorelbine and melphalan in anthracycline-refractory advanced breast cancer. *J Clin Oncol* 1995;13:2567–2574.

103. Degardin M, Bonneterre J, Hecquet B, et al. Vinorelbine (Navelbine) as a salvage treatment for advanced breast cancer. *Ann Oncol* 1994; 15:423–426.

104. Gasparini G, Caffo O, Barni S, et al. Vinorelbine is an active antiproliferative agent in pretreated advanced breast cancer patients: a phase II study. *J Clin Oncol* 1994;12:2094–2101.

105. Stoger H, Schmid M, Bauernhofer T, et al. A phase II trial of weekly high-dose folinic acid and 5-fluorouracil in combination with epirubicin as salvage chemotherapy in advanced breast cancer. *Oncology* 1994;51:518–522.

106. Ingle JN, Mailliard JA, Schaid DJ, et al. Randomized trial of doxorubicin alone or combined with vincristine and mitomycin-C in women with metastatic breast cancer. *Am J Clin Oncol* 1989;12:474–480.

107. Sedlacek SM. First-line and salvage therapy of metastatic breast cancer with mitomycin/vinblastine. *Oncology* 1993;50:16–23.

108. Francini G, Petrioli R, Aquino A, et al. Advanced breast cancer treatment with folinic

acid, 5-fluorouracil, and mitomycin C. *Cancer Chemother Pharmacol* 1993;32:359–364.

109. Konits PH, Aisner J, Van Echo DA, et al. Mitomycin C and vinblastine chemotherapy for advanced breast cancer. *Cancer* 1981;48: 1295–1298.

110. Garewal HS, Brooks RJ, Jones SE, et al. Treatment of advanced breast cancer with mitomycin C combined with vinblastine or vindesine. *J Clin Oncol* 1983;1:772–775.

111. Radford JA, Knight RK, Rubens RD. Mitomycin C and vinblastine in the treatment of advanced breast cancer. *Eur J Cancer Clin Oncol* 1985; 21:1475–1477.

112. Cameron DA, Gabra H, Leonard RC. Continuous 5-fluorouracil in the treatment of breast cancer. *Br J Cancer* 1994;70:120–124.

113. Reichman BS, Seidman AD, Crown JPA, et al. Paclitaxel and recombinant human granulocyte colony-stimulating factor as initial chemotherapy for metastatic breast cancer. *J Clin Oncol* 1993;11:1943–1951.

114. Mamounas E, Brown A, Fisher DL, et al. Three-hour high-dose taxol infusion in advanced breast cancer: an NSABP phase II study. *Proc Am Soc Clin Oncol* 1995;14:127. Abstract.

115. Seidman AD, Tiersten C, Hudis M, et al. Phase II trial of paclitaxel by 3-hour infusion as initial and salvage chemotherapy for metastatic breast cancer. *J Clin Oncol* 1995;13:2575–2581.

116. Wilson WH, Berg SL, Bryant G, et al. Paclitaxel in doxorubicin-refractory breast cancer: a phase I/II trial of 96-hour infusion. *J Clin Oncol* 1994; 12:1621–1629.

117. Abrams JS, Vena DA, Baltz J, et al. Paclitaxel activity in heavily pretreated breast cancer: a National Cancer Institute treatment referral center trial. *J Clin Oncol* 1995;13:2056–2065.

118. Ten Bokkel Huinink WW, Prove AM, Piccart M, et al. A phase II trial with docetaxel (Taxotere) in second line treatment with chemotherapy for advanced breast cancer. *Ann Oncol* 1994;5: 527–532.

119. Valero V, Holmes FA, Walters RS, et al. Phase II trial of docetaxel: a new highly effective antineoplastic agent in the management of patients with anthracycline resistant metastatic breast cancer. *J Clin Oncol* 1995;13:2886–2894.

120. Gianni L, Munzone E, Capri G, et al. Paclitaxel by 3-hour infusion in combination with bolus doxorubicin in women with untreated metastatic breast cancer: high antitumor efficacy and cardiac effects in a dose-finding and sequence-finding study. *J Clin Oncol* 1995;13:2688–2699.

121. Slichenmeyer WJ, Rowinsky EK, Donehower RC, et al. The current status of camptothecin analogues as antitumor agents. *J Natl Cancer Inst* 1993;85:271–291.

122. Chang AY, Garrow G, Boros L, et al. Clinical and laboratory studies of topotecan in breast cancer. *Proc Am Soc Clin Oncol* 1995;14:105. Abstract.

123. Bonneterre J, Pion JM, Adenis A, et al. A phase II study of a new camptothecin analogue CPT-11 in previously treated advanced breast cancer patients. *Proc Am Soc Clin Oncol* 1993;12:94. Abstract.

124. Carmichael J, Possinger K, Philip P, et al. Difluorodeoxycytidine (gemcitabine): a phase II study in patients with advanced breast cancer. *Proc Am Soc Clin Oncol* 1993;12:64. Abstract.

125. Hryniuk WM, Bush H. The importance of dose intensity in chemotherapy of metastatic breast cancer. *J Clin Oncol* 1984;2:1281–1287.

126. Bruce WR, Meeker BE, Valeriote FA. Comparison of the sensitivity of normal hematopoietic and transplanted lymphoma colony-forming cells to chemotherapeutic agents administered in vivo. *J Natl Cancer Inst* 1966;37:233–245.

127. Bonadonna G, Valagussa P. Dose-response effect of adjuvant chemotherapy in breast cancer. *N Engl J Med* 1981;304:10–15.

128. Lazarus HM, Herzig RH, Graham-Pole J, et al. Intensive melphalan chemotherapy and cryopreserved autologous bone marrow transplantation for the treatment of refractory cancer. *J Clin Oncol* 1983;2:359–367.

129. Peters WP, Ross M, Vredenburgh JJ, et al. High-dose chemotherapy and autologous bone marrow support as consolidation after standard-dose adjuvant therapy for high-risk primary breast cancer. *J Clin Oncol* 1993;11:1132–1143.

130. Peters WP, Jones RB, Vredenburgh J, et al. A large, prospective, randomized trial of high-dose combination alkylating agents (CPB) with autologous cellular support (ABMS) as consolidation for patients with metastatic breast cancer achieving complete remission after intensive doxorubicin-based induction therapy (AFM). *Proc Am Soc Clin Oncol* 1996;15:149. Abstract.

131. Falkson G, Holcroft C, Gelman RS, et al. Ten-year follow-up study of premenopausal women with metastatic breast cancer: an Eastern Coop-

erative Oncology Group study. *J Clin Oncol* 1995;13:1453–1458.

132. Diamandidou E, Buzdar AU, Smith T, et al. Treatment-related leukemia in breast cancer patients treated with 5-fluorouracil, doxorubicin, cyclophosphamide (FAC) combination adjuvant chemotherapy. *J Clin Oncol* 1996;14:2722–2730.

133. Carter C, Allen C, Henson D. Relation of tumor size, lymph node status, and survival in 24,740 breast cancer cases. *Cancer* 1989;56:181–187.

134. Sedlacek SM, Horowitz KB. The role of progestins and progesterone receptors in the treatment of breast cancer. *Steroids* 1984;44:467–484.

135. Buchanan RB, Blamey RW, Durrant KR, et al. A randomized comparison of tamoxifen with surgical oophorectomy in premenopausal patients with advanced breast cancer. *J Clin Oncol* 1986;4:1326–1330.

136. Ingle JN, Krook JE, Green SJ, et al. Randomized trial of bilateral oophorectomy versus tamoxifen in premenopausal women with metastatic breast cancer. *J Clin Oncol* 1986;4:178–185.

137. Escher GC, Heber JM, Woodard HQ, et al. Newer steroids in the treatment of advanced mammary carcinoma. In: White A, ed. *Symposium on steroids in experimental and clinical practice.* Philadelphia: P Blakiston, 1951:375–378.

138. Nathanson IT, Engel LL, Kennedy BJ, et al. Screening of steroids and allied compounds in neoplastic disease. In: White A, ed. *Symposium on steroids in experimental and clinical practice.* Philadelphia: P Blakiston, 1951:379–405.

139. Lundgren S. Progestins in breast cancer treatment. A review. *Acta Oncol* 1992;31:709–722.

140. Kaufmann M, Jonat W, Kleeberg U, et al. Goserelin, a depot gonadotropin-releasing hormone agonist in the treatment of premenopausal patients with metastatic breast cancer. German Zoladex Trial group. *J Clin Oncol* 1989;7:1113–1119.

141. Kaufmann M, Jonat W, Schachner-Wunschmann E, et al. The depot GnRH analogue goserelin in the treatment of premenopausal patients with metastatic breast cancer—a 5-year experience and further endocrine therapies. Cooperative German Zoladex Study group. *Onkologie* 1991;14:22–24.

142. Jonat W, Howell A, Blomqvist C, et al. A randomized trial comparing two doses of the new selective aromatase inhibitor anastrozole (Arimidex) with megestrol acetate in postmenopausal patients with advanced breast cancer. *Eur J Cancer* 1996;32A:404–412.

143. Buzdar AU, Jonat A, Howell A, et al. Anastrozole, a potent and selective aromatase inhibitor, versus megestrol acetate in postmenopausal women with advanced breast cancer: results of an overview analysis of two phase III trials. *J Clin Oncol* 1996;14:2000–2011.

CHAPTER *11*

Inflammatory Breast Cancer

S. EVA SINGLETARY
AMAN U. BUZDAR

*I*nflammatory breast cancer (IBC) is a highly malignant form of breast cancer. As early as 1814, Sir Charles Bell (1) said that "When a purple color is on the skin over the tumor it is a very unpropitious beginning." The term *inflammatory breast cancer* was initially used in 1924 by Lee and Tannenbaum (2), who likened the appearance of the inflamed areas to erysipelas. Others have since confirmed the unique, rapidly fatal nature of IBC (3–7). Today, with prompt diagnosis and multimodality therapy, the outlook for patients with IBC has improved and 30% to 48% remain free of disease for more than 10 years (8).

Epidemiology

IBC represents 1% to 6% of all cases of breast cancer in the United States (3,4,9). Studies showed that the median age of women with this disease is 52 years, which is similar to the average age for women with invasive ductal breast cancer in general (2–4,6,10,11). Rarely, IBC is found in men. Treves (12) reported that 3 (2%) of 131 men with breast cancer had features consistent with IBC.

Pregnancy and lactation were thought to be associated with IBC in some early studies (13–15). However, Taylor and Meltzer (3) found that only 1 of 38 patients with IBC developed the disease during pregnancy, and Haagensen (4) reported that only 4 of 89 patients with IBC were pregnant or lactating.

Staging System

The most widely used cancer staging system is the tumor-node-metastasis (TNM) system of the American Joint Committee on Cancer (16) and the International Union Against Cancer (17), which designates IBC as a T4 (stage IIIB) breast carcinoma. In the Columbia Clinical Classification System (4), stage C disease is defined by edema of less than one third of the breast skin, skin ulceration, chest wall fixation, axillary node fixation, or axillary nodes larger than 2.5 cm in diameter; and stage D disease is characterized by two or more of these "grave signs." The Institut Gustave-Roussy has used its own system (18), Poysee Evolutive (PEV), which differs from the TNM staging system by including tumor growth characteristics and signs of inflammation. The PEV categories are described as follows: PEV 0, a tumor without recent increase in volume and without inflammatory signs; PEV 1, a tumor showing marked increase in volume for a period of 2 months but without inflammatory signs; PEV 2, a tumor in which the overlying breast tissue, particularly the skin, is affected by subacute inflammation and edema involving less than half of the breast surface; and PEV 3, a tumor with acute or subacute inflammation and edema involving more than half of the breast surface.

Diagnosis

The diagnosis of IBC continues to be based on three clinical findings: 1) erythema (associated with increased heat), 2) skin edema or peau d'orange (exaggerated hair follicle pits secondary to tumor blockage of the lymphatics), and 3) wheals or ridging of the skin (indicating that the lymphatics have filled with tumor cells) (Fig. 11-1). A history of rapid onset (within 3 months) is often used to distinguish IBC from locally advanced breast carcinoma with secondary clinical lymphatic invasion.

The description of primary IBC versus secondary IBC is controversial. Taylor and Meltzer (3) defined primary IBC as the simultaneous development of inflammatory skin changes and carcinoma in a previously normal breast, whereas secondary IBC was referred to as the development of inflammatory changes in a breast that already contained cancer. Haagensen (4) and Sherry et al (10) urged colleagues to discontinue using the term *secondary IBC* because neglected locally advanced breast carcinoma may have a better clinical course than true IBC. However, the results of retrospective studies by Piera et al (19) and others (20,21) suggest that primary and secondary IBC patients may have similar outcomes when treated with the same modalities.

Another controversy concerns whether histologic evidence of dermal lymphatic involvement is necessary for the diagnosis of IBC. Anecdotal reports (22,23) indicate that patients with documented histologic dermal lymphatic invasion have a worse prognosis than do those

F I G U R E **11-1**

Clinical signs of inflammatory carcinoma in situ of the breast include rapid onset of (*A*) subtle erythema or (*B*) violaceous erythema, (*C*) skin ridging, and (*D*) peau d'orange secondary to dermal lymphatic tumor involvement.

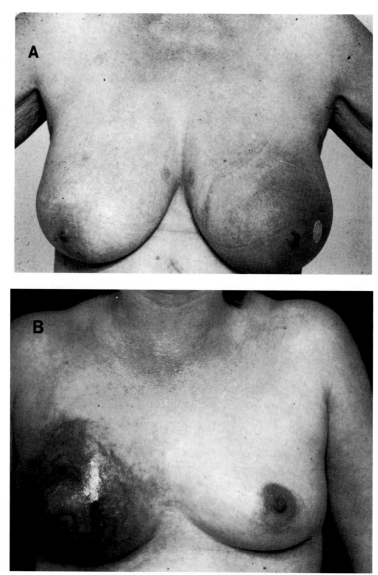

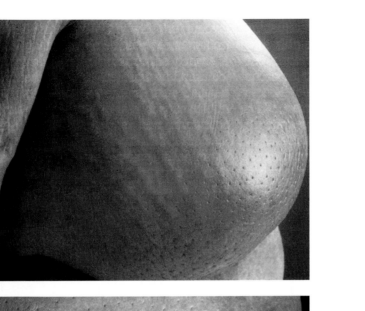

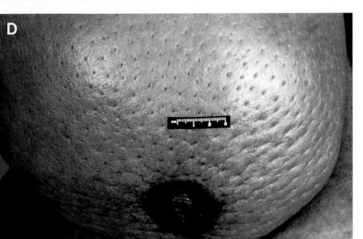

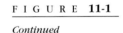

F I G U R E **11-1**

Continued

without such histologic findings. In contrast, Lucas and Mesa-Perez (24) found that patients with clinical signs of IBC had a median survival time of 14 months regardless of histologic skin involvement. In that study, a subset of patients with occult IBC (histologic evidence of dermal lymphatic disease without clinical signs) had the best median survival time (40 months). Unfortunately, this study also included locally advanced breast carcinomas, and patients were treated with a variety of modalities. Analysis of Surveillance, Epidemiology, and End Results (SEER) program data for patients who received chemotherapy plus surgery and radiation therapy revealed that those who had both clinical and pathologic diagnoses of IBC had a 3-year survival rate of 34%, compared with a 60% rate for patients with only clinical features of IBC

and 52% for those with only a histologic diagnosis (9). To resolve this issue, future studies should include a skin biopsy before therapy to assess whether dermal lymphatic invasion has occurred. In addition, even though IBC is more likely than other types of breast cancer to test negative for estrogen and progesterone receptors (25–28), receptor status should also be assessed to identify patients who may benefit from hormonal therapy.

Treatment

The dismal results of surgical treatment alone for IBC (Table 11-1) (2–4,29–33) led to the philosophy that surgery was contraindicated for this disease. Thus, the policy on treatment of

T A B L E **11-1**

Five-Year Survival Rate and Median Duration of Survival for Patients with Inflammatory Breast Cancer Treated by Radical or Simple Mastectomy Alone

Authors	Total No. of Patients	5-Year Survival Rate (%)	Median Survival Duration (mo)
Lee and Tannenbaum (2)	4	0	15
Taylor and Meltzer (3)	6	0	21
Treves (29)	114	3.5	NA
Byrd and Stevenson (30)	12	0	16
Donegan (31)	12	0	18.5
Haagensen (4)	30	3	19
Robbins et al (32)	4	0	12
Bozzetti et al (33)	8	0	12

NA = not available.

T A B L E **11-2**

Five-Year Survival Rate and Median Duration of Survival for Patients with Inflammatory Breast Cancer Treated by Combined Radiation Therapy and Surgery

Authors	Total No. of Patients	5-Year Survival Rate (%)	Median Survival Duration (mo)
Lee and Tannenbaum (2)	4	0	24
Meyer et al (36)	47	2	28
Chris (37)	7	0	13
Rogers and Fitts (38)	20	5	21
Dao and McCarthy (39)	6	0	13
Richards and Lewison (40)	11	0	14
Barber et al (41)	50	10	25
Donegan (31)	9	0	16
Droulias et al (7)	5	20	29

IBC has evolved to radical irradiation alone. From 1948 to 1972 at The University of Texas M. D. Anderson Cancer Center, a protracted irradiation technique, first with orthovoltage and subsequently with cobalt-60 irradiation, was used to deliver doses up to 100 Gy over 10 to 14 weeks. This experience was first reported in 1965 (34). In 47 treated patients, a locoregional recurrence rate of 40.5% and a 5-year survival rate of 12% were observed (34). An updated report in 1976 (35) showed only 7 (10%) of 69 patients were alive at 5 years. In 1972, an accelerated fractionation technique was introduced; it delivered 74 Gy to the breast over 5.5 weeks in twice-daily treatments. Of 11 patients treated with irradiation alone, the locoregional failure rate was 27%, and the disease-free survival rate at 24 months was 27%.

The disappointing survival results associated with irradiation alone or irradiation combined with surgery (Table 11-2) (4,7,31,36–41) provided the rationale for using systemic chemotherapy as the first-line approach in IBC patients as soon as active drugs became available. The regimen used at M. D. Anderson Cancer Center from 1973 to 1981 was a combination of 5-fluorouracil, doxorubicin, and cyclophosphamide (FAC). After a median of three courses of chemotherapy, a mastectomy or definitive irradiation (twice-daily fractionation) was performed; maintenance chemotherapy continued for 2 years. In 63 patients with a recorded response, induction chemotherapy resulted in a complete response in 13%, a partial response in 57%, and a minor response in 23%. The 5-year disease-free survival rate was 25%, and the overall survival rate was 33% (8).

Because of a locoregional relapse in 25% of these patients and an interruption of systemic therapy for 9 to 10 weeks in patients treated with irradiation only, a standard mastectomy was included beginning in 1982 for all patients with operable disease. Vincristine and prednisone (VP) were added to the FAC combination chemotherapy (FACVP). After three cycles of FACVP, patients underwent mastectomy, which was followed by eight cycles of FACVP and then irradiation. In 1987 at M. D. Anderson, we began using an alternative chemotherapy regimen of methotrexate and vinblastine (MV) before surgery if the patient's disease did not respond to three cycles of FACVP (42). If the tumor still had not responded after two cycles of MV, irradiation was performed followed by mastectomy. If the tumor responded to MV, the patient underwent a mastectomy followed by four more cycles of MV chemotherapy.

A recent analysis of the combined experience (1973–1993) of 172 consecutive patients at M. D. Anderson who received induction chemotherapy for IBC demonstrated that the clinical response to chemotherapy is significantly related to disease-free and overall survival rates (43). The 5-year disease-free and overall survival rates were 63% and 70%, respectively, for the 21 patients who had a complete response, and 37% and 44% for the 106 patients with a partial response, and only 7% and 12% for the 45 patients with a nonsignificant response. The amount of residual tumor found on histologic examination of the mastectomy specimen was also highly predictive of overall and disease-free survival. For the 38 patients with less than 1 cm³ of residual tumor in the mastectomy specimen after induction chemotherapy, the 5-year disease-free and overall survival rates were 59% and 71%, respectively, as compared to 27% and 31% in 87 patients with more than 1 cm³ of remaining tumor. Factors that did not affect survival were age (≤50 years versus >50), estrogen receptor status, initial nodal stage, biopsy-proved dermal lymphatic invasion, and specific chemotherapy protocol.

The effect of the addition of mastectomy to chemotherapy plus radiation therapy on overall and disease-free survival depended on the patient's response to induction chemotherapy. Patients who had a clinical complete response or partial response to induction chemotherapy and were treated with mastectomy in addition to chemotherapy and irradiation had improved overall and disease-free survival rates compared with those patients with a complete or partial response who underwent only chemotherapy plus irradiation. Five-year overall and disease-free survival rates were 60% and 53%, respectively, for patients treated with mastectomy compared to 34% and 31% for patients who were treated with only chemotherapy and irradiation. Patients who had no significant response to induction chemotherapy demonstrated no improvement in overall or disease-free survival rates when mastectomy was added to chemotherapy plus irradiation (43).

Fields et al (44) also reported an improvement in relapse-free survival rates in 53 patients undergoing mastectomy as part of their treatment compared with 52 patients having no surgery. Locoregional recurrences occurred in 45% overall (19% of patients treated with mastectomy versus 70% of patients without surgery), with 90% of these relapses occurring within 2 years of treatment. Similarly, the results of the study by Brun et al (45) of attempts to conserve the breast by substituting interstitial irradiation for mastectomy in patients who experienced substantial tumor reduction with chemotherapy showed that local recurrence occurred in 7 of 13 patients treated conservatively, as compared with only two local relapses in 10 patients who had a mastectomy. Other advantages of including mastectomy as part of the combined-modality therapy are the abilities to obtain important information on histologic response to induction chemotherapy and to allow the use of a lower dose of radiation afterward (46–49). In patients who have a good tumor response to chemotherapy and who may attain long-term survival, avoiding late complications from high-dose radiation is of substantial benefit. For patients who fail to respond to chemotherapy, mastectomy serves only as a palliative tumor-debulking measure.

The major obstacle in improvement of survival has been the large percentage of patients who have a poor response to chemotherapy (25% of 172 patients in the M. D. Anderson series [43]). An analysis of 45 patients with IBC from a National Cancer Institute study indicated that a higher number of chemotherapy cycles combined with hormonal synchronization until maximal clinical response was achieved resulted in a 98% response rate and that 55% of patients had a clinically complete response (50). Thus far, relapses have occurred in 21 patients (47%), with a median time to progression of 23 months and a median survival duration of 36 months. This survival duration is similar to that observed in other studies that used chemotherapy before local therapy (Table 11-3) (1,28,45,51–58).

Our current protocol is to evaluate whether paclitaxel (Taxol), which has demonstrated activity against metastatic breast disease despite a history of prior anthracycline chemotherapy exposure, can provide a better crossover tumor response (Fig. 11-2).

Another strategy in the treatment of IBC explores the use of high-dose chemotherapy

T A B L E **11-3**

Five-Year Survival Rate and Median Duration of Survival for Patients with Inflammatory Breast Cancer Treated by Initial Chemotherapy and Local Modalities

Authors	Treatment	Total No. of Patients	5-Year Survival Rate (%)	Median Survival Duration (mo)
DeLena et al (50)	CT + RT ± CT	36	NA	25
Krutchik et al (51)	CT + RT + CT	32	NA	24
Pouillart et al (52)	CT + RT + CT	77	NA	34
Zylberberg et al (53)	CT + S + CT ± RT	15	70	>56
Keiling et al (54)	CT + S + CT	41	63	NA
Israel et al (55)	CT + S + CT	25	62	NA
Brun et al (44)	CT + RT + S + CT	26	NA	31
Thoms et al (11)	CT + S + CT + RT	61	35	NA
Fields et al (56)	CT + S + RT + CT	37	44	49
Rouesse et al (57)	CT + RT + CT + H	91	40	36
	CT + RT + CT + H	97	55	NA
Maloisel et al (28)	CT + S + CT + RT + H	43	75	46

CT = chemotherapy; RT = radiation therapy; S = surgery; H = hormonal therapy; NA = not available.

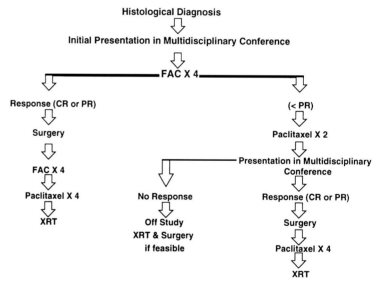

INFLAMMATORY CARCINOMA OF BREAST

FIGURE **11-2**

M. D. Anderson Cancer Center's current strategy for the treatment of patients with inflammatory carcinoma of the breast. CR = complete response; PR = partial response; <PR = less than partial response; FAC = 5-fluorouracil, doxorubicin, and cyclophosphamide; XRT = radiation therapy.

and autologous stem cell support. In a review of five trials (a total of 56 women) of either single- or multiple-drug chemotherapy followed by autologous bone marrow transplantation (ABMT) for IBC and other stage III breast cancers, Antman et al (59) reported that 79% (44/56) of the patients had achieved a complete response after induction chemotherapy but before ABMT and that 89% were in complete remission after ABMT. Complete remission was maintained in 54% (30/56 patients); follow-up duration was 1 to 37 months. The mortality rate associated with the treatment was 4%. In a review of four studies of combination chemotherapy plus ABMT in 53 previously untreated IBC and metastatic breast cancer patients (some of whom had adjuvant therapy), 47% (25/53) of the patients achieved a complete response either before or after ABMT, and the overall response rate was 75%. The complete remission rate was maintained in 17% (9/53 patients) for 4 to 86 months following ABMT.

The mortality rate associated with the treatment was 9%.

The ABMT approach is still investigational, but these limited data indicate that it warrants further evaluation. A randomized study is under way at M. D. Anderson for IBC patients who have four or more positive axillary lymph nodes after preoperative chemotherapy but are rendered disease free by surgery. The trial involves the use of standard FAC or FAC followed by two cycles of high-dose chemotherapy (cyclophosphamide, etoposide, and cisplatin) and either ABMT or peripheral stem cell support.

The need to develop more effective treatment strategies for patients with IBC is clear. Because there is urgent need to further improve therapy for IBC, patients should be treated as part of clinical studies whenever feasible.

The current recommendation for patients not treated in research studies includes preoperative FAC for three cycles followed by mastectomy in patients with tumor downstaging, then postoperative FAC for six cycles, followed by radiation therapy (60).

REFERENCES

1. Bell C. *A system of operative surgery*, vol. 2. Hartford, CT: Hale & Hosmer, 1814:136.

2. Lee B, Tannenbaum N. Inflammatory carcinoma of the breast: a report of twenty-eight (28) cases from the breast clinic of Memorial Hospital. *Surg Gyncol Obstet* 1924;39:580–595.

3. Taylor G, Meltzer A. Inflammatory carcinoma of the breast. *Am J Cancer* 1938;33:33–49.

4. Haagensen C. Inflammatory carcinoma. In: Haagensen C, ed. *Diseases of the breast.* 2nd ed. Philadelphia: WB Saunders, 1971:576–584.

5. Lucas F, Perez-Mesa C. Inflammatory carcinoma of the breast. *Cancer* 1978;41:1595–1605.

6. Stocks L, Patterson FMS. Inflammatory carcinoma of the breast. *Surg Gynecol Obstet* 1976; 143:885–889.

7. Droulias S, Sewell C, McSweeney M, Powell RW. Inflammatory carcinoma of the breast: a correlation of clinical, radiologic, and pathologic findings. *Ann Surg* 1976;184:217–222.

8. Singletary SE, Ames FC, Buzdar AU. Management of inflammatory breast cancer. *World J Surg* 1994;18:87–92.

9. Levine PH, Steinhorn SC, Ries LG, Aron JL. Inflammatory breast cancer: the experience of the Surveillance, Epidemiology, and End Results (SEER) program. *J Natl Cancer Inst* 1985; 74:291–297.

10. Sherry M, Johnson D, Page DI, et al. Inflammatory carcinoma of the breast: clinical review and summary of the Vanderbilt experience with multimodality therapy. *Am J Med* 1985;79: 355–364.

11. Thoms WN, McNeese MD, Fletcher GH, et al. Multimodal treatment for inflammatory breast cancer. *Int J Radiat Oncol Biol Phys* 1989;17: 739–745.

12. Treves N. Inflammatory carcinoma of the breast in the male patient. *Surgery* 1953;34:810–820.

13. Klotz ID. *Uber mastitis carcinomatosa gravidarum et lactantium.* Halle, Germany: Lyske, 1869:30.

14. Von Volkmann R. *Brust Krebse. Beitrage Zur Chirugie.* Leipzig, Germany: Breitkopf & Hartel, 1875:319–334.

15. Schumann EA. A study of carcinoma mastitoides. *Ann Surg* 1911;54:69–77.

16. Beahrs O, Henson D, Hatter R, eds. *Manual for staging of cancer.* 3rd ed. Philadelphia: JB Lippincott, 1988:145–150.

17. Hermanek P, Sobin LH, eds. *TNM classification of malignant tumors: UICC international union against cancer.* 4th ed. Berlin: Springer, 1987: 93–99.

18. Denoix P. The Institut's contribution to the definition of factors guiding the choice of treatment and phase I development. *Recent Results Cancer Res* 1970;32:3–11.

19. Piera J, Alonso M, Ojeda M. Locally advanced breast cancer with inflammatory component: a clinical entity with poor prognosis. *Radiat Oncol* 1986;7:199–204.

20. McBride C, Hortobagyi G. Primary inflammatory carcinoma of the female breast: staging and treatment possibilities. *Surgery* 1985;98:792–797.

21. Henderson M, McBride C. Secondary inflammatory breast cancer: treatment options. *South Med J* 1988;81:1512–1516.

22. Ellis DL, Teitelbaum SL. Inflammatory carcinoma of the breast: a pathologic definition. *Cancer* 1974;33:1045–1047.

23. Saltzstein SL. Clinically occult inflammatory carcinoma of the breast. *Cancer* 1974;34:382–388.

24. Lucas FV, Mesa-Perez C. Inflammatory carcinoma of the breast. *Cancer* 1978;41:1595–1605.

25. DeLarue JC, May-Levin F, Mouriesse H, et al. Oestrogen and progesterone cytosolic receptors in clinically inflammatory tumors of the human breast. *Br J Cancer* 1981;44:911–916.

26. Harvey H, Lipton A, Lawrence BV, et al. Estrogen receptors in inflammatory breast carcinoma. *J Surg Oncol* 1982;21:42–44.

27. Paradiso A, Tommasi S, Brandi M, et al. Cell kinetics and hormonal receptor status in inflammatory breast carcinoma: comparison with locally advanced disease. *Cancer* 1989;64:1922–1927.

28. Maloisel F, Dufour P, Bergerat JP, et al. Results of initial doxorubicin, 5-fluorouracil, and cyclophosphamide combination chemotherapy for inflammatory carcinoma of the breast. *Cancer* 1990;65:851–855.

29. Treves N. The inoperability of inflammatory carcinoma of the breast. *Surg Gynecol Obstet* 1959;109:240–242.

30. Byrd B Jr, Stevenson S Jr. Management of inflammatory breast cancer. *South Med J* 1960;53:945–948.

31. Donegan W. Staging and end results. In: JS Spratt, WL Donegan, eds. *Cancer of the breast.* Philadelphia: WB Saunders, 1967:117–161.

32. Robbins GF, Shah J, Rosen P, et al. Inflammatory carcinoma of the breast. *Surg Clin North Am* 1974;54:801–810.

33. Bozzetti F, Saccozzi R, DeLena M, Salvadori B. Inflammatory cancer of the breast: analysis of 114 cases. *J Surg Oncol* 1981;18:355–361.

34. Fletcher GH, Montague ED. Radical irradiation of advanced breast cancer. *J Roentgenol* 1965;93:573–584.

35. Barker JL, Nelson JA, Montague ED. Inflammatory carcinoma of the breast. *Radiology* 1976;121:173–176.

36. Meyer AC, Dockerty MB, Harrington SW. Inflammatory carcinoma of the breast. *Surg Gynecol Obstet* 1948;87:417–424.

37. Chris SM. Inflammatory carcinoma of the breast: a result of 20 cases and a review of the literature. *Br J Surg* 1950;38:163–174.

38. Rogers CS, Fitts WT. Inflammatory carcinoma of the breast: a critique of therapy. *Surgery* 1956;39:367–370.

39. Dao TL, McCarthy JD. Treatment of inflammatory carcinoma of the breast. *Surg Gynecol Obstet* 1957;105:289–294.

40. Richards G, Lewison E. Inflammatory carcinoma of the breast. *Surg Gynecol Obstet* 1961;113:729–732.

41. Barber KW, Dockerty MB, Clagett OT. Inflammatory carcinoma of the breast. *Surg Gynecol Obstet* 1961;112:406–410.

42. Koh EH, Buzdar AU, Ames FC, et al. Inflammatory carcinoma of the breast: result of a combined-modality approach—M. D. Anderson Cancer Center experience. *Cancer Chemother Pharmacol* 1990;27:94–100.

43. Fleming RYD, Asmar L, Buzdar AU, et al. Effectiveness of mastectomy by response to induction chemotherapy for control in inflammatory breast cancer. *Ann Surg Oncol* 1997;4:452–461.

44. Fields JN, Kuske RR, Perez CA, et al. Prognostic factors in inflammatory breast cancer, univariate and multivariate analyses. *Cancer* 1989;63:1225–1232.

45. Brun B, Otmezguine Y, Feuilhade F, et al. Treatment of inflammatory breast cancer with combination chemotherapy and mastectomy versus breast conservation. *Cancer* 1988;161:1096–1103.

46. Hagelberg RS, Jolly PC, Anderson RP. Role of surgery in the treatment of inflammatory breast carcinoma. *Am J Surg* 1984;148:125–131.

47. Moore MP, Ihde JK, Crowe JP, et al. Inflammatory breast cancer. *Arch Surg* 1991;126:304–306.

48. Schafer P, Alberto P, Forni M, et al. Surgery as part of a combined modality approach for inflammatory breast carcinoma. *Cancer* 1987;59:1063–1067.

49. Knight CD, Martin JK, Welch JS, et al. Surgical considerations after chemotherapy and radiation therapy for inflammatory breast cancer. *Surgery* 1986;99:385–391.

50. Swain SM, Lippman ME. Treatment of patients with inflammatory breast cancer. In: DeVita V Jr, Hellman S, Rosenberg S, eds. *Cancer: principles and practice of oncology.* Philadelphia: JB Lippincott, 1989:129–150.

51. DeLena M, Zucali R, Viganotti G, et al. Combined chemotherapy-radiotherapy approach in a locally advanced (T3-T4) breast cancer. *Cancer Chemother Pharmacol* 1978;1:53–59.

52. Krutchik AN, Buzdar AU, Blumenschein GR, et al. Combined chemoimmunotherapy and radiation therapy of inflammatory breast cancer. *J Surg Oncol* 1979;11:325–332.

53. Pouillart P, Palangie T, Joure M. Cancer inflammatoire du sein traite par une association de chimotherapie et d'irradiation. *Bull Cancer (Paris)* 1981;68:171–196.

54. Zylberberg B, Salat-Baroux J, Ravina JH, et al. Initial chemoimmunotherapy in inflammatory carcinoma of the breast. *Cancer* 1982;49: 1537–1543.

55. Keiling R, Guiochot N, Calderoli H, et al. Preoperative chemotherapy in the treatment of inflammatory breast cancer. In: Wagener DJT, Blijham GH, Smeets JBE, Wils JA, eds. *Primary chemotherapy in cancer medicine.* New York: Alan R. Liss, 1985:95–104.

56. Israel L, Breau JL, Morere J-F. Two years of high dose cyclophosphamide and 5-fluorouracil followed by surgery after three months for acute inflammatory breast carcinomas: a phase II study

of 25 cases with a median follow-up of 35 months. *Cancer* 1986;57:24–28.

57. Fields JN, Perez C, Kuske R, et al. Inflammatory carcinoma of the breast: treatment results in 107 patients. *Int J Radiat Oncol Biol Phys* 1989; 17:249–255.

58. Rouesse J, Sarrazin D, Spielman M, et al. Treatment of inflammatory cancer of the breast: combined chemotherapy and radiotherapy—a study of 270 women treated at the Institut Gustave-Roussy. *Bull Cancer (Paris)* 1989;76:87–92.

59. Antman K, Bearman SI, Davidson N, et al. Dose intensive therapy in breast cancer: current status. In: Gale RP, Champlin RE, eds. *New strategies in bone marrow transplantation.* New York: Alan R. Liss, 1990:423–426.

60. Singletary SE. Inflammatory breast cancer. In: Cameron JL, ed. *Current surgical therapy.* St Louis: Mosby Year Book, 1992:608–611.

CHAPTER *12*

Lobular Carcinoma In Situ

S. EVA SINGLETARY

*D*escribed histologically in 1941 by Foote and Stewart (1), lobular carcinoma in situ (LCIS) develops from the inner cuboidal cell layer of the terminal duct–lobular acini (2,3). Microscopically, LCIS is defined by the disorderly proliferation of epithelial cells to the extent that more than 50% of the acini are filled and distended (4,5). Although the proliferating cells are usually enlarged and have loss of cohesion, these cells have a bland, homogeneous appearance with rarely any mitosis or necrosis. When these changes are less developed with no more than 50% of the acini involved or incompletely filled, the term *atypical lobular hyperplasia* should be used (5). LCIS is usually associated with diploid DNA morphology (6), low proliferative rates (7), and the lack of amplification or overexpression of c-*erb* B-2 (8,9). Because of its low-grade nature and anticipated favorable clinical outcome, the term *lobular neoplasia* has been advocated. However, this term is imprecise and unclear in meaning, so today use of the original terminology of LCIS is preferred (10).

The diagnosis of LCIS is usually made incidentally from a biopsy specimen obtained from a patient with a palpable mass or a mammographic abnormality. When discovered within biopsy specimens of tissue containing microcalcifications, LCIS is often adjacent to, but not necessarily contained within, the area of calcifications (11–13). Because routine screening mammography has become more accepted as a standard of care, the number of diagnostic biopsies has also increased, leading to a slight increase in the incidence of LCIS (14). LCIS has been detected in approximately 2.5% of all breast biopsy specimens (14–16).

At the time of diagnosis, most patients with LCIS are premenopausal and in their late 40s (17–22). This finding suggests the hypothesis that LCIS is estrogen dependent and may regress after menopause. Although LCIS may be more likely to be estrogen receptor positive (23,24), approximately one fourth to one third of cases are found in postmenopausal women, including those not on estrogen replacement therapy (25,26).

LCIS occurs 12 times more frequently in white women than in black women, whereas Japanese women have a much lower incidence (21,27,28). Similar to invasive breast carcinoma, a family history of breast cancer is found in 15% to 20% of women with LCIS (17,22,27–29). No relationship to a history of abortion and LCIS has been confirmed (30).

In the past, treatment of the ipsilateral breast in patients with LCIS alone has varied from biopsy only to total mastectomy, sometimes including axillary node dissection (22). Today, LCIS is considered to be a marker of increased risk for the development of breast cancer rather than necessarily as a site of origin for cancer. This philosophy is based on the following observations: 1) The lifetime risk of subsequent development of an invasive breast carcinoma following a biopsy revealing LCIS is as high as 20% to 30% overall; 2) this risk is equally divided between the two breasts (10%–15% risk per breast, or approximately 0.5%–1.0% per year from the time of the initial diagnosis of LCIS) (Table 12-1) (5,10,20,22,30–35); and 3) 50% to 65% of invasive carcinomas subsequent to a diagnosis of LCIS are ductal rather than lobular in histology (30). Further evidence that LCIS itself is not always a precursor to an invasive process is that

T A B L E   **12-1**

Risk and Mortality of Subsequent Invasive Breast Carcinoma
Following Diagnosis of Lobular Carcinoma In Situ

Series	No. of Evaluable Patients	Mean Follow-up (yr)	Ipsilateral Carcinoma Intact Breast	Contralateral Carcinoma Intact Breast	No. of Deaths
Page et al (5)	39	18	6/39 (15%)	4/39 (10%)	3
Haagensen et al (10)	295	16.3	33/281 (12%)	27/276 (10%)	11
McDivitt et al (20)	48	—	9/40 (23%)	4/47 (9%)	2
Singletary (22)	45	10	2/13 (15%)	1/27 (4%)	2
Rosen et al (30)	84	24	19/83 (23%)	19/83 (23%)	16
Wheeler et al (31)	35	15.7	1/25 (4%)	3/32 (9%)	2
Andersen (32)	52	15	9/46 (20%)	4/47 (9%)	6
Carson et al (33)	65	6.9	3/51 (6%)	0/60 (0%)	0
Hutter and Foote (34)	49	—	10/40 (25%)	4/46 (9%)	2
Salvadori et al (35)	99	4.8	5/78 (6%)	0/99 (0%)	0
Total	811	13.8	97/696 (14%)	66/756 (9%)	44 (5%)

most subsequent carcinomas occur 10 to 15 years after the initial diagnosis, with 40% detected more than 20 years later (30). The extent of LCIS within the biopsy specimen (17,30) or a personal or family history of breast carcinoma (5,30) has not been conclusively shown to add further to this risk. In contrast, a family history of breast cancer doubles the risk of breast cancer following a biopsy revealing atypical lobular hyperplasia (eight times the risk of the general population), approaching the risk of LCIS alone (5).

LCIS represents a bilateral diffuse process, with multicentricity noted in more than 60% of mastectomy specimens (18,36–38) and bilaterality in 18% to 69% (21,27,36–41). LCIS treatment options include lifelong observation of both breasts with mammography and physical examination, bilateral total mastectomies with consideration of breast reconstruction (Fig. 12-1), or participation in clinical prevention trials such as hormone/growth factor regulation with tamoxifen or retinoid analogues (22,42). Ipsilateral total mastectomy, radiation therapy, and re-excision of the original biopsy site to obtain clear margins are not indicated because all genetically identical breast tissue (i.e., both breasts) is at increased risk for breast carcinoma. Routine contralateral biopsy in the absence of standard indications, such as an abnormal finding on physical examination or by mammography, is not justified because the likelihood of finding a lesion requiring treatment (invasive carcinoma or ductal carcinoma in situ)

is small (<5%). The clinical significance of contralateral LCIS may be negligible, and negative biopsy results have never been clearly shown to be associated with reduced risk (43–45). As with excisional biopsy, subcutaneous mastectomy that leaves significant residual breast tissue may not reduce the risk substantially and may, in fact, give a false sense of security to the patient and physician (46). Thus, if surgery is elected for LCIS alone, the preferred choice is bilateral total mastectomy (22,39,47–49). Because the incidence of axillary nodal metastases associated with LCIS alone is less than 1%, an axillary node dissection offers no benefit (22,36,50). With major advances in breast reconstruction, particularly the use of autogenous flaps, reconstructive surgery at the time of mastectomy should be considered for most patients, unless the additional procedure increases the operative risk or the patient has already indicated that the procedure is unnecessary for her quality of life (51).

With the option of nonoperative observation, it is imperative that both the patient and the physician fully understand the lifelong commitment to careful surveillance of the breasts with physical examinations and yearly mammography (17,22,33,52). The combined data from 811 patients with LCIS in 10 follow-up series showed a 5% mortality rate from breast cancer with mean time intervals from the diagnosis of LCIS of 5 to 24 years (see Table 12-1). Thus, the purpose of observation is to detect a subsequent breast carcinoma at an early stage

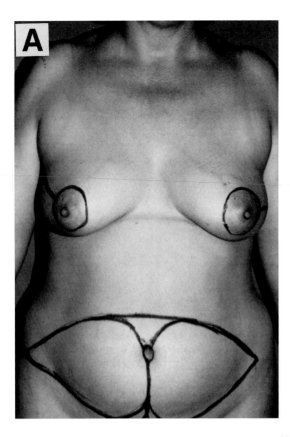
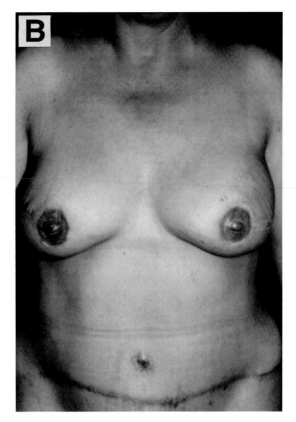

F I G U R E   **12-1**

A. A 50-year-old woman with lobular carcinoma in situ of the right breast chose to have bilateral prophylactic total mastectomies with immediate reconstruction. *B.* The breast mounds were created with autogenous tissue using the transverse rectus abdominis myocutaneous flap (TRAM), the so-called "tummy tuck" method. With this technique, a large area of the abdominal skin and fat is outlined and raised with a portion of the rectus muscle and its blood supply. The flap can then be tunneled under the skin or directly transferred by a free microvascular anastomosis of the inferior epigastric to the axillary thoracodorsal vessels. Nipple reconstruction was performed 3 months later using double-opposing tab flaps from nearby skin of the breast mound. The areola was created by tattooing.

so that the diagnosis will not significantly have an adverse affect on the patient's chances of survival. The decreased breast cancer mortality observed in mammographic screening trials supports this approach (53–55).

For patients in whom LCIS is associated with another primary ipsilateral breast carcinoma, treatment is based on the stage and histology of the non-LCIS breast carcinoma (22). Local recurrence rates after breast preservation surgery and irradiation reveal no significant difference by histology of the primary tumor and may instead be related to whether histologically clear margins of the non-LCIS lesion were

actually achieved (56–58). Prophylactic mastectomy of the contralateral breast may be appropriate in a very select group of patients, such as those who need or elect to have an ipsilateral mastectomy and desire to remove the other breast for their perceived emotional well-being (22,59).

R E F E R E N C E S

1. Foote FW, Stewart FW. Lobular carcinoma in situ: a rare form of mammary carcinoma. *Am J Pathol* 1941;17:491–495.

2. Tobon H, Price HM. Lobular carcinoma in situ: some ultrastructural observations. *Cancer* 1972; 30:1082–1091.

3. Gad A, Azzopardi JG. Lobular carcinoma of the breast: a special variant of mucin-secreting carcinoma. *J Clin Pathol* 1975;28:711–716.

4. Rosen PP. Lobular carcinoma in situ and intraductal carcinoma of the breast. *Monogr Pathol* 1984;25:59–105.

5. Page DL, Kidd TE, Dupont WD, et al. Lobular neoplasia of the breast: higher risk for subsequent invasive cancer predicted by more extensive disease. *Hum Pathol* 1991;22:1232–1239.

6. Ludwig AS, Okagaki T, Richart RM, Lattes R. Nuclear DNA content of lobular carcinoma in situ of the breast. *Cancer* 1973;31:1553–1560.

7. Meyer JS. Cell kinetics of histologic variants of in situ breast carcinoma. *Breast Cancer Res Treat* 1986;7:171–180.

8. Porter PL, Garcia R, Moe R, et al. c-*erb* B-2 oncogene protein in situ and invasive lobular breast neoplasia. *Cancer* 1991;68:331–334.

9. Schimmelpenning H, Eriksson ET, Pallis L, et al. Immunohistochemical c-*erb* B-2 proto-oncogene expression and nuclear DNA content in human mammary carcinoma in situ. *Am J Clin Pathol* 1992;97(suppl 1):S48–S52.

10. Haagensen CD, Lane N, Lattes R, Bodian C. Lobular neoplasia (so-called lobular carcinoma in situ) of the breast. *Cancer* 1978;42:737–769.

11. Hutter RVP, Snyder RE, Lucas JC, et al. Clinical and pathologic correlation with mammographic findings in lobular in situ. *Cancer* 1969; 23:826–839.

12. Pope TL, Fechner RE, Wilhelm MC, et al. Lobular carcinoma in situ of the breast: mammographic features. *Radiology* 1988;168:63–66.

13. Beute BJ, Kalisher L, Hutter RVP. Lobular carcinoma in situ of the breast: clinical, pathologic, and mammographic features. *AJR* 1991;157: 257–265.

14. Mackarem G, Yacoub LK, Lee AKC, et al. Effects of screening on detection of lobular carcinoma in situ of the breast: nonspecificity of mammography and physical examination. *Breast Dis* 1994;7:339–345.

15. Schwartz GF, Feig SA, Rosenberg AL, et al. Staging and treatment of clinically occult breast cancer. *Cancer* 1984;53:1379–1384.

16. Giordano JM, Klopp CT. Lobular carcinoma in situ: incidence and treatment. *Cancer* 1973;31: 105–109.

17. Haagensen CD. Lobular neoplasia (lobular carcinoma in situ). In: Haagensen CD, ed. *Diseases of the breast.* 3rd ed. Philadelphia: WB Saunders, 1986:192–241.

18. Benfield JR, Jacobson M, Warner NE. In situ lobular carcinoma of the breast. *Arch Surg* 1965;91:130–135.

19. Farrow JH. Clinical considerations and treatment of in situ lobular breast cancer. *AJR Am J Roentgenol* 1968;102:652–656.

20. McDivitt RW, Hutter RVP, Foote FW Jr, Stewart FW. In situ lobular carcinoma. *JAMA* 1967; 201:96–100.

21. Newman W. In situ lobular carcinoma of the breast. *Ann Surg* 1963;157:591–599.

22. Singletary SE. Lobular carcinoma in situ of the breast: a 31-year experience at The University of Texas M. D. Anderson Cancer Center. *Breast Dis* 1994;7:157–163.

23. Giri DD, Dundas SAC, Nottingham JF, Underwood JCE. Oestrogen receptors in benign epithelial lesions and intraductal carcinomas of the breast. *Histopathology* 1989;15:575–584.

24. Bur ME, Zimarowski MJ, Schnitt SJ, et al. Estrogen receptor immunohistochemistry in CIS of the breast. *Cancer* 1992;69:1174–1181.

25. Hutter RVP. The management of patients with lobular carcinoma in situ of the breast. *Cancer* 1984;53:798–802.

26. Rosen PP, Senie RT, Farr GH, et al. Epidemiology of breast carcinoma: age, menstrual status, and exogenous hormone usage in patients with lobular carcinoma in situ. *Surgery* 1979;85: 219–224.

27. Farrow JH. Current concepts in the detection and treatment of the earliest of early breast cancers. *Cancer* 1970;25:468–477.

28. Rosner D, Bedwani RN, Vana J, et al. Noninvasive breast carcinoma: results of a national survey by the American College of Surgeons. *Ann Surg* 1980;192:139–147.

29. Davis N, Baird RM. Breast cancer in association with lobular carcinoma in situ: clinicopathologic review and treatment recommendation. *Am J Surg* 1984;147:641–645.

30. Rosen PP, Lieberman PH, Braun DW, et al. Lobular carcinoma in situ of the breast: detailed analysis of 99 patients with average follow-up of 24 years. *Am J Surg Pathol* 1978;3:225–251.

31. Wheeler JE, Enterline HT, Roseman JM, et al. Lobular carcinoma in situ of the breast: long-term follow-up. *Cancer* 1974;34:554–563.

32. Andersen JA. Lobular carcinoma in situ of the breast: an approach to rational treatment. *Cancer* 1977;39:2597–2602.

33. Carson W, Sanchez-Forgach E, Stomper P, et al. Lobular carcinoma in situ: observation without surgery as an appropriate therapy. *Ann Surg Oncol* 1994;1:141–146.

34. Hutter RVP, Foote FW. Lobular carcinoma in situ. *Cancer* 1969;24:1081–1085.

35. Salvadori B, Bartoli C, Zurrida S, et al. Risk of invasive cancer in women with lobular carcinoma in situ of the breast. *Eur J Cancer* 1991; 27:35–37.

36. Carter D, Smith RRL. Carcinoma in situ of the breast. *Cancer* 1977;40:1189–1193.

37. Dall'Olmo CA, Ponka JL, Horn RC, Rui R. Lobular carcinoma of the breast in situ: are we too radical in its treatment? *Arch Surg* 1975; 110:537–542.

38. Ringberg A, Palmer B, Linell F. The contralateral breast at reconstructive surgery after breast cancer operation: a histopathological study. *Breast Cancer Res Treat* 1982;2:151–161.

39. Urban JA. Biopsy of the "normal" breast in treating breast cancer. *Surg Clin North Am* 1969; 49:291–301.

40. Rosen PP, Braun DW, Lyngholm B, et al. Lobular carcinoma in situ of the breast: preliminary results of treatment by ipsilateral mastectomy and contralateral breast biopsy. *Cancer* 1981;47:813–819.

41. Sunshine JA, Moseley HS, Fletcher WS, Krippaehne WW. Breast carcinoma in situ: a retrospective review of 112 cases with a minimum of 10 year follow-up. *Am J Surg* 1985;150:44–51.

42. Nayfield SG, Karp LG, Dorr FA, Kramer BS. Potential role of tamoxifen prevention of breast cancer. *J Natl Cancer Inst* 1991;83:1450–1459.

43. Balch CM, Singletary SE, Bland KI. Clinical decision-making in early breast cancer. *Ann Surg* 1993;217:207–225.

44. Baker RR, Kuhajda FP. The clinical management of a normal contralateral breast in patients with lobular breast cancer. *Ann Surg* 1989;210: 444–448.

45. Walt AJ, Simm M, Swanson GM. The continuing dilemma of lobular carcinoma in situ. *Arch Surg* 1992;127:904–916.

46. Goodnight JE, Quagliana JM, Morton DL. Failure of subcutaneous mastectomy to prevent the development of breast cancer. *J Surg Oncol* 1984;26:198–201.

47. Osborne MP, Hoda SA. Current management of lobular carcinoma in situ of the breast. *Oncology* 1994;8:45–54.

48. Frykberg ER, Santiago F, Betsill WL, O'Brien PH. Lobular carcinoma in situ of the breast. *Surg Gynecol Obstet* 1987;164:285–301.

49. Swain SM. Lobular carcinoma in situ: incidence, presentation, guidelines to treatment. *Oncology* 1989;3:35–51.

50. Rosen PP. Axillary lymph node metastases in patients with occult noninvasive breast carcinoma. *Cancer* 1980;46:1298–1306.

51. Singletary SE. Surgical concepts in lobular carcinoma in situ. *Breast Surg Index Rev* 1993;1:1, 19.

52. Frykberg ER, Bland KI. Management of in situ and minimally invasive breast carcinoma. *World J Surg* 1994;18:45–57.

53. Shapiro S, Venet W, Strax P, et al. Ten-to-fourteen year effect of screening on breast cancer mortality. *J Natl Cancer Inst* 1982;46: 1298–1303.

54. Tabar L, Fagerberg CJG, Gad A, et al. Reduction in mortality from breast cancer after mass screening with mammography. *Lancet* 1985; 1:829–832.

55. Seidman H, Gelb SK, Silverberg E, et al. Survival experience in the Breast Cancer Detection Demonstration Project. *CA Cancer J Clin* 1987;37:258–290.

56. Kurts JM, Jacquamier J, Torhorst J, et al. Conservation therapy for breast cancers other than infiltrating ductal carcinoma. *Cancer* 1989; 63:1630–1635.

57. Schnitt SJ, Connolly JL, Recht A, et al. Influence of infiltrating lobular histology on local tumor control in breast cancer patients treated with conservative surgery and radiotherapy. *Cancer* 1989;64:448–454.

58. Schnitt SJ, Abner A, Gelman R, et al. The relationship between microscopic margins of resection and the risk of local recurrence in patients with breast cancer treated with breast conserving surgery and radiation therapy. *Cancer* 1994;74:1746–1751.

59. Singletary SE, Taylor SH, Guinee VF. Occurrence and prognosis of contralateral carcinoma of the breast. *J Am Coll Surg* 1994;178:390–396.

CHAPTER 13

Breast Cancer in the Elderly

S. EVA SINGLETARY

he probability of breast cancer developing is highest in older women. Data from the Surveillance, Epidemiology, and End Results study (1) reveal that for women 80 to 84 years old, the breast cancer incidence is as high as 435 per 100,000; in contrast, the incidence is 212 per 100,000 in women 50 to 54 years old. Whether a woman survives breast cancer depends on the biology of the tumor, the immune defenses of the patient, and the appropriateness of the intervention by the physician. Controversy over the management of breast cancer in the elderly has been generated by the following ingrained beliefs:

1. Elderly patients more often have locally advanced disease at the time of initial presentation.
2. Elderly patients have more indolent disease.
3. Elderly patients have a limited life expectancy from comorbid conditions other than breast cancer.
4. Elderly patients cannot tolerate standard treatment.

However, in a review of 184 women older than 69 years who received treatment for locoregional breast cancer between 1976 and 1985 at The University of Texas M. D. Anderson Cancer Center, the majority of elderly women whose breast cancer had been treated appropriately remained free of disease and maintained a good quality of life (2). Therefore, the myths surrounding the treatment of the elderly need to be examined.

Myth 1. Elderly Patients More Often Have Locally Advanced Disease at the Time of Initial Presentation

Mueller et al (3), in a review of 3558 breast cancer patients, reported that stage I disease was equally common in all age groups. The limitation of the study was that 25% of the elderly patients did not undergo staging at the time of diagnosis. Other investigators noted a higher proportion of locally advanced tumors among elderly patients (4–6). Most patients in these series were classified as having stage III disease because of the large size of the primary tumor rather than the presence of regional (matted axillary nodes) or positive supraclavicular nodes. In the M. D. Anderson Cancer Center series (2), on clinical examination, 66 (36%) of the elderly patients had primary tumors 2 cm or smaller (T1), 81 (44%) had tumors larger than 2 cm but no larger than 5 cm (T2), and 15 (8%) had tumors larger than 5 cm (T3). Only 22 (12%) had skin ulceration or dermal lymphatic involvement (peau d'orange) of the breast (T4). The axilla was described as clinically negative (N0) in 131 (71%), contained palpable, movable lymph nodes (N1) in 35 (19%), and contained fixed or matted lymph nodes (N2) in only 18 (10%). Based on the current American Joint Committee on Cancer staging system (7), 61 (33%) of patients had stage I disease (T1, N0), 85 (46%) had stage II (T1, N1; T2, N0-1; T3, N0-1), and 38 (21%) had stage III (T3, N2; T4, N0-2).

Presentation with a locally advanced tumor is often attributed to a delay in seeking treatment by an individual. However, recent studies indicated that the medical profession also may substantially contribute to this delay. In a review of 1680 women with breast cancer treated in 17 community hospitals, Chu et al (8) found that elderly patients with breast lumps were less likely to undergo mammography or biopsy or to be referred for consultation. Makuc et al (9) found that older women were also less likely than younger women to have had a recent clinical examination of their breasts by their physician or to have been instructed in breast self-examination. In the M. D. Anderson Cancer Center series (2), 157 (85%) of the women detected their breast cancer by self-examination; only 22 (12%) of tumors were discovered by a physician. Only 5 (3%) of the women had a screening mammogram with a positive result. Although elderly women are often accused of delaying seeking a diagnosis, 78% sought medical attention within 2 months of the onset of symptoms.

Myth 2. Elderly Patients Have More Indolent Disease

The presumption that elderly patients have less aggressive biologic forms of breast cancer has been based on reports of a higher frequency of low-grade tumors (10,11); of more indolent histologic subtypes such as medullary, colloid, and tubular carcinomas (12); and of estrogen receptor–positive lesions in elderly patients (13). It has also been postulated that the gradual involution of immunity that occurs with aging may offer an immunologic advantage in reducing the likelihood of immunofacilitating mechanisms of tumor enhancement (suppressor T cells) (14).

Other studies challenged this concept of indolent disease in the elderly (3,15). Although 80% of breast cancers in women over age 75 have been reported to be estrogen receptor positive (13), the prognostic significance of this is uncertain. In patients with axillary nodal metastases or locally advanced disease, estrogen receptor status has been observed to have no prognostic significance (15,16). Furthermore, data suggest that estrogen receptor positivity in node-negative breast cancer may reflect growth rate rather than metastatic potential, and therefore serves as a predictor only of the pattern of

recurrence (predominantly bone) and a longer disease-free interval (15,16). In addition, the growth rate of a breast cancer (tumor doubling time) may not remain constant over time.

In the M. D. Anderson Cancer Center series (2), of 104 women with known estrogen receptor status, 82 (79%) were estrogen receptor positive (≥10 fmol). Invasive ductal carcinoma was the predominant histologic type (84%). Pure noninvasive disease was detected in 5 patients and other histologic types in 24 (colloid or mucinous, 13; invasive lobular, 5; Paget's disease, 3; papillary, 2; and tubular, 1). Recurrent breast cancer occurred in 47 patients (26%); 10 experienced locoregional relapse (on the chest wall or within the intact breast) only, 24 had distant metastases only, and 13 had both. The median interval between diagnosis and distant relapse was 33 months. The most common presentations or sites of distant metastases were simultaneous multiple sites in 40%, bone in 27%, and visceral organs in 24%. After distant recurrence, the median survival time was 11 months.

Stoll (17) defined "shower of metastases" as the involvement in rapid succession of at least two or three major sites of recurrence or metastasis (local, osseous, or visceral), followed by death within 18 months of the appearance of the first metastasis. In his series of 1141 breast cancer patients, recurrence developed in 755 patients. A "shower of metastases" occurred in 55% (50/91) of all women with recurrences before the age of 40 but in only 26% (23/90) of women older than 70. However, the proportion of patients whose first recurrence occurred at least 3 years after treatment was similar in all age groups.

Myth 3. Elderly Patients Have a Limited Life Expectancy from Comorbid Conditions Other Than Breast Cancer

Satariano et al (18) reported that the comorbid conditions present in elderly women with breast cancer are similar to those found in women in the general population. Arthritis, cardiovascular disease, and hypertension were the predominant health problems for women with or without breast cancer in their study. Similarly, Koch et al (19) found the likelihood of patients with breast cancer dying of other causes similar to that of the sex-matched and age-matched population.

The assumption that elderly patients have concurrent health problems that override the life-threatening risks from breast cancer has frequently resulted in less aggressive treatment of breast cancer. Greenfield et al (20) discovered that only 58.9% of women over age 50 with moderate to severe comorbid conditions received appropriate therapy for breast cancers, whereas 81.3% of women with no or only minor comorbidity received appropriate therapy. After adjustment for stage of disease and comorbidity, age remained a significant predictor of treatment. Only 83% of patients aged 70 or older with stage I or II disease and minimal comorbidity were treated appropriately, whereas 95.6% of similar patients aged 50 to 69 received appropriate treatment (20).

At the time of breast cancer diagnosis in the M. D. Anderson Cancer Center series (2), the most frequent comorbid conditions under active treatment were hypertension (48%), cardiovascular disease (23%), and arthritis (26%). Although 27% of elderly patients had no other major health problems requiring treatment and 91% were totally mobile, two or more comorbid conditions were present in 29%. Over a 16-year follow-up period (median, 106 months for living patients), there were 101 deaths. Forty percent of these deaths were from breast cancer and 60% from other causes (Fig. 13-1). The breast cancer–specific survival rate was 79% at 7 years. The most common known cause of non-cancer-related death was cardiovascular disease.

As life expectancy increases in the elderly population, physicians must recognize that physiologic and chronologic age often do not coincide. Treatment should be guided by an acceptable benefit-risk ratio that allows for quality and quantity of life.

Myth 4. Elderly Patients Cannot Tolerate Standard Treatment

Based on the assumption that older individuals cannot tolerate surgery, surgeons may be reluctant to perform standard surgical procedures on the elderly. In a study of 4050 operations, Turnbull et al (21) found the operative mortality rate in patients over age 70 (4.8%) to be similar to that in patients of all ages (3.4%). For breast cancer surgery in elderly patients, most series reported an operative mortality rate of 1% or less, and the primary morbidity appears to be related to short-term wound complications that respond to conservative management (6,22–24). In the M. D. Anderson Cancer Center series (2), total mastectomy with axillary node dissection (including three radical mastectomies) was performed in 82% of elderly patients. Only 18 patients had breast preservation surgery. Seven patients had total mastectomy without node dissection for debulking, and nine patients received no surgical intervention because of advanced disease and poor performance status. Only three postoperative deaths occurred (at 5 days, 7 days, and 23 days). Each of these deaths was related to myocardial infarction. Only 24% of the remaining patients who had surgery

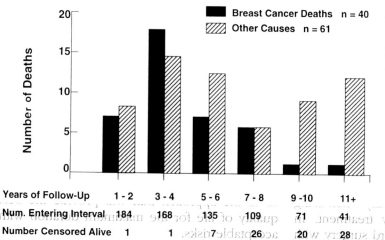

FIGURE 13-1

Cause of 101 deaths by years of follow-up in 184 women age 70 years or older with locoregional breast cancer.

experienced complications. The most common postsurgical problems were related to the wound: infection in 14 patients, hematoma in 5, and minor flap necrosis in 8.

As randomized clinical trials have not shown a survival difference between standard mastectomy and breast preservation surgery plus radiotherapy, the option to preserve the breast should also be discussed with the elderly patient (25,26). Radiation can decrease the likelihood of local recurrence following breast preservation and is well tolerated by the elderly (27). In the M. D. Anderson Cancer Center study, radiation therapy was given to 30% of patients: 10 preoperatively and 44 postoperatively. Complications from the radiation were recorded in fewer than 5%.

As indicated, elderly patients with breast cancer treated by standard therapy can attain a survival rate equal to that of younger patients with breast cancer. The physician must remember, however, to treat the patient and not just the disease. In elderly patients with significant comorbid conditions and limited life expectancy, the magnitude of the surgical procedure must be adjusted. The randomized National Surgical Adjuvant Breast and Bowel Project trial B-04 showed that axillary node dissection in patients with clinically negative axillae does not affect survival (28). Only 20% of patients in the non-axillary-dissection group required a subsequent therapeutic node dissection for clinical evidence of axillary disease. Thus, in elderly patients with operable tumors who are at high risk for complications of general anesthesia, a partial or total mastectomy under local anesthesia without axillary dissection is appropriate.

Recently, the antiestrogen tamoxifen was proposed as an alternative to surgery. Overall response rates to tamoxifen have ranged from 49% to 68%; complete responses were noted in 27% to 40% of patients (29–31). Clinical trials that compared tamoxifen to surgery did not show a survival difference (32–34). However, the median follow-up time for these studies was short (≤3 years). Horobin et al (31) demonstrated that at a minimum follow-up time of 5 years, 70 (62%) of 113 patients aged 70 or older with locoregional breast cancer did not achieve disease control with tamoxifen alone. The incidence of local relapses continued to increase over time; thus, caution is necessary when using tamoxifen as the sole primary treatment. In patients able to undergo standard surgery with acceptable risks, tamoxifen may be more appropriate in the adjuvant setting (35) or as a preoperative induction therapy for those with locally advanced disease.

The role of chemotherapy in elderly breast cancer patients has yet to be fully explored. Most chemotherapy protocols have had age limits of 65 or 70 years, the requirement of normal renal function, or an arbitrary dose reduction in patients older than 60 (36,37). Nineteen studies conducted by the Eastern Cooperative Oncology Group (ECOG) of cancer chemotherapy for eight tumor types (breast cancer excluded) demonstrated that toxicity and response rates were identical in younger patients and in those 70 years or older (38). A subsequent ECOG study of 92 patients aged 65 to 90 who had advanced breast carcinoma and were treated with combination cyclophosphamide, methotrexate, and 5-fluorouracil with dose adjustments based on creatinine clearance revealed no significant age trends in toxicity, response, or cycle-by-cycle reduction of chemotherapy dose (39). In the M. D. Anderson Cancer Center series of elderly patients (2), combination chemotherapy was used as an adjuvant in only eight patients (4%). Eleven additional patients (6%) received preoperative chemotherapy for initially unresectable disease. Seven of the 11 patients were disease free at the time of writing. No major toxicities from the chemotherapy occurred in any of the 19 patients. Thus, for elderly patients with estrogen receptor–negative or hormone-resistant breast carcinomas, the use of chemotherapy should be based on physiologic parameters (renal, liver, and marrow function) and performance status rather than on chronologic age (40–42).

Conclusions

Elderly women have the same right as their younger counterparts to take part in decisions about their health care. Women with breast cancer, regardless of age, should be informed of treatment options and the advantages and disadvantages of each choice as it applies to their individual circumstance. In patients with poor performance status and known limited life expectancy, clinical judgment should be used as to the approach that will provide the best quality of life for the maximum duration with acceptable risks.

REFERENCES

1. Ries LAB, Hankey BF, Edwards BK, eds. *Cancer statistics review, 1973-1987*. NIH publication no. 90-2789. Washington, DC: National Cancer Institute, 1990.

2. Singletary SE, Shallenberger R, Guinee VF. Breast cancer in the elderly. *Ann Surg* 1993; 218:667–671.

3. Mueller CB, Ames F, Anderson GD. Breast cancer in 3558 women: age as significant determinant in the rate of dying and causes of death. *Surgery* 1978;83:123–131.

4. Davis SJ, Karrer FW, Moor BJ, et al. Characteristics of breast cancer in women over 80 years of age. *Am J Surg* 1985;150:655–658.

5. Herbsman H, Feldman J, Seldera J, et al. Survival following breast cancer surgery in the elderly. *Cancer* 1981;47:2358–2363.

6. Hunt KE, Fry DE, Bland KI. Breast carcinoma in the elderly patient. *Am J Surg* 1980;140: 339–342.

7. Chu J, Diehr P, Feigl P, et al. The effect of age on the care of women with breast cancer in community hospitals. *J Gerontol* 1987;42:185–190.

8. Makuc DM, Fried VM, Kleinman JC. National trends in the use of preventive health care by women. *Am J Public Health* 1989;79:21–26.

9. American Joint Committee on Cancer. *Manual for staging of cancer*. 3rd ed. Philadelphia: JB Lippincott, 1988:145–150.

10. Berg JW, Robbins GF. Modified mastectomy for older poor risk patients. *Surg Gynecol Obstet* 1961;11:631–634.

11. Taylor SG, Gelman RS, Falkson G, Cummings FJ. Combination chemotherapy compared to tamoxifen as initial therapy for stage IV breast cancer in elderly women. *Ann Intern Med* 1986; 104:455–461.

12. Rosen PP, Lesser ML, Kinne DW. Breast carcinoma at the extremes of age: a comparison of patients younger than 35 years and older than 75 years. *J Surg Oncol* 1985;28:90–96.

13. Von Rosen A, Gardelin A, Auer G. Assessment of malignancy potential in mammary carcinomas in elderly patients. *Am J Clin Oncol* 1987; 10:61–64.

14. Ershler WB. Why tumors grow more slowly in old people. *J Natl Cancer Inst* 1986;77:837–839.

15. Adami H-O, Graffman S, Lindgren A, Sallstrom J. Prognostic implications of estrogen receptor content in breast cancer. *Breast Cancer Res Treat* 1985;5:293–300.

16. Qazi R, Chuang J-LC, Drobyski W. Estrogen receptors and the pattern of relapse in breast cancer. *Arch Intern Med* 1984;144:2365–2367.

17. Stoll BA. Does the malignancy of breast cancer vary with age? *Clin Oncol* 1976;2:73–80.

18. Satariano WA, Ragheb NE, Dupuis MH. Comorbidity in older women with breast cancer: an epidemiologic approach. In: Yancik R, Yates JW, eds. *Cancer in the elderly: approaches to early detection and treatment*. New York: Springer, 1989:71–103.

19. Koch M, Hanson J, Gaedke H, Wilson D. Competing causes of death in breast cancer patients. In: Paterson AHG, Lees AW, eds. *Proceedings of the second international symposium on fundamental problems in breast cancer*. Alberta, Canada: 1986:265–272. Norwell, MA: Kluwer, 1986.

20. Greenfield S, Blanco DM, Elashoff RM, Ganz PA. Patterns of care related to age of breast cancer patients. *JAMA* 1987;20:2766–2770.

21. Turnbull AD, Gundy E, Howland WS, Beattie EJ Jr. Surgical mortality among the elderly. An analysis of 4050 operations (1970–1974). *Clin Bull* 1978;8:139–142.

22. Amsterdam E, Birkenfeld S, Gilad A, Krispin M. Surgery for carcinomas of the breast in women over 70 years of age. *J Surg Oncol* 1987;35: 180–183.

23. Kesseler HJ, Seton JZ. The treatment of operable breast cancer in the elderly female. *Am J Surg* 1978;135:664–666.

24. Svastics E, Sulyok Z, Besnyak I. Treatment of breast cancer in women older than 70 years. *J Surg Oncol* 1989;41:19–21.

25. Fisher B, Redmond C, Poisson R, et al. Eight-year results of a randomized clinical trial comparing total mastectomy and lumpectomy with or without irradiation in the treatment of breast cancer. *N Engl J Med* 1989;320:822–828.

26. Veronesi U, Salvadore B, Luini A, et al. Conservative treatment of early breast cancer. Long-term results of 1232 cases treated with quadrantectomy, axillary dissection and radiotherapy. *Ann Surg* 1990;211:250–259.

27. Kantorowitz DA, Poulter CA, Sischy B. Conservative surgery and radiotherapy in elderly women. *Int J Radiat Oncol Biol Phys* 1988;15: 263–270.

28. Fisher B, Redmond C, Fisher ER, et al. Ten-year results of a randomized clinical trial comparing radical mastectomy and total mastectomy with or without radiation in the treatment of breast cancer. *N Engl J Med* 1985;312:665–673.

29. Akhtar SS, Allan SG, Rodger A, et al. A 10-year experience of tamoxifen as primary treatment of breast cancer in 100 elderly and frail patients. *Eur J Surg Oncol* 1991;17:30–35.

30. Bradbeer JW, Kyngdon J. Primary treatment of breast cancer in elderly women with tamoxifen. *Clin Oncol* 1983;9:31–34.

31. Horobin JM, Preece PE, Dewar JA, et al. Long-term follow-up of elderly patients with locoregional breast cancer treated with tamoxifen only. *Br J Surg* 1991;78:213–217.

32. Bates T, Riley DL, Houghton J, et al. Breast cancer in elderly women: a Cancer Research Campaign trial comparing treatment with tamoxifen and optimal surgery with tamoxifen alone. *Br J Surg* 1991;78:591–594.

33. Gazet J-C, Ford HT, Coombes RC, et al. Prospective randomized trial of tamoxifen versus surgery in elderly patients with breast cancer. *Eur J Surg Oncol* 1994;20:207–214.

34. Robertson JFR, Todd JH, Ellis IO, et al. Comparison of mastectomy with tamoxifen for treating elderly patients with operable breast cancer. *BMJ* 1988;297:511–514.

35. Castiglione M, Gelber RD, Goldhirsch A (International Breast Cancer Study Group). Adjuvant systemic therapy for breast cancer in the elderly: competing causes of mortality. *J Clin Oncol* 1990;8:519–526.

36. Bonadonna G, Valagussa P. Dose response effect of adjuvant chemotherapy in breast cancer. *N Engl J Med* 1981;304:10–15.

37. *Compilation of experimental cancer therapy protocol summaries*. NIH publication no. 81-1116. Washington, DC: National Cancer Institute, 1981:1–51.

38. Begg CB, Carbone PP. Clinical trials and drug toxicity in the elderly. *Cancer* 1983;2:1986–1992.

39. Gelman RS, Taylor SG IV. Cyclophosphamide, methotrexate, and 5-fluorouracil chemotherapy in women more than 65 years old with advanced breast cancer. The elimination of age trends in toxicity by using doses based on creatinine clearance. *J Clin Oncol* 1984;2:1404–1413.

40. Christman K, Muss HB, Case DL, Stanley V. Chemotherapy of metastatic breast cancer in the elderly. The Piedmont Oncology Association experience. *JAMA* 1992;268:57–62.

41. Martin LM, Le Pechoux C, Calitchi E, et al. Management of breast cancer in the elderly. *Eur J Cancer* 1994;30A:590–596.

42. Muss HB. The role of chemotherapy and adjuvant therapy in the management of breast cancer in older women. *Cancer* 1994;74:2165–2171.

CHAPTER 14

Pregnancy, Hormone Replacement Therapy, and Reproductive Factors

FRANKIE ANN HOLMES

The pregnant patient newly diagnosed with breast cancer never fails to emotionally affect even the most seasoned oncologist. Although pregnant breast cancer patients require highly specialized, integrated multidisciplinary care, all physicians—generalists as well as specialists—should be aware of the current options for therapy. It is the generalist physicians to whom these women first turn, and the generalists often influence which subspecialists the women see.

Incidence of Breast Cancer During Pregnancy: Good News and Bad News

The good news is that breast cancer during pregnancy is rare. Table 14-1 shows results from some of the reported series in which incidence figures were calculated (1–15). The most widely quoted series is White's review of the world literature (4), showing an incidence of 2.8% of all breast cancers and about 1 of every 3333 deliveries. Others looked at the incidence of breast cancer during pregnancy by focusing on only fertile patients younger than 40 years who are at risk for both pregnancy and breast cancer. In that subset, the incidence of breast cancer

during pregnancy or lactation is higher, ranging from 1.5% to 26% (5,8–12). This wide range is the result of differences in the cutoff age chosen by various authors. In these historical series, the younger the cutoff age, the more likely a woman with breast cancer was to be pregnant. If breast cancer occurred at a young age, the likelihood of a concurrent pregnancy was high. *Lactation* is defined as the period from delivery to 6 to 12 months after delivery regardless of whether the patient actually breast-feeds. As Donegan (16) observed, in view of the known long natural history of breast cancer, 1 year to several years for a tumor to reach 1 cm in diameter, the distinction between breast cancers diagnosed during pregnancy and those diagnosed during lactation is somewhat arbitrary. One can assume that in all lactating women in these series, the tumor was present during pregnancy.

The bad news is that breast cancer during pregnancy is certain to become more common. The incidence of breast cancer increased 32% from 1980 to 1987. Recently, this trend has stabilized or even reversed (17). In 1994 there were approximately 182,000 new cases of breast cancer and 46,000 deaths from breast cancer, the same as in 1993 (18). However, increasing numbers of women defer or delay childbearing (19). Both of these reproductive behaviors increase the risk of breast cancer (20,21). In addition, the incidence of breast cancer increases with age. While breast cancer is distinctly uncommon in women in their 20s

---

Portions of this chapter are reprinted from Holmes FA. Breast cancer during pregnancy. *Cancer Bull* 1994;46: 400–411. Copyright 1994, The University of Texas M. D. Anderson Cancer Center, Houston, Texas. Used with permission.

and 30s, a substantial majority of patients are affected in their 40s (22,23). Many career women will be in their 40s during their first pregnancy. Cognizant of these data, even perinatal nursing journals are addressing the issue of breast cancer during pregnancy (24).

Diagnosis and Staging

Two cardinal rules must be followed in the evaluation of a breast problem in a pregnant patient: First, ignore the pregnancy and evaluate the problem; second, keep the fetus out of the evaluations. During pregnancy, the physiologic changes in the breast are almost as striking as those in the uterus. The nipple enlarges, and the glandular tissue of the breast increases and begins to differentiate. The breast feels engorged and is tender on pal-

pation. Against this background, examination of the breast is difficult. However, the most common presentation of breast cancer during pregnancy is a painless lump discovered by the patient.

Differential Diagnosis

The differential diagnosis of a breast mass in a pregnant woman is similar to that in a nonpregnant patient. In one illuminating series, Byrd et al (6) reviewed 134 pregnant or lactating women who had undergone surgery for a mass in the breast. Pregnant women accounted for 86 patients (64%) in the series. Of the 134 tumors, 105 (78%) were benign. Of the benign tumors, 37% were nonmalignant neoplasms, such as adenofibroma, lipoma, papilloma, or cystosarcoma phyllodes; 34% were cystic disease; 22% were other breast

T A B L E **14-1**

Incidence of Breast Cancer During Pregnancy and Lactation from Selected Series

Study[a]	Years Accrued	No. of Patients	Average Age, Yr (Range)[b]	Percentage of All Breast Cancers	Percentage of All Breast Cancers Occurring During Pregnancy or Lactation in Potentially Fertile Women	Incidence per Number of Deliveries
Harrington (1937)	1910–33	92	37	2.0	NA	NA
Lewison (1954)	1932–51	46	NA	NA	NA	1/1360
White (1955)[a]	1850–1953	1413	38[c]	2.8	NA	1/3333
Treves (1958)[a]	1937–49	108	≤35	NA	19.6	NA
Byrd (1962)	1925–60	29	34	2.5	NA	NA
Rissanen (1968)[a]	1940–61	33	34.6 (25–42)	0.9	NA	NA
Crosby (1971)[a]	1932–65	29 135 <35 yr	38 (26–54)	1.1	NA 1.5	NA NA
Applewhite (1973)[a]	1948–67	2689 (655 <45 yr)	34	2.0	8.3 (in women ≤45 yr)	NA
Riberio (1977)	1941–69	88	? (21–47)	0.3	2.8 (in women ≤45 yr)	NA
Noyes (1982)[a]	1945–77	32	≤30	0.9	26 (in women ≤30 yr)	NA
Nugent (1985)	1970–80	19	32 (26–37)	1.4	11 (in women <40 yr)	NA
King (1985)	1950–80	60	35 (22–44)	NA	NA	NA

Modified from Wallach et al (14) and van der Vange et al (15).

NA = not available.

[a] Denotes that both pregnant and lactating patients were included.

[b] Age range not available for all series.

[c] Age known in 55% of series of 1375 patients [White 1955 (4)].

changes of pregnancy, such as lobular hyperplasia or galactocele; and 7% were inflammation or abscess. Not noted in Byrd's series, but reported by others, is the phenomenon of infarction of a fibroadenoma or hyperplastic breast tissue stimulated to grow rapidly during pregnancy (25). Only 22% of the tumors in Byrd et al's series were malignant. This percentage was identical to the percentage of malignant tumors among all the breast masses removed during the 5-year period preceding publication of Byrd et al's results (1956–1961). Thus, a breast lump in a pregnant woman is not more likely to be malignant than is a breast lump in a nonpregnant woman.

Complete Physical Examination and Biopsy

Standard evaluation of a breast mass in a pregnant woman begins with a complete examination of the breast and the lymph node basins of the breast. Complete breast examination is a standard part of all gynecologic and obstetric evaluations. If a painless mass alone is discovered, it should be evaluated by fine-needle aspiration or ultrasonography to determine whether it is cystic or solid (26,27). If the mass is cystic, it should be aspirated and the aspirate should be sent for cytologic evaluation. While the occurrence of intracystic carcinomas (28) is infrequent, so is breast cancer during pregnancy. If no fluid is obtained or a mass persists after aspiration, an incisional or excisional biopsy should be performed, and the tissue should be sent for histopathologic evaluation and estrogen (ER) and progesterone receptor (PR) assays. Biopsy is necessary because although fine-needle aspiration is a reliable method of diagnosing malignancy, it cannot differentiate invasive from noninvasive masses (29).

Hormone Receptor Determination

Only limited studies of hormone receptor data are available in the literature (11,27,30–32). The majority of young patients have hormone receptor–negative tumors (33). When determination of ER status is performed by the ligand-binding method, there is a concern that false-negative results may occur in premenopausal women because of competitive inhibition by the high circulating levels of endogenous estrogens (34). However, determination of ER by

enzyme immunoassay (EIA) (35) or immunocytochemical assay (ICA) (36) avoids this problem by using a monoclonal antibody that recognizes both the occupied and the unoccupied form of the receptor. A second theoretical concern is that the high levels of circulating estrogens will downregulate ERs and PRs. Other evaluations for research purposes include flow cytometry with determination of DNA index and S-phase fraction and evaluation for HER-2/*neu* oncogene (37). However, these latter data do not contribute information necessary for decisions about treatment.

Diagnostic Imaging and Laboratory Studies

The use of mammography for evaluation of breast masses in pregnant women is somewhat controversial. Liberman et al (38) noted that the exposure to the human embryo from a standard bilateral mammography study with craniocaudal and mediolateral oblique views of both breasts using low-dose screen-film technique and shielding of the pelvis is less than 50 mrad (500 μGy). In contrast the dose estimated to cause intrauterine death in preimplantation mouse embryos is 10 rad (100 mGy) or higher, that is, 200-fold higher. Thus, the radiation risk to the fetus is minimal (39). However, the increased density of the breast makes accurate interpretation difficult (40). Even when the mammogram shows no signs of cancer, the physician should obtain an accurate histopathologic diagnosis. Thus, obtaining a mammogram may only delay appropriate management. Mammography, may, however, be useful to document occult disease in the contralateral breast.

Metastatic Workup

If invasive malignancy is confirmed, the patient needs evaluation for systemic disease as a prelude to initiation of local therapy. Evaluation for systemic disease includes a thorough physical examination with attention to the contralateral breast and all draining nodal basins. Standard laboratory evaluations include a hemogram, liver function studies, and cancer markers such as carcinoembryonic antigen (CEA) and CA 15-3. Radiographic and scintigraphic imaging should be done only if justified by clinical and laboratory findings. A chest radiograph may be safely performed, since the maximum dose to the uterus will be less than

50 mrad (reported doses range from 0.2–43.0 mrad) (39). If blood test results are abnormal, an ultrasound of the liver or radiographs of specific symptomatic bones may be obtained. Radiographs of the lumbosacral spine will expose the uterus to 51 to 126 mrad (41). Although a bone scan may be performed in a pregnant patient by using special precautions such as hydration and insertion of a Foley catheter (42), bone scans rarely provide evidence of metastases in an asymptomatic patient with normal laboratory findings.

Dental Evaluation

The patient's dentition should always be evaluated. Pregnancy causes hypertrophy of the gums, and the ensuing periodontal disease that occurs in some patients—not the loss of calcium—is the basis for the "old wives' tale" about loss of one tooth for each live birth. In a patient who may need chemotherapy, good dental health is important to prevent oral complications of chemotherapy.

Effect of Concomitant Pregnancy and Breast Cancer on Outcome—The Basis for Selection of Therapy

Effect on the Patient

In 1880, Samuel Gross's vivid description of breast cancer during pregnancy entrenched the notion that pregnancy has a negative effect on the course of breast cancer (43): "When, however, carcinoma appears during pregnancy or during lactation, its growth is wonderfully rapid and its course is excessively malignant. . . ." Beatson's treatise on castration as an effective therapy undoubtedly galvanized this notion (44). However, critical review of the available data in the literature does not support the concept of a uniformly dismal outcome.

Tables 14-2 and 14-3 show the 5- and 10-year survival rates from reported series by nodal status (Table 14-2) and stage (Table 14-3) (1,3,6–10,12,13,45–50). Note that most series include both pregnant and lactating patients. Only total survival, not disease-free survival, rates are reported. Three conclusions are obvious from Table 14-2. First, patients with nodal involvement had dismal outcomes. Second, for patients without nodal involvement,

5- and 10-year survival rates were reasonable in most series. Third, the majority of patients in most series, 60% to 85%, had nodal involvement. A number of authors commented on the unusually high percentage of pregnant patients with involved lymph nodes compared to their nonpregnant patients. Delay in diagnosis may explain this.

Delay in Diagnosis

Table 14-4 (6,8,10,15,51) shows results from selected series in which the timeliness of diagnosis and treatment of patients with breast cancer was reviewed. Delays of 6 months to 1 year were common and were the result of both patient and physician judgments. Zemlickis et al (52), in a 1992 case-control study from the Princess Margaret Hospital in Canada, compared the stage at presentation of breast cancers in a group of 118 pregnant patients to a control group of 3949 women younger than 48 years diagnosed during the same time period. The pregnant patients were less likely to have stage I or II disease and more likely to have stage IV disease (52). In Canada, unlike the United States, access to medical care is universal, so delays were probably not due to problems accessing medical care. The authors concluded that pregnant patients are at a higher risk of presenting with advanced disease because pregnancy impedes early detection.

Overall Outcome Is Similar

Peters (51), Nugent and O'Connell (12), Petrek (49), and Zemlickis et al (52) compared outcomes in pregnant patients with those in control patients matched by age and stage and found no differences. Nugent and O'Connell (12) and others (8,11,23,51) suggested that the worse outcome of pregnant patients is related to the young age of the patients and not to pregnancy. Earlier series unfairly compared young pregnant women with series that included predominantly postmenopausal women, the majority of whom have more indolent disease.

Three series found worse outcomes for pregnant patients than for nonpregnant patients even when patients were matched by age and stage (15,50,53). Guinee et al (50) reviewed records of 407 patients who were 20 to 29 years old at the time of diagnosis of breast cancer and who were treated at one of nine cancer centers in the United States or Europe collaborating in

T A B L E **14-2**

Five and 10-Year Survival Rates for Pregnant or Lactating[a] Breast
Cancer Patients in Selected Series by Nodal Status

Study	Years Accrued	No. of Patients	Survival Rate			Comments
			Overall	Node Neg	Node Pos	
Harrington (1937)	1910–33	92 P + L	5yr: NA 10yr: NA	62% 40%	6% 3%	N0 = 14 (15%) N+ = 78 (85%)
Haagensen (1967)	1915–50	48 P + L	5yr: 31% 10yr: 0%	83% NA	NA NA	N0 = 6: 31 patients had radical mastectomy
White (1955)	≤1948	27 P + L	5yr: NA 10yr: NA	73% 26%	6% 0%	N0 = 11 (41%); N+ = 16 (59%); personal series
Byrd (1962)	1925–60	24 P + 5 L	5yr: 55% 10yr: NA	100% 80%	28% 6%	N0 = 11 (38%) N+ = 18 (62%); 3 had metastases
Holleb and Farrow (1962)	1920–53	45 P 72 L	5yr: NA 5yr: NA	58% 68%	21% 13%	N0: P = 26%, L = 28% vs 54% N0 in subsequent pregnancy
Miller (1962)	1921–55	45	5yr: NA 10yr: NA	47% 20%	16% 3%	N0 = 15 (33%) N+ = 30 (67%)

Crosby (1971)	1932–65	29 P + L	5yr: 46%
			10yr: 36%
				NA
				NA
					NA
					NA
						5-yr survival: P = 33%, L = 50%;
						  5 patients (17%) had
						  metastases; 0 aborted

Applewhite (1973)	1948–67	48 P + L	5yr: 25% 10yr: 15%	56% 22%	18% 13%	N0 = 9 (19%) N+ = 39 (81%)
Clark (1978)	1931–75	121 P 80 L	10yr: 22% 10yr: 32%	35% 69%	22% 18%	Total series: N0 = 25%, N+ = 39%, N? = 36%
Nugent (1985)	1970–80	19 P	5yr —	100%	50%	N0 = 4 (21%); N+ = 14 (74%); stage IV = 1 (5%) w/ 0% 5yr S
King (1985)	1950–80	63 P	5yr: 53% 10yr: 49%	82% 71%	33% 33%	N0 = 24 (38%); N+ = 39 (62%); includes stage IV
Petrek (1991)	1960–80	12 P + 44 L	5yr: 61% 10yr: 45%	82% 77%	47% 25%	N0 = 22 (39%); N+ = 34 (61%); 30% had adj chemo
Guinee (1994)	1978–88	26 P	5yr: 40%	NA	NA	N0 = 9 (35%); N = 11 (42%); N? = 6 (23%) 50% had adj chemo; 11 had abortions

P = pregnant; L = lactating; NA = not available; N0 = node negative; N+ = node positive; N? = unknown nodal
  status; adj chemo = adjuvant chemotherapy; S = survival.

[a]Lactation refers to the period from delivery until 6–12 months after delivery regardless of whether the patient actually
  breast-fed.

the International Cancer Patient Data Exchange Systems between January 1, 1978, and December 31, 1988 (Table 14-5) (50). Only 26 patients were pregnant at the time of diagnosis. Complete data were available for only 291 patients, 20 of whom were pregnant at the time of diagnosis of breast cancer. These data show that the risk of dying from breast cancer was inversely related to the length of time between diagnosis of breast cancer and date of the most recent previous pregnancy, with the highest risk in patients who were pregnant at diagnosis. For each additional year up to 4 years between the most recent previous pregnancy and the diagnosis of breast cancer, the risk of dying of breast cancer decreased by 15%. Patients diagnosed with breast cancer 4 or more years after the most recent pregnancy had a risk of dying of breast cancer not statistically different from that for patients who had never been pregnant. While the authors did not speculate on possible causes for these findings, subsequent letters (54,55) and a report (56) suggested that some aspect of the immunosuppressive effects of pregnancy may be contributory.

On balance, most of the available data support the conclusion that, when matched by age and stage with nonpregnant breast cancer patients, pregnant patients with breast cancer do not have worse outcomes.

TABLE **14-3**

Five and 10-year Survival Rates for Pregnant or Lactating[a] Breast Cancer Patients in Selected Series by TNM Staging[b]

Study	Years Accrued	No. of Patients	Survival Rate				Comments
			Stage I	Stage II	Stage III	Stage IV	
Rissanen (1968)	1940–61	33	5yr: 80%	8/10[c]	2/13[c]	0%	Only 2 patients were lactating
			10yr: 80%	7/9[c]	2/9[c]	0%	
Riberio (1977)	1941–69	88	5yr: 90%	37%	15%	0%	% Survival matched by age and stage *Pregnant* v *Not*
			10yr: 90%	21%	10%	0%	5yr: 38 45
							10yr: 24 29

[a]Lactation refers to the period from delivery until 6–12 months after delivery regardless of whether or not the patient actually breast-fed.

[b]In this staging system, stage I means tumor confined to breast; II, breast and lymph nodes; III, any T4 regardless of nodes; IV, distant metastases.

[c]Data presented as number of living patients at specified time interval versus those at risk.

TABLE **14-4**

Delays in Diagnosis of Breast Cancer in Selected Series

Study	Delays in Pregnant Patients (Months)			Delays in Nonpregnant Patients			Difference in Total Delay Between Pregnant and Nonpregnant Patients
	Total	Patient	Doctor	Total	Patient	Doctor	
Westberg (1946)	9	6	3	6	4	2	3
Applewhite (1973)	11	>6 (in 36%)	2.2	4	18% > 6	0.6m	7
Byrd (1962)	6 (average)						range: 2 days to 24 months
Bunker, Peters (1962)[a]	>6 (in 50%)						
Peters (1968)	15 (stage IV)			9 (stage IV)			
Riberio (1977)	10						

[a]Data from van der Vange and van Donegan.

Other Myths About Pregnancy and Breast Cancer

Some authors suggested an increased incidence of inflammatory cancer in pregnancy. However, a review of available data by Zinns (57) and other more recent reports (27,31) showed no differences in reported histologic types between pregnant and nonpregnant patients. Peters (51) initiated the concept of worse prognosis in the second trimester of pregnancy. No other studies, however, replicated this finding (52).

Effect on the Fetus

Metastases to the placenta or fetus are uncommon. A 1989 review found only 45 documented cases of placental metastases and 7 cases of fetal metastases. None of these seven were in patients with breast cancer (58). In 1994, Salamon et al (59) described microscopic metastases to the placenta that were not detectable on gross examination, in a patient with brain and liver metastases from an invasive ductal carcinoma diagnosed approximately 12.5 months earlier. This pattern of normal findings on gross

T A B L E   **14-5**

Tumor Size, Nodal Status, Chemotherapy, 5-Year Overall Survival, and Risk of Breast Cancer in 291 Patients by Time from Most Recent Pregnancy to Diagnosis of Breast Cancer[a]

Risk factor	Time from Most Recent Pregnancy to Diagnosis of Breast Cancer				
	Never Pregnant (n = 139)	Pregnant at Diagnosis (n = 26)	0–12 Months (n = 40)	13–48 Months (n = 51)	≥49 Months (n = 35)
Tumor size, cm					
≤2	36%	8%	17%	34%	37%
>2–5	27%	35%	35%	29%	31%
>5	7%	19%	10%	8%	31%
Unknown	30%	38%	38%	29%	29%
No. of Positive Lymph Nodes					
0	47%	35%	28%	35%	37%
1–3	26%	19%	22%	26%	29%
≥4	20%	23%	35%	27%	17%
Unknown	7%	23%	15%	12%	17%
Received Chemotherapy, %	50%	50%	65%	53%	49%
5-yr Overall Survival	74%	40%	n	65%	n
RR of Breast Cancer Death (95% CI)					
Unadjusted	1.0	3.26 (1.81–5.87)	1.89 (1.09–3.29)	1.59 (0.96–2.63)	0.66 (0.31–1.39)
Adjusted[b]	1.0	2.83 (1.24–6.45)	1.88 (0.88–3.98)	1.09 (0.54–2.19)	0.54 (0.19–1.54)

RR = relative risk; CI = confidence interval.

[a] Modified from Guinee et al.[50] (50)

[b] Adjusted for tumor size and number of involved axillary lymph nodes.

examination but extensive microscopic disease is reminiscent of the behavior of the lobular subtype of carcinoma in the breast, although this patient apparently did not have this subtype. Detailed sectioning revealed that adenocarcinoma was present only within the intervillous (maternal) space, not in the chorionic villi (fetal space). Salamon et al (59) recommended careful evaluation of the placenta for evidence of invasion of the chorionic villi. They postulated a higher risk of neonatal metastatic disease if invasion of the chorionic villi is observed.

Zemlickis et al (52) at the Princess Margaret Hospital assessed fetal outcomes by evaluation of detailed delivery records available for 62 of 85 deliveries (83 live births, 2 stillbirths) from patients diagnosed with breast cancer between 1958 and 1987 (out of a total of 118 pregnant patients with breast cancer). Sixty of the 62 deliveries were live births. Of these 60, there was a statistically lower mean birth weight compared to matched control birth weights. The mean gestational age was also lower

because of preterm deliveries (22 cesarean sections, 18 of which were to expedite cancer treatment), compared to matched control ages. The ratio of stillbirths to live births (2/85, 2.4%) was numerically greater than the general figure in Ontario (11.1 stillbirths/1000 total births, 1.1%). However, the small sample size precludes any meaningful conclusions. Earlier, Clark and Reid (48) observed a higher incidence of spontaneous abortions in patients with breast cancer diagnosed during pregnancy than in patients with breast cancer diagnosed during lactation or later (14% versus 1% and 7%, respectively).

Therapy Decisions

Local Therapy

In 1943, when Haagensen and Stout developed their criteria for operability of breast cancer, they noted that none of the 20 patients who developed breast cancer during pregnancy or lactation were cured and declared this subset of patients categorically inoperable (45). However, after several subsequent pregnant or lactating patients who had mastectomy performed by Haagensen and Stout's colleagues during pregnancy or lactation were observed to have longer survival times, Haagensen reversed his decision (45).

For pregnant patients with localized breast cancer (stages I–III) the usual criteria for conservative therapy versus modified radical mastectomy pertain (60). Both standard modified radical mastectomy and lumpectomy with axillary dissection are acceptable methods of local control. However, if the patient chooses lumpectomy, definitive local irradiation should be deferred until after delivery. The doses of internally scattered radiation have been calculated in experimental situations (15). Throughout the initial 12 weeks of pregnancy, when the fetus is still within the true pelvis, a tumor dose of 5000 cGy will expose the fetus to 10 to 15 cGy. Later in gestation, when the fetus is high in the abdomen, some fetal areas may receive as much as 200 cGy. Although some authors question whether there is any safe dose of radiation to the fetus, Brent (61) extensively reviewed this area and defined 5 cGy as a relatively safe upper limit of fetal exposure. There is no reason to risk exposure to the embryo or fetus in a non-life-threatening situation.

Anesthetic Considerations

In experienced hands, general anesthesia can be safely administered to the pregnant patient (62–64). When surgery is performed in the second and third trimesters, careful attention must be paid to proper positioning of the patient so as to avoid uterine compression of the vena cava. Other effects of pregnancy include increased blood volume and coagulability, decreased lung capacity, and slow gastric emptying (64). In Byrd et al's classic surgical series (6) of 86 pregnant patients, all patients had general anesthesia for breast biopsy, and a radical mastectomy was performed if the diagnosis was carcinoma. There were no maternal deaths, and only one fetal death occurred. They reported this as a 0.75% mortality. (However, in the denominator they erroneously included 48 women who were lactating. The actual rate should have been reported as 1.2% or 1 of 86 pregnant women, which is not

significantly different.) Even that one death, however, seems somewhat peripherally related to the procedure since it occurred 3 weeks after the biopsy when the patient, who was perimenopausal and who had a negative pregnancy test twice before excision of a cystic lesion, had a spontaneous abortion.

"Therapeutic" Abortion?

As noted earlier, Gross's (43) description of breast cancer during pregnancy led to a general principle that the hormonal changes of pregnancy must contribute to the cancer's rapid growth. The apparently worse outcome of this subset of patients with breast cancer supported a consensus for therapeutic abortion. However, although controlled clinical trials are not possible in this situation, most published series did not consistently show improved survival rates for patients who had spontaneous or therapeutic abortion (see Addendum) (7,13,46,48,65). Adair's study (65), which showed an apparent benefit for therapeutic abortion, considered both patients who were pregnant at the time of diagnosis and patients who subsequently became pregnant after treatment of breast cancer. These are entirely different patient groups, as discussed later. In some series, patients who continued the pregnancy fared better than did those who terminated the pregnancy. Although Clark and Reid (48) and King et al (13) specifically stated that selection of abortion was not biased for patients with more advanced disease, this bias is a valid concern in the interpretation of retrospective study results. However, two other issues are relevant to the question of therapeutic abortion: the age of the patient, discussed already, and the hormone receptor status of the tumor.

Hormone Receptor Determination

Since the late 1970s tumors have been analyzed for hormone receptors as a guide to prognosis and therapy. As noted earlier, women younger than 50 years tend to have hormone receptor–negative tumors (33). Initially this finding was thought to reflect limitations of the ligand-binding technique in which endogenous estrogen blocked the ability of the radiolabeled ligand to bind to and "detect" the receptor. However, as discussed previously, the more modern EIAs and ICAs use monoclonal antibodies that detect the receptor whether or not it is bound by endogenous estrogen. Earlier studies by the ligand-binding technique (12), as well as more recent studies using the ICA (30), confirmed the excess of estrogen receptor–negative tumors in women younger than 50 years. Thus, there is no justification for termination of pregnancy or castration as an adjunct to therapy.

When Is Abortion Indicated?

Abortion may be indicated in patients with rapidly progressive disease, such as inflammatory breast cancer or metastatic breast cancer. In the case of inflammatory cancer, the chance for long-term survival depends on immediate initiation of combination chemotherapy. As discussed later, the use of combination chemotherapy in the second and third trimesters is associated with a low to absent probability of fetal malformations or death (66,67). In the first trimester, however, the risks are higher. In the case of metastatic disease, the goal of therapy is effective palliation. While 3% to 5% of patients with metastatic disease continue unmaintained remissions for 10 or more years, the median survival time in large series is 2 to 3 years (68). The patient and the child's father must consider the probability that the mother will not live to parent her child.

In summary, except in unique circumstances, Byrd et al's advice (6) continues to be timely: "better terminate the disease than terminate the pregnancy."

Chemotherapy

In an era when health professionals advise most pregnant patients to limit caffeine consumption and abstain from alcohol and nicotine, it is paradoxical for other health professionals to talk about the use of antineoplastic agents during pregnancy. In the early years of our chemotherapy program for pregnant patients with breast cancer, some nurses refused to administer antineoplastic agents to pregnant patients. However, despite solid theoretical reasons for avoiding these agents during pregnancy, the incidence of serious complications from administration of chemotherapy during pregnancy is quite low.

Effects of Chemotherapy on the Fetus

Doll et al (66) extensively reviewed the literature of fetal injury related to intrauterine expo-

sure and found that, except for aminopterin, the use of chemotherapy agents was not associated with the frequency of adverse outcomes that would be predicted. One special problem with aminopterin and other analogues of methotrexate is sequestration in third spaces such as ascites, pleural effusions, and amniotic fluid. However, there are only limited data about the extent to which chemotherapy drugs cross the placenta and enter the fetal circulation (69,70). It is known, however, that the expression of P-glycoproteins is high in uterine and placental tissue. These proteins function as drug efflux pumps for xenobiotic substances and may exclude many drugs from the fetus (71,72). The experience at M. D. Anderson Cancer Center with administration of chemotherapy to pregnant patients shows that fetal hair growth is normal even though the mother has alopecia (73). The risk of major teratogenesis is highest during the first trimester, when organogenesis occurs. The most critical portion of this trimester, when the embryo is exquisitely sensitive to multiple system malformation, is from the week 2 to week 4 (days 14–28) from conception, only 5% of the total duration of pregnancy (61). Major malformations in this period are often spontaneously aborted, as noted by Doll et al (66), because of the narrow range between lethal fetal toxicity and no discernible effect. In the second and third trimesters, there is little risk of serious teratogenicity; however, there is a risk of impaired fetal growth and functional development, spontaneous abortion, premature labor, and major organ toxicity. Note that in the normal population of pregnant patients without cancer, the background incidence of spontaneous abortion is 30% to 50%, and the incidence of major and minor congenital malformations is 3% and 9%, respectively (61).

Clinical Studies

For the adjuvant or palliative treatment of patients with breast cancer, the Breast Medical Oncology Department of The University of Texas M. D. Anderson Cancer Center uses the standard combination of fluorouracil, doxorubicin, and cyclophosphamide (FAC) (67). Although antimetabolites such as fluorouracil are generally believed to be associated with a higher risk for fetal complications than are alkylators, we have not observed complications. We never administer methotrexate to pregnant patients. Other centers also utilize doxorubicin-based combinations (74,75). Preliminary results of our small series have been presented in abstract form (67). From 1989 to 1992, we treated 11 patients who had concomitant breast cancer and pregnancy. The median age was 34 years (range, 24–37). The distribution of patients by stage was as follows: stage II, 4 patients; stage III, 5; and stage IV, 2. Three patients had preoperative chemotherapy followed by mastectomy; six patients had postmastectomy chemotherapy. The remaining two patients had metastatic disease at the time of presentation so mastectomy was not indicated. The maximum number of chemotherapy courses given was 7; the median was 4 (range, 1–7). Ten normal infants were delivered. The eleventh infant was spontaneously delivered during a period of maternal neutropenia and fever and experienced respiratory distress. However, his peripheral blood counts were normal (i.e., appropriately elevated), and he recovered uneventfully. At the time of this writing two children were older than 4 years; all children had reached normal developmental milestones.

Aviles et al (76) at the University of Mexico evaluated long-term outcomes of 43 children of mothers with hematologic malignancies who were treated with chemotherapy during pregnancy. At the time of the report, the median age of the children was 9 years (range, 3–19). Nineteen mothers (44%) received chemotherapy during the first trimester, and most received antimetabolites and alkylators. Comprehensive evaluations of the children included physical examination, hemogram, cytogenetic studies, bone marrow aspiration and biopsy, determination of immunoglobulin levels and stimulated lymphocyte responses to various mitogens, Wechsler intelligence testing, and the Bender-Gestalt test. There were no instances of physical or intellectual dysfunction or cytogenetic abnormalities.

In 1985, Mulvihill at the University of Pittsburgh Genetics Institute established a national registry for patients exposed to chemotherapy in utero (77). The database also includes a summary of all cases published in all languages since 1950. Although data on the initial patients are scanty, more complete data have been obtained on recent patients. These data show that many pregnant women exposed to chemotherapy, particularly if within the second and third trimesters, generally had normal children. This registry provides an important opportunity to document outcomes in these patients. I strongly recommend that all physicians who administer chemotherapy to pregnant patients register their patients.

Management of Chemotherapy Complications in the Pregnant Patient

The usual acute and subacute complications of chemotherapy include nausea, vomiting, stomatitis, neutropenia with fever, and alopecia.

Emesis can be effectively prevented by a number of agents. We used diphenhydramine, promethazine (Phenergan), and lorazepam in our series. However, ondansetron (Zofran) was used to control hyperemesis gravidarum without adverse consequences in two patients in weeks 11 and 30 to 33 of pregnancy (78,79). Ondansetron is classified as pregnancy category B, which means that no teratogenicity has been seen in animal studies and isolated human cases but that controlled studies in humans have not been done. Prevention of nausea and vomiting is important because dehydration, especially in the last trimester, is permissive for preterm labor.

Accurate dosing of the patient becomes difficult as the patient's body weight increases during pregnancy. We generally use body weight at the time of diagnosis to calculate the initial chemotherapy dose and adjust dose on the basis of nadir granulocyte counts on day 14. We aim for a nadir granulocyte count between 500 and 1000 cells/μL and the absence of fever, infection, serious stomatitis, or other gastrointestinal symptoms such as diarrhea or abdominal cramping. Unless patients have metastatic disease with involvement of the bone marrow, thrombocytopenia is not a serious concern. Anemia may be important if the patient had anemia before pregnancy. However, a physiologic anemia occurs during the first trimester as a result of the increased plasma volume and should not alarm the oncologist.

In all patients, prompt management of fever during neutropenia is important. For pregnant patients whose chemotherapy will continue after delivery, the timing of the last cycle before delivery is important. We generally administer the last chemotherapy treatment before delivery, no later than 6 weeks before the estimated due date (at 32–33 weeks). In the one patient in our series who was neutropenic, the neonate experienced respiratory distress that resolved completely; his white blood cell count was appropriately elevated (67).

For patients whose chemotherapy continues postpartum, special arrangements are needed to help the patient deal with the newborn's around-the-clock needs. Although many patients tolerate chemotherapy quite well, some patients receiving chemotherapy experience chronic fatigue, which will be exacerbated in the pregnant patient if sleep is limited and irregular.

Lactation

If chemotherapy is initiated in the second trimester, patients are not usually able to breast-feed. For patients who must continue to receive chemotherapy after delivery, lactation is contraindicated. Antineoplastic agents are excreted in the milk. There is one case report of cytopenia in a breast-fed neonate whose mother was receiving cyclophosphamide (80,81).

Fertility

The ovary appears to be more resistant to chemotherapy than the testes do (82,83). However, in both sexes, the incidence of chemotherapy-induced sterility increases with age and cumulative dose of alkylating agents (83,84). Shalet (85) observed the following correlation between the age of the patient and the total dose of cyclophosphamide received before the onset of amenorrhea: older than 40 years, 5.2 g; 30 to 39 years, 9.3 g; and 20 to 29 years, 20.4 g. Doxorubicin probably contributes to the risk of infertility, but the antimetabolite fluorouracil does not. Richards et al (86) reported that 37% and 97%, respectively, of patients

younger than and older than 40 years became amenorrheic after adjuvant cyclophosphamide, methotrexate, and fluorouracil. Hortobagyi et al (87) reported the age-related incidence of amenorrhea during chemotherapy as well as the probability of resumption of menses after completion of chemotherapy in a subset of premenopausal patients treated with adjuvant FAC at M. D. Anderson Cancer Center (Table 14-6). Over half of all patients younger than 40 who became amenorrheic resumed menses after completion of chemotherapy. In a 1990 review of 227 consecutive patients who were 35 years or younger and were treated with the same doxorubicin-based combination for a median of 12 months, the status of menstrual function was known in 56%. Of these, 59% had no amenorrhea, 32% had temporary amenorrhea, and 11% had permanent amenorrhea (31). In pregnant patients with breast cancer, in whom the median age is approximately 32 to 34 years, a majority of patients will retain fertility after chemotherapy treatment with standard doses of FAC. However, all patients must be cautioned about the possibility of permanent amenorrhea and premature menopause.

Two pharmacologic strategies to prevent chemotherapy-induced sterility have been evaluated: oral contraceptives and the gonadotropin agonists. The working hypothesis was that the ovary would be suppressed in a manner similar to suppression of the adrenal gland during administration of exogenous corticosteroids. Neither of these approaches was completely protective (88).

The science of infertility medicine has advanced considerably, and a number of options may be available in the future for the patient who becomes infertile because of

T A B L E **14-6**

Incidence of Amenorrhea by Age in Patients Treated with FAC Adjuvant Chemotherapy at M. D. Anderson Cancer Center

Age, Years	Percentage Patients Who Became Amenorrheic During Chemotherapy	Percentage of Patients Who Resumed Menses After Chemotherapy
<30	0	—
30–39	33	50
40–49	96	"few"
≥50	100	

Data from Hortobagyi GN, Buzdar AU, Marcus CE, et al. Immediate and long-term toxicity of adjuvant chemotherapy regimens containing doxorubicin in trials at M. D. Anderson Hospital and Tumor Institute. *Monogr Natl Cancer Inst* 1986;1:105–109.

F = fluorouracil; A = doxorubicin; C = cyclophosphamide.

chemotherapy but who wants to become pregnant. First, efforts are ongoing to develop techniques to harvest and cryopreserve the patient's own oocytes, analogous to sperm banking (88). Second, if the patient's own ova are no longer available, ova may be donated by family or others. The patient is given hormonal stimulation to prepare the uterus, and the donor ova are fertilized in vitro with the husband's (or other donor) sperm. The viable 8- to 12-cell preembryos are transferred to the patient's uterus. Successful pregnancy with this technique was achieved in a patient rendered menopausal from her adjuvant chemotherapy (89). In 1994, investigators in London discussed the use of fetal ova as a donor source (90).

Pregnancy After Breast Cancer

Effect of Pregnancy on Risk of Recurrence

The recommendations about pregnancy after breast cancer emanate from the same "forces of intuitive conviction" (91) who advocate therapeutic abortion as an adjuvant to treatment of breast cancer. The obvious concern is that the significant rise in sex hormones, particularly estrogen, during pregnancy will stimulate recurrent cancer.

Most of the historical series of patients with breast cancer antedate the use of cytotoxic chemotherapy, and most institutes do not routinely employ castration as a therapeutic maneuver. Thus, there is substantial information on the outcome of patients who become pregnant after a diagnosis of breast cancer. Danforth (92) reviewed this issue in detail in 1991, with critical commentary by Epstein and Henderson (91) and Wood (93). Approximately 25% of women who develop breast cancer are of reproductive age. Nearly one third (7% of all women who develop breast cancer) of these women of reproductive age will have one or more pregnancies subsequently, and 70% of these pregnancies will occur within 5 years of treatment. The available data do not show that subsequent pregnancy hastens or induces recurrence. Epstein and Henderson (91) noted that the numbers of patients are too small to rule out an effect, but the studies do suggest that if there is any effect, it is very small. In two series, patients who had subsequent pregnancies had higher survival rates than those who did not. The most important prognostic factors were the nodal status and the stage.

How Reliable Are Available Data?

Conversely, Petrek (94) argued that the available data are based on only a small subset of patients who become pregnant after a diagnosis of breast cancer. First, she noted that as pregnancy is not a disease, it is not coded in hospital or tumor registries. Patients may not always report a subsequent pregnancy to the physician who treated the breast cancer. Thus, it may be difficult to determine the total number of patients at risk. Second, Petrek reviewed the data from her own institution, Memorial Sloan-Kettering Cancer Center, over a 30-year period. She found only 41 patients with stage I and II cancer who became pregnant after a diagnosis of breast cancer. Assuming the above estimate of a 7% pregnancy rate for women younger than 40 years, and accounting for the age distribution of patients seen during that era, Petrek estimated that at least 450 women would have had a subsequent pregnancy. She concluded that while existing data do not suggest that subsequent pregnancy increases the risk of recurrence, these data are based on a nonrandom, and perhaps positively biased sampling of 10% or fewer of the total patients at risk who did have a good outcome.

The Finnish Studies: Population Registry Data—Complete, Accurate

However, subsequent to these two reviews, Sankila et al (95) from Finland reported the results of a population-based matched survival study designed to assess the risk of death from breast cancer in breast cancer patients relative to whether they did or did not have a subsequent pregnancy producing a live birth. Because medicine is socialized, reports of all diagnoses of cancer and all death certificates in which cancer is mentioned are required to be sent to the centralized Finnish Cancer Registry. Additionally, since 1967, all citizens have been given a unique personal identification number. This study used the Finnish Cancer Registry to identify 2536 women who were diagnosed with breast cancer between 1967 and 1990 and were younger than 40 years at the time of diagnosis. Linking the patients' unique personal identification numbers to the Central Population Register, Sankila et al determined the dates of births of the patients' biologic children. Information on abortions and stillbirths was not available. Of these 2536 women, 95 (3.7%) had a child before the end of

1990. These 95 patients were matched for stage, age, and year of diagnosis with one to six control subjects chosen from the remaining patients. Appropriate control subjects could not be found for four patients. The results showed that control patients had a 4.8-fold higher risk of death compared with patients who had a subsequent pregnancy. The authors acknowledged one possible confounding issue. Patients were matched with data from the time of diagnosis. However, to assess the actual effect of the pregnancy on survival, it would have been more accurate to match patients at the time of delivery, which ranged from 10 to 154 months after diagnosis. This was not possible with their database. The authors hypothesized that patients who felt and did well had children, whereas those who were affected by recurrence did not. They termed this the "healthy mother effect." Note that the rate of pregnancy in this group of women was accurately determined and was approximately 4%. There are at least two possible explanations for this relatively low rate. Patients with breast cancer may not decide to have children at the same rate as those who have not had breast cancer. In addition, in earlier eras physicians usually cautioned against subsequent pregnancy.

M. D. Anderson Cancer Center's Experience

Sutton et al (31) reviewed the M. D. Anderson experience with patients who were 35 or younger at the time of diagnosis and became pregnant after adjuvant chemotherapy with FAC. Of 227 consecutive breast cancer patients, 25 patients had 33 pregnancies. The median interval between the completion of chemotherapy and pregnancy was 12 months (range, 0–87). Ten pregnancies were terminated, 2 spontaneously aborted, and 19 resulted in normal, full-term infants; 2 patients were still pregnant at the time of the report. The incidence of recurrence was 46% and 28%, respectively, in patients who did not become pregnant and those who had subsequent pregnancies. Similarly, 38% of patients without subsequent pregnancies, but only 12% of subsequently pregnant patients had died at the time of publication.

Conclusion: Should I? When?

The two questions all patients ask are "Should I become pregnant?" and "When?" (92). Given the lack of any demonstrable effect of pregnancy on the risk of recurrence, the "Should I?" question compels the patient and physician to address openly the probability of recurrence and to consider how recurrence would affect any future children. Patients with a low risk of recurrence (those with stage I or II disease with fewer than three involved axillary lymph nodes) can be advised that because of their favorable prognosis, it is probable that if they do conceive, they will live to mother their children. Patients with high-risk breast cancer (stage II with four or more involved axillary lymph nodes, stage III, and stage IV) have a less favorable prognosis and should be advised that the probability of living to parent their children is low.

As regards "When?," Danforth endorsed the standard 2- to 3-year waiting period after diagnosis before conceiving. Epstein and Henderson (91) disagreed and suggested that for patients with low-risk breast cancers, waiting only wastes time. In the current therapeutic era, many patients receive adjuvant chemotherapy for early-stage breast cancer. Certainly this will impose a minimum 6-month interval between the end of treatment and conception.

Lactation After Previous Breast Surgery and Irradiation

Harris's group (96) noted that the usual administered radiation dose of 4600 cGy injures the glandular and ductal tissue, causing atrophy of the lobules and perilobar and periductal fibrosis which inhibit the normal physiology of lactation. They noted reports of successful lactation in 24% of a sample of 52 patients who became pregnant after conservative surgery and breast irradiation. However, in their own experience at the Joint Center for Radiation Therapy in 23 patients with 30 live births after surgery and irradiation for breast cancer, few women reported being able to lactate. Dow et al (96) advised patients not to attempt breastfeeding because they fear that the disruptions of the ductal system will cause mastitis.

Two other investigators, however, observed lactation in a few patients who had lumpectomy and irradiation (97,98). Location of the incision was important. Not surprisingly, circumareolar incisions are associated with absence of lactation, because they interrupt multiple ducts. Radial incisions may disrupt fewer ducts but may be cosmetically inferior.

Pregnancy After Transverse Rectus Abdominis Myocutaneous Flap Breast Reconstruction

Many women opt for breast reconstruction after mastectomy. The use of autogenous tissue for reconstruction has become a particularly attractive alternative because of recent reports of adverse consequences of silicone-filled breast implants. The transverse rectus abdominis myocutaneous (TRAM) flap, which uses skin and muscle from the abdominal area to reconstruct a breast, is one approach to breast reconstruction. Since patients who undergo a TRAM flap reconstruction lose an important component of abdominal support, concerns are raised when these patients become pregnant. In 1993, surgeons at M. D. Anderson reported a pregnancy that occurred after TRAM flap reconstruction, and reviewed the literature about this situation (99). Nine cases of pregnancy after TRAM flap breast reconstruction have been reported since the technique was first described in 1981. None of the patients had problems with abdominal wall integrity during pregnancy, and all but one patient had full-term spontaneous vaginal deliveries. One patient had a spontaneous abortion at 6 weeks' gestation unrelated to the abdominal-wall integrity. Two patients, including the patient in the case report, had postpartum abdominal bulges that did not require repair. These limited data indicate that normal pregnancy and delivery are possible after TRAM flap breast reconstruction.

Hormone Replacement Therapy

Hormone Replacement Therapy After Breast Cancer

An even more difficult question than pregnancy after breast cancer in this era is the question of hormone replacement therapy after menopause, whether natural or chemotherapy induced, for patients with a history of breast cancer. Hormone replacement therapy should address the four major areas affected by estrogen deficiency: vasomotor and neurocognitive/neuropsychiatric function, genitourinary tract (dyspareunia and frequent urinary tract infections), bones, and the cardiovascular system (100). A full review of this topic is beyond the scope of this chapter. A comprehensive review

by a proponent of hormone replacement therapy was published in 1993 (101). Since then, a handful of papers have addressed this issue. Eden et al (102) performed a case-control study of combined estrogen-progestin replacement therapy in 90 women who had been treated for breast cancer, most of whom had node-negative disease. The median time from diagnosis to initiation of estrogens was 5 years (range, 0–25 years). The ER status of the primary tumor was known in only 22 patients (24%); 12 tumors were ER positive and 10 were ER negative. In this select group, only 6 patients had a recurrence (7%) compared to 30 (17%) of 180 control subjects who did not use estrogens. The ER status of the primary was known in only 2 of the 6 patients whose disease recurred. One tumor was ER negative; one was ER positive. The median duration of estrogen use was only 1.5 years (range, 0.3–12.0). Despite the small numbers of patients and the limited follow-up time, the authors concluded that short-term use of estrogens posed little risk of breast cancer recurrence.

Is Previous Hormone Replacement Therapy a Risk Factor for Development of Breast Cancer?

Two trials comparing the use of hormone replacement therapy in women with and without breast cancer were published in 1995. The trials reached opposite conclusions.

Population Case-Control Study: No

Stanford et al (103) performed a population-based case-control study comparing 537 patients with breast cancer diagnosed between January 1 and June 30, 1988, with a random control group of 492 women without a history of breast cancer. These authors found no association between breast cancer risk and the use of either estrogen alone or estrogen with progestin. In addition, long-term use from 8 to 20 years was not associated with an increased risk of breast cancer. In an accompanying editorial, Adami and Persson (104) noted two limitations of this study. First, patients with in situ carcinoma were included. In situ disease was not used as an end point in most other studies because it does not inevitably progress to invasive disease. Second, the power of the study was only sufficient to reveal a substantially increased risk of 2.5-fold or higher after long-term therapy, so although there was certainly no major excess risk, a small but biologically illuminating and clinically important excess risk could not be ruled out. Adami and Persson noted that a Swedish study, to be completed by 1996, of over 3000 women who were given combined estrogen and progestin replacement therapy should provide additional information. These authors also referenced a report suggesting that breast cancer occurring in patients receiving estrogen replacement therapy has a more favorable prognosis than do tumors that arise in the absence of hormone replacement therapy. The reader is cautioned that this concept that tumors arising during hormone replacement therapy are less aggressive was also erroneously believed to be true of the initial endometrial cancers induced by tamoxifen.

Cohort Study: Yes, Increased Risk

In contrast to the findings of Stanford et al (103), Colditz et al (105) reported a 30% to 46% increase in the risk of breast cancer in women receiving hormone replacement therapy in a cohort of nurses registered in the Nurses' Health Study followed from 1976 through 1992. The report was based on 725,550 person-years of follow-up of menopausal women. Risk increased by age and number of years of hormone use after 5 years of use. Moreover, this study excluded cancer in situ, and as noted in the accompanying editorial by Davidson (106), the death rate from breast cancer paralleled the incidence of it. This suggested that these cancers were clinically important, that is, not less aggressive. Little increase in risk was noted for women of any age who used estrogen or estrogen and progestin for less than 5 years. Both the Stanford and the Colditz studies observed that the addition of progestin did not neutralize the increased risk of breast cancer. Colditz et al (105) noted that the lack of an increased risk of breast cancer in younger women might relate only to the short time since menopause and the correspondingly shorter periods of use.

Breast Cancer During Estrogen Replacement Therapy: Therapeutic Withdrawal

For patients diagnosed with stage I, II, or III breast cancer who decide to use hormone replacement therapy and subsequently develop metastatic disease, estrogen withdrawal may provide clinically meaningful palliation. Dhodapkar et al (107) evaluated and Pritchard and Sawaka (108) reviewed the use of withdrawal as a therapeutic manipulation in three patients with a history of primary breast cancer who developed metastatic disease while using estrogens and a fourth patient who was using estrogens who presented with diffuse bone metastases and a breast mass. Withdrawal of estrogens caused disease regression lasting 2 to 3 years in all four patients.

Use of Megestrol Acetate for Tamoxifen-Induced Hot Flashes

Loprinzi et al (109) evaluated the use of a 6-week course of megestrol acetate to ameliorate climacteric symptoms in a double-blind, randomized, placebo-controlled study of 97 women with a history of breast cancer who had "bothersome" hot flashes. Eighty-one percent of the patients were receiving tamoxifen. They found an 83% reduction in hot flash scores with megestrol acetate compared with a 27% reduction with placebo. However, this study was not designed to look at long-term consequences such as disease recurrence and effect on lipid profile. Progestins can "blunt, block, or even overwhelm estrogenic effects, particularly on lipoproteins" (110). Conversely, Powles et al (111) gave conjugated estrogens (Premarin, 0.625 mg daily) to 35 women experiencing menopausal symptoms caused by adjuvant tamoxifen for stage I, II, or III primary breast cancer. In five women, the dose needed to control hot flashes was 1.25 mg daily. Nearly 70% (24/35) of the women had total or partial relief of symptoms. At a mean follow-up time of 43 months, one patient each had a relapse with local and distant metastases at 68 and 27 months, respectively. Powles et al (111) concluded that concomitant use of tamoxifen and estrogens did not compromise the effectiveness of either treatment.

Need for Further Data

All of the previously mentioned investigators and many practicing oncologists echo Epstein and Henderson's thoughts that "the jury is not in" (91) on the relationship between hormone replacement therapy and breast cancer risk. A large-scale randomized (inter)national trial should be designed to answer this question. At the National Cancer Institute of the United States, an open meeting was held in November 1993 to address this issue. In a succinct review of this meeting, Cobleigh et al (112) made a clarion call for a national trial. As of late 1995, no national protocol has emerged. Since 1993, investigators at the M. D. Anderson Cancer Center have been conducting a randomized, placebo-controlled trial using conjugated estrogens (Premarin) 0.625 mg daily for 5 years with escalation of the dose to 1.25 mg daily based on serum follicle-stimulating hormone (FSH) levels. Patients must be confirmed to be postmenopausal by serum FSH levels and must have had either stage I or II breast cancer. Patients for whom the hormonal status of the original tumor was ER negative or unknown are eligible at 2 and 10 years after diagnosis, respectively. Unfortunately, patients whose original tumor was ER positive are not eligible. This study has two objectives: first, to evaluate the effect of estrogen replacement therapy on maintenance of bone mineral density, and second, to evaluate the effect of estrogen replacement therapy on recurrence rates. Lipid profiles and fibrinogen levels will also be followed serially. Because this issue is emotionally charged for both physicians and patients, accrual has been very slow. The issue of hormone replacement therapy after breast cancer challenges the international oncology community to address the other side of the coin, the consequences of adjuvant therapies in women whose lives have been spared or prolonged.

Reproductive Factors and the Risk of Breast Cancer

Pregnancy Before Age 30

The landmark study of the International Union Against Cancer (UICC) in 1962 (113) showed an increased incidence of breast cancer in nulliparous patients and in patients who became pregnant after age 30. Layde et al (20) confirmed the importance of age at first full-term pregnancy but showed that the increased risk of breast cancer was confined only to premenopausal breast cancer. After age 50, women who had had a full-term pregnancy at any age had a lower risk of breast cancer than nulliparous women had. Vatten and Kvinnsland (114) showed that parity of four or more pro-

vided a lifelong protective effect against breast cancer [relative risk (RR) adjusted for age and age at first birth, 0.73; 95% confidence interval (CI), 0.54–0.98] independent of the protection afforded by early first term birth. However, they showed that the effects of parity varied by age. Nulliparous women had a lower risk (RR, 1.65; 95% CI, 1.18–2.31) of breast cancer than did women whose first pregnancy occurred after age 34 (RR, 1.77; 95% CI, 1.04–3.00) even after adjustment for parity. Nulliparous women also had a lower risk of breast cancer than did women of low parity (one to three births) before age 45. However, sometime between ages 45 and 49, these risks reversed, and women of any parity had a lower risk of breast cancer than did nulliparous women, an occurrence Vatten and Kvinnsland (114) termed a "crossover effect." Kalache et al (115) suggested that the age of the most recent pregnancy is more important than the age at the first pregnancy. However, Vatten and Kvinnsland's data (114) did not support this. While reproductive decisions will not be made on the basis of these data, health-care providers should be aware of this information in light of recent trends in breast cancer incidence and age at the time of first pregnancy.

Does Pregnancy Cause a Transient Increase in the Risk of Developing Breast Cancer?

Guinee et al's study discussed earlier (50) suggested that recent pregnancy adversely affects the survival of women diagnosed with breast cancer. Bruzzi et al (116) and Williams et al (117) observed that a full-term pregnancy causes a short-term increase in the risk of developing breast cancer. However, Williams et al (117) acknowledged that both their and Bruzzi's results could have been influenced by selection bias in the control groups. Vatten and Kvinnsland (114), in a prospective cohort study of 29,981 Norwegian women, found no evidence of a transient increase in the risk of developing breast cancer subsequent to pregnancy.

Proposed Protective Alternative to Early Pregnancy

Based on data showing that combination oral contraceptives have reduced the risk of endometrial and ovarian cancer, Pike's group (118) developed a contraceptive program to reduce breast cell proliferation, and thus limit the opportunities for the occurrence and accumulation of potentially neoplastic genetic damage, by reducing the sex steroid levels that stimulate breast cell proliferation. The gonadotropin-releasing hormone agonist leuprolide acetate in depot form is given monthly to suppress ovarian hormone production. To prevent menopausal symptoms, a low dose of conjugated estrogens (Premarin, 0.625 mg) is used orally for 6 of every 7 days. Every fourth 28-day cycle, medroxyprogesterone acetate, 10 mg, is given orally for 13 days to protect the uterus from the potentially neoplastic effects of unopposed estrogen. The estimated benefit from 10 years of this is a greater than 50% reduction in the lifetime risk of breast cancer.

In a pilot study to test the tolerability and other metabolic effects of this regimen, 21 patients with a fivefold or greater risk of breast cancer were randomized to either the control arm, 7 patients, or the treatment arm, 14 patients (118). Only two side effects required medication changes: Vaginal dryness was relieved by increasing the conjugated estrogen dose to 0.9 mg, and loss of bone mineral density was stopped by addition of low doses of androgen. Although the study is too small and premature, a marked reduction in mammographic parenchymal density was observed after 12 months in the patients in the treatment arm. This was interpreted as an intermediate end point, that is, obvious evidence of reduced breast cell proliferation. From the clinician's perspective, this decrease in mammographic parenchymal density would also translate into more effective detection of any new mass by physical and radiographic examination of the breast.

Lactation

Early study findings suggested that lactation is protective against breast cancer (119). However, later studies showed that it is the pregnancy, not the lactation, that had the protective effect. A 1994 analysis (120) showed that lactation provides a small measure of protection against breast cancer. The benefits of breast-feeding to the newborn and mother are well described. This is one more reason to recommend it.

Oral Contraceptive Use

A related issue is whether oral contraceptive use is a risk factor for subsequent breast cancer. In a review of 44 epidemiologic studies conducted from 1974 through 1991, La Vecchia (121) showed there was no consistent association for "ever use" of oral contraceptives and breast cancer risk. However, in 19 of the 20 trials that focused on long-term use in "young" (defined heterogeneously as 20–34 years, 30–44 years, "premenopause," or younger than 35, 40, or 45 years) women, he noted an increased relative risk of breast cancer. Two meta-analyses evaluating duration-related effects of oral contraceptive use before first full-term pregnancy reached the same conclusions (122,123). However, in their compendious analysis, Prentice and Thomas (122) reviewed all aspects of collateral effects of oral contraceptives in nine trials addressing oral contraceptive use before first full-term pregnancy and found inconsistent results precluding any definitive conclusions in this area. The most dramatic and well-characterized studies are from Sweden, where Olsson et al (124,125) found a significant relationship between early use of oral contraceptives and increased risk of breast cancer in women aged 30 to 40 years. These women tended to have larger tumors with more frequent lymph node involvement and higher indices of cell proliferation (124). Of interest, in women who had used oral contraceptives at an early age who had a history of breast cancer in first-degree relatives, indices of cell proliferation (S-phase fraction and ploidy) were not higher than those in similar women without a family history. Olsson et al (125) independently showed that HER-2/*neu* oncogene is amplified more frequently in women who used oral contraceptives at an early age.

However, there are a number of confounding factors. The most obvious is that early use of oral contraceptives delays the age of first childbirth and decreases parity, two known risk factors for breast cancer (126). Herbst and Berek (126) further showed that in women aged 20 to 44 years, the apparent increase in risk of breast cancer with extended use of oral contraceptives before the first pregnancy is directly related to parity. Only the nulliparous women have an increased relative risk of breast cancer. Second, the formulations of the agents used before 1980 contained higher doses of steroid hormones than do preparations currently used. Thus, results from an earlier era may not be applicable. This is an area that merits continued evaluation.

Abortions: No Convincing Data

In 1981, Pike et al (127) reported that women younger than 33 years who had a first-trimester abortion before the first full-term pregnancy had a 2.4-fold greater risk of breast cancer compared with women who had not had spontaneous or induced abortions. Since that time, a number of studies supporting and refuting Pike et al's finding have appeared (124,128–132). These studies also addressed other aspects of this issue such as spontaneous versus induced abortions and abortions in women with a family history of breast cancer. The case-control study from Rosenberg et al (132) at Boston University compared 3200 women with breast cancer with 4844 control subjects and found that the risk of breast cancer was not related to the number of spontaneous or induced abortions. In 1993, Louise Brinton (128) at the National Cancer Institute's Division of Cancer Etiology concluded that the available data on the relationship between abortion and breast cancer were not convincing. Her own study of breast cancer risk factors including abortion was nearing completion in 1993 but no results have been published as of December 1995.

Lehrer et al (133) noted an interesting twist to this issue, however. They identified a polymorphism in the ER gene that, in association with a history of spontaneous abortion, is correlated with an increased incidence of ER-positive breast cancer in middle-aged and older women. The incidence of ER-negative breast cancers is not affected. The single point mutation in the B allele of the ER gene does not result in an amino acid change in the ER protein, so the investigators interpreted this to mean that another mutation that segregates with the mutated allele is responsible for the spontaneous abortions in these patients.

Conclusions

Review of the available data suggests that the outcome of breast cancer occurring during pregnancy is not worse than the outcome in the nonpregnant patient. The options for treatment of breast cancer during pregnancy are somewhat limited. Radiotherapy should not be given during pregnancy; however, chemotherapy may be administered after the first trimester with reasonable safety to mother and fetus. Surgery may be performed safely at any time. All therapies require close coordination of care between the medical oncologist, surgeon, and maternal-fetal specialist. Abortion has not been shown to improve outcomes. The relationship of previous and subsequent reproductive events and hormonal therapies to outcomes was reviewed. Pregnancy after the diagnosis of breast cancer does not worsen survival. Conflicting data exist regarding the influence of hormone replacement therapy after breast cancer on the risk of recurrence. A national or international trial is sorely needed to address this issue.

Acknowledgments

The author appreciates the secretarial assistance of Judy Dillon and editorial assistance of Stephanie Deming.

REFERENCES

1. Harrington SW. Carcinoma of the breast: results of surgical treatment when the carcinoma occurred in the course of pregnancy or lactation and when pregnancy occurred subsequent to operation (1910–1933). *Ann Surg* 1937;106: 690–700.

2. Lewison EF. Breast cancer and pregnancy or lactation. *Surg Gynecol Obstet* 1954;99:417–424.

3. White TT. Prognosis of breast cancer for pregnant and nursing women. Analysis of 1,413 cases. *Surg Gynecol Obstet* 1955;100:661–666.

4. Treves N, Holleb AI. A report of 549 cases of breast cancer in women 35 years of age or younger. *Surg Gynecol Obstet* 1958;107:271–283.

5. White TT. Carcinoma of the breast in the pregnant and the nursing patient. Review of 1375 cases. *Am J Obstet Gynecol* 1955;69:1277–1286.

6. Byrd BF, Bayer DS, Robertson JC, Stephenson SE. Treatment of breast tumors associated with pregnancy and lactation. *Ann Surg* 1962;155: 940–947.

7. Rissanen PN. Carcinoma of the breast during pregnancy and lactation. *Br J Cancer* 1968;22: 663–668.

8. Crosby CH, Barclay THC. Carcinoma of the breast: surgical management of patients with special conditions. *Cancer* 1971;28:1628–1636.

9. Applewhite RR, Smith LR, DiVincenti F. Carcinoma of the breast associated with pregnancy and lactation. *Ann Surg* 1973;39:101–104.

10. Riberio GG, Palmer MK. Breast carcinoma associated with pregnancy: a clinician's dilemma. *BMJ* 1977;2:1524.

11. Noyes RD, Spanos WJ, Montague ED. Breast cancer in women aged 30 and under. *Cancer* 1982;49:1302–1307.

12. Nugent P, O'Connell TX. Breast cancer and pregnancy. *Arch Surg* 1985;120:1221–1224.

13. King RM, Welch JH, Martin JK Jr, Coulam CB. Carcinoma of the breast associated with pregnancy. *Surg Gynecol Obstet* 1985;160:228–232.

14. Wallach MK, Wolf JA Jr, Bedwinek J, et al. Gestational carcinoma of the female breast. *Curr Probl Cancer* 1983;7:1–58.

15. van der Vange N, van Donegan JA. Breast cancer and pregnancy. *Eur J Surg Oncol* 1991;17:1–8.

16. Donegan WL. Breast cancer and pregnancy. *Obstet Gynecol* 1977;50:244–252.

17. Garfinkel L. Evaluating cancer statistics. *CA Cancer J Clin* 1994;44:5–6.

18. Boring CC, Squires TS, Tong T, Montgomery S. Cancer statistics 1994. *CA Cancer J Clin* 1994;44:7–27.

19. National Center for Health Statistics. *Advance report of final natality statistics, 1989. Monthly vital statistics report*, vol. 50 (suppl). Publication no. (PHS) 92-1120. Washington, DC: Government Printing Office, 1991:1.

20. Layde PM, Webster LA, Baughman AL, et al. The independent associations of parity, age at first full term pregnancy, and duration of breast-feeding with the risk of breast cancer. Cancer and Steroid Hormone Study Group. *J Clin Epidemiol* 1989;42:963–973.

21. White E. Projected changes in breast cancer incidence due to the trend toward delayed childbearing. *Am J Public Health* 1987;77:495–497.

22. Mueller CB, Ames F, Anderson GD. Breast cancer in 3558 women: age as a significant determinant in the rate of dying and causes of death. *Surgery* 1978;83:123–132.

23. Adami H-O, Malker B, Holmberg L, et al. The relation between survival and age at diagnosis in breast cancer. *N Engl J Med* 1986;315:559–563.

24. Preftakes DK. Breast cancer and pregnancy: implications for perinatal care and fetal outcomes. *J Perinat Neonat Nurs* 1994;7:31–41.

25. Jimenez JF, Ryals RO, Cohen C. Spontaneous breast infarction associated with pregnancy presenting as a palpable mass. *J Surg Oncol* 1986;32:174–178.

26. Bottles K, Taylor RN. Diagnosis of breast masses in pregnant and lactating women by aspiration cytology. *Obstet Gynecol* 1985;66(3 suppl):76S–78S.

27. Tobon H, Horowitz LF. Breast cancer during pregnancy. *Breast Dis* 1993;6:127–134.

28. Roth JA, Feinberg M, McAvoy JM. Carcinoma arising in the wall of a breast cyst during pregnancy. *Ann Surg* 1977;185:247–250.

29. Bibbo M, Underhill S. Cytology of fine needle aspiration. In: Harris JR, Hellman S, Henderson IC, Kinne DW, eds. *Breast diseases*. 2nd ed. Philadelphia: JB Lippincott, 1991:297–300.

30. Elledge RM, Ciocca DR, Langone G, McGuire WL. Estrogen receptor, progesterone receptor, and HER-2/neu protein in breast cancers from pregnant patients. *Cancer* 1993;71:2499–2506.

31. Sutton R, Buzdar AU, Hortobagyi GN. Pregnancy and offspring after adjuvant chemotherapy in breast cancer patients. *Cancer* 1990;65:847–850.

32. Wolin M, Giuliano A, Glaspy J. Breast cancer in pregnancy: the UCLA experience. *Proc Am Soc Clin Oncol* 1990;9:45. Abstract 171.

33. Clark GM, Osborne CK, McGuire WL. Correlations between estrogen receptor, progesterone receptor, and patient characteristics in human breast cancer. *J Clin Oncol* 1984;2:1102–1109.

34. Sarrif AM, Durant JR. Evidence that estrogen-receptor-negative, progesterone-receptor-negative breast and ovarian carcinoma contain estrogen receptor. *Cancer* 1981;48:1215–1220.

35. Holmes FA, Fritsche HA, Loewy JW, et al. Measurement of estrogen and progesterone receptors in human breast tumors: enzyme immunoassay versus binding assay. *J Clin Oncol* 1990;8:1025–1035.

36. McClelland RA, Berger U, Millar LS, et al. Immunocytochemical assay for estrogen receptor in patients with breast cancer: relationship to a biochemical assay and to outcome of therapy. *J Clin Oncol* 1986;4:1171–1176.

37. McGuire WL, Tandon AK, Allred DC, et al. How to use prognostic factors in axillary node-negative breast cancer patients. *J Natl Cancer Inst* 1990;82:1006–1015.

38. Liberman L, Giess CS, Dershaw DD, et al. Imaging of pregnancy-associated breast cancer. *Radiology* 1994;191:245–248.

39. Wagner LK, Lester RG, Saldana LR. The amount of radiation absorbed by the conceptus. In: *Exposure of the pregnant patient to diagnostic*

radiations. A guide to medical management. Philadelphia: JB Lippincott, 1985:52.

40. Max MH, Lamer TW. Breast cancer in 120 women under 35 years old. *Am Surg* 1984;50: 23–25.

41. Imaging modalities during pregnancy. In: Cunningham FG, MacDonald PC, Leveno KJ, et al, eds. *Williams obstetrics.* 19th ed. Norwalk, CT: Appleton & Lange, 1993:981–989.

42. Baker J, Ali A, Groch MW, et al. Bone scanning in pregnant patients with breast carcinoma. *Clin Nucl Med* 1987;12:519–524.

43. Gross SW. *A practical treatise on tumors of the mammary gland: embracing their histology, pathology, diagnosis, and treatment.* New York: D Appleton, 1880:146.

44. Beatson GT. On the treatment of inoperable cases of carcinoma of the mamma: suggestions for a new method of treatment with illustrative cases. *Lancet* 1886;2:104–107.

45. Haagensen CD. Cancer of the breast in pregnancy and during lactation. *Am J Obstet Gynecol* 1967;98:141–149.

46. Holleb AI, Farrow JH. The relation of carcinoma of the breast and pregnancy in 283 patients. *Surg Gynecol Obstet* 1962;115:65–71.

47. Miller HK. Cancer of the breast during pregnancy and lactation. *Am J Obstet Gynecol* 1962; 83:602–611.

48. Clark RM, Reid J. Carcinoma of the breast in pregnancy and lactation. *Int J Radiat Oncol Biol Phys* 1978;4:693–698.

49. Petrek JA, Dukoff R, Rogatko A. Prognosis of pregnancy-associated breast cancer. *Cancer* 1991;67:869–872.

50. Guinee VF, Olsson H, Möller T, et al. Effect of pregnancy on prognosis for young women with breast cancer. *Lancet* 1994;343:1587–1589.

51. Peters MV. The effect of pregnancy in breast cancer. In: Forrest APM, Kunkler PB, eds. *Prognostic factors in breast cancer.* Edinburgh: E & S Livingstone, 1968:65–81.

52. Zemlickis D, Lishner M, Degendorger P, et al. Maternal and fetal outcome after breast cancer in pregnancy. *Am J Obstet Gynecol* 1992;166: 781–787.

53. Tretli S, Kvalheim G, Thoresen S, Host H. Survival of breast cancer patients diagnosed during pregnancy or lactation. *Br J Cancer* 1988;58: 382–384.

54. Oliver RTD. Pregnancy and breast cancer. *Lancet* 1994;344:471–472. Letter.

55. Stewart THM. Pregnancy and breast cancer. *Lancet* 1994;344:1235–1236. Letter.

56. Tafuri A, Alterink J, Moller P, et al. T cell awareness of paternal alloantigens during pregnancy. *Science* 1995;270:630–633.

57. Zinns JS. The association of pregnancy and breast cancer. *J Reprod Med* 1979;22:297–301.

58. Dildy G, Moise K, Carpenter R, et al. Maternal malignancy metastatic to the products of conception: a review. *Obstet Gynecol Surv* 1989;44: 535–540.

59. Salamon MA, Sherer DM, Devereux N, et al. Placental metastases in a patient with recurrent breast carcinoma. *Am J Obstet Gynecol* 1994;171: 573–574.

60. Kinne DW. Primary treatment of breast cancer. In: Harris JR, Hellman S, Henderson IC, Kinne DW, eds. *Breast diseases.* 2nd ed. Philadelphia: JB Lippincott, 1991:356–359.

61. Brent RL. The effect of embryonic and fetal exposure to x-ray, microwaves, and ultrasound: counseling the pregnant and nonpregnant patient about these risks. *Semin Oncol* 1989;16: 347–368.

62. Kim Y, Pomper J, Goldberg ME. Anesthetic management of the pregnant patient with carcinoma of the breast. *J Clin Anesth* 1993;5:76–78.

63. Diaz JH. Perioperative management of the pregnant patient undergoing nonobstetric surgery. Part I. Indications for surgery and direct and indirect effects of anesthetics on fetal well-being. *Anesth Rev* 1991;18:21–22.

64. Saunders CM, Baum M. Breast cancer and pregnancy: a review. *J R Soc Med* 1993;86:162–165.

65. Adair EA. Cancer of the breast. *Surg Clin North Am* 1953;33:313–327.

66. Doll DC, Ringenberg S, Yarbro JW. Antineoplastic agents and pregnancy. *Semin Oncol* 1989; 16:337–346.

67. Theriault R, Walters R, Holmes F, et al. Management of breast cancer (BC) during pregnancy. *Proc Am Soc Clin Oncol* 1992;11:86. Abstract 171.

68. Hortobagyi GN, Frye D, Buzdar AU, et al. Complete remissions in metastatic breast cancer: a thirteen year follow-up report. *Proc Am Soc Clin Oncol* 1988;7:37. Abstract 143.

69. Roboz J, Gleicher N, Wu K, et al. Does doxorubicin cross the placenta? *Lancet* 1979;2: 1382–1383. Letter.

70. Karp GI, von Oeyen P, Valone F, et al. Doxorubicin in pregnancy: possible transplacental passage. *Cancer Treat Rep* 1983;67:773–777.

71. Arceci RJ, Croop JM, Horwitz SB, Housman D. The gene encoding multidrug resistance is induced and expressed at high levels during pregnancy in the secretory epithelium of the uterus. *Proc Natl Acad Sci USA* 1988;85:4350–4354.

72. Weinstein RS, Kuszak JR, Kluskens LF, Coon JS. P-glycoproteins in pathology: the multidrug resistance gene family in humans. *Hum Pathol* 1990;21:34–48.

73. Theriault RL, Stallings CB, Buzdar AU. Pregnancy and breast cancer: clinical and legal issues. Clinical case reports from MD Anderson Cancer Center. *Am J Clin Oncol* 1992;15:535–539.

74. Willemse PHB, van der Sijde R, Sleijfer DTh. Combination chemotherapy and radiation for stage IV breast cancer during pregnancy. *Gynecol Oncol* 1990;36:281–284.

75. Barni S, Ardizzola A, Zanetta G, et al. Weekly doxorubicin chemotherapy for breast cancer in pregnancy. A case report. *Tumori* 1992;78:349–350.

76. Aviles A, Diaz Maqueo JC, Talavera A. Growth and development of children of mothers treated with chemotherapy during pregnancy: current status of 43 children. *Am J Hematol* 1991;36:243–248.

77. Randall T. National registry seeks scarce data on pregnancy outcomes during chemotherapy (News). *JAMA* 1993;269:323.

78. Guikontes E, Spantideas A, Diakakis J. Ondansetron and hyperemesis gravidarum. *Lancet* 1992;340:1223. Letter.

79. World MJ. Ondansetron and hyperemesis gravidarum. *Lancet* 1993;341:185. Letter.

80. Beely L. Drugs and breast feeding. *Clin Obstet Gynecol* 1981;8:291–295.

81. Sutcliffe SB. Treatment of neoplastic disease during pregnancy: maternal and fetal effects. *Clin Invest Med* 1985;8:333–338.

82. Klein CE, Glode M. Options for preserving fertility in the chemotherapy patient. *Contemp Oncol* 1993;48–56.

83. Gradishar WJ, Schilsky RL. Ovarian function following radiation and chemotherapy for cancer. *Semin Oncol* 1989;16:425–436.

84. Damewood MD, Grochow LB. Prospects for fertility after chemotherapy or radiation for neoplastic disease. *Fertil Steril* 1986;45:443–459.

85. Shalet SM. Effects of cancer chemotherapy on gonadal function of patients. *Cancer Treat Rev* 1980;7:1419–1520.

86. Richards MA, O'Reilly SM, Howell A, et al. Adjuvant cyclophosphamide, methotrexate, and fluorouracil in patients with axillary node-positive breast cancer: an update of the Guy's/Manchester trial. *J Clin Oncol* 1990;8:2032–2039.

87. Hortobagyi GN, Buzdar AU, Marcus CE, Smith TE. Immediate and long-term toxicity of adjuvant chemotherapy regimens containing doxorubicin in trials at M. D. Anderson Hospital and Tumor Institute. *Monogr Natl Cancer Inst* 1986;1:105–109.

88. Jones SE, Stringer CA, Dorr RT, Senzer NN. Cancer and pregnancy. In: *American Society of Clinical Oncology (ASCO) educational book.* Chicago: ASCO and Bostrom Corp, 1991:228–236.

89. Sauer MV, Paulson RJ, Lobo RA. Successful pre-embryo donation in ovarian failure after treatment for breast carcinoma. *Lancet* 1990;335:723. Letter.

90. Farley JC, Gregory SS, Quinn M, et al. Harvesting fetal ovaries. *Time* 1994;143:19.

91. Epstein RJ, Henderson IC. The Danforth article reviewed: the jury is in. *Oncology* 1991;5:30–31.

92. Danforth DN Jr. How subsequent pregnancy affects outcome in women with a prior breast cancer. *Oncology* 1991;11:21–30.

93. Wood WC. The Danforth article reviewed. *Oncology* 1991;5:35.

94. Petrek JA. Pregnancy safety after breast cancer. *Cancer* 1994;74:528–531.

95. Sankila R, Heinävaara S, Hakulinen T. Survival of breast cancer patients after subsequent term pregnancy: "healthy mother effect." *Am J Obstet Gynecol* 1994;170:818–823.

96. Dow KH, Harris JR, Roy C. Pregnancy after breast-conserving surgery and radiation therapy for breast cancer. *Monogr Natl Cancer Inst* 1994;16:131–137.

97. Higgins S, Haffty B. Pregnancy and lactation after breast-conserving therapy for early stage breast cancer. *Cancer* 1994;73:2175–2180.

98. Tralins A. Is lactation possible after breast irradiation? *Proc Am Soc Clin Oncol* 1993;12:77. Abstract 109.

99. Miller MJ, Ross ME. Pregnancy following breast reconstruction with autogenous tissue (case report). *Cancer Bull* 1993;45:546–548.

100. Theriault RL, Sellin RV. Estrogen-replacement therapy in younger women with breast cancer. *Monogr Natl Cancer Inst* 1994;16:149–152.

101. DiSaia PJ. Hormone-replacement therapy in patients with breast cancer. A reappraisal. *Cancer* 1993;71(4 suppl):1490–1500.

102. Eden JA, Bush T, Nand S, et al. A case-control study of combined continuous estrogen-progestin replacement therapy among women with a personal history of breast cancer. *Menopause* 1995;2:67–72.

103. Stanford JL, Weiss NS, Voigt LF, et al. Combined estrogen and progestin hormone replacement therapy in relation to risk of breast cancer in middle-aged women. *JAMA* 1995;274:137–142.

104. Adami HO, Persson I. Hormone replacement and breast cancer. A remaining controversy? *JAMA* 1995;274:178–179. Editorial.

105. Colditz GA, Hankison SE, Hunter DJ, et al. The use of estrogens and progestins and the risk of breast cancer in postmenopausal women. *N Engl J Med* 1995;332:1589–1593.

106. Davidson NE. Hormone-replacement therapy—breast versus heart versus bone. *N Engl J Med* 1995;332:1638–1639. Editorial.

107. Dhodapkar MV, Ingle JN, Ahmann DL. Estrogen replacement therapy withdrawal and regression of metastatic breast cancer. *Cancer* 1995;75:43–46.

108. Pritchard KI, Sawaka CA. Menopausal estrogen replacement therapy in women with breast cancer. *Cancer* 1995;75:1–3.

109. Loprinzi CL, Michalak JC, Quella SK, et al. Megestrol acetate for the prevention of hot flashes. *N Engl J Med* 1994;331:347–352.

110. Effects of estrogen or estrogen/progestin regimens on heart disease risk factors in postmenopausal women. The Postmenopausal Estrogen/Progestin Interventions (PEPI) Trial. The Writing Group for the PEPI Trial. *JAMA* 1995;273:199–208.

111. Powles TJ, Hickish T, Casey S, et al. Hormone replacement after breast cancer. *Lancet* 1993; 342:60–61. Letter.

112. Cobleigh MA, Berris RF, Bush T, et al. Estrogen replacement therapy in breast cancer survivors. A time for change. *JAMA* 1994;272:540–545.

113. MacMahon B, Cole P, Lin TM, et al. Age at first birth and breast cancer risk. *Bull World Health Organ* 1970;43:209–221.

114. Vatten LJ, Kvinnsland S. Pregnancy-related factors and risk of breast cancer in a prospec-tive study of 29,981 Norwegian women. *Eur J Cancer* 1992;28A:1148–1153.

115. Kalache A, Maguire A, Thompson SG. Age at last full-term pregnancy and risk of breast cancer. *Lancet* 1993;341:33–36.

116. Bruzzi P, Negri E, La Vecchia C, et al. Short term increase in risk of breast cancer after full term pregnancy. *BMJ* 1988;297:1096–1097.

117. Williams EMI, Jones L, Vessey MP, McPherson K. Short term increase in risk of breast cancer associated with full term pregnancy. *BMJ* 1990; 300:578–579.

118. Spicer DV, Krecker EA, Pike MC. The endocrine prevention of breast cancer. *Cancer Invest* 1995; 3:495–504.

119. MacMahon B, Lin TM, Lowe CR, et al. Lactation and cancer of the breast. A summary of an inter-national study. *Bull World Health Organ* 1970; 42:185–194.

120. Newcomb PA, Storer BE, Longnecker MP, et al. Lactation and a reduced risk of premenopausal breast cancer. *N Engl J Med* 1994;330:81–87.

121. La Vecchia C. Oral contraceptives and breast cancer. Review article. *Breast* 1992;2:76–81.

122. Prentice RL, Thomas DB. On the epidemiology of oral contraceptives and disease. *Adv Cancer Res* 1987;49:285–401.

123. Romieu I, Berlin JA, Colditz G. Oral contra-ceptives and breast cancer. *Cancer* 1990;66: 2253–2263.

124. Olsson H, Ranstam J, Baldetorp B, et al. Prolif-eration and DNA ploidy in malignant breast tumors in relation to early oral contraceptive use and early abortions. *Cancer* 1991;67:1285–1290.

125. Olsson H, Borg A, Fernö M, et al. Her-2/neu and INT2 proto-oncogene amplification in malignant breast tumors in relation to repro-ductive factors and exposure to exogenous hormones. *J Natl Cancer Inst* 1991;83:1483–1487.

126. Herbst AL, Berek JS. Contraceptive choices for women with medical problems. Impact of con-traception on gynecologic cancers. *Am J Obstet Gynecol* 1993;168:1980–1985.

127. Pike MC, Henderson BE, Casagrande JT, et al. Oral contraceptive use and early abortion as risk factors for breast cancer in young women. *Br J Cancer* 1981;43:72–76.

128. Parkins T. Does abortion increase breast cancer risk? (News). *J Natl Cancer Inst* 1993;35:1987–1988.

129. Andrieu N, Clavel F, Gairard B, et al. Familial risk of breast cancer and abortion. *Cancer Detect Prev* 1994;18:51–55.

130. Parazzini F, La Vecchia C, Negri E. Spontaneous and induced abortions and risk of breast cancer. *Int J Cancer* 1991;48:816–820.

131. Parazzini F, La Vecchia C, Negri E, et al. Menstrual and reproductive factors and breast cancer in women with family history of the disease. *Int J Cancer* 1992;51:677–681.

132. Rosenberg L, Palmer JR, Kaufman DW, et al. Breast cancer in relation to the occurrence and time of induced and spontaneous abortion. *Am J Epidemiol* 1988;127:981–989.

133. Lehrer S, Schmutzler RK, Rabin JM, et al. An estrogen receptor genetic polymorphism and a history of spontaneous abortions—correlation with estrogen receptor positive breast cancer but not in women with estrogen receptor negative breast cancer or women without cancer. *Breast Cancer Res Treat* 1993;26:175–180.

Addendum: Effect of Interruption of Pregnancy on Outcome of Breast Cancer

Study	Years Accrued	No. of Patients	Normal Delivery No. of Patients	% Survival 5 Yr	10 Yr	Therapeutic Abortion No. of Patients	% Survival 5 Yr	10 Yr	Comments
Adair (1953)	NA	59	36	44	NA	23	70	NA	25 pregnant at diagnosis, 34 pregnant after treatment for cancer. Only node-positive patients benefited from abortion
Holleb (1962)	1962	24	12	33	NA	12	17	NA	Patients operated on during first trimester
Rissanen (1968)	1940–61	31	20*	50	NA	7*	43	NA	*4 other patients (totalling 31) were stage IV (1 aborted, 3 delivered); all were dead at 5 yr
Clark (1978)	1931–75	121	93	29	23	13	15	8	12% spontaneously aborted; 1 infant was stillborn. Abortion was not biased for more advanced disease
King (1985)	1950–80	63	35*	67	NA	18*	53	NA	*10 other patients (4 normal delivery, 6 aborted) were stage IV; only 1 alive at 5 yr. For stage I patients: 5-yr survival rate = 88% for normal delivery (n = 18) and 33% for abortion (n = 4)

NA = not available.

SECTION 2

Cervix

CHAPTER *15*

Secondary Prevention Screening for Carcinoma of the Cervix

FOLKE PETTERSSON

A little more than 100 years ago (1889), Tait stated, "Cancer of the cervix is the most painful and terrible disease inflicted on humanity, because there is no way to cure or even relieve it" (1). A few decades later the picture had changed completely. The introduction of ionizing irradiation from radium and other radioactive isotopes as well as from x-ray beams in the treatment of cervical carcinomas gave curative effects. The development of surgical techniques that became possible through advancements in anesthesiology and postoperative care was also an important contribution to the treatment of carcinoma of the uterine cervix. Screening with Papanicolaou's (Pap) smear has reduced the incidence and mortality rates in many countries. However, cancer of the uterine cervix is still the second most common cancer in women worldwide. In developing countries it is the most common cancer in women. In some of the Nordic countries, it has disappeared from the list of the 10 most common cancers. The losses from this disease are comparable only to deaths from complications of childbearing and delivery, as it often strikes women in younger age groups.

A screening program with the aim to detect precancerous stages of cervical cancer should be based on knowledge of the natural history and the epidemiology of the disease. Many details are still unknown but we have to consider that the majority of invasive carcinomas of the uterine cervix have a long precancerous stage, starting with atypical changes in the epithelium that progress over a long time toward more severe dysplasias, in situ carcinomas, and ultimately invasive carcinomas. In most patients these precancerous stages are detectable by an exfoliative cytology test. The treatment of the preinvasive disease in most women is easily and safely performed. The result should be a reduction in the incidence rate and a reduction in the mortality rate of invasive cervical carcinoma.

In almost 100% of patients, untreated invasive carcinoma of the uterine cervix leads to death. With local brachytherapy with radium or cesium and external radiation and, in suitable patients, radical operation, it is possible to obtain an overall 5-year survival rate of about 60%. The results of treatment highly depend on the stage in which the tumor is treated and are far better for the early stages compared with the more advanced stages of disease. There is a need for expensive, specialized, and well-equipped clinics for treatment.

There is no doubt that carcinoma of the uterine cervix is an important health-care problem. Thus, this disease fulfills the first condition claimed for a disease suited for secondary prevention by screening. The second main condition is that patients in the precancerous stage can be offered a treatment that is more successful than the treatment given when the disease is invasive and symptomatic. A third condition is that the prevalence of the preclinical disease should be fairly high; otherwise the cost for finding precancerous cases will be too high.

Epidemiology

A number of observations provide evidence that the risk of developing carcinoma of the uterine cervix is not evenly distributed among the female population. Thus, women living under severe socioeconomic circumstances, especially in large cities, run a higher risk for this disease. Factors connected with sexual activity influence the risk of this disease. Carcinoma of the uterine cervix is practically unknown among women without sexual contacts but is more common among women with several partners and several pregnancies. Early sexual debut increases the risk. Early on, there was suspicion that some infectious agent, and more specifically, a sexually transmitted infection, was responsible for the disease. Since the late 1960s, many observations pointed out an infection with herpes virus as a possible cause. Recent studies indicated that an infection with human papillomavirus (HPV), together with some cofactors, leads to the development of cervical intraepithelial neoplasia (CIN) and cervical cancer (2,3). Cigarette smoking as well as vitamin deficiencies seem to play a role in the genesis of this disease (4).

Natural History

The common belief about the natural history of carcinoma of the uterine cervix is that there is a slowly progressing process from early precancerous stages in the form of dysplasia via carcinoma in situ over to the invasive carcinoma of the uterine cervix. A few classic works (5,6) observed a number of carcinoma in situ cases during the course of several years and found that after 10 years' observation, this lesion had

evolved to invasive carcinoma of the cervix in 30% to 70% of patients. Many sources of error are connected with this type of study. On the one hand, repeat biopsies in some patients may have cured the precancerous disease and stopped it. On the other hand, it is not impossible that there might have been invasive carcinomatous changes in connection with the precancerous lesion from the beginning. Mean intervals between the time of detection of in situ carcinoma and invasive carcinoma of the cervix ranged from 8 to 20 years in different studies. It is possible that the latency period from the preinvasive to the invasive carcinoma varies with age, and the progress may be more rapid in elderly women compared with younger women. An important number of these precancerous stages probably regress. There is also a possibility that a number of cancers have a very short precancerous stage.

The mean age according to stage and histologic type of carcinoma of the uterine cervix from the Annual Report is presented in Table 15-1 (7). The age span between stage I and stage IV epidermoid carcinoma was almost 12 years. The mean age for the total series was 52.5 years. Only when we can show that the diagnosis in precancerous stages or early stages of invasive carcinoma results in a decreased cumulative incidence and mortality rate over a longer period, can we talk about the benefit of screening. It is not necessarily so that treatment in earlier stages will be beneficial in the long term. An investigation in Wales (8) showed that the mean age of patients with stage I cervical carcinoma was 51 years; with stage II, 54.5 years; with stage III, 58 years; and with stage IV, 58.9 years. The mean age at death for patients with cancer diagnosed in stage I was 57.7 years; in stage II, 57.4 years; in stage III, 59.1 years; and in stage IV, 60.4 years. This study included all patients with carcinoma of the cervix registered in South Wales from 1960 to 1974. In

Histologic Type	Stage I	Stage II	Stage III	Stage IV	Total
Epidermoid	47.2	54.6	57.2	59.1	52.8
Adenocarcinoma	46.4	55.6	60.6	64.8	52.2
Adenosquamous	44.9	52.2	54.9	64.1	46.9
Clear cell	47.3	55.3	54.4	48.5	51.1
Other	46.1	52.1	57.3	56.9	52.1

T A B L E **15-1**

Mean Age for Invasive Cervical Carcinoma by Stage and Histopathologic Type

Source: Pettersson F, ed. *Annual report on the results of treatment in gynecological cancer*, vol. 22. Stockholm: Editorial Office, Radiumhemmet, 1995.

addition, the investigation, which was performed in 1975, showed that 48% of the women diagnosed in stage I were alive in 1975, whereas 30% of stage II, 12% of stage III, and only 6% of stage IV patients survived 1975. One conclusion from this study was that an important part of the observed improved healing for the earlier stages compared with the advanced stages may be explained by a more favorable age distribution for the early stages. Not less than 50% of the observed benefit of early diagnosis disappeared in the long term according to this study. It could be concluded that our common knowledge on the epidemiology as well as of the natural history of carcinoma of the cervix is still incomplete, which will influence the preventive measures undertaken. It is also necessary to take into account the different histopathologic types of carcinoma of the cervix.

The overwhelming literature dealing with the natural history and the epidemiology of cervical carcinoma is based on experiences from squamous epithelial carcinoma, which in different hospital materials represents 80% to 95% of the total number of cervical carcinomas (9). Above all, it is the squamous epithelial carcinomas that are apt to be diagnosed

T A B L E **15-2**

Percentage of Adenocarcinomas Including Mucoepidermoid Carcinomas by Birth Cohorts and Age Groups

Years of Birth	Age (yr)						
	25–29	30–34	35–39	40–44	45–49	50–54	55–59
1905–09	—	—	—	—	—	—	6.1
1910–14	—	—	—	—	—	6.8	4.8
1915–19	—	—	—	—	5.4	6.7	7.1
1920–24	—	—	—	5.4	5.1	9.3	18.9
1925–29	—	—	5.8	6.4	10.3	15.2	—
1930–34	—	4.6	7.5	11.5	12.4	—	—
1935–39	10.6	7.1	11.3	13.0	—	—	—
1940–44	5.3	10.8	15.4	—	—	—	—
1945–49	9.2	11.5	—	—	—	—	—
1950–54	12.3	—	—	—	—	—	—

Source: Pettersson F. Adenocarcinoma of the uterine cervix. Changes in incidence. Presented at the 38th annual meeting of the Society of Pelvic Surgeons, Toronto, Ontario, Canada, October 5–8, 1988.

T A B L E **15-3**

Adenocarcinoma and Mucoepidermoid Carcinomas of the Uterine Cervix in Sweden per 100,000 Women, by Year of Birth Cohorts and 5-Year Age Groups

Years of Birth	Age (yr)						
	25–29	30–34	35–39	40–44	45–49	50–54	55–59
1905–09	—	—	—	—	—	—	2.4
1910–14	—	—	—	—	—	3.2	1.9
1915–19	—	—	—	—	2.9	2.8	2.0
1920–24	—	—	—	3.0	2.3	2.4	2.9
1925–29	—	—	2.4	2.9	2.8	2.4	—
1930–34	—	1.0	2.4	2.4	2.6	—	—
1935–39	0.7	1.3	2.2	2.5	—	—	—
1940–44	0.4	1.7	2.8	—	—	—	—
1945–49	0.9	1.8	—	—	—	—	—
1950–54	1.2	—	—	—	—	—	—

Source: Pettersson F. Adenocarcinoma of the uterine cervix. Changes in incidence. Presented at the 38th annual meeting of the Society of Pelvic Surgeons, Toronto, Ontario, Canada, October 5–8, 1988.

early, in precancerous stages, with the Pap test. Screening works as a selective process, causing a relative increase in the number of the adenocarcinomatous cases. Data from the Swedish National Cancer Registry illustrate this selection.

Table 15-2 shows a successive relative increase in the percentage of adenocarcinomas among all cervical carcinomas. It should be noted that the true incidence of adenocarcinomas of the cervix was practically unchanged during this period whereas the incidence of squamous epithelial carcinomas decreased considerably (Table 15-3).

The Pap Test

The tool for cervical cancer screening, the exfoliative cytology test, was described by George Papanicolaou (10) and by Babés in 1928 (11). The accuracy of the Pap smear technique for early detection of cervical cancers and its precursors has been evaluated by various means and with differing results. False-negative rates ranging from 5% to 40% have been reported. Some of the reports showed that the majority of the false-negative results could be attributed to sampling error. Different changes in smear techniques and quality control have been proposed to improve the accuracy of the screening test (12–15).

Strategies for Evaluation of the Impact of Screening

For different reasons, the pioneers of cervical cancer screening did not undertake any randomized study to evaluate cervical cancer screening. Later this was considered unethical.

Considerable efforts have been directed toward studies on the incidence and mortality trends within circumscribed geographic regions or populations characterized by different screening intensities. Other efforts take into account clinical data, detection rates of preinvasive disease, incidence, and mortality data for invasive disease in order to create mathematical models simulating the effect of different screening strategies.

Prescreening Trends

The last century's expanding and improving medical facilities within the industrialized world gave women easier access to gynecologic service, which meant earlier clinical diagnosis of malignant tumors. This is evident from data gathered in the FIGO Annual Report (7). Altogether 537,553 cases of carcinoma of the uterine cervix treated in the years 1913 to 1989 (inclusive) have been reported to the editorial office for the Annual Report. These data in the Annual Report illustrate the trends in stage distribution and in survival rates after treatment of cervical carcinoma.

Figure 15-1 reviews the changes in stage distribution as reported in the periods 1950 to 1954 (volume 12), to 1987 to 1989 (volume 22) (7). The proportion of stage I cervical carcinomas continuously increases from 23% in the period 1950 to 1954 to 38% in 1987 to 1989. During the same period the proportion of stage II cervical carcinomas decreases from 38% to 33% and for stage III from 33% to 25%. The proportion of stage IV cervical carcinomas decreases from 6.5% to 4.5%.

The results in terms of 5-year survival of patients with stage I carcinoma improved from

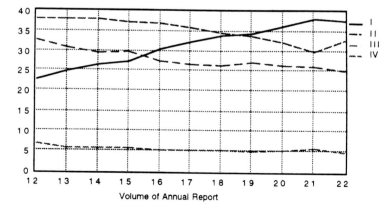

F I G U R E   **15-1**

Carcinoma of the uterine cervix. Distribution by stage (percentage) and by period of treatment (volume 12 = 1950-1954 and volume 22 = 1987-1989). (From Pettersson F, ed. *Annual report on the results of treatment in gynecological cancer*, vol. 22. Stockholm: Editorial Office, Radiumhemmet, 1995.)

75% to 85% and for those with stage II from 53% to 66%. For stage III cervical carcinoma, the change was from 26% to 39% and for stage IV from 6% to 11% (Fig. 15-2) (7).

Improvement in treatment results by stage contributed to changes in mortality rates. The overall 5-year survival rate for patients with cervical cancer treated at Radiumhemmet in Stockholm from 1915 to 1930 was less than 30%, while those treated after 1955 had a 60% 5-year survival rate (Table 15-4). The corresponding figures for 10-year survival were 19% compared to 52%. This improvement, along with stable incidence rates over the period, should result in a 50% reduction in mortality rate for carcinoma of the uterine cervix.

Early Reports on the Efficacy of Cervical Cancer Screening

Screening programs for precancerous stages of cervical cancer were organized in the province of British Columbia, Canada, 1949, and in Louisville, Jefferson County, Kentucky, 1956. Early optimistic reports provided evidence of reduced mortality from cancer of the uterine cervix in these screened regions (16–18). Other authors, referring to prescreening trends and weakness in notification and registration of incidence data as well as mortality data, severely criticized these reports. Furthermore, there seemed to be problems with the calculated population at risk (14,15,19–21).

Measures for Efficacy of Screening

The effect of a screening program must be evaluated in terms of its impact on the mortality rate of carcinoma of the uterine cervix within the whole population. Owing to the special case with cervical carcinoma, where the disease is detected in a preinvasive stage and treated before development of invasive carcinoma, the incidence of invasive cervical carcinoma also

T A B L E   **15-4**

Carcinoma of the Uterine Cervix: Treatment Results, Radiumhemmet, Stockholm, Sweden

Years	5-Year Survival Rate (%)	10-Year Survival Rate (%)
1915–30	25	19
1935–50	44	39
1955–70	60	52

Source: Internal statistics, Radiumhemmet, Stockholm, Sweden.

F I G U R E   **15-2**

Carcinoma of the uterine cervix. Five-year survival rates by stage and by period of treatment (volume 12 = 1950-1954 and volume 22 = 1987-1989). Data for the two last volumes are given as corrected actuarial survival and for the previous volumes as crude direct 5-year survival rates. (Pettersson F, ed. *Annual report on the results of treatment in gynecological cancer*, vol. 22. Stockholm: Editorial Office, Radiumhemmet, 1995.)

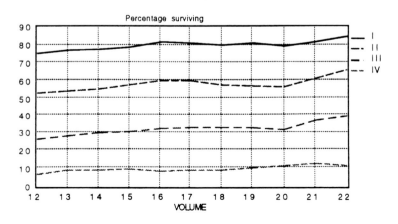

serves as a good measure of the effect of screening. A good parallel between incidence rate reduction and mortality rate reduction has been shown (22).

Critical Viewpoints on Given Incidence and Mortality Rates for Carcinoma of the Uterine Cervix

Incidence as well as mortality rates derive from a numerator giving the number of cancer cases or deaths and a denominator giving the female population within which the cancers occurred. The difficulties studying incidence and mortality rates in different parts of the world are as follows:

1. Lack of national cancer registries covering the whole population
2. Changes in reporting and registration routines
3. Changes in definitions and nomenclature
4. Difficulties defining and delineating the population from which the cases are recruited—problems with migration

Many examples in the literature illustrate these problems. Additional problems affecting mortality rates are reliability of death certificates and, in earlier periods, difficulties distinguishing death from carcinoma of the uterine cervix from that of endometrial carcinoma (23).

Studies on the Sensitivity of the Screening Procedure, Optimal Intervals, and Ages to Be Screened

The International Agency for Research on Cancer (IARC) collaborative study on the eval-uation of cervical cancer screening programs made use of data from organized screening programs in many European and North American states (24). The study concentrated on the questions of whom to screen (i.e., whom to invite initially for screening) and how often to rescreen those with negative results on screening tests. The comparison of different screening strategies can be made in terms of the reduction in risk of invasive disease that each strategy might be expected to produce. The risk associated with a particular screening pattern is given by the cumulative incidence of invasive disease during each interscreening interval, together with the risks that accumulate before the first screening test and after the last screening test. The individual screening programs and their results were analyzed either as case-control studies done with the records of a centrally organized screening program or cohort studies done with the records of a centrally organized program or case-control studies done in areas without a mass screening program.

Table 15-5 summarizes the relative protection (geometric means) calculated from the different data from the centers. Table 15-6 gives the percentage reduction in the cumulative rate of invasive cervical cancer over the age range 35 to 65 years, according to different frequencies of screening. It is obvious that good results can be obtained with screening intervals ranging from 1 to 5 years. A 3-year interval may be optimal. The additional gain with shorter intervals is marginal and is connected with considerably higher costs.

The developed countries with good screening programs have decreasing incidence and mortality rates for cervical carcinoma, but even

Time Since Last Negative Smear (mo)	Relative Protection (No. of Cases)	95% Confidence Intervals
0–11	15.3 (25)	10.0–22.6
12–23	11.9 (23)	7.5–18.3
24–35	8.0 (25)	5.2–11.8
36–47	5.3 (30)	3.6–7.6
48–59	2.8 (30)	1.9–4.0
60–71	3.6 (16)	2.1–5.9
72–119	1.6 (6)	0.6–3.5
120+	0.8 (7)	0.3–1.6
Never screened	1.0	

T A B L E **15-5**

Summary of Relative Protections (Geometric Mean Values) over the Centers

Source: Hakama M, Miller AB, Day NE. Screening for cancer of the uterine cervix. *IARC Sci Publ* 1986;76:133–142.

here still a great number of women get this disease and die from it.

Why Does Carcinoma of the Uterine Cervix Occur Within Screened Populations?

1. It is important to realize that the screening with the Pap smear is efficient in catching the precancerous stages of squamous epithelial cell carcinomas but less efficient catching those of other histopathologies. Therefore, a relative increase in the proportion of adenocarcinomas among remaining cases of cervical cancer is seen (9,25).

2. For more or less clear-cut reasons, a number of women avoid screening voluntarily or are not reached by the screening programs. One category of women who more or less escape screening activities are those who are older than the proposed target group for screening. The category of women who, in spite of invitations to screening, still avoid participation includes not only women who are socially bad off but also women with higher social

T A B L E   **15-6**

Percentage Reduction in the Cumulative Rate of Invasive Cervical Cancer over the Age Range 35 to 65, With Different Frequencies of Screening*

Screening Frequency	% Reduction in the Cumulative Rate	No. of Tests
1 yr	93.3	30
2 yr	92.5	15
3 yr	91.4	10
5 yr	83.9	6
10 yr	64.2	3

*Assuming a screening occurs at age 35, and that a previous screening test had been performed.

Source: Hakama M, Miller AB, Day NE. Screening for cancer of the uterine cervix. *IARC Sci Publ* 1986;76: 133–142.

status who do not recognize themselves as at risk for this disease. Furthermore, there are groups of immigrants for whom screening was not possible in their countries of origin. More than 15% of newly diagnosed carcinomas of the uterine cervix treated at Radiumhemmet, Stockholm, from 1987 to 1988 were in women belonging to immigrant groups, especially those from non-Nordic countries (26). Within the age group 47 years and younger, 25% were immigrants.

3. Another group of women who develop invasive cervical cancer are those who were treated previously for precancerous stages, carcinoma in situ, or different degrees of dysplasia—the treatment may have been conization with cold knife, laser, or diathermy. Even after hysterectomy, recurrences occur in the top of the vagina and are often labeled carcinoma of the vagina but should be viewed as carcinoma of the uterine cervix. Thus, this group of women treated for precancerous disease still constitute a high-risk group and should be carefully monitored (Table 15-7) (27). As Table 15-7 shows, from the time of treatment of the precancerous stage and for as long as the cohort was followed (20 years), the risk of developing an invasive carcinoma of the uterine cervix is still two to three times the expected risk. A subgrouping by age into those younger than 50 years and those 50 years and older at the time of treatment for the precancerous stages shows that the risk is considerably higher among the older age group (Table 15-8).

4. "False-negative" screening results constitute a category of disease that sometimes is mislabeled as rapidly generated and rapidly growing tumors. More thorough investigation may reveal that some of the patients with rapidly growing tumors have a history of less successfully treated precancerous stages. In other cases negative screening results are due to cell samples that are too sparse to permit diagnosis.

T A B L E   **15-7**

Annual Incidence Rates of Invasive Carcinoma of the Uterine Cervix per 100,000 Among 56,116 Women Treated in 1958 to 1977 for In Situ Cancer in Sweden, and Observed to Expected (O/E) Rates by Time Since Treatment

	Years Since Treatment					
	<1	1–4	5–9	10–14	15–19	20+
Incidence per 100,000	21.4	51.4	53.4	60.0	35.5	84.1
O/E rates	0.98	2.28	2.43	2.84	1.61	3.85

Pettersson F, Malker B. Invasive carcinoma of the uterine cervix following diagnosis and treatment of in situ carcinoma. Record linkage within a National Cancer Registry. *Radiother Oncol* 1989;16:115–120.

T A B L E   **15-8**

Invasive Carcinoma of the Uterine Cervix Occurring 1 to 20 Years After In Situ Carcinoma by Age at Treatment of In Situ Carcinoma

Age Group	Observed (O)	Expected (E)	O/E
≤49 yr	145	77.4	1.9
≥50 yr	66	10.7	6.2

Pettersson F, Malker B. Invasive carcinoma of the uterine cervix following diagnosis and treatment of in situ carcinoma. Record linkage within a National Cancer Registry. *Radiother Oncol* 1989;16:115–120.

To conclude, the distribution of new cases of carcinoma of the uterine cervix within the female population is strongly influenced by screening activities. Efficient use of resources for screening necessitates continuous monitoring of incidence and mortality trends within different population strata.

Advantages of Controlled Screening Programs

Controlled screening programs are defined as programs organized through official health authorities and with the goal to cover all women at risk within a circumscribed society. Women at risk for developing a malignant disease of the uterine cervix include all sexually active women within that population. Epidemiologic research points at high-risk factors such as early sexual debut, multiple partners, and cigarette smoking, among others. Any attempt to save resources through a restriction of the screening efforts to selected high-risk groups of women has, however, failed. Thus, it is important to cover the whole population at risk. When resources are restricted, however, screening certain age groups should be discussed. The nearer the age of the maximum incidence of disease that the screening is undertaken, the more cost-effective results will probably be achieved. When screening is organized in that way, the probability of detecting precancerous stages and preventing invasive growth and death of the cancer should be highest (28).

The philosophy behind the organization of health care and hospital administration differs between different countries. In some countries there is a long tradition of a responsibility for the government and state to provide health-care facilities for the whole population and furthermore to economize the facilities so as to cover all strata within the population. In other societies the freedom and responsibility of each individual to take care of his or her own business gives rise to other kinds of organizations with more pronounced private practice, private insurance, and so on. These basic differences in organization of health-care systems naturally influence the possibilities to organize screening programs. Whatever type of organization there is for screening, some demands remain similar.

1. The result of the screening must be viewed in relation to its impact on the incidence of invasive carcinoma and mortality rate of carcinoma of the uterine cervix within the whole population.

2. There must be an organization for dealing with cervical abnormalities of different degrees as well as follow-up after treatment of such lesions.

3. In order to evaluate the effect, it is necessary to have regional national cancer registries with good coverage. In the Nordic countries, Norway, Finland, Denmark, Sweden, and Iceland, national cancer registries have been in function for more than 30 years and the populations in these countries have been well registered for a long time. Screening programs were organized in these countries but with some differences in design. Finland, Iceland, and Sweden organized nationwide population-based screening programs in the early 1970s. The target group included women aged 30 to 55 years in Finland, 25 to 69 years in Iceland, and 30 to 49 years in Sweden. Screening intervals in the three countries differed: 2 to 3 years in Iceland, 4 years in Sweden, and 5 years in Finland. In Denmark, target groups and ages to be screened varied by counties. Norway started with an ambitious pilot study covering only one county (22,24,29).

Experiences from the Scandinavian countries provide some basis for evaluation of the efficiency of controlled screening programs compared to Pap smears taken outside the organized programs. Denmark, starting with the highest incidence rate in the Nordic countries, showed a moderate reduction corresponding to the proportion of the population screened. Finland, with screening programs directed to women aged 30 to 55 years and with a 5-year screening interval, and Sweden, with a target population 30 to 50 years old and a screening interval of 4 years, had a similar reduction in incidence and mortality in cervical carcinoma; however, the reduction was even more pronounced in Finland (22,29) (Figs. 15-3 and 15-4).

In Norway, which had organized screening in only one county until recently, the findings are totally different. The incidence rose steadily until recent years when a moderate reduction occurred. However, it must be noted that in Norway, as in the other Nordic countries, considerable numbers of smears are taken outside screening programs (28–30). The different findings in the Nordic countries have been interpreted as evidence of the efficacy of organized as compared to unorganized screening for cervix cancer. In analyses of Swedish data, we found that the detection rate of precancerous lesions in the part of the female population that did not attend the organized screening equaled that within the part that attended

the organized screening. However, the cost of this was that several times more smears were obtained outside the organized screening program than within the organized program. Thus, some 200,000 smears were taken annually within the organized screening program and about four times as many outside the programs (29,30).

The advantages of organized screening programs are as follows: The cost-effectiveness of organized programs will prove to be superior. Coverage of the population at risk will be more complete. Uniform organization and uniform education of the nurses or midwives who take the smears probably result in better samples of smears than those taken by physicians. Uniform organization will also permit better quality control at all levels of the chain, from the sampling to the preparation at the laboratory, the laboratory routine, and the laboratory report. Routines for dealing with different kinds of cervical abnormalities will be more efficient if they are organized for a larger group of patients. A computerized system for

FIGURE **15-3**

Carcinoma of the uterine cervix in Sweden. Trends in age-specific incidence rates. The Swedish Cancer Registry, 1965 to 1990. (Organized screening was developed 1964–1973. Target population of women aged 30–50 years.)

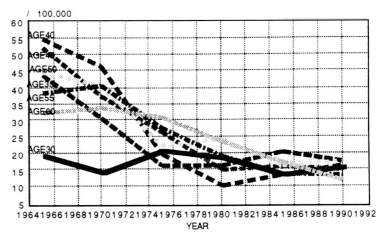

FIGURE **15-4**

Carcinoma of the uterine cervix. Trends in mortality rates in Sweden, 1973 to 1992, based on the Swedish Cause of Death Register.

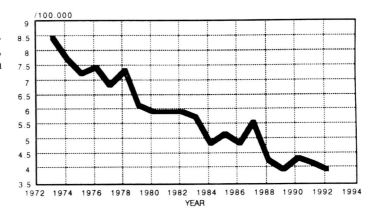

inviting women from the population register will facilitate the work of checking the population covered. A computerized follow-up system for women with different degrees of cervical abnormalities in the smears will prevent women who should be treated from being lost.

In order to evaluate the effect of an organized screening program, it is necessary to have regional or national cancer registries with as complete registration of precancerous stages and invasive carcinomas of the uterine cervix as possible. It should be possible to link screening registries to cancer registries and population registries.

Current Dilemmas with Cervical Cancer Screening

There is no doubt that a large number of lives have been saved and will be saved through good screening programs (22,31). In addition, a vast amount of suffering will be avoided. With successful screening programs, fewer and fewer cases of cervical cancer will be left to catch at later stages. As a consequence, the cost per capita to find these remaining cases will increase. In a shrinking economy for public health affairs, this situation will tempt health-care administrators and politicians to withdraw support for screening programs. Furthermore, a decreasing number of positive smears will be a danger to the laboratories reading the smears as they will be less experienced, necessitating continuous quality control. Also among physicians, nurses, and midwifes obtaining smears, a reduced number of positive findings may tempt them to sample the cervical tissue less carefully. It is of paramount importance to realize that screening must be a continuing process; otherwise the gains will soon be lost.

Conclusions

The goal of screening is to influence the health within the whole population by sorting out women with precancerous lesions that should be treated. The ideal model for screening programs must be tailored for each country and population with respect to tradition and health-care organization. For the Scandinavian countries, the officially organized screening program, inviting all women at risk by means of computerized population registries, has proved to be a potent method of influencing

the incidence of invasive carcinoma of the uterine cervix as well as the mortality of the disease. Even better results can be achieved by coordination between the organized screening and Pap smears taken outside the programs.

REFERENCES

1. Uttenbroeck F. *Past and present of radical surgery in gynaecological and mammary cancerology.* Leuven: Peeters, 1987.

2. Wright TC, Richart RM. Role of papillomavirus in the pathogenesis of genital tract warts and cancer. *Gynecol Oncol* 1990;37:151–164.

3. Munoz N, Bosch FX, Jensen OM. Human papillomavirus and cervical cancer. *IARC Sci Publ* 1989;94:1–8.

4. Hellberg D, Valentin J, Nilsson S. Smoking and cervical intra-epithelial neoplasia. An association independent of sexual or other risk factors. *Acta Obstet Gynecol Scand* 1986;65:625–631.

5. Pedersen O. Precancerous stages of the cervical epithelium in relation to manifest cervical carcinoma. *Acta Radiol Suppl* 1955;127.

6. Kottmeier HL. Evolution et traitement des epitheliomas. *Rev Fr Gynecol Obstet* 1961;56:821.

7. Pettersson F, ed. *Annual report on the results of treatment in gynecological cancer*, vol. 22. Stockholm: Editorial Office, Radiumhemmet, 1995.

8. West RR. Cervical cancer: age at registration and age at death. *Br J Cancer* 1977;35:236–241.

9. Pettersson F. Adenocarcinoma of the uterine cervix. Changes in incidence. Presented at the 38th annual meeting of the Society of Pelvic Surgeons, Toronto, Ontario, Canada, October 5–8, 1988.

10. Papanicolaou GN. New cancer diagnosis. In: Third race betterment conference. 1928:538. Reprinted in *Cancer* 1973;23:171.

11. Babés A. Cancer du col uterin par Les-Frottis. *Presse Med* 1928;29:451.

12. Näslund I, Auer G, Pettersson F, Sjövall K. Evaluation of the pulse wash sampling technique for screening of uterine cervical carcinoma. *Acta Radiol Oncol* 1986;25:131–136.

13. Stenkvist B, Bergström R, Eklund G, Fox CH. Papanicolaou smear screening and cervical cancer. What can you expect? *JAMA* 1984;252: 1423–1426.

14. Shulman JJ, Leyton M, Hamilton R. The Papanicolaou smear: an insensitive case-finding procedure. *Am J Obstet Gynecol* 1974;120:446.

15. Sigurdsson K. Quality assurance in cervical cancer screening: the Icelandic experience 1964–1993. *Eur J Cancer* 1995;31A:728–734.

16. Christopherson WM, Parker JE, Mendez WM, Lundin FE Jr. Cervix cancer death rates and mass cytologic screening. *Cancer* 1970;26:808–811.

17. Boyes DA, Knowelden J, Phillips AJ. The evaluation of cancer control measures. Summary of the conclusion of UICC Symposium held in Sheffield in September 1972. *Br J Cancer* 1973;28:105.

18. Christopherson WM, Lundin FE Jr, Mendez WM, Parker JE. Cervical cancer control. A study of morbidity and mortality trends over a twenty-one-year period. *Cancer* 1976;38:1357–1366.

19. Martin PL. How preventable is invasive cervical cancer? A community study of preventable factors. *Am J Obstet Gynecol* 1972;113:541–548.

20. Cramer DW. The role of cervical cytology in the declining morbidity and mortality of cervical cancer. *Cancer* 1974;34:2018–2027.

21. Sackett DL. Can screening programs for serious diseases really improve health? *Sci Forum* 1970;15:9.

22. Hakama M, Magnus K, Pettersson F, et al. Effect of the organized screening in the Nordic countries on the risk of cervical cancer. In: *Cancer screening. International Union Against Cancer.* Cambridge, UK: Cambridge University Press, 1991:153–162.

23. Saxén EA. Trends: facts or fallacy. In: Magnus K, ed. *Trends in cancer incidence. Causes and practical implications.* New York: Hemisphere Publishing, 1982:5–16.

24. Hakama M, Miller AB, Day NE. Screening for cancer of the uterine cervix. *IARC Sci Publ* 1986;76:133–142.

25. Boon ME, de Graaff Guilloud JC, Kok LP, et al. Efficacy of screening for cervical squamous and adenocarcinoma. The Dutch experience. *Cancer* 1987;59:862.

26. Pettersson F. Vem får cervixcancer? Nordisk Förening för Obstet. och Gynecol. Kongress, Reykjavik, Island, 9–12 Juni 1992.

27. Pettersson F, Malker B. Invasive carcinoma of the uterine cervix following diagnosis and treatment of in situ carcinoma. Record linkage within a National Cancer Registry. *Radiother Oncol* 1989;16:115–120.

28. Knox EG. Ages and frequencies for cervical cancer screening. *Br J Cancer* 1976;34:444–452.

29. Pettersson F, Björkholm E, Näslund I. Evaluation of screening for cervical cancer in Sweden: trends in incidence and mortality 1958–1980. *Int J Epidemiol* 1985;14:521–527.

30. Pettersson F, Näslund I, Malker B. Evaluation of the effect of Papanicolaou screening in Sweden: record linkage between a central screening registry and the National Cancer Registry. *IARC Sci Publ* 1986;76:91–105.

31. Guzick DS. Efficacy of screening for cervical cancer: a review. *Am J Public Health* 1978;68:125–134.

CHAPTER 16

Cervical Intraepithelial Neoplasia

EVA RYLANDER

*C*ancer of the cervix uteri is the second most common female cancer in the world and the most frequent in the Third World. An estimated 480,000 new cases of cervical cancer arise annually (1). Screening programs to prevent the development of this disease have been carried out to a larger extent than for any other type of cancer. Cervical cancer is a disease suitable for screening because of its well-defined, generally long-lasting precancerous phase, which is rather easy to detect and which is possible to eradicate in an uncomplicated and quick way (2). In some Nordic countries (Finland, Iceland, Sweden), nationwide population-based cytologic screening has been performed for more than 30 years. The incidence and the mortality of the disease have decreased among women who have been subjected to screening during a substantial period of their lives. In Norway, however, the reduction is less pronounced, probably due to the fact that until recently only a small proportion of the female population was covered by the organized screening program (3).

Etiology

Certain epidemiologic conditions are associated with a risk for developing cervical cancer. Such factors are low age at first sexual intercourse, multiple male sexual partners, and multiple pregnancies (4).

It has long been recognized that some kind of chemical or infectious carcinogenic agent is transferred at intercourse. It is now clear that some of the approximately 30 identified genital papillomaviruses [mainly human papillomavirus (HPV) 16 and 18] are able to act on imma-

ture epithelial cells and transform them into potentially malignant ones (5). Their viral proteins E6 and E7 are able to bind and inactivate the host's tumor suppressor proteins p53 and Rb. High-risk papillomaviruses are considered necessary but not sufficient for the development of invasive cervical cancer—other concurrent factors are required. Immunodeficiency [e.g., due to human immunodeficiency virus (HIV) infection] may hasten the progression of a precancerous to an invasive stage. Women positive for HIV have an increased risk for developing cervical cancer compared to women positive for HPV only (6). Factors such as smoking, long-term use of oral contraceptives, and mutagene metabolites appearing in connection with chronic cervical infections have also been suggested as cofactors (7). Since the major risk factors predisposing to the development of invasive cervical cancer are strongly correlated to sexual behavior, this cancer may be regarded as a late consequence of a sexually transmitted disease.

Pathophysiology

To understand the development of cervical cancer, it is important to know about the process going on in the affected tissue (8). The vaginal wall is covered by stratified, squamous epithelium consisting of several layers of cells. The cervical canal is lined by a one-layered columnar epithelium. Somewhere at the outer cervical os, these two tissues meet. The position of the boundary varies depending on age and hormonal influence. An increase in sexual hormones, that is, at puberty, during pregnancy, and during oral contraceptive use, may cause hypertrophy and eversion of the columnar epithelium. The area of the ectocervix that is covered by columnar epithelium is named *ectropion*. Approximately 65% of women younger than 25 years have an ectropion. The border between the squamous and the original columnar epithelia is called the *squamocolumnar junction* (SCJ).

The acidity of the vaginal secretion and the presence of many different bacteria as well as mechanical friction are factors that stimulate the development of a new epithelium (metaplasia), initiated at the SCJ. Gradually the ectropion will be substituted or covered by the metaplastic epithelium, which finally will differentiate into squamous epithelium. The process of differentiation sometimes continues for years. This area is named the *transformation zone* (TZ). It may be covered partly by immature and partly by fully differentiated squamous epithelium. In this area cysts caused by retained secretion (nabothian cysts) may appear. They may vary in size and are easy to recognize owing to their yellow content and very distinguished capillaries. With time, the SCJ advances into the cervical canal and from the age of 50 it may be impossible to identify the TZ, because it is out of reach for colposcopic inspection.

Morphology and Terminology

Metaplastic cells, being immature, are especially sensitive to the influence of HPV, which may turn them into malignant ones. In differentiated squamous epithelium, cells with atypical features may first appear in the lower part, consisting of immature (i.e., parabasal) cells. This degree of atypia is called *mild cervical intraepithelial neoplasia* (CIN 1) (Fig. 16-1). Simultaneously, the upper layers may show koilocytosis (cells with perinuclear halos, thickened cell borders, and mild nuclear atypia). These cells reflect cellular degeneration due to replication of viral particles in the nuclei. When two thirds of the epithelial thickness is covered by more atypical cells with or without simultaneous koilocytosis, the atypia is referred to as *moderate* (CIN 2). If the whole thickness of the epithelium is full of immature abnormal cells and mitosis, *severe intraepithelial neoplasia* (CIN 3) is present (Fig. 16-2). With increasing severity, the nuclei of the cells become more irregular and hyperchromatic. As long as the malignant cells do not penetrate the basal membranes into the stromal tissue, the lesion is precancerous. Such a lesion is possible to eradicate by simple surgical techniques.

Mild atypical changes due to infections other than HPV infections or due to reparative processes in the epithelium may be difficult to distinguish from CIN 1. Lesions with HPV-associated changes are equivalent to CIN 1 because the definition of koilocytosis includes the presence of somewhat atypical nuclei. Such lesions will often regress spontaneously. However, epidemiologic studies showed that abut 25% of women who turned HPV DNA positive after being HPV DNA negative did develop CIN 2 or 3 within 2 years (9). Based on a review of the literature, Ostor (10) reported that 11%

FIGURE **16-1**

Low-grade (mild) cervical intraepithelial neoplasia. The epithelium is thickened and there are cytologically atypical and multinucleated cells present. In addition, many cells have a perinuclear halo (koilocytosis), a cytopathologic effect associated with a productive human papillomavirus infection. (Courtesy of Ralph Richart.)

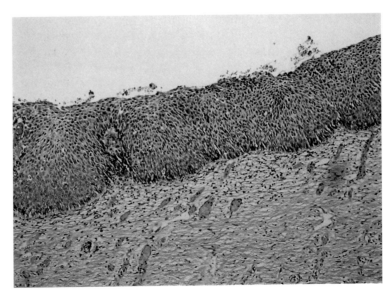

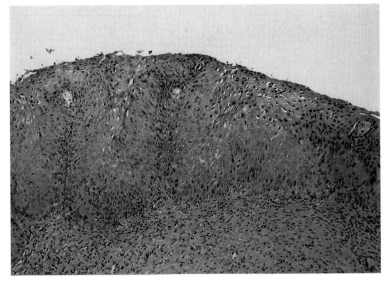

F I G U R E **16-2**

The pleomorphic cells are "undifferentiated" through the full thickness of the epithelium and there is little or no koilocytosis. This is consistent with high-grade (severe) intraepithelial neoplasia. (Courtesy of Ralph Richart.)

of CIN 1 lesions progress to CIN 3. However, as many as 57% of CIN 1 lesions do regress.

The progression from mild to more severe neoplasia is often a long-lasting process and the average time for CIN 3 to turn into invasive carcinoma has been calculated to be 10 years. More than 30% of carcinomas in situ, when left untreated, turn into invasive carcinoma after 13 years or longer (11).

HPV identification by polymerase chain reaction (PCR) and typing by hybridization are being tested as tools for identifying lesions that are prone to progress (12). Still the techniques are laborious and the validity is not optimal. Moreover, it is not possible to foresee which cofactors influence the behavior of the lesions.

Precursor lesions in the cervical epithelium, nowadays mostly known as intraepithelial neoplasia, were earlier classified as dysplasia and carcinoma in situ (i.e., mild dysplasia = CIN 1, moderate dysplasia = CIN 2, and severe dysplasia–cancer in situ = CIN 3).

A simplified terminology for cytology was proposed in 1988 (Bethesda nomenclature), namely, low- and high-grade intraepithelial lesions (SILs). Low-grade SILs include HPV infection and CIN 1 (i.e., generally virulent infection). High-grade SILs correspond to preinvasive epithelial lesions. Uncharacteristic atypia that cannot be categorized among these grades is instead referred to as *atypical squamous cells of uncertain significance* (ASCUS) (13).

It should be borne in mind that precancerous lesions do not give rise to any symptoms, contrary to invasive cervical cancer, which initially causes postcoital vaginal bleeding.

Natural History of HPV Infection and Intraepithelial Neoplasia

In 1932, carcinoma in situ was identified as a precursor of invasive cervical cancer (14), but not until the 1950s was moderate intraepithelial neoplasia regarded as a precursor of in situ carcinoma. DNA ploidy analysis helped establish the biologic continuum (15).

With exfoliative cervical cytology used as a screening tool, CIN has been detected in an increasing number of women (16). All screening program data show that CIN 1 and 2 are more prevalent than CIN 3, and CIN 3 is more prevalent than invasive carcinoma. The age at the maximal incidence of CIN 1 and 2 is about 25 years; of CIN 3, about 35 years; and of invasive carcinoma, between 50 and 65 years (17).

Knowledge of the natural history of CIN derives from follow-up studies of untreated women or patients lost for follow-up and also through mathematical models based on results of screening programs (18). Studies of more than 6000 women with CIN have elucidated the natural history. One drawback with studies of untreated women is that a biopsy has to be obtained to get a reliable initial diagnosis. Such a minor surgical procedure may either totally remove the lesion or change the natural history. According to studies on women in whom the only intervention was the target biopsy, approximately 25% of the precancerous lesions progress, whereas the remaining lesions either persist or regress (19). Studies of women who were lost for follow-up showed higher rates of progression (about 50%) (20).

In spite of treatment, the risk of developing new lesions remains. Kolstad and Klem (21) found a recurrence rate of 3.3% within 5 to 15 years among more than 1000 women with carcinoma in situ treated by cone biopsy or hysterectomy. However, McIndoe et al (22) observed a much higher recurrence rate (20%) after the same treatment modalities in a similar number of patients.

Screening Tool

A Pap smear may indicate that some part of the cervical or vaginal epithelium is atypical. For a proper diagnosis, it is essential to identify and evaluate the area of abnormality by means of a colposcope and also to obtain target biopsy specimens for histopathology. Moreover, with the colposcope it is important to localize the borders of the TZ, especially the proximal borderline (SCJ).

It is essential to point out that screening by Pap smears may not help to prevent adenocarcinoma. This type of cancer, which derives from columnar epithelium, is said not to pass through a long-standing phase similar to the one of squamous cervical carcinoma. Moreover, columnar cells do not exfoliate as easily as squamous and metaplastic cells.

Diagnostic Tools

Certain diagnostic tools improve the accuracy of the identification.

Colposcopy

Adequate magnification and a good light source are required for identification of the TZ. The colposcope should have a magnifying capacity of 10 to 40 times.

Capillary Patterns

Through magnification, various capillary patterns may be distinguished. Neoplastic areas often contain vessels with a punctate, mosaic, or atypical formation. To sum up, the coarser the capillaries, the wider the distance between them, and the more atypical the vessels, the more probable is the presence of severe precancerous lesions. Micropapillary HPV lesions also contain capillaries but the pattern is symmetrical and orderly, forming hairpin loops and corkscrew formations.

Surface Configuration

It is possible to identify lesions because of their surface structure. There may be micropapillary or microconvoluted areas, with various degrees of hyperkeratosis. The lesions are generally sharply demarcated.

Acetic Acid Test

Application of 5% acetic acid will induce a whitish color and swelling of atypical epithelium due to a relatively high DNA content of the abnormal cells (high nuclear-cytoplasmic ratio). The surface configuration and the margins will be distinctly outlined. There is some correlation between the degree of whiteness and swelling and the level of histopathologic abnormality.

Iodine Staining

Fully differentiated squamous epithelium of the cervix and the vagina stains dark brown with iodine. This effect is due to the presence of glycogen in the superficial epithelial cells. Because of the absence of glycogen, columnar and immature epithelia remain colorless. Moreover, in papillomavirus-infected epithelium as well as in neoplastic epithelium, the glycogen content is reduced or absent. When 5% iodine solution (Lugol's solution) is applied, such tissue will become yellowish and sharply demarcated.

If microinvasive or invasive cervical cancer is present, neither acetic acid nor iodine is of any help. Instead, the presence of severely atypical vessels, uneven surface, and hemorrhage would confirm the diagnosis.

Target Biopsies and Cervical Curettage

A positive outcome of the acetic acid and iodine tests represents an indication for subsequent histologic evaluation of biopsy specimens.

Samples should be obtained from areas appearing most abnormal. The ectocervical area is rather painless and analgesia is not required. Generally, biopsy specimens can be obtained without the complication of uncontrolled hemorrhage.

However, to obtain reliable material at cervical curettage, it is necessary to have a potent analgesia, because the endocervix is very sensitive, in contrast to the ectocervix.

Different opinions exist concerning the need for cervical curettage in all young women. A reason against such a diagnostic interference is the assumption that all lesions appear in the TZ, and if this area is situated entirely outside the external cervical os, there is no need for curettage. Moreover, the material obtained by curettage is often scarce and seldom includes tissue from the cervical crypts. A reason in favor of performing endocervical curettage in all women with high-grade lesions, as determined by Pap smear, is the fact that the rate of adenocarcinoma seems to have increased lately and this malignancy may develop in the columnar epithelium of the cervical canal (23).

Treatment

Since there are currently no methods to determine which of the approximately 10% to 20% of all precancerous lesions will progress into invasive carcinoma, it is obvious that a certain number of patients will be treated for safety reasons. There are three key issues for the clinician to address:

1. A microinvasive cancer must be ruled out.
2. Will treatment diminish the risk of developing cervical cancer in the future?
3. The reproductive situation of the woman must be taken into consideration.

The clinician must have adequate knowledge of the colposcopic appearance of the cervix and the natural history of CIN.

An important concept to keep in mind is that CIN is confined to the TZ and the whole of this area is at risk despite the presence of a limited lesion. Thus, the entire TZ, including the atypical cervical epithelium, should be eradicated to prevent development of invasive cancer. However, it is very important that treatment be carried out with caution, especially in women of childbearing age.

All methods of treatment are nearly equivalent in outcome and approximately 90% of the patients are cured (24,25). The recurrence rate ranges from 10% to 30% if CIN is present at the margin of the excision (21,22).

Treatment should be based on two principles:

1. Destruction. Destruction of the TZ is determined on the basis of well-documented biopsy and often endocervical curettage findings. The destructive methods used are cryosurgery, electrocoagulation, and laser vaporization.
2. Excision. Excision of the TZ is either performed after diagnosis has been made by biopsies and cervical curettage or as a simultaneous diagnostic and therapeutic approach. The advantage of excisional treatment is that the whole tissue can be histopathologically evaluated. Excision can be performed by laser, by diathermy, or by conventional knife. To a great extent, the latter method has been replaced by the outpatient procedures. Sometimes hysterectomy is performed, mainly when there are other reasons to eradicate the uterus, for example, in women with fibroids or in older women in whom the TZ has reached the internal os of the cervix uteri.

Excision rather than destruction should be performed

1. When the area of atypical epithelium is very large (also when CIN 2 only is suspected), because in a large area it is more likely that some part contains severe neoplasia.
2. When the SCJ is localized in the cervical canal and not visible with colposcopy.
3. When the lesion corresponds to CIN 3. An exception to this rule is permitted if the atypical area is very small and the woman is young ($\leq$35 years).

All women who have had CIN 3 should be checked regularly after the lesions have been eradicated because they still have an increased risk for malignant development in the lower genital tract (21,22).

The depth of treatment from the ectocervical surface as well as from the endocervical lining should always be at least 5mm. This is because the precancerous epithelium may penetrate 2mm into endocervical crypts that protrude into the stromal tissue beneath the epithelial lining, which has a depth of 0.5mm (26).

Cryotherapy

Cryotherapy was the first outpatient modality for destructive treatment of CIN (27). The advantages of this technique are the low cost and no need of anesthesia. One disadvantage is a profuse long-standing discharge and another, more important, is the risk of inaccurate treatment. The depth of destruction cannot be controlled in the same way as with the CO_2 laser or the excisional diathermia loop. Cryosurgery should be used only if the entire TZ is situated on the ectocervix and there are minor lesions only, and if the cryosurgery is preceded by satisfactory colposcopically directed biopsies. The entire TZ, including the atypical area, should be covered by the probe tip. A double freeze-thaw cycle is preferable. The destruction should reach at least 5mm beyond the surface. If the lesion or TZ extends toward the cervical canal, cryosurgery should be avoided.

CO_2 Laser

One advantage of the CO_2 laser technique is that the equipment is connected to a colposcope and thus offers a microsurgical procedure (28). Moreover, the laser can be used either for destruction or for excision, when tissue is required for complete histopathologic evaluation. The laser has the advantage of allowing a colposcopically tailored approach with minimal injury of the surrounding normal tissue. As a matter of fact, if the smallest spot size is used, the zone of thermal injury outside the excision is exceptionally narrow, which makes this technique outstanding compared to all other techniques except use of the cold knife.

The treatment is an outpatient procedure and generally requires local anesthetics only. However, owing to local traditions the treatment is quite often performed with general anesthesia. The disadvantage with this laser technique is primarily the cost of the equipment. An effective smoke evacuator system is required.

Loop Excision

The introduction of diathermia loop excision has resulted in a substantial shift from laser excision (29). The prime reason for this is that loop excision is quicker and easier to perform for unskilled physicians. The loop treatment is often more painful than laser treatment, probably because the conduction of heat into the surrounding tissues may be higher than that during laser treatment. As with laser treatment the smoke has to be evacuated.

Primarily loop excision was to replace destructive therapies, to obtain a large piece of tissue for analysis. Currently, loop excision is often used not only for superficial tissue removal but also for higher cone biopsies as well. However, unlike the laser procedure, all tissue cannot be removed in one piece. Instead, two or more pieces are obtained and the specimen including the lining of the cervical canal is taken with a smaller loop.

The loop has been used as a "see and treat" modality. To obtain a diagnosis and to treat at the same time, the procedure is often performed at the time of the first consultation for an atypical Pap smear. However, there is a risk of overtreatment with this approach.

Cold-Knife Cone Biopsy

For many years, a large cone biopsy by means of a knife has been a routine to treat carcinoma in situ. Although it is mostly replaced by the modern outpatient techniques, it still has a role in the management of certain selected patients. Thus, cold-knife excision may be preferable when a deep cone specimen with intact margins is required, for example, when microinvasion or adenocarcinoma is suspected.

Treatment Complications

Complications can be divided into acute and long-term side effects and are rather similar regardless of the treatment method. All techniques except cryosurgery can cause bleeding, which requires intervention in about 3% of the patients. Cervical stenosis may affect a few women, more often after cryosurgery compared to other modalities. Treatment using any technique in an estrogen-deficient woman (postpartum or postmenopausal) can cause cervical stenosis. Estrogen replacement is advisable to avoid such a complication.

There is a slight risk of premature delivery in women who have undergone a high cone biopsy (30). It is of utmost importance to take into consideration the fertility aspect in connection with the degree of abnormality and the size of the lesion, and to remove the smallest possible volume of tissue along the cervical canal.

REFERENCES

1. Boffetta P, Parkin DM. Cancer in developing countries. *CA Cancer J Clin* 1994;44:81–90.

2. Ferenczy A, Winkler B. Cervical intraepithelial neoplasia. In: Kurman RJ, ed. *Blaustein´s pathology of the female genital tract.* 3rd ed. New York: Springer, 1987:184–191.

3. Hakama M. Trends in the incidence of cervical cancer in the Nordic countries. In: Magnus K, ed. *Trends in cancer incidence.* Washington, DC: Hemisphere, 1992:279–292.

4. Munoz N, Bosch FX, Shah KV, Meheus A, eds. The epidemiology of human papillomavirus and cervical cancer. *IARC Sci Publ* 1992;119.

5. Pecoraro G, Lee M, Morgan D, Defendi V. Evolution of in vitro transformation and tumorigenesis of HPV 16 and HPV 18 immortalized primary cervical epithelial cells. *Am J Pathol* 1991;138:1–8.

6. Maiman M, Fruchter RG, Guy L, et al. Human immunodeficiency virus infection and invasive cervical carcinoma. *Cancer* 1993;71:402–406.

7. Brinton LA, Reeves WC, Brenes MM, et al. Oral contraceptive use and risk of invasive cervical cancer. *Int J Epidemiol* 1990;19:4–11.

8. Singer A, Monaghan JM. *Lower genital tract precancer: colposcopy, pathology and treatment.* Boston: Blackwell Science, 1994.

9. Koutsky LA, Holmes KK, Critchlow CW, et al. A cohort study of the risk of cervical intraepithelial neoplasia grade 2 or 3 in relation to papillomavirus infection. *N Engl J Med* 1992;327: 1272–1278.

10. Ostor AG. Natural history of cervical intraepithelial neoplasia: a critical review. *Int J Gynecol Pathol* 1993;12:186–192.

11. Petersen O. Spontaneous course of cervical precancerous conditions. *Am J Obstet Gynecol* 1956;72:1063–1071.

12. Lörincz AT, Reid R, Jenson AB, et al. Human papillomavirus infection of the cervix: relative risk associations of 15 common anogenital types. *Obstet Gynecol* 1992;79:328–337.

13. Kurman RJ, Henson DE, Herbst AL, et al. Interim guidelines for the management of abnormal cervical cytology. *JAMA* 1994;271:1866–1869.

14. Broder AC. Carcinoma in situ contrasted with benign penetrating epithelium. *JAMA* 1932;99: 1670–1674.

15. Fu YS, Reagan JW, Richart RM. Definition of cervical precursors. *Gynecol Oncol* 1981;12S: 220–231.

16. Carson HJ, DeMay RM. The mode ages of women with cervical dysplasia. *Obstet Gynecol* 1993;82:430–434.

17. DeVesa SS, Young JL Jr, Brinton LA, Fraumeni J. Recent trends in cervix uteri cancer. *Cancer* 1989;64:2184–2190.

18. Barron BA, Cahill MD, Richart RM. A statistical model of the natural history of cervical neoplastic disease: the duration of carcinoma in situ. *Gynecol Oncol* 1978;6:196–205.

19. Kinlen LJ, Spriggs AI. Women with positive cervical smears but without surgical intervention. *Lancet* 1978;2:463–465.

20. Spriggs AI. Natural history of cervical dysplasia. *Clin Obstet Gynecol* 1981;8:65–79.

21. Kolstad P, Klem W. Long-term follow-up of 1121 cases of carcinoma in situ. *Obstet Gynecol* 1976;48:125–129.

22. McIndoe WA, McLean MR, Jones RW, Mullins PR. The invasive potential of carcinoma in situ of the cervix. *Obstet Gynecol* 1984;64:451–458.

23. Miller BE, Flax SD, Arheart K, Photopulos G. The presentation of adenocarcinoma of the uterine cervix. *Cancer* 1993;72:1281–1285.

24. Benedet JL, Miller DM, Nickerson KG. Results of conservative management of cervical intraepithelial neoplasia. *Obstet Gynecol* 1992;79: 105–110.

25. Luesley DM, Cullimore J, Redman CWE. Loop diathermy of the cervical transformation zone in patients with abnormal cervical smears. *BMJ* 1990;300:1690–1693.

26. Abdul-Karim FW, Fu YS, Reagan JW, Wentz WB. Morphometric study of intraepithelial neoplasia of the uterine cervix. *Obstet Gynecol* 1982;60: 210–214.

27. Hemmingsson E, Stendahl U, Stenson S. Cryosurgical treatment of cervical intraepithelial neoplasia with follow up of 5 to 8 years. *Am J Obstet Gynecol* 1981;139:144–147.

28. Wright VS, Davies E, Riopelle MA. Laser surgery for cervical intraepithelial neoplasia: principles and results. *Am J Obstet Gynecol* 1983;145:181–184.

29. Prendiville W, Cullimore J, Norman S. Large loop excision of the transformation zone (LLETZ). A new method of management for women with cervical intraepithelial neoplasia. *Br J Obstet Gynaecol* 1989;96:1054–1060.

30. Kristensen J, Langhoff-Roos J, Wittrup M, Bock JE. Cervical conization and preterm delivery/low birth weight. A systematic review of the literature. *Acta Obstet Gynecol Scand* 1993;72:640–644.

Invasive Carcinoma of the Cervix: Evaluation

NINA EINHORN

RALPH M. RICHART

*T*he aim of the evaluation of all tumors is to establish the diagnosis, the tumor's volume, and the probability of dissemination in order to decide the appropriate therapeutic strategy. In the evaluation process, staging of the disease is important, but the strategy of therapy is not necessarily clear once the stage is established. Carcinoma of the cervix was the first tumor for which a staging procedure was proposed and decided on. In 1928 the Cancer Commission of the Health Organization of the League of Nations met to discuss the treatment of carcinoma of the cervix. When reports of treatment from different clinics were discussed, it became clear that the results could be evaluated only if they were recorded in a uniform way, and it became evident that a common language was needed, along with acceptable guidelines for diagnostic workups. In 1937 the first rules for staging procedures were published (1). The following rules, which were established at that time, are still valid today:

1. When it is doubtful to which stage a given tumor is to be allocated, the lower stage should be chosen.
2. The fact that a single tumor presents two or more of the conditions that characterize a particular stage does not affect the staging.
3. The stage of each tumor should be decided by examination before treatment, and this classification should not be altered retrospectively.
4. When one is allocating a tumor to a stage, nothing but the data established by examination should be taken into account.

A study of the evolution of the staging systems for carcinoma of the cervix reveals that the principal objectives of staging have changed over the years. Initially the aim of establishing a staging system was to facilitate the exchange of information among treatment centers to permit the greatest possible comparability. It was stated very firmly that the staging procedure should be used in all hospitals and by all physicians who treated the disease. Sophisticated methods were not available for most staging systems, and simplicity was one of the more important issues. Over the years the staging system was modified to take into account prognostic factors and to use those factors in planning treatment. The current objectives of staging is well described by the International Union Against Cancer (UICC) guidelines (2):

1. Aiding the clinician in planning treatment
2. Giving some indication of prognosis
3. Assisting in the evaluation of end results
4. Facilitating the exchange of information among treatment centers
5. Assisting in the continuing investigation of cancer

To strive for simplicity and to encourage all centers to participate in the same staging procedure, it is important to recognize that methods for establishing tumor volume and the probability of dissemination have to be limited to those that can be used by all centers dealing with invasive carcinoma of the cervix. The physical examination is essential, but it must be performed with the patient under anesthesia. The following examinations are permitted procedures to be used in staging: palpation, inspection, colposcopy, endocervical curettage, hysteroscopy, cystoscopy, proctoscopy, intravenous urography, and x-ray examinations of the lungs and the skeleton. Suspected bladder or rectal involvement should be confirmed by biopsy and histologic examination. Other procedures such as magnetic resonance imaging (MRI), lymphography, computed tomography (CT), arteriography, venography, and laparoscopy may be of value in planning therapy but may not generally be available. Their use for staging would make the interpretation of results variable. The findings derived from those procedures should not change the clinical staging (3).

Even if it is obvious that clinical staging has its pitfalls and that differences will be found between clinical staging and surgical findings, staging laparotomy has not found many advocates. The issue has been extensively discussed over the years, but surgical staging is not used in many centers nowadays (4–7). With the development of noninvasive techniques allowing better diagnosis of disseminated disease, there is really no place for surgical staging in carcinoma of the cervix. Nuclear MRI has been very well investigated as a method for establishing the volume of cervical carcinoma, and several studies found a strong correlation between MRI findings preoperatively and the volume of the tumor found during surgery (8,9). The study by Hricak (9) indicated that MRI is especially useful in determining tumor volume in patients whose tumor diameter exceeds 4 cm. A study performed by Ryberg et al (10) concluded that MRI estimates tumor size better than CT. These investigators found a poor correlation between International Fed-

eration of Gynecology and Obstetrics (FIGO) stages and MRI findings for cancers in the lower clinical stages but a significant correlation when the tumor invaded the parametrial tissue and side wall (10). Compared to MRI, CT appears to be a better diagnostic tool in recognizing lymph node metastasis. A positive predictive value as high as 96% for CT detecting lymph node metastasis has been documented (11).

Over the years there has been considerable controversy over the definition of *microinvasive carcinoma* (12,13), with the FIGO classification swinging from a depth-of-penetration definition to a volume-based definition back to depth of penetration. In the present FIGO classification, *microinvasion* is defined as a lesion in which neoplastic epithelium invades the stroma in one or more places to a depth of 5 mm or less below the basement membrane of the epithelium and is no wider than 7 mm (Figs. 17-1 and 17-2). Microinvasive carcinoma can be suspected but not definitively diagnosed by punch biopsy to rule out invasive cancer of greater dimensions and definitively make a diagnosis of microinvasion. Lesions that are 3 mm or less in greatest depth of penetration are classified as stage Ia1; those with 3.1 to 5.0 mm of stromal invasion are classified as stage Ia2. It is important to note that the definition of microinvasive cancer was derived empirically from observations that patients with invasion to a depth of less than 3.1 mm are at an extremely low risk of developing metastases (14). In fact, the risk is virtually nonexistent when invasion is 1 mm or less; the risk of metastatic disease is small when

FIGURE **17-1**

Microinvasive cervical carcinoma.

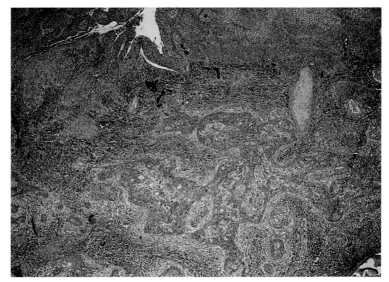

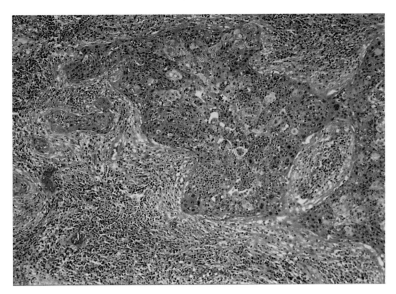

F I G U R E **17-2**

Frankly invasive squamous cell cancer.

invasion is between 2 and 3 mm, but invasion can occur. The reason patients with microinvasive cancer can be treated more conservatively than patients with frank invasion is because the risk of radical treatment exceeds the risk of metastases in patients whose lesions measure less than 3.1 mm in greatest depth of penetration.

Although the relationship between depth of penetration and risk of metastasis is clear-cut, the same cannot be said for the relationship between lymph-vascular space involvement and metastatic disease. Although the percentage of cases with lymph-vascular space involvement increases with depth of penetration, the clinical significance of lymph-vascular space involvement is still controversial, with some authors finding such involvement to be an adverse prognostic indicator and others finding no influence on prognosis. Nonetheless, the prevailing opinion is that patients who have demonstrable lymph-vascular space involvement should not be classified as having stage Ia disease (15).

Burghardt and Holzer (16) championed the importance of tumor volume in defining microinvasive cancer and preferred to measure not only depth of penetration but also volume by serially sectioning cone specimens. Others (17) suggested that the lateral spread of the microinvasive cancer can be substituted for volume measurements based on serial sections. Although there are data to support using a volume measurement for prognostic purposes, the methodology is time-consuming

and difficult to apply on a routine basis, and few laboratories use such procedures for diagnosis.

Because microinvasive carcinoma is associated with a low risk of metastatic disease in the absence of lymph-vascular space involvement (and even under those conditions, the risk is low) and because larger numbers of young women are being diagnosed with this condition, it is becoming increasingly common to treat women who wish to become pregnant in the future by conization alone. Although very long-term follow-up data are not available, there is sufficient information to recommend a less radical procedure than conization for women in the reproductive-age group who wish to preserve their childbearing capacity.

The significance of tumor volume in the staging of cervical cancer is controversial. Pierquin et al (18) addressed this issue and claimed that dimensions of the tumor have a major prognostic impact and that stage IIb should be subdivided into small or proximal lesions in immediate proximity to the cervix both in the vagina and in the parametrium, and larger, more distal lesions beyond the upper third of the vagina or the medial third of the parametrium. They also suggested the division of stage IIb into involvement of one versus both parametria. Investigators at the M. D. Anderson Hospital in Houston also suggested substaging within the FIGO classification based on the volume of cancer. The main criticism was that barrel-shaped lesions were ignored (18). Other

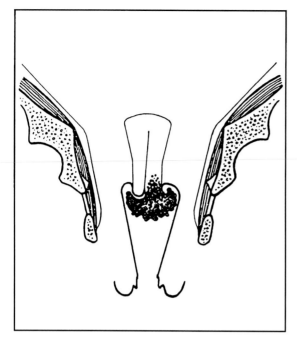

FIGURE **17-3**

Stage Ib, involving cervix.

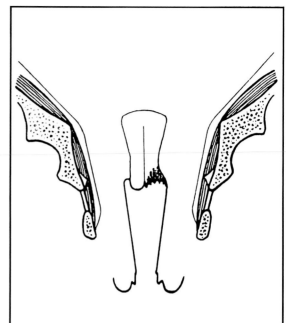

FIGURE **17-4**

Stage IIa, involving the left fornix.

TABLE **17-1**

Cervical Cancer Staging (1995 FIGO System)

Stage I. The carcinoma is strictly confined to the cervix (extension to the corpus should be disregarded).
    Stage Ia. Invasive cancer identified only microscopically. All gross lesions, even with superficial invasion, are stage Ib cancers.
        Invasion is limited to measured stromal invasion with a maximum depth of 5 mm and no wider than 7 mm.*
      Stage Ia1. Measured invasion of stroma no greater than 3 mm in depth and no wider than 7 mm.
      Stage Ia2. Measured invasion of stroma greater than 3 mm and no greater than 5 mm in depth and no wider than 7 mm.
    Stage Ib. Clinical lesions confined to the cervix or preclinical lesions greater than stage Ia lesions.
      Stage Ib1. Clinical lesions no greater than 4 cm.
      Stage Ib2. Clinical lesions greater than 4 cm.
Stage II. The carcinoma extends beyond the cervix, but has not extended to the pelvic wall. The carcinoma involves the vagina, but not as far as the lower third.
    Stage IIa. No obvious parametrial involvement.
    Stage IIb. Obvious parametrial involvement.
Stage III. The carcinoma has extended to the pelvic wall. On rectal examination there is no cancer-free space between the tumor and the pelvic wall. The tumor involves the lower third of the vagina. All patients with hydronephrosis or nonfunctioning kidney should be included, unless it is known to be due to other causes.
    Stage IIIa. No extension to the pelvic wall, but involvement of the lower third of the vagina.
    Stage IIIb. Extension to the pelvic wall or hydronephrosis or nonfunctioning kidney.
Stage IV. The carcinoma has extended beyond the true pelvis or has clinically involved the mucosa of the bladder or rectum.
    Stage IVa. Spread of the growth to adjacent organs.
    Stage IVb. Spread to distant organs.

*The depth of invasion should not be more than 5 mm taken from the base of the epithelium, either surface or glandular, from which it originates. Vascular space involvement, either venous or lymphatic, should not alter the staging.

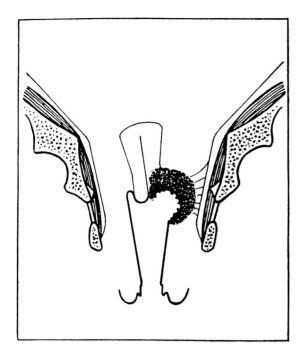

FIGURE **17-5**
Stage IIb, involving the left parametrium.

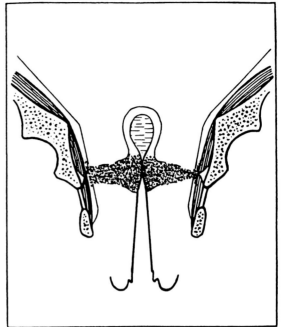

FIGURE **17-7**
Stage IIIb, involving both pelvic walls.

FIGURE **17-6**
Stage IIIa, involving more than two thirds of the vagina.

FIGURE **17-8**
Stage IVa, involving the bladder.

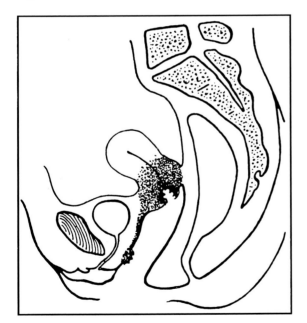

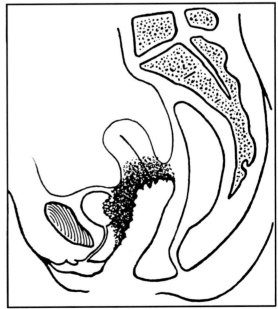

studies documented significant differences in the recurrence rate between patients with a tumor smaller than 3 cm and those with a tumor larger than 3 cm in diameter (19). It has also been documented that the incidence of lymph node metastasis in stage I disease is associated with tumor size (20–23). The same applies for stage IIa disease where survival rates for patients with a tumor smaller in size than 1 cm and those with a tumor 5 to 8 cm are 80%

and 60%, respectively (24). There is no doubt that the prognostic significance of tumor volume has to be taken into consideration in management strategies and therapeutic planning.

Invasive squamous cell carcinomas can be subclassified according to their histologic type. Wentz and Reagan (25) classified these neoplasms into large-cell keratinizing, large-cell nonkeratinizing, and small-cell nonkeratinizing types, and reported that there was a survival difference between these types, with the best survival being associated with the large-cell nonkeratinizing group and the poorest survival with the small-cell nonkeratinizing group. More recently, in the World Health Organization (WHO) classification, the small-cell neuroendocrine-type tumors were placed in a separate category and the remaining tumors were subdivided between keratinizing and nonkeratinizing. Another classification system— the so-called Broder system (26)—divides squamous cell cancers into grades 1 (well differentiated) to 3 (poorly differentiated). As anticipated, there is still controversy concerning the degree to which Broder's differentiation can be used to predict clinical outcome. One of the problems in all histologic classification systems is the high degree of variability among pathologists in assigning tumors to the various grades and subtypes. Indeed, intraobserver variability may be so great as to preclude using histologic subclassification systems to determine therapy or to predict outcome.

The 1995 FIGO clinical staging system (Table 17-1) is based on distinct anatomic differences (Figs. 17-3 to 17-8). To be able to perform satisfactory clinical staging, it is of vital importance that the examination be done by an experienced physician and with anesthesia.

After the staging procedure is performed, the decision regarding treatment has to be made. In the following process, not only results of other noninvasive methods such as CT, lymphography, and MRI, but also all other factors such as the microscopic appearance of the tumor and the patient's age and general condition have to be taken into consideration.

REFERENCES

1. Heyman J, ed. *Annual report on the results of radiotherapy in cancer of the uterine cervix*, vol. 1. Stockholm, 1937.

2. Spress LB, Bealers OH, Hermanek P, et al. *International Union Against Cancer: illustrated guide to the classification of malignant tumours*. Heidelberg: Springer, 1982.

3. Pettersson F, ed. *Annual report on the results of treatment in gynecological cancer*, vol. 22. Stockholm, 1995.

4. Brunschwig A. Surgical treatment of carcinoma of the cervix stages I and II. *AJR Am J Roentgenol* 1968;102:147–151.

5. Kaideman MT, Bosch A. Is staging laparotomy in cervical cancer justifiable? *Int J Radiat Oncol Biol Phys* 1977;2:1235–1238.

6. Averette HE, Dudan R, Ford JH. Exploratory celiotomy for surgical staging of cervical cancer. *Am J Obstet Gynecol* 1972;113:1090–1096.

7. Wharton JT, Jones HS III, Day TGJ, et al. Preirradiation celiotomy and extended field irradiation for invasive carcinoma of the cervix. *Obstet Gynecol* 1977;49:333–338.

8. Burghardt E, Hofmann HMH, Ebner F, et al. Magnetic resonance imaging in cervical cancer: a basis for objective classification. *Gynecol Oncol* 1989;33:61–67.

9. Hricak H. Cancer of the uterus: the value of MR imaging in primary and recurrent disease and its potential impact on patient management. Dissertation, Karolinska Institute, Stockholm, 1992.

10. Ryberg M, Blomqvist L, Göranson H, Hellström AC, et al. A study comparing the tumour extension shown by MRI and CT with the clinical staging of cervical carcinoma according to FIGO. Presented at the meeting of the International Gynecologic Cancer Society, Philadelphia, 1995. Abstract 223.

11. Piver MS, Barlow JJ. Para-aortic lymphadenectomy, aortic node biopsy, and aortic lymphangiography in staging patients with advanced cervical cancer. *Cancer* 1973;32:367–370.

12. Benson WL, Norris HJ. A critical review of the frequency of lymph node metastasis and death from microinvasive carcinoma of the cervix. *Obstet Gynecol* 1977;49:632–636.

13. Christophersen WM, Parker JE. Microinvasive carcinoma of the uterine cervix: a clinical-pathological study. *Cancer* 1964;17:1123–1131.

14. Averette HE, Nelson JH, Ng AP, et al. Diagnosis and management of microinvasive (stage IA) carcinoma of the uterine cervix. *Cancer* 1976; 38:414–425.

15. Wright TC, Ferenczy A, Kurman RJ. Carcinoma and other tumors of the cervix. In: Kurman RJ,

ed. *Blaustein's pathology of the female genital tract.* 4th ed. New York: Springer, 1994:279–326.

16. Burghardt E, Holzer E. Diagnosis and treatment of microinvasive carcinoma of the cervix uteri. *Obstet Gynecol* 1977;49:641.

17. Sedlis A, Sall S, Tsukada Y, et al. Microinvasive carcinoma of the uterine cervix: a clinical-pathologic study. *Am J Obstet Gynecol* 1979;133:64–74.

18. Pierquin BK, Wilson JF, Chassagne D, eds. *Modern brachytherapy.* 2nd ed. New York: Masson, 1987.

19. Piver MS, Chung WS. Prognostic significance of cervical lesion size and pelvic node metastases in cervical carcinoma. *Obstet Gynecol* 1975;46:507.

20. Fuller AF, Elliott N, Kosloff BSC, et al. Determinants in increased risk for recurrence in patients undergoing radical hysterectomy for stage IB and IIA carcinoma of the cervix. *Gynecol Oncol* 1989;33:34–39.

21. Chung CK, Nahhas WA, Stryker JA, et al. Analysis of factors contributing to treatment failures in stage IB and IIA carcinoma of the cervix. *Am J Obstet Gynecol* 1980;138:550–556.

22. Hopkins MP, Morley GW. Stage IB squamous cell cancer of the cervix: clinicopathologic features related to survival. *Am J Obstet Gynecol* 1991;164:1520–1529.

23. Einhorn N, Patek E, Sjöberg B. Outcome of different treatment modalities in cervix carcinoma stage IB and IIA. *Cancer* 1985;55:949–955.

24. Kovalic JJ, Perez CA, Grigsby PW, et al. The effect of volume of disease in patients with carcinoma of the uterine cervix. *Int J Radiat Oncol Biol Phys* 1991;21:905–910.

25. Wentz WB, Reagan JW. Survival in cervical cancer with respect to cell type. *Cancer* 1959;12:384–388.

26. Broders AC. Squamous-cell epithelioma of the lip: a study of 537 cases. *JAMA* 1920;74:656–664.

CHAPTER 18

Treatment of Invasive Carcinoma of the Cervix

NINA EINHORN
A. DENNY DEPETRILLO

Treatment of carcinoma of the cervix has undergone refinement during the years but the main methods still used are surgery and radiotherapy. Chemotherapy is usually reserved for palliative treatment but investigative approaches using combined-modality regimes are currently being studied.

Freund, in 1878, made the first attempt to treat cervical carcinoma with surgery, but today we recognize Wertheim as the father of radical surgery. He performed his first surgery in 1898, the same year that radium was discovered by the Curies. Because surgery had extremely high mortality and morbidity rates, with the discovery of radium, radiation therapy became the accepted treatment for cervical carcinoma during the first 50 years of the century. With improvements in anesthesia as well as general surgical care, higher success rates and fewer complications have been achieved by surgery and surgery has become an important part of the therapy. As a rule surgery is reserved for patients with limited disease, especially younger patients for whom it is important to maintain ovarian function.

Radiotherapy can be used for treatment of all patients and stages, and as a result, the selection of treatment depends on the stage, age, and general condition of the patient.

For women with early-stage disease, guidelines for treatment include the pathology and the morbidity of the treatment regime. For women with advanced-stage disease, decision-making factors include the use of radiotherapy and perhaps combined-treatment modalities.

The pattern of spread of cervical cancer has been well studied. This tumor spreads primarily by local extension and through lymphatic channels. Hematogenous spread seldom occurs. Because of the high tendency to involve the lymph nodes relatively early in the course of the disease, the primary nodes (external iliac, hypogastric, paracervical, and obturator) have to be treated either with surgery or with radiotherapy. It is only in stage Ia1 disease where the incidence of lymph node metastasis is so low that treatment to the pelvic nodes can be avoided (Fig. 18-1).

Early Disease

Stage Ia

Stage Ia represents a lesion where invasion is identified only microscopically. Invasion is limited to stromal invasion with a maximum depth of 5 mm and no wider than 7 mm. Vascular space involvement, either venous or lymphatic, does not alter the staging.

Stage Ia1

Stage Ia1 is a condition where stromal invasion is not more than 3 mm in depth and not wider than 7 mm. This diagnosis should be based on cone biopsy, not punch biopsy, with careful

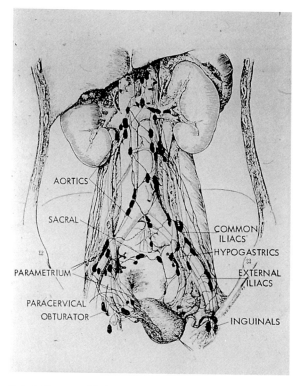

F I G U R E **18-1**

The pelvic and para-aortic lymph nodes.

pathologic evaluation of the cone specimen. Several studies documented that such invasion presents virtually no risk of lymph node metastasis and the trend during recent years has moved toward conservative therapy with treatment options being simple hysterectomy or conization of the cervix, depending on the patient's desire to preserve fertility (1–7). Several studies now confirmed that conization is effective (8–13) but it is important to note that conization should be done under colposcopic guidance and that the margin of the cone specimen should be free of atypical change.

Vascular space invasion is not included in the International Federation of Gynecology and Obstetrics (FIGO) staging of carcinoma of the cervix. The prognostic significance of lymph vascular involvement in stage Ia1 carcinoma of the cervix remains controversial (14–17). For this reason, conservative treatment in patients with evident vascular space invasion is generally not accepted.

There is no definition as yet of microinvasive adenocarcinoma (adenocarcinoma of the cervix) and as a result conservative treatment of early adenocarcinoma of the cervix requires further confirmation.

Stage Ia2

The FIGO staging system for cervical carcinoma adopted in 1994 defines stage Ia2 as stromal invasion of more than 3mm, but not more than 5mm and not wider than 7mm. The frequency of lymph node metastasis for patients with invasion of 3.1 to 5.0mm collected from several studies indicates that the risk of pelvic lymph node metastasis ranges from 4% to 10% (2,6,12,15). With this in mind, treatment options included modified radical hysterectomy with bilateral pelvic node dissection or primary radiation therapy.

A new method of conservative treatment in patients who have a strong desire to preserve fertility is under investigation at several centers. Laparoscopic pelvic lymphadenectomy with vaginal trachelectomy has been pioneered by Dargent et al (18) and supported by others (19,20), with satisfactory results. In the future, trachelectomy and laparoscopic lymphadenectomy may be used for treatment in this select group of women, even with early stage Ib disease.

Stages Ib and IIa

By the FIGO staging system definition, stage Ib includes lesions confined to the cervix or preclinical lesions greater than stage Ia lesions. In stage IIa the lesion involves the vagina, but not as far as the lower third, and there is no obvious parametrial involvement. Patients with this entity can be treated by either radical hysterectomy and bilateral pelvic node dissection or radiation therapy, with similar results. Selection should be based on size of lesion, age, preservation of ovarian function, habitus of the patient, and expertise available in the cancer center. The annual report on the results of treatment of gynecologic cancer (21) shows that the incidence of stage I disease has increased from 23% in the period 1950 to 1954 to 38% in 1982 to 1986. During the period 1986 to 1989, 43% of patients with stage I disease were treated by surgery alone, 17% by radiotherapy alone, and 13% by a combination of radiation and surgery. These results include both stage Ia and Ib disease. Very few randomized trials have compared radiation therapy and radical surgery in patients with cervical cancer of various stages, and as a consequence our knowledge is mostly based on retrospective data. Most of the randomized studies showed comparable survival rates for treatment of stage Ib disease with either surgery or radiation therapy (22–25). Some historical control studies—not randomized—showed superiority of combined therapy over radiotherapy alone (26,27).

Proper selection of patients with stage Ib and IIa disease depends on the factors mentioned above but the most important indicator for selection is the volume of the tumor. Some authors consider the limit for radical surgery to be a cervical tumor 3 cm in diameter (28,29). Some reports indicate that careful observation during radiotherapy for bulky disease in stage Ib or IIa can contribute to a proper decision in adding surgery to the treatment (30–33).

Patients with small lesions in stage Ib or IIa disease are mostly treated by radical hysterectomy and in select patients, a modified radical hysterectomy and bilateral pelvic node dissection. According to a recent study by Kinney et al (34), patients with a tumor size less than 2 cm and no tumor emboli in vascular spaces may be treated with modified hysterectomy.

Radiotherapy for early invasive carcinoma of the cervix is differentiated according to stage. For stage Ia1 and some patients with stage Ia2 disease, radiotherapy consists of intracavitary brachytherapy. For stages Ib and IIa, treatment should consist of external-beam therapy and brachytherapy.

The North American school favors treatment by either surgery or radiation therapy but rarely both. However, some European centers such as the Radiumhemmet and the Gustave-Roussy Institut employ combined therapy for large-volume tumors.

In summary, patients with FIGO stage Ib or IIa disease may be treated by either radiotherapy or surgery or on occasion by combined treatment. Selection of proper patients is crucial and the most important factor in selection is the volume of the tumor. With these selection criteria, survival rates of 70% to 85% are expected.

Surgical Procedure

Modifications in the surgical treatment of early invasive carcinoma of the cervix (stages Ia2, Ib, and IIa) have taken place throughout the years since Wertheim first described the procedure in 1898. Pelvic lymph node dissection was not included in his original description but was pioneered by Meigs in 1944. The procedure of choice today is either a radical or a modified radical hysterectomy including bilateral pelvic node dissection. Modification of the radicalness of the procedure depends on the amount of parametrium removed and the posterior extent of dissection on the uterosacral ligaments. This varies in extent according to the philosophy of the operating surgeon. Nevertheless, the magnitude of bladder and bowel dysfunction following radical hysterectomy depends on parasympathetic denervation, which increases with the amount of tissue removed. In selected patients, a radical vaginal procedure is done depending on the physical habitus of the patient and the pelvic lymphadenectomy technique. Simple hysterectomy is never an option for patients with invasive carcinoma of the cervix because of the inherent risk of a "cutthrough" procedure. Patients who have undergone a simple hysterectomy for presumed nonmalignant conditions and are found to have invasive cancer are usually treated with postoperative radiation therapy.

Pelvic lymphadenectomy always accompanies the radical hysterectomy approach. A complete pelvic lymphadenectomy usually includes removal of the paracervical, obturator, internal iliac, and external iliac nodes to the common iliac chain. Some centers include the para-aortic and common iliac nodes with their initial dissection. Others treat these last two segments surgically only if the lower nodes are involved with tumor. There is controversy at the present time regarding whether excision of grossly involved lymph nodes improves local control or whether the procedure should be abandoned if grossly positive nodes are found (35,36). Laparoscopic lymphadenectomy in the management of cervical cancer is currently gaining favor and acceptance (19,20,37). This is either combined with a laparoscopic radical hysterectomy or a radical vaginal trachelectomy or hysterectomy. Indeed, the role of laparoscopy in gynecologic oncologic surgery is now being defined, with further indications for its role being accepted as investigative studies are completed.

Complications of Radical Hysterectomy

The mortality rate is less than 1%. More serious complications include ureteral fistulae (1%–2%), pulmonary embolism (1%–2%), small-bowel obstruction (1%), and vesicovaginal fistulae (<1%). Wound infection can occur in less than 5% of patients. Hypertonic dysfunction of the bladder can be seen in up to 20% of patients depending on the extent of the parametrial dissection. Obstipation of the bowel is seen in 5% of patients, the morbidity again depending on the amount of dissection (38–40).

Postoperative Radiation after Surgery

High-risk patients primarily treated with radical hysterectomy often undergo postoperative radiation. High-risk factors include positive pelvic nodes, positive surgical margins, involvement of the paracervical tissue, increasing lesion size, deeper stromal invasion, lymphatic-vascular invasion, and unfavorable histopathologic type (41).

The value of postoperative pelvic irradiation for positive pelvic nodes is still controversial. The pelvic recurrence rate is reduced but survival rates have not been affected. Morrow (42) found no difference in survival when the number of positive nodes was three or less. Other authors (43) found significantly higher survival rates after radiotherapy in microscopically positive nodes. There seems to be agreement regarding the role of postoperative radiation therapy in high-risk patients in reducing the rate of pelvic recurrences, and even to prevent bleeding, pelvic pain, leg edema, and other local complications (42–46).

Para-aortic Node Treatment

There is ongoing discussion regarding whether resection of bulky positive lymph nodes, especially in the para-aortic area, improves survival compared with radiation therapy alone. A study of 23 patients with bulky positive lymph nodes showed that resection of these nodes followed by external-beam radiation therapy can result in a 3-year survival rate of 68% (47). Other authors reported 5-year survival rates ranging from 40% to 50% (48–50). In one randomized study, patients at high risk for para-aortic lymph node involvement were randomized to receive either radiotherapy of the pelvis or extended-field irradiation. No statistical difference in survival was found after 4 years of observation (51). In a second study, patients in stage Ib, IIa, or IIb with a tumor larger than 4 cm were randomized to receive either pelvic radiation or extended-field therapy. In this study a significant difference favoring irradiation of the extended field was found (52). Several retrospective studies

claimed that the value of radiotherapy is uncertain whereas others reported a 30% to 50% benefit (53–57). Fletcher (58) found that a dose of 40 to 45 Gy to the para-aortic nodes given electively can be expected to control 70% to 80% of subclinical disease and therefore can be curative.

Advanced Disease—Stages IIb, III, and IV

Radiotherapy is generally accepted as the primary treatment of choice in advanced carcinoma of the cervix. Five-year survival rates in the range of 40% to 60% are reported. Failures are attributed to large tumor volume, side-wall disease, and nodal metastases. Studies are now under way to determine the optimal dose rate for brachytherapy, with an increasing shift from low-dose-rate brachytherapy to high-dose-rate brachytherapy. Further studies are needed to determine the best fractionation scheme (59–61).

Principles of Radiation Therapy

The fundamental objective of radiotherapy is to deliver a dose of radiation sufficient to destroy all malignant tissue without injury to normal tissue. The principle of irradiation therapy is based primarily on extensive empiric experience, as the method has been applied since the beginning of this century. Later, the physical principles of ionization became better understood and factors that play a role in the cell and tissue responses to irradiation have been identified. Still, the extensive radiobiologic knowledge that we have access to today did not change very much the empiric radiotherapeutic approach.

Carcinoma of the cervix was the first solid tumor treated successfully by radiation therapy. The first successfully treated carcinoma of the cervix with intracavitary radium therapy was described as early as 1905 (62). The anatomy of the cervix makes the organ suitable for intracavitary radiation therapy. The sac form of the uterus and vagina allows for high-dose irradiation, and the resistance of the uterus and vaginal normal tissue to irradiation is an additional advantage.

During the early years of the century, three intracavitary brachytherapy methods were developed: the Stockholm, Paris, and Manchester techniques. Later, Fletcher and Suit at the M. D. Anderson Cancer Center modified the Manchester system and this modification became very popular in the United States. All these techniques differ with regard to the applicators as well as the amount of the radioactive source and the exposure time (Figs. 18-2 to 18-4). The bladder and rectum are dose-limiting organs, and many of these techniques estimate the treatment time on the basis of maximal doses to the rectum and bladder. Other groups rely on the estimation of so-called milligram hours, which is a multiplication of the milligrams of radium or radium equivalent by the total number of hours that the patient is exposed. Two anatomic points are defined for prescribing purposes: point A located 2 cm superior to the mucosal membrane of the lateral fornix and 2 cm lateral to the cervical canal, and point B located on the same transverse axis as point A but 5 cm lateral to the cervical canal.

In 1984, the International Commission on Radiation Units (ICRU) recommended a new principal measurement for dose and volume specifications. Many of the dose and volume specifications offered in the ICRU report (63) are redefinitions and standardizations of conventional terminology and are still of very little use. A clinically used prescription based on the anatomic points A and B for dose definition, milligram hours, and doses to the bladder and rectum is still the most used specification in brachytherapy.

From the beginning, the intracavitary devices were manually loaded and manually placed in the cavities. During the late 1950s and the beginning of the 1960s, afterloading techniques were developed. The factors initiating this development were the increasing consciousness of the effects of radiation exposure and the wish to minimize exposure to the staff. Manual afterloading is performed in empty applicators, where placement in the cavities has been proved satisfactory by x-ray before deposition of the radioactive sources. The later development of a remote afterloading system can totally protect the staff from irradiation exposure. The radioactive sources are stored in a radiation-protected safe and connected to the hollow applicator in the vagina and uterus. The sources can then automatically pass to the patient after the staff has left the room. One of the important developments in the remote afterloading technique is the high-dose-rate technique. High-dose intracavitary irradiation can

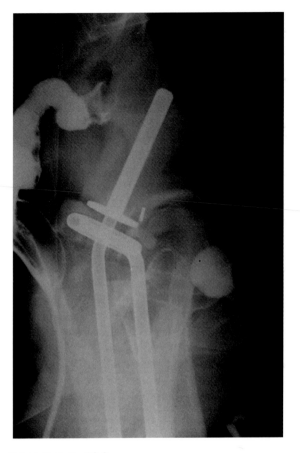

F I G U R E   **18-2**

Stockholm afterloading applicators with contrast medium in the bladder and rectum.

shorten the treatment time from hours to minutes, but has to be given in a larger number of fractions. The radiobiologic differences between a high dose and a low dose rate have not been fully explored; no randomized trial has compared these two techniques. The low-dose afterloading system is more protracted and usually takes several hours. The high-dose-rate afterloading system can be applied during a few minutes but requires several fractions of treatment, which creates practical problems regarding the patient's comfort. The high-dose-rate system can be used in the outpatient setting, which spares hospital beds. Some authors claim that the high-dose-rate system is economically cost beneficial while others claim that several treatment fractions are as expensive as hospital beds to the patients (64,65).

As the dose of radiation given at a point is inversely proportional to the square of the distance from the source of radiation, it is important to have accurate positioning of the

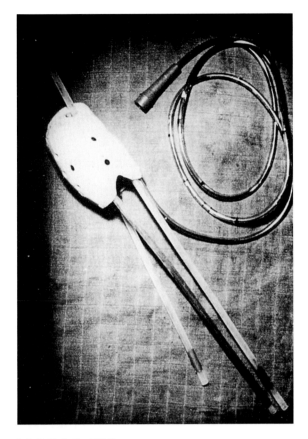

FIGURE **18-3**

Paris moulage system with three source tubes—two for the vagina, one for the uterus—and a lavage catheter for irrigation of the interior of the moulage during the treatment.

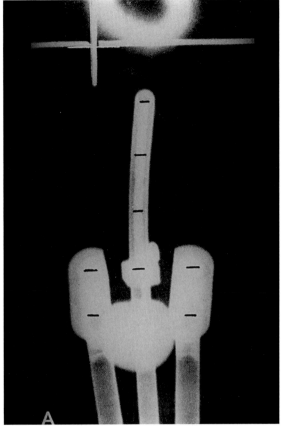

FIGURE **18-4**

Fletcher-Suit applicators with two ovoid and intrauterine tandem with tungsten shields to decrease the dose to the bladder and rectum.

intracavitary sources. On the other hand, the rapid fall of the dose means that many of the sensitive normal tissues within the pelvis, particularly the rectum and bladder, may be spared an excessive radiation dose.

Planning Treatment

High-quality planning for the treatment of carcinoma of the cervix is crucial as often the combination of brachytherapy and external therapy is needed (Fig. 18-5).

The first step in planning external therapy is to establish the target volume and treatment dose, with special consideration given to the doses given before or planned to be given to the critical organs during brachytherapy. These critical organs are the bladder and rectum, with tolerable radiation limits of about 60 Gy. Partial shielding is often necessary during external treatment.

Dose planning should start with computed tomography (CT) or magnetic resonance imaging (MRI) of the relevant anatomic parts. With CT or MRI, multiple image data sets can be obtained and the target area and critical organs can be defined in each plane. There are several documentations regarding the improvement in target volume localization achieved with anatomic data from CT compared with previous conventional radiographic methods.

The position of the patient during CT and treatment planning has to be identical with the position during treatment. This can cause problems in obese patients. It is possible today to improve the localization of the field and reproduction of the position. Special on-line systems have been recently developed based on different principles, e.g., filming light from a fluorescent screen placed under the patient or measuring signals from a large number of detectors placed in a matrix behind the patient.

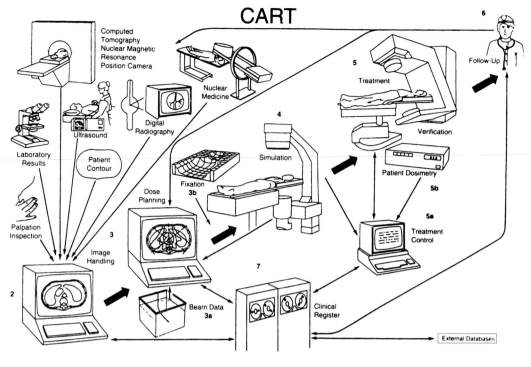

F I G U R E **18-5**

Overview of dose-planning procedure. [From CART (Computer Aided Radiotherapy), a Nordic RLD project referred to in SBU report (Swedish Council on Technology Assessment in Health Care) *Acta Oncologica* 1996;35(suppl 6):31.]

Visible skin marks are required to reproduce the position.

The target volume as well as correlation to critical organs can be exactly established directly in the dose-planning computer. In conjunction with the responsible radiophysicist, the treatment technique is chosen. The position of the irradiation field needed to reach the required dose as well as the fractionation scheme is established (Fig. 18-6).

When dose planning is finished, the next step is simulation of treatment on a simulator. With the patient placed in the treatment position and treatment margins marked on the patient's skin, an x-ray control picture is made, and any corrections instituted (Fig. 18-7).

After the simulation, treatment can start. X-ray control of the first treatment is especially important. If brachytherapy has been given primarily, shielding may be applied to the critical organs. It is important that calculations for shielding be done for each patient.

The treatment-planning technique is changing quickly. Conformal therapy, taking into consideration the exactness of the target volume contour as well as the sensitivities of the criti-

cal organs, is developing. With conformal therapy, irradiation fields can be better formed. With better concentration of the beam to the target volume, there is the possibility of giving higher doses to the tumor and decreasing the side effects in the critical organs (Fig. 18-8). Three-dimensional dose calculation algorithms have already been developed and with them it is possible to reach the target volume with very good precision (Fig. 18-9). Still, it is important to remember that the reproducibility of treatment in conformal therapy is crucial.

How to fractionate external irradiation is still under investigation even though development in this area has been going on for the last 20 years. With hypofractionation, hyperfractionation, and accelerated fractionation, different programs have been used for different tumor types and intense investigations are ongoing to optimize these fractionation schemes for the different tumors.

With high-quality dose planning, better fractionation patterns, and improved techniques, especially conformal therapy, in the future radiotherapy may be easier and more accurate to administer, with an increased possibility of

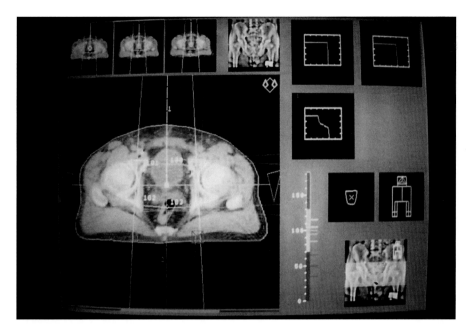

FIGURE **18-6**

Dose planning using computed tomography.

FIGURE **18-7**

Simulation radiography for the treatment of pelvis and para-aortic lymph nodes with shielding of the bladder and rectum.

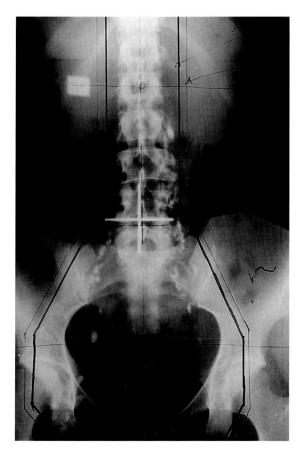

giving higher doses to the target volumes and increasing the cure rate.

Complications of Irradiation Treatment

The rate of major complications of irradiation therapy given alone or in combination with surgery ranges between 1.9% to 5.3% (66,67). Most of them are rectal complications in the form of stricture and more seldom, fistula. Most of the complications from the rectum occur during the first 2 years. Urinary tract complications are seen more frequently 3 to 4 years after treatment (68,69).

Chemotherapy

The use of cytotoxic chemotherapy in patients with advanced cervical cancer is currently under investigation. In one major randomized study performed in Argentina, chemotherapy was used in half of the patients in an adjuvant setting before surgery for bulky stage Ib carcinoma of the cervix. The treatment was completed with whole-pelvic external irradiation at 50 Gy to all patients. Preliminary results showed statistically better survival in patients treated with neoadjuvant chemotherapy (70). Randomized studies for high-risk patients with early-stage disease comparing radiotherapy treatment

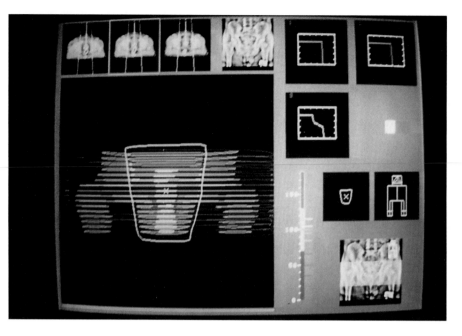

F I G U R E   **18-8**

Example of planning for conformal therapy, taking into consideration the target volume and different sensitivities of the organs.

F I G U R E   **18-9**

Three-dimensional dose calculations using a computed tomography data set.

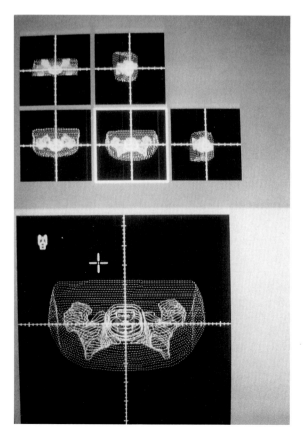

alone with radiotherapy in combination with chemotherapy are ongoing.

Several studies used chemotherapy in patients with advanced disease. Two different approaches can be identified:

1. *Neoadjuvant chemotherapy.* Several studies used neoadjuvant chemotherapy before radiotherapy for advanced carcinoma of the cervix. None of these studies demonstrated any superiority of neoadjuvant chemotherapy before irradiation (71–74).

2. *Concurrent irradiation and chemotherapy.* A Gynecologic Oncology Group randomized trial with hydroxyurea demonstrated superiority of the treatment in which chemotherapy was included, but this study was criticized for the low irradiation dose, small port size, and lack of follow-up in one half of the patients (75). A subsequent study by the Gynecologic Oncology Group with irradiation and hydroxyurea failed to show any significant difference in survival (76). A Radiation Therapy Oncology Group study of irradiation versus irradiation and misonidazole showed no difference in survival (77). A study on the feasibility of rapidly alternating chemotherapy with accelerated radiotherapy in 8 patients with advanced-stage carcinoma was performed. The findings are very preliminary, with short observation times and a small patient sample, but are promising (78).

In summary, several phase I and II studies and some phase III studies using neoadjuvant and concomitant chemotherapy with irradiation were performed in patients with advanced carcinoma of the cervix. Most of them failed to show any benefit of the use of chemotherapy for patients with cervical cancer. At present, irradiation alone is the standard treatment for advanced carcinoma of the cervix.

Recurrence of Cervical Carcinoma

One third of the patients treated for cervical cancer will have a recurrence of the disease within the first 3 years. The recurrence may develop in the vagina, in the central pelvis and more laterally on the pelvic wall, and also as distant metastases. Symptoms may be localized to the pelvis and include bleeding and pain. Especially in the presence of lymph node metastases on the pelvic wall, a very characteristic pain of the back and leg occurs during the night when the patient is in a horizontal position. Most common distant metastases are in the lungs and bone, but even liver and brain localizations are not uncommon. Ureteral obstruction is one of the symptoms of pelvic recurrence. In 50% of patients, the recurrence will be confined to the pelvis.

In patients with pelvic recurrence, it is mandatory to confirm the disease cytologically or histologically. One of the best methods of diagnosing recurrence deep in the pelvis is aspiration biopsy. The procedure can be performed either transvaginally or transrectally with a fine needle 20 cm long. A ringlike holder is attached to the distal end of the index finger, which

makes it possible to guide the insertion of the needle (79,80) (Fig. 18-10). With this procedure, a specimen can be obtained even from deep localized metastases in the pelvis. Ultrasound or CT often can be helpful in localizing the pathologic change. A guided thin-needle biopsy can be performed easily.

In patients who primarily underwent surgical treatment alone, external irradiation of at least 50 Gy can be given to the pelvis. For metastases localized to the vagina, intracavitary or interstitial treatment can be used. Salvage rates to 40% have been achieved with irradiation for recurrence after primary surgery (81). For central pelvic recurrence after radical irradiation therapy, surgery may be performed as either a radical hysterectomy, in a very small number of patients with lesions smaller than 2 cm, or by pelvic exenteration as the accepted surgical approach. The operative mortality is an acceptable 5% with a survival rate as high as 60% in some series (82,83). Physical, psychosocial, and psychosexual rehabilitation of these patients has been greatly enhanced by advances in urinary, rectal, and vaginal reconstruction techniques (84–86).

Chemotherapy has not proved to be of any curative importance in the treatment of recurrent cervical cancer. Palliation of distant metastases, especially in the lungs and soft tissues, not previously irradiated, has been observed, but unfortunately not of any long duration (87,88).

Adenocarcinoma of the Cervix

For many years there has been an ongoing controversy regarding the prognostic importance of adenocarcinoma of the cervix. Some authors

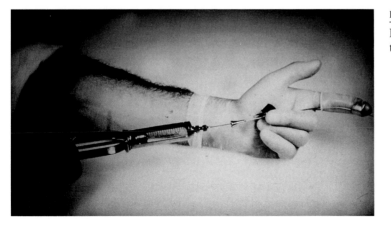

F I G U R E **18-10**

Instrument for transvaginal or transrectal aspiration biopsy.

concluded that adenocarcinoma in the same stage of disease has a worse prognosis than does squamous carcinoma. Others claimed there is no real difference. The most recent volume of the annual report on the results of treatment of gynecological cancer (21) gives actual survival rates according to stage and histology, and for each stage the squamous carcinoma was associated with better survival than was adenocarcinoma. A recent M. D. Anderson study comparing squamous carcinoma of the cervix with adenocarcinoma, treated by irradiation, demonstrated a statistically significant better survival for patients with squamous cell carcinoma, with tumors larger than 4 cm in diameter. The adenocarcinoma patients had a higher risk of developing distant metastases than did those with squamous cell carcinoma (89). A comparative study between adenocarcinoma patients treated with radiotherapy and a combination of radiotherapy and surgery at the Radiumhemmet demonstrated significantly better survival for patients treated with combination therapy (90). Several other studies reported poor survival for adenocarcinoma patients with stage Ib disease. Still some others failed to demonstrate the influence of histology on prognosis (91–100).

In summary, adenocarcinoma of the cervix in early stages has a poorer prognosis than does comparable-stage squamous cell carcinoma.

Cervical Cancer During Pregnancy

Cervical cancer seldom complicates pregnancy, 0.2% to 4.0% of deliveries according to the literature (101). How cervical cancer associated with pregnancy is defined differs in the literature. Mostly, it means that the tumor was diagnosed during the pregnancy and 6 months after the pregnancy was completed. Usually there is a lack of symptoms and a Pap smear should be taken routinely at the first physical examination during pregnancy. Histopathologic findings in the specimen and staging are important elements in decision making. Early microscopically invasive cancer of the cervix can be treated conservatively, even during pregnancy, with conization. In women with cancer of all other stages during the first and second trimesters, the pregnancy should be terminated and treatment started. Only in the last trimester is delay acceptable, but delivery of the fetus should be achieved as soon as possible, when the fetus is viable. This can be performed simultaneously with primary Wertheim operation in women with early-stage cancer, or before radiotherapy commences in those with advanced-stage cancer. Stage for stage, however, there is no difference in the outcome of pregnant versus nonpregnant patients after treatment.

REFERENCES

1. Averette HE, Nelson JH, Ng AG, et al. Diagnosis and management of microinvasive (stage Ia) carcinoma of the uterine cervix. *Cancer* 1976;38:414–425.
2. Fouchee JH, Greiss FC, Lock FR. Stage Ia squamous cell carcinoma of the uterine cervix. *Am J Obstet Gynecol* 1969;105:46–58.
3. Leman MH, Benson WL, Kurman RJ, Park RC. Microinvasive carcinoma of the cervix. *Obstet Gynecol* 1976;48:571–578.
4. Roch WD, Norris HJ. Microinvasive carcinoma of the cervix: the significance of lymphatic invasion and confluent patterns of stromal growth. *Cancer* 1975;36:180–186.
5. Seski JC, Abell MR, Morley GW. Microinvasive squamous carcinoma of the cervix: definition, histologic analysis, late results of treatment. *Obstet Gynecol* 1977;50:410–414.
6. Simon NL, Gore H, Shingleton HM, et al. Study of superficially invasive carcinoma of the cervix. *Obstet Gynecol* 1986;68:19–24.
7. Yajima A, Noda K. The results of treatment of microinvasive carcinoma (stage Ia) of the uterine cervix by means of simple and extended hysterectomy. *Am J Obstet Gynecol* 1979;135:685–688.
8. Kolstad P. Carcinoma of the cervix. Stage Ia. Diagnosis and treatment. *Am J Obstet Gynecol* 1969;104:1015–1022.
9. Richart RM, Townsend D, Crisp W. An analysis of long term follow-up results in patients with cervical intraepithelial neoplasia treated by cryosurgery. *Am J Obstet Gynecol* 1980;137:823–826.
10. Coppleson M. Management of preclinical carcinoma, early invasive squamous and adenocarcinoma of the cervix. In: Coppleson M, ed. *Gynecologic oncology.* London: Churchhill Livingstone, 1992:631–648.
11. Andersen E, Husth M, Joerjenson A, Nielsen K. Laser conization microinvasive carcinoma of the

cervix: short-term results. *Int J Gynecol Cancer* 1993;3:183–185.

12. Kolstad P. Follow-up of 232 patients with stage Ia1 and 411 patients with stage Ia2 squamous cell carcinoma of the cervix (microinvasive carcinoma). *Gynecol Oncol* 1988;33:265–272.

13. Morris M, Follen Mitchell M, Silva EG, et al. Cervical conization as definitive therapy for early invasive squamous carcinoma of the cervix. *Gynecol Oncol* 1993;51:193–196.

14. Boyce J, Fruchter R, Nicastri A. Prognostic factors in stage I carcinoma of the cervix. *Gynecol Oncol* 1981;12:154–165.

15. Simon NL, Gore H, Shingleton HM, et al. Study of superficially invasive carcinoma of the cervix. *Obstet Gynecol* 1986;68:19–24.

16. Nelson JH, Averette HE, Richart RM. Cervical intraepithelial neoplasia and early invasive cervical carcinomas. *Cancer* 1989;39:157–178.

17. Tsukamoto N, Kaku T, Matsukuma T, et al. The problem of stage Ia (FIGO, 1985) carcinoma of the uterine cervix. *Gynecol Oncol* 1989;34:1–6.

18. Dargent D, Brun JL, Roy M, Rémy I. Pregnancies following radical trachelectomy for invasive cervical cancer. Abstract presented at the meeting of the Society of Gynecologic Oncologists, Orlando, Florida, February 6–9, 1994.

19. Childers J, Hatch K, Surwit E. The role of laparoscopic lymphadenectomy in the management of cervical carcinoma. *Gynecol Oncol* 1992;47:38–43.

20. Querleu D, LeBlanc E, Castelain B. Laparoscopic pelvic lymphadenectomy in the staging of early carcinoma of the cervix. *Am J Obstet Gynecol* 1991;164:579–581.

21. Pettersson F, ed. *Annual report on the results of treatment in gynecological cancer*, vol. 22. Stockholm: 1995.

22. Creasman WT, Soper JT, Clarke-Pearson D. Radical hysterectomy as therapy for early carcinoma of the cervix. *Am J Obstet Gynecol* 1986; 155:964–969.

23. Morley GW, Seski JC. Radical pelvic surgery versus radiation therapy for stage I carcinoma of the cervix (exclusive of microinvasion). *Am J Obstet Gynecol* 1976;126:785–798.

24. Newton M. Radical hysterectomy or radiotherapy for stage I cervical cancer: a prospective comparison with 5 and 10 year follow-up. *Am J Obstet Gynecol* 1975;123:535–542.

25. Perez CA, Grigsby PW, Camel H, et al. Irradiation alone or combined with surgery in stage IB, IIA and IIB carcinoma of the uterine cervix; update of a non-randomized comparison. *Int J Radiat Oncol Biol Phys* 1995;31:703–716.

26. Einhorn N, Bygdeman M, Sjöberg B. Combined radiation and surgical treatment for carcinoma of the uterine cervix. *Cancer* 1980;45:720–723.

27. Einhorn N, Patek E, Sjöberg B. Outcome of different treatment modalities in cervix carcinoma stage Ib and IIa. *Cancer* 1985;55:949.

28. Knapp RC, Berkowitz RS, eds. *Gynecologic oncology.* New York: McGraw-Hill, 1993:202.

29. Fuller A, Elliott N, Kosloff C, et al. Determinants of increased risk for recurrence in patients undergoing radical hysterectomy for stage IB and IIA carcinoma of the cervix. *Gynecol Oncol* 1989;33:34–39.

30. Gallion HH, van Nagell JR Jr, Donaldson ES, et al. Combined radiation therapy and extrafascial hysterectomy in the treatment of stage Ib barrel-shaped cervical cancer. *Cancer* 1985;56:262–265.

31. Rutledge FN, Wharton JT, Fletcher GH. Clinical studies with adjunctive surgery and irradiation therapy in the treatment of carcinoma of the cervix. *Cancer* 1976;38:596–602.

32. Marcial VA, Bosch A. Radiation-induced tumor regression in carcinoma of the uterine cervix: prognostic significance. *AJR Am J Roentgenol* 1970;108:113–128.

33. Hardt N, van Nagell JR Jr, Hanson MB, et al. Radiation-induced tumor regression as a prognostic factor in patients with invasive cervical cancer. *Cancer* 1982;49:35–39.

34. Kinney WK, Hodge DO, Egorshin EV, et al. Identification of a low-risk subset of patients with stage Ib invasive squamous cancer of the cervix possibly suited to less radical surgical treatment. *Gynecol Oncol* 1995;57:3–6.

35. Delgado G, Bundy BN, Zaino R, et al. Prospective surgical-pathological study of disease-free interval in patients with stage IB squamous cell carcinoma of the cervix: a Gynecologic Oncology Group study. *Gynecol Oncol* 1990;38:352–357.

36. Kjorstad KE, Kolbenstvedt A, Strickert T. The value of complete lymphadenectomy in radical treatment of cancer of the cervix, stage IB. *Cancer* 1984;54:2215–2219.

37. Fowler J, Carter J, Carlson J, et al. Lymph node yield from laparoscopic lymphadenectomy in cervical cancer: a comparative study. *Gynecol Oncol* 1993;51:187–192.

38. Mann WJ Jr, Orr JW Jr, Shingleton HM, et al. Perioperative influences on infectious morbidity in radical hysterectomy. *Gynecol Oncol* 1981;11: 207–212.

39. Lowe J, Mauger G, Carmichael J. The effect of Wertheim hysterectomy upon bladder and urethral function. *Am J Obstet Gynecol* 1981;139: 826–834.

40. Hatch KD, Parham G, Shingleton HM, et al. Ureteral strictures and fistulae following radical hysterectomy. *Gynecol Oncol* 1984;19:17–23.

41. Eifel PJ, Morris M, Wharton JT, Oswald MJ. The influence of tumour size and morphology on the outcome of patients with FIGO stage IB squamous cell carcinoma of the uterine cervix. *Int J Radiat Oncol Biol Phys* 1994;29:9–16.

42. Morrow P. Panel report. Is pelvic irradiation beneficial in the postoperative management of stage Ib squamous cell carcinoma of the cervix with pelvic node metastases treated by radical hysterectomy and pelvic lymphadenectomy? *Gynecol Oncol* 1980;10:105–110.

43. Nahhas WA, Sharkey FE, Whitney CW, et al. The prognostic significance of vascular channel involvement and deep stromal invasion in early cervical cancer. *Am J Clin Oncol* 1983;6:259–264.

44. Inoue T, Okumura M. Prognostic significance of parametrial extension in patients with cervical carcinoma stage Ib, IIa, and IIIb. *Cancer* 1984;54:1714–1719.

45. Bleker O, Ketting B, Wayjean-eecen B, Kloosterman G. The significance of microscopic involvement of the parametrium and/or pelvic lymph nodes in cervical cancer stages Ib and IIa. *Gynecol Oncol* 1983;16:56–62.

46. Shingleton HM, Orr JW Jr. Primary surgical and combined treatment. In: Singe A, Jordan J, eds. *Cancer of the cervix.* New York: Churchill Livingstone, 1983:79.

47. Hacker NF. Resection of bulky positive lymph nodes in patient with cervical carcinoma. *Int J Gynecol Cancer* 1995;5:250–256.

48. Potish R, Adcock L, Jones T, et al. The morbidity and utility of para-aortic radiotherapy in cervical carcinoma. *Gynecol Oncol* 1983;15: 1–9.

49. Lepanto P, Littman P, Mukuto J, et al. Treatment of para-aortic nodes in carcinoma of the cervix. *Cancer* 1975;35:1510–1513.

50. Rubin SC, Brookland R, Mikuta JJ, et al. Para-aortic nodal metastases in early cervical carcinoma: long term survival following extended field radiotherapy. *Gynecol Oncol* 1984;18:213–217.

51. Haie C, Pejovic MH, Gerbaulet A, et al. Is prophylactic para-aortic irradiation worthwhile in the treatment of advanced cervical carcinoma? Results of a controlled clinical trial of the EORTC radiotherapy group. *Radiother Oncol* 1988;11: 101–112.

52. Rotman M, Choi K, Guze C, et al. Prophylactic irradiation of the para-aortic lymph node chain in stage IIb and bulky stage Ib carcinoma of the cervix, initial treatment results of RTOG 7920. *Int J Radiat Oncol Biol Phys* 1990;19:513–521.

53. Cunningham MJ, Dunton CJ, Corn B, et al. Extended-field radiation therapy in early-stage cervical carcinoma: survival and complications. *Gynecol Oncol* 1991;43:51–54.

54. Vigliotti AP, Wen B-C, Hussey DH, et al. Extended field irradiation for carcinoma of the uterine cervix with positive para-aortic nodes. *Int J Radiat Oncol Biol Phys* 1992;23:501–509.

55. Nori D, Valentine E, Hilaris BS. The role of paraaortic node irradiation in the treatment of cancer of the cervix. *Int J Radiat Oncol Biol Phys* 1985;11:1469–1473.

56. Inoue T, Morita K. 5-Year results of postoperative extended-field irradiation of 76 patients with nodal metastases from cervical carcinoma stages Ib to IIIb. *Cancer* 1988;61:2009–2014.

57. Lovecchio JL, Averette HE, Donato D, Bell J. 5-Year survival of patients with para-aortic nodal metastases in clinical stage Ib and IIa cervical carcinoma. *Gynecol Oncol* 1989;34:43–44.

58. Fletcher GH. Elective irradiation of the para-aortic nodes in squamous cell carcinoma of the uterine cervix. *Int J Radiat Oncol Biol Phys* 1990;19:799–780.

59. Patel FD, Sharma SC, Pritam SN, et al. Low dose rate vs high dose rate brachytherapy in the treatment of carcinoma of the uterine cervix; a clinical trial. *Int J Radiat Oncol Biol Phys* 1993; 28:335–341.

60. Perez CA, Fox S, Lockett MA, et al. Impact of dose in outcome of irradiation alone in carcinoma of the uterine cervix; analysis of two different methods. *Int J Radiat Oncol Biol Phys* 1991;21:885–898.

61. Perez CA, Grigsby PW, Castro-Vita H, Lockett MA. Carcinoma of the uterine cervix. II. Lack of impact of prolongation of overall treatment time on morbidity of radiation therapy. *Int J Radiat Oncol Biol Phys* 1996;34:3–11.

62. Abbe R. The use of radium in malignant disease. *Lancet* 1913;2:524.

63. *International Commission on Radiation Units report 38: dose and volume specifications for reporting intracavitary therapy in gynecology.* Baltimore: International Commission on Radiation Units, 1985:1–16.

64. Orton CG, Seyedsadr M, Somney A. Comparison of high and low dose rate remote afterloading for cervix cancer and the importance of fractionation. *Int J Radiat Oncol Biol Phys* 1991;21:1425–1434.

65. Stitt JA, Thomadsen BR, Fowler JF. High-dose-rate brachytherapy for carcinoma of the cervix. High tech or high risk? *Int J Radiat Oncol Biol Phys* 1992;24:383–386.

66. Einhorn N. Frequency of severe complications after radiation therapy for cervical carcinoma. *Acta Radiol* 1975;14:42–48.

67. Van Nagall JR Jr, Parker JC Jr, Maruyama Y, et al. Bladder or rectal injury following radiation therapy for cervical cancer. *Am J Obstet Gynecol* 1974;119:727–732.

68. Kottmeier HL. Complications following radiation therapy in carcinoma of the cervix and their treatment. *Am J Obstet Gynecol* 1964;88:854.

69. Perez CA, Kuske RR, Camel HM, et al. Analysis of pelvic tumour control and impact on survival in carcinoma of the uterine cervix with radiation therapy alone. *Int J Radiat Oncol Biol Phys* 1987;14:613–621.

70. Sardi J, Sananes C, Giaroli A, et al. Results of a prospective randomized trial with neoadjuvant chemotherapy in stage Ib, bulky, squamous carcinoma of the cervix. *Gynecol Oncol* 1993;49: 156–165.

71. Chauvergne J, Rohart J, Heron JF, et al. Randomized phase II trial of neoadjuvant chemotherapy (CT) + radiotherapy (RT) vs. RT in stage IIb, III carcinoma of the cervix (CACS): a cooperative study of French oncology centers. *Proc Am Soc Clin Oncol* 1988;7:136.

72. Souhami L, Gil RA, Allan SE, et al. A randomized trial of chemotherapy followed by pelvic irradiation therapy in stage IIIb carcinoma of the cervix. *J Clin Oncol* 1991;9:970–977.

73. Tattersall MHN, Ramirez C, Coppleson M. A randomized trial of adjuvant chemotherapy after radical hysterectomy in stage Ib-IIa cervical cancer patients with pelvic lymph node metastases. *Gynecol Oncol* 1992;46:176–181.

74. Cardenas J, Olguin A, Figucroa F, et al. Randomized neoadjuvant chemotherapy in cervical carcinoma stage IIb. PEC + RT versus RT. *Proc Am Soc Clin Oncol* 1991;10:620.

75. Hrechchyshyn MM, Aron BS, Boronow RC, et al. Hydroxyurea or placebo combined with radiation to treat stages IIIb and IV cervical cancer confined to the pelvis. *Int J Radiat Oncol Biol Phys* 1979;5:317–322.

76. Stehman FB, Bundy BN, Keys H, et al. A randomized trial of hydroxyurea versus misonidazole adjunct to radiation therapy in carcinoma of the cervix. A preliminary report of GOG study. *Am J Obstet Gynecol* 1988;159:87–94.

77. Leibel S, Bauer M, Wasserman T, et al. Radiotherapy with or without misonidazole for patients with stage IIIb or stage IV squamous cell carcinoma of the uterine cervix. Preliminary report of a Radiation Therapy Oncology Group randomized trial. *Int J Radiat Oncol Biol Phys* 1987;13:451–459.

78. Chadha M, Lacobs AJ, Stenson R. Chemotherapy rapidly alternating with accelerated radiotherapy for advanced carcinoma of the uterine cervix. *Int J Gynecol Cancer* 1995;5:257–261.

79. Einhorn N, Zajicek J. Aspiration biopsy of intrapelvic metastases of cervical carcinoma. *Acta Radiol* 1978;17:257–262.

80. Linsk JA, Franzen S, eds. *Clinical aspiration cytology.* Philadelphia: JB Lippincott, 1983:247.

81. Thomas GM, Dembo AJ, Myhr T, et al. Long-term results of concurrent radiation and chemotherapy for carcinoma of the cervix recurrent after surgery. *Int J Gynecol Cancer* 1993;3: 193–198.

82. Morley GW. Pelvic exenteration in the treatment of recurrent cervical cancer. In: Heintz APM, Griffiths CT, Trimbos JB, eds. *Surgery in gynecological oncology.* The Hague: Martinus Nijhoff, 1984:174.

83. Averette HE, Lichtinger M, Sevin BU, Girtanner RE. Pelvic exenteration: a 15 year experience in general metropolitan hospital. *Am J Obstet Gynecol* 1984;150:179–184.

84. Lockhart JL. Remodeled right colon: an alternative urinary reservoir. *J Urol* 1987;138:730–734.

85. Wheeless CR, Hempling RE. Rectal J pouch reservoir to decrease the frequency of tenesmus and defecation in low coloproctostomy. *Gynecol Oncol* 1989;35:136–138.

86. Andersen BL, van der Does J. Sexual morbidity following gynecologic cancer: an international problem. *Int J Gynecol Cancer* 1994;4:225–240.

87. Muscato MS, Perry MC, Yarbro JW. Chemotherapy of cervical carcinoma. *Semin Oncol* 1982;9: 373–387.

88. Thigpen JT. Single agent chemotherapy in carcinoma of the cervix. In: Surwit EA, Alberts DS, eds. *Cervical cancer.* Boston: Martinus Nijhoff, 1987:119–136.

89. Eifel PJ, Burke TW, Morris M, Smith TL. Adenocarcinoma as an independent risk factor for disease recurrence in patients with stage Ib cervical carcinoma. *Gynecol Oncol* 1995;59:38–44.

90. Moberg P, Einhorn N, Silfverswärd C, Söderberg G. Adenocarcinoma of the uterine cervix. *Cancer* 1986;57:407–410.

91. Kleine W, Rau K, Schwoerer D, Pfleiderer A. A prognosis of adenocarcinoma of the cervix uteri: a comparative study. *Gynecol Oncol* 1989;35: 145–149.

92. Hopkins M, Morley GW. A comparison of adenocarcinoma and squamous cell carcinoma of the cervix. *Obstet Gynecol* 1991;77:912–917.

93. Grigsby PW, Perez CA, Kuske RR, et al. Adenocarcinoma of the uterine cervix: lack of evidence for a poor prognosis. *Radiother Oncol* 1988;12:289–296.

94. Kilgore LC, Soong SJ, Gore H, et al. Analysis of prognostic features in adenocarcinoma of the cervix. *Gynecol Oncol* 1988;31:137–153.

95. Kjörstad KE. Adenocarcinoma of the uterine cervix. *Gynecol Oncol* 1977;5:219–223.

96. Miller BE, Flax SD, Arheart K, Photopulos G. The presentation of adenocarcinoma of the uterine cervix. *Cancer* 1993;72:1281–1285.

97. Shingleton HM, Gore H, Bradley DH, Soong SJ. Adenocarcinoma of the cervix. I. Clinical evaluation and pathologic features. *Obstet Gynecol* 1981;139:799–814.

98. Vesterinen E, Forss M, Nieminen U. Increase of cervical adenocarcinoma: a report of 520 cases of cervical carcinoma including 112 tumors with glandular elements. *Gynecol Oncol* 1989;33: 49–53.

99. Eide TJ. Cancer of the uterine cervix in Norway by histologic type, 1970–1984. *J Natl Cancer Inst* 1987;79:199–205.

100. Milsom I, Friberg LG. Primary adenocarcinoma of the uterine cervix: a clinical study. *Cancer* 1983;52:942–947.

101. Hacker NF, Berek JS, Lagasse LJ, et al. Carcinoma of the cervix associated with pregnancy. *Obstet Gynecol* 1982;59:735–746.

SECTION 3

Corpus

CHAPTER *19*

Precancerous Lesions of the Endometrium: Pathology, Etiology, and Treatment

KJELL E. KJØRSTAD
VERA M. ABELER

*E*ndometrial carcinomas of the endometrioid type (common adenocarcinoma, adenosquamous carcinoma, and adenoacanthoma) constitute the vast majority of malignancies found in the uterine corpus. They have recognizable precursors characterized by hyperproliferative changes of the endometrium typically caused by hormonal imbalance, with a disturbed ratio between estrogens and gestagens.

The most common reaction of the endometrium to prolonged estrogen overstimulation is commonly known as *cystic hyperplasia.* This is not a premalignant condition. Polyps as such have no malignant potential, but can be involved in atypical processes.

Until recently, no generally agreed classification of the different types of endometrial hyperplasias existed. Terms such as *adenomatous hyperplasia, atypical adenomatous hyperplasia,* and *carcinoma in situ* have been used by different pathologists for the same lesions, and conversely, clinical investigators have used the same terms to describe different lesions. A committee appointed by The International Society of Gynecological Pathologists recently agreed on a classification of tumors, which subsequently was adopted by the World Health Organization (Table 19-1) (1,2). This classification is presently the most widely accepted.

Definition

Endometrial hyperplasia is a noninvasive abnormal proliferation of the endometrial glands and stromal cells that results in a morphologic pattern of glands of varying shape and size with an increase in the gland-stroma ratio compared with proliferative endometrium.

Current Classification

Hyperplasia comprises a spectrum of histologic appearances, from the mildest form of simple hyperplasia without atypia to severe complex hyperplasia with atypia. Endometrial hyperplasia is subdivided into two main groups: hyperplasias with and those without atypia. These lesions are further divided into simple and complex hyperplasia according to the extent of glandular growth.

Macroscopic Features

Contrary to common belief, hyperplastic endometrium is not distinctive macroscopically. The volume of dilation and curettage specimens is usually increased, but it may vary considerably. In perimenopausal and postmenopausal

T A B L E   **19-1**

World Health Organization Classification of Endometrial Hyperplasia

Hyperplasia (without atypia)
   Simple
   Complex (adenomatous)

Atypical hyperplasia
   Simple
   Complex (adenomatous with atypia)

women, it may actually be less than that of specimens obtained during the late proliferative or secretory phase of a normal cycle. In hysterectomy specimens it may be inconspicuous, or it may show considerable diffuse or polypoid thickening. The consistency is usually soft and sometimes spongy and the color is grayish.

Microscopic Features

Simple Hyperplasia

Simple hyperplasia is characterized by great variability in glandular size (Fig. 19-1). Some glands may be very large and cystically dilated and lined by flattened inconspicuous epithelium. Some glands are small like proliferative glands of the normal cycle and lined by tall, frequently pseudostratified cylindrical cells. Normal mitotic figures may be abundant or sparse and are seen both in the epithelium and in the stroma. There is no evidence of cytologic atypia. In simple hyperplasia, the stroma takes

part in the hyperplastic process and the normal gland-stroma ratio is maintained. The stroma is usually focally hypercellular.

Complex Hyperplasia

Complex hyperplasia is characterized by crowded glands with little intervening stroma (Fig. 19-2). Back-to-back glands with glandular outpouchings or buddings and papillary intraluminal infoldings are typical features. The epithelium is pseudostratified and proliferative with abundant mitoses. Cytologic atypia is absent. The stroma is cellular and foci with lipid-laden stromal cells may be seen. The process at times involves the entire endometrium or may be focal. Frequently, complex hyperplasia is intermingled with normal endometrium or foci with simple hyperplasia.

Atypical Hyperplasia

In contrast to endometrial hyperplasia without atypia, most cases of atypical hyperplasia have a complex pattern with crowding of the glands (Fig. 19-3). Atypical hyperplasia is restricted to the glands and is mostly focal. The glands tend to be highly irregular in size and shape with a back-to-back pattern and papillary intraluminal tufts and infoldings. Although they are tightly packed, the glands in atypical hyperplasia are surrounded by stroma. The diagnosis of atypia is based on the cytologic appearance. The nuclei are enlarged and rounded rather than oval (Fig. 19-4). They may be vesicular and have prominent nucleoli. The nuclei often show

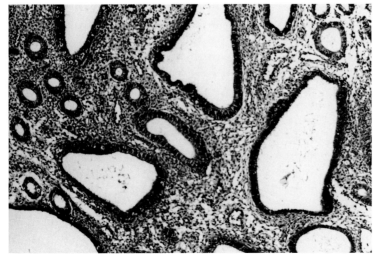

F I G U R E   **19-1**

Simple hyperplasia. Some glands are cystically dilated while others are of normal proliferative size. The stroma is cellular. The normal gland-to-stroma ratio is maintained.

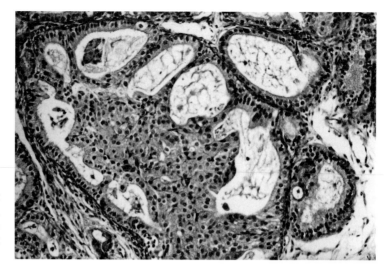

FIGURE **19-2**

Complete hyperplasia without atypia. The glands are crowded and partially filled with a non-keratinizing squamous epithelium that bridges the lumen.

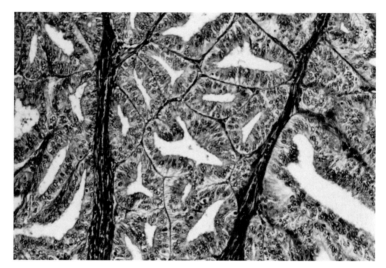

FIGURE **19-3**

Complex atypical hyperplasia. The glands are closely packed, "back to back" with little intervening stroma.

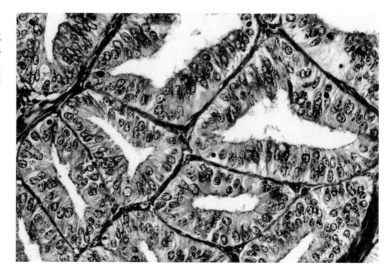

FIGURE **19-4**

Same patient as Fig. 19-3. The lining epithelium shows atypia. The glands are closely packed and lined by tall atypical cells. The nuclei are round to oval with small nucleoli.

stratification with loss of polarity in relation to the basement membrane. This contrasts with the pseudostratification seen in nonatypical hyperplasia. Atypical mitotic figures may be present.

Metaplasia

Any of the hyperplasias may be accompanied by metaplastic changes. The most common change is squamous metaplasia, particularly the morular variant. Extensive squamous metaplasia should not lead to a diagnosis of adenocarcinoma with squamous differentiation unless the glandular component fulfills the criteria of adenocarcinoma. Ciliated cells are frequently seen. Secretory or mucinous metaplasia is occasionally found.

Differential Diagnosis

Simple and complex hyperplasia without atypia must be distinguished from a disordered proliferative phase, polyps, and cystic atrophy; simple atypical hyperplasia, from atypical polypoid adenomyoma; and atypical complex hyperplasia, from complex hyperplasia without atypia and well-differentiated adenocarcinoma of the endometrioid type.

Precursors of malignancy for the other histologic variants of endometrial carcinoma (papillary serous and clear-cell type) are less well known and described. Spiegel (3) observed changes of what he described as carcinoma in situ in a large proportion of these tumors. He postulated that many of these malignancies develop directly in the surface epithelium without an intervening phase of atypical hyperplasia.

If there is a continuum between precancerous lesions and clearly invasive cancer, the same risk factors should apply to both conditions. Age, obesity, diabetes, and hypertension are all associated with a higher than normal incidence of endometrial cancer. The theory of MacDonald and Siiteri (4) from 1973 explains why obesity is a risk factor. The estrogen precursor androstenedione, which is produced by the adrenal cortex, is converted to estrone in peripheral fatty tissue, leading to a constant overexposure to estrogenic substances, of which estrone is the more harmful in these women. This results in the development of complex hyperplasia, possibly with atypia. It is

not established that isolated hypertension per se is an independent risk factor. Thus, the number of well-established risk factors are reduced to two—age and hormonal imbalance. The latter can also be induced by exogenous overexposure to estrogens alone, as was the case in the United States during the 1970s when an increase in endometrial cancer incidence was believed to be caused by unopposed estrogen hormone replacement therapy.

Tamoxifen, frequently used in treating breast cancer, is an antiestrogenic substance, but also exerts a weak estrogenic effect. There is evidence that tamoxifen can be used in treating disorders of the endometrium caused by estrogen overexposure. On the other hand, the results of long-term use of the drug, as in primary breast cancer patients, strongly suggest that the estrogenic effect causes endometrial cancer. In one case-control study by Robinson et al (5), the risk of cancer development was increased by a factor of 15.

Diethylstilbestrol (DES) exposure in utero is associated with the subsequent development of clear-cell adenocarcinoma of the cervix in young women. However, the disease is not unknown in nonexposed women. Therefore, in utero exposure may well be an associated factor that leads to a higher than expected incidence. DES was used from the early 1950s to the mid-1970s. Consequently, the first women exposed in utero now approach the age when clear-cell adenocarcinoma of the uterus is most prevalent. Whether a rise in the incidence of this disease will occur is purely speculative.

The second most common cause of endogenous relative overexposure to estrogenic substances is the polycystic ovarian syndrome, which occasionally leads to the development of cancer in the endometrium at an age when the endometrioid type of adenocarcinoma is extremely rare. Granulosa cell tumors, whether benign or malignant, also produce estrogens. Endometrial hyperplasia, usually nonatypical, is almost invariably found in patients with these conditions.

Symptoms and Diagnosis

A precancerous condition in most instances does not give rise to any symptoms. Longstanding hyperplasia will cause endometrial shedding and the most common reason for seeking medical attention is postmenopausal bleeding. In all such patients whose last menstrual period was more than 6 months ago, a sample of the endometrium must be obtained. There are numerous reports of the use of methods other than dilation and curettage to obtain an endometrial sample, by either aspiration, washing, or introducing a brush or other device to obtain a cytologic specimen. Clinical observations show that as much as 40% of the endometrium is not removed even after what the clinician believes is a thorough scraping of the uterine cavity. Schei et al (6) found that particularly in patients younger than 50 years, a high percentage of endometrial pathology remains undetected after so-called microcurettage with a disposable plastic curette. Therefore, in our opinion, minimally invasive techniques, even if successful in the hands of dedicated investigators, cannot completely replace dilation and curettage as a diagnostic tool in ruling out cancer or precancerous lesions of the uterine cavity in any age group.

Treatment

Hyperplasia occurs in many phases of a woman's life as a result of functional or dysfunctional changes of the endocrine system and is particularly frequent in adolescents and perimenopausal women. A discussion of the treatment of these conditions is outside the scope of this presentation, but the administration of progestogens with or without estrogens is recommended as the first step and is very often successful. There is a lack of agreement as to the malignant potential of the different hyperplasias described here. The reason for this is that a condition that causes abnormal bleeding is nearly always treated and prolonged observation without intervention is unusual.

Some authors tried to estimate the risk of cancer development in patients with untreated atypical hyperplasia (7,8) and gave figures varying from 23% to 88%. There is little disagreement that simple or complex hyperplasia without atypia constitutes a very small risk of rapid cancer development.

Is Atypical Hyperplasia Reversible?

Kjørstad et al (9) published the results of high-dose progestogen treatment in 32 women with atypical hyperplasia who were given 6000 mg of hydroxyprogesterone caproate intramuscularly

in the course of 1 week. Thereafter, 1000 mg was given weekly for 6 weeks and a new dilation and curettage was performed. In patients showing total or partial regression, the same schedule was repeated for another 6 weeks; otherwise, a hysterectomy was performed. Pharmacodynamic studies showed that these women achieved a high and stable level of hydroxyprogesterone caproate and there were no immediate harmful side effects.

The end results were as follows: six patients developed evidence of invasive disease despite the heavy hormonal treatment. These women underwent hysterectomy and evaluation of the uterine specimen confirmed the diagnosis of cancer. In 1 patient more than minimal invasion into the endometrial stroma was found, thus indicating that at least in this patient the pretreatment diagnosis of atypical hyperplasia was an underestimation of the actual severity of the process. Another 14 patients had hysterectomy performed within the next 3 years, either because the condition recurred or because of abnormal bleeding. Among these patients another 4 were shown to have invasive cancer.

In the remaining 12 patients the atypical hyperplasia regressed completely and no further treatment was indicated. It is of interest that 10 of these women were premenopausal or perimenopausal and comprised the youngest women in this series.

In conclusion, it seems that very high doses of progestogens may revert approximately 30% of premalignant lesions of the endometrium, but there is no evidence that invasive disease can be cured by hormonal treatment. The fact that the treatment was only effective in premenopausal and perimenopausal women gives rise to speculations as to whether cyclic treatment with or without estrogens would have caused a more complete shedding of the endometrium and a faster recovery. It is quite clear that hormonal manipulation of precancerous lesions with a curative intent should only be undertaken in relatively young women.

In the absence of endocrine disorders, endometrial adenocarcinoma is an extremely rare disease in women under the age of 40. Therefore, conservative treatment, even in the event of atypia, is warranted in this age group.

From a clinical viewpoint, atypical hyperplasia in the postmenopausal woman is a serious condition and hysterectomy should be performed to rule out or confirm the diagnosis of endometrial carcinoma.

Screening and Atypical Hyperplasia

Unlike screening for cervical cancer, there is no evidence that mass screening for endometrial cancer is cost-effective. At the Norwegian Radium hospital, simple sampling of endometrial material with a thin blunt cannula was performed at the same time that a cervical smear was obtained, as part of a regional mass screening program. Among 4000 specimens from asymptomatic women, a single case of endometrial adenocarcinoma was detected (unpublished material).

Grønroos et al (10) in Finland conducted a study aimed at risk groups. Women with a known diagnosis of diabetes or hypertension were invited to participate in a program that used an aspiration device to obtain material from the endometrium. Of 1332 patients who fulfilled the criteria of being between 45 and 70 years old and with a confirmed diagnosis of hypertension, diabetes, or both, 620 refused to participate and in 115 women the procedure could not be performed owing to insertion difficulties. This occurred in 19% of the postmenopausal women (N = 101), opposed to only 3% in the premenopausal group (N = 496). In the whole study group, 8 patients were found to have adenocarcinoma in situ or atypical hyperplasia and all of these patients were diabetic. No significant pathology was found in the 139 women in this series who had hypertension alone. Grönroos concluded that mass screening programs probably are warranted for diabetic women over the age of 45. His results, however, indicate major problems with attendance and with adequacy of the samples obtained, two factors of paramount importance in the architecture of successful screening programs.

REFERENCES

1. Scully RE, Bonfiglio TA, Kurman RJ, et al. *International histological classification and typing of female genital tract tumours.* Berlin: Springer, 1994.

2. Silverberg SG, Kurman RJ. *Atlas of tumor pathology. Tumors of the uterine corpus and gestational trophoblastic disease.* Washington, DC: Armed Forces Institute of Pathology, 1992.

3. Spiegel GW. Endometrial carcinoma in situ in postmenopausal women. *Am J Surg Pathol* 1995;19:417–432.

4. MacDonald PC, Siiteri PK. The relationship between the extraglandular production of estrone and the occurrence of endometrial neoplasia. *Gynecol Oncol* 1974;2:259–263.

5. Robinson DC, Bloss JD, Schiano MA. A retrospective study of tamoxifen and endometrial cancer in breast cancer patients. *Gynecol Oncol* 1995;59:186–190.

6. Schei B, Bang TF, Halgunset J, et al. Microcurettage sampling of the endometrium for histopathological examination—simpler but not safe? Comparison of endometrial histopathology in samples obtained by a disposable mechanical curette and by traditional curettage. *Acta Obstet Gynecol Scand* 1994;73:497–501.

7. Wentz WB. Progestin therapy in endometrial hyperplasia. *Gynecol Oncol* 1974;2:362–367.

8. Kurman RJ, Kaminski PF, Norris HJ. The behavior of endometrial hyperplasia. A long term study of "untreated" hyperplasia in 170 women. *Cancer* 1985;56:403–411.

9. Kjørstad KE, Welander C, Halvorsen T, et al. Progestogens as primary treatment in premalignant changes of the endometrium. In: Bush, King, Taylor, eds. *Endometrial cancer.* London: Bailliere Tindal, 1978:188.

10. Grönroos M, Salmi T, Vuento MH, et al. Mass screening for endometrial cancer directed in risk groups of patients with diabetes and patients with hypertension. *Cancer* 1993;71:1279–1282.

CHAPTER 20

Evaluation, Diagnosis, and Treatment of Corpus Cancer

C. PAUL MORROW
HAROLD FOX

Epidemiology and Screening

Epidemiology

Endometrial carcinoma is the most common invasive neoplasm of the female genital tract in the United States. According to the American Cancer Society, 34,000 new cases were expected to be diagnosed in the United States in 1996 (1). The incidence doubled in the early 1970s, presumably related to the widespread use of unopposed estrogen replacement therapy, although part of the increase may have been related to decreased childbearing (2). The incidence of endometrial cancer has remained stable over the past 10 to 12 years.

The average age at diagnosis of endometrial carcinoma is 58 years. Only 2% to 5% of all cases occur in women less than age 40, and the disease is rare before age 30. In the United States white women have a 2.4% lifetime risk of developing endometrial carcinoma as compared to a 1.3% risk for black women. A number of constitutional factors have been identified in women who develop endometrial carcinoma (Table 20-1) (3–5). In addition to race and postmenopausal status, additional associated factors are reported to be tallness; a history of ovarian, colon, or breast cancer; and a family history of endometrial carcinoma, polycystic ovarian disease, estrogen-producing ovarian stromal tumors, and hypothyroidism. Pelvic irradiation therapy, especially low-dose radiation therapy,

is a risk factor for both endometrial adenocarcinoma and carcinosarcoma (6). In these patients endometrial carcinoma tends to be less well differentiated and is associated with a poorer outcome compared to endometrial carcinoma in patients without prior pelvic radiation. Protective factors include cigarette smoking and the use of progestational or combination oral contraceptives. Worldwide, the variable incidence of endometrial cancer is most strongly associated with socioeconomic status, fertility, and total dietary fat consumption (7).

Many studies confirmed the increased rate of endometrial carcinoma in women who take *medicinal estrogens*. This risk is related to the dose of estrogen, the duration of therapy, and possibly the schedule of administration, that is, continuous versus cyclic. Women with presumed estrogen-induced endometrial cancer typically have a well-differentiated, superficially invasive tumor, although the increased risk is not limited to the favorable types (8). Nevertheless, the overall survival rate of women developing endometrial carcinoma during estrogen replacement therapy exceeds that of all women with endometrial cancer. Women who stop estrogen replacement continue to have an increased risk of endometrial cancer for several years. There is considerable evidence that progestins alone or combined with estrogen reduce the risk of endometrial carcinoma. However, since this protection is not absolute, some women who take both estrogen and progestin will still develop the disease (9).

T A B L E   **20-1**

Estimate of Risk Ratios for Certain Factors Associated with Endometrial Carcinoma

Risk Factor	Reported Range of Relative Risk
Overweight (lb)	1.9–11.0
20–50	3
>50	9
Parous vs. nulliparous	0.1–0.9
Late menopause (age ≥52 yr)	1.7–2.4
Diabetes mellitus	1.3–2.7
Pelvic radiation (low dose)	8
Estrogen replacement therapy	1.6–12.0
Oral contraceptive use	
Sequential	0.9–7.3
Combined	0.1–1.0
Hypertension	1.2–2.1

Sources: MacMahon B. Risk factors for endometrial cancer. *Gynecol Oncol* 1974;2:122; Parazzini F, LaVecchia C, Bocciolone L, Franceschi S. The epidemiology of endometrial cancer. *Gynecol Oncol* 1991;41:1; Wynder EL, Escher GC, Mantel N. An epidemiologic investigation of cancer of the endometrium. *Cancer* 1966; 19:489.

Recent investigations highlighted two additional populations of women at increased risk for the development of endometrial cancer. The first group consists of those women who take *tamoxifen* following breast cancer therapy. Tamoxifen is a hormone that has a weak stimulatory effect on the endometrium. In a literature review, Barakat (10) noted marked inconsistencies in the effects of tamoxifen on the endometrium. The reported incidence of endometrial polyps varies from 8% to 36% [relative risk (RR) range, 1–4]; endometrial hyperplasia, from 2% to 20% (RR range, 1–16); and endometrial cancer, from 0% to 8% (RR range, 1–7). High-risk histology (papillary serous, clear cell, carcinosarcoma) was observed in 25% of patients but the type varied among the studies, and grade 3 adenocarcinoma was noted in 27% of patients. Other reports showed no difference in the histology of tamoxifen- and non-tamoxifen-associated cases. Based on randomized trials of breast cancer treatment, it is estimated that the annual risk for endometrial cancer is 0.006 (11) after an average of 5 years of tamoxifen exposure. Ultrasound evaluation of women taking tamoxifen has led to the observation that the thickness of the endometrial "stripe" is more than 5 mm in 50% of these women (normal in non-tamoxifen-exposed patients is <5 mm), and values up to 8 mm are considered to be normal. Despite the concern that these women have an increased risk for uterine cancer, the recommended monitoring program is an annual gynecologic examination. Further studies are reserved for the symptomatic patient (e.g., those with uterine bleeding).

The second group of women recently identified as having an increased risk for endometrial carcinoma are those members of a *hereditary non-polyposis colon cancer* (HNPCC) family. Typically members of families with this genetic cancer syndrome present with colon cancer. Among women in HNPCC families the most common noncolon cancer is uterine. As is true of hereditary cancer in general, the cancers in the HNPCC families tend to occur at a younger age than the sporadic cases in the general population.

Screening

No satisfactory technique is available for the routine screening of large populations of women for endometrial carcinoma and its precursors. Because the majority of endometrial cancers are stage I at diagnosis and the outcome for these patients is relatively favorable, mass screening is unlikely to be cost-effective or to improve survival. Thus, routine endometrial cytology, biopsy, or ultrasound evaluation cannot be recommended for all women. Routine evaluation of the endometrium on an annual basis may be appropriate, however, for postmenopausal women who are taking estrogen without progestin, and whenever unscheduled bleeding occurs. Symptomatic patients must have a prompt evaluation including biopsy.

There are numerous devices for obtaining endometrial specimens in the outpatient setting, and biopsy has proved to be more accurate than cytology in detecting endometrial carcinoma and hyperplasia. Complications are unusual but the failure rate, which increases with the age of the patient, averages 10% to 15%.

Ultrasonic measurement of the thickness of the endometrium may be an adjunct to endometrial biopsy in the evaluation of a patient with symptoms or when endometrial biopsy is not feasible. If the endometrial stripe is less than 5 mm thick, the incidence of endometrial neoplasia in postmenopausal women is very low (12). Conversely, when the endometrium is thicker than 10 mm, 10% to 20% of patients will have hyperplasia or carcinoma. Any patient who is noted to have a thickened endometrium on ultrasound scans should have an endometrial biopsy.

Routine cervical cytology occasionally leads to the diagnosis of endometrial cancer. Findings suspicious for endometrial pathology are 1) numerous histiocytes in the postmenopausal smear; 2) normal-appearing endometrial cells obtained during the second half of the menstrual cycle or anytime after the menopause except in women taking estrogens [while Cherkis et al (13) reported that 13% of postmenopausal women with normal endometrial cells on routine Pap smears had endometrial cancer, Yancey et al (14) found none]; and 3) atypical or malignant glandular cells in any age group. These findings are an indication for endocervical or endometrial sampling.

Diagnosis and Evaluation

Symptoms

The preeminent symptom of endometrial carcinoma is abnormal uterine bleeding. Approximately three fourths of cases occur in the perimenopausal or postmenopausal age group, and in more than 90% the initial complaint is vaginal bleeding. Other important initial symptoms are a purulent, sometimes blood-tinged discharge and pain. The latter is often the result of metastases. Only 1% to 5% of endometrial carcinomas are diagnosed while the patient is asymptomatic. This most often results from investigation of a Pap smear showing atypical or malignant endometrial cells, or the discovery of cancer in a uterus removed for benign gynecologic indications.

The causes of postmenopausal bleeding are numerous, but 10% to 20% of patients with this complaint have a gynecologic malignancy, usually endometrial carcinoma. Common physician errors in managing these patients are the assumption that the bleeding is due to medicinal estrogens or to atrophic vaginitis, that the bleeding is insufficient to warrant investigation, that the cervical os is stenotic and therefore bleeding from the uterus could not have occurred, or that a Pap smear is adequate evaluation for postmenopausal bleeding. Although a single episode of spotting or bleeding is most likely due to causes such as an atrophic vaginal mucosa, in the study of Hawwa et al (15) 7% of these patients had carcinoma, approximately the same percentage as for patients with spotting or bleeding for 2 to 6 days. The older the patient with bleeding, the greater the risk of cancer.

Women with endometrial carcinoma who are premenopausal or perimenopausal invariably have abnormal uterine bleeding, often characterized as menometrorrhagia or oligomenorrhea. A variation of this pattern is cyclic bleeding, which may persist after the expected age of the menopause. This is often misinterpreted as ovulatory bleeding. For this reason, periodic endometrial evaluation is recommended for women still "menstruating" after age 52. Most premenopausal women with corpus cancer are in the over-40 age group, but the disease must also be considered in younger women with abnormal bleeding that is persistent or recurrent, or at any time if obesity and chronic anovulation (oligomenorrhea) are present.

Physical Examination

Clues to the presence of endometrial carcinoma are seldom found on general examination, although obesity, diabetes, and hypertension are commonly associated constitutional factors. Rarely, peripheral lymph gland metastases or metastases to the vaginal introitus and suburethral area are present. On bimanual rectovaginal palpation the uterus is frequently enlarged by fibroids, myometrial hypertrophy, hematometra or pyometra, and occasionally, tumor bulk; however, in some instances the uterus is atrophic. The adnexa may contain metastatic disease or a concurrent primary ovarian carcinoma. Often the results of the entire examination are normal.

Differential Diagnosis

The more common conditions that must be considered when evaluating the patient suspected of having endometrial cancer are those that cause abnormal bleeding, especially postmenopausal bleeding: vaginal, cervical, tubal, and ovarian carcinoma; benign and malignant myometrial tumors; endometrial polyps; and endometrial hyperplasia. Metastasis to the endometrium causing vaginal bleeding is rarely the first sign of an extrapelvic carcinoma.

Diagnosis

Microscopic analysis of endometrial tissue is required to make the diagnosis of endometrial carcinoma. The classic means for obtaining the tissue specimen is fractional curettage. This consists of a circumferential endocervical scrape followed by systematic, comprehensive endometrial curettage. The two specimens are submitted to the laboratory separately. Fractionation of the curettage sample serves to detect an occult endocervical carcinoma and to determine whether the endometrial carcinoma involves the cervix. Naturally, biopsies should be performed for any suspicious lesion of the lower genital tract.

Office endometrial biopsy (EMB) with endocervical curettage (ECC), rather than a formal curettage in the operating room, is the accepted first step for evaluating postmenopausal bleeding or whenever endometrial pathology is suspected. EMB consists of multiple strokes with a curette, sampling as much of the uterine cavity as feasible. Frequently the procedure is tantamount to a formal curettage. Office biopsy is generally well tolerated, accurate, and cost-effective (16). Unless the results of these studies are negative, it is not appropriate to attribute postmenopausal bleeding to benign causes such as atrophic vaginitis, hormone therapy, or urethral caruncle. Fibroids should never be accepted as a cause of postmenopausal bleeding. When the cervical canal is stenotic or patient tolerance does not permit adequate office evaluation of the endometrium and endocervix, an ultrasound examination, or curettage under anesthesia is necessary.

Granberg et al (12) proposed using vaginal ultrasound to screen women with postmenopausal bleeding prior to performing uterine curettage. They pointed out that fewer than 10% of women with postmenopausal bleeding have endometrial carcinoma. If a cutoff limit of 5 mm for the thickness of the normal endometrial stripe is used, 80% of curettages could be avoided. Thus, if office evaluation of the woman with postmenopausal bleeding is unsatisfactory or inconclusive, transvaginal ultrasound can be used to select patients for formal uterine curettage. Ultrasound does not, however, evaluate the cervix. Thus, ECC or endocervical cytology is necessary. Recurrent bleeding is an indication for dilatation and curettage and hysteroscopy even if the ultrasound scan appears normal (17,18). Patients with postmenopausal bleeding whose pelvic examination is unsatisfactory should also be evaluated with ultrasound.

Clinical Staging

In 1988 the International Federation of Gynecology and Obstetrics (FIGO) staging for endometrial carcinoma was changed from clinical to surgical (Table 20-2) (19). However, clinical staging is still important in terms of preoperative evaluation and planning for surgery, and still correlates well with prognosis (Table 20-3). The most important elements are the physical examination and the fractional curettage. The uterine size and the status of the parametrial tissues, adnexa, and the peripheral lymph nodes should be noted. Particular attention should be given also to the vagina and suburethral area. In more than 75% of patients there is no clinical evidence of extrauterine involvement (clinical stage I). The most common site of extension is the cervix (clinical stage II). For stage I and II patients the only additional studies

T A B L E   20-2

FIGO Surgical Staging for Carcinoma of the Corpus Uteri (1988)

Stage*	Definition
I	The cancer is limited to the corpus uteri.
Ia	Tumor limited to the endometrium.
Ib	Invasion to <50% of the myometrium.
Ic	Invasion to >50% of the myometrium.
II	The cancer involves the cervix.
IIa	Endocervical glandular involvement only.
IIb	Cervical stromal invasion.
III	The cancer extends outside the uterus to the pelvis or retroperitoneal lymph nodes.
IIIa	Tumor invades serosa and/or adnexa, and/or positive peritoneal cytology.
IIIb	Vaginal metastases.
IIIc	Metastases to pelvic and/or aortic lymph nodes.
IV	The cancer involves the bladder, bowel, or DM.
IVa	Tumor invasion of bladder and/or bowel mucosa.
IVb	Distant metastases including intra-abdominal and/or inguinal lymph nodes.

*The stage is not affected by the tumor grade.

Source: Pettersson F, ed. FIGO annual report. *Int J Gynecol Obstet* 1991;36:S1.

TABLE   **20-3**

Endometrial Carcinoma: Actuarial Survival According to Clinical Stage, 1982–1986, FIGO Annual Report 1991

Clinical Stage	Total No. of Patients	Stage (%)	5-year Survival Rate (%)
I	7092	70.2	76.3
II	1803	17.8	59.2
III	818	8.1	29.4
IV	364	3.6	10.3

Source: Pettersson F, ed. FIGO annual report. *Int J Gynecol Obstet* 1991;36:S1.

required are chest x-ray, electrocardiography, and the usual preoperative blood tests. Measurement of serum CA-125 level can also be of value, especially for high-risk histologies. About 20% of patients with clinical stage I or II endometrial carcinoma have an elevated serum CA-125 value: 80% of surgically upstaged patients but only 8% of patients without surgical-pathologic evidence of extrauterine disease (20,21).

Clinical staging has proved to be unreliable in assessing the patient for many important prognostic factors including cervix/isthmic invasion, histologic grade and type of cancer, depth of myometrial invasion, lymph-vascular space invasion (LVSI), and the presence of nodal, adnexal, and intraperitoneal metastases. The presence of malignant tissue in the ECC is commonly a "contaminant" from the endometrial lesion. Thus, a "positive" ECC does not confirm cervical involvement unless there is demonstrable endocervical gland replacement or cervical stromal invasion (22). The prognostic importance of stromal invasion in the endocervical curettage sample has been well documented (23,24). Furthermore, gross cervical involvement augers a worse prognosis than does microscopic disease [60% versus 75% 5-year survival rate (25)]. The lesion grade, however, more strongly influences the outcome in patients with endometrial carcinoma than does the presence of cervical invasion (26).

Cone biopsy has been used to improve the accuracy of determining cervical invasion, but when the involvement is preclinical, this information is of little value. Conization is recommended only when one is uncertain that a malignancy exists or when one is uncertain as to whether the cancer is endometrial or endocervical in origin. Hysteroscopy and hysterography have been used to determine the extent of tumor and its proximity to the cervix, but both have the potential to push cancer cells through the fallopian tubes and into uterine

vascular spaces. Their use should be limited to patients in whom a diagnosis is not forthcoming by the usual procedures. Occasionally, both the cervix and the endometrium are overtly involved with adenocarcinoma, and it is impossible to determine whether the origin is from the cervix, isthmus, or corpus. This is the classic *corporis et colli* (body and cervix) lesion and should be considered endometrial in origin.

A spate of reports has appeared since 1985 concerning transvaginal ultrasound and magnetic resonance imaging (MRI) determination of myoinvasion. Because the probability of extrauterine metastases correlates with the depth of myoinvasion, this is potentially important information in planning surgery, especially if the patient with deep myoinvasion will require referral to a tertiary center for treatment. In brief, it appears that both methods can measure the depth of myoinvasion in about 80% of patients, but the accuracy is poorer for deeply invasive lesions. The studies are somewhat less reliable for detecting cervical invasion, and unreliable for determining the presence of lymph node and intraperitoneal metastases (27–30). Since MRI is much more expensive than ultrasound, the latter is the method of choice for assessing myometrial invasion preoperatively.

More extensive preoperative evaluation is indicated for patients whose disease has features that put them at high risk for metastases. When the lesion is poorly differentiated, papillary serous, clear cell, or sarcomatous, computed tomography (CT) of the abdomen and pelvis is warranted to evaluate the liver and retroperitoneal nodes. CT should also be performed on patients who have abnormal liver function, an elevated serum CA-125 value, clinical evidence of metastases, and parametrial or vaginal extension. Adnexal pathology is common in patients with endometrial carcinoma because the tube and ovary are frequent sites of metastases. Furthermore, endometrial carcinoma tends to occur in conjunction with certain ovarian malignancies (endometrioid adenocarcinoma, clear-cell carcinoma, and granulosa cell tumors), particularly in pre-menopausal women (31). Ultrasound is the study of choice to evaluate the adnexa. For locally advanced disease, cystoscopy, barium enema, or sigmoidoscopy may be necessary to accurately stage the patient. Bone and brain scans are not indicated in the absence of symptoms or evidence of hematogenous metastases.

Pathology

The pathologic variables in any patient with endometrial neoplasia are of importance as prognostic criteria and it is from that particular viewpoint that they are discussed here.

Histologic Type

The histologic classification of epithelial tumors of the endometrium is detailed in Table 20-4. The classification is somewhat complex and only the major tumor categories are considered here. Endometrioid adenocarcinomas are those that show some degree of endometrial differentiation and bear a resemblance, albeit an anarchic one, to normal proliferative endometrium. These account for about 80% of endometrial neoplasms and are therefore "the usual type of endometrial adenocarcinoma"; this form of nomenclature is clearly too unwieldy and hence the term *endometrioid adenocarcinoma* is preferred, and although this nomenclature is not to everyone's taste, it is semantically, even pedantically, correct. Most endometrioid adenocarcinomas are reasonably well differentiated (Fig. 20-1) and easily recognizable as such, with irregular architecturally complex glands lined by cuboidal or columnar epithelium of recognizably endometrial type. The tumor cells show cytologic atypia and mitotic activity: Papillary infoldings, multilayering, intraluminal tufting, and the formation of intraglandular epithelial bridges are common. The glandular acini are often separated from each other only by a thin wisp of stroma or show a true "back-to-back" pattern. A minority of endometrioid adenocarcinomas are less well differentiated and have a partly solid and partly acinar growth pattern (Fig. 20-2) while occasional endometrioid adenocarcinomas are so poorly differentiated (Fig. 20-3) that they can

T A B L E **20-4**

Classification of Primary Epithelial Neoplasms of the Endometrium

1. Endometrioid adenocarcinoma
   Variants
      With squamous metaplasia
      Papillary
      Secretory
      Ciliated
      Sertoliform
2. Adenosquamous carcinoma
3. Serous papillary adenocarcinoma
4. Clear-cell adenocarcinoma
5. Mucinous adenocarcinoma
6. Squamous cell carcinoma
7. Undifferentiated carcinoma

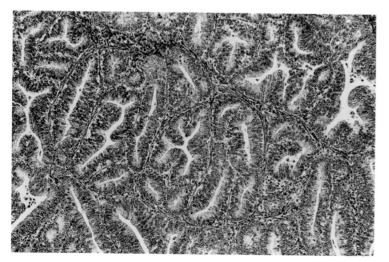

F I G U R E **20-1**

A well-differentiated endometrioid adenocarcinoma of the endometrium. The tumor is composed of closely packed, well-formed glandular acini lined by a stratified columnar epithelium, set in a fibrous stroma.

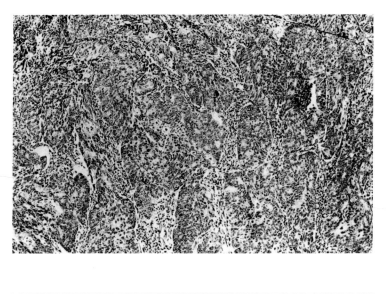

FIGURE 20-2

A moderately differentiated end-ometrioid adenocarcinoma of the endometrium. Glandular acini are poorly formed, though approximately 50% of the neoplasm has a glandular/acinar pattern.

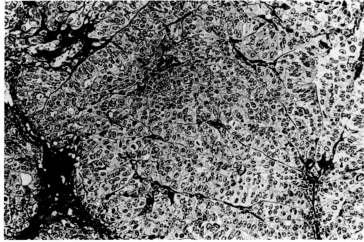

FIGURE 20-3

Poorly differentiated carcinoma of the endometrium. The neoplasm is composed almost entirely of sheets and nests of cells.

only be identified as being of endometrioid type if there is, in some areas, a tentative attempt at formation of endometrial glandular acini.

Squamous metaplasia is very common in endometrioid adenocarcinomas and may be a conspicuous feature. There may be foci of bland, well-differentiated squamous tissue that are wholly within the neoplastic acini and have a fully benign appearance or "morules" that consist of nests of spindly cells with small bland nuclei; the morules are also intraglandular but can expand to compress, and sometimes mask, the surrounding glandular cells. Endometrioid adenocarcinomas showing extensive squamous metaplasia are often put into a separate diagnostic category of "adenoacanthoma," it being believed that such neoplasms are a distinct entity with an unusually good prognosis. However, the criterion for recognition of such a tumor (i.e., the presence of "extensive" meta-

plasia) is both imprecise and subjective; further, it has been clearly demonstrated that, stage for stage and grade for grade, endometrioid adenocarcinomas showing a striking degree of squamous metaplasia have a prognosis that does not differ significantly from that for those in which there is little or no squamous metaplasia (32). Therefore, there seems little justification for considering "adenoacanthoma" as a distinct entity or for retaining this diagnostic category.

It is important to distinguish between the bland squamous metaplasia seen in many endometrioid adenocarcinomas and the malignant squamous epithelium that is present in an adenosquamous carcinoma of the endometrium. Tumors of this latter type account for about 5% of endometrial neoplasms and contain both malignant glandular and malignant squamous components (Fig. 20-4) that are admixed but discrete from each other (33–35). The glandular element is usually an endometrioid adenocarcinoma while the squamous component is clearly malignant and infiltrates the stroma in an invasive fashion. Adenosquamous carcinomas are aggressive neoplasms with a relatively poor prognosis. It is only fair to note that some pathologists do not agree with the concept of endometrial adenosquamous carcinoma, arguing that there is a continuous spectrum of malignancy in squamous differentiation within endometrioid adenocarcinomas, that the division between benign squamous metaplasia and infiltrating malignant squamous epithelium is far from clear-cut, and that the prognosis always depends on the degree of differentiation of the glandular component (36,37). This may well turn out to be true but in most cases the squamous component does seem to fit rather

clearly into either a metaplastic or a malignant category.

The serous papillary adenocarcinoma of the endometrium (Fig. 20-5) is histologically identical to a serous papillary adenocarcinoma of the ovary (38–41). These neoplasms have a papillary architecture with tumor cells covering broad fibrovascular stalks: The tumor cells show high-grade atypia and are markedly pleomorphic. These neoplasms invade uterine lymphatic and vascular channels at an early stage in their evolution and are associated with an extremely gloomy prognosis. However, some papillary serous adenocarcinomas have been confined to a polyp at the time of initial diagnosis (42) and even these have a poor prognosis. Indeed, all the classic prognostic factors for endometrial carcinoma do not seem to be applicable to serous papillary carcinomas (43). The serous

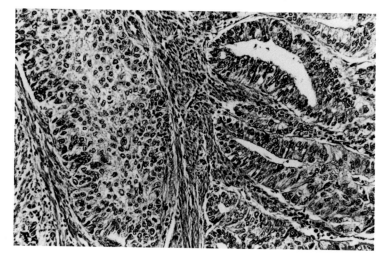

F I G U R E **20-4**

Adenosquamous carcinoma of the endometrium. Well-formed malignant glandular acini lie to the right of the field and a sheet of infiltrating, nonkeratinizing, squamous carcinoma lies to the left.

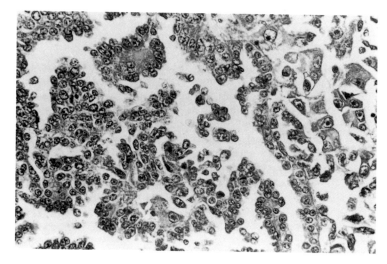

F I G U R E **20-5**

Serous papillary carcinoma of the endometrium. The well-formed papillary processes are covered by cells showing high-grade atypia.

papillary adenocarcinoma has to be distinguished from the papillary form (Fig. 20-6) of an endometrioid adenocarcinoma (villoglandular endometrioid adenocarcinoma), which is generally considered to have an excellent prognosis (39,44), though dissenting voices, claiming either that all papillary neoplasms of the endometrium have a poor prognosis (45) or that papillary endometrioid tumors have a worse prognosis than the typical endometrioid adenocarcinoma but a better prognosis than papillary serous tumors (46), have been raised.

The clear-cell adenocarcinoma of the endometrium (Fig. 20-7) is identical histologically to the clear-cell adenocarcinoma of the ovary and shows a complex permutation of tubulocystic, solid, papillary, and glandular patterns: "Hob-nail" cells tend to be a prominent feature, these being admixed with clear cells containing abundant cytoplasmic glycogen. These neoplasms tend to show high-grade atypia and also invade lymphatic and vascular spaces at an early stage, with a resulting extremely poor prognosis (47–50), though it should be noted that low-stage clear-cell carcinoma has a rather better prognosis than does low-stage 1 serous papillary serous adenocarcinoma (51,52).

Mucinous adenocarcinomas of the endometrium, identical histologically to well-differentiated mucinous adenocarcinomas of the ovary and well-differentiated endocervical adenocarcinomas, have a prognosis similar to that of endometrioid adenocarcinomas of the same grade, this being generally very good (53).

Pure squamous cell carcinomas of the endometrium are very rare (54) and tend to arise in endometria showing ichthyosis uteri; they have a poor prognosis (55).

Some carcinomas of the endometrium are "undifferentiated," to the extent that their carcinomatous nature can only be recognized with

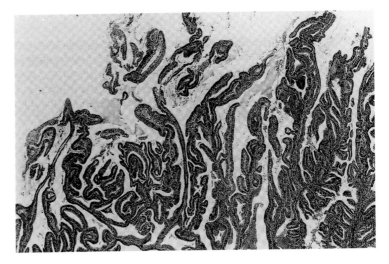

FIGURE 20-6
A papillary endometrioid adenocarcinoma of the endometrium. The papillae are delicate and covered by cells of endometrioid type showing only low-grade atypia.

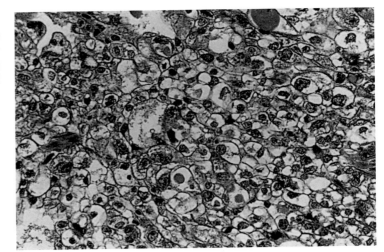

FIGURE 20-7
Clear-cell adenocarcinoma of the endometrium. In this field the tumor has a solid pattern and is composed of large cells with well-defined margins and clear cytoplasm.

the aid of epithelial markers such as those for cytokeratins. These also have a relatively poor prognosis, though not as gloomy as that for serous papillary or clear-cell neoplasms (56). Undifferentiated carcinomas should be distinguished from the highly aggressive small-cell carcinoma of the endometrium that is a neuroendocrine neoplasm (57,58).

Tumor Grade

Grading is probably only of prognostic value in endometrioid adenocarcinomas of the endometrium. Architectural grading is certainly of no value in serous papillary or clear-cell adenocarcinomas and there is considerable doubt as to whether nuclear grading is of any value either in these tumors. The currently recommended FIGO grading system is as follows:

Grade 1. Five percent or less of the tumor shows a solid growth pattern.

Grade 2. Between 6% and 50% of the tumor is growing in a solid fashion.

Grade 3. More than 50% of the tumor shows a solid growth pattern.

In making this grading, solid sheets of metaplastic squamous epithelium are ignored. Significant cytologic atypia in grade 1 or 2 tumors raises the grading by one grade.

This grading system can, in terms of the proportion of the tumor growing in a solid fashion, be applied in a consistent fashion by pathologists and has proved to be prognostically valid in terms of predicting both lymph node involvement and survival rate (59), but problems have arisen as to the exact meaning of the phrase "significant cytologic atypia." In view of this, a nuclear grading system has now been clearly defined (60). In this, nuclear grade 1 is defined as rounded nuclei with even chromatin and inconspicuous nucleoli whereas grade 2 nuclei are irregularly oval with even chromatin and evident nucleoli and grade 3 nuclei are large, irregular, and pleomorphic with coarse chromatin and prominent nucleoli. A moderate degree of diagnostic consistency could be attained using this nuclear grading system and only the presence of grade 3 nuclei was taken to be "significant atypia" in terms of raising the architectural grade.

Whether this grading system requires further refinement is a matter of debate and it should be noted that no distinction is drawn between tumors that have no areas of solid growth and those that have a solid growth pattern that constitutes up to 5% of the neoplasm. This distinction may be important for it has been claimed that even the presence of small areas of solid growth, constituting less than 5% of the tumor, have an independent adverse prognostic impact (61).

Depth of Invasion

There is general agreement that the depth of invasion of the myometrium by adenocarcinomatous cells is of considerable prognostic significance, increasing depth of invasion being associated with increasing rates of recurrence and death (62,63). Exactly why this should be so is uncertain but stage I invasive carcinomas are currently subdivided into those invading into the inner half of the myometrium and those extending into the outer half. It should be noted that naked-eye estimation of depth of invasion, while quite good for well-differentiated neoplasms, is highly inaccurate when dealing with poorly differentiated tumors (64).

Lymphatic-Vascular Space Invasion

LVSI by tumor cells is an independent prognostic factor of considerable importance, being associated with markedly reduced survival rates (65,66).

State of Nonneoplastic Endometrium

Assessment of the state of any nonneoplastic endometrium that is present in a uterus harboring an endometrial adenocarcinoma is important. It has been clearly shown that adenocarcinomas arising from a background of atypical endometrial hyperplasia are associated with a much higher 5-year survival rate than are those developing in an endometrium that is normally cycling or atrophic (67).

Receptor Status, Ploidy, Oncogene Expression, Tumor Suppressor Genes

Estrogen and progesterone receptors can be demonstrated immunocytochemically and, in general, are found most frequently and in greatest density in well-differentiated endometrioid adenocarcinomas. There is a correlation between high tumor content of steroid hormone receptors and a good prognosis (68) but on multivariate analysis it is only a high content of progesterone receptor that survives as an independent prognostic variable (69).

The many studies of DNA ploidy in endometrial adenocarcinoma have shown that, unsurprisingly, aneuploidy correlates with poor tumor differentiation, vascular space involvement, and deep myometrial invasion and is an independent indicator of a poor prognosis (70–72).

Studies of the expression in endometrial adenocarcinomas of proto-oncogenes, such as c-*myc* and c-*ras*, and growth factors, such as c-Erb B-2 and epidermal growth factor receptor, and of the tumor suppression gene p53 yielded results that are currently inconclusive in terms of their status as independent prognostic variables (73).

Staging

Comments

The inherent inaccuracy of clinical staging for endometrial carcinoma is a serious impediment to the selection of optimal therapy, and over the years has resulted in both overtreatment and undertreatment. Several systematic, surgical-pathologic investigations of clinical stage I and II endometrial carcinomas documented that the incidence of pelvic and aortic node metastases is clinically significant (62,74,75). The rate of node metastasis increases with the depth of myoinvasion, loss of tumor differentiation, and extension to the isthmus or cervix. One third to one half of the patients with pelvic node involvement also have aortic node spread, but the aortic glands are seldom a solitary site of metastasis. Thus, surgical staging studies are in agreement with the long-recognized correlation between tumor grade, myoinvasion, and prognosis. The overall magnitude of understaging is 15% to 25% (62,74–78) (Table 20-5).

Intraoperative Staging Procedure

An examination under anesthesia should always precede surgical staging to assess the status of the vagina, the parametrium, and the paracolpium. In the typical patient the abdomen is opened with a vertical, lower abdominal incision. For all patients intraoperative staging includes peritoneal washings from the pelvis

T A B L E   **20-5**

Surgical-Pathologic Risk Factors Determined at Staging Laparotomy on 222 Patients with Clinical Stage I Endometrial Carcinoma

Risk Factor	N	% of Total Cases
Outer one-third myoinvasion	33	15
Positive pelvic cytology	26	12[a]
Pelvic node metastases	23	10
Extension to the cervix/isthmus	18	8
Aortic node metastases	17	7.5[b]
Adnexal metastases	16	7
LVSI	16	7
Peritoneal tumor implants	6	3

LVSI = lymph-vascular space invasion.

[a] Percent of all 222 patients. Results not available on 51 patients.

[b] Percent of all 222 patients. Results not available on 65 patients.

Source: Boronow RC, Morrow CP, Creasman WT, et al. Surgical staging in endometrial cancer: clinicopathological findings of a prospective study. *Obstet Gynecol* 1984;63:825.

and abdomen, a careful visual and palpatory exploration of the abdominal contents, especially both leaves of the diaphragm, Morison's pouch, the liver, aortic nodes, omentum, the pelvic peritoneum, and pelvic nodes. Evaluation of nodal areas is done preferably with the peritoneum opened. In all patients suspicious lymph nodes should be removed and submitted for frozen-section evaluation. Similarly suspicious adnexal and peritoneal lesions should be subjected to intraoperative pathologic study. Whenever feasible, all enlarged, tumor-bearing nodes are removed to optimize the patient's status for postoperative adjuvant therapy. The documentation of nodal metastases in the pelvic or aortic chain makes diagnostic node dissection in that area unnecessary.

For "high-risk" patients a selective aortic node dissection is performed. Patients at high risk for aortic node metastases have one or more of the following features (62): 1) grossly suspicious aortic nodes, pelvic nodes, or adnexa; 2) adverse histology (papillary serous carcinoma, clear-cell carcinoma); 3) grade 2 or 3 endometrioid adenocarcinoma with more than 50% myometrial invasion; 4) more than 50% of the uterine cavity involved by tumor; and 5) elevated serum CA-125 value. When it is deemed infeasible or unsafe to remove aortic nodes, and whenever there is a contraindication

Maximum Myoinvasion	Histologic Grade		
	1 (N = 180) Pelvic/Aortic	2 (N = 288) Pelvic/Aortic	3 (N = 153) Pelvic/Aortic
None	0/0	3/3	0/0
Inner one third	3/1	5/4	9/4
Middle one third	0/5	9/0	4/0
Outer one third	11/6	19/14	34/24

T A B L E   **20-6**

Percent of Pelvic and Aortic Node Metastases in 621 Patients with Clinical Stage I Endometrial Carcinoma

Source: Creasman WT, Morrow CP, Bundy BN, et al. Surgical-pathologic spread patterns of endometrial cancer: a Gynecologic Oncology Group study. *Cancer* 1987;60:2035.

to postoperative pelvic radiation therapy, a selective pelvic node dissection should be done. In the latter case a therapeutic node dissection is advisable. As Table 20-6 reveals, the risk of pelvic node metastases is 5% or greater for grade 1 cancers invading deeper than the middle one third of the myometrium, and for grade 2 and 3 cancers with any degree of myometrial invasion. Certainly pelvic node dissection is warranted in all patients with apparent surgical stage Ic endometrial cancer when there is a contraindication to adjuvant pelvic radiation therapy.

The method of selective pelvic node dissection for uterine cancer consists of excising the node-bearing tissue on the medial face of the external iliac artery and vein, and clearing the obturator fossa superior to the obturator nerve. The method of selective aortic node dissection involves the removal of the precaval nodes and left lateral aortic nodes from the origin of the IMA to the midpoint of the common iliac vessels. Although the lymphatics of the uterine fundus, at least the subserosal lymphatics, drain to the infrarenal lymph nodes in the manner of ovarian carcinoma (79), the frequency of metastases to this area in the absence of more distal aortic nodal involvement has not been demonstrated in surgical-pathological studies. In addition to the node sampling, the infracolic omentum should be removed from patients with clear-cell or papillary serous carcinoma, because of their proclivity for intraperitoneal metastases.

Laparoscopic staging in conjunction with laparoscopic assisted vaginal hysterectomy and adnexectomy has been performed in selected patients with endometrial carcinoma (80). It appears to be a reliable method of surgical staging and therapy, and, as expected for minimally invasive surgery, the patient's post-

operative recovery is more rapid than that which occurs after a laparotomy.

Results of Surgical Staging

The 222 patient Gynecologic Oncology Group (GOG) pilot surgical-pathologic staging study of endometrial carcinoma (74) is more representative of the frequency of the various findings than the group-wide GOG study (75), because the latter study admitted patients more selectively. In the pilot study 18% of the subjects had demonstrable evidence of extrauterine spread, including 10% with pelvic and 7% with aortic node metastases. Some patients had multiple-site involvement. Table 20-6 correlates the frequency of pelvic and aortic node metastases with histologic grade and myometrial invasion as determined by the larger, group-wide GOG staging study. The highest rates of metastasis to the pelvic and aortic node chains, ranging from 14% to 34%, are reported for grade 2 and 3 lesions with outer one-third myometrial invasion. Other results reported in the literature are in harmony with these findings (77,81–83).

The prognostic value of the surgical-pathologic staging data has been quantified for the group-wide GOG study (62). There is a 60% recurrence risk at 5 years for patients with aortic node metastasis as the only extrauterine disease, 35% for patients with LVSI, 25% for patients with documented pelvic node or adnexal metastasis, and 22% for those patients with positive pelvic cytology. Nearly 45% of patients with two or more sites of extrauterine metastases had a recurrence. Involvement of the isthmus/cervix was not a statistically significant factor, but the varying degrees of cervical involvement as incorporated in the 1988 FIGO staging system were not assessed separately.

LVSI, which is diagnosed in 15% of stage I patients, is the most important adverse prognostic feature after aortic node metastases. Other investigators also noted a high recurrence rate in patients with LVSI (65,66,84). The frequency of LVSI increases with advancing age, grade, and muscle invasion, and not surprisingly, the time to recurrence is shorter in patients with LVSI. The depth of myometrial invasion and histologic grade have prognostic import even in the absence of other adverse features. This is clearly demonstrated in the 390 GOG surgically staged patients without aortic node, pelvic node, or adnexal metastases, with negative peritoneal cytology, no LVSI, and no extension to the cervix (62). Altogether 5% of the 390 patients experienced recurrence at 3 years' follow-up, but the failure rate varied with adverse histologic findings and treatment. Only 3.8% of patients having grade 1 tumors with less than middle third myoinvasion had a relapse compared to 19% of patients having grade 3 cancers with invasion in the mid to outer one third. Other tumor factors are also prognostic although their role in treatment planning remains uncertain. Schink et al (85) reported that the rate of pelvic node metastases correlates with tumor size in endometrial carcinoma (<2 cm, 4%; >2 cm, 15%; entire cavity involved, 35%). These investigators found that no patient with a grade 2 lesion and less than 50% myoinvasion had pelvic node involvement provided that the tumor was less than 2 cm in diameter; 18% of patients with a tumor more than 2 cm in diameter had pelvic node metastases.

Complications of Surgical Staging

For endometrial cancer patients the risk from surgical therapy (i.e., simple hysterectomy) is quite low and primarily due to associated morbidity such as obesity, diabetes, cardiovascular disease, and other age-related conditions. These comorbid factors may be additive such that the obese patient may be at significantly increased risk if she is also hypertensive and diabetic (86). The safety of surgically staging patients with endometrial cancer is a reasonable concern considering the good prognosis of the group as a whole, their age, and the frequency with which these patients have complicating medical problems. This issue has been addressed by a number of authors (78,87–91). To a large degree, the outcome with respect to operating time, blood loss, and complications depends on the weight and age of the patients, and the

operator. Although infrequent, the most significant risks of surgical staging are increased blood loss, venous thromboembolism, and perhaps small-bowel obstruction. The reported rate of thromboembolic events in the larger series is 5% for the surgically staged patients, approximately twice the rate for the patients who did not undergo pelvic and aortic node sampling. Small-bowel obstruction is primarily encountered in patients undergoing radiation therapy after surgery. In a study of 235 endometrial carcinoma patients receiving postoperative pelvic radiotherapy, the actuarial risk of a severe bowel complication was 3%. This risk was increased to 11% when surgical staging was performed (92). If the node dissection is extensive, chronic lymphedema may develop in some patients, particularly those who also receive whole-pelvic radiation therapy.

Management of Early-Stage Endometrial Carcinoma

Stage I and Occult Stage II

Comments

After the workup is completed, the patient with clinical stage I or occult stage II (positive ECC findings with no clinical evidence of cervical involvement) endometrial carcinoma of any grade or histology is subjected to surgery as the first step in the treatment program. This approach reflects the generally accepted evidence that most patients with endometrial carcinoma do not need adjuvant radiation therapy, that preoperative radiotherapy can obscure important surgical-pathologic information about the cancer, and that postoperative radiation is as effective as preoperative radiation therapy in reducing the risk for local/regional recurrence. The objective is to obtain, as accurately as feasible, the surgical-pathologic staging data concurrent with the hysterectomy. The surgical-pathologic staging data provide the information for the selection of postoperative adjuvant therapy.

Operative Management

Abdominal Hysterectomy; Risk Assessment
In the typical case the abdomen is opened

through a midline suprapubic incision, washings of the pelvic cavity for cytology are obtained, the abdomen is carefully explored, and then an extrafascial, total hysterectomy with bilateral salpingo-oophorectomy is performed. Removal of the adnexa, even in the premenopausal woman, is part of the therapy because they may contain microscopic metastases or a primary ovarian tumor, or the ovaries may be the source of estrogen production which could stimulate the progression of residual, occult endometrial cancer. These patients also have an increased lifetime risk for developing ovarian carcinoma. The recommendation to remove the apparently normal ovaries is supported by the study of Gitsch et al (31) in which 8 of 17 women 45 years or younger with endometrial carcinoma had either a concomitant primary ovarian cancer (N = 5) or metastases to the ovaries.

The uterus is opened off the field to determine the extent of the growth. If there is obvious adnexal involvement, gross pelvic node involvement, or myoinvasion of more than 50% in a patient with a grade 2 or grade 3 lesion, a selective left and right aortic/common iliac node dissection is performed as previously discussed. These criteria are based on the group-wide GOG study (62) in which 47 of 48 patients with aortic node involvement had one or more of these findings at staging laparotomy. Pelvic and aortic node sampling, and infracolic omentectomy are recommended for patients with high-risk histology: papillary serous carcinoma and clear-cell carcinoma. Hormone receptor status of the primary or metastatic tumor is determined to assist in the selection of postoperative treatment and advise the patient with regard to hormone replacement therapy.

When the depth of invasion is not grossly evident, it is determined by frozen-section analysis, which is about 95% reliable versus 80% for gross inspection (64,93). If the frozen-section analysis of suspicious pelvic nodes reveals cancer, then selective pelvic node dissection is not necessary, but all enlarged nodes should be removed. Similarly selective aortic node dissection is unnecessary if frozen-section analysis of a suspicious aortic node discloses metastases. When the patient is known to have a high risk for pelvic node metastases or pelvic recurrence and will be receiving pelvic radiation therapy, assessing the state of the aortic nodes becomes the most important determinant of prognosis and the extent of postoperative treatment. Both the left and right sides should

be sampled (94). Overall, less than 25% of an average population of endometrial cancer patients will have an indication for aortic node sampling. Pelvic node sampling is most valuable when the aortic node dissection may be unduly hazardous or there is some contraindication to postoperative radiation therapy, but pelvic node sampling should not routinely replace the aortic node dissection in view of the fact that 40% of patients with aortic node metastases have negative pelvic nodes (62).

A few surgeons (78) advocate an alternative to this approach to surgical staging. The argument is that in view of the low incidence of complications attending selective node sampling, it is justified even when the risk of metastases is low, because the failure to identify extrauterine disease will result in undertreatment. Furthermore, the added surgery will not prolong the operation as it can be accomplished during the time required to obtain the frozen-section evaluation of the uterus.

Transverse Incision There are situations in which the low transverse incision is a reasonable choice, such as for the young woman with a grade 1 adenocarcinoma. However, the surgeon who selects this incision should be prepared to make a separate vertical incision if it is required to carry out the proper surgical procedure. The disease, not the incision, must dictate the scope of the operation. In endometrial cancer, the probability that a low transverse incision will prove to be inadequate is substantial in the presence of a moderately to poorly differentiated malignancy, an enlarged uterus, cervical extension, an adnexal tumor, advanced age, or an elevated serum CA-125 value.

Vaginal Hysterectomy The vaginal approach to removing the uterus is useful in certain patients with endometrial carcinoma even though it may not be feasible to remove the adnexa or explore the pelvis and abdomen (95,96). The most frequently cited indication for the vaginal approach to hysterectomy in endometrial cancer is marked obesity. However, vaginal hysterectomy is often more imposing than abdominal hysterectomy in the obese woman, especially if she is nulliparous. Consequently, the vaginal approach is often not an easy solution to this problem. Furthermore, most obese women are in generally good health, so they should get optimal therapy. The most convincing indication for vaginal hysterectomy as definitive surgical therapy for endometrial carcinoma is the existence of a comorbid condition, such as severe cardiopulmonary disease, which is a contraindication to an abdominal operation but an acceptable risk for vaginal surgery. Thus, the vaginal approach becomes a choice intermediate between optimal surgery and no surgery.

Minimal access surgery is another approach to the management of endometrial carcinoma that minimizes or eliminates the disadvantages of vaginal hysterectomy. Laparoscopy is used to examine the peritoneal cavity, remove the adnexa, and sample the retroperitoneal nodes prior to vaginal hysterectomy (76). Portions of the hysterectomy, such as division of the round ligaments and ovarian vessels, can be carried out to facilitate the vaginal procedure.

Postoperative Management

The pathologist's evaluation of the specimen is extremely important if optimal treatment results are to be obtained. The least-differentiated area of the tumor, the greatest depth of myometrial invasion, the presence of LVSI, the histologic subtype, and the proximity of the tumor to the isthmus or cervix need to be defined. Each of these factors has prognostic as well as therapeutic implications. In addition, accurate study of the peritoneal cytology, lymph nodes, and adnexa is necessary.

Postoperatively patients can be divided into three groups based on the expected recurrence rate (97).

1. Low risk (<5% recurrence): grade 1 or 2 endometrioid or adenosquamous lesions confined to the upper two thirds of the corpus, no evidence of extrauterine spread, no LVSI, and less than one third myoinvasion. These patients require no further treatment.
2. Intermediate risk (5%–10% recurrence): grade 1 or 2 endometrial carcinoma confined to the upper two thirds of the corpus, no evidence of extrauterine spread, with middle third myoinvasion and no LVSI. Grade 1 or 2 lesions with less than one third myoinvasion and extension to the cervix or isthmus also fall into this group. These patients should have postoperative intravaginal ovoid brachytherapy.
3. High risk (>10% recurrence): all other cases. These patients are candidates for postoperative pelvic radiation (4000–5000

cGy at 170–180-cGy daily fraction). If metastases to the aortic nodes are documented, extended-field radiation therapy is recommended in the absence of more widespread metastases because approximately 40% of these patients are expected to survive 5 years or longer (62,92,98,99). If the aortic node metastases are large or multiple, a scalene fat pad dissection may be warranted, because node metastasis at this level would be a contraindication to aortic-field radiation therapy. The morbidity of extended-field radiation therapy after surgery precludes the use of aortic radiation therapy solely on the basis of uterine risk factors. Thus, the emphasis in this protocol is on surgical documentation of nodal involvement.

In this scheme 50% to 75% of patients will receive no postoperative therapy. Vaginal-cuff irradiation has traditionally been delivered via applicators loaded with low-dose-rate radium or cesium sources 4 to 6 weeks postoperatively, allowing the cuff to heal completely. The applicators are typically inserted under general anesthesia, with the total time of the application lasting 36 to 48 hours. Recently high-dose-rate brachytherapy utilizing either iridium-92 or cobalt-60 sources has been gaining in popularity because of the short treatment time (15–30 minutes) and general anesthesia is not required (100). Multiple applications are necessary, however. A common schedule is to administer 700 cGy to the vaginal apex per application for a total dose of 2100 cGy. If the patient has received whole-pelvic radiotherapy, the high-dose-rate boost to the cuff is 500 cGy per fraction (total of 1500 cGy). Vaginal-cuff radiation, however, adds little to the local control benefit of external-beam therapy and increases the risk of complications, especially after the extra dissection required by the surgical staging procedure. Therefore, vaginal-cuff radiation therapy is not recommended in conjunction with postoperative external-beam radiation in these patients. Prophylactic treatment of the entire vagina in early endometrial carcinoma is unwarranted.

Adjuvant systemic therapy with progestins, cytotoxic chemotherapy, and radiation therapy have all been tested in early-stage endometrial carcinoma (the latter two modalities for patients at high risk for recurrence) with no obvious patient benefit in the trials reported to date

(101–104). In an ongoing randomized trial, the GOG is comparing postoperative whole-pelvic radiation therapy to six cycles of cisplatin plus doxorubicin chemotherapy in patients with intermediate-risk stage I endometrial carcinoma. The results of this study will determine whether radiation therapy can be replaced by chemotherapy in this situation.

Overt Stage II

Comments

The reported survival rate of stage II patients varies widely, but there is considerable agreement that occult cervical involvement is attended by a better 5-year survival rate (75%) than is overt cervical invasion (55%) (25). Patients with occult cervical stromal invasion have a worse prognosis than do patients with involvement of the endocervical glands only (23,24). Nevertheless, patients with clinically occult stage II endometrial cancer (a clinically normal cervix with microscopic cervical invasion) can be managed the same as stage I patients, except that no intraoperative frozen section is needed to document the need for selective pelvic and aortic node dissection. On the other hand, when cervical involvement is extensive, surgical therapy should be a radical hysterectomy, or pelvic irradiation followed by an adjuvant simple hysterectomy and aortic node sampling.

Radiation and Adjuvant Simple Hysterectomy

When the cervix is clinically involved by tumor, whole-pelvic radiation plus intracavitary brachytherapy followed by adjunctive simple hysterectomy and selective aortic/common iliac node dissection is usually the treatment of choice. As in stage I endometrial carcinoma, the addition of hysterectomy substantially improves the survival of patients with stage II disease (105). Pretreatment CT is advised in addition to the routine chest x-ray study to search for extrapelvic disease. This is especially important in patients with high-risk histology. At the time of laparotomy the same procedures are followed as described earlier in the chapter. When there is obvious residual disease in the cervix at the completion of radiation therapy, an adjuvant hysterectomy should be performed with the degree of radicalness tailored to obtain an adequate margin of excision. The aortic node sampling should not be omitted, but the pelvic nodes that have already been treated are removed only if there is evidence of residual tumor. The outcome for stage II patients treated in this manner is similar to that for patients with stage II disease treated by surgery first (106).

Radical Hysterectomy

Radical hysterectomy, at first glance, seems to be well suited to encompass the known spread pattern of stage I and II endometrial carcinoma. However, the patient population tends to be obese, elderly, and diabetic, and to suffer from cardiovascular disease—all conditions that increase the risks of extended pelvic surgery. Even in well-selected patients, however, there are problems with the use of radical hysterectomy for endometrial cancer therapy. Many, if not most, patients would be seriously overtreated by such surgery. Identifying the patients requiring more than a simple hysterectomy is not readily done preoperatively, even after excluding grade 1 cases, although ultrasound can identify some of the patients with deep myoinvasion. The reported cure rate achieved by simple hysterectomy and selective postoperative radiation therapy is often as good as that reported for treatment by radical hysterectomy. Furthermore, many of the patients who may benefit from radical hysterectomy and pelvic lymphadenectomy on the basis of the risk of lymphatic spread will already have extrapelvic spread, as evidenced by positive peritoneal cytology or the presence of aortic node metastases. Intensifying regional therapy in patients with extraregional metastases is not likely to improve survival.

Therefore, the role of radical hysterectomy must remain a minor one in endometrial carcinoma management (107). The most suitable candidates are patients 1) with gross cervical involvement who are physically and medically suited to radical hysterectomy; 2) who, subsequent to radiation therapy for cervical cancer, developed endometrial cancer—unfortunately, these patients usually have extrauterine disease (108); 3) who exhibit appropriate risk factors and refuse radiation therapy; and 4) who have a relative contraindication to radiation therapy (e.g., concomitant ovarian cancer; pelvic kidney).

Optimal surgical treatment of endometrial carcinoma with clinically overt cervical involvement requires a Wertheim radical hysterectomy, bilateral pelvic lymphadenectomy, and selective aortic node dissection. If the pelvic and aortic nodes, surgical margins, and the peritoneal washings are negative for cancer, no further treatment is needed. Otherwise, pelvic or extended-field radiation may be appropriate, especially for hormone receptor–poor tumors.

Management of Advanced-Stage Endometrial Carcinoma

Stage III

The current FIGO stage III is surgical-pathologic and includes patients with disease involving the adnexa, pelvic lymph nodes, aortic lymph nodes, vagina, pelvic peritoneum, or malignant peritoneal cytology, a very heterogeneous prognostic group (e.g., pelvic lymph node metastasis as the only adverse feature is associated with a 75% five-year survival). Although parametrial disease is not mentioned in the new staging system, presumably this would also qualify a patient for stage III grouping. Patients who have clinical stage III endometrial carcinoma by virtue of vaginal or parametrial extension are given pelvic radiation therapy after a thorough metastatic survey (chest x-ray study, CT, CA-125 measurement). When the therapy is complete, exploratory laparotomy is recommended for patients whose disease seems to be resectable. Along with the hysterectomy and adnexectomy, surgical-pathologic staging is carried out to determine the extent of residual disease. Extended-field radiation therapy or systemic therapy with cytotoxic drugs or hormones is warranted in the presence of extrapelvic metastases. If tumor tissue is obtained for hormone receptor analysis, the choice between chemotherapy and hormone therapy can be facilitated.

After proper evaluation, patients placed in the clinical stage III category on the basis of an adnexal mass should undergo surgery without preoperative radiation therapy to determine the nature of the mass (inflammatory, pedunculated myoma, adnexal neoplasm, metastasis to the ovary), to perform surgical-pathologic staging, and to carry out tumor reductive surgery. If the uterus is resectable, hysterectomy and adnexectomy should also be done. Traditionally patients with adnexal involvement have been managed by postoperative pelvic radiation therapy. However, adjuvant systemic therapy may be warranted in view of the fact that only 50% are expected to survive 5 years. Certainly patients with gross adnexal involvement are candidates for a systemic treatment protocol. Patients who are stage III by virtue of clinically evident inguinal node metastases should have the suspicious nodes excised prior to irradiation. Patients with microscopic stage III disease have a 40% to 80% five-year survival rate compared to 10% to 30% for those with gross extrauterine pelvic extension. Survival of the latter group, however, correlates strongly with resectability (109–111). A large component of the current FIGO stage III cancers will be apparent stage I disease with a positive cytology or retroperitoneal node metastases.

The GOG is conducting a trial of stage III endometrial carcinoma randomizing patients to either whole abdominal radiation or cisplatin plus doxorubicin chemotherapy. In an antecedent phase II study of whole abdominal radiation for stage III/IV patients with residual disease less than 2 cm in maximum diameter, 3-year survival rates of 31% and 33% were reported for patients with endometrioid adenocarcinoma and patients with papillary serous carcinoma, respectively (112).

Stage IV

Endometrial cancer patients with clinical evidence of intra-abdominal or distant metastasis are most often suitable for systemic hormonal therapy or chemotherapy. Local irradiation, however, may be beneficial in special patients such as those with brain or bone metastases. Occasionally, pelvic radiotherapy or hysterectomy will be indicated to provide local tumor control and prevent bleeding or complications from pyometra, especially in the patient who is to undergo chemotherapy. Hysterectomy, whenever it is feasible, is the preferred method for controlling the primary tumor and its symptoms. The efficacy of whole-abdomen radiation in endometrial carcinoma involving the peritoneal cavity is uncertain. Some authors reported that patients with macroscopic metastasis cannot be cleared with whole abdominal radiation (113), while others reported good success in patients with residual disease of less than 2 cm (114). Nevertheless, it is a good practice to reserve whole-abdomen radiation therapy for those patients having neither macroscopic abdominal disease nor distant metastases at the time of laparotomy (115). The remaining patients are managed the same as those with ovarian cancer: tumor reductive surgery and chemotherapy, unless the metastases contain high levels of hormone receptor protein, in which case progestin or antiestrogen therapy is indicated.

REFERENCES

1. Parker SL, Tong T, Bolden S, Wingo PA. Cancer statistics 1996. *CA Cancer J Clin* 1996;46:5–27.

2. Tretli S, Haldorsen T. A cohort analysis of breast cancer, uterine corpus cancer, and childbearing pattern in Norwegian women. *J Epidemiol Commun Health* 1990;44:215–219.

3. MacMahon B. Risk factors for endometrial cancer. *Gynecol Oncol* 1974;2:122–129.

4. Parazzini F, LaVecchia C, Bocciolone L, Franceschi S. The epidemiology of endometrial cancer. *Gynecol Oncol* 1991;41:1–16.

5. Wynder EL, Escher GC, Mantel N. An epidemiologic investigation of cancer of the endometrium. *Cancer* 1966;19:489.

6. Meredith RF, Eisert DR, Kaka Z, et al. An excess of uterine sarcomas after pelvic irradiation. *Cancer* 1986;58:2003–2007.

7. Tropé CG, Makar A. Epidemiology, etiology, screening, prevention, and diagnosis in female genital cancer. *Curr Opin Oncol* 1991;3: 908–919.

8. Rubin GL, Peterson HB, Lee NC, et al. Estrogen replacement therapy and the risk of endometrial cancer: remaining controversies. *Am J Obstet Gynecol* 1990;162:148–154.

9. McGonigle KF, Karlan BY, Barbuto DA, et al. Development of endometrial cancer in women on estrogen and progestin hormone replacement therapy. *Gynecol Oncol* 1994;55:126–132.

10. Barakat RR. The effect of tamoxifen on the endometrium. *Oncology* 1995;9:129–134.

11. Fisher B. Endometrial cancer risk from tamoxifen, an NSABP study. *J Natl Cancer Inst* 1994;86:527–537.

12. Granberg S, Wikland M, Karlsson B, et al. Endometrial thickness as measured by endovaginal ultrasonography for identifying endometrial abnormality. *Am J Obstet Gynecol* 1991;164: 47–52.

13. Cherkis RC, Patten SF Jr, Andrews TJ. Significance of normal endometrial cells detected by cervical cytology. *Obstet Gynecol* 1988;71: 242–244.

14. Yancey M, Magelssen D, Demaurez A, Lee RB. Classification of endometrial cells on cervical cytology. *Obstet Gynecol* 1990;76:1000–1005.

15. Hawwa ZM, Nahhas WA, Copenhaver EH. Postmenopausal bleeding. *Lahey Clin Found Bull* 1970;19:61–70.

16. Feldman S, Berkowitz RS, Tosteson AN. Cost-effectiveness of strategies to evaluate postmenopausal bleeding. *Obstet Gynecol* 1993;81: 968–975.

17. De Jong P, Doel F, Falconer A. Outpatient diagnostic hysteroscopy. *Br J Obstet Gynaecol* 1990; 97:299–303.

18. Gimpelson RJ, Rappold HO. A comparative study between panoramic hysteroscopy with directed biopsies and dilation and curettage: a review of 276 cases. *Am J Obstet Gynecol* 1988; 158:489–492.

19. Pettersson F, ed. FIGO annual report. *Int J Gynecol Obstet* 1991;36:S1.

20. Duk JM, Aalders JG, Fleuren GJ, deBruijn HWA. CA-125: a useful marker in endometrial carcinoma. *Am J Obstet Gynecol* 1986;155: 1097–1102.

21. Patsner B, Mann WJ, Cohen H, Loesch M. Predictive value of preoperative serum CA125 levels in clinically localized and advanced endometrial carcinoma. *Am J Obstet Gynecol* 1988;158: 399–402.

22. Chen SS, Lee L. Reappraisal of endocervical curettage in predicting cervical involvement by endometrial carcinoma. *J Reprod Med* 1986; 31:50.

23. Fanning J, Alvarez PM, Tsukada Y, Piver MS. Prognostic significance of the extent of cervical involvement by endometrial cancer. *Gynecol Oncol* 1991;40:46–47.

24. Kadar N, Malfetano JH, Homesley HD. Determinants of survival of surgically staged patients with endometrial carcinoma histologically confined to the uterus: implications for therapy. *Obstet Gynecol* 1992;80:655–659.

25. Homesley HD, Boronow RC, Lewis JL Jr. Stage II endometrial adenocarcinoma: Memorial Hospital for Cancer, 1949–1965. *Obstet Gynecol* 1977; 49:604.

26. Wallin TE, Malkasian GD Jr, Gaffey TA, et al. Stage II cancer of the endometrium: a pathologic and clinical study. *Gynecol Oncol* 1984; 18:1.

27. Belloni C, Vigano R, del Maschio A, et al. Magnetic resonance imaging in endometrial carcinoma staging. *Gynecol Oncol* 1990;37:172–177.

28. Cacciatore B, Lehtovirta P, Wahlström T, Ylöstalo P. Preoperative sonographic evaluation of endometrial cancer. *Am J Obstet Gynecol* 1989;160:133–137.

29. Gordon AN, Fleischer AC, Reed GW. Depth of myometrial invasion in endometrial cancer: preoperative assessment by transvaginal ultrasonography. *Gynecol Oncol* 1990;39:321–327.

30. Hricak H, Rubinstein LV, Gherman GM, Karstaedt N. MR imaging evaluation of endometrial carcinoma: results of an NCI cooperative study. *Radiology* 1991;179:829–832.

31. Gitsch G, Hanzal E, Jensen D, Hacker NF. Endometrial cancer in premenopausal women 45 years and younger. *Obstet Gynecol* 1995;85: 504–508.

32. Barrowclough H, Jaarsma KW. Adenoacanthoma of the endometrium; a separate entity or a histological curiosity? *J Clin Pathol* 1980;33: 1064–1067.

33. Ng ABP, Reagan JW, Storaasli JP, Wentz WG. Mixed adenosquamous carcinoma of the endometrium. *Am J Clin Pathol* 1973;59: 765–781.

34. Haqquani MT, Fox H. Adenosquamous carcinoma of the endometrium. *J Clin Pathol* 1976;29: 959–966.

35. Alberhasky RC, Connelly PJ, Christopherson WM. Carcinoma of the endometrium. IV. Mixed adenosquamous carcinoma: a clinicopathological study of 68 cases with long term follow up. *Am J Clin Pathol* 1982;77:655–664.

36. Zaino RJ, Kurman RJ. Squamous differentiation in carcinoma of the endometrium: a critical appraisal of adenoacanthoma and adenosquamous carcinoma. *Semin Diagn Pathol* 1988; 5:154–171.

37. Abeler VM, Kjorstad KE. Endometrial adenocarcinoma with squamous cell differentiation. *Cancer* 1992;69:488–495.

38. Hendrickson MR, Ross J, Eiffel P, et al. Uterine papillary serous carcinoma: a highly malignant form of endometrial carcinoma. *Am J Surg Pathol* 1982;6:93–108.

39. Chen JL, Trost DC, Wilkinson EJ. Endometrial papillary adenocarcinomas: two clinicopathological types. *Int J Gynecol Pathol* 1985;4: 279–288.

40. Abeler VM, Kjorstad KE. Serous papillary carcinoma of the endometrium: a histopathological study of 22 cases. *Gynecol Oncol* 1990;39: 266–271.

41. Lee KR, Belinson JL. Papillary serous adenocarcinoma of the endometrium; a clinicopathologic study of 19 cases. *Gynecol Oncol* 1992;46: 51–54.

42. Carcangiu ML, Chambers JT. Uterine papillary serous carcinoma: a study of 108 cases with emphasis on the prognostic significance of associated endometrioid carcinoma, absence of invasion and concomitant carcinoma. *Gynecol Oncol* 1992;47:207–217.

43. Kato DT, Ferry JA, Goodman A, et al. Uterine papillary serous carcinoma (UPSC): a clinicopathologic study of 30 cases. *Gynecol Oncol* 1995;59:384–389.

44. Ward BG, Wright RG, Free K. Papillary carcinomas of the endometrium. *Gynecol Oncol* 1990;39:347–351.

45. O'Hanlan KL, Levine PA, Harbatkin D, et al. Virulence of papillary endometrial adenocarcinoma. *Gynecol Oncol* 1990;37:112–119.

46. Ambros RA, Ballouk F, Maljetano HJ, et al. Significance of papillary (villoglandular) differentiation in endometrioid carcinoma of the uterus. *Am J Surg Pathol* 1994;18:569–575.

47. Kurman RJ, Scully RE. Clear cell carcinoma of the endometrium: an analysis of 21 cases. *Cancer* 1976;37:872–882.

48. Christopherson WM, Alberhasky RC, Connelly PJ. Carcinoma of the endometrium. I. A clinicopathologic study of clear cell carcinoma and secretory carcinoma. *Cancer* 1982;69:1511–1523.

49. Abeler VM, Kjorstad KE. Clear cell carcinoma of the endometrium: a histopathological study of 97 cases. *Gynecol Oncol* 1991;40:207–217.

50. Kanbour-Shakir A, Tobon H. Primary clear cell carcinoma of the endometrium: a clinicopathologic study of 20 cases. *Int J Gynecol Pathol* 1991;10:67–78.

51. Carangiu ML, Chambers JT. Early pathologic stage clear cell carcinoma and uterine papillary serous carcinoma of the endometrium: comparison of clinicopathologic features and survival. *Int J Gynecol Pathol* 1995;14:30–38.

52. Malpica A, Tornos C, Burke TW, Silva EG. Low-stage clear-cell carcinoma of the endometrium. *Am J Surg Pathol* 1995;19:759–774.

53. Ross JC, Eiffel PJ, Cox RS, et al. Primary mucinous adenocarcinoma of the endometrium: a

clinicopathologic and histochemical study. *Am J Surg Pathol* 1983;7:715–729.

54. Jeffers MD, McDonald GS, McGuinness EP. Primary squamous cell carcinoma of the endometrium. *Histopathology* 1991;19:177–179.

55. Bibro MC, Kapp DS, LiVolsi VA, Schwartz PE. Squamous carcinoma of the endometrium with ultrastructural observations and review of the literature. *Gynecol Oncol* 1980;10:217–223.

56. Abeler VM, Kjorstad KE, Nesland JM. Undifferentiated carcinoma of the endometrium: a histopathological study of 31 cases. *Cancer* 1991;68:98–105.

57. Huntsman DG, Clement PB, Gilks CB, Sculy RE. Small cell carcinoma of the endometrium: a clinicopathological study of sixteen cases. *Am J Surg Pathol* 1994;18:364–375.

58. van Hoeven KH, Hudock JA, Woodruff JM, Sutherland DJ. Small cell neuroendocrine carcinoma of the endometrium. *Int J Gynecol Pathol* 1995;14:21–29.

59. Zaino RJ, Silverberg SG, Norris HJ, et al. The prognostic value of nuclear versus architectural grading in endometrial adenocarcinoma: a Gynecologic Oncology Group study. *Int J Gynecol Pathol* 1994;13:29–36.

60. Zaino RJ, Kurman RJ, Diana KL, Morrow CP. The utility of the revised International Federation of Gynecology and Obstetrics histologic grading of endometrial adenocarcinoma using a defined nuclear grading system: a Gynecologic Oncology Group study. *Cancer* 1995;75: 81–86.

61. Alm P, Gudmundsson T, Martenssons R, et al. Identification of small areas of solid growth has a strong prognostic impact in differentiated endometrial carcinomas: a histopathologic and morphometric study. *Int J Gynecol Cancer* 1995;5:87–93.

62. Morrow CP, Bundy BN, Kurman RJ, et al. Relationship between surgical-pathological risk factors and outcome in clinical stage I and II carcinoma of the endometrium: a Gynecologic Oncology Group study. *Gynecol Oncol* 1991;40: 55–65.

63. Ambros RA, Kurman RJ. Identification of patients with stage I uterine endometrioid adenocarcinoma at high risk of recurrence by DNA ploidy, myometrial invasion, and vascular invasion. *Gynecol Oncol* 1992;45:235–239.

64. Goff BA, Rice LW. Assessment of depth of myometrial invasion in endometrial adenocarcinoma. *Gynecol Oncol* 1990;38:46–48.

65. Hanson MB, van Nagell JR, Powell DE, et al. The prognostic significance of lymph vascular invasion in stage I endometrial cancer. *Cancer* 1985;55:1753–1757.

66. Sivridis E, Buckley CH, Fox H. The prognostic significance of lymphatic vascular space invasion in endometrial adenocarcinoma. *Br J Obstet Gynaecol* 1987;94:984–991.

67. Beckner ME, Mori I, Silverberg SG. Endometrial carcinoma: non-tumor factors in prognosis. *Int J Gynecol Pathol* 1985;4:131–145.

68. Creasman WT. Prognostic significance of hormone receptors in endometrial cancers. *Cancer* 1993;71:1467–1470.

69. Kerner H, Sabo E, Friedman M, et al. An immunohistochemical study of estrogen and progesterone receptors in adenocarcinoma of the endometrium and in the adjacent mucosa. *Int J Gynecol Cancer* 1995;5:275–281.

70. Ikeda M, Watanabe Y, Nanjoh T, Noda K. Evaluation of DNA ploidy in endometrial cancer. *Gynecol Oncol* 1993;50:25–29.

71. Sorbe B, Risberg B, Thomthwaite J. Nuclear morphometry and DNA flow cytometry as prognostic methods for endometrial carcinoma. *Int J Gynecol Cancer* 1994;4:94–100.

72. Nordstrom B, Strang P, Lindgren A, et al. Carcinoma of the endometrium: do the nuclear grade and DNA ploidy provide more prognostic information than do the FIGO and WHO classifications? *Int J Gynecol Pathol* 1996;15: 191–201.

73. Nogales FF. Prognostic factors in endometrial neoplasia: old and new. *Curr Opin Obstet Gynecol* 1996;8:74–78.

74. Boronow RC, Morrow CP, Creasman WT, et al. Surgical staging in endometrial cancer: clinicopathologic findings of a prospective study. *Obstet Gynecol* 1984;63:825.

75. Creasman WT, Morrow CP, Bundy BN, et al. Surgical pathologic spread patterns of endometrial cancer: a Gynecologic Oncology Group study. *Cancer* 1987;60:2035.

76. Chuang L, Burke TW, Tornos C, et al. Staging laparotomy for endometrial carcinoma: assessment of retroperitoneal lymph nodes. *Gynecol Oncol* 1995;58:189.

77. Cowles TA, Magrina JF, Masterson BJ, Capen CV. Comparison of clinical and surgical staging in patients with endometrial carcinoma. *Obstet Gynecol* 1985;66:413.

78. Orr JW Jr, Holloway RW, Orr PF, Holimon JL. Surgical staging of uterine cancer: an analysis of perioperative morbidity. *Gynecol Oncol* 1991; 42:209.

79. Burke TW, Levenback C, Tornos C, et al. Intraabdominal lymphatic mapping to direct selective pelvic and paraaortic lymphadenectomy in women with high-risk endometrial cancer: results of a pilot study. Presented at the 27th annual meeting of the Society of Gynecologic Oncologists, New Orleans, Feb. 10–14, 1996.

80. Childers JM, Brzechffa PR, Hatch KD, Surwit EA. Laparoscopically assisted surgical staging (LASS) of endometrial cancer. *Gynecol Oncol* 1993;51:33.

81. Chen SS, Lee L. Retroperitoneal lymph node metastases in stage I carcinoma of the endometrium: correlation with risk factors. *Gynecol Oncol* 1983;16:319.

82. Figge DC, Otto PM, Tamimi HK, Greer BE. Treatment variables in the management of endometrial cancer. *Am J Obstet Gynecol* 1983; 146:495.

83. Piver MS, Lele SB, Barlow JJ, Blumenson L. Paraaortic lymph node evaluation in stage I endometrial carcinoma. *Obstet Gynecol* 1982; 59:97.

84. Ambros RA, Kurman RJ. Combined assessment of vascular and myometrial invasion as a model to predict prognosis in stage I endometrioid adenocarcinoma of the uterine corpus. *Cancer* 1992;69:1424.

85. Schink JC, Rademaker AW, Miller DS, Lurain JR. Tumor size in endometrial cancer. *Cancer* 1991; 67:2791.

86. Foley K, Lee RB. Surgical complications of obese patients with endometrial carcinoma. *Gynecol Oncol* 1990;39:171.

87. Clarke-Pearson DL, Cliby WA, Dodge R, et al. Morbidity and mortality associated with selective pelvic and para-aortic lymphadenectomy in the surgical staging of endometrial adenocarcinoma. Presented at the 24th annual meeting of the Society of Gynecologic Oncologists, Feb 7–10, 1993.

88. Homesley HD, Kadar N, Barrett RJ, Lentz SS. Selective pelvic and periaortic lymphadenectomy does not increase morbidity in surgical staging of endometrial carcinoma. *Am J Obstet Gynecol* 1992;167:1225.

89. Larson DM, Johnson K, Olson KA. Pelvic and para-aortic lymphadenectomy for surgical staging of endometrial cancer: morbidity and mortality. *Obstet Gynecol* 1992;79:998.

90. Lewandowski G, Torrisi J, Potkul RK, et al. Hysterectomy with extended surgical staging and radiotherapy versus hysterectomy alone and radiotherapy in stage I endometrial cancer: a comparison of complication rates. *Gynecol Oncol* 1990;36:401.

91. Moore DH, Fowler WC Jr, Walton LA, Droegemueller W. Morbidity of lymph node sampling in cancers of the uterine corpus and cervix. *Obstet Gynecol* 1989;74:180.

92. Corn BW, Lanciano RM, Greven KM, et al. Endometrial cancer with para-aortic adenopathy: patterns of failure and opportunities for cure. *Int J Radiat Oncol Biol Phys* 1992;24:223.

93. Noumoff JS, Menzin A, Mikuta J, et al. The ability to evaluate prognostic variables on frozen section in hysterectomies performed for endometrial carcinoma. *Gynecol Oncol* 1991; 42:202.

94. Flanagan CW, Maannel RS, Walker JL, Johnson GA. Incidence and location of para-aortic lymph node metastases in gynecologic malignancies. *J Am Coll Surg* 1995;181:72.

95. Bloss JD, Berman ML, Bloss LP, Buller RE. Use of vaginal hysterectomy for the management of stage I endometrial cancer in the medically compromised patient. *Gynecol Oncol* 1991; 40:74.

96. Lellé RJ, Morley GW, Peters WA. The role of vaginal hysterectomy in the treatment of endometrial carcinoma. *Int J Gynecol Cancer* 1994;4:342.

97. *Carcinoma of the endometrium.* ACOG technical bulletin, no. 162. The American College of Obstetricians and Gynecologists, December 1991.

98. Feuer GA, Calanog A. Endometrial carcinoma: treatment of positive paraaortic nodes. *Gynecol Oncol* 1987;27:104.

99. Potish RA. Radiation therapy of periaortic node metastases in cancer of the uterine cervix and endometrium. *Radiology* 1987;165:567.

100. Reisinger SA, Staros EB, Feld R, et al. Preoperative radiation therapy in clinical stage II endometrial cancer. *Gynecol Oncol* 1992;45:174.

101. Martinez A, Schray M, Podratz K, et al. Postoperative whole abdomino-pelvic irradiation for

patients with high risk endometrial cancer. *Int J Radiat Oncol Biol Phys* 1989;17:371.

102. Moore TD, Phillips PH, Nerenstone SR, Cheson BD. Systemic treatment of advanced and recurrent endometrial carcinoma: current status and future directions. *J Clin Oncol* 1991;9:1071.

103. Stringer CA, Gershenson DM, Burke TW, et al. Adjuvant chemotherapy with cisplatin, doxorubicin, and cyclophosphamide (PAC) for early-stage high-risk endometrial cancer: a preliminary analysis. *Gynecol Oncol* 1990;38:305.

104. Vergote I, Kjorstad K, Abeler V, Kolstad P. A randomized trial of adjuvant progestagen in early endometrial cancer. *Cancer* 1989;64:1011.

105. Cox JD, Komaki R, Wilson JF, Greenberg M. Locally advanced adenocarcinoma of the endometrium: results of irradiation with and without subsequent hysterectomy. *Cancer* 1980;45:715.

106. Ahmad K, Kim YH, Deppe G, et al. Radiation therapy in stage II carcinoma of the endometrium. *Cancer* 1989;63:854.

107. Rutledge F. The role of radical hysterectomy in adenocarcinoma of the endometrium. *Gynecol Oncol* 1974;2:331.

108. Kwon TH, Prempree T, Tang C-K, et al. Adenocarcinoma of the uterine corpus following irradiation for cervical cancer. *Gynecol Oncol* 1981;11:102.

109. Aalders JG, Abeler V, Kolstad P. Clinical (stage III) as compared to subclinical intrapelvic extrauterine tumor spread in endometrial carcinoma: a clinical and histopathological study of 175 patients. *Gynecol Oncol* 1984;17:64.

110. Genest P, Drouin P, Girard A, Gerig L. Stage III carcinoma of the endometrium: a review of 41 cases. *Gynecol Oncol* 1987;26:77.

111. Mackillop WJ, Pringle JF. Stage III endometrial carcinoma: a review of 90 cases. *Cancer* 1985;56:2519.

112. Axelrod J, Bundy B, Roy T, et al. Advanced endometrial carcinoma treated with whole abdominal irradiation: a Gynecologic Oncology Group study. *Gynecol Oncol* 1995;56:135. Abstract.

113. Potish RA, Twiggs LB, Adcock LL, Prem KA. Role of whole abdominal radiation therapy in the management of endometrial cancer: prognostic importance of factors indicating peritoneal metastases. *Gynecol Oncol* 1985;21:80.

114. Greer BE, Hamberger AD. Treatment of intraperitoneal metastatic adenocarcinoma of the endometrium by the whole-abdomen moving-strip technique and pelvic boost irradiation. *Gynecol Oncol* 1983;16:365.

115. Loeffler JS, Rosen EM, Niloff JM, et al. Whole abdominal irradiation for tumors of the uterine corpus. *Cancer* 1988;61:1332.

CHAPTER *21*

Pathology of Uterine Sarcomas

HAROLD FOX

*U*terine sarcomas can be pure, containing only a malignant mesenchymal component, or mixed, containing a malignant mesenchymal component admixed with an epithelial element, which can be either benign or malignant. Pure sarcomas may be homologous, differentiating into mesenchymal tissues normally present in the uterus such as smooth muscle or endometrial stroma, or heterologous, differentiating into mesenchymal tissues normally alien to the uterus such as striated muscle or cartilage. In reality, pure heterologous sarcomas of the uterus, such as rhabdomyosarcomas and chondrosarcomas, are so rare that for practical clinical purposes, they can be ignored. The only pure sarcomas that are encountered are leiomyosarcomas and endometrial stromal sarcomas (1). Among the mixed sarcomas there are various permutations but the only malignant entities to be firmly established are those with a benign epithelial component and a malignant mesenchymal component, adenosarcomas, and those in which both epithelial and mesenchymal components are malignant, carcinosarcomas. There exists a third theoretical possibility, the carcinofibroma, in which the epithelial component is malignant and the mesenchymal component is benign, but such neoplasms have not been convincingly documented.

Very little is known about the etiology or pathogenesis of uterine sarcomatous neoplasms, though prior uterine irradiation has been implicated as a possible etiologic factor in a proportion of patients with carcinosarcoma.

Pure Sarcomas

Leiomyosarcoma

Uterine smooth muscle tumors are extremely common and the vast majority are clearly benign while a few are clearly malignant and pose little in the way of a diagnostic challenge.

Overtly malignant smooth muscle neoplasms, leiomyosarcomas, present as solitary, poorly demarcated intramural masses that often bulge into the uterine cavity. On section the cut surface is usually soft, fleshy, and grayish-yellow to pink with areas of hemorrhage and necrosis. Histologically these neoplasms are highly cellular and contain pleomorphic spindle-shaped smooth muscle cells with hyperchromatic nuclei (Fig. 21-1). Mitotic figures are numerous and not uncommonly of abnormal form. Multinucleated cells are often seen and there is irregular and extensive invasion of the adjacent myometrium.

It is only a small minority of uterine smooth muscle neoplasms, those that occupy the gray area between the controlled orderly growth pattern of a benign neoplasm and the cellular anarchy of a sarcoma, that cause confusion in the minds of many gynecologic pathologists and pose therapeutic problems to the gynecologist. The criteria for the recognition of malignancy in such tumors are still far from being cast in concrete and remain a controversial subject for debate and for nomenclatural argu-

310

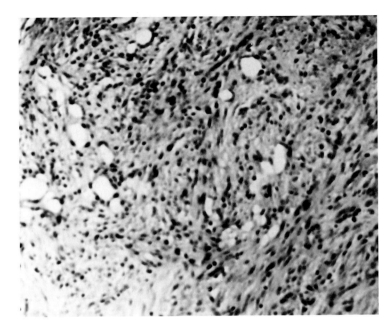

ment. The traditional approach to this problem was established in the classic paper of Taylor and Norris in 1966 (2), which placed great emphasis on the importance of mitotic counts in the diagnosis of malignancy in uterine smooth muscle neoplasms. To some extent, this was seized upon by pathologists who saw this as a relatively easy technique for differentiating between benign and malignant neoplasms. Hence, the mitotic count achieved paramount status and neoplasms with a mitotic count of more than 10 mitotic figures per 10 high-power fields (10 mf/10 hpf) were routinely classified as leiomyosarcomas, irrespective of any other attributes of the tumor. It is now realized that the mitotic count alone is not an indication of malignancy and that neoplasms with mitotic counts as high as 20 mf/10 hpf, or even higher, can and do behave in a benign manner (3–5). This is not to deny that mitotic counts are an important factor in the assessment of malignancy in uterine smooth muscle tumors but to emphasize that they are only one factor and that their importance must be assessed in combination with other histopathologic aspects of the neoplasm. An absolute mitotic count is, by itself, of no importance. Thus, for instance, a mitotic count of 12 mf/10 hpf may indicate malignancy when allied to some histopathologic features of a tumor but can equally be considered as being fully compatible with a benign process when associated with other histologic findings.

Currently two approaches to the diagnosis of malignancy in uterine smooth muscle neoplasms are advocated, one employing two variables and the other three variables. O'Connor and Norris (5) considered that the diagnosis of malignancy depends on a combination of a mitotic count and an assessment of the degree of atypia of the tumor cells; no attention is paid to the degree of cellularity of the neoplasm. Hence, in their categorization, if the tumor has a mitotic count of 1 to 4 mf/10 hpf, the diagnosis is leiomyoma, irrespective of the degree of atypia within the neoplasm. If the tumor contains 5 to 9 mf/10 hpf and there is grade 1 atypia, a diagnosis of smooth muscle tumor of uncertain malignant potential is made; a similar mitotic count in association with grade 2 or 3 atypia indicates a diagnosis of leiomyosarcoma as does a mitotic count of more than 10 mf/10 hpf in association with any degree of atypia. It will be noted that in this schema there are only three diagnostic outcomes, benign, malignant, or of uncertain malignant potential.

Hendrickson and Kempson and their group at Stanford (1,6) advocate an alternative, and more complex approach. They consider three factors to be important, each of which must be titrated against each other, these being the mitotic count, the presence of either focal or diffuse atypia of significant degree, and the presence or absence of coagulative necrosis of tumor cells; again, the cellularity of the neoplasm is not thought to be relevant. This group has evolved a rather complex terminology to replace the designation *smooth muscle tumor of uncertain malignant potential*, largely because they believe that this diagnosis does not in itself convey to the clinician any impression of the magnitude of the risk of the neoplasm behaving in a malignant fashion. They consider that a "low-risk" diagnosis indicates a less than 10% chance of malignant behavior and that a "high-risk" diagnosis is indicative of a risk of malignancy that is above 10%. Therefore, they subdivide smooth muscle tumors of the conventional type (i.e., not showing an epithelioid or myxoid pattern) into the following groups:

1. Tumors with no atypia and no coagulative necrosis are classed as leiomyomas, irrespective of the mitotic count; if, however, the mitotic count is higher than 5 mf/10 hpf, the tumor is regarded as a leiomyoma with increased mitotic count.

2. Tumors with diffuse significant atypia and no coagulative necrosis. If such a neoplasm has a mitotic count of less than 10 mf/10 hpf, it is classed as an atypical leiomyoma with low risk. If the mitotic count is above 10 mf/10 hpf, a neoplasm of this type is classed as a leiomyosarcoma.

3. Tumors with diffuse significant atypia and coagulative necrosis. All neoplasms showing both these features should be regarded as leiomyosarcomas.

4. Tumors with no significant atypia but with coagulative necrosis. Tumors of this type with a mitotic count of more than 10 mf/10 hpf are classed as leiomyosarcomas while those with lesser counts are categorized as smooth muscle tumors of low malignant potential.

5. Tumors with focal significant atypia but with no coagulative necrosis are classed as atypical leiomyomas, irrespective of mitotic count.

It should be added that the Stanford group attach the caveat "with limited experience" to some of their subcategories, indicating that they have seen too few cases for a risk factor to be clearly defined.

Whether the diagnostic schema advocated by the Stanford workers gives therapeutically more valid results than that employed by O'Connor and Norris must await the passage of time and the accumulation of more data. The Stanford study was, however, based on a very large group of neoplasms and there is little doubt in the minds of most experienced pathologists that their third variable, the presence of coagulative tumor cell necrosis, is an important diagnostic and prognostic feature.

It should be noted that the Stanford workers put all their high-risk problematic smooth muscle tumors into the single category of leiomyosarcoma, a reasonable stratagem in therapeutic terms because in most of these groups the malignant behavior rate was about 40% to 50%. However, they put their low-risk tumors into three diagnostic categories: atypical leiomyoma with low risk of recurrence, atypical leiomyoma, and tumors of low malignant potential. Given the present state of knowledge, there does not seem to be any very obvious or compelling reason why all these neoplasms should not be grouped together into a single category of "smooth muscle tumor of low malignant potential." It is true that this does introduce the word *malignant* into the terminology with all the conscious or subconscious biases and connotations it carries; it may therefore be better to use the term *atypical leiomyoma*.

Certain categories of smooth muscle tumors of the uterus merit special attention and fall outside the decision-making process and categorization just described. Some smooth muscle tumors are formed, entirely or largely, of cells that have an epithelioid appearance and the criteria for the recognition of malignancy in these rare epithelioid neoplasms differ from those outlined for tumors showing a more conventional pattern of smooth muscle differentiation. In these neoplasms a mitotic count of more than 5 mf/10 hpf is cause for some alarm even in the absence of significant atypia or coagulative necrosis (1).

Myxoid change can occur in fully benign leiomyomas and such neoplasms have to be distinguished from a myxoid leiomyosarcoma. The latter is a treacherous neoplasm that tends to have infiltrative margins and to show some degree of nuclear hyperchromatism. These features may not be striking but nevertheless these tumors behave in a malignant fashion even when the mitotic count is less than 2 mf/10 hpf (7,8).

Endometrial Stromal Sarcoma

The basic diagnostic criterion for recognition of an endometrial stromal neoplasm is that it is formed of cells that resemble those of the endometrial stroma during the proliferative phase of the menstrual cycle (Fig. 21-2). Endometrial stromal sarcomas have traditionally been divided into low-grade and high-grade categories, this subdivision being based solely on the mitotic count of the tumor. Thus neoplasms with a mitotic count of less than 10 mf/10 hpf were considered to be low-grade sarcomas while those with higher counts were regarded as high-grade sarcomas (9). More recently it was pointed out that many, indeed most, of the tumors categorized as high-grade endometrial stromal sarcomas do not merit this designation for they are formed of cells that are anaplastic and show no evidence of endometrial stromal cell differentiation (10). There are usually no morphologic features within such neoplasms that allow for any indication of their histogenesis (Fig. 21-3) and these tumors are best classified as undifferentiated uterine sarcomas; they are aggressive neoplasms that respond poorly to treatment and are associated with an extremely poor prognosis.

If undifferentiated uterine sarcomas are excluded, as they should be, from the category of endometrial stromal sarcomas, does the traditional subdivision into high-grade and low-grade neoplasms based on mitotic counts still hold true? A large study of tumors that met the diagnostic criteria of an endometrial stromal neoplasm showed that within stage I neoplasms the mitotic count was not a prognostic feature and that patients whose neoplasms had a mitotic count of more than 10 mf/10 hpf fared no worse than did those whose tumors showed a mitotic count of less than 10 mf/10 hpf (11). Hence, in tumors that meet the diagnostic criteria for an endometrial stromal sarcoma the distinction between high-grade and low-grade neoplasms is no longer valid. Stage is the most important prognostic factor for endometrial

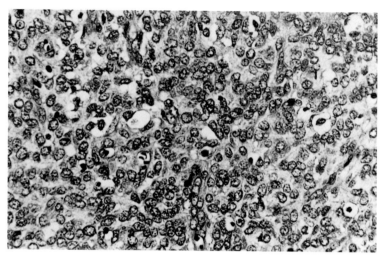

F I G U R E **21-2**

An endometrial stromal sarcoma formed of sheets of cells that resemble those of normal endometrial stroma during the proliferative phase of the cycle. (Reproduced by permission from Buckley CH, Fox H. *Biopsy pathology of the endometrium.* London: Chapman and Hall, 1989.)

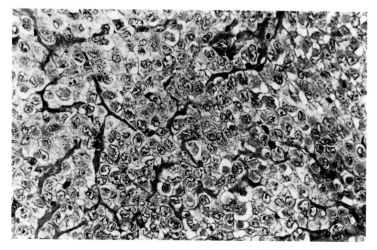

F I G U R E **21-3**

An undifferentiated sarcoma; this bears no resemblance to the stromal cells of the normal proliferative endometrium and should not be classed as a high-grade endometrial stromal sarcoma. (Reproduced by permission from Buckley CH, Fox H. *Biopsy pathology of the endometrium.* London: Chapman and Hall, 1989.)

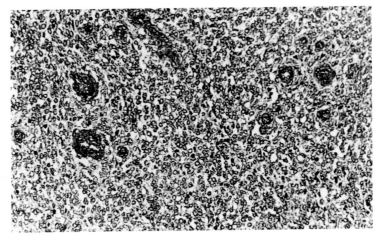

FIGURE **21-4**

An endometrial stromal sarcoma with a prominent vascular component. (Reproduced by permission from Buckley CH, Fox H. *Biopsy pathology of the endometrium.* London: Chapman and Hall, 1989.)

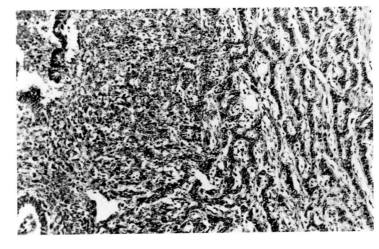

FIGURE **21-5**

An endometrial stromal sarcoma infiltrating the endometrium and showing (on the right) a sex cord–like pattern. (Reproduced by permission from Buckley CH, Fox H. *Biopsy pathology of the endometrium.* London: Chapman and Hall, 1989.)

stromal sarcomas and, indeed, the clinical course pursued by endometrial stromal sarcomas indicates that all are low-grade neoplasms.

An endometrial stromal sarcoma is formed of sheets of generally uniform cells with darkly staining, small, round or ovoid nuclei, scanty cytoplasm, and ill-defined limiting membranes. Nuclear pleomorphism and cytologic atypia are absent or minimal but focal hyaline change is common and sometimes a predominant feature. There is a rich ramifying vascular network within these neoplasms (Fig. 21-4), the vessels sometimes resembling the spiral arterioles of the normal uterus.

Some endometrial stromal sarcomas show unusual patterns that may cause diagnostic confusion. A few have, either in part or in whole, a sex cord–like pattern (Fig. 21-5) with cells arranged in nests, trabeculae, cords, or tubules (12); others can show endometrial glandular differentiation that is usually focal but may be extensive (13). If these patterns are known, they are usually easily recognized but endometrial stromal sarcomas showing extensive glandular differentiation can be confused with adenomyosis and sometimes distinguishing between these two conditions can be extremely difficult.

Endometrial stromal sarcomas have infiltrating margins and vascular invasion is a frequent, and often prominent, feature.

Mixed Sarcomas

Adenosarcoma

These tumors (14) occur predominantly, but by no means solely, in postmenopausal women. They present as solitary, smooth, fleshy polypoid masses that usually arise in the uterine fundus and often fill the uterine cavity. Histologically an adenosarcoma is characterized by benign müllerian epithelium admixed with a sarcomatous stroma (Fig. 21-6). There is a pattern of broad papillary structures, clefts, glands, and cystic spaces covered and lined most commonly by endometrial-type epithelial cells. Other müllerian-type epithelia are usually also present and a coexistence of several types of epithelium is a characteristic feature (15,16). The epithelium often shows a minor degree of focal cytologic atypia while there may be glandular crowding and budding (17). The mesenchymal component of adenosarcomas tends to be predominant and commonly resembles an endometrial stromal sarcoma. Less frequently it has the appearance of a low-grade fibromyosarcoma or leiomyosarcoma. The sarcomatous tissue is of variable cellularity and compactness but is characteristically condensed beneath the surface epithelium and around the contained glands or cysts to form a hypercellular "cambium" layer (Fig. 21-7). The stromal element shows pleomorphism and atypia, though this is rarely of a striking degree, and there is commonly a generous sprinkling of mitotic figures. In a few tumors a sex cord–like pattern is seen in the stroma (18) while heterologous elements such as rhabdomyoblasts, cartilage, and fat are present in the stroma in about 25% of tumors.

Adenosarcomas are of low-grade malignancy and rarely metastasize but show a ten-

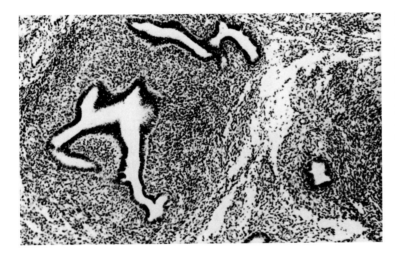

F I G U R E **21-6**

A uterine adenosarcoma. Benign glandular elements of endometrioid type are set in a stroma that shows the features of a low-grade sarcoma. (Reproduced by permission from Buckley CH, Fox H. *Biopsy pathology of the endometrium.* London: Chapman and Hall, 1989.)

F I G U R E **21-7**

A uterine adenosarcoma. Condensation of the sarcomatous stroma, forming a cambium layer, is seen around the gland to the right, which is lined by stratified squamous epithelium. The gland to the left is lined by endocervical-type epithelium and the cambium layer here is less striking. (Reproduced by permission from Buckley CH, Fox H. *Biopsy pathology of the endometrium.* London: Chapman and Hall, 1989.)

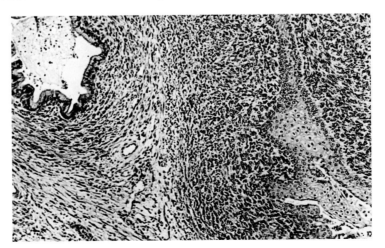

dency to recur after surgical therapy, probably in about 20% of patients, with many such recurrences developing more than 5 years after initial therapy (17). The only indicator of an increased risk of recurrence is deep myometrial invasion. In a few adenosarcomas there is an overgrowth of a poorly differentiated, highly pleomorphic sarcoma with a subsequently poor prognosis (16,19,20).

Carcinosarcoma

These tumors, often also known as *malignant mixed müllerian tumors*, contain morphologically admixed carcinomatous and sarcomatous elements. Tissue culture and immunocytochemical studies tend to suggest, however, that they are metaplastic carcinomas rather than true mixed tumors (21–24) and it has been proposed that they should be classed as *sarcomatoid carcinomas* (25,26); while the scientific evidence for adopting this terminology is quite persua-

sive, some pathologists have been reluctant to make this terminologic change and in this account such tumors will still be considered as carcinosarcomas.

Uterine carcinosarcomas occur predominantly in elderly women and form bulky polypoid masses that usually fill the uterine cavity and may extend into, and even through, the endocervical canal. Histologically the epithelial and mesenchymal components of the neoplasm are intimately admixed. The carcinomatous component is commonly endometrioid in type but it can be, either in whole or part, serous papillary, clear cell, or squamous in nature. Not uncommonly, the adenocarcinomatous element is too poorly differentiated to be specifically identified (Fig. 21-8). The nonepithelial component may resemble an endometrial stromal sarcoma while, infrequently, a leiomyosarcomatous or fibrosarcomatous pattern predominates. Often, however, the appearances are those of a sarcoma of indeterminate type with

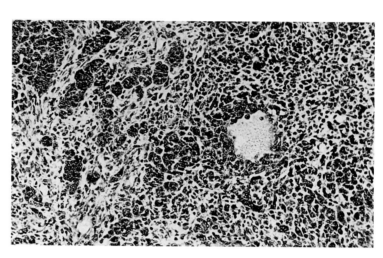

FIGURE **21-8**

A uterine carcinosarcoma. Poorly differentiated carcinomatous elements, to the left, are set in a sarcomatous stroma. (Reproduced by permission from Buckley CH, Fox H. *Biopsy pathology of the endometrium.* London: Chapman and Hall, 1989.)

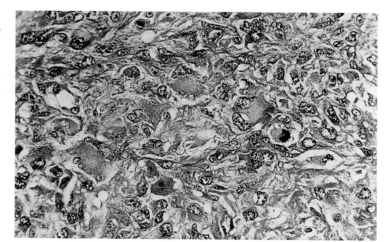

FIGURE **21-9**

Rhabdomyoblasts in the stroma of a uterine carcinosarcoma. (Reproduced by permission from Buckley CH, Fox H. *Biopsy pathology of the endometrium.* London: Chapman and Hall, 1989.)

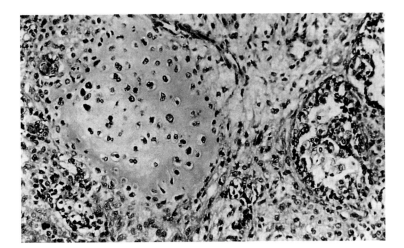

F I G U R E **21-10**

A uterine carcinosarcoma with heterologous elements. The malignant glands to the right are lined by clear cells similar to those seen in a clear-cell carcinoma whereas the cartilaginous tissue, to the left, shows pleomorphism. (Reproduced by permission from Buckley CH, Fox H. *Biopsy pathology of the endometrium.* London: Chapman and Hall, 1989.)

sheets of fusiform or polygonal cells. The nonepithelial component is usually highly cellular, commonly lacks the cambium-layer formation that characterizes mixed tumors of lesser malignancy, and shows conspicuous pleomorphism, atypia, and mitotic activity. Bizarre tumor giant cells with atypical nuclei are often present and heterologous components are present in about 50% of tumors, striated muscle (Fig. 21-9), cartilage (Fig. 21-10), bone, and fat being the alien tissues most frequently encountered; neuroectodermal or neuroendocrine differentiation may occasionally be apparent (27,28).

The initial spread of carcinosarcomas is to locoregional lymph nodes whereas peritoneal and hematogenous spread is also common. There has been much debate about prognostic pathologic features in carcinosarcoma, though it is now widely agreed that neither the presence nor the absence of heterologous elements is of prognostic import and that vascular space invasion is an adverse prognostic factor (29–32). In one large study the biologic behavior of these neoplasms depended largely, if not solely, on the histologic type and grade of the carcinomatous element (30). In another study, however, the grade of the sarcomatous element appeared to be an important prognostic guide (32) and certainly the biologic dominance of the

carcinomatous element has been brought into question by the demonstration that carcinosarcomas are more aggressive neoplasms than are high-grade endometrial tumors (33).

R E F E R E N C E S

1. Hendrickson MR, Kempson RL. Pure mesenchymal tumours of the uterine corpus. In: Fox H, ed. *Haines and Taylor: textbook of obstetrical and gynecological pathology.* 4th ed. Edinburgh: Churchill Livingstone, 1995:519–577.

2. Taylor HB, Norris HJ. Mesenchymal tumors of the uterus. IV. Diagnosis and prognosis of leiomyosarcomas. *Arch Pathol* 1966;82:40–44.

3. Perrone T, Dehner LP. Prognostically favourable "mitotically active" smooth muscle tumors of the uterus: a clinicopathologic study of ten cases. *Am J Surg Pathol* 1988;12:1–8.

4. Prayson RA, Hart WR. Mitotically active leiomyomas of the uterus. *Am J Clin Pathol* 1992; 97:14–20.

5. O'Connor DM, Norris HJ. Mitotically active leiomyomas of the uterus. *Hum Pathol* 1990; 21:223–227.

6. Bell SW, Kempson RL, Hendrickson MR. Problematic uterine smooth muscle neoplasms: a

clinicopathologic study of 213 cases. *Am J Surg Pathol* 1995;18:535–558.

7. King ME, Dickersin GR, Scully RE. Myxoid leiomyosarcoma of the uterus: a report of six cases. *Am J Surg Pathol* 1982;6:589–598.

8. Peacock G, Archer S. Myxoid leiomyosarcoma of the uterus: case report and review of the literature. *Am J Obstet Gynecol* 1989;160:1515–1518.

9. Norris HJ, Taylor HB. Mesenchymal tumors of the uterus. I. A clinical and pathological study of 53 endometrial stromal tumors. *Cancer* 1966;19:755–766.

10. Evans HL. Endometrial stromal sarcoma and poorly differentiated endometrial sarcoma. *Cancer* 1982;50:2170–2182.

11. Chang KL, Crabtree GS, Lim-Tan SK, et al. Primary uterine endometrial stromal neoplasms: a clinicopathologic study of 117 cases. *Am J Surg Pathol* 1990;14:415–438.

12. Clement PB, Scully RE. Uterine tumors resembling ovarian sex-cord tumors: a clinicopathologic analysis of fourteen cases. *Am J Clin Pathol* 1976;66:512–525.

13. Clement PB, Scully RE. Endometrial stromal sarcomas of the uterus with extensive endometrioid glandular differentiation: a report of three cases that caused problems in differential diagnosis. *Int J Gynecol Pathol* 1992;11:163–173.

14. Clement PB, Scully RE. Müllerian adenosarcoma of the uterus: a clinicopathologic analysis of ten cases of a distinct type of müllerian mixed tumor. *Cancer* 1974;34:1138–1149.

15. Clement PB, Scully RE. Uterine tumors with mixed epithelial and mesenchymal elements. *Semin Diagn Pathol* 1988;5:199–222.

16. Kaku T, Silverberg SG, Major FJ, et al. Adenosarcoma of the uterus: a Gynecologic Oncology Group clinicopathologic study of 31 cases. *Int J Gynecol Pathol* 1992;11:75–88.

17. Clement PB, Scully RE. Müllerian adenosarcoma of the uterus: a clinicopathologic analysis of 100 cases with a review of the literature. *Hum Pathol* 1990;21:363–381.

18. Clement PB, Scully RE. Müllerian adenosarcoma of the uterus with sex cord-like elements: a clinicopathologic analysis of eight cases. *Am J Clin Pathol* 1989;91:664–672.

19. Clement PB. Müllerian adenosarcoma of the uterus with sarcomatous overgrowth: a clinico-pathological analysis of ten cases. *Am J Surg Pathol* 1989;13:28–38.

20. Zanotti F, Mussida M, Merlo D, et al. High-grade sarcoma with areas of müllerian adenosarcoma of the uterus. *Ann Ostet Ginecol Med Perinatale* 1991;112:29–35.

21. George E, Manivel JC, Dehner LP, Wick MR. Malignant mixed müllerian tumors: an immuno-histochemical study of 47 cases, with histogenetic considerations and clinical correlation. *Hum Pathol* 1991;22:215–223.

22. Gorai I, Doi C, Minaguchi H. Establishment and characterization of carcinosarcoma cell line of the human uterus. *Cancer* 1993;71:775–786.

23. Emoto M, Iwasaki H, Kikuchi M, Shirakawa K. Characteristics of cloned cells of mixed müllerian tumor of the human uterus: carcinoma cells showing myogenic differentiation in vitro. *Cancer* 1993;71:3065–3075.

24. DeBrito PA, Silverberg SG, Orenstein JM. Carcinosarcoma (malignant mixed müllerian [mesodermal] tumor) of the female genital tract: immunohistochemical and ultrastructural analysis of 28 cases. *Hum Pathol* 1993;24:132–142.

25. Wick MR, Swanson PE. Carcinosarcomas: current perspectives and an historical review of nosological concepts. *Semin Diagn Pathol* 1993;10:118–127.

26. Colombi RP. Sarcomatoid carcinomas of the female genital tract (malignant mixed müllerian tumors). *Semin Diagn Pathol* 1993;10:169–175.

27. Gersell DJ, Duncan DA, Fulling KH. Malignant mixed müllerian tumor of the uterus with neuroectodermal differentiation. *Int J Gynecol Pathol* 1989;8:169–178.

28. Manivel C, Wick MR, Sibley RK. Neuroendocrine differentiation in müllerian neoplasms: an immunohistochemical study of a "pure" endometrial small cell carcinoma and a mixed müllerian tumor containing small cell carcinoma. *Am J Clin Pathol* 1986;86:438–443.

29. Gagne E, Tetu B, Blondeau L, et al. Morphologic prognostic factors for malignant mixed müllerian tumor of the uterus: a clinicopathologic study of 58 cases. *Mod Pathol* 1989;2:433–438.

30. Silverberg SG, Major FJ, Blesing JA, et al. Carcinosarcoma (malignant mixed mesodermal tumor) of the uterus: a Gynecologic Oncology Group pathologic study of 203 cases. *Int J Gynecol Pathol* 1990;9:1–19.

31. Larsen B, Silfversward C, Nilsson B, Petterson F. Mixed müllerian tumours of the uterus—prognostic factors: a clinical and histopathological

study of 147 cases. *Radiother Oncol* 1990;17: 123–132.

32. Major FJ, Blessing JA, Silverberg SG, et al. Prognostic factors in early-stage uterine sarcoma: a Gynecologic Oncology Group study. *Cancer* 1993;71:1702–1709.

33. George E, Lillemoe TJ, Twigs LB, Perrone T. Malignant mixed müllerian tumor versus high grade endometrial carcinoma and aggressive variants of endometrial carcinoma: a comparative analysis of survival. *Int J Gynecol Pathol* 1995;14:39–44.

CHAPTER 22

Treatment of Uterine Sarcomas

NINA EINHORN

*A*lready at the time of Hippocrates, sarcomas had been distinguished from carcinomas by the distinction of a "fleshy tumor" in contrast to "crab like" tumors. These descriptions also provided the basis for the names, as *sarcoma* means "fleshy tumor" in Greek and *cancer* means "crab."

Uterine sarcomas belong to the group of soft tissue sarcomas in which the gynecologic sarcomas in parenchymal organs differ from the other soft tissue sarcomas that usually are found in the extremities and retroperitoneum.

The treatment of uterine sarcomas and especially adjuvant treatment have not been well standardized, as uterine sarcomas represent a heterogeneous group of tumors and the experience with this group is limited. Very few randomized studies have been performed and the guidelines for treatment basically derive from retrospective studies. Unfortunately many of the retrospective studies analyzed all subgroups together, which gives quite confusing and often controversial results.

Staging

In 1978 Salazar and the Gynecologic Oncology Group (GOG) suggested use of the International Federation of Gynecology and Obstetrics (FIGO) clinical staging classification for endometrial carcinoma even for the uterine sarcomas. They suggested excluding the division of stage I into Ia and Ib because the difference in uterine depth was of no prognostic significance. In uterine sarcomas no formal attempt has yet been made to base the staging of sarcomas on surgical findings, in spite of the fact that a modified scheme of endometrial cancer surgical staging has been suggested, even for uterine sarcomas (1).

Etiology and Incidence

The only documented etiologic factor in gynecologic sarcomas is prior radiotherapy for the subgroup of mixed mesodermal tumors. No association has been found between sarcomas and the use of hormones, either birth control pills or postmenopausal hormone replacement treatment.

The incidence of uterine sarcomas varies in the literature from 2.4% to 6.2% of all uterine malignancies. Altogether uterine sarcomas represent 1% of all gynecologic malignancies. There are very few population-based estimations of the incidence (2–5). One of the latest and largest studies presents the incidence of uterine sarcomas in Sweden during the years 1958 to 1984 (5). Two thousand cases of uterine sarcoma were registered during this period. Among them, 62% were recorded as leiomyosarcoma; 20%, as mixed müllerian sarcomas; 10.5%, as endometrial stromal sarcomas; and 7.5%, as sarcomas NOS (without definition). During the observation time the leiomyosarcoma incidence decreased annually by 2.1% and the incidence of mixed müllerian sarcomas increased annually by 5% (5).

The mean age for all patients with uterine sarcomas is 58 years; for leiomyosarcoma, 48 years; and for mixed müllerian sarcomas and endometrial stromal sarcoma, 63 years (1).

The most common associated diseases are

obesity and hypertension, which occur in less than 40% of all patients.

The treatment of uterine sarcomas is described according to the three largest subgroups.

Leiomyosarcomas

Leiomyosarcomas arise from uterine smooth muscle, but rarely from leiomyoma. Less than 1% of leiomyosarcomas arise from preexisting myoma. Still rapid enlargement of myomas is a possible sign of malignant degeneration. Common symptoms of leiomyosarcoma are abnormal uterine bleeding and lower abdominal pains. Clinically it is very difficult to distinguish leiomyosarcomas from leiomyomas. The Papanicolaou smear is of no use and uterine curettage can diagnose only 10% of uterine leiomyosarcomas.

The primary treatment is surgery but the important question is whether oophorectomy should be done together with hysterectomy. One study demonstrated better survival for premenopausal than for postmenopausal women (6). Some authors expressed suspicion that good survival in younger patients can be explained by their inclusion of somewhat benign cellular or atypical myomas (7,8). Larsson et al (9), in a large series of 143 uterine leiomyomas, found that the premenopausal women had a better survival than did postmenopausal women even after they allowed for stage and mitotic count. In addition, premenopausal women with residual ovarian tissues seem to have better survival than do women whose primary treatment is bilateral salpingo-oophorectomy (10–12), which suggests that the presence of retained ovaries may improve the prognosis in patients with leiomyosarcoma. In the same series no metastases to the ovaries were found. Several other authors concluded that leaving the ovaries in situ does not alter the survival for patients with leiomyosarcoma. This fact may advocate that the preservation of the ovaries in premenopausal women with leiomyosarcoma is the right approach.

Clinical stage at the time of diagnosis is one of the most important prognostic factors (6,10,13,14). At the time of diagnosis leiomyosarcomas are more often in stage I, with the tumor confined to the corpus, compared to other uterine sarcomas. In the series of Salazar et al (13), 80% of the leiomyosarcomas were in stage I at the time of diagnosis.

Prognostic Factors

In a French comparative study 81 patients with leiomyosarcoma were studied with respect to prognostic factors. In this study the strongest predictors for survival were menopausal status as well as stage and World Health Organization (WHO) performance status. Unfortunately in this study the results were based on all types of uterine sarcomas (15). In another study from Israel, once again based on all uterine sarcomas, the prognostic factors were clinical stage, histologic type, and method of treatment. There was better survival for patients without adjuvant therapy, which probably could be explained by the selection of patients (16).

In studies on prognostic factors for leiomyosarcoma based on 143 patients from Stockholm, mitotic count was the strongest predictor of survival (9). Recently a study from Linköping, Sweden, presented results of 51 patients with uterus leiomyosarcoma for whom the independent prognostic factors in multivariate analysis were DNA ploidy, S-phase fraction, and surgical stage (17).

The 5-year survival rate for patients with stage I leiomyosarcoma varied in different series, probably due to different classifications, between 20% and 67%. For the total population of patients with leiomyosarcoma including all stages the survival rate varied between 17% and 37%.

Treatment

The most important primary curative measure is surgery. Adjuvant treatment of leiomyosarcomas is controversial.

Adjuvant Radiotherapy

To date, the place of radiotherapy in leiomyosarcoma treatment is controversial and based only on the results of retrospective studies, where the patient subgroups for the different histology are small.

Salazar and Dunne (18) were probably the first to claim that adjuvant irradiation increases the ability to control the disease in the pelvis but others were also of the same opinion (19), showing that postoperative radiotherapy improves 5- and 10-year survival rates, although the differences are not statistically significant (6).

A GOG study analyzing the use of radiation therapy for stage I and II uterine sarcomas was published in 1986 (20). In this study initiated in 1982, radiation therapy was optional and because of that the radiation doses and techniques were not standardized. Of 48 patients with leiomyosarcoma, only 11 received radiation therapy, whereas 49 (45%) of 109 non-leiomyosarcoma patients underwent adjuvant radiation therapy. For the leiomyosarcoma patients with no adjuvant treatment, the survival rate was 37%, which could be compared with 56% for patients treated with radiation and chemotherapy. A 50% survival rate was achieved in the radiation therapy–alone group and a 67% rate was achieved in the chemotherapy-alone group. All these groups of patients with leiomyosarcoma were very small (20). In the Stockholm series presented by Larsson et al (9), of patients treated with surgery alone, 42% had a recurrence in the pelvis, compared with a 16% recurrence rate for patients treated with surgery and radiotherapy. On the other hand, distant metastases were found in 19% of patients treated with surgery alone and in 40% of patients treated with surgery and radiotherapy. This series did not show that adjuvant radiotherapy for leiomyosarcoma is related to better survival (9).

Adjuvant Chemotherapy

Few chemotherapeutic trials distinguishing between leiomyosarcomas and other forms of uterine sarcomas have been performed. Most of the trials were done on recurrent or metastatic leiomyosarcomas, showing some response of short duration. The drugs investigated were doxorubicin with or without dacarbazine (21), ifosfamide (22,23), and paclitaxel (24). A GOG study of doxorubicin versus doxorubicin plus dacarbazine for the treatment of uterine sarcomas showed no advantage for the two-drug regime versus the one-drug regime, but did show a significantly longer survival time for patients with leiomyosarcomas than for those with sarcomas with other cell types (21). In another GOG randomized study of doxorubicin versus no adjuvant treatment after total abdominal hysterectomy and bilateral salpingo-oophorectomy for stage I and II uterine sarcomas, neither survival nor progression-free interval was prolonged by adjuvant chemotherapy (25).

Mixed Mesodermal Tumors

Mixed mesodermal tumors containing both carcinomatous and sarcomatous elements have to be distinguished from the much more benign type of tumor with benign epithelial malignant stromal elements. The mixed mesodermal tumors were often associated with previous irradiation to the pelvis but only about 5% to 15% of them have been related to previous irradiation (7,26–28).

The most common symptom in mixed müllerian sarcomas is vaginal bleeding, usually postmenopausal since most of the patients are over 60 years old. Mixed müllerian sarcomas are very aggressive tumors and lymphatic or hematogenous spread occurs early in the disease. In a series presented by DiSaia et al (29), more than 60% of the patients at the time of diagnosis had the disease outside the uterus. In the Stockholm series presented by Larsson et al (30) on 147 mixed müllerian sarcoma patients treated between 1969 and 1981, patients with homologous tumors were younger and more often had early-stage disease and a normal-size uterus compared to patients with heterologous tumors.

Adjuvant Radiotherapy

For many years preoperative irradiation had been supported by many authors (14,28,31,32). Perez et al (31) noted a 17% recurrence rate in patients with mixed müllerian sarcomas receiving preoperative irradiation compared with a 50% recurrence rate in patients treated with surgery alone. In a GOG study patients who received radiotherapy to the pelvis postoperatively for stage I or II mixed müllerian sarcoma had a significant reduction in the rate of recurrence within the irradiation treatment field (20). Kohorn et al (28) found a correlation with residual tumor after preoperative irradiation, demonstrating a 10% two-year survival rate when residual tumor was found in the specimen, compared with a 70% survival rate in patients with no residual tumor found during surgery. In the same series the best survival rate—82%—was obtained in patients who received a combination of intracavitary and external irradiation and surgery. In 5 patients a combination of radiation, surgery, and adjuvant chemotherapy resulted in an 80% five-year survival rate (28). In the Stockholm series presented by Larsson et al (30), most of the patients were treated with a combination of surgery and irradiation. The best 5-year survival rate after surgery was reached when both intracavitary radium and external irradiation were added to the treatment. In the multivariate analysis, early stage, absence of abdominal pain, and low age were predictors of a favorable prognosis (30).

Even if preoperative irradiation is considered of value in the management of mixed müllerian sarcomas, the latest trend is to do primary surgery for uterine malignancy and that includes even mixed müllerian sarcomas, although a study using randomization to treatment with or without preoperative irradiation would probably help us learn more about the validity of previous observations.

Adjuvant Chemotherapy

Adjuvant chemotherapy was used in the previously mentioned GOG studies for completely resected stage I or II disease (25). Doxorubicin versus no further therapy was studied and no statistical difference was found for progression-free interval and recurrence rate. The number of patients in each histologic subgroup was too small to permit statistical significance, although 39% of the mixed müllerian sarcoma patients receiving doxorubicin had a recurrence, compared with 51% for patients who received no further therapy (25). Further trials on chemotherapy regimes have been opened for patients with completely resected stage I or II disease.

For the more advanced and recurring mixed müllerian sarcomas, several agents such as cyclophosphamide, doxorubicin, cisplatin, and dacarbazine have been found to be active, but the duration of their activities is not too long. Ifosfamide is the single most active agent (33), but cisplatin also provides some response in patients with advanced disease (34,35). It is no doubt that the combination of surgery, radiotherapy, and chemotherapy should be evaluated in this group of very malignant tumors.

The survival rate for patients with mixed müllerian sarcomas is poor. In the Swedish study, the 5-year survival rate for the homogeneous type of mixed müllerian sarcomas was 60% and the 10-year survival rate was 35%; for the heterogeneous type the 5-year survival rate was 19%; for the undifferentiated type the 5-year survival rate was 26% and the 10-year rate was 21% (30). For patients with completely resected stage I or II disease the recurrence rate varied between 40% and 60% (20,36). It has also been reported that up to 45% of patients with stage I disease have retroperitoneal lymph node metastases (37,38).

Endometrial Stromal Sarcomas

To describe the epidemiologic and clinical aspects of endometrial stromal sarcoma presents some difficulties, as the studies presented in the literature mostly are related to the traditional categorization of low- and high-grade sarcomas based on mitotic count. In light of the result from the study of Chang et al (39), which found the mitotic count of no prognostic value, and taking into consideration the views presented in Chapter 21, it is difficult to translate the results of the published reports.

Until now, all literature concerning endometrial stromal sarcoma is based on the classic pathologic classification; therefore, the description on the results of treatment of patients with low-grade and high-grade disease are done in accordance with the old classification.

Endolymphatic Stromal Myosis— Low-Grade Stromal Sarcoma

According to several authors, endolymphatic stromal myosis has a much more protracted clinical course compared with high-grade endometrial stromal sarcoma. Local recurrences are typical, often sometimes as late as 25 years after the primary diagnosis. As much as 50% of the patients have a recurrence after initial therapy. Interestingly, curettage does not always give the correct diagnosis. Two Finnish studies showed that only in 70% and 83% of patients can the correct diagnosis be made by curettage (6,40). The reason for this is that probably endometrial stromal sarcomas in some patients are not connected to the endometrium.

In the Swedish series presented by Larsson et al (41), 28 patients with endometrial stromal sarcoma were treated between 1936 and 1981 at Radiumhemmet. The histopathologic review done in 1987 to 1988 classified 16 stromal sarcomas as high grade and 12 as low grade. A significant relation between mitotic count and relative survival within 10 years of diagnosis was found, showing a more favorable outcome for patients with a low mitotic count compared with those with higher counts (41).

Fifty-two patients with low-grade stromal sarcoma, also called endolymphatic stromal myosis, were studied by a group of oncologists trained at the M. D. Anderson Cancer Center (42). The criteria for being included in the study was a mitotic count in the specimen of less than 10 mitotic figures per 10 high-power fields. All slides have been reviewed. Twenty-nine patients in stage I had a recurrence, many of them as long as 25 years after diagnosis.

DNA ploidy as a prognostic factor was studied by a few groups with different results. According to Lurain and Piver (43), flow cytometric analysis was useful in distinguishing between endometrial stromal sarcoma of high and low malignancy. A Norwegian group found contradictory results; in their study DNA ploidy was not significantly correlated to prognosis (44).

As early as 1968, Pelillo (45) documented activity of gestagens in the treatment of low-grade stromal sarcomas. Later, Krumholtz et al (46), Piver et al (42), as well as other investigators (47–51) confirmed these findings. Because of its less toxic side effects, progestin has been recommended for use in endometrial stromal sarcoma prior to chemotherapy. The role of progestins as adjuvant therapy should, if possible, be investigated in prospective studies.

High-Grade Endometrial Stromal Sarcoma

In series where endolymphatic stromal myosis was distinguished from pure stromal sarcoma, the reported survival rate for the latter was poor, with the 5-year survival rate varying between 0% and 26%. In series where radiotherapy was used, a favorable response was found both in patients with recurrence and in patients with extrauterine growth (52,53). Some retrospective studies also reported a favorable response to radiotherapy given as adjuvant therapy (19,54). It is of interest that in the Swedish study presented by Larsson et al (41), 11 patients with stage I high-grade tumors received adjuvant therapy and 8 (73%) of them survived 5 years.

It is also of interest to mention that Belgrad et al (55), combining results from several institutions, found that the 2-year survival rate was improved by postoperative irradiation for endometrial stromal sarcomas (57% versus 37%) and mixed müllerian sarcomas (35% versus 20%) but not for leiomyosarcomas.

The role of chemotherapy in endometrial stromal sarcomas has not been well documented. Sporadic reports described antitumor activities with treatment with doxorubicin as well as doxorubicin plus cyclophosphamide (56) and others showed activities when a variety of chemotherapeutic agents were used (57–60). Recently, a GOG report (61) demonstrated ifosfamide as an active drug for metastatic or recurrent endometrial stromal sarcomas.

Conclusions

Frankly malignant uterine sarcomas generally have a much worse prognosis than does adenocarcinoma of the endometrium. The most important therapeutic tool is surgery; if the tumor is still confined to the uterus, the survival rate after surgery may be 50%. For patients in other stages of the disease, the prognosis is extremely poor.

Adjuvant radiotherapy seems to play a role in the treatment of mixed müllerian sarcomas and endometrial stromal sarcoma, but probably less of one in leiomyosarcoma. Adjuvant chemotherapy has until now not shown any promising results. There are ongoing trials regarding both adjuvant chemotherapy and radiotherapy.

REFERENCES

1. Salazar OM, Bonfiglio TA, Patten SF, et al. Uterine sarcomas. *Cancer* 1978;42:1152–1160.

2. Harlow BL, Weiss NS, Lofton S. The epidemiology of sarcomas of the uterus. *Natl J Cancer Inst* 1986;76:399–402.

3. Christopherson WM, Williamson EO, Gray LA. Leiomyosarcoma of the uterus. *Cancer* 1972; 29:1512–1517.

4. Schwartz Z, Dgani R, Lancet M, Kessler I. Uterine sarcoma in Israel: a study of 104 cases. *Gynecol Oncol* 1985;20:354–363.

5. Larsson B. Uterine sarcoma: an epidemiological and clinicopathological study. Dissertation. Karolinska Institute, Stockholm, 1989.

6. Kahanpää KV, Wahlström T, Gröhn P, et al. Sarcomas of the uterus: a clinicopathologic study of 119 patients. *Obstet Gynecol* 1986;67:417–424.

7. Bartsich EG, O'Leary JA, Moore JG. Carcinosarcoma of the uterus: a 50-year review of 32 cases. *Obstet Gynecol* 1967;30:518–523.

8. Hart RW, Billman JK. A reassessment of uterine neoplasms originally diagnosed as leiomyosarcomas. *Cancer* 1978;41:1902–1910.

9. Larsson B, Silfverswärd C, Nilsson B, Pettersson F. Prognostic factors in uterine leiomyosarcoma. *Acta Oncol* 1990;29:185–191.

10. Aaro LA, Symmonds RE, Docherty MD. Sarcoma of the uterus: a clinical and pathologic study of 177 cases. *Am J Obstet Gynecol* 1966;94:101–109.

11. Bass JC, O'Leary JA. Leiomyosarcoma of the uterus. *South Med J* 1970;63:473–478.

12. Taylor HB, Norris HJ. Mesenchymal tumors of the uterus. IV. Diagnosis and prognosis of leiomyosarcomas. *Arch Pathol* 1966;82:40–44.

13. Salazar OM, Bonfiglio TA, Patten SF, et al. Uterine sarcomas. Natural history, treatment and prognosis. *Cancer* 1978;3:1152–1160.

14. Badib AO, Vongtama V, Kurohara SS, Webster JH. Radiotherapy in the treatment of sarcomas of the corpus uteri. *Cancer* 1969;24:724–729.

15. George M, Pejovic MH, Kramar A, et al. Uterine sarcomas: prognostic factors and treatment modalities—study on 209 patients. *Gynecol Oncol* 1986;24:58–67.

16. Schwartz Z, Dgani R, Lancet M, Kessler I. Uterine sarcoma in Israel: a study of 104 cases. *Gynecol Oncol* 1985;20:354–363.

17. Blom R, Guerrieri C, Malmström H. Prognostiska faktorer för uterusleiomyosarcom. Svenska Läkarsällskapets Rikstämma, Stockholm, 1996. Abstract, 34P.

18. Salazar OM, Dunne ME. The role of radiation therapy in the management of uterine sarcomas. *Int J Radiat Oncol Biol Phys* 1980;6:899–902.

19. Rose PG, Boutselis JG, Sachs L. Adjuvant therapy for stage I uterine sarcoma. *Am J Obstet Gynecol* 1987;156:660–662.

20. Hornback NB, Omura G, Major FJ. Observations on the use of adjuvant radiation therapy in patients with stage I and II uterine sarcoma. *Int J Radiat Oncol Biol Phys* 1986;12:2127–2130.

21. Omura GA, Major FJ, Blessing JA, et al. A randomized study of Adriamycin with and without dimethy triazenoimidazole carboxamide in advanced uterine sarcomas. *Cancer* 1983;52:626–632.

22. Sutton GP, Blessing JA, Barrett RJ, McGehee R. Phase II trial of ifosfamide and mesna in leiomyosarcoma of the uterus: a Gynecologic Oncology Group study. *Am J Obstet Gynecol* 1992;166:556–559.

23. Sutton GP, Blessing JA, Malfetano JH. Ifosfamide and doxorubicin in the treatment of advanced leiomyosarcomas of the uterus: a Gynecologic Oncology Group study. *Gynecol Oncol* 1996;62:226–229.

24. Sutton GP, Blessing JA, Ball HG. Advanced or recurrent uterine leiomyosarcomas unexposed to other chemotherapy: a Gynecologic Oncology Group study. Abstract presented at the Society of Gynecologic Oncologists meeting, New Orleans, February 10–14, 1996.

25. Omura GA, Blessing JA, Major E, Silverberg S. A randomized trial of Adriamycin versus no adjuvant chemotherapy in stage I and II uterine sarcomas. *J Clin Oncol* 1985;9:1240–1245.

26. Norris HJ, Taylor HB. Mesenchymal tumors of the uterus. III. A clinical and pathologic study of 31 carcinosarcomas. *Cancer* 1966;19:1459–1465.

27. Peters WA, Kumar NB, Fleming WP, Morley GW. Prognostic features of sarcomas and mixed tumors of the endometrium. *Obstet Gynecol* 1984;63:550–556.

28. Kohorn EI, Schwartz PE, Chambers JT, et al. Adjuvant therapy in mixed müllerian tumors of the uterus. *Gynecol Oncol* 1986;23:212–221.

29. DiSaia PJ, Castro JR, Rutledge FN. Mixed mesodermal sarcoma of the uterus. *Obstet Gynecol* 1976;177:632–636.

30. Larsson B, Silfverswärd C, Nilsson B, et al. Mixed müllerian tumours of the uterus—prognostic factors: a clinical and histopathological study of 147 cases. *Radiother Oncol* 1990;17:123–132.

31. Perez CA, Askin F, Baglan RJ, et al. Effects of irradiation on mixed müllerian tumors of the uterus. *Cancer* 1979;43:1274–1284.

32. Salazar OM, Bonfiglio TA, Patten SF, et al. Uterine sarcomas: analysis of failures with special emphasis on the use of adjuvant radiation therapy. *Cancer* 1978;42:1161–1170.

33. Sutton GP, Blessing JA, Homesley HD, Malfetano JH. A phase II trial of ifosfamide and mesna in patients with advanced or recurrent mixed mesodermal tumors of the ovary previously treated with platinum-based chemotherapy: a

Gynecologic Oncology Group study. *Gynecol Oncol* 1994;53:24–26.

34. Thigpen JT, Blessing JA, Orr JW Jr, et al. Phase II trial of cisplatin in the treatment of patients with advanced or recurrent mixed mesodermal sarcomas of the uterus. *Cancer Treat Rep* 1986; 70:271–274.

35. Gershenson DM, Kavanagh JJ, Copeland IJ, et al. Cisplatin therapy for disseminated mixed mesodermal sarcoma of the uterus. *J Clin Oncol* 1987;5:618–621.

36. Meredith RF, Eisert DR, Kaka Z, et al. An excess of uterine sarcomas after pelvic irradiation. *Cancer* 1986;58:2003–2007.

37. Silverberg SG, Major FJ, Blessing JA, et al. Carcinosarcoma (malignant mixed mesodermal tumor) of the uterus. A Gynecologic Oncology Group pathologic study of 203 cases. *Int J Gynecol Pathol* 1990;9:1–18.

38. Costa MJ, Khan R, Judd R. Carcinosarcoma (mixed müllerian (mesodermal) tumor) of the uterus and ovary. *Arch Pathol Lab Med* 1991; 115:583–590.

39. Chang CL, Crabtree GS, Lim-Tan SK, et al. Primary uterine endometrial stromal neoplasms: a clinicopathologic study of 117 cases. *Am J Surg Pathol* 1990;14:415–438.

40. Taina E. Mäenpää J, Erkkola R, et al. Endometrial stromal sarcoma: a report of nine cases. *Gynecol Oncol* 1989;32:156–162.

41. Larsson B, Silfverswärd C, Nilsson B, Pettersson F. Endometrial stromal sarcoma of the uterus. *Eur J Obstet Gynecol* 1990;35:239–249.

42. Piver MS, Rutledge FN, Copeland L, et al. Uterine endolymphatic stromal myosis: a collaborative study. *Obstet Gynecol* 1984;64:173–178.

43. Lurain JR, Piver MS. Uterine sarcomas: clinical features and management. In: Coppleson M, ed. *Gynecologic oncology.* 2nd ed. London: Churchill Livingstone, 1992.

44. Nordal RR, Kristensen GB, Kaern J, et al. The prognostic significance of surgery, tumor size, malignancy grade, menopausal status, and DNA ploidy in endometrial stromal sarcoma. *Gynecol Oncol* 1996;62:254–259.

45. Pelillo D. Proliferative stromatosis of the uterus with pulmonary metastases. Remission following treatment with a long-acting synthetic progestin. A case report. *Obstet Gynecol* 1968;31:33.

46. Krumholz BA, Lobovsky FY, Halitsky V. Endolymphatic stromal myosis with pulmonary metastasis, remission with progestin therapy: report of a case. *J Reprod Med* 1973;10:85–89.

47. Tsukamoto N, Kamura T, Matsukuma K, et al. Endolymphatic stromal myosis: a case with positive estrogen and progestogen receptors and good response to prognosis. *Gynecol Oncol* 1985;20:120–128.

48. Lantta M, Kahanpää K, Karkkainen J, et al. Estradiol and progesterone receptors in two cases of endometrial stromal sarcoma. *Gynecol Oncol* 1984;18:233–239.

49. Gloor E, Schynder P, Cites M, et al. Endolymphatic stromal myosis: surgical and hormonal treatment of extensive abdominal recurrence 20 years after hysterectomy. *Cancer* 1982;50:1880–1893.

50. Katz L, Merino MJ, Sakamato H, Schwartz PE. Endometrial stromal sarcoma: a clinicopathologic study of 11 cases with determination of estrogen and progestin receptor levels in three tumors. *Gynecol Oncol* 1987;26:87–97.

51. Baggish M, Woodruff D. Uterine stromatosis. Clinicopathologic features and hormone dependency. *Obstet Gynecol* 1972;40:487–498.

52. Koss LG, Spiro RH, Brunschwig A. Endometrial stromal sarcoma. *Surg Gynecol Obstet* 1965; Sept:531.

53. Yoonessi M, Hart WR. Endometrial stromal sarcomas. *Cancer* 1977;40:898.

54. Vongtama V, Karlen JR, Piver SM, et al. Treatment, results and prognostic factors in stage I and II sarcomas of the corpus uterine. *Am J Roentgenol Radiat Ther Nucl Med* 1976; 126:139–147.

55. Belgrad R, Elbadawi N, Rubin P. Uterine sarcomas. *Radiology* 1975;114:181.

56. Muss HB, Bundy B, Disia PJ, et al. Treatment of recurrence of advanced uterine sarcoma: a randomized trial of doxorubicin versus doxorubicin and cyclophosphamide (a phase III trial of the Gynecologic Oncology Group). *Cancer* 1985;55:1648–1653.

57. Adducci JE. Doxorubicin (Adriamycin) therapy of uterine sarcoma without surgery in an elderly patient. *J Am Geriatr Soc* 1976;24:473–475.

58. Lehrner LM, Miles PA, Enck RE. Complete remission of widely metastatic endometrial stromal sarcoma following combination chemotherapy. *Cancer* 1979;43:1189–1194.

59. Mansi JL, Ramachandra S, Wiltshaw E, Fisher C. Endometrial stromal sarcoma. *Gynecol Oncol* 1990;36:113–118.

60. Yung-Chang L, Kudelka AP, Tresukosol D, et al. Case report. Prolonged stabilization of progressive endometrial stromal sarcoma with prolonged oral etoposide therapy. *Gynecol Oncol* 1995;58:262–265.

61. Sutton GP, Blessing JA, Park R, et al. Ifosfamide treatment of recurrence of metastatic endometrial stromal sarcomas previously unexposed to chemotherapy: a study of the Gynecologic Oncology Group. *Obstet Gynecol* 1996;87:747–750.

CHAPTER 23

Gestational Trophoblastic Diseases

GORDON J. S. RUSTIN
RICHARD H. J. BEGENT

The first use of cytotoxic chemotherapy for choriocarcinoma in the 1950s changed the outlook of women with this rapidly growing cancer from almost certain death to high chance of cure. It is now apparent that the spectrum of trophoblastic diseases extends from benign hydatidiform moles, which usually resolve spontaneously, to life-threatening choriocarcinoma. Provided that patients are correctly diagnosed and the appropriate therapy is administered early enough in the course of disease, the trophoblastic diseases are almost all curable. Only physicians in specialist centers gain adequate experience in treating these rare tumors. However, with the incidence of hydatidiform mole ranging from 0.5 to 2.5/1000 pregnancies, most obstetric units will see at least one case per year. A woman who has had a hydatidiform mole has approximately a 1000-fold higher chance of developing choriocarcinoma than one who has had a live birth. Continued awareness and education are required not only so that management and follow-up of molar pregnancy are optimal but also so that choriocarcinoma developing after nonmolar pregnancy is detected as early as possible.

Pathology

A World Health Organization (WHO) scientific group (1) clarified the clinical and pathologic definitions of the various conditions that make up gestational trophoblastic disease (GTD). This term includes the diseases detailed here as well as two conditions that are not followed by malignant sequelae: hydropic degeneration—an aborted conceptus with no evidence of fetal development containing excessive fluid or liquefaction of placental villous stroma without undue trophoblastic hyperplasia, also called *blighted ovum*—and placental site reaction—the presence of trophoblastic cells and leukocytes in a placental bed. The histology of GTD has been well reviewed (2,3) and brief definitions are given here.

Complete Hydatidiform Mole

The term *hydatidiform mole* is derived from the Greek word *hydatis* meaning a "drop of water" and the Latin word *mola* meaning "a mass." Complete hydatidiform mole is defined as an abnormal conceptus without an embryo, with gross hydropic swelling of the placental villi and usually pronounced trophoblastic hyperplasia, having both cytotrophoblastic and syncytial elements. The villous swelling leads to central cistern formation with a concomitant compression of the maturing connective tissue that has lost its vascularity. A classic mole resembles a bunch of grapes. The use of early pregnancy ultrasound can lead to the diagnosis of mole and those pregnancies that lack a fetal pole are electively terminated. The lack of trophoblastic hyperplasia on histology leads to their reclassification as hydropic abortuses.

Partial Hydatidiform Mole

This is an abnormal conceptus with an embryo or fetus that tends to die early, with a placenta subject to focal and villous swelling leading to cistern formation and focal trophoblastic hyperplasia, usually involving the syncytiotrophoblast only. The unaffected villi appear normal and vascularity of the villi disappears following fetal death. Unequivocal choriocarcinoma has only rarely been recorded after the occurrence of partial hydatidiform mole. Chemotherapy has been given to about 1% of women following a partial mole because of metastases or elevated human chorionic gonadotropin (hCG) levels. The results of most studies suggest that complete hydatidiform mole is more common than partial hydatidiform mole.

Invasive Mole

This is a tumor invading the myometrium and is characterized by trophoblastic hyperplasia and persistence of placental villous structures. It results from complete hydatidiform or partial hydatidiform mole and progresses to choriocarcinoma in about 15% of patients. It may metastasize, with villi apparent in the metastases, but does not progress like a true cancer unless the histologic picture changes to that of choriocarcinoma, and it may regress spontaneously.

Gestational Choriocarcinoma

This is a carcinoma arising from the trophoblastic epithelium that shows both cytotrophoblastic and syncytiotrophoblastic elements. It may arise from conceptions that result in a live birth, a stillbirth, an abortion at any stage, an ectopic pregnancy, or a hydatidiform mole. The lack of villous structures distinguishes choriocarcinoma morphologically from invasive mole. Over 50% of choriocarcinomas are preceded by hydatidiform mole in most series.

Placental Site Trophoblastic Tumor

This tumor arises from intermediate trophoblast of the placental bed and is composed mainly of cytotrophoblastic cells. This accounts for the relatively low level of hCG associated with this condition. About one case of this tumor is seen for every 100 cases of invasive mole and choriocarcinoma. Pathologists may initially consider it as atypical choriocarcinoma. It was earlier called *trophoblast pseudotumor of the uterus* but the term *placental site trophoblastic tumor* is now preferred because of the malignant behavior reported in some tumors. Complete surgical excision is the preferred treatment as these tumors are not as chemosensitive as choriocarcinoma (4).

Gestational Trophoblastic Tumors

The term *gestational trophoblastic tumor* (GTT) is used to denote those conditions that require more active intervention, usually chemotherapy, and includes invasive mole, choriocarcinoma, and placental site tumors. The reliance on persistently elevated hCG levels for diagnosis and the frequent absence of tissue for histology make it often impossible to differentiate between invasive mole and choriocarcinoma, so the designation GTT covers both diseases.

Histologic Grading

There has been considerable debate among pathologists as to whether histologic features of the complete hydatiform moles are of prognostic significance. Hertig and Mansell (5) proposed a grading system in the prechemotherapy era but Elston and Bagshawe (6) and Genest et al (7) clearly showed it to have no efficacy for grading moles with contemporary clinical management. An absence of fibrinoid in the implantation site, now recognized as largely consisting of fibronectin secreted by the trophoblast, has been correlated with an adverse outcome (8). Theoretically fibrinoid could act as a barrier to trophoblast invasiveness but is difficult to grade.

Epidemiology

The very high incidence of hydatidiform mole in Asia, parts of Africa, and South and Central America may have been exaggerated because complicated births are more likely to be managed in hospitals. Therefore, hospital-based studies are likely to overestimate the true incidence, owing to selection bias (9,10). Population studies in Japan reported an average incidence of about 2.5/1000 pregnancies, compared to a nationwide Chinese incidence of 0.78/1000 pregnancies. Studies in the United States reported incidence rates of 0.5 to 1.08/1000 pregnancies, while a study from England and Wales showed an incidence of 1.54/1000 live births. Large differences in incidence in different racial groups have not been confirmed (9,10).

Studies from many countries showed that the risk of hydatidiform mole increases progressively in women older than 40, reaching almost 1 in 3 live births in those older than 50 (11). The risk is also slightly higher in pregnancies of those younger than 15 years. One study showed a relative risk of 2.9 in pregnancies fathered by men older than 45 (12).

Increasing gravidity does not appear to increase the risk of hydatidiform mole. However, a woman who has had a hydatidiform mole has a more than 20-fold increased chance of having a further one; the rate for a second hydatidiform mole ranges from 0.8% to 2.9% and for a third mole from 15% to 28% (11). Among the 6842 women from England and Wales in the study from Bagshawe et al (11), 1.4% had more than one molar pregnancy.

A case-control study suggested that low estrogen levels may be associated with a disruption of normal ovulation and predispose to choriocarcinoma (13). Other reported weak associations include prior miscarriages, artificial insemination by donor, longer duration of smoking, and reduced carotene intake. Oral contraception appears to be unrelated.

The incidence of choriocarcinoma in the United States has been reported to be 1/24,096 pregnancies or 1/19,920 live births (14). The incidence in Asia is higher. Choriocarcinoma is preceded by a hydatidiform mole in 29% to 83% of patients. Among 602 patients treated for GTT at the Charing Cross Hospital over a 10-year period, 83% of the tumors followed hydatidiform mole, 10% followed normal term delivery, 1% occurred after a live birth preceded by a molar pregnancy, and 5% followed an abortion (15). Maternal age over 40 is a significant risk factor for choriocarcinoma and the risk is also increased in the 15- to 19-year age group. Other factors such as diet, estrogen levels, oral contraception, and histocompatibility are not well established (16).

Genetics

Complete hydatidiform mole appears to result from fertilization of an egg from which the nucleus has been lost or inactivated. The chromosomal complement arises by androgenesis and there are no maternal chromosomes, although the mitochondrial DNA is of maternal origin (17). At least 75% to 85% of complete moles are homozygous 46,XX; in most cases the paternal contribution stems from a duplication of a haploid sperm or from two different sperm. Approximately 15% to 25% of complete moles are heterozygous, predominantly 46,XY, but some 46,XX complete heterozygous moles have been reported. These heterozygous moles do not appear to have a higher chance of progressing to choriocarcinoma than do the homozygous ones.

DNA fingerprinting can be used to show the presence of paternal chromosomal DNA in trophoblast tissue (18). The absence of a paternal contribution in a representative tumor sample indicates that it is nongestational, either an ovarian teratoma or trophoblast differentiation of, most commonly, lung or stomach cancer, and can explain why drug resistance develops in these patients.

Genetic studies show partial hydatidiform mole to be triploid with one maternal and two paternal chromosome sets. It is thought to arise by dispermy. Flow cytometry on nuclei prepared from fresh or formalin-fixed paraffin-embedded tissue is very useful in confirming the triploid nature of partial hydatidiform mole.

Investigations

Human Chorionic Gonadotropin

hCG is a placental hormone that is secreted by the syncytiotrophoblast and serves to maintain corpus luteum function and preserve progesterone secretion during the early stages of gestation. In a normal pregnancy it can be detected about 5 days after conception and reaches its peak at 8 to 10 weeks of pregnancy. Although syncytiotrophoblast is the physiologic source of hCG, an hCG-like substance has been detected in a wide variety of normal human tissues and low levels can be measured in normal human plasma.

The α-subunit of hCG is nearly identical to the α-units of thyroid-stimulating hormone, follicle-stimulating hormone, and luteinizing hormone. The β-subunit shares many similarities with the β-subunits of other glycoprotein hormones, but the carboxyl-terminal end contains unique amino acid sequences giving distinct antigenic characteristics. Immunoassays that utilize the intact hCG molecule as immunogen may be influenced by luteinizing hormone levels. Single-step assay kits may dangerously underestimate hCG levels if large amounts are present, owing to the "high-dose hook" effect. This can be avoided by doing assays at two dilutions or by incorporating a washing step. A good assay detects levels as low as 2 IU/L in serum. Assays on urine are useful in the long-term follow-up of patients, although the background noise on urine assays tends to be higher than that in serum so that values up to the equivalent of 30 IU/L may not be significant. Urine estimations should be based on timed collections or be related to creatinine concentration. The preferred preservative for immunoassay is thiomersal (Merthiolate, 100 mg/24-hr collection). Pregnancy test results will be positive in most patients with trophoblastic diseases but the test may miss some cases due to the lower sensitivity.

Nicked β-subunit of hCG and the β-core fragment may account for a high proportion of total hCG in trophoblastic tumors. In an attempt to distinguish between normal placenta and trophoblastic tumors, hCG fragments and many placental proteins, including pregnancy-specific B1 glycoprotein, human placental lactogen, and inhibin, have been investigated. Higher levels of serum progesterone have been found prior to evacuation of hydatidiform moles that require chemotherapy compared to those that spontaneously remit. The clinical value of measuring compounds in addition to hCG remains unclear.

Use in Establishing the Diagnosis and Monitoring Therapy

It is not possible to differentiate between a molar and normal pregnancy based on hCG measurement. Elevated serum levels will be present until fewer than 10^5 trophoblast cells remain.

Choriocarcinoma may be excluded by the presence of a normal serum hCG level (<2 IU/L). An elevated level could be due to pregnancy, residual placental elements, ovarian germ cell tumor, placental site tumor, trophoblast differentiation in a carcinoma, or ectopic production from a variety of different tumors. Nontrophoblastic tumors are rarely associated with hCG levels higher than 1000 IU/L.

The close linear relationship between the number of choriocarcinoma cells present and the serum concentration of hCG allows for a more accurate assessment of response than for any other tumor. Levels of hCG can sometimes rise during the early days of drug therapy even though the tumor is chemosensitive. This is thought to be related to tumor lysis. Serum hCG levels should be measured prior to evacuation and monitored at least weekly during therapy.

A plateau above the normal range may be due to cross reaction of the assay with luteinizing hormone if the patient has become menopausal. However, a plateau or rising levels usually indicate drug resistance. Owing to the accuracy of hCG monitoring, repeat x-ray studies and scans are required only to confirm resolution of metastases or uterine or ovarian abnormalities at the end of treatment or to detect surgically resectable masses in patients with drug-resistant disease. Radiologic abnormalities may persist for some time after the hCG has become normal before finally resolving.

Other Investigations

Hydatidiform Mole

Ultrasound In a woman thought to be pregnant, ultrasound scanning of the pelvis is the investigation most likely to confirm the presence of hydatidiform mole (Table 23-1). Hydatidiform mole produces a characteristic pattern of echoes that appear like a snowstorm due to echogenicity of the walls of molar vesicles. The diagnosis of hydatidiform mole normally depends on exclusion of a normal pregnancy, although twin gestations with one mole and one normal pregnancy are reported. Lutein cysts of the ovary are common and generally resolve with resolution of the trophoblastic disease, but it is wise to repeat ultrasound examination after the hCG level has returned to normal to exclude other pathology. Ultrasound can be used to determine uterine volume, which is more accurate than the value obtained by palpation, and this is useful in assessing prognosis. Ultrasound is helpful in showing invasion of tumor through the myometrium and in identifying extrauterine masses. Doppler ultrasound can show the characteristic abnormalities of blood flow in the uterine artery. These are due to the large vascular channels that form in trophoblastic disease

TABLE 23-1

Differential Diagnosis and Distinguishing Investigations of Molar Pregnancy

Diagnosis	Investigation
Pregnancy	Ultrasound
Abortion	Ultrasound
Partial hydatidiform mole	Histology, genetics
Toxemia of pregnancy	Ultrasound
Hyperemesis gravidarum	Ultrasound
Ovarian cysts	Ultrasound, hCG measurement
Invasive mole	Histology, hCG measurement (persistently elevated)

hCG = human chorionic gonadotropin.

in the myometrium. They change the waveform in the uterine artery, which may be expressed as an altered pulsatility index (19).

Chest Radiographs A chest x-ray study should be performed to exclude trophoblastic emboli or metastases of invasive mole or choriocarcinoma (Fig. 23-1).

Biopsy The products obtained at evacuation are usually the only tissue available for histol-

FIGURE 23-1

Example of classic cannonball metastases on a chest x-ray film of a woman with choriocarcinoma.

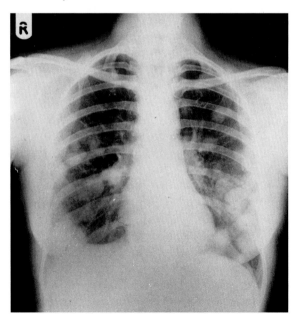

ogy. Biopsy of vaginal metastases should not be performed as this frequently leads to profuse bleeding that may be difficult to control.

Laboratory Tests A full blood cell count is required to check for anemia and 2 units of blood should be cross-matched prior to evacuation. Triiodothyronine and thyroxine should be measured prior to surgery if there is any suspicion of thyrotoxicosis.

Invasive Mole and Choriocarcinoma

Histologic confirmation of the diagnosis is not required if there is a history of a recent molar pregnancy, the hCG level is grossly elevated, and the distribution of disease is typical of choriocarcinoma (Table 23-2). Provided pregnancy has been excluded in patients with grossly elevated levels of hCG, even without a history of a mole, it is safer to treat them as having choriocarcinoma than to risk performing a biopsy on a metastasis. Needle biopsies of the liver or other sites have resulted in fatal hemorrhage, and delay in starting therapy while recovering from surgical biopsies allows the tumor to grow.

Clinical examination should include inspection of the vagina for metastases. The only routine staging investigations required are posteroanterior and lateral chest x-ray studies and pelvic ultrasound. Cerebrospinal fluid

TABLE 23-2

Differential Diagnosis of Gestational Trophoblastic Disease

Diagnosis	Investigation
Abortion	Ultrasound, histology
Menorrhagia	hCG measurement
Amenorrhea, infertility	hCG measurement
Hydatidiform mole	History, histology, hCG measurement (persistently elevated)
Metastases from any tumor	hCG measurement, color, histology (if safe)
Common sites	Vagina and lung
Rare sites	Bone and lymph nodes
Pulmonary hypertension	hCG measurement

hCG = human chorionic gonadotropin.

levels of hCG should be measured if the patient fits into the high-risk prognostic group (see later) or has lung metastases. Cerebrospinal fluid levels of hCG that are more than one sixtieth of the serum level indicate the presence of brain metastases, though a normal ratio does not exclude them.

A computed tomography (CT) or magnetic resonance imaging (MRI) scan of the brain is only required if there is clinical suspicion of brain metastases or the serum–cerebrospinal fluid hCG ratio is abnormal. MRI sometimes detects lesions in the brain missed on CT scans, especially in the posterior fossa. MRI is the investigation of choice if spinal metastases are suspected. CT of the chest will detect metastases missed on chest x-ray films but in our experience this has not led to a change in management and CT is not performed routinely for initial investigation. Scans of the abdomen are only performed if there is clinical suspicion of disease there. Pelvic arteriography is rarely performed now except in patients who have severe vaginal hemorrhage after eradication of the mole. Radioimmunolocalization using radiolabeled antibody against hCG can locate drug-resistant deposits of tumor that may then be resected. This method of imaging can sometimes detect deposits missed on CT or ultrasound scans and may differentiate between viable and necrotic deposits (20).

Prior to the start of therapy, a full blood cell count is required and renal and hepatic function must be assessed. Thyroid function should be measured. The blood group of the patient and her partner responsible for the most recent or molar pregnancy is required for the prognostic score (see later).

Presentation

Hydatidiform Mole

The great majority of hydatidiform moles are detected between 8 and 24 weeks of gestation, with a peak around 14 weeks. Vaginal bleeding is the most common presenting symptom. Many women pass molar tissue mixed with blood clot by way of the vagina. A fluid like prune juice, consisting of old blood, may be seen. This blood loss can lead to severe anemia, especially in malnourished women. Acute life-threatening hemorrhage can occasionally occur. The uterus is large for dates in approximately half the patients at presentation but may also be small for dates. Partial moles are rarely associated with excessive uterine enlargement. Theca lutein cysts are also common. These cysts can cause abdominal pain due to torsion or rupture and commonly take up to 4 months to regress following evacuation. Pre-eclampsia and hyperemesis gravidarum are seen in about one fourth of these patients.

Clinical hyperthyroidism is uncommon, although increased thyroid function may be detected biochemically. This is probably due to the high levels of hCG, which is thyrotropic in bioassays. The possibility of thyrotoxicosis must be mentioned to an anesthetist prior to evacuation because of the danger of precipitating a thyroid crisis.

Symptoms due to uterine perforation, pelvic sepsis, and disseminated intravascular coagulopathy can occur. Severe symptoms due to trophoblastic pulmonary embolization sometimes develop after evacuation but these usually resolve with supportive care. The major long-term risk after molar pregnancy is the development of either invasive mole or choriocarcinoma. In the prechemotherapy era the risk of choriocarcinoma after hydatidiform mole was estimated to be less than 3%. The risk of developing invasive mole depends on the criteria used for its identification, but probably 90% of hydatidiform moles resolve spontaneously.

Twin pregnancy consisting of hydatidiform mole and a coexisting fetus occurs in 1/22,000 to 100,000 pregnancies (21). About 20% of the fetuses survive.

Several factors are associated with an increased risk of GTT (22) (Table 23-3). The lack of relationship between histologic grading of hydatidiform mole and subsequent clinical course was discussed in the pathology section.

T A B L E   **23-3**

Features of Hydatidiform Moles That Increase the Chances of Requiring Chemotherapy

Pre-evacuation human chorionic gonadotropin level >100,000 IU/L
Uterine size > gestational age
Large (>6 cm) theca lutein cysts
Maternal age >40 yr
Medical induction hysterectomy or hysterotomy

Invasive Mole and Choriocarcinoma

Invasive mole is seen in the early months following the evacuation of hydatidiform mole and is only rarely recognized in the absence of such a history. Some centers diagnose invasive mole if the hCG level is still elevated at 8 to 10 weeks, giving an incidence of about 25%. Using raised levels at 6 months gives an incidence of about 7%. A few metastatic invasive moles with characteristic villi on histology have been seen in deposits in the lungs, cervix, vagina, vulva, and even the brain. Apart from problems associated with these metastases, the symptoms of invasive mole are due to the invasive trophoblast. These include vaginal bleeding, amenorrhea, infertility, abdominal pain, and intraperitoneal bleeding resulting from uterine perforation.

Histology is the only way of differentiating invasive mole from choriocarcinoma. The symptoms may be identical but while all invasive moles are preceded by a hydatidiform mole, only about 50% of choriocarcinomas have a history of prior molar pregnancy. Those patients whose GTT did not follow a mole must have choriocarcinoma rather than invasive mole. The time interval between antecedent pregnancy and onset of treatment ranged in one series from 0.5 to 58.0 months (15).

The most frequent symptom of choriocarcinoma is vaginal bleeding. The most common site of metastasis is the lungs, where it is usually asymptomatic until it becomes very advanced. On chest x-ray films, the metastases classically appear like cannonballs but there may be widespread small nodules. Pleuritic pain and hemoptysis can occur owing to tumor invasion or following pulmonary infarction. Dyspnea is seen with more extensive metastases. Dyspnea and signs of pulmonary hypertension can also result from the rare growth of choriocarcinoma in the pulmonary artery.

The vagina is the next most common site of metastases. Their great vascularity makes them appear densely reddened. They bleed easily and may be missed without careful visual inspection.

Cerebral metastases may present suddenly as a cerebrovascular accident; hCG levels should always be measured in women of childbearing age presenting with this syndrome. It is also essential to check hCG levels after a cerebral event in women considered as organ transplant donors, as the event may have been due to choriocarcinoma and several cases of graft recipients developing choriocarcinoma have been recorded. Symptoms such as headache and fits or loss of consciousness or those related to the site of neurologic damage may be nonspecific. Liver metastases are usually now discovered incidentally on scans. Purple skin deposits are sometimes seen. Lymph node and bone deposits are so rare that histologic review is advisable if they are suspected (see Table 23-2).

Staging and Prognostic Factors

The spectrum of GTD extends from persistence of a small focus of trophoblast in the uterus to widespread metastases. In an attempt to tailor the intensity of therapy to the expected prognosis, Hammond (23) devised the first classification of GTT and split patients into low- and high-risk metastatic disease groups (24). This was later designated the National Cancer Institute classification but has been superseded by a new staging system proposed by the International Federation of Gynecology and Obstetrics (25) (Table 23-4). These systems are based on the anatomic distribution of tumor deposits, which do not give a particularly useful indication of the likelihood of response to chemotherapy. They would be appropriate when the management of these tumors is surgical, depending for good prognosis on complete surgical excision. Prognostic systems that depend on factors predicting for resistance to cytotoxic drugs are much more useful and most major trophoblastic disease centers use an adaptation of a prognostic scoring system originally devised by Bagshawe (26) and adopted by the WHO (Table 23-5) (1). This system was based on retrospective analysis which showed that various factors were related to survival. To stratify treatment according to prognostic factors, a weighting was applied for each prognostic factor. Each was assumed to act as an independent variable and the sum of the scores is used to split patients into low-, medium-, and high-risk groups. Slight alterations by various centers to the score of certain factors can make comparisons between results of different treatments difficult to interpret. Between 1958 and 1982, of the 860 patients treated for GTTs at the Charing Cross Hospital, 223 were in the high-risk group and 105 (47%) died; 232 fit into the middle-risk group, and 3 (1.3%) died; and 405 fell into the low-risk group and 1 died from an intercurrent tumor. The overall incidence of "high-risk" disease is probably exaggerated in

Stage	Site of Disease	Number of Risk Factors*
Ia	Uterus	None
b	"	1
c	"	2
IIa	Extrauterine but limited to adnexa vagina, or broad ligament	None
b	"	1
c	"	2
IIIa	Lungs with or without sites of stage I or II	None
b	"	1
c	"	2
IVa	Other metastatic sites	None
b	"	1
c	"	2

T A B L E **23-4**

Staging of Gestational Trophoblastic Tumors (International Federation of Gynecology and Obstetrics, 1991)

*Risk factors human chorionic gonadotropin level >100,000 IU/L; interval from antecedent pregnancy >6 mo.

T A B L E **23-5**

World Health Organization Scoring System Based on Prognostic Factors

Prognostic Factors	Score[a]			
	0	**1**	**2**	**4**
Age (yr)	≤39	>39		
Antecedent pregnancy	Hydatidiform mole	Abortion	Term	
Interval[b]	4	4–6	7–12	>12
hCG (IU/L)	$<10^3$	10^3–10^4	10^4–10^5	$>10^5$
ABO groups (female × male)		O × A	B	
		A × O	AB	
Largest tumor, including uterine tumor		3–5 cm	>5 cm	
Site of metastases		Spleen, kidney	GI tract, liver	Brain
No. of metastases identified		1–4	4–8	>8
Prior chemotherapy			Single drug	2 or more

[a] The total score for a patient is obtained by adding the individual scores for each prognostic factor. Total score: <4 = low risk; 5–7-middle risk; >7 = high risk.

[b] Interval time (in months) between the end of antecedent pregnancy and start of chemotherapy.

this series because the center receives many referrals of patients with drug-resistant disease previously treated elsewhere.

Treatment

Evacuation of Hydatidiform Mole

Patients with clinical and ultrasound features suggestive of hydatidiform mole should have any significant blood loss replaced and the uterus evacuated by suction. Even a large hydatidiform mole can usually be evacuated

with little blood loss. The need for chemotherapy after evacuation of hydatidiform mole is twofold to threefold greater in patients who underwent a medical induction, hysterectomy, or hysterotomy compared with those whose hydatidiform mole was evacuated by vacuum or surgical curettage or who aborted spontaneously (27). If bleeding is severe after uterine evacuation, use of ergometrine is sometimes unavoidable. The single contraction produced by this agent appears to be less likely to produce embolization of trophoblast than are the repeated contractions induced by oxytocin or prostaglandin. Many gynecologists perform a second dilation and curettage routinely 2 weeks later or if there is persistent bleeding following the initial evacuation. Because curettage cannot remove invasive mole from the myometrium, further dilation and curettage is of no value. Hysterectomy should be avoided because of the intense vascularity and high risk of uncontrollable bleeding and frequent failure to eliminate the disease as well as the need to preserve fertility.

Prophylactic Chemotherapy

Certain centers have abandoned the use of prophylactic chemotherapy following evacuation of a hydatidiform mole because of unacceptable toxicity in women who had a high chance of never requiring chemotherapy. The results of nonrandomized studies suggest that patients who received prophylaxis had less chance of requiring subsequent chemotherapy than did patients not given prophylactic chemotherapy. Goldstein and Berkowitz (28) proposed using actinomycin D, $1.25\,mg/m^2$, or methotrexate, $50\,mg/m^2$, following evacuation for women who fit into their high-risk group after the hydatidiform mole was evacuated (see Table 23-3). The major attraction of prophylactic chemotherapy is for patients in whom follow-up is likely to be difficult.

Selection of Patients for Chemotherapy

Chemotherapy is obviously required for choriocarcinoma or persistent invasive mole but various criteria have been used to define persistence of mole that requires therapy (29). A WHO scientific group (1) agreed that treatment should be started if any of the following applies after evacuation of a hydatidiform mole:

1. High level of hCG more than 4 weeks after evacuation (serum level >20,000 IU/L, urine level >30,000 IU/L)
2. Progressively increasing hCG values at any time after evacuation
3. Histologic identification of choriocarcinoma at any site or evidence of central nervous system, renal, hepatic, or gastrointestinal metastases, or pulmonary metastases larger than 2 cm in diameter or more than three in number

Persistent uterine hemorrhage in the presence of an elevated hCG level is an indication for therapy in most centers. The major risk in delaying treatment in the patient with very high levels of hCG is uterine perforation. There is considerable disagreement about management of patients with persisting hCG levels. Some centers give chemotherapy to patients in whom hCG is detectable at a defined time, such as 8 to 10 weeks after evacuation. Others treat all patients who have a stationary hCG level for 2, 3, or more consecutive weeks. This results in approximately 27% of molar patients receiving chemotherapy. The policy at the Charing Cross Hospital since 1973 has been to allow hCG to remain detectable for up to 4 to 6 months after evacuation, as spontaneous disappearance of hCG can take that long. This results in less than 8% of molar patients requiring chemotherapy.

Surgery

Surgery has only a limited role apart from evacuation of hydatidiform mole, as discussed already. Uterine perforation is best managed by local resection of tumor and uterine repair. Hysterectomy may be required for persistent heavy bleeding but this usually settles with chemotherapy. Angiographic embolization may be used to control bleeding if uterine preservation is desired. Surgical removal of drug-resistant disease has a curative role in the rare patient in whom the disease is limited to resectable sites.

Elective hysterectomy has been used in the hope of reducing the need for or the duration of chemotherapy in patients not wishing to retain their reproductive potential. However, many such patients still require a full course of chemotherapy.

Chemotherapy

The three drugs with the greatest activity against GTTs are methotrexate, actinomycin D, and etoposide. 6-Mercaptopurine, vincristine, cyclophosphamide, cisplatin, and hydroxyurea also have proven activity. 5-Fluorouracil has been used successfully in China but not elsewhere (30). Primary drug resistance has been seen only rarely after treatment with methotrexate and actinomycin D but not yet after etoposide therapy. Drug resistance developing during treatment is a problem, especially in patients with a high prognostic score (see above). The prognostic group must be determined so that patients at higher risk of developing drug resistance are given combination chemotherapy from the start.

Low-Risk Patients

There is general agreement that methotrexate followed by folinic acid is the preferred treatment for the low-risk group, provided renal and hepatic functions are normal. The most proven regimen is given over 8 days (Table 23-6). To prevent relapse, treatment should be repeated every 14 days and continued until the hCG level is undetectable (<2 IU/L) for about 6 weeks. Provided patients drink at least 2 liters of fluid a day, they are unlikely to develop mucositis. Apart from the occasional occurrence of chemical pleurisy, other side effects are very uncommon. Of 347 low-risk patients treated at the Charing Cross Hospital between 1974 and 1986, all entered complete remission and only 1 died from intercurrent lymphoma (31). However 69 (20%) had to change treatment because of drug resistance and 23 (6%) needed to change treatment because of drug-induced toxicity (Fig. 23-2).

Complete sustained remissions have been observed in 87% of patients given methotrexate, 0.4 mg/kg intravenously daily for 5 days, repeated every 14 days (32); in 84% of patients given methotrexate, 1000 mg, followed by folinic acid every 7 to 10 days (33); and in 78% given weekly methotrexate, 30 mg/m² intramuscularly (34). Differences in prognostic criteria make it impossible to compare these results with each other. It is even more difficult to compare them with the Charing Cross results because more than 50% of the American patients probably would have had spontaneous remission if the Charing Cross criteria for initiating treatment were applied. Actinomycin D, 1.25 mg/m², has been recommended but nausea, vomiting, alopecia, skin rashes, and myelosuppression become problems with repeated courses. Etoposide cannot be recommended in this patient group as it invariably causes alopecia and is carcinogenic.

T A B L E   **23-6**

Regimen for Low-Risk Patients

Day	Treatment
1	Methotrexate (MTX), 50 mg IM at noon
2	Folinic acid (FA), 6 mg IM at 6.00 P.M. (30 hr later)
3	MTX, 50 mg IM at noon
4	FA, 6 mg IM at 6.00 P.M.
5	MTX, 50 mg IM at noon
6	FA, 6 mg IM at 6.00 P.M.
7	MTX, 50 mg IM at noon
8	FA, 6 mg IM at 6.00 P.M.

Note: Courses are repeated after an interval of 6 days. Start each course on the same day of the week.

F I G U R E   **23-2**

Log graph of urine and serum human chorionic gonadotropin (hCG) demonstrating rising levels of urine hCG following evacuation of mole as a reason for therapy. This patient received six courses of low-risk methotrexate (MTX) plus folinic acid but then developed resistance as shown by rising hCG levels. The middle-risk regime was then started and sensitivity to etoposide (EP) was apparent by a rapid fall in hCG levels. Other drugs in the middle-risk regimen include actinomycin D (AD) and vincristine and cyclophosphamide (VC). BHCG = β-human chorionic gonadotropin.

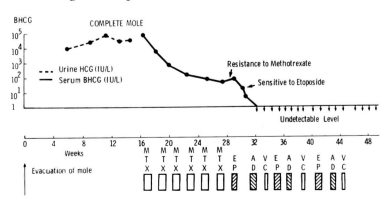

Medium-Risk Patients

This group has a greater tendency to develop drug resistance and the regimen was designed to introduce a range of drugs sequentially, reserving the more toxic high-risk regimens for patients with a higher score of adverse prognostic factors. Many centers divide their patients into only low- and high-risk groups because the high-risk regimens have become less toxic. The middle-risk regimen is maintained at the Charing Cross Hospital because it allows for the introduction as a single agent of new drugs shown to be active in resistant patients. This regimen, which is continued for 8 to 10 weeks after hCG has become undetectable, starts with etoposide, 250 mg/m² on days 1 and 3. Etoposide alternates every 14 days with either the low-risk methotrexate regimen with added hydroxyurea, 500 mg orally twice on day 1, and 6-mercaptopurine, 75 mg orally on the same days as folinic acid, or with actinomycin, 0.5 mg daily for 5 days. At the Charing Cross Hospital 103 patients were treated in the medium-risk group between 1973 and 1980. There have been three deaths, all due to drug resistance.

High-Risk Patients

Only 31% of patients in this group survived when given single-agent methotrexate (31). Several intensive multidrug regimens including CHAMOCA (cyclophosphamide, hydroxyurea, adriamycin, methotrexate, vincristine, and actinomycin D) developed at the Charing Cross Hospital and MAC III (methotrexate, actinomycin D, cyclophosphamide) used in the United States (35) have now been superseded. Since 1979, patients in the high-risk group at the Charing Cross Hospital have received a weekly alternating regimen called EMA/CO (etoposide, methotrexate, actinomycin D, cyclophosphamide, and vincristine) (Table 23-7, Fig. 23-3). This regimen is given on the same day each week unless the total white blood cell count falls below 1.5 × 10⁹/L or the platelet count falls below 75 × 10⁹/L or mucosal ulceration develops. Of 151 patients who received EMA/CO as initial therapy, 129 (85%) survived and 8 patients had a relapse; of 121 who received EMA/CO after prior therapy, 109 (90%) survived and 12 patients had a relapse (36). In patients who develop drug resistance, cisplatin, 75 mg/m², and etoposide, 100 mg/m², can lead

T A B L E   23-7

EMA/CO Regimen for High-Risk Patients

Course *1 EMA*

Day 1
  Actinomycin D, 0.5 mg IV stat
  Etoposide, 100 mg/m² in 200 mL N/S over 30 min
  Methotrexate, 300 mg/m² IV 12-hr infusion

Day 2
  Actinomycin D, 0.5 mg stat
  Etoposide, 100 mg/m² IV in 200 mL N/S over 30 min
  Folinic acid, 15 mg PO or IM bid. for 4 doses starting 24 hr after the start of methotrexate
  5-day drug-free interval to course 2

Course *2 CO*

Day 1
  Vincristine, 1.0 mg/m² IV stat (maximum 2.0 mg)
    Cyclophosphamide, 600 mg/m² IV infusion over 20 min
  6-day drug-free interval

If there is no mucositis, patients normally start each course on the same day of the week.

Note: Intervals between courses should not be increased unless white blood cell count <1.5 × 10⁹/L or platelets <75 × 10⁹/L or mucositis develops.

If mucositis develops, delay next course until it has healed. Continue alternating courses 1 and 2 until the patient is in complete remission or there is evidence of drug resistance.

N/S = 150 mmol NaCl.

to a durable remission when substituted for the CO course of EMA/CO. Improved management is required for patients with liver metastases who only have a 27% five-year survival expectation.

In patients with extensive pulmonary metastases, deaths can occur owing to respiratory failure, which can be exacerbated by initial therapy that is too aggressive. Ventilation or high-dose steroids have not been shown to be of any value in this situation; extracorporeal membrane oxygenation is now being assessed.

Central Nervous System Metastases

In countries without adequate follow-up after treatment for hydatidiform mole and in patients presenting with choriocarcinoma following an abortion or term delivery, there is an incidence of central nervous system metastases of 3% to 15%. The EMA/CO regimen should be modified for these patients, with the dose of methotrex-

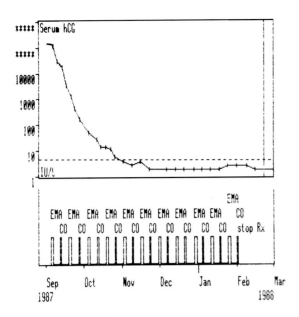

F I G U R E **23-3**

Log graph of serum human chorionic gonadotropin (hCG) levels in a 26-year-old woman who presented with pleuritic chest pains and shortness of breath due to choriocarcinoma in the pulmonary artery causing pulmonary hypertension. There was an excellent response to EMA/CO chemotherapy with good recovery of pulmonary function.

ate in the EMA course increased to 1 g/m² and folinic acid rescue to 30 mg every 6 hours for 3 days. Also 12.5 mg of methotrexate is given intrathecally with each course of CO. Eighteen patients who presented with central nervous system metastases were so treated and 13 (72%) were disease free at the time of the report (37). Because of the vascular nature of these tumors, early surgical excision to prevent early death from intracerebral hemorrhage should be considered. Although radiotherapy has been used in other centers, the reported results do not approach the 72% survival rate obtained without radiotherapy.

Follow-up

After Molar Pregnancy

Following the diagnosis of a molar pregnancy, follow-up by measurement of hCG levels in serum or urine is essential to detect the women who require chemotherapy for invasive mole or choriocarcinoma based on a plateau or rise of hCG levels. The serum half-life of hCG is approximately 24 to 36 hours. After a full-term normal delivery, serum and urine hCG levels become undetectable (<2 IU/L) within 10 to 20 days, but a small proportion of women have detectable hCG for longer periods. After a nonmolar abortion, hCG takes a few days longer to become undetectable, partly because the level is higher early in pregnancy and possibly because of retained products of conception. In a series of patients who did not require chemotherapy following evacuation of a hydatidiform mole, hCG levels were still detectable in 3% until 20 to 22 weeks following evacuation (11). In 42% of the patients hCG levels had become undetectable by 7 weeks following evacuation of a mole and none of this group required chemotherapy, suggesting they require a shorter follow-up.

A national follow-up service for hydatidiform mole patients has been in operation in the United Kingdom since 1972. Patients are registered centrally and then are automatically sent boxes with prepaid returnable postage containing tubes and a letter requesting urine or serum samples, which are to be returned to one of three assay centers. It is recommended that hCG measurements be performed every 2 weeks until the limit of detection is reached, monthly during the first year after evacuation, and every 3 months during the second year. Measurements should continue for at least 6 months after the hCG has been undetectable because of the occasional late recrudescence. It is advisable to confirm that hCG is undetectable for 6 months before starting another pregnancy.

The values for hCG must be monitored after all further pregnancies because of the 2% chance of a second hydatidiform mole developing and the slightly increased risk of choriocarcinoma arising either from a subsequent mole or from a normal pregnancy. Follow-up is not necessary after hydropic degeneration because of the low risk of malignant sequelae, but when the diagnosis is in doubt, it is prudent to monitor hCG levels.

After Chemotherapy

There is a strong case for continuing hCG follow-up for life because of the potential of choriocarcinoma to recur after several years.

Future Pregnancies and Contraception

Patients are advised against pregnancy for a year after chemotherapy. The main reason for this advice is that most relapses occur during this period and there is the risk of delayed teratogenicity. It is difficult initially to differentiate between a relapse and a new pregnancy because both lead to a rise in hCG levels. It is possible that a relapse with metastatic disease could become apparent during a subsequent pregnancy, though we have not seen this.

Some but not other series found that women who take exogenous hormones while hCG levels are still elevated have an increased chance of requiring chemotherapy (38,39). We therefore advise patients not to take an oral contraceptive until the hCG level has been normal for 3 months after molar evacuation. Intrauterine devices are also best avoided until the uterine size has returned to normal and there is less risk of hemorrhage.

Subsequent Fertility

The largest study of women treated with chemotherapy for GTT showed that among 455 women, 187 of those 217 women (86%) wishing to have a further pregnancy succeeded in having at least one live birth (40). The incidence of congenital abnormalities was not higher than expected. There is a risk of an early menopause occurring following chemotherapy, and especially the older women should be warned of the possible need for hormone replacement therapy after chemotherapy.

Second Tumors

It has been clearly shown that there is no increased incidence of second tumors in patients who just received methotrexate (41). A recent analysis of 1394 women treated between 1958 and 1990 found 37 second cancers when only 24.45 were expected ($p < 0.011$) and confirmed that there was no increased risk among the 554 women receiving single agent therapy (42). There were significantly increased standardized incidence ratios of myeloid leukemia (16.6), colon cancer (4.6), melanoma (3.4), and breast cancer but only in those followed more than 25 years (5.8). All those who developed leukemia received etoposide as well as other cytotoxic drugs. The observation that 1.5% of women who received etoposide developed leukemia demonstrates the danger of giving this drug as initial therapy to women with GTT who are in the low-risk prognostic group.

REFERENCES

1. World Health Organization Scientific Group. *Gestational trophoblastic diseases.* Technical report series 692. Geneva: WHO, 1983.

2. Paradinas FJ. The histological diagnosis of hydatidiform moles. *Curr Diagn Pathol* 1994; 1:24–31.

3. Redline RW, Abdul-Karim FW. Pathology of gestational trophoblastic disease. *Semin Oncol* 1995;22:96–109.

4. Dessau R, Rustin GJS, Dent J, et al. Surgery and chemotherapy in the management of placental site tumour. *Gynecol Oncol* 1990;39:56–59.

5. Hertig AT, Mansell H. Tumors of the female sex organs. Part 1. Hydatidiform mole and choriocarcinoma. In: *Atlas of tumor pathology.* Series 1, fascicle 33. Washington, DC: Armed Forces Institute of Pathology, 1956.

6. Elston CW, Bagshawe KD. The value of histological grading in the management of hydatidiform mole. *J Obstet Gynaecol Br Commonw* 1972;79:717–724.

7. Genest DR, Laborde O, Berkowitz RS, et al. A clinicopathologic study of 153 cases of complete hydatidiform mole (1980–1990): histologic grade lacks prognostic significance. *Obstet Gynecol* 1991;78:402–409.

8. Rice LW, Genest DR, Berkowitz RS, et al. Pathologic features of sharp curettings in complete hydatidiform mole: predictors of persistent gestational trophoblastic disease. *J Reprod Med* 1991;36:17–20.

9. Bracken MB. Incidence and aetiology of hydatidiform mole: an epidemiological review. *Br J Obstet Gynaecol* 1987;94:1123–1135.

10. Rustin GJS, Bagshawe KD. Gestational trophoblastic tumours. *Crit Rev Oncol Hematol* 1984;3:103–142.

11. Bagshawe KD, Dent J, Webb J. Hydatidiform mole in England and Wales 1973–83. *Lancet* 1986;2:673–677.

12. Parazzini F, La Vecchia C, Pampallona S. Parental age and risk of complete and partial hydatidiform mole. *Br J Obstet Gynaecol* 1986;93:582–585.

13. Buckley JD, Henderson BE, Morrow CP, et al. Case-control study of gestational choriocarcinoma. *Cancer Res* 1988;48:1004–1010.

14. Brinton LA, Bracken MB, Connelly RR. Choriocarcinoma incidence in the United States. *Am J Epidemiol* 1986;123:1094–1100.

15. Tidy JA, Rustin GJS, Newlands ES, et al. Presentation and management of choriocarcinoma after nonmolar pregnancy. *Br J Obstet Gynaecol* 1995;102:715–719.

16. Semer DA, Macfee MS. Gestational trophoblastic disease: epidemiology. *Semin Oncol* 1995;22: 109–113.

17. Lawler SD, Fisher A. Genetic studies in hydatidiform mole with clinical correlations. *Placenta* 1987;8:77–88.

18. Fisher RA, Newlands ES, Jeffreys AJ, et al. Gestational and nongestational trophoblastic tumors distinguished by DNA analysis. *Cancer* 1992;69: 839–845.

19. Long MG, Boultbee JE, Langley R, et al. Doppler assessment of the uterine circulation and the clinical behaviour of gestational trophoblastic tumours requiring chemotherapy. *Br J Cancer* 1992;66:882–887.

20. Begent RHJ, Bagshawe KD, Green AJ, Searle F. The clinical value of imaging with antibody to human chorionic gonadotrophin in the detection of residual choriocarcinoma. *Br J Cancer* 1987; 55:657–660.

21. Steller MA, Genest DR, Bernstein MR, et al. Clinical features of multiple conception with partial or complete molar pregnancy and coexisting fetuses. *J Reprod Med* 1994;39:147–154.

22. Goldstein DP, Berkowitz RS, Bernstein MR. Management of molar pregnancy. *J Reprod Med* 1981;26:208–212.

23. Hammond CB, Borchert LG, Tyrey L, et al. Treatment of metastatic gestational trophoblastic disease: good and poor prognosis. *Am J Obstet Gynecol* 1973;115:451–457.

24. Kohorn EI. The trophoblastic tower of Babel: classification systems for metastatic gestational trophoblastic neoplasia. *Gynecol Oncol* 1995;56: 280–288.

25. Einhorn N. Evolution and current status of gynecologic cancer staging. *Curr Probl Obstet Gynecol Fertil* 1992;15:251–268.

26. Bagshawe KD. Risk and prognostic factors in trophoblastic neoplasia. *Cancer* 1976;38:1373–1385.

27. Stone M, Bagshawe KD. An analysis of the influences of maternal age, gestational age, contraceptive method, and the mode of primary treatment of patients with hydatidiform moles on the incidence of subsequent chemotherapy. *Br J Obstet Gynaecol* 1979;86:782–792.

28. Goldstein DP, Berkowitz RS. Prophylactic chemotherapy of complete molar pregnancy. *Semin Oncol* 1995;22:157–160.

29. Kohorn EI. Evaluation of the criteria used to make the diagnosis of nonmetastatic gestational trophoblastic neoplasia. *Gynecol Oncol* 1993;48: 139–147.

30. Song H, Xia Z, Wu B, Wang Y. 20 Years' experience in chemotherapy of choriocarcinoma and malignant mole. *Chin Med J* 1979;92:677–687.

31. Bagshawe KD, Dent J, Newlands ES, et al. The role of low-dose methotrexate and folinic acid in gestational trophoblastic tumours (GTT). *Br J Obstet Gynaecol* 1989;96:795–802.

32. Lurain JR, Elfstrand EP. Single-agent methotrexate chemotherapy for the treatment of nonmetastatic gestational trophoblastic tumors. *Am J Obstet Gynecol* 1995;172:574–579.

33. Elit L, Covens A, Osborne R, et al. High-dose methotrexate for gestational trophoblastic disease. *Gynecol Oncol* 1994;54:282–287.

34. Homesley HD, Blessing JA, Rettenmaier M, et al. Weekly intramuscular methotrexate for nonmetastatic gestational trophoblastic disease. *Obstet Gynecol* 1988;72:413–418.

35. Berkowitz RS, Goldstein DP, Bernstein MR. Modified triple chemotherapy in the management of high-risk metastatic gestational trophoblastic tumours. *Gynecol Oncol* 1984;19:173–181.

36. Bower M, Newlands ES, Holden L, et al. EMA/CO for high-risk gestational trophoblastic tumors: results from a cohort of 272 patients. *J Clin Oncol* 1997;15:2636–2643.

37. Rustin GJS, Newlands ES, Begent HJ, et al. Weekly alternating chemotherapy (EMA/CO) for treatment of central nervous system metastases of choriocarcinoma. *J Clin Oncol* 1989;7:900–903.

38. Berkowitz RS, Goldstein DP. Presentation and management of molar pregnancy. In: Hancock BW, Newlands ES, Berkowitz RS, eds. *Gestational trophoblastic disease*, vol. 8. London: Chapman and Hall, 1997:127–142.

39. Newlands ES. Presentation and management of persistent gestational trophoblastic diseases and gestational trophoblastic tumors in the UK. In:

Hancock BW, Newlands ES, Berkowitz RS, eds. *Gestational trophoblastic disease*, vol. 9. London: Chapman and Hall, 1997:143–156.

40. Rustin GJS, Booth M, Dent J, et al. Pregnancy after cytotoxic chemotherapy for gestational trophoblastic tumours. *BMJ* 1984;288:103–106.

41. Rustin GJS, Rustin F, Dent J, et al. No increase in second tumors after cytotoxic chemotherapy for gestational trophoblastic tumours. *N Engl J Med* 1983;308:473–477.

42. Rustin GJS, Newlands ES, Lutz JM, et al. Combination but not single agent methotrexate chemotherapy for gestational trophoblastic tumors (GTT) increases the incidence of second tumors. *J Clin Oncol* 1996;14:2769–2773.

SECTION 4

Vagina and Vulva

CHAPTER 24

Vaginal Intraepithelial Neoplasia: Clinical Features and Treatment

JOHN L. BENEDET

*C*arcinoma in situ and dysplasia, or vaginal intraepithelial neoplasia (VAIN), is uncommon and occurs much less frequently than the corresponding cervical and vulvar lesions. Despite its uncommon nature, VAIN is being diagnosed with increasing frequency (1,2). As a result of the widespread use of colposcopy to assess lower genital tract problems, it seems likely that even more of these lesions will be identified (3). Most patients with VAIN are asymptomatic (1–5) and are discovered during investigation of abnormal Papanicolaou test results or incidentally during evaluation for other gynecologic complaints. VAIN has been studied less extensively and as a result our knowledge is much less precise than it is for the analogous preinvasive changes in other lower genital tract sites.

Terminology

There is no agreed-upon terminology to describe and classify intraepithelial neoplastic lesions of the vagina. Historically carcinoma in situ of the vagina was essentially the only preinvasive lesion described and discussed. More recently, however, terminology similar to that used to categorize cervical cancer precursors has been utilized to describe similar lesions of the vagina and vulva. Various degrees of atypicality are thus described, that is, VAIN I, II, and III, with most attention being directed to the VAIN III lesions. This newer terminology may also be partially responsible for the apparent increase in the frequency of VAIN, as in the past many of the lower-grade lesions were usually not treated or reported. With the use of the VAIN terminology, most series (6–11) combined patients with all three grades, without a clear understanding of the biologic potential of the subgroups, which makes it difficult to assess the appropriateness of various therapies.

It should also be noted that there have been no designed prospective observational studies with regard to many of the lower-grade lesions, so that it is only by inference that the ultimate relationship to invasive disease has been made. In one of the few observational studies reported, Aho et al (12) studied 23 patients with VAIN who were followed untreated for 3 to 15 years. Progression to invasive vaginal carcinoma occurred in 2 patients with a further 3 patients having persistence of their lesions; in the remainder the lesions regressed. Of the two lesions that progressed, one was graded VAIN III and the other VAIN I-II. Of the 18 patients (78%) in whom the lesion regressed, 14 lesions were VAIN I or II and the remaining 4 were VAIN III. This study did show that appreciable numbers of lesions may spontaneously regress if left untreated, although it must be noted that the diagnostic biopsy may have affected their natural history. This study (12), like other studies (4,10) that have recorded the subsequent development of invasive carcinoma in patients with VAIN III, indicates our inability to clearly predict and identify the subsequent behavior and potential of any individual lesion diagnosed.

Incidence and Etiology

The true incidence of VAIN is unknown but has been estimated at 0.2/100,000 women (13). Hummer et al (14), in 1970, reporting on the Mayo Clinic experience, noted that the first case of vaginal carcinoma in situ recorded at the clinic occurred in 1933 and the second case was not described until 1946. In 1981, Woodruff (15) reported that fewer than 300 cases of carcinoma in situ of the vagina had been documented in the literature.

Nwabineli and Monaghan (16) noted that of more than 4000 women who had cervical intraepithelial neoplasia (CIN) and were treated by laser vaporization, 2.5% had a coexisting VAIN that represented extension of the lesions involving both the cervix and the upper vagina. The reported age distribution for patients with VAIN has ranged from the late teens to the ninth decade of life. The average age, from most literature reports (2,4,7,14), has generally been in the 50- to 55-year range but more recent reports (8,11,17,18) noted a younger mean age. Audet-Lapointe et al (9) noted a 15-year age difference between individuals with VAIN I and II as compared to those with VAIN III. It has been postulated that this might reflect either different diseases or etiologic agents for the lesions in these age groups.

The specific causes of these lesions remain obscure but it is likely that the same predisposing factors and agents responsible for CIN and vulvar intraepithelial neoplasia (VIN) are also involved in the causation of these lesions. Current thinking (19–21) is that infection by certain strains of the human papillomavirus (HPV) is the most likely causal agent for the majority of these lesions. The less common occurrence of VAIN as compared to CIN has been explained by the general lack of an active transformation zone within the vagina as is seen in the cervix. The cervical transformation zone is likely much more susceptible to HPV influence than is mature squamous epithelium and may be one of the major factors that account for the relative greater frequency of cervical as compared to vaginal lesions.

It is thought that similar to other HPV-related precancers of the lower genital tract, the development of VAIN is most likely a multistep process involving other cofactors. The cofactors that have been usually associated with CIN such as smoking, the immune status of the patient, as well as nutritional factors may also be important in the development of VAIN. Several earlier reports (21–23) documented an increased incidence of VAIN in diethylstilbestrol (DES)-exposed individuals but more recent literature (20) would suggest that this trend is unsubstantiated.

Radiation treatment to the pelvis may also be a cause of VAIN. The association of the two is not uncommon and the lesions usually occur 10 to 15 years after radiotherapy.

Individuals on immunosuppressive therapy as well as those who are genetically immunosuppressed have a reported (19) increased incidence of VAIN. These individuals, in particular, often have multifocal lesions that may be persistent and are often difficult to eradicate. HPV may well play a major role in these particular situations.

Finally, it would appear that the majority of cases are those in individuals who have undergone prior hysterectomy for CIN or cervical neoplasia. Virtually all reported series confirmed the association of VAIN with prior concomitant or subsequent lower genital tract neoplasia. The exact relationship of VAIN to the preceding pathology of the cervical lesion is not always clear but undoubtedly many of these cases represent extension of disease from the cervical lesions onto the vagina that were not recognized at the time of the original surgery. Nonetheless the occurrence of many cases several years after hysterectomy with an interval of normal cytologic follow-up would suggest that VAIN does arise de novo from the vaginal epithelium and may have a different pathophysiologic basis in some of these instances. In many series, 30% to 40% of patients had a hysterectomy for a benign condition. Although it is not unusual to see discrete lesions of VAIN in the vagina with concomitant cervical lesions separated by what appears to be colposcopically and histologically normal epithelium, the occurrence of primary vaginal lesions without corresponding cervical lesions is extremely uncommon. In some of the reported series (3–5,7–10) the interval between hysterectomy and subsequent VAIN ranged from a few months to over 20 years.

Pathology

The concept of VAIN suggests a continuum with three specific histologic categories defined to reflect the severity of the histologic abnormality. VAIN I is like a mild dysplasia where the cellular atypia is confined to the lower one third of the epithelium. VAIN II similarly reflects changes consistent with a moderate dysplasia and would involve the lower one half to two thirds of the vaginal epithelium. Finally, VAIN III is used to describe histologic changes compatible with severe dysplasia or carcinoma in situ, or both, involving essentially the full thickness of the epithelium. Individual microscopic features are similar to those noted for cervical lesions with an increased nuclear-cytoplasmic ratio, loss of polarity, nuclear pleomorphism, and also abnormal mitoses.

More recently it was suggested, as has become the practice with cervical lesions, that it might be simpler to divide the vaginal lesions into low-grade (VAIN I) and high-grade (VAIN II and III) lesions.

Intraepithelial lesions of glandular epithelium are rare (24). The association of intrauterine exposure to DES with vaginal adenosis and clear-cell carcinoma of the vagina is well documented but the evolution of these malignancies from adenosis has remained elusive. Robboy et al (25) believed that atypical adenosis is the transitional lesion as evidenced by the frequency and proximity of atypical tubo-endometrial-type epithelium to the clear-cell adenocarcinomas.

Clinical Features

VAIN is essentially an asymptomatic condition, with the majority of patients discovered as a result of the investigation of an abnormal-appearing Papanicolaou smear or during follow-up for other genital tract neoplasms. Colposcopy has revolutionized the management of these individuals and is considered indispensable for proper assessment.

A good understanding of the anatomy and histology of the vagina is fundamental to optimally evaluating and managing VAIN. The vagina is a fibromuscular tube measuring approximately 7 to 8 cm in length and extends from the vaginal introitus to the uterine cervix. The walls of the vagina consist of an outer fibrous layer, a muscular layer, and an inner epithelial lining. The vaginal epithelium is composed of stratified squamous epithelium and this lining blends with that covering the surface of the cervix. In women in the younger repro-

ductive age group the lining of the vagina is also composed of numerous folds called *rugae*. In women with normal estrogen levels the vaginal epithelium is thick and is a continuous surface unbroken by glandular openings, but at times embryonic remnants can produce glandular structures or cysts in the vaginal epithelium or subepithelial spaces. Vaginal adenosis is perhaps the best-known example of persistence of embryonic glandular elements occupying the vaginal epithelium or subepithelial layer. Normally the estrogenized vaginal epithelium is soft and pliable and can be examined in a thorough fashion with the proper technique and care.

In approximately 3% to 4% of women the original squamocolumnar junction of the cervix may be found in the upper vagina. Most commonly this will be noted in the anterior or posterior fornix. There is evidence that in these situations müllerian-derived epithelium forms part of the vaginal lining. This transformation zone may on occasion show evidence of persisting columnar epithelium or small mucus-retention cysts that may be the only evidence that this area was once originally lined with a columnar-type, mucus-producing epithelium. In most instances, however, no specific features will be noted to suggest to the colposcopist that the epithelium in the vaginal fornices was müllerian in origin. However, if Schiller's test is performed, nonstaining areas may be seen in the upper anterior or posterior vaginal fornix as the only evidence or indication that this was indeed a vaginal transformation zone. Often biopsies of the nonglycogenated nonstaining areas in these patients will invariably show only metaplastic-type epithelium.

The area more commonly involved with VAIN is the upper third of the vagina, although involvement of the middle and lower thirds can also occur. In addition, in some uncommon situations, the entire vaginal length may be involved. Lesions that involve the entire length of the vagina are often HPV related and may represent lower grades of VAIN.

Although the technique of vaginal colposcopy is similar to that used for the colposcopic evaluation of the cervix, there are some important differences and modifications. Colposcopic examination of the vagina is generally more tedious and time-consuming. Essentially the entire vaginal epithelium must be examined and this is accomplished by slowly withdrawing and rotating the vaginal speculum so all of the epithelial surfaces can be visualized.

Table 24-1 lists the essential elements of the vaginal colposcopic examination.

It is recommended that prior to the commencement of any colposcopic examination, a gentle digital examination be carried out with careful palpation of the entire circumference of the vaginal tube and all of the fornices. This might alert the colposcopist to lesion locations and findings that otherwise may not be evident or that may be obscured by the speculum itself. This is particularly important in detecting subepithelial nodularity and thickening that might represent occult lesions, either of a DES nature or from obliterated or buried vaginal epithelium, following a previous hysterectomy. A digital examination also helps in determining the optimum size of the speculum that should be used during the colposcopic examination. Selection of the appropriate-size speculum for each patient is one of the most crucial steps in performing vaginal colposcopy. Unlike cervical colposcopy where a large speculum is helpful in keeping the vaginal walls apart to enable good visualization of the entire cervical circumference and fornices, the use of a similar approach in performing vaginal colposcopy in the posthysterectomy patient will often produce tears in the lateral vaginal walls that may confuse and interfere with proper assessment. A narrower Pedersen-type speculum is extremely helpful, particularly in postmenopausal patients or in women who have undergone prior vaginal surgery or radiation therapy.

Women who are postmenopausal will also benefit from a 10- to 14-day course of either oral or topical estrogen administration. This medication will help thicken the vaginal epithelium and facilitate the examination for both the patient and the colposcopist. The use of hormonal therapy in these situations will also ultimately help in the recognition of any abnormal areas. Most importantly this will also ensure more accurate differential staining with Schiller's test, which is an essential part of vaginal colposcopic assessment as in estrogen-deficient postmenopausal patients the entire vaginal epithelium is usually nonstaining.

Once the speculum has been inserted, careful inspection should be carried out to see if any obvious vascular patterns or lesions are visible. Once this has been completed, the area should be gently cleansed with a 3% to 5% acetic acid solution and time taken to enable the acetic acid to have its effect on the epithelium. With this approach the entire vaginal epithelium can be carefully examined. Once lesions have been identified and their extent and characteristics determined, Schiller's test should also be used to confirm the boundaries of the lesion and to ensure that no previously unrecognized nonstaining areas are present.

Most vaginal lesions are confined to the upper third of the vagina and usually at the apex or in the areas of the lateral vaginal fornices. In patients who have previously undergone hysterectomy, certain types of vaginal suspension may lead to deep lateral angles, the recesses of which may be difficult to completely visualize. The use of endocervical specula or small skin hooks or even fine tissue forceps as retractors may help to expose the depths of these crypts and facilitate visualization. In some instances this may not be possible, and if a clear source of the abnormal cells seen on cytology is not identified in these posthysterectomy patients, examination under anesthesia may be necessary to properly visualize these deep tunnels.

Biopsy of vaginal lesions may be difficult, particularly in individuals with atrophic epithelium. In such patients the use of a small skin hook to study the epithelium or slight retraction of the speculum to produce a vaginal fold with punch biopsy across a fold is useful to help obtain specimens. In most patients biopsy will produce minimal discomfort; however, if lesions lie along a vaginal vault suture line they may

T A B L E   **24-1**

Vaginal Colposcopic Examination

Digital examination prior to speculum insertion
Select appropriate-size speculum
Saline solution or warm water as speculum
   lubricant
Avoid lateral vaginal tears
Look before as well as after applying acetic acid
   (3%–5%)
Gently withdraw and rotate speculum to visualize
   entire vagina
Schiller's or Lugol's iodine test
Perform biopsy across a fold
Hemostasis, silver nitrate, or Monsel's solution with
   or without tampon
Carefully record findings

be not only difficult to biopsy but also quite uncomfortable owing to the proximity of the peritoneum.

Hemostasis is achieved in the usual manner, with the use of either silver nitrate or Monsel's solution and with pressure placed on the biopsy site with a vaginal tampon.

Colposcopic patterns seen in the presence of VAIN are similar to those noted for lesions of the cervix. Aceto-white epithelium with fine punctation and sharp borders are the basic patterns most often seen. Mosaic patterns, however, are extremely uncommon, even with the higher grades of VAIN. Most lesions will tend to produce a fairly flat or slightly raised surface without much irregularity. Lesions that do produce a markedly irregular surface or that have a yellowish-gray appearance are suggestive of early invasion. In general, the features of VAIN will not be as pronounced as for a CIN lesion of similar histology. Invasive carcinomas tend to have a clearly abnormal vascular pattern with an irregular surface contour. It should be noted that other lesions can coexist with intraepithelial neoplasia, particularly HPV infection. Liberal and judicious use of biopsy should help distinguish VAIN from other lesions that may involve the vagina such as endometriosis, vaginal vault recurrence, endometrial or ovarian carcinoma, and melanoma.

Patients who had prior pelvic irradiation may be particularly challenging. The epithelium is usually thin and atrophic, responds poorly to hormonal stimulus, and often has telangiectatic and bizarre blood vessel patterns. Biopsy is also difficult because of epithelial atrophy and loss of tissue elasticity.

Treatment

Numerous different treatment methods ranging from various methods of local tissue destruction or ablation through to more extensive surgery including total vaginectomy as well as intracavitary radiotherapy have been used to treat VAIN and are listed in Table 24-2. Selection of the appropriate treatment should be based on a careful study of many factors including the general medical condition of the patient, the histologic degree of the abnormality, the location and extent of lesions, and the experience and expertise of the treating physician with the specific treatment methods. In addition, the proximity of the urethra,

T A B L E   **24-2**

Treatment Modalities for Vaginal Intraepithelial Neoplasia

Observation only
Surgical
Local excision
Partial vaginectomy
Total vaginectomy
Ablative
Cryosurgery
CO_2 laser
Electrocautery
Electrosurgical excision
Chemical
Topical 5-fluorouracil
Estrogen
Radiation

bladder, and rectum to the vaginal epithelium must be remembered, particularly when local destructive, ablative methods or surgical excision is considered. Damage or injury to these structures can occur with potentially disastrous effects, particularly in women who had prior radiation therapy.

Observation

In elderly patients with low-grade lesions or in individuals who are frail or in poor medical health, observation with careful colposcopic examination and assessment on a 4- to 6-month basis is an acceptable form of management. This may be desirable particularly for low-grade lesions. If there is evidence of progression, then re-evaluation and consideration of a more aggressive approach is warranted.

Topical 5-Fluorouracil

The use of topical 5-fluorouracil (5-FU), a cytotoxic antimetabolite, to treat VAIN was first reported by Woodruff et al (26) in 1975. They noted a complete response in 8 of 9 patients so treated. Since then, several reports on the efficacy of 5-FU as primary treatment for VAIN have appeared in the literature, with a combined success rate of approximately 83% (Table 24-3) (9,11,18,26–29). Topical 5-FU treatment has the theoretical advantage of permitting more comprehensive treatment of the entire vaginal mucosa. Therapy is ambulatory and does not require an anesthetic or complicated, expensive equipment. This therapy may be particularly suitable for patients with widespread or multifocal lesions for which the more extensive surgical procedures that would be required for excision of all of the disease would result in functional compromise.

Several different treatment protocols for the use of this medication (see Table 24-3) have been reported, without a clear consensus as to what the optimal dose and application schedule should be. Nonetheless, results with these approaches have generally been quite good. Townsend (20) advocated the use of one fourth of a vaginal applicator (approximately 1.5–2.0 g) of 5% 5-FU cream for 5 consecutive nights. Stokes et al (30) suggested the use of a similar amount once weekly at bedtime for 10 consecutive weeks. Krebs (18) also used various treatment schedules and advocated using 5-FU once every 2 weeks for 3 months after initial treatment to minimize treatment failure. With this regimen he found that up to 95% of individuals remained free of disease for up to 7 years. All authors advocate using a protective ointment such as petroleum jelly or zinc oxide to the introitus and the vulva just prior to the application of 5-FU, which can cause painful burns and ulcerations to the vulvar and perineal skin if prolonged contact with these tissues occurs. Also, having the patient insert the 5-FU at bedtime can minimize the chances for prolonged contact with vulvar skin; such contact can result if the patient is up walking about with this medication in place intravaginally. In addition, some individuals recommended dividing a tampon in half and inserting the lower half with the attached string into the vagina after the application of the 5-FU cream, to further protect the vulvar structures from spillage of this material.

Sexual intercourse is contraindicated at the time of 5-FU usage. Side effects during treatment are generally minimal and the medication is usually well tolerated by patients, the most common complaints being vaginal irritation and a burning sensation. With repeated treatments, however, sloughing of the vagina with ulceration may occur. There have also been reports (31,32) of vaginal adenosis occurring in some women with frequent and prolonged use of intravaginal 5-FU with and without combined CO_2 laser therapy. This particular complication can be quite difficult to manage and also be quite uncomfortable and distressing to the patient.

Sillman et al (33) reported on what he called 5-FU/chemosurgery. With this approach 5-FU is used for approximately 1 week and is then followed by removal of the affected

T A B L E   **24-3**

Topical 5-Fluorouracil Treatment of Vaginal Intraepithelial Neoplasia (VAIN): Collected Literature Results

Principal Author	Year	No. Treated	No. With VAIN III	Outcome Success/ Treated	Follow-up Mean	Follow-up Range	Treatment Protocol
Woodruff (26)	1975	9	9	8/9	N.R.	6 wk–6 yr	1/4 applicator bid × 1 mo
Ballon (27)	1979	12	6	9/12	13 mo	6–30 mo	Tampon applicator bid × 2 wk
Petrilli (28)	1980	15	9	12/15	N.R.	2–60 mo	5 mL daily × 5 days
Caglar (29)	1981	25	9	25/25	N.R.	3–48 mo	1/4 applicator daily for 5–10 days every wk × 2
Kirwan (11)	1985	10	7	8/10	15 mo	4–42 mo	2.5 g once weekly × 10 wk
Krebs (18)	1989	58	38	47/58	32 mo	12–84 mo	1/4 applicator × 7 days, 1 wk apart × 3 or 1/3 applicator once/wk × 10 wk
Audet-Lapointe (9)	1990	9	2	7/9	20 mo	9–42 mo	5 g/day × 5 days

N.R. = not reported.

epithelium. 5-FU apparently loosens the epithelial-stromal bond, enabling the diseased epithelium to be easily stripped off without risk to underlying tissues.

Local Destructive Therapies

Cryosurgery, electrocautery, and CO_2 laser therapy have all been used to treat VAIN. CO_2 laser is undoubtedly superior to both cryosurgery and electrocauterization because of its precision in determining the extent of disease destroyed or treated. Extensive destruction by any of these methods, particularly with electrocautery, has the potential for inducing fistula formation, either immediately or later as a result of thermal necrosis.

If cryotherapy is used, a probe tip of a size similar to the lesion should be selected and a single freeze-thaw cycle is recommended. Trying to produce an iceball that will extend 2 to 3mm beyond the margins of all lesions is also desirable.

Stafl et al (23) were the first to report use of the CO_2 laser to treat VAIN. Since then, numerous reports have appeared in the literature, showing success rates in the 80% to 85% range.

It would appear that multifocal lesions and those involving the deep recesses of the vaginal fornices are more likely to require repeated laser treatments to eradicate the disease. Table 24-4 summarizes the results and experience with the CO_2 laser described in selected literature reports, together with the basic technical

recommendations (6–10,17,18,23,28,34,35). It should be noted that as with 5-FU, most series are small and the length of follow-up short. The reported success rates with CO_2 laser therapy were obtained with repeated treatments in all but three of the series.

Sherman (36), in one of the largest series reported, treated 143 patients with the CO_2 laser from 1975 to 1990. Twenty-three patients required retreatment, one developed a vesicovaginal fistula, and 28 had bleeding that required some intervention. Unfortunately, information regarding patient histopathology, length of follow-up, and the specific technical aspects of the laser treatment are lacking. He did, however, report that the use of subepithelial saline or 0.5% procaine hydrochloride solution and the use of wire sutures to elevate the mucosa, particularly in areas that were often difficult to access, helped to make laser therapy easier and safer.

In a study (37) of 56 patients with VAIN, colleagues and I measured the thickness of the involved and noninvolved epithelium and found that the range of involved epithelium varied from 0.1 to 1.4mm. There was also no statistically significant difference in the epithelial thickness in lesions in premenopausal and postmenopausal women with VAIN. Information from this study led us to recommend tissue destruction to a depth of 1.0 to 1.5mm as being sufficient to destroy the epithelium without damaging surrounding structures.

For most lesions, laser vaporization is best performed under general anesthesia, particu-

T A B L E 24-4

Laser Treatment Results for Vaginal Intraepithelial Neoplasia (VAIN): Collected Literature Reports

Principal Author	Year	No. Treated	No. with VAIN III	Outcome Success/ Treated	Recommended Depth of Ablation	Power in Watts (W) or Power Density (W/cm²)	Follow-up	
							Mean	Range
Stafl (23)	1977	6	5	5*/6	1.5–2.0mm	7 W	N.R.	3–12 mo
Petrilli (28)	1980	10	9	9*/10	3–4mm	20 W	6 mo	2–12 mo
Townsend (6)	1982	36	18	28*/36	Lamina propria	300–1100 W/cm²	N.R.	N.R.
Jobson (34)	1983	24	15	24*/24	1.5–2.5	900 W/cm²	15 mo	6–27 mo
Woodman (7)	1984	14	N.R.	6*/14	2–4mm	20 W	30 mo	6–60 mo
Curtin (17)	1985	27	N.R.	24*/27	3–5mm	500–800 W/cm²	15.6 mo	6–42 mo
Lenehan (10)	1986	22	19	11/22	2–4mm	20 W	18 mo	6–27 mo
Stuart (8)	1988	27	8	21*/27	2–3mm	1130 W/cm²	14.4 mo	6–38 mo
Krebs (18)	1989	22	12	16/22	2–3mm	400–1200 W/cm²	30 mo	12–84 mo
Audet-Lapointe (9)	1990	34	22	24*/34	2–4mm	1500 W/cm²	39.2 mo	7–85 mo
Hoffman (35)	1991	26	26	15/26	1–2mm	500–1000 W/cm²	27 mo	11–56 mo

N.R. = not reported.

*Included repeat treatments.

larly in patients with lesions at the apex of the vagina and those with extensive involvement in the vaginal fornices. Some authors also recommended injection of the mucosa with local anesthetic or saline solution in an attempt to raise or separate the epithelium of the lesions from the underlying basement membrane, with the objective being to protect the deeper underlying tissues and structures from damage. In postmenopausal patients, a 10-day to 2-week course of intravaginal estrogen cream is helpful to improve the thickness of the epithelium and also to better outline and visualize any lesions that are present prior to laser application.

In some postmenopausal patients the use of intravaginal estrogen cream may eliminate some VAIN lesions, particularly lower-grade changes. In order to be effective, this may require prolonged use for several months and patients should be monitored carefully over this period of time.

More recently, Patsner (38) reported using loop excision of VAIN in 5 patients without problems, and as enthusiasm for loop excision of cervical lesions is now widespread, it seems likely that this will lead to more VAIN being treated in this way.

Surgical Excision

Several different surgical procedures ranging from simple local excision of lesions through to partial or total vaginectomy (39–41) are available for the treatment of VAIN. Surgical excision has the advantage of producing additional tissue for histologic assessment as well as being among the most effective methods for eradicating VAIN. Surgery in the form of local excision is most useful for individuals with one or two discrete lesions located at the apex of the vagina. In women treated by local surgical excision, narrowing and shortening of the vagina can occur, particularly if one attempts to close the defects by approximating the mucosal edges. Stenosis and stricture formation can be avoided by simply inserting a vaginal pack and allowing the areas to re-epithelialize from the existing mucosal margins. Healing is usually complete within a 6-week period and generally produces a most satisfactory functional result. We also adopted this approach with partial upper vaginectomy, with good success.

A particularly difficult group of lesions to treat are those noted after hysterectomy that involve the deep vaginal fornices or so-called dog ears. During surgical removal of these affected areas, care must be taken not to injure the adjacent bladder or ureters that are in close proximity. Also, one needs to be sure that all buried epithelium from the previous vault closure is removed. Many of these particular problems are undoubtedly related to the method of vaginal vault closure and suspension used during the hysterectomy. These arise because involved epithelium extending from the cervix or from the cervicovaginal margin may have been included in the vault closure and is then responsible for the subsequent appearance of these lesions. Much debate took place, particularly in the older literature, regarding the amount of vaginal cuff that should be removed at the time of hysterectomy for cervical lesions. Creasman and Rutledge (42) noted that the recurrence rate of CIS following hysterectomy was independent of the amount of cuff removed.

It may also be possible to prevent some of these situations from occurring by some slight modifications to the basic surgical techniques of hysterectomies.

In patients in whom the vaginal route was used for hysterectomy, careful staining of the cervix and upper vagina with Schiller's or Lugol's iodine prior to the start of the procedure permits one to see the precise amount of tissue that needs to be removed. Conversely, at the time of abdominal hysterectomy, once the specimen has been removed, the cervical surface and attached vaginal tissue can be stained in a similar fashion to see if any non-staining areas extend to resection margins, which would indicate possible incomplete excision.

Finally, when one is performing abdominal hysterectomy and applying upward traction on the uterus, it should be remembered that the fornices tend to be stretched upward and it is quite easy to include or pinch outer cervical or vaginal tissue from the fornices with the forceps or clamps that are placed in close approximation to the cervix during the final steps of the hysterectomy. An approach that may help prevent this from happening is as follows: Just prior to the application of the surgical clamps to secure the vaginal angles and the lower surgical pedicles, the vagina is first entered anteriorly and the circumferential mucosal incision made and then the vaginal angles are individually secured. This will ensure that the lateral cervical and vaginal mucosa is not clamped and buried with the final application of surgical forceps or hemostatic clamps to these last two pedicles.

The use of total vaginectomy is rarely necessary to treat intraepithelial lesions of the vagina. However, where extensive disease exists, involving virtually the entire length of the vaginal tube, and conservative measures have failed, this may be necessary. Fortunately this is a very rare occurrence. When total vaginectomy is performed, a neovagina, using split-thickness skin grafts applied over a mold (McIndoe procedure), can be created concomitantly or more extensive surgery with the use of myocutaneous flaps may be done either at the time of surgery or after an interval of time.

Radiotherapy

Intercavitary radiation with various techniques has been used to treat major grades of VAIN with good results in some centers. Problems that can occur with radiotherapy are scarring and stenosis as well as vaginal shortening. This not only may preclude satisfactory sexual intercourse but also may make subsequent follow-up and assessment extremely difficult. This is particularly true if the patients are not sexually active and are not well motivated to use vaginal dilators regularly. Radiotherapy also can result in permanent injury and disability of the bladder, rectum, and small bowel.

Conclusions

VAIN is fortunately an uncommon condition but one that appears to be increasing in frequency, particularly in young women. Our knowledge regarding the epidemiology and etiology of this condition is incomplete and much of our current understanding and concepts are based on an extrapolation of data and information from CIN to these vaginal lesions. Colposcopy has revolutionized the assessment of individuals with abnormal-appearing vaginal Papanicolaou smears and is essential for the proper evaluation and management of VAIN. Various treatment modalities are available for successful therapy and careful evaluation and individualization of treatment are recommended. Local therapy such as ablative or local excision usually will produce good results in younger individuals without compromise of sexual func-

tion. Older patients may respond best to local surgical excision or laser vaporization after a short course of topical estrogen therapy. 5-FU is also a useful therapeutic modality in women with extensive and multifocal disease. Any woman who has had a hysterectomy for cervical neoplasia or vulvar preneoplasia requires ongoing follow-up of the vagina as well. Similarly, in most series of VAIN that developed after hysterectomy, at least one fourth of cases occurred in women who had their surgery for benign conditions, so that even these women should continue with periodic cytologic surveillance.

The true potential of many of these lesions is not clearly understood and individuals treated require indefinite ongoing assessment to ensure that any recurrence or progression is promptly diagnosed and managed.

REFERENCES

1. Gallup DG, Morley GW. Carcinoma in situ of the vagina. *Obstet Gynecol* 1975;46:334–340.
2. Lee RA, Symmonds RE. Recurrent carcinoma in situ of the vagina in patients previously treated for in situ carcinoma of the cervix. *Obstet Gynecol* 1976;48:61–64.
3. Benedet JL, Boyes DA, Nichols TM, Millner A. The role of colposcopy in the evaluation of abnormal vaginal vault smears. *Gynecol Oncol* 1977;5:338–345.
4. Benedet JL, Sanders BH. Carcinoma in situ of the vagina. *Am J Obstet Gynecol* 1984;148:695–700.
5. Hernandez-Linares W, Puthawala A, Nolan JF, et al. Carcinoma in situ of the vagina: past and present management. *Obstet Gynecol* 1980;56:356–359.
6. Townsend DE, Levine RU, Crum CP, Richart RM. Treatment of vaginal carcinoma in situ with the carbon dioxide laser. *Am J Obstet Gynecol* 1982;143:565–568.
7. Woodman CBJ, Jordan JA, Wade-Evans T. The management of vaginal intraepithelial neoplasia after hysterectomy. *Br J Obstet Gynaecol* 1984;91:707–711.
8. Stuart GCE, Flagler EA, Nation JG, et al. Laser vaporization of vaginal intraepithelial neoplasia. *Am J Obstet Gynecol* 1988;158:240–243.
9. Audet-Lapointe P, Body G, Vauclair R, et al. Vaginal intraepithelial neoplasia. *Gynecol Oncol* 1990;36:232–239.

10. Lenehan PM, Meffe F, Lickrish GM. Vaginal intraepithelial neoplasia: biologic aspects and management. *Obstet Gynecol* 1986;68:333–337.

11. Kirwan P, Naftalin NJ. Topical 5-fluorouracil in the treatment of vaginal intraepithelial neoplasia. *Br J Obstet Gynaecol* 1985;92:287–291.

12. Aho M, Vesterinen E, Meyer B, et al. Natural history of vaginal intraepithelial neoplasia. *Cancer* 1991;68:195–197.

13. Cramer DW, Cutler SJ. Incidence and histopathology of malignancies of the female genital organs in the United States. *Am J Obstet Gynecol* 1974;118:443–460.

14. Hummer WK, Mussey E, Decker DG, Dockerty MB. Carcinoma in situ of the vagina. *Am J Obstet Gynecol* 1970;108:1109–1116.

15. Woodruff JD. Carcinoma in situ of the vagina. *Clin Obstet Gynecol* 1981;24:485–501.

16. Nwabineli NJ, Monaghan JM. Vaginal epithelial abnormalities in patients with CIN: clinical and pathological features and management. *Br J Obstet Gynaecol* 1991;98:25–29.

17. Curtin JP, Twiggs LB, Julian TM. Treatment of vaginal intraepithelial neoplasia with the CO_2 laser. *J Reprod Med* 1985;30:942–944.

18. Krebs HB. Treatment of vaginal intraepithelial neoplasia with laser and topical 5-fluorouracil. *Obstet Gynecol* 1989;73:657–660.

19. Sillman F, Stanek A, Sedlis A, et al. The relationship between human papillomavirus and lower genital intraepithelial neoplasia in immunosuppressed women. *Am J Obstet Gynecol* 1984;150:300–308.

20. Townsend DE. Intraepithelial neoplasia of vagina. In: Coppleson M, ed. *Gynecologic oncology. Fundamental principles and clinical practice.* Edinburgh: Churchill Livingstone, 1992: 493–499.

21. Bornstein J, Kaufman RH, Adam E, Adler-Storthz K. Human papillomavirus associated with vaginal intraepithelial neoplasia in women exposed to diethylstilbestrol in utero. *Obstet Gynecol* 1987;70:75–80.

22. Robboy SJ, Noller KL, O'Brien P, et al. Increased incidence of cervical and vaginal dysplasia in 3980 diethylstilbestrol-exposed young women. *JAMA* 1984;252:2979–2983.

23. Stafl A, Wilkinson EJ, Mattingley RF. Laser treatment of cervical and vaginal neoplasia. *Am J Obstet Gynecol* 1977;128:128–136.

24. Clement PB, Benedet JL. Adenocarcinoma in situ of the vagina. *Cancer* 1979;43:2479–2485.

25. Robboy SJ, Young RH, Welch WR, et al. Atypical vaginal adenosis and cervical ectropion. Association with clear cell adenocarcinoma in diethylstilbestrol-exposed offspring. *Cancer* 1984;54:869–875.

26. Woodruff JD, Parmley TH, Julian CG. Topical 5-fluorouracil in the treatment of vaginal carcinoma-in-situ. *Gynecol Oncol* 1975;3:124–132.

27. Ballon SC, Roberts JA, Lagasse LD. Topical 5-fluorouracil in the treatment of intraepithelial neoplasia of the vagina. *Obstet Gynecol* 1979;54: 163–166.

28. Petrilli ES, Townsend DE, Morrow CP, Nakao CY. Vaginal intraepithelial neoplasia: biologic aspects and treatment with topical 5-fluorouracil and the carbon dioxide laser. *Am J Obstet Gynecol* 1980;138:321–328.

29. Caglar H, Hertzog RW, Hreshchchyshyn MM. Topical 5-fluorouracil treatment of vaginal intraepithelial neoplasia. *Obstet Gynecol* 1981;58: 580–583.

30. Stokes IM, Sworn MJ, Hawthorne JHR. A new regimen for the treatment of vaginal carcinoma in situ using 5-fluorouracil. *Br J Obstet Gynaecol* 1980;87:920–921.

31. Bornstein J, Sova Y, Atad J, et al. Development of vaginal adenosis following combined 5-fluorouracil and carbon dioxide laser treatments for diffuse vaginal condylomatosis. *Obstet Gynecol* 1993;81:896–898.

32. Goodman A, Zuckerberg LR, Nikrui N, Scully RE. Vaginal adenosis and clear cell carcinoma after 5-fluorouracil treatment for condylomas. *Cancer* 1991;68:1628–1632.

33. Sillman FH, Boyce JG, Macasaet MA, Nicastri AD. 5-Fluorouracil/chemosurgery for intraepithelial neoplasia of the lower genital tract. *Obstet Gynecol* 1981;58:356–360.

34. Jobson VW, Homesley HD. Treatment of vaginal intraepithelial neoplasia with the carbon dioxide laser. *Obstet Gynecol* 1983;62:90–93.

35. Hoffman MS, Roberts WS, LaPolla JP, et al. Laser vaporization of grade 3 vaginal intraepithelial neoplasia. *Am J Obstet Gynecol* 1991;165:1342–1344.

36. Sherman AI. Laser therapy for vaginal intraepithelial neoplasia after hysterectomy. *J Reprod Med* 1990;35:941–944.

37. Benedet JL, Wilson PS, Matisic JP. Epidermal thickness measurements in vaginal intraepithelial neoplasia. A basis for optimal CO_2 laser vaporization. *J Reprod Med* 1992;37:809–812.

38. Patsner B. Treatment of vaginal dysplasia with loop excision: report of five cases. *Am J Obstet Gynecol* 1993;169:179–180.

39. Hoffman MS, DeCesare SL, Roberts WS, et al. Upper vaginectomy for in situ and occult, superficially invasive carcinoma of the vagina. *Am J Obstet Gynecol* 1992;166:30–33.

40. Curtis P, Shepherd JH, Lowe DG, Jobling T. The role of partial colpectomy in the management of persistent vaginal neoplasia after primary treatment. *Br J Obstet Gynaecol* 1992;99:587–589.

41. Ireland D, Monaghan JM. The management of the patient with abnormal vaginal cytology following hysterectomy. *Br J Obstet Gynaecol* 1988;95:973–975.

42. Creasman WT, Rutledge F. Carcinoma in situ of the cervix: an analysis of 861 patients. *Obstet Gynecol* 1972;39:373–380.

CHAPTER *25*

Malignant Tumors of the Vagina

LUIS DELCLOS
J. TAYLOR WHARTON
CREIGHTON L. EDWARDS

Malignant tumors of the vagina are rare. Sixty percent occur in patients between the ages of 50 and 70; 25% of the patients are older and 15% are younger. The majority of tumors are squamous cell carcinomas; adenocarcinomas are less frequent. Rare tumors include sarcomas and melanomas in the adult female and clear-cell carcinoma in the young female. Table 25-1 shows the distribution by histology of the tumors found in 411 patients seen and treated by irradiation at M. D. Anderson Cancer Center between January 1954 and December 1990. In addition, there are some rare tumors like the sarcoma botryoides and endodermal sinus tumor in the child; these two tumors are not treated by irradiation modalities. Metastatic tumors may also occur in the vagina, with the primary tumor being in the endometrium, uterine cervix (squamous carcinomas or adenocarcinomas), or gastrointestinal tract. Direct extension and recurrences in the vagina may occur from any of the above-mentioned sites and also from the urinary bladder and urethra or paraurethral glands including the Bartholin glands. Primary tumors can also be found in breasts or lungs.

Patterns of Spread

The lymphatic drainage of the upper and lower halves of the vagina is divided into two main groups, although there is communication between the two. One group extends along the uterine artery and the other along the vaginal artery. The first group drains the upper vagina into the external iliac nodes. The second group drains the lower vagina into the interiliac (or hypogastric) node chain. The upper vagina anastomoses with the lymphatic system of the uterine cervix and the lower vagina anastomoses with the lymphatics of the vulva. Some may anastomose with the perirectal lymphatics. These drainage differences as well as the results of a lower extremity lymphangiogram are important to know when treatment is planned. For instance, when the results of the lymphangiogram are negative, there is no need to include the common iliac lymphatics, even for tumors of the proximal vagina, as in our experience there is a low incidence of pelvic node failures (Table 25-2) in patients treated with small-field irradiation that did not include even the lateral pelvic walls (1). For tumors of the distal half, however, it is important to include the midupper femoral nodes in the radiation field because tumors in this lower location can metastasize first to this lymphatic area.

Staging Workup

Baseline studies should include a lower extremity lymphangiogram. The lymphangiogram is particularly important when the findings are positive because it provides the location and

355

T A B L E   **25-1**

Malignant Tumors of the Vagina Treated by Radio-therapy: January 1954 to December 1990

Squamous cell carcinoma	302
Atypical squamous carcinoma	3
Adenocarcinoma	34
Clear-cell carcinoma	28
Subtotal	367
Others	
Melanomas	8
Sarcomas	10
Unclassified	22
Rare*	4
Subtotal	44
Total	411

*Neuroblastoma, lymphoma, transitional, adenoid cystic.

volume of the peripheral positive nodes; visibly positive nodes require a higher dose of irradiation. The lymphangiogram, however, does not visualize the interiliac (hypogastric) or the perirectal and presacral nodes, but these lymphatics are always included in the volume irradiated.

The International Federation of Gynecology and Obstetrics (FIGO) staging system (2) (Table 25-3) accepted by the American Joint Committee on Staging is not useful for planning therapy because it does not take into account the extent, volume, or location of the tumor. The FIGO staging system is used to report broad results and there is a strong correlation with survival;

however, we and others recommend including other factors (3–5).

Treatment Planning

Conservation of the bladder, urethra, rectum, and vagina becomes an important factor in the treatment decision. Anatomic limitations do not allow for conservative surgery because a sufficient surgical margin cannot be obtained. Therefore, irradiation is generally the treatment of choice.

For treatment planning, the importance of knowing the tumor volume and the tumor location, mainly whether it is in the upper or lower half of the vagina, must be emphasized (1,3–5). In addition, knowing whether the tumor is in anterior, posterior, or lateral locations is also important because of the proximity of the bladder and urethra to the anterior wall and the rectum and anus to the posterior wall. Another important factor is the presence or absence of a uterus, as the presence of a uterus allows for treatment of some tumors of the upper vagina like tumors of the uterine cervix, by inserting radioactive sources into the uterus and vagina (Fig. 25-1). It must be stressed that treatment of these tumors is highly individualized, as many factors must be considered. Some of these tumors occur in patients treated earlier by surgery or irradiation for cancer of the uterine cervix (40%) (1) and treatment must also take this into consideration.

T A B L E   **25-2**

Sites of Failure Related to Disease Stage*

	Stages				
	I	**II**	**III**	**IVa**	**Total**
No. of patients treated	71	42	38	11	162
Failures					
Central only	13 (18%)	6 (14%)	9 (24%)	3	31 (19%)
Pelvic only	1	1	1	—	3 (<2%)
Central + pelvic	1	—	—	—	1 (<1%)
Inguinal nodes	5 (7%)	—	—	1	6 (<4%)
Distant metastasis	2	2	5	—	9 (<6%)
Central + distant metastasis	2	—	—	1	3 (<2%)
Pelvic + distant metastasis	—	1	—	—	1 (<1%)
Central + pelvic + distant metastasis	—	—	1	—	1 (<1%)

*For period of January 1955 to December 1982; time of analysis December 1986.

Source: Reprinted by permission of the publisher from Frank Dancuart et al. Primary squamous cell carcinoma of the vagina treated by radiotherapy: a failures analysis—the M. D. Anderson hospital experience 1955–1982. *Int J Radiat Oncol Biol Phys* 14:747, 1988 (Table 3).

T A B L E **25-3**

FIGO Classification and Staging of Malignant Tumors in the Female
Pelvis (Approved by UICC and AJC)

Site	Classification
Carcinoma of the vagina	Cases should be classified as carcinoma of the vagina when the primary site of the growth is in the vagina. Tumors present in the vagina as secondary growths from either genital or extragenital sites should be excluded from registration
	A growth that has extended to the portio *and reached the area of the external os* should always be allotted to carcinoma of the cervix.
	A growth that is limited to the urethra should be classified as carcinoma of the urethra.

Definitions of the clinical stages in carcinoma of the vagina

Preinvasive carcinoma	Carcinoma in situ.
Stage 0	Intraepithelial carcinoma.
Invasive carcinoma	
Stage I	The carcinoma is limited to the vaginal wall.
Stage II	The carcinoma has involved the subvaginal tissues but has not extended to the pelvic wall.
Stage III	The carcinoma has extended to the pelvic wall.
Stage IV	The carcinoma has extended beyond the true pelvis or has involved the mucosa of the bladder and rectum.
Stage IVa	The growth has spread to adjacent organs.
Stage IVb	The growth has spread to distant organs.

FIGO = International Federation of Gynecologists and Oncologists; UICC = Committee of the International Union Against Cancer; AJC = American Joint Committee for Cancer Staging Results Report.

Source: Reproduced by permission from *Annual report on the results of treatment in gynecological cancer*, vol. 18. Radiumhemmet. Stockholm: 1988:13–18.

T A B L E **25-4**

Primary Squamous Cell Carcinoma of the Vagina: the M. D. Anderson
Cancer Center, 1948 to 1972

Stage	No. of Patients Treated	No. of Patients Alive 5 Years and NED (%)	Therapy Failure Sites Within 5 Years		
			Recurrences in Treated Area	Distant Metastases	Unknown
I	25	16 (64%)	4	2	1
II	39	23 (59%)	6	1	1
III	28	10 (36%)	6	—	—
IV	20	8 (40%)	6	5	—
Total	112	57 (50%)	22	8	2

NED = no evidence of disease.

The use of external-beam irradiation alone or in combination either 1) with intracavitary (see Fig. 25-1) or transvaginal irradiation (see Fig. 25-10) for tumors of the upper half of the vagina or 2) with interstitial irradiation with stainless-steel needle guides (Fig. 25-2) afterloaded with iridium wires or seed chains has enhanced the outlook for patients with vaginal cancer (6). Table 25-4 gives the survival data for a group of patients treated at M. D. Anderson Cancer Center in the last three decades.

Treatment Technique

External-beam irradiation in patients whose lymphangiogram showed no disease is given with portals that extend from the midsacrum to the vaginal introitus, which has been marked with a silver seed that will be visualized on the simulation films (Fig. 25-3). Laterally the portals extend about 1.5 cm lateral to the pelvic brim. These portals will include the whole vagina and

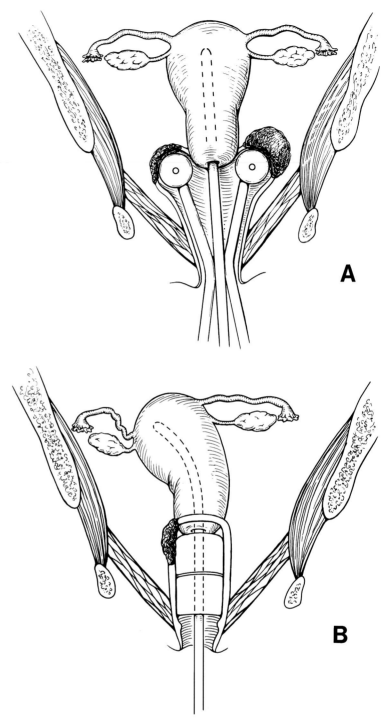

FIGURE **25-1**

When the uterus is present, tumors of the upper vagina are treated by external irradiation (4000 cGy in 20 fractions in 4 weeks for small tumors or 5000 cGy in 25 fractions in 5 weeks for larger tumors) followed by placement of intrauterovaginal radioactive sources in a "tandem" and in "colpostats." Colpostats are of the Fletcher type for use against the lateral fornices (*A*) or are cylindrical (*B*) for when irradiation along the vagina is needed. The intrauterine tandem can be tilted to the site of the tumor to increase the dose to the tumor.

the lymphatics of the pelvis [paracolpal and parametrial channels, interiliac (hypogastric), perirectal, presacral, external iliac, and junctional nodes]. The common iliac nodes will not be included unless the lymphangiogram shows positive pelvic nodes, in which case the fields will be extended to the top of L5 or 4 cm above the highest positive node. If the tumor is located in the lower (distal) half of the vagina, then the fields have to be extended down to include the vaginal introitus and therefore some of the vulva, and also laterally to include the midupper femoral nodes (around the midinguinal ligament, "groin"). The midupper femoral nodes are located by clinical examination. We use an 18-MeV photon beam unless the midupper femoral nodes are clinically involved, in which case we use a laterally larger anterior portal

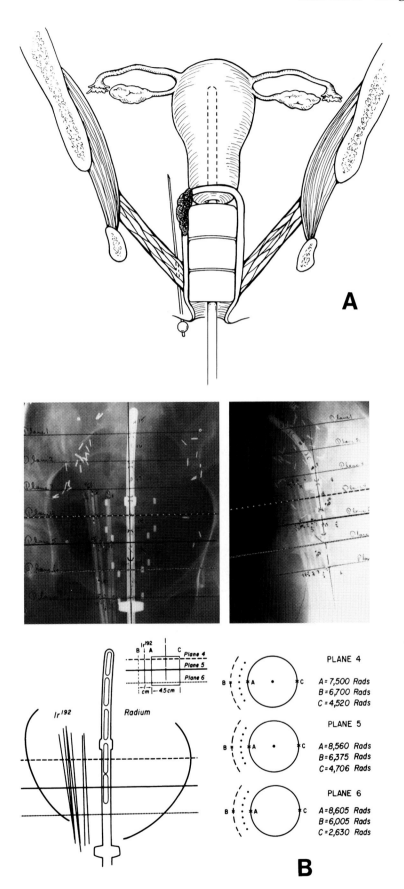

FIGURE **25-2**

A. The addition of interstitial irradiation to intracavitary irradiation. *B–D.* Radiographs and isodoses of the combination, after external irradiation, of an intrauterine tandem, Fletcher colpostats, and an iridium-192 implant. (B, C, D from Delclos L, Flectcher H, Moore EB, Sampiere VA. Minicolpostats, dome cylinders, and other additions and improvements of the Fletcher-Suit afterloading system: indications and limitations of their use. *Int J Radiat Oncol Biol Phys* 1980;6:1203. Reproduced with permission from Pergamon Press, Ltd.)

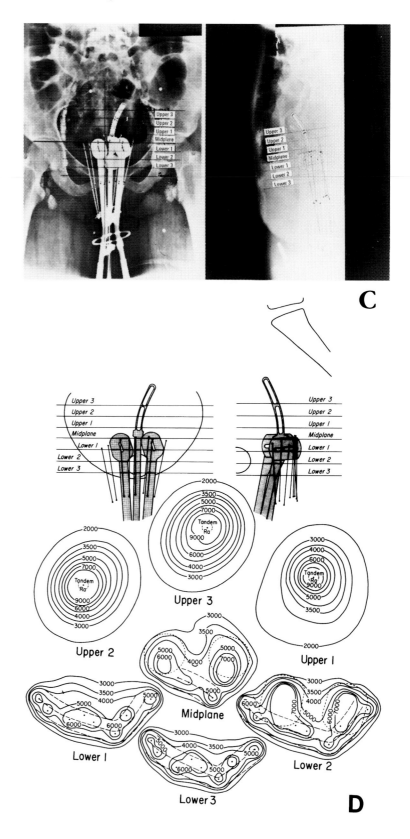

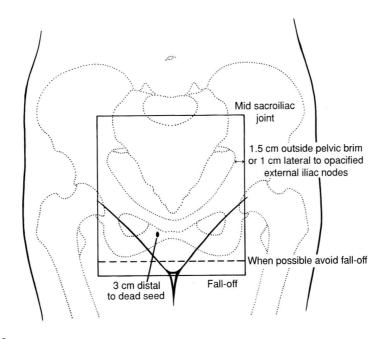

F I G U R E **25-3**

Diagram of the anteroposterior-posteroanterior pelvic portals employed to treat tumors of the vagina when a lower extremity lymphangiogram shows no disease involvement. The portal will extend from the middle of the sacroiliac joint to 3 cm below a silver seed marker placed at the lowermost extension of the tumor; this distal edge of the portal may have to fall off the vulva to obtain adequate margin. Laterally the portals extend 1.5 cm outside the pelvic bream. When the tumor extends or is located in the lower one half of the vagina, special care is taken to include the "groin" (upper midfemoral nodes) around the midinguinal ligament. Lateral portals are not recommended for tumors of the vagina.

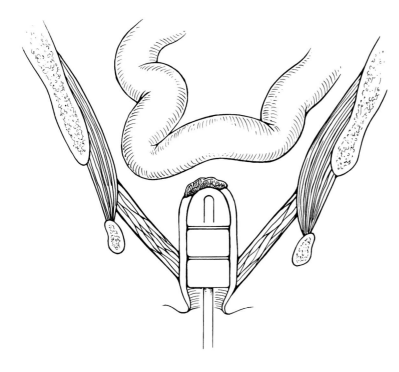

F I G U R E **25-4**

When there is no uterus, a "dome cylinder" will treat adequately superficial tumors of the vaginal vault, employing a "point" source alone or in combination with a "linear" source below. A thick tumor may require an implant.

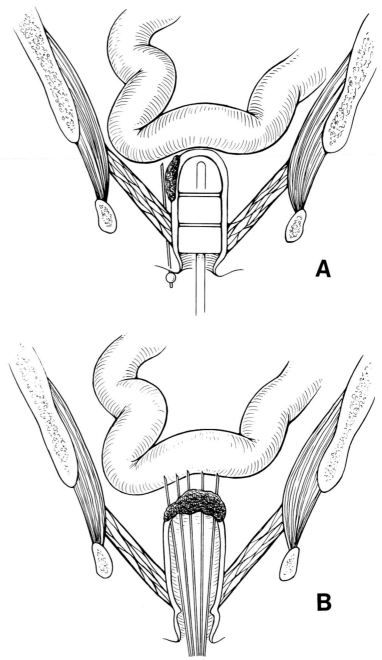

FIGURE **25-5**

When there is no uterus, thick tumors involving the upper vagina should preferably be treated by external irradiation plus interstitial irradiation. Most patients who had the uterus removed have small bowel adherent to the vaginal cuff and therefore interstitial irradiation should be carried out with laparotomy or laparoscopy guidance; adhesions are sectioned during the procedure, leaving the small intestine free. Either of the two procedures allows the placing of omentum between the vaginal cuff and the bowel, reducing the chances of damage to the bowel.

with 6-MeV photon beam and a smaller posterior 18-MeV photon beam; the treatment portals are then similar to the ones employed for preoperative or postoperative treatment of carcinoma of the vulva.

Initially, a dose of 4000 cGy is given in 20 fractions in 4 weeks to the midline of the pelvis, employing parallel opposed portals. For tumors of the upper half (proximal) of the vagina, when the uterus is present, we generally add intracavitary irradiation with intrauterine and vaginal sources (see Fig. 25-1). Several colpostats are available, and generally we use two insertions of 48 hours each, 2 weeks apart. If the tumor extends to the middle one third of the vagina, the addition of interstitial irradiation to external and intracavitary irradiation may be required (see Fig. 25-2) (6). In the absence of a uterus, we may continue with external-beam irradiation and reduce the size of the portals, delivering a total midline dose of 6400 to 6600 cGy at 200 cGy per fraction. The use of two

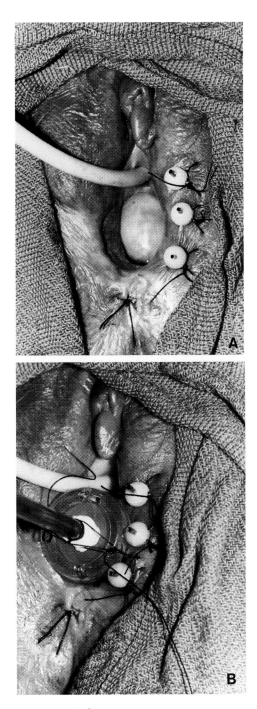

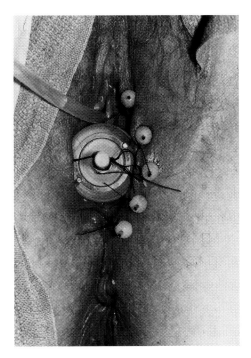

F I G U R E **25-7**
A larger (five needles in this case) implant is also maintained in place with an empty cylinder. During placement of the implant, the most anterior needles could enter the urinary bladder; therefore, we fill the bladder with a solution of methylene blue diluted in water or saline solution, as explained in the text. The posterior needles are guided with the index finger of the opposite hand in the rectum. At completion of implant placement, cystoscopy and proctoscopy are recommended to ensure that the needles did not penetrate the bladder or rectum. (Reproduced by permission from Delclos L. Afterloading interstitial irradiation techniques. In: Levitt SH, Khan FM, Potish RA, eds. *Levitt-Tapley technological basis of radiation therapy: practical clinical applications.* 2nd ed. Philadelphia: Lea & Febiger, 1992.)

F I G U R E **25-6**

Example of three needle implants along the left lateral wall of the vagina. *A.* Without the empty vaginal cylinder, the opposite wall is prolapsing. *B.* With the cylinder the vagina is maintained distended, sparing the opposite wall from the high dose delivered to the tumor site. The cylinder also keeps the needles parallel. (Reproduced by permission from Delclos L. Afterloading Interstitial irradiation techniques. In: Levitt SH, Khan FM, Potish RA, eds. *Levitt-Tapley technological basis of radiation therapy: practical clinical applications.* 2nd ed. Philadelphia: Lea & Febiger, 1992.)

parallel opposed portals (anteroposterior-posteroanterior) or the addition of lateral portals depends on tumor extension and individual anatomic variations. Lateral portals should only be used when there is a possibility of reducing irradiation to the small bowel, bladder, and rectum. To this, we may add a "dome colpostat" (Fig. 25-4), "Bloedorn colpostat" or "ovoidal colpostats" (without shielding) to deliver a higher dose to the upper vagina. In selected patients, we use interstitial irradiation with stainless-steel needle guides (7) loaded with iridium wires or iridium seed chains. Laparoscopy or laparotomy is required to guide the needles (Fig. 25-5). We add 4000 cGy to the

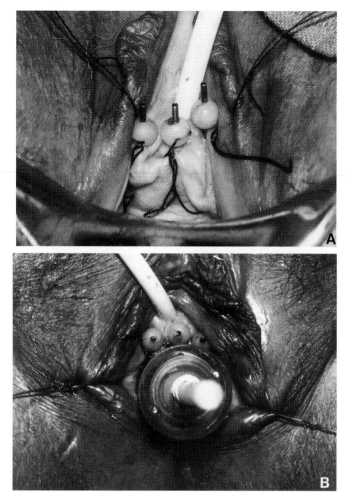

FIGURE **25-8**

Implant of the anterior vaginal wall (suburethral area) (*A*) without and (*B*) with a vaginal cylinder. For implant placement along the anterior vaginal wall, the bladder is filled with methylene blue diluted in water or saline solution. The needles are open at the end, so that if the bladder or urethra is entered during placement of the needle implant, the tinted fluid flows through the needle, alerting the clinician. If this happens, the needle is withdrawn and reimplanted.

periphery of the tumor in 3 to 5 days from the implant to the 4000 cGy delivered from the external beam, or 3000 cGy in 2 to 4 days if pelvic irradiation has been increased to 5000 cGy. For lesions of the lower half of the vagina (distal), after external irradiation, we use interstitial irradiation. This area is vulnerable to radiation reactions, sequelae, and complications because the tissues of the vaginal introitus, vulva, and perineal area tolerate radiation poorly and they are exposed to constant irritation from perspiration, urine, and soiling. Therefore, it is paramount to minimize radiation to the normal surrounding areas.

Interstitial Irradiation

Examples of implants of the lateral wall are shown in Figures 25-6 and 25-7 (7). An empty plastic cylinder is always used not only to spare

the uninvolved areas of the vagina but also to maintain the needles in a parallel position.

For placement of implants along the anterior vaginal wall, the bladder is filled with methylene blue diluted in water or saline solution. Since the needles are open at the end, if the bladder or urethra is entered during placement of the needle implant, the tinted fluid flows through the needle and the clinician is alerted to the situation. The needle is then withdrawn and reimplanted. An example of an implant of the anterior vaginal wall is shown in Figure 25-8 (7).

Although the majority of implants are placed in a single plane, occasionally for larger tumors we use more than one plane. An example is shown in Figure 25-9 (6). Placement of implants in the upper vagina requires laparoscopy or laparotomy to visualize the tip of the needles and minimize the chances of entering the peritoneal cavity.

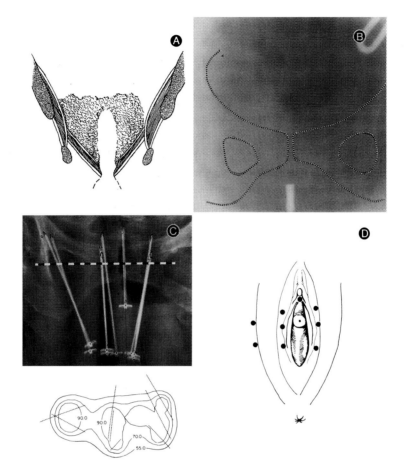

F I G U R E **25-9**

In 1961, a 71-year-old woman underwent a total abdominal hysterectomy and bilateral salpingo-oophorectomy for carcinoma in situ of the uterine cervix. She did well for 9 years. In May 1970, she was found to have an extensive squamous cell carcinoma of the vagina. *A*. The lesion involved the entire vagina and extended to both paracolpal areas, being fixed to the right pelvic wall. There was a crater at the apex of the vagina. The patient was treated by a combination of external and interstitial irradiation. *B*. From May 13, 1970, to June 9, 1970, she received 4000 rads in 20 fractions by means of a 22-MeV photon beam and parallel opposed fields. On June 17, 1970, an iridium-192 implant was placed with an open bladder. *C, D*. Anteroposterior x-ray film and diagram and the isodose distribution of the implant. A dose of 4000 rads was given in 73 hours (55 rads/hour isodose). The patient showed no evidence of disease in July 1975. (Reproduced by permission from Fletcher GH, Delclos L, Wharton JT, Rutledge FN. Tumors of the vagina and female pelvis. In: Fletcher GH, ed. *Textbook of radiotherapy*. 3rd ed. Philadelphia: Lea & Febiger, 1980.)

Clear-Cell Carcinoma in the Young Female

Adenocarcinoma may occur in young females, in the vagina or uterine cervix. Some adenocarcinomas have been associated with maternal use of diethylstilbestrol (DES) early in gestation. However, identical cancers can occur in patients with no exposure.

Small tumors, 2.5 cm or less in diameter, may be treated with interstitial or transvaginal radiation alone (Fig. 25-10) and spare the uterus and ovaries, maintaining fertility. Figure 25-11

F I G U R E   **25-10**

Transvaginal cone for orthovoltage (kilovoltage) irradiation (250-kV photons) is indicated for small well-differentiated tumors of the upper vagina (<2.5 cm in diameter) in the younger female, in an attempt to preserve the uterus and the ovaries.

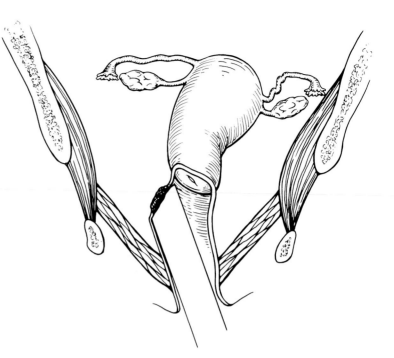

F I G U R E   **25-11**

Equipment for transvaginal irradiation with orthovoltage. *A.* Transvaginal cone mounted on the periscope attached to a kilovoltage therapy unit. *B.* Transvaginal treatment cones of different diameters.

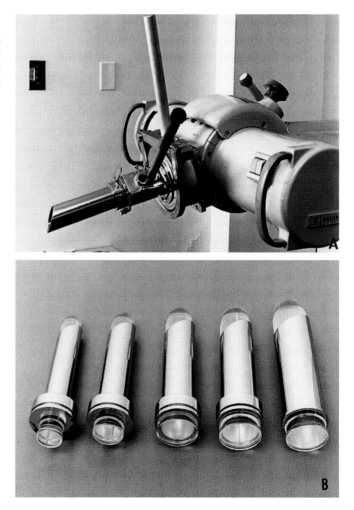

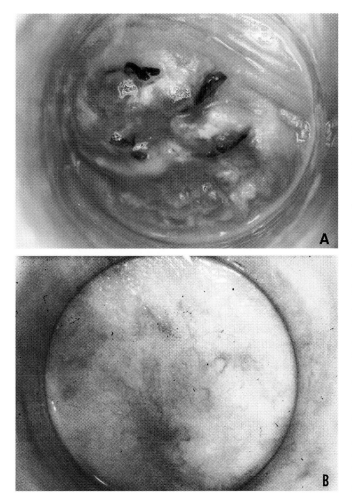

F I G U R E **25-12**
A 22-year-old white woman was first seen in March 1981 with a clear-cell carcinoma of the upper third of the vagina, located in the posterior wall near the uterine cervix. The uterine cervix was not involved. The tumor was flat and slightly less than 2 cm in diameter in an area of adenosis. Results of all pertinent studies were normal (intravenous pyelography, chest x-ray, lymphangiography, barium enema, and cystoscopy). Treatment involved transvaginal irradiation through a 3-cm transvaginal cone (125-kV beam, HVL 3.4 mm of aluminum delivering a "given dose" of 5400 rads divided into 15 fractions) (treatment started on March 26, 1981, and ended on April 15, 1981). *A.* The tumor. It should be noted that black silk sutures are used to outline the tumor, to guide daily placement of the transvaginal cone. *B.* The irradiated area 2 years later is completely healed. She was well in 1992 when she became pregnant and in December 1992 she delivered a normal baby after an uneventful pregnancy.

Minimal and moderate reactions (treated conservatively)	
Cystitis	6 (4/6 developed vaginal fibrosis)*
Proctitis	6
Vaginal necrosis	2 14/115 (12%)
Sequalae	
Vaginal fibrosis*	11 (2/11 urethral stenosis) 11/115 (10%)
Severe complications	
Rectosigmoid stenosis	4
Rectosigmoid hemorrhage	
Multiple fistulae	1 1 6/115 (5%)

T A B L E **25-5**

Complications in Patients Without Recurrent Disease: The M. D. Anderson Cancer Center, January 1955 to December 1982, 115 Patients

*All vaginal fibrosis = 15/115 (13%).

Source: Reprinted by permission of the publisher from Frank Dancuart et al. Primary squamous cell carcinoma of the vagina treated by radiotherapy: a failures analysis—the M. D. Anderson Hospital Experience 1955–1982. *Int J Radiat Oncol Biol Phys* 14:747, 1988 (Table 6).

shows the equipment used for transvaginal irradiation. Figure 25-12 shows a tumor treated by transvaginal cone irradiation. Conservative treatment was possible in 8 of 28 patients with clear-

cell carcinoma of the vagina (all with stage I disease). Four of the 8 patients were able to conceive, and they delivered normal babies. Large lesions are treated like carcinomas in the older female. Again the volume, location, and extent of the tumor are the primary factors in planning treatment. The treatment techniques and doses are the same as for squamous cell carcinomas.

Complications

Treatment complications are shown in Table 25-5 (1). Some vaginal stenosis may occur, but since large portions of the vagina are treated to lower doses (4000–5000 cGy), the vagina retains considerable elasticity and compensates for the radiation-induced scarring. Delayed healing must be treated conservatively, avoiding the temptation of repeat biopsies of the area that may promote a painful and slow-healing necrosis.

REFERENCES

1. Dancuart F, Delclos L, Wharton JT, Silva EG. Primary squamous cell carcinoma of the vagina treated by radiotherapy: a failures analysis—the M. D. Anderson experience 1955–1982. *Int J Radiat Oncol Biol Phys* 1988;14:745–749.

2. *Annual report on the results of treatment in gynecological cancer*, vol. 18. Radiumhemmet. Stockholm: 1988:13–18.

3. Perez CA, Arneson AN, Dehner LP, Galakatos A. Radiation therapy in carcinoma of the vagina. *Obstet Gynecol* 1974;44:862–872.

4. Peters WA, Kumar NB, Morley GW. Carcinoma of the vagina. Factors influencing treatment outcome. *Cancer* 1985;55:892–897.

5. Prempree T, Amornharn R. Radiation treatment of primary carcinoma of the vagina. *Acta Radiol Oncol* 1985;24:51–56.

6. Fletcher GH, Delclos L, Wharton JT, Rutledge FN. Tumors of the vagina and female urethra. In: Fletcher GH, ed. *Textbook of radiotherapy.* 3rd ed. Philadelphia: Lea & Febiger, 1980:812–828.

7. Delclos L. Afterloading interstitial irradiation techniques. In: Levitt SH, Khan FM, Potish RA, eds. *Levitt-Tapley technological basis of radiation therapy: practical clinical applications.* 2nd ed. Philadelphia: Lea & Febiger, 1992:123–154.

CHAPTER 26

Preinvasive Vulvar Cancer

JOHN E. CULLIMORE

*V*ulvar intraepithelial neoplasia (VIN) is a condition in which neoplastic cells are present within the boundaries of the surface epithelium and its adnexal structures. VIN can be subdivided into squamous VIN, Paget's disease of the vulva, and in situ melanoma. Because of the comparative rarity of the latter two lesions, this review concentrates mainly on squamous VIN.

Squamous Vulvar Intraepithelial Neoplasia

In 1986, the 8th World Congress of the International Society for the Study of Vulvar Disease (ISSVD) recommended a revised classification of VIN (Table 26-1). Since then, this classification has been confirmed by the International Society of Gynaecological Pathologists (1,2). Like cervical intraepithelial neoplasia (CIN), VIN has been divided into three categories dependent to a major extent on the level of epithelial involvement by undifferentiated cells.

Grading of VIN, therefore, is based on morphologic criteria, and the risk of invasive disease may not be related to grade. There is inevitably some subjectivity in diagnosis. These observations led one author (3) to the comment that grading of VIN is ". . . arbitrary, artificial, non-reproducible and for all purposes clinically meaningless." There are two distinct histologic varieties of VIN 3, notably "basaloid" VIN and "warty" VIN. These subtypes can be seen in different areas of the same lesion. The ISSVD committee recommended that the presence of condyloma or koilocytosis should not influence the diagnosis or grading of VIN (1).

Issues Influencing the Classification of Intraepithelial Squamous Lesions of the Vulva

The clinical and pathologic spectrum of VIN is broad and encompasses diverse clinical presentations and pathologic appearances. The terms *Bowen's disease, bowenoid papulosis,* and *erythroplasia of Queyrat* have been applied until recently to atypical vulval squamous epithelial lesions. These conditions are clinical variants of one histologic process, that is, VIN. There is no reason to believe that diversifying the terminology of VIN to take into account clinical and histopathologic variation will contribute to better understanding or improved management. However, some of these descriptive clinical terms (e.g., bowenoid papulosis) are still encountered, particularly in the dermatologic literature.

Clinical Features

Symptoms

1. Pruritus, present in 38% to 73% of patients.
2. Vulvodynia (i.e., pain, soreness, stinging, or rawness).
3. A lump or lesion; only a minority of patients present in this way.
4. Asymptomatic; these patients make up the majority of some series with many lesions detected at "routine" gynecologic examination.

T A B L E   **26-1**

International Society for the Study of Vulvar Disease Classification of Vulvar Intraepithelial Neoplasia (VIN)

VIN 1
  Mild dysplasia; nuclear hyperchromasia, cellular disarray involving lower one third of vulvar squamous epthelium, with or without normal or abnormal mitosis in lower one third

VIN 2
  Moderate dysplasia; extension of abnormal epithelium into middle one third of epithelium, mitoses within lower two thirds, usually abnormal

VIN 3
  Severe dysplasia; more than lower two thirds occupied by abnormal epithelium, mitoses throughout epithelium, usually abnormal
  VIN-3–carcinoma in situ; full-thickness/nearly full-thickness epithelial abnormality

Physical Signs

Clinical manifestations are highly variable. Lesions can be papular with rough surfaces resembling genital warts, or they may be macular with indistinct or irregular borders. Lesions with micropapillary or granular surfaces reflect underlying acanthosis. Pigmentation yielding brown or black lesions is common. White lesions reflect underlying hyperkeratosis and are commonly seen in the keratinized portion of the vulva. Diffuse erythematosus and vulval ulceration have been described. Recognition is facilitated by the application of 2% to 5% acetic acid to the vulva. After 3 to 4 minutes some VIN lesions become colposcopically detectable. Acetic acid should not be applied to areas of ulceration or excoriation.

Distribution of VIN; Associated Lesions

There is no site of predilection for VIN. Lesions can occur in hair-bearing and nonhairy skin. In hairy skin, underlying sebaceous glands or dermal hair follicles can be involved. Most lesions (approximately 60%) involve nonhairy skin exclusively (4,5). The most common site for VIN is the posterior one third of the medial aspect of the labium minus extending to the frenulum of the fourchette. It is unusual to find VIN solely in hair-bearing areas (6). VIN lesions may be unifocal (33%) or multifocal (66%). Multifocal disease is the norm in women under 40

years old (7–9). Unifocal lesions are more common in postmenopausal women (10).

Contiguous structures—the anus (22%), the clitoral glans (18%), and the vagina (10%)—are commonly involved (11). Abell and Gosling (12) highlighted the frequency of multicentric neoplastic disease in the lower genital tract, postulating a "common field of reaction . . . to either hormonal or infectious agents." CIN can be found in approximately one third and condylomas in one half of women with VIN (6).

Diagnosis

VIN is diagnosed by microscopy and therefore a biopsy is always required. Biopsies can be performed under local anesthesia. Discomfort during infiltration of a local anesthetic can be avoided by prior application of lidocaine–prilocaine hydrochloride (Emla) cream. Small biopsy samples can be taken using a cervical punch forceps, a "Keyes punch," or a scalpel. Preliminary infiltration with local anesthetic elevates the skin off underlying tissues and makes the biopsy specimen easier to take.

Colposcopy

Colposcopic examination is of uncertain value in the assessment of VIN and early invasive lesions of the vulva. Labial epithelium is thick, cornified, and often hyperkeratotic, rendering the underlying terminal vasculature invisible. Only on the medial aspect of the labia minora and in the region of the urethral orifice is the vascular pattern clearly visible, and in these areas mosaicism and punctation are easily recognized. Inflammation and microulceration due to scratching can produce acetowhitening and obscure the colposcopic picture of VIN. VIN involvement of hair follicles cannot be identified colposcopically.

Use of toluidine blue, a nuclear stain, has been recommended (13). False-positive results occur with acute excoriative lesions, and false-negative results with hyperkeratotic lesions (14). With these reservations, staining with toluidine blue has the capacity for defining abnormal areas for further assessment by biopsy. Colposcopy may be helpful in the identification of early invasive lesions devoid of hyperkeratosis, where irregularities of the surface epithelium and abnormal vascular patterns are recognizable. Areas suspicious of invasion should be excised.

Thorough assessment of the whole lower genital tract, including cervical cytology and colposcopy, is mandatory for patients with VIN.

Circumstances where excisional biopsy rather than limited sampling should be considered are as follows:

1. Elevated lesions, irregular surfaces
2. Areas with distinct vascular patterns, for example, mosaic, abnormal vessels
3. Excessive hyperkeratosis in hair-bearing areas
4. Pigmented lesions
5. Elderly women with unifocal lesions

Is the Incidence Increasing?

VIN is uncommon although it is believed that its incidence is increasing, particularly in young women. It is not unusual to see women in their 20s with VIN and it is described in prepubertal girls with a history of sexual abuse. The U.S. Third National Cancer Survey (15) estimated the incidence rate for vulvar carcinoma in situ to be 0.53/100,000 white women based on a sample of 157 reported cases. Reported increases may be due solely to increased awareness mediated through more widespread application of colposcopy.

Etiology

There are strong associations between sexually transmitted diseases and VIN. The most commonly associated are condyloma, herpes simplex, gonorrhea, syphilis, trichomoniasis, and *Gardnerella vaginalis* infection. It seems likely, given the available evidence, that human papillomavirus (HPV) is of overriding etiologic significance.

Women with clinical condyloma and those with a marked koilocytosis are significantly younger than those with little or no koilocytosis. Hence, two populations distinguishable by age may be affected by VIN (16,17). The potential for malignant progression appears much lower for the younger age group.

In situ hybridization and the polymerase chain reaction have identified HPV-DNA (predominantly HPV-16) in 43% to 79% of lesions and commonly patients with HPV-positive lesions are found to be younger than those with virus-negative lesions (18–20). HPV was present in 61% of vulval malignancies associated with VIN 3 but in only 13% of tumors without VIN

3, whereas no HPV-DNA was detected in the vulvar tissues of 101 normal control subjects (21). HPV was found more often in young women with multifocal disease and VIN 3–associated tumors. This supports the concept of a subset of vulval malignancies preceded by VIN with HPV as a major associated factor in carcinogenesis (21,22). Therefore, squamous carcinomas of the vulva appear to be etiologically diverse, with a small proportion being HPV related. Histologic subtypes of invasive disease are described (21); basaloid and warty subtypes showing a strong association with HPV, young age, VIN 3, and metachronous squamous lesions; the common type of well-differentiated keratinizing squamous carcinoma, usually seen in older women, is associated with adjacent squamous hyperplasia but not HPV. Such findings suggest that VIN is a precursor of basaloid and warty carcinomas and HPV appears to have a role in the development of these tumors. Buscema et al (14) noted that on analyzing invasive cancers, only one fourth to one third showed evidence of classic VIN in adjacent epithelium (14), while more than 50% were associated with vulvar nonneoplastic disorders, that is, lichen scle-rosus and squamous hyperplasia. Again, this implies that many invasive lesions do not evolve from long-standing preinvasive lesions and there may be two varieties of vulval cancer:

1. Negatively associated with VIN or HPV and positively associated with nonneoplastic inflammatory conditions such as lichen sclerosus (23)
2. Positively associated with smoking, HPV, young age, and related VIN 3 (24,25)

The likely pathogenetic mechanism appears to be via integration of HPV-DNA into the host genome, resulting in insertional mutagenesis and interference with normal function of the tumor suppressor gene.

Smokers are at higher risk of developing VIN and invasive carcinoma (25,26).

Natural History

There has been no comprehensive study of the behavior of VIN, and therefore there are no accepted rates of progression or regression.

The natural history of VIN 1 and 2 lesions is poorly documented, and most information on VIN derives from retrospective studies of vulvar carcinoma in situ.

Regression of VIN can occur. In 1980, Friedreich et al (11) reported regression in 5 of 9 untreated patients with VIN 3, and of those in whom regression occurred, 4 (80%) were pregnant when diagnosed. In 1983 Bernstein et al (8) observed that in 5 of 13 patients with VIN 3, the lesion regressed within 6 months. Regression is most likely to occur in young women with multifocal disease.

The risk of invasive disease after the diagnosis of VIN is small and impossible to quantify precisely. The clinician needs to be aware that there are caveats associated with any data suggesting progression rates for VIN. Hence, it is not possible to say with 100% certainty whether preinvasive changes "progressed" or early invasive lesions were overlooked or occurred de novo after treatment. Studies have indicated that in 6% to 9% of patients whose diagnosis was based on a limited biopsy, subsequent excisional treatments confirmed the presence of early invasion (11,27–29).

Secondly, it is impossible to calculate the risk associated with any particular VIN 3 lesion as it appears that the risk is governed by the circumstances under which it occurs. For instance, VIN is usually multicentric, yet patients with this subtype of disease are usually 30 years younger than patients with invasion (18). Moreover, unifocal disease is associated with a higher risk of progression. In a recent retrospective series of 60 patients, 57 (95%) of whom had prior treatment, invasive disease subsequently developed in 3 (5%) (4) after a mean follow-up of 31 months. The subjects who developed invasive disease were 58, 69, and 74 years old. The most comprehensive follow-up of VIN 3 to date concerned 83 women whose management was reviewed retrospectively over an observation period of 32 years (30). The majority of women (90.6%) were treated by either surgery or laser vaporization. In 4 patients in the treated group, the disease progressed to invasion. Of these, 1 was immunosuppressed; the remaining 3 were over 40 years old when diagnosed. Invasion developed at intervals varying between 7 and 18 years after treatment. Eight women with VIN 3 were untreated, and 7 developed invasive disease at intervals of 2 to 8 years after the initial diagnosis (median interval, 5 years). However, in this subgroup of 7 patients, 5 had a previously diagnosed invasive cancer of the lower genital tract (cervix or vagina) and 4 had received radiotherapy. One other woman had multifocal lower genital tract intraepithelial neoplasia (30).

The precise relationship between VIN and invasion remains obscure. An increased risk of invasive disease is associated with postmenopausal presentation and unifocal lesions (10,17). VIN and invasive cancer may not necessarily be causally related conditions, but could represent differing responses to an identical stimulus that leads to invasive neoplasia in the older woman or a field effect of intraepithelial change in the younger woman in response to viral infection (28).

For the practicing clinician, these observations indicate that management should be individualized when a woman presents with VIN. Some helpful indicators are described below.

Age

The risk of invasion seems largely to be restricted to those patients who are over 45 years old (4,11,14,17,20).

Immunosuppression

Those with evidence of immunosuppression, that is, patients with renal transplants, systemic lupus erythematosus, immunoproliferative disorders, Fanconi's anemia, Sjögren's syndrome, lymphoma, or human immunodeficiency virus (HIV) infection, seem to be at higher risk of invasive disease (17,31,32). Immunocompromised patients have a higher than expected incidence of neoplasms and HPV-induced lesions (33,34). It is likely that immunosuppression is associated with an increased burden of sexually acquired infectious agents. The precise size of the risk is impossible to define.

Multifocal Lower Genital Tract Neoplasia

Those who have multifocal lower genital tract neoplasia (i.e., not merely multifocal vulvar disease), either invasive or preinvasive, seem to be at higher risk of vulval invasion (30,35).

Management

The above-mentioned observations have justified an increasingly conservative approach to the management of this condition in young women (Table 26-2). There have been no randomized prospective comparisons of any treatment modality to guide the clinician. A problem arises when VIN is detected in asymptomatic young patients. It is difficult to justify interven-

T A B L E **26-2**

Management Decisions in Vulvar Intraepithelial Neoplasia

The following may provide guidance on individualization of management in certain patients. It is not meant to represent an absolute protocol.

Factors favoring a policy of:

OBSERVATION	TREATMENT
Asymptomatic	Distressing symptoms
Age <40 yrs	Age >40 yrs
Multifocal disease	Unifocal disease
Pregnant when diagnosed	Evidence of chronic
Short-term reversible	immunosuppression
immunosuppression	(see text)
Unfit/poor general	Previous LGT
condition	neoplasia/CIN
Reassuring colposcopic	Colposcopic suspicion
findings	of invasion
Likely to attend follow-up	Problems achieving
Ability to accurately	follow-up
document lesion	
characteristics, e.g.,	
photography	

LGT = lower genital tract; CIN = cervical intraepithelial neoplasia.

tion because the risk of invasion is extremely small, and VIN is notoriously liable to recur despite treatment. Recurrence rates of up to 84% have been reported (20). The performance of radical procedures offers no guarantee against recurrence or development of invasion. In 1984, Wolcott and Gallup (36) reported that 21.1% of patients had recurrent disease after simple vulvectomy for VIN. Early invasive disease subsequently developed in 2 of 4 patients with VIN treated by simple vulvectomy (20).

Who Should Be Treated?

Under certain specified circumstances it is permissible to observe VIN in anticipation of regression, for example, in young women who are pregnant when diagnosed. In this situation, VIN is likely to have developed during a period of reversible immunosuppression. Hence, it is reasonable to observe the patient and defer any interventions until a postpartum reassessment has been made. In 1980, Friedreich and Wilkinson (11) observed that spontaneous regression occurred in 4 of 5 pregnant women with VIN who were followed prospectively.

Apart from these special circumstances, treatment of VIN is recommended, but this

should be individualized, taking into consideration the presence or absence of symptoms and whether risk factors are present, that is:

Postmenopausal presentation

Immunosuppression/immunodeficiency

Presence of histologically progressive lesions on serial biopsy

Excessively hyperkeratotic lesions

In patients for whom the risk of invasion is thought to be low, and in those for whom colposcopy, biopsy, and histologic examination excluded malignancy, a form of treatment that avoids major mutilating surgery should be selected.

Treatment Techniques

Treatment techniques for VIN include vulvectomy (37), skinning vulvectomy and split skin graft to the denuded site (38), wide local excision (39), topical 5-fluorouracil (40), dinitrochlorobenzene (41), cryosurgery (39), carbon dioxide laser ablation (42), ultrasonic aspiration (43), and topical interferon alfa gel (44).

Radical surgery is rarely employed because it is disfiguring, invariably results in impairment of sexual function, and produces serious psychological sequelae. Skinning vulvectomy carries with it the need to remove a graft from the thigh or buttock. In 1987, Rettenmaier et al (29) reported a recurrence rate of 27% after such surgery, and recurrence has been observed in grafted areas.

The results of 5-fluorouracil are disappointing. Persistence and recurrence of lesions are common, failure rates vary between 38% and 100%, and severe pain and itching frequently accompany treatment, often leading to discontinuation of therapy. Dinitrochlorobenzene is a topical immunotherapeutic agent which induces a delayed hypersensitivity response that may reverse vulvar atypia. Limited successes have been described. However, a high incidence of severe reactions often leads to discontinuation.

Interferons are cellular proteins that have an inhibitory effect on viral replication, and may therefore have a role in HPV-related disorders such as VIN. Twenty-one women, the majority of whom had previous treatment for VIN, were administered topical interferon alfa (44). Fifty percent showed a complete response and a further 28% showed a reduction in the size of the lesions. However, there was no untreated control group. Only 28% of patients reported minor discomfort in association with therapy, which was continued in all of them.

Carbon dioxide laser surgery for VIN is well described. After colposcopic assessment including biopsy, VIN can be localized and vaporized with preservation of as much normal tissue as possible.

Destruction of abnormal areas to a depth of 3 mm was initially advocated (42) but this was prior to any morphometric studies of the distribution of VIN into adnexal structures of the skin, that is, hair follicles, their associated sebaceous ducts, and eccrine sweat glands. There are practical difficulties in destroying the vulva to a predetermined depth. Multifocal lesions vary in thickness, making such an approach illogical (45). In 1985, Reid (46) advocated a technique of assessing depth of destruction during laser vulvectomy, by recognition of colposcopically identifiable surgical planes determined by the appearance of the tissue vaporized at that level. Tissue is destroyed to the third surgical plane, which constitutes the upper reticular dermis. This is the deepest level from which optimal healing will occur. Vaporization extending to a deeper level leads to a third-degree burn, with slow healing, fibrosis, and contracture.

None of the above recommendations were supported by systematic measurement of the depth of involvement of VIN lesions. In 1989, Shatz et al (5) measured the thickness of VIN lesions and the extent of involvement of VIN in the adnexal structures. This involvement consisted of extension into sebaceous glands (21%) and hair follicles (32%). For VIN in nonhairy skin, with the potential for extension into sebaceous glands, ablation to a 1-mm depth (below the surface of adjacent normal epithelium) will destroy in excess of 99% of these lesions without sacrificing the entire gland, the distal portion of which is rarely involved with VIN. Eradication of all sebaceous glands leads to dry skin and dyspareunia. In hairy skin, ablation to a depth of 2 mm will remove more than 99% of VIN that extends along hair follicles.

Small lesions can be dealt with on an outpatient basis using local anesthesia. Large areas of VIN require general anesthesia for laser treatment. The main disadvantage of laser therapy is postoperative pain. This can be managed with analgesics and the application of 5% lignocaine ointment. Urinary contamination of the area is prevented by suprapubic catheterization. Some advocate routine twice-daily application of silver sulfadiazine cream to the treated area. Success rates quoted for laser procedures vary from 90% to 97%, although multiple treatments were commonly required (7,42,47,48). Long-term follow-up studies are lacking.

Although use of lasers has been advocated for destructive therapy, lasers have generally been in declining use for the management of premalignancy in the United Kingdom since the early 1990s and there is no reason to believe that simpler and less-expensive destructive methods (e.g., ball-end electrocautery using a Valleylab Force 2 electrosurgical generator at 30 W, or simple point electrocautery) used in association with the above guidelines will be any less successful or be associated with higher morbidity.

Surgical management may still be appropriate for VIN, notably in middle-aged and elderly patients in whom the risk of invasion may dictate that a complete excision biopsy be done. Wide local excision of lesions can be performed, taking an 8-mm margin of normal tissue (36). Although recurrence rates may be higher than with radical surgery, recurrence can be managed with further conservative surgery, and the limited evidence available points to there being no excess risk of malignancy in patients managed this way (36). Procedures employing vaginal undercutting and advancement can be used simultaneously to cover denuded areas (49).

Histologic examination of the margins of resection is advocated. Recurrence seems less likely if lesions are excised completely (36). However, others (29) reported that recurrence rates were not related to surgical margins. Such "recurrences" could represent new disease in a susceptible patient.

Combination treatment, that is, excision of lesions in hair-bearing areas with laser destruction in non-hair-bearing areas, has been advocated (6). The argument is that in nonhairy areas, VIN is essentially a surface epithelial lesion that is easily destroyed, with good cosmetic and functional results. In hair-bearing areas, deeper destruction would sacrifice many adnexal structures, and there is a risk of failing to sample hyperkeratotic lesions adequately by directed biopsy. Conservative excision of VIN in these areas seems reasonable.

Paget's Disease of the Vulva

In 1874, Sir James Paget described the original cases of the disease bearing his name (50), which affected the nipple and areola and were associated with an underlying carcinoma of the breast. Extramammary Paget's disease (EMPD) is much rarer, arising from apocrine gland–bearing areas. While there are reports of disease affecting the axilla, umbilicus, and anus, the majority of cases of EMPD arise in the vulva and occur classically in white postmenopausal women. It is notable that in most women with mammary Paget's disease there is extension of cancer cells from an underlying mammary cancer via the lactiferous ducts (a phenomenon known as *epidermotropic metastasis*). However, the histogenesis of vulvar Paget's disease is more complex (51).

Histopathologic Features

There are usually "nests" of Paget's cells found close to the basal epithelial layer. The cells are large, pale, vacuolated, and oval, with large ovoid nuclei and abundant cytoplasm. Mitotic figures are rare. Paget's cells can also be found in hair follicles, apocrine and eccrine ducts, and sebaceous glands. Paget's cells may be seen distributed throughout the epithelium. Dermal invasion with Paget's cells, sometimes forming glandlike structures, has been described (51–54).

Immunohistochemistry may help when a differential diagnosis of Paget's disease and melanoma merits consideration. Paget's disease exhibits positive staining with periodic acid–Schiff (PAS) and alcian blue by staining intracytoplasmic mucin. In addition, Paget's cells fail to stain with S100 protein, but stain positively for carcinoembryonic antigen (CEA) (55,56).

Adnexal Involvement with Paget's Disease

Simple extension of Paget's cells into adnexal structures is a well-recognized phenomenon analogous to adnexal involvement with VIN, and should not be misdiagnosed as adnexal carcinoma (53,57,58). Adnexal involvement has been noted in 35% of patients with anogenital Paget's disease (57).

Histogenesis of Vulval Paget's Disease

Although the histogenesis of vulval Paget's disease is a complex and controversial subject, clinicians should have some understanding of this issue because it will facilitate the assess-

ment and management of women under their care.

The controversy relates to whether Paget's disease is a primary epithelial disturbance with the potential to invade or whether it represents secondary spread from an underlying adnexal or more remote adenocarcinoma. The short answer is that Paget's disease of the vulva can arise via both mechanisms, but the most common presentation is with intraepithelial disease.

Subjacent Apocrine Carcinoma

Paget's disease can be associated with a subjacent apocrine carcinoma. The true incidence of this association is disputed, but contemporary literature indicates that such an association is uncommon. In an early (1963) study of anogenital disease in both men and women (57), evidence of apocrine cancer was found in 32.5%. In 1975, Creasman et al (59) reported on 15 patients with vulval Paget's disease. Adenocarcinoma was present in the subjacent tissues in 5 (33%) yet other authors found no evidence of subjacent carcinoma (60–63).

In patients with subjacent apocrine cancer, Paget's disease results from epidermotropic spread. This is also the mechanism by which adjacent organ cancers manifest cutaneous Paget's disease.

The Invasive Potential of Intraepithelial Paget's Disease

It seems likely that the majority of cases of Paget's disease are primary intraepithelial adenocarcinomas derived from pluripotential stem cells in the basal layers of the epidermis. Evidence relating to the invasive potential of the disease is increasing. Several authors (52–54,60,64) documented dermal invasion arising from intraepithelial disease. Some authors reported dermal invasion in association with inguinal node metastasis and death from disseminated carcinomatosis, suggesting that some invasive lesions may carry a poor prognosis (54,64). The incidence of progression from Paget's disease to invasion is unclear, although dermal invasion was reported in 20% of patients in one clinical series (53). There are no adequate data to guide the clinician on the risk of lymph node metastasis in association with dermal invasion, although the impression generated by the rather sparse literature is that the prognosis is likely to be poor (51,65).

Association with Other Malignancy

Paget's disease may also be a marker for invasive disease near to or remote from vulval epithelium and malignancy may be synchronous or metachronous in its occurrence. Helvig and Graham (57) recorded Paget's disease in 98 patients; in 25 the disease was associated with or preceded an invasive malignancy. While the most common association was with vulval subjacent/Bartholin gland cancers, of the more remote sites the breast was most common, followed by the vulva, cervix, and vagina. More recent opinions do not confirm such a high incidence of associated malignancy, but acknowledge that there is a rare association (66). Anorectal cancers have been reported in association with Paget's disease involving the perianal skin (67). Vulval Paget's disease has been associated with VIN (68), basal cell carcinoma of the skin, bladder cancer, and gallbladder cancer (62).

Incidence

In 1955, the accumulated world literature amounted to 23 cases (69). In a series from a tertiary referral center, one case of Paget's disease was found for every 53 vulval cancers (62).

Symptoms

Intense soreness and irritation are common, as is itching. The patient may have noticed the presence of a weepy lesion. Considerable delay in diagnosis is common, with the average interval from symptom onset to histologic diagnosis being 3 years (59,70).

Clinical Features

The clinical features can vary, and a firm diagnosis can only be made after microscopy of a representative biopsy specimen. The lesion is classically hyperemic, well demarcated, weepy, and moist. Patches of white (hyperkeratosis) alternate with raw reddened weepy areas, sometimes described as a "cake-icing" effect. The lesion may have focal areas of ulceration in addition to hyperkeratosis. The disease commonly begins in the hair-bearing areas of the vulva and is often multifocal. While Paget's disease is usually an intraepithelial lesion, evidence of thickening on palpation of the lesion may indicate the presence of a subjacent adenocarcinoma. It is not uncommon for Paget's disease to be initially misdiagnosed as eczema or chronic candidiasis. Eventually, vulval biopsy yields the diagnosis.

Management

Initial assessment should include a thorough examination to exclude carcinomas for which cutaneous Paget's disease may be a marker. Treatment of any invasive disease discovered during investigation naturally takes precedence over the treatment of Paget's disease itself. Hence, every woman should have a thorough pelvic and breast examination, and consideration should be given to cervical cytology/colposcopy, mammography, and sigmoidoscopy/barium studies.

Disease that is considered to be exclusively intraepithelial can be managed by wide local excision. More radical procedures than this offer no advantage when recurrence rates are assessed in relation to extent of surgery (70). The deep margins of the resection should reach subcutaneous fat, in view of possible adnexal involvement. Resection into the upper layer of subcutaneous fat should yield an operative specimen that is approximately 6 mm thick. Because Paget's cells can be found on microscopy more than 2 cm beyond the macroscopic extent of the lesion (71), a 2.5-cm margin of apparently normal skin beyond the margins of the visible Paget's disease should be obtained. Intraoperative assessment of surgical margins by frozen-section histology is an option (70). If the margins are positive for the disease, additional skin can be excised. However, frozen-section analysis reportedly has false-negative rates ranging between 25% and 43% (70,72,73) and marginal status is not predictive of disease recurrence (70,72,73), reported recurrence rates being of the order of 30% to 55% (57,58,73). There are data to support the contention that clinical assessment is no less efficient than frozen-section analysis for assessing the extent of Paget's disease (73). Thus, on the basis of this evidence it seems difficult to justify the extra costs incurred by frozen-section analysis. However, a randomized study has not been carried out. Preoperative intravenous injection of 2 mL of 10% fluorescein sodium has been advocated as a useful adjunct to facilitate decisions on the site of surgical margins. It is believed that the compound concentrates in dilated blood vessels underlying areas of Paget's disease. Subsequently, when viewed under ultraviolet light, a fluorescent area is demonstrated. A study of two patients reported 99.8% sensitivity and 98% specificity (74).

Even with wide local excision, large defects may be created and may require skin grafting. Grafted areas are not immune to recurrence.

The whole of the specimen removed should be subjected to detailed histopathologic assessment to exclude the presence of an underlying adenocarcinoma, to exclude dermal invasion, and to assess the surgical margins. Routine hematoxylin and eosin staining seems adequate for the latter purpose, as none of the immunocytochemical markers tested in this disease provide any additional sensitivity in identifying residual Paget's cells at the surgical margins (75).

The recurrence rate after treatment is of the order of 30% to 55% (57,58,73), and provided adenocarcinoma has been confidently excluded by primary therapy, management can be conservative, by wide local excision. The same surgical principles apply to the management of recurrent disease.

Women in whom an underlying adenocarcinoma is found should be managed in the same manner as any other woman with invasive vulvar carcinoma, that is, usually by radical vulvectomy and groin node dissection.

Pigmented Vulvar Lesions

Vulvar Intraepithelial Neoplasia 3

Pigmentation may arise from VIN 3, often clinically manifesting as multicentric pigmented Bowen's disease or bowenoid papulosis. In this clinical variant, there is often a uniform configuration of neoplastic cells. Melanin synthesis is increased in VIN 3, the excess melanin being extruded into the papillary dermis where it is phagocytosed by melanophages.

Melanoma or Its Precursors

Melanomas constitute 10% of all vulvar neoplasms. Of these, 10% may be nonpigmented.

Lesions usually arise in the non-hair-bearing areas, especially the labia minora and clitoris. Most vulval nevi show junctional activity and have the potential for malignancy. They should be removed prophylactically with a margin of normal skin. Features indicative of an increased possibility of malignant change are recent rapid growth, color change, bleeding or itching, diameter of lesion larger than 7 mm, and a family history of melanoma (76,77). Where disease has extended beyond the stage of melanoma in situ, prognosis is related to the depth of cutaneous invasion and tumor thickness (78–80).

REFERENCES

1. Wilkinson EJ, Kneale B, Lynch PJ. Report of the ISSVD Terminology Committee. *J Reprod Med* 1986;31:973–974.

2. Ridley M, Frankman O, Jones ISC, et al. New nomenclature for vulvar disease. Report of the committee on terminology. *Am J Obstet Gynecol* 1989;160:769.

3. Ferenczy A. Intraepithelial neoplasia of the vulva. In: Coppleson M, ed. *Gynaecologic oncology*, vol. 1. Edinburgh: Churchill Livingstone, 1992:443–456.

4. Barbero M, Micheletti L, Preti M, et al. Vulvar intraepithelial neoplasia. A clinicopathologic study of 60 cases. *J Reprod Med* 1990;35:1023–1028.

5. Schatz P, Bergeron C, Wilkinson EJ, et al. Vulvar intraepithelial neoplasia and skin appendage involvement. *Obstet Gynecol* 1989;74:769–774.

6. Wright VC, Chapman WP. Colposcopy of intraepithelial neoplasia of the vulva and adjacent sites. *Obstet Gynecol Clin North Am* 1993;20:231–253.

7. Townsend DE, Levine RU, Richart RM, et al. Management of vulvar intraepithelial neoplasia by carbon dioxide laser. *Obstet Gynecol* 1982; 60:49–52.

8. Bernstein SG, Kovacs BR, Townsend DE, Morrow CP. Vulvar carcinoma in-situ. *Obstet Gynecol* 1983;61:304–307.

9. Husseinzadeh N, Newman NJ, Wesseler TA. Vulvar intraepithelial neoplasia. A clinicopathological study of carcinoma in-situ of the vulva. *Gynecol Oncol* 1989;33:157–163.

10. Wilkinson EJ. Normal histology and nomenclature of the vulva, and malignant neoplasms including VIN. *Dermatol Clin* 1992;10:283–296.

11. Freidrich EG, Wilkinson EJ, Fu YS. Carcinoma in-situ of the vulva. A continuing challenge. *Am J Obstet Gynecol* 1980;136:830–838.

12. Abell MR, Gosling JRG. Intraepithelial and infiltrative carcinoma of the vulva; Bowens type. *Cancer* 1961;14:318–329.

13. MacLean AB, Reid WMN. Benign and premalignant disease of the vulva. *Br J Obset Gynaecol* 1995;102:359–363.

14. Buscema J, Woodruff JD, Parmley TH, Genandry R. Carcinoma in-situ of the vulva. *Obstet Gynecol* 1980;55:225–230.

15. Cutler S, Young J. *Third national cancer survey: incidence data.* National Cancer Institute monograph no. 41. 1975.

16. Crum CP, Fu FS, Levine RU, et al. Intraepithelial squamous lesions of the vulva: biologic and histologic criteria for the distinction of condylomas from vulvar intraepithelial neoplasia. *Am J Obstet Gynecol* 1982;144:77–83.

17. Crum CP, Liskow A, Petras P, et al. Vulvar intraepithelial neoplasia (severe atypia and carcinoma in situ). *Cancer* 1984;54:1429–1434.

18. Park JS, Jones RW, McLean MR, et al. Possible etiologic heterogeneity of vulvar intraepithelial neoplasia. A correlation of pathologic characteristics with human papillomavirus detection by in-situ hybridization and polymerase chain reaction. *Cancer* 1991;67:1599–1607.

19. Rusk D, Sutton GP, Look KY, Roman A. Analysis of invasive squamous cell carcinoma of the vulva and vulvar intraepithelial neoplasia for the presence of human papillomavirus DNA. *Obstet Gynecol* 1991;77:918–922.

20. Hording V, Dangaard S, Iversen AKN, et al. Human papillomavirus type 16 in vulvar carcinoma, vulvar intraepithelial neoplasia, and associated cervical neoplasia. *Gynecol Oncol* 1991; 42:22–26.

21. Hording U, Kringsholm B, Andreasson B, et al. HPV in vulvar squamous carcinoma and in normal vulvar tissues. A search for a possible impact of HPV on vulvar cancer prognosis. *Int J Cancer* 1993;55:394–396.

22. Andersen WA, Franquemont DW, Williams J, et al. Vulvar squamous cell carcinoma and papillomaviruses: two separate entities? *Am J Obstet Gynecol* 1991;165:329–336.

23. Neill SM, Leibowitch M, Pelisse M, Moyal-Barracco M. Lichen sclerosus, invasive squamous cell carcinoma and human papillomavirus. *Am J Obstet Gynecol* 1990;162:1633–1634.

24. Liao SY, Wilczynski SP, Bloss JD, et al. Clinical and histologic features of vulvar carcinomas analyzed for HPV status. *Lab Invest* 1990;335A.

25. Brinton LA, Nasca PC, Mallin K, et al. Case control study of cancer of the vulva. *Obstet Gynecol* 1990;75:859–866.

26. Wilkinson EJ, Cook JC, Friedrich EG, Massey JK. Vulvar intraepithelial neoplasia, association with cigarette smoking. Colposc Gynecol Laser Surg 1988;4:143–145.

27. Collins CG, Roman-Lopez JJ, Lee FY. Intraepithelial carcinoma of the vulva. *Am J Obstet Gynecol* 1970;108:1187–1191.

28. Woodruff JD, Julian C, Puray T, et al. The contemporary challenge of carcinoma in situ of the vulva. *Am J Obstet Gynecol* 1973;115:677–68.

29. Rettenmaier MA, Berman ML, DiSaia PJ. Skinning vulvectomy for the treatment of multifocal vulval intraepithelial neoplasia. *Obstet Gynecol* 1987;69:247–250.

30. Jones RW, Rowan DM. Vulvar intraepithelial neoplasia III: a clinical study of the outcome in 113 cases with relation to the later development of invasive vulvar carcinoma. *Obstet Gynecol* 1994;84:5, 741–745.

31. Choo YC. Invasive squamous carcinoma of the vulva in young patients. *Gynecol Oncol* 1982;13: 158–164.

32. Becagli L, Cadore L. Sjögren's syndrome and vulvar cancer. *Clin Exp Obstet Gynecol* 1987;14: 69–71.

33. Koranda FC, Dehmel EM, Kahn G, Penn I. Cutaneous complications in immunosuppressed renal homograft recipients. *JAMA* 1974;229: 419–424.

34. Marshburn PB, Trofatter KF. Recurrent condyloma acuminatum in women over age 40; association with immunosuppression and malignant disease. *Am J Obstet Gynecol* 1988;159:429–433.

35. Jones RW, McLean MR. Carcinoma in situ of the vulva: a review of 31 treated and five untreated cases. *Obstet Gynecol* 1986;68:499–503.

36. Wolcott HD, Gallup DG. Wide local excision in the treatment of vulvar carcinoma in situ: a reappraisal. *Am J Obstet Gynecol* 1984;150:695–698.

37. Parry-Jones E. The management of premalignant and malignant conditions of the vulva. *Clin Obstet Gynecol* 1976;3:217–227.

38. Rutledge F, Sinclair M. Treatment of intraepithelial carcinoma of the vulva by skin excision and graft. *Am J Obstet Gynecol* 1968;102:806–818.

39. Forney JP, Morrow CP, Townsend DE, DiSaia PJ. Management of carcinoma in situ of the vulva. *Am J Obstet Gynecol* 1977;127:801–806.

40. Carson TE, Hoskins WJ, Wurzel JF. Topical 5-fluorouracil in the treatment of carcinoma in situ of the vulva. *Obstet Gynecol* 1976;47(suppl):59–62.

41. Weintraub I, Lagasse LD. Reversibility of vulvar atypia by DNCB-induced delayed hypersensitivity. *Obstet Gynecol* 1973;41:195–199.

42. Baggish MS, Dorsey JH. CO_2 laser for the treatment of vulvar carcinoma in situ. *Obstet Gynecol* 1981;57:371–375.

43. Rader JS, Leake JF, Dillon MB, Rosenhein NB. Ultrasonic surgical aspiration in the treatment of vulvar disease. *Obstet Gynecol* 1991;77:573–576.

44. Spirtos NM, Smith LH, Teng NNH. Prospective randomized trial of topical alfa-interferon (alfa-interferon gels) for the treatment of vulvar intraepithelial neoplasia III. *Gynecol Oncol* 1990; 37:34–38.

45. Dorsey J. Skin appendage involvement and vulval intraepithelial neoplasia. In: *Gynaecological laser surgery. Proceedings of the 15th study group of the RCOG. October 1985*. Ithaca, NY: Perinatology Press, 1985:193–195.

46. Reid R. Superficial laser vulvectomy; a new surgical technique for appendage conserving ablation of refractory condylomas and vulvar intraepithelial neoplasia. *Am J Obstet Gynecol* 1985;152:504–509.

47. Wright VC, Davies E. Laser surgery for vulval intraepithelial neoplasia; principles and results. *Am J Obstet Gynecol* 1987;156:374–378.

48. Ferenczy A. Using the laser to treat vulvar condylomata acuminata and intradermal neoplasia. *Can Med Assoc J* 1983;128:135–137.

49. Singer A, Monahan JM. Vulvar intraepithelial neoplasia. In: *Lower genital tract pre cancer*. Oxford: Blackwell Scientific, 1994:214–218.

50. Paget J. On disease of mammary areola preceding cancer of mammary gland. *St Bartholomew Hosp Rep* 1874;10:86–94.

51. Evans AT, Neven P. Invasive adenocarcinoma arising in extramammary Paget's disease of the vulva. *Histopathology* 1991;18:355–360.

52. Parmley TH, Woodruff JD, Julian CG. Invasive vulvar Paget's disease. *Obstet Gynecol* 1975;46: 341–346.

53. Jones RE, Austin C, Ackerman AB. Extramammary Paget's disease. A critical re-examination. *Am J Dermatopathol* 1979;1:101–132.

54. Feuer GA, Shevchuk M, Calanog A. Vulvar Paget's disease, the need to exclude an invasive lesion. *Gynecol Oncol* 1990;38:81–89.

55. Ohiji M, Furue M, Tamaki K. Serum carcinoembryonic antigen level in Paget's disease. *Br J Dermatol* 1984;110:211–213.

56. Furakawa F, Kashihara M, Miyauchi H, et al. Evaluation of carcinoembryonic antigen in extramammary Paget's disease. *J Cutan Pathol* 1984; 11:558–561.

57. Helvig EB, Graham JH. Anogenital (extramammary) Paget's disease. *Cancer* 1963;16:387–388.

58. Lee SC, Roth LM, Ehrlich C, Hall JA. Extramammary Paget's disease of the vulva. *Cancer* 1977;39:2540–2549.

59. Creasman WG, Gallagher HS, Rutledge F. Paget's disease of the vulva. *Gynecol Oncol* 1975;3:133–148.

60. Fenn ME, Morley GW, Abell MR. Paget's disease of the vulva. *Obstet Gynecol* 1971;38:660–670.

61. Fetherston WCC, Friedreich EG. The origin and significance of vulvar Paget's disease. *Obstet Gynecol* 1972;39:735.

62. Friedreich EG. Intraepithelial neoplasia of the vulva. In: Coppleson M, ed. *Gynecologic oncology; fundamental principles and clinical practice*. New York: Churchill Livingstone, 1981: 303.

63. Kaufmann RH, Boice EH, Knight WR. Paget's disease of the vulva. *Am J Obstet Gynecol* 1960; 79:451–453.

64. Hart WR, Millman JB. Progression of intraepithelial Paget's disease of the vulva to invasive carcinoma. *Cancer* 1977;40:233–237.

65. Fine BA, Fowler LJ, Valente PT, Gaudet T. Minimally invasive Paget's disease of the vulva with extensive lymph node metastases. *Gynecol Oncol* 1995;57:262–265.

66. DiSaia PJ, Creasman WJ. Invasive carcinoma of the vulva. In: *Clinical gynecologic oncology*. 4th ed. New York: Mosby Year Book, 1993:263–272.

67. Ferenczy A, Richart RM. Ultrastructure of perianal Paget's disease. *Cancer* 1972;20:1141–1149.

68. Hawley IC, Husain F, Pryse Davies J. Extramammary Paget's disease of the vulva with dermal invasion and vulval intraepithelial neoplasia. *Histopathology* 1991;18:374–376.

69. Woodruff JD. Paget's disease of the vulva. *Obstet Gynecol* 1955;5:175–179.

70. Bergen S, DiSaia PJ, Liao SY, et al. Conservative management of extramammary Paget's disease of the vulva. *Gynecol Oncol* 1989;33:151–156.

71. Adamsons K, Reisefield D. Observations on intradermal migration of Paget cells. *Am J Obstet Gynecol* 1964;90:1274.

72. Curtin PJ, Rubin SC, Jones WB, et al. Paget's disease of the vulva. *Gynecol Oncol* 1990;39:374–377.

73. Fishman DA, Setsuko K, Chambers MD, et al. Extramammary Paget's disease of the vulva. *Gynecol Oncol* 1995;56:266–270.

74. Misas JE, Cold CJ, Weley Hall F. Vulvar Paget disease; fluorescein aided visualisation of margins. *Obstet Gynecol* 1991;77:156–159.

75. Ganjei P, Gueraldo KA, Lampe B, Nadji M. Vulvar Paget's disease. Is immunohistochemistry helpful in assessing the surgical margins? *J Reprod Med* 1990;35:1002–1004.

76. Curtin JP, Morrow CP. Melanoma of the female genital tract. In: Coppleson M, ed. *Gynecologic oncology.* 2nd ed. Edinburgh: Churchill Livingstone, 1992:1059–1068.

77. Mackie RM. Clinical recognition of early invasive malignant melanoma. *BMJ* 1990;301:1005–1006.

78. Chung AF, Woodruff JM, Lewis TL. Malignant melanoma of the vulva: a report of 44 cases. *Obstet Gynecol* 1975;45:638–646.

79. Clark WH, From L, Bernardino EA, Mihm MC. The histogenesis and biological behaviour of primary human malignant melanomas of the skin. *Cancer Res* 1969;29:705–727.

80. Breslow A. Thickness, cross sectional areas, and depth of invasion in the prognosis of cutaneous melanoma. *Ann Surg* 1970;172:902–908.

CHAPTER 27

Vulvar Cancer

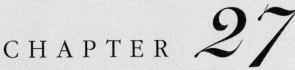

PETER T. GRANT
NEVILLE F. HACKER

he treatment of vulvar cancer has been the focus of considerable change over the past 10 to 15 years. It has evolved from a routine en bloc dissection of the vulvar tumor and inguinofemoral lymph nodes as described by Taussig (1) and Way (2), to individualized treatment for patients, often combining surgery, radiation therapy, and chemotherapy.

Many of the changes in management have resulted from an increasing awareness of the morbidity of standard therapy, both physical and psychological (3–5). Unlike other radical gynecologic procedures, the results of surgery are evident to the patient and her partner, and understandably profound psychosexual consequences can follow the treatment of vulvar cancer. The physical morbidity of conventional therapy is also significant, with rates of 40% to 85% for wound breakdown, 10% to 69% for chronic lymphedema, and 10% to 15% for recurrent lymphangitis or cellulitis, and an operative mortality of 1% to 2%.

The option of less radical surgery can be offered to the majority of patients with vulvar cancer without jeopardizing survival but at the same time reducing the morbidity previously associated with this disease (4,6–9).

Epidemiology

Until recently, vulvar cancer made up 3% to 5% of all gynecologic malignancies; however, this rate has now increased to nearly 8% (10). The incidence of vulvar cancer varies considerably from one country to another, but lies within the range of 0.5 to 3.0 cases/100,000 women-years (11). The majority (>85%) are squamous cell cancers, with melanoma making up approximately 5% to 6% of cases and Bartholin gland carcinoma 4% to 5% (11). Other malignancies on the vulva are rare (Table 27-1).

The association of vulvar cancer with medical disorders such as obesity, hypertension, cardiovascular disease, diabetes, and syphilis has been postulated but recent case-control studies did not confirm these as significant factors in the development of this disease (12–14). Sherman et al (15), in a case-control study of 330 patients with invasive or in situ lesions, confirmed that hormonal factors were not important in the development of vulvar cancer.

Other risk factors that have been identified include a history of genital warts, a history of cervical cancer, smoking, and immune suppression (16–18). Human papillomavirus (HPV)–DNA has been detected in many vulvar cancers, particularly in patients younger than 60 years (19–21). This younger group of patients typically have 1) HPV type 16 or 18 (in as many as 70% of patients), 2) associated vulvar intraepithelial neoplasia (VIN), 3) a high incidence of smoking, 4) a high incidence of cervical neoplasia, and 5) a lesion with a baseloid or warty histologic appearance.

The association of chronic pruritus and particularly lichen sclerosus with vulvar cancer is well documented but its relationship as a causal factor is unclear. The majority of vulvar cancers found in association with lichen sclerosus occur in older patients (>60 years), are likely to be HPV negative, and frequently do not demonstrate any VIN changes (16,21–23).

T A B L E   **27-1**

Vulvar Malignancy

Histologic Type	%
Squamous carcinoma	85
Melanoma	5–6
Bartholin gland carcinoma	4–5
Basal cell carcinoma	2–3
Adenocarcinoma (skin appendage, Paget's)	1–2
Sarcoma	1–2
Verrucous carcinoma	<1

T A B L E   **27-2**

Intraepithelial Neoplastic Disorders of Vulvar Skin

A. Squamous vulvar intraepithelial neoplasia (VIN)
    VIN 1 (formerly mild dysplasia)
    VIN 2 (formerly moderate dysplasia)
    VIN 3 (formerly severe dysplasia)
B. Nonsquamous intraepithelial neoplasia
    Paget's disease
    Tumors of melanocytes, noninvasive

The median age at the time of diagnosis of vulvar cancer is 60 to 65 years but most series report that at least 30% of cases will occur in women over 70 years old (16,24). Elliott et al (25) reported that the average age at diagnosis of vulvar cancer is falling and the condition is now being seen more frequently in women in their 20s and 30s (11,21).

T A B L E   **27-3**

Nonneoplastic Disorders of Vulvar Skin

Lichen sclerosus
Squamous hyperplasia (formerly hyperplastic dystrophy without atypia)
Other dermatoses

Preinvasive Disease

The classification of benign and preinvasive vulvar disease has been simplified by recent changes. In particular, the separation of vulvar dermatoses into those with and those without atypia no longer exists, as any vulvar skin condition with associated cellular atypia is now included under the classification VIN (Table 27-2).

Vulvar Intraepithelial Neoplasia

The true prevalence and incidence of VIN are unclear; however, it does appear to be increasingly recognized, particularly in young women. Sturgeon (11) reported a doubling in the incidence of VIN 3 between 1973 and 1987. The mean age at the time of diagnosis in series prior to 1975 was greater than 50 years while recent publications reported an average age of 35 to 38 years (21,24).

There is a strong association between cervical intraepithelial neoplasia (CIN), not necessarily a synchronous one, and the diagnosis of VIN. Campion et al (26) identified CIN in 40% of patients with VIN whereas other authors quoted figures as high as 75% to 80% (16,27). HPV type 16 and less frequently type 18 can be identified in 80% to 90% of VIN 3 lesions (28,29). VIN in older patients (>60 years) is more likely to be HPV negative, unifocal, and associated with lichen sclerosus (30,31). A history of genital warts is associated with a 15 times increase in the risk of VIN 3 and subsequent vulvar cancer (17).

The risk of progression of VIN 3 to invasive malignancy occurs in 5% to 10% of patients (21,28,32). These reports frequently included patients who were treated for VIN and then followed. Recently, Jones and Rowan (33) reported that 90% of a group of patients with untreated VIN 3 developed cancer within 8 years.

Vulvar Dystrophies

In 1987 the International Society for the Study of Vulvar Disease simplified the classification of vulvar dystrophies (Table 27-3). These are nonneoplastic epithelial disorders without any evidence of cellular atypia. If atypia is present, then the disorder should be classified as a VIN lesion. For many years, the presence or absence of atypia has confused the clinician's ability to determine the premalignant potential of vulvar dystrophies. Vulvar dystrophy has been associated with 60% to 100% of vulvar cancers but follow-up studies showed a low progression rate of lichen sclerosus to vulvar cancer (16,23). Overall, the rate of progression of lichen sclerosus would appear to be less than 5% (30,32).

Paget's Disease of the Vulva

Paget's disease of the vulva typically presents as an erythematous, eczematous eruption, often with areas of hyperkeratosis. Pruritus, vulvar pain, and burning are common symptoms and the average age at presentation ranges from 65 to 70 years (34,35). This slowly progressive intraepithelial neoplasm is characterized by large, clear, mucin-containing Paget's cells in the epidermis and is associated with an underlying skin adenocarcinoma in 20% to 25% of patients (21,35,36). A synchronous or metachronous carcinoma elsewhere in the genital tract, breast, or bowel is found in 20% to 30% of women with this disease, and 70% of women with Paget's disease involving the anal canal will have a rectal cancer (28,36,37).

Because of the significant incidence of underlying invasive adenocarcinoma, the optimal treatment is excision of the involved skin. The clinical limit of disease frequently underestimates the pathologic lateral extent to which Paget's cells can be found in the epidermis. Adamsons and Reisfield (38) found Paget's cells up to 2 cm beyond the clinical edge of the disease and numerous series reported recurrence rates of 12.5% to 40.0% (21,34,36,39). Recurrences of noninvasive Paget's disease tend to occur late and if small, may be treated by ablative means or re-excision.

Vulvar Squamous Cell Carcinoma

Clinical Presentation and Diagnosis

The typical presentation of a patient with vulvar cancer is the presence of a lump or ulcer that has often been associated with prolonged itching or vulval irritation. Presentation with symptoms of abnormal bleeding or discharge is infrequent, particularly as women are now presenting with disease at an earlier stage. Despite earlier presentation, there is still a mean delay of 10 months between the onset of symptoms and the diagnosis and this is often a physician-related delay (4). Clinical examination frequently reveals an exophytic, ulcerated area but condylomatous or hyperkeratotic lesions are also seen. The tumor is most commonly found on the labia majora but any region of the vulva can be involved and approximately 10% of vulvar cancers are multifocal (28,36,40).

The diagnosis is easily made where there is a typical raised, ulcerated lesion, providing the vulva is actually examined and a biopsy performed on any suspicious lesion. However, the diagnosis of early cancer in association with other underlying vulvar pathology such as condylomata and lichen sclerosus is often difficult to make.

Any vulvar lesion that has an atypical appearance requires a biopsy before treatment. To obtain a diagnosis, a wedge or punch biopsy of the vulvar lesion can usually be done under local anesthesia. For some small lesions, it may be appropriate to perform an excisional biopsy but generally a small diagnostic biopsy is preferable.

As part of the general assessment of a patient with vulvar cancer, a careful specimen for a Papanicolaou smear should be obtained from the endocervix and ectocervix and the cervix and vagina examined through a colposcope for any associated lower genital tract intraepithelial neoplasia.

Patterns of Spread

Vulvar cancer typically spreads by the following routes:

1. Direct growth to involve the vagina, urethra, anus, and other contiguous structures
2. Lymphatic spread to regional lymph glands
3. Hematogenous spread to distant sites, which is a late phenomenon

The lymphatic drainage of the vulva is an important factor to consider while planning treatment for patients with squamous cancer. The groin lymph nodes consist of two groups:

1. The superficial or inguinal group of lymph nodes lies above the fascia lata and cribriform fascia. They lie along the inguinal ligament and saphenous vein, but nodes are rarely found on the lateral 15% of the inguinal ligament. A recent study by Nicklin et al (41) using lymphangiography showed that the lateral extent of the superficial node dissection can be reduced by 15% to 20%, with a complete nodal clearance rate of 99.8% being achieved. This may be important in terms of further reducing the surgical morbidity encountered during treatment of this disease.
2. A femoral group of nodes lies within the fossa ovalis. This group usually consists of

one to four lymph glands and they lie on or medial to the femoral vein, cephalad to the distal margin of the fossa ovalis (42). This limits the dissection needed to remove the deep femoral nodes, and the fascia lata lateral to the fossa ovalis can be left intact (43).

The vulvar lymphatics run anteriorly, medial to the labiocrural fold, before turning laterally at the mons veneris to reach the inguinal lymph glands (44). Iversen and Aas (45) showed that lymphatic drainage from the clitoris and perineum is bilateral and that there is also significant bilateral flow from the anterior labium minus. They found no direct drainage from the vulva or clitoris to the pelvic lymph glands (45).

While it appears that the primary lymphatic drainage is to the superficial or inguinal group of glands, there does appear to be direct lymphatic drainage to the deep or femoral node group through the cribriform fascia. Involved femoral nodes without involvement of inguinal nodes has been reported and recurrence in the femoral glands where findings of an inguinal lymphadenectomy were previously negative has been frequently documented (46–50). Lymphatic mapping recently confirmed these observations (51).

The overall incidence of lymph node involvement in vulvar cancer is about 30% (52,53). Clinical evaluation of groin lymph nodes is inaccurate, as approximately 25% of clinically normal glands will have metastatic tumor present (53,54). Pelvic lymph node involvement occurs in about 10% of patients with vulvar cancer but is rare when there is no macroscopic nodal involvement or there are fewer than three nodes involved with microscopic tumor (53–56).

The major risk factor identified in many reports that predicts for inguinofemoral node involvement is depth of invasion (52–59) (Table 27-4). Sedlis et al (57) identified histologic

TABLE 27-4

Incidence of Positive Lymph Nodes Versus Depth of Invasion

Depth of Invasion (mm)	Positive Nodes (%)
<1	<1
1–3	10
3.1–5.0	25
>5	33

TABLE 27-5

Incidence of Lymph Node Metastases Versus Size of Lesion

Size of Lesion (cm)	Positive Nodes (%)
<1	5
1–2	15
2.1–4.0	30
>4	50

grade, capillary-like space invasion, clitoral or perineal location, and clinically suspicious nodes as other major risk factors. Binder et al (52) also showed that clinical tumor size is a significant predictor of lymph node involvement (Table 27-5).

Treatment

The introduction of en bloc radical vulvectomy and bilateral inguinofemoral lymphadenectomy resulted in a significant improvement in survival for patients with carcinoma of the vulva (1,2). However, as many patients (>50%) now present with stage I disease (Table 27-6), the routine use of this operation for all patients with vulvar cancer is unsatisfactory. Concerns about the long-term physical and psychosexual morbidity, together with a better understanding of the spread and recurrence patterns of vulvar cancer, have resulted in major treatment modifications over the past 15 years (3,60–63).

Early Vulvar Cancer (T1, N0-1)

In planning the treatment for a patient with vulvar cancer, it is necessary to consider the management of the primary lesion and the regional lymph nodes.

Primary Lesion The extent of vulvar excision for early cancers is largely determined by the size of the lesion and by the presence or absence of associated vulvar skin conditions. If the remainder of the vulva is healthy, then radical local excision of the lesion is appropriate but lateral and deep margins should be at least 10 mm (64–66). The local recurrence rates reported with either radical vulvectomy or radical local excision are very similar (6%–10%) (60,65,67–70).

If the vulvar cancer arises in association with widespread VIN or vulvar dystrophy, then

T A B L E   **27-6**

Revised FIGO Staging for Vulvar Cancer, 1988

FIGO Stage	TNM	Clinical/Pathologic Findings
Stage 0	Tis	Carcinoma in situ, intraepithelial carcinoma
Stage I	T1, N0, M0	Tumor confined to the vulva or perineum, <2 cm in greatest dimension, nodes are negative
Ia		Invasion not >1 mm
Ib		Invasion >1 mm
Stage II	T2, N0, M0	Tumor confined to the vulva and/or perineum, >2 cm in greatest dimension, nodes are negative
Stage III	T3, N0, M0	Tumor of any size with
	T3, N1, M0	1. Adjacent spread to the lower urethra or the anus
	T1, N1, M0	2. Unilateral regional lymph node metastasis
	T1, N1, M0	
Stage IVa	T1, N2, M0	Tumor invades any of the following:
	T2, N2, M0	Upper urethra, bladder mucosa, rectal mucosa, pelvic bone, or bilateral regional nodes
	T3, N2, M0	
	T4, N0–2, M0	
Stage IVb	T1–4, N0–2, M1	Any distant metastases including pelvic lymph nodes

a radical vulvectomy may be appropriate. However, it is often possible, even in these situations, to perform a radical local excision of the cancer and treat the remaining nonmalignant skin condition appropriately.

Surgical Technique The skin incision margin should extend at least 10 mm beyond the tumor and the deep margin should extend to the inferior fascia of the urogenital diaphragm. Lesions adjacent to the urethra can be removed by mobilizing and resecting the lower 1 cm of the urethra without affecting continence. For perineal lesions that extend onto or near the anus, preoperative or postoperative radiotherapy may be considered in order to allow more conservative resection margins and preservation of normal anal function.

Anterior lesions involving or adjacent to the clitoris present a problem in that resection of the clitoris will have major effects on sexual function. Alternative management strategies such as combining local radiotherapy, either teletherapy or interstitial therapy, with conservative resection of any remaining skin abnormality may allow preservation of normal anatomy.

Management of Groin Lymph Nodes The use of separate groin incisions has significantly reduced the incidence of wound breakdown, which was seen in more than 50% of patients treated with the traditional en bloc procedure (1,2,71). Unfortunately, the problems associated

with leg edema still persist but modifications to the extent of dissection in the groin may reduce this complication (41).

Despite the complications associated with inguinofemoral node dissection, it is an essential part of treatment for most squamous cancers of the vulva. The only T1 vulvar cancer with a negligible risk of involved lymph nodes is that with a depth of invasion of less than 1 mm, and it is only in these patients that a lymphadenectomy can be omitted. If a biopsy shows less than 1-mm invasion, then the entire lesion needs to be excised to accurately define the depth of tumor. Wilkinson et al (72) proposed that depth of invasion should be measured from the most superficial dermal papilla adjacent to the tumor to the deepest point of invasion. Many reports quote tumor thickness rather than depth of invasion and the estimated difference between the two measures is 0.3 mm (25,40).

Lateral lesions are suitable for ipsilateral lymph node dissection as the incidence of contralateral lymph node involvement in T1 lesions is less than 1% (50,55,68,73,74). In patients with clitoral, midline perineum, or anterior labium minus lesions, both inguinofemoral lymph node areas should be dissected because of the bilateral lymphatic drainage that has been identified from these regions (44).

Berman et al (67) recommended that a superficial inguinal lymph node dissection is sufficient for T1 lesions with no clinically suspicious nodes. However, there have been several reports of recurrences in the groin of patients who had undergone superficial node dissection only, the findings of which were negative (48,49,75). Stehman et al (50), in a Gynecologic Oncology Group study, found that 9 of 121 patients with negative superficial lymph nodes had a recurrence in the groin. Therefore, if node dissection is indicated, it should be a thorough inguinofemoral lymphadenectomy (76,77). The mortality rate associated with recurrence in an undissected groin is 90% (78).

Technique for Groin Dissection An oblique incision is made just above or below the groin crease down to the level of the superficial (Camper's) fascia. The fascia is carefully mobilized from the overlying subcutaneous tissue from the incision to the apex of the femoral triangle and superiorly to 1 to 2 cm above the inguinal ligament. In the lateral extent of the dissection, the outer 15% to 20% of the tissue

FIGURE 27-1

Inguinofemoral lymph nodes. Dissection of the superficial node group extends from just above the inguinal ligament to the apex of the femoral triangle. The lateral 15% to 20% of the inguinal area is left intact. The deep node group lies within the fossa ovalis. The inguinal ligament forms the superior border of the femoral triangle. The saphenous vein runs through the superficial node group and then through the cribriform fascia to the femoral vein. It may be left intact.

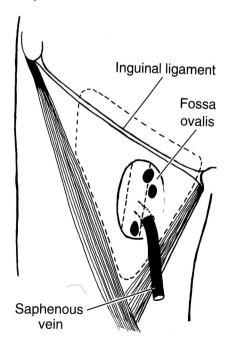

Inguinal ligament

Fossa ovalis

Saphenous vein

between the pubic tubercle and anterior superior iliac spine should be left undissected (Fig. 27-1). The saphenous vein should be identified coursing through the superficial fat and nodal tissue and can be preserved or ligated near the apex of the femoral triangle. Once the superficial nodal tissue is freed from the subcutaneous fat, it is then mobilized on its deep margin from the fascia lata, which remains intact. The fossa ovalis and cribriform fascia can then be identified and the small group of deep inguinal (femoral) nodes removed medial to the femoral vein. If needed, the saphenous vein can be ligated where it joins the femoral vein (Fig. 27-2).

A suction drain is routinely placed under the skin flap and postoperatively low-dose heparin is administered and pneumatic calf compression maintained to reduce the incidence of deep venous thrombosis. To prevent lymphocysts from forming in the groin, a soft gauze roll can be taped over the femoral triangle to maintain pressure between the superficial fascia and the fascia lata (79).

T2 and T3 Vulvar Cancer

Radical vulvectomy and bilateral groin lymph node dissection using a traditional en bloc resection with a butterfly-type incision has been regarded as standard therapy for T2 and some T3 tumors. While radical local excision achieves equivalent local control rates in T1 tumors, whether or not this approach is appropriate for these larger lesions has not been clear. Modified radical resection for larger vulvar tumors still requires surgical margins of at least 10 mm and must extend down to the deep fascia. Tumor involvement of the distal urethra does not preclude resection, as up to 1 cm of the mobilized urethra can be removed without compromising continence.

Siller et al (64) reported on 27 patients with T2-3 tumors treated by radical vulvectomy and separate groin incisions and showed no difference in local recurrence rates and overall survival when compared to 20 patients who were treated by conventional surgery. Hacker et al (4) treated a similar group of 51 patients with advanced disease using the triple-incision technique and no patient developed an isolated skin bridge recurrence. Burke et al (48) treated 43 women with T2 tumors by radical local excision and inguinal node dissection. Nine had recurrence on the vulva. All were controlled by

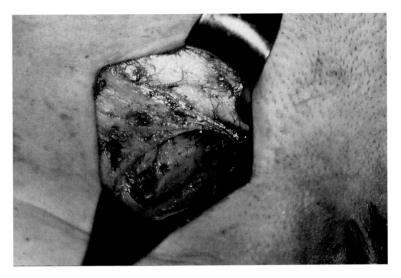

FIGURE **27-2**
Groin lymph node dissection. Groin anatomy following the removal of superficial and deep inguinofemoral lymph nodes. The fascia lata is intact and the fossa ovalis cleared of nodal tissue. The long saphenous vein has been ligated and excised.

further local excision. The postoperative morbidity reported for the modified vulvar resection and separate groin incision is significantly less than that seen with the conventional en bloc resection (4,70).

For patients with a T2 and some with T3 vulvar cancers and otherwise normal vulvar skin, a modified radical vulvectomy and separate inguinofemoral lymphadenectomy would appear to offer equivalent tumor control with significant reduction in morbidity.

Radical Vulvectomy: Surgical Technique
Typically the incision for a radical vulvectomy starts over the mons pubis, extending laterally in an arc to enter the labiocrural fold on each side and then continuing across the perineum. For large lesions the lateral line of the incision may need to be widened to ensure an adequate (>10mm) tumor-free margin. The incision needs to be carried down to the fascia over the pubic symphysis anteriorly and then down to the deep fascia in each labiocrural fold. Some branches of the pudendal vessels posteriorly may need to be individually ligated but the remaining lateral dissection can be achieved using diathermy. The bulbocavernosus muscles and clitoral crura need to be identified and ligated where they pass under the pubic symphysis.

The inner or medial margin again needs to be fashioned to ensure adequate tumor clearance. For lesions encroaching on the lower vagina or urethra, mobilization of these structures is essential and if necessary some of the distal urethra can be removed. Dividing the

vulvar bridge posteriorly will often allow more accurate and easier fashioning of the medial resection margins.

When one is closing vulvar defects, it is essential that the epithelial edges be opposed without tension and that there is adequate hemostasis. Lateral skin margins can be undermined along the plane of the deep fascia to achieve this tension-free closure but on occasions the defect is too large to close primarily and other techniques need to be used. Some of the more commonly used techniques for vulvar reconstruction are as follows:

1. Full-thickness skin flaps such as a rhomboid flap are particularly useful in closing the posterior vulva, or perineal defects (80).
2. Myocutaneous grafts that bring in vascularized pedicles are occasionally required to bridge large anterior and lateral vulval defects or to close areas previously treated with radiotherapy. The most frequently used grafts utilize the gracilis, rectus abdominis, or tensor fascia lata muscles (81–83).

Locally Advanced Vulvar Cancer
(Large T3 or T4)

Locally advanced squamous carcinoma of the vulva has usually been treated by radical surgical procedures that frequently require the creation of one or more stomas. Overall survival rates have been poor, with only 37% of patients with clinical stage III and 21% with stage IV disease surviving 5 years (84,85). Even with highly selected patients undergoing exenterative therapy for T3 or T4 tumors, survival rates range from 40% to 60% (86–88). Operative mortality rates of up to 10% have been reported in what is usually an elderly group of patients, and postoperative morbidity is significant (89,90).

Following the initial reports of Boronow (91), a combined radiotherapy-surgical approach for these locally advanced vulvar cancers is now recommended. He initially recommended treatment with brachytherapy and then radical vulvectomy, but subsequently modified this to external-beam radiotherapy and then limited excision of the vulvar tumor bed (92,93). Boronow reported a 5-year survival rate for the treatment of primary disease of 75.6% and a recurrence rate of 62.6%. Hacker et al (94) reported the use of preoperative external-beam radiotherapy and local excision of the tumor bed; no patient developed a fistula and 50% had no evidence of persisting tumor in the vulvar skin following excision of the tumor bed. Similar changes in the management of squamous cancer of the anus have resulted in abdominoperineal resection being reserved for salvage therapy in this disease (95). Survival and local control rates with chemoradiotherapy are better than those achieved with primary surgery (96).

Patients with advanced vulvar cancer should initially undergo a bilateral groin dissection to determine the status of the lymph nodes. If the results are negative, the inguinofemoral area may be omitted from the radiation fields. If there are bulky, positive nodes, the enlarged nodes should be removed and the groin and pelvis then included in the treatment fields (97). Over the last decade, many investigators also reported on the use of chemoradiotherapy (98–100). Whether this improves local control or survival compared to preoperative radiotherapy alone is unclear. The addition of chemotherapy certainly increases the acute vulvar morbidity and a 1- to 2-week break in the treatment is almost invariably required. The use of radiotherapy or chemoradiotherapy alone is associated with a local recurrence rate of up to 50% (99).

Preoperative radiotherapy with or without concurrent chemotherapy should be regarded as the treatment of choice for patients with locally advanced vulvar cancer who would otherwise require some form of exenterative surgery.

Management of Patients with Positive Groin Nodes

The presence of inguinofemoral lymph node metastases has been identified as the most important determinant of survival in patients with vulvar cancer. These patients usually fall into one of two groups:

1. Those with microscopically positive groin nodes found after complete inguinofemoral node resection
2. Those with macroscopically involved nodes evident before or during surgery

Patients with one microscopically positive lymph node would appear not to require adjuvant radiotherapy to the groin and pelvis (73,101). Survival rates of 80% to 94% have been observed in this group of patients (68,73). The Gynecologic Oncology Group performed a randomized study of either ipsilateral pelvic lymphadenectomy or groin and pelvic radiotherapy for patients with positive groin nodes. Compared to pelvic lymphadenectomy, postoperative radiotherapy resulted in improved survival and a reduced incidence of groin recurrence for patients with more than one microscopically involved node (102).

Van der Velden et al (103) identified extracapsular tumor in lymph nodes as a major predictor of survival, independent of the number of nodes involved. They reported that 9 (55%) of 16 patients with a single positive node and extracapsular tumor died of recurrent disease. There are no studies as yet to show whether adjuvant therapy will influence survival when extracapsular tumor has been found, but it is logical to add radiation therapy, as many of the recurrences are in the groin.

Henderson et al (104) reported on 91 patients treated with ilioinguinal irradiation instead of groin dissection for N0 and N1 tumors. There were no recurrences within the treatment field. A similar Gynecologic Oncology Group study, however, showed a significant frequency (5/27) of groin recurrence in patients receiving radiotherapy, which resulted in early closure of the trial (105). It has since been identified that the dose of radiotherapy to the lymph nodes was subtherapeutic, and therefore, the efficacy of this form of treatment is still unclear (106).

The presence of macroscopically involved inguinofemoral lymph glands is associated with a high risk of pelvic lymph node involvement (25%–46%) (53,54,73,102). In the past, these patients would have undergone a full inguino-femoral and pelvic lymphadenectomy followed by pelvic radiotherapy. However, resection of only macroscopically enlarged nodes, either in the groin or in the pelvis, followed by radio-therapy to both the groin and pelvis is an alter-native that appears to reduce the risk of chronic leg edema. Patients with N2 or N3 groin lymph nodes warrant a preoperative computed tomog-raphy (CT) scan of the pelvis to determine whether there are also enlarged pelvic nodes that should be removed before radiotherapy is started.

Recurrent Vulvar Cancer

Local recurrences on the vulva occur in 6% to 23% of patients following treatment (66,85). Heaps et al (66) identified the best predictors for local recurrence as surgical margin less than 1 cm, depth of invasion of more than 5 mm, presence of lymph-vascular invasion, and infil-trative growth pattern.

Isolated recurrences on the vulva are usually amenable to further resection although preoperative radiotherapy should be appropri-ate where resection would require an exenter-ative procedure (107,108). The majority of patients with isolated vulvar recurrence can be cured by these means.

The most accurate predictor of regional and distant recurrence is the number of involved groin nodes. Patients with three or more involved nodes have a distal recurrence rate of 50% to 75% (73,102,109). These patients are rarely cured but local control may be achieved with radiotherapy, chemotherapy, or both. The rate of response to chemotherapy alone is low and the response is of short duration.

Prognosis

The presence of inguinofemoral lymph node metastases is the single most important predic-tor of recurrence and death from vulvar cancer (54,69,73,97,101,110,111). The 5-year survival rate for patients with no lymph node spread is about 90% and is only marginally lower for patients with microscopic involvement of one node, providing there is no extracapsular tumor. Patients with two or three involved nodes have a survival rate of 66% while those with more

than three positive groin nodes have only a 30% survival rate (101,112,113).

Melanoma

Malignant melanoma is the second most common malignancy of the vulva and accounts for 5% to 10% of all cases of melanoma (114). It is seen predominantly in postmenopausal white women and usually presents as a raised pigmented lump on the vulva. It is found most commonly on the labia minora, near the vul-vovaginal junction, or in the periclitoral area (115). A large number of malignant melanomas appear to arise de novo; however, some do appear in conjunction with a dysplastic nevus, lentigo maligna, or benign nevus.

The two most common clinical pictures on the vulva are as follows:

1. Superficial spreading melanoma—often a 1- to 3-cm, well-defined pigmented plaque usually brown-black in color
2. Nodular melanoma—frequently a deeply pigmented, raised tumor although amelan-otic varieties are occasionally seen on the vulva.

Staging and Prognosis

Depth of invasion appears to be the single most important prognostic indicator for melanoma (114–117). The commonly used staging sys-tems for vulvar melanoma are those of Clark et al (118) and of Breslow (119) (Table 27-7). Breslow's classification seems to have the better association with survival when applied to vulvar melanoma.

Lesions with invasion of less than 1 mm have a good prognosis, with survival rates of 95% to 100% being reported (114,117,120). The

T A B L E   **27-7**

Staging of Vulvar Melanoma

	Clark's Levels	Breslow*
I	Intraepithelial	<0–0.76 mm
II	Into papillary dermis	0.76–1.50 mm
III	Filling dermal papillae	1.51–2.25 mm
IV	Into reticular dermis	2.26–3.00 mm
V	Into subcutaneous fat	>3 mm

*Breslow depth of invasion measured from the surface of intact epithelium to the deepest point of invasion.

survival rate for patients with a depth of invasion up to 4 mm is 40%, while invasion beyond 4 mm is associated with survival rates of only 15% to 20%. Phillips (117) suggested that central tumor location is also associated with a poorer survival.

Treatment

The definitive treatment for vulvar melanoma is surgery. Lesions with less than 1 mm of invasion require radical local excision only (121). More advanced tumors have been treated with en bloc radical vulvectomy and groin node dissection, but a recent publication by Davidson (122) showed no advantage for this treatment over radical local excision. The place of lymph node dissection in the treatment of melanoma is unclear. Nonrandomized series suggest that patients undergoing inguinofemoral lymphadenectomy have improved survival rates compared to patients in whom this is omitted (114,121). However, a recent study by Phillips et al (123) showed no difference in survival rates when lymphadenectomy was not performed. The few randomized studies on lymph node dissection for cutaneous melanoma elsewhere on the body did not show any advantage for lymph node dissection over observation (124,125). However, it is difficult to recommend omission of groin dissection at this stage in view of the fact that some patients with positive groin nodes do survive following removal of the glands.

Bartholin Gland Carcinoma

Bartholin gland carcinoma is a rare condition making up less than 5% of vulvar malignancies. According to Copeland et al (126), for a definitive diagnosis of Bartholin gland carcinoma to be made, transition from normal duct or gland tissue to neoplastic tissue must be identified. It is difficult to identify this transition if the tumor is extensive. The presence of an adenocarcinoma or transitional cell carcinoma in the region of Bartholin's gland should suffice. The tumors may arise in either duct or gland tissue and so may present as either squamous carcinoma, adenocarcinoma, adenosquamous carcinoma, or adenoid cystic carcinoma (127).

The tumors typically present as a slowly enlarging mass in the posterior vulva and delay in diagnosis is common, particularly in pre-menopausal women. The overall 5-year survival rates are reported as 50% to 80% (27,126,128).

Copeland et al (126) reported good results with radical local excision or hemivulvectomy and unilateral inguinofemoral lymph node dissection. Because many of these lesions invade deeply into the ischiorectal fossa, postoperative vulvar radiotherapy is recommended and can reduce the local recurrence rate from 27% to 7%. Patients with positive ipsilateral groin nodes should receive postoperative pelvic and groin radiotherapy.

Basal Cell Carcinoma

Most basal cell carcinomas of the vulva arise in the labia majora and appear as a raised pigmented or red nodule that may exhibit central ulceration. They are rare and make up less than 2% of all vulvar malignancies (27,28,40). These tumors are locally aggressive and wide local excision is usually adequate treatment. Lymph node metastases are extremely rare and groin lymph node dissection is not required in the absence of suspicious glands (129).

Basosquamous carcinoma is a variant of basal cell carcinoma that is more locally aggressive and more likely to metastasize. These lesions warrant treatment along the same lines as a squamous cancer of the vulva.

Verrucous Carcinoma

Verrucous carcinoma is an extremely rare variant of a squamous cell carcinoma seen mainly in postmenopausal women. It usually presents as a "condylomatous-like lesion" (giant condyloma of Buschke-Löwenstein) that has frequently been unsuccessfully treated with local surgery, laser, diathermy, or topical agents.

Unless biopsy specimens include the base of the lesion and underlying dermis the diagnosis will be missed.

The tumors tend to be slow growing and locally invasive. Metastases to local lymph glands are rare and if present, are usually due to the association with areas of true squamous cell carcinoma in the verrucous carcinoma (130,131). Treatment is radical local excision of the lesion. Aspiration cytology or excisional biopsy of inguinofemoral lymph nodes is required only if there are suspicious glands.

Radiation therapy is contraindicated in the treatment of verrucous carcinoma. Crowther et al (131), in their review of 102 patients, found only 1 patient with a vulval lesion who was cured with radiotherapy and a further 4 patients who appeared to undergo anaplastic change. The survival rate for patients treated with surgery alone is higher than 90%, although local recurrence requiring re-excision is not uncommon (131–133).

Vulvar Sarcomas

Primary sarcomas of the vulva are rare and represent only 1% to 2% of all vulvar malignancies (27,40). Leiomyosarcoma is the most common vulvar sarcoma, usually presenting as an enlarging painful mass in the labium majus. Lymphatic metastases are uncommon and radical local excision appears to be appropriate treatment.

Kaposi's sarcoma is a slowly progressive angiosarcoma that has been rarely found in women, but with the increasing incidence of the acquired immunodeficiency syndrome (AIDS), this condition is likely to be seen more frequently on the vulva (27). Dermatofibrosarcoma protruberans is occasionally found in the vulva or labiocrural folds, as a slowly expanding violaceous tumor that may eventually ulcerate. Wide local excision is usually all that is required, although recurrence and death occur in about 5% of patients (27).

Rhabdomyosarcoma occurs mainly during childhood and can involve the vulva. Since the advent of chemoradiation and conservative surgery the extremely poor survival rates have improved markedly. Hays et al (134) used combined chemotherapy, surgery, and radiotherapy, and 8 of 9 patients were free of disease at 4 years.

REFERENCES

1. Taussig FJ. Cancer of the vulva. An analysis of 155 cases (1911–1940). *Am J Obstet Gynecol* 1940;40:764–779.

2. Way S. Carcinoma of the vulva. *Am J Obstet Gynecol* 1960;79:692–697.

3. Cavanagh D, William S, Roberts WS, et al. Changing trends in the surgical treatment of invasive carcinoma of the vulva. *Surg Gynecol Obstet* 1986;162:164–168.

4. Hacker NF, Leuchter RS, Berek JS, et al. Radical vulvectomy and bilateral inguinal lymphadenec-tomy through separate groin incisions. *Obstet Gynecol* 1981;58:574–579.

5. Anderson BL, Hacker NF. Psychological adjustment after vulvar surgery. *Obstet Gynecol* 1983; 62:457–462.

6. Kneale BL. Carcinoma of the vulva then and now. *J Reprod Med* 1988;33:496–499.

7. Grant PT. Vulvar cancer. *Aust N Z J Obstet Gynaecol* 1995;35:70.

8. Podratz KC, Symmonds RE, Taylor WF, Williams TJ. Carcinoma of the vulva. Analysis of treatment and survival. *Obstet Gynecol* 1983;61:63–74.

9. Cavanagh D, Hoffman MS. Controversies in the management of vulvar carcinoma. *Br J Obstet Gynaecol* 1996;103:293–300.

10. Keys H. Gynecologic Oncology Group randomized trials of combined therapy for vulvar cancer. *Cancer* 1993;71:1691–1696.

11. Sturgeon SR, Brinton LA, Devesa SS, Kurman RJ. In situ and invasive vulvar cancer incidence trends (1973 to 1987). *Am J Obstet Gynecol* 1992; 166:1482–1485.

12. Mabuchi K, Bross DS, Kessler I. Epidemiology of cancer of the vulva. A case-control study. *Cancer* 1985;55:1843–1848.

13. Daling JR, Sherman KJ, Hislop TG, et al. Cigarette smoking and the risk of ano-genital cancer. *Am J Epidemiol* 1992;135:180–189.

14. Parazzini F, La Vecchia C, Garsia S, et al. Determinants of invasive vulvar cancer risk: an Italian case-control study. *Gynecol Oncol* 1993;48:50–55.

15. Sherman KJ, Daling JR, McKnight B, Chu J. Hormonal factors in vulvar cancer. A case-control study. *J Reprod Med* 1994;39:857–861.

16. Crum CP. Carcinoma of the vulva: epidemiology and pathogenesis. *Obstet Gynecol* 1992;79: 448–454.

17. Brinton LA, Nasca PC, Mallin K, et al. Case-control study of cancer of the vulva. *Obstet Gynecol* 1990;75:859–865.

18. Carter J, Carlson J, Fowler J, et al. Invasive vulvar tumors in young women—a disease of the immunosuppressed? *Gynecol Oncol* 1993;51: 307–310.

19. Monk BJ, Burger RA, Lin F, et al. Prognostic significance of human papillomavirus DNA in vulvar cancer. *Obstet Gynecol* 1995;85:709–715.

20. Jones RW, Park JS, McLean MR, Shah KV. Human papillomavirus in women with vulvar

intraepithelial neoplasia III. *J Reprod Med* 1990; 35:1124–1126.

21. Ferenczy A. Intraepithelial neoplasia of vulva. In: Coppleson M, ed. *Gynecologic oncology*, vol. 1. 2nd ed. Edinburgh: Churchill Livingstone, 1992:443–464.

22. Toki T, Kurman RJ, Park JS, et al. Probable nonpapillomavirus etiology of squamous cell carcinoma of the vulva in older women. A clinicopathologic study using in situ hybridization and polymerase chain reaction. *Int J Gynecol Pathol* 1991;10:107–125.

23. Rodke G, Friedrich EG, Wilkinson EJ. Malignant potential of mixed vulvar dystrophy (lichen sclerosus associated with squamous cell hyperplasia). *J Reprod Med* 1988;33:545–550.

24. Giles GG, Kneale LG. Vulvar cancer: the Cinderella of gynaecological oncology. *Aust N Z J Obstet Gynaecol* 1995;35:71–75.

25. Elliott PM. Early invasive cancer of vulva: definition, clinical findings and management. In: Coppleson M, ed. *Gynecologic oncology*, vol. 1. 2nd ed. Edinburgh: Churchill Livingstone, 1992: 465–478.

26. Campion MJ, Franklin CW, Burrell MO, Cregier MA. Vulvar dysplasia in relation to other genital tract dysplasia: a regional disease. *Colposc Gynecol Laser Surg* 1988;4:111–114.

27. Hewitt J, Pelisse M, Paniel BJ. *Malignant diseases of the vulva.* London: McGraw-Hill, 1991:171–197.

28. Ng ABP. Histopathology of premalignant and malignant tumors of the vulva. In: Knapstein PG, di REF, DiSaia P, et al, eds. *Malignancies of the vulva.* New York: Thieme Medical, 1991:1–24.

29. Hording U, Junge J, Poulsen H, Lundvall F. Vulvar intraepithelial neoplasia III. A viral disease of undetermined progressive potential. *Gynecol Oncol* 1995;56:276–279.

30. Ansink AC, Krul MRL, De Weger RA, et al. Human papillomavirus, lichen sclerosus and squamous cell carcinoma of the vulva: detection and prognostic significance. *Gynecol Oncol* 1994;52:180–184.

31. Bloss JD, Liao SY, Wilczynski SP, et al. Clinical and histologic feature of vulva carcinoma analyzed for human papilloma virus status: evidence that squamous cell carcinoma of the vulva has more than one etiology. *Hum Pathol* 1991;22:711–718.

32. Kaufman RH, Friedrich EG, Gardner HL. Intraepithelial neoplasia of the vulva and vagina. Benign diseases of the vulva and vagina. Chicago: Year Book Medical, 1989:159–193.

33. Jones RW, Rowan DM. Vulvar intraepithelial neoplasia III: a clinical study of the outcome in 113 cases with relation to the later development of invasive vulvar carcinoma. *Obstet Gynecol* 1994;84:741–745.

34. Fishman DA, Chambers SK, Schwartz PE, et al. Extramammary Paget's disease of the vulva. *Gynecol Oncol* 1995;56:266–270.

35. Kodano S, Kaneko T, Saito M, et al. A clinicopathologic study of 30 patients with Paget's disease of the vulva. *Gynecol Oncol* 1995;56:63–70.

36. Jones RE, Austin C, Ackerman AB. Extra mammary Paget's disease: a critical re-examination. *Am J Dermatopathol* 1979;1:101–132.

37. Chandra JJ. Extramammary Paget's disease: prognosis and relationship to internal malignancy. *J Am Acad Dermatol* 1985;13:1009–1014.

38. Adamsons K, Reisfield D. Observation on intradermal migration of Paget cells. *Am J Obstet Gynecol* 1964;90:1274–1280.

39. Stacy D, Burrell MO, Franklin EW III. Extramammary Paget's disease of the vulva and anus. Use of intraoperative frozen-section margins. *Am J Obstet Gynecol* 1986;155:519–522.

40. Ferenczy A. Pathology of malignant tumors of vulva and vagina. In: Coppleson M, ed. *Gynecologic oncology*, vol 1. 2nd ed. Edinburgh: Churchill Livingstone, 1992:419–442.

41. Nicklin JL, Hacker NF, Heintze SW, et al. An anatomical study of inguinal lymph node topography and clinical implications for the surgical management of vulval cancer. *Int J Gynecol Cancer* 1995;5:128–133.

42. Borgno G, Micheletti L, Barbero M, et al. Topographic distribution of groin lymph nodes. A study of 50 female cadavers. *J Reprod Med* 1990;35:1127–1129.

43. Micheletti L, Borgno G, Barbero M, et al. Deep femoral lymphadenectomy with preservation of the fascia lata. Preliminary report on 42 invasive vulvar carcinomas. *J Reprod Med* 1990;35: 1130–1133.

44. Parry-Jones E. Lymphatics of the vulva. *J Obstet Gynaecol Br Emp* 1963;70:751–765.

45. Iversen T, Aas M. Lymph drainage from the vulva. *Gynecol Oncol* 1983;16:179–189.

46. Chu J, Tamimi HK, Figge DC. Femoral node metastases with superficial inguinal nodes in early vulvar cancer. *Am J Obstet Gynecol* 1981; 140:337–338.

47. Hacker NF, Nieberg RK, Berek JS, et al. Superficially invasive vulvar cancer with nodal metastases. *Gynecol Oncol* 1983;15:65–77.

48. Burke TW, Levenback C, Coleman RL, et al. Surgical therapy of T1 and T2 vulvar carcinoma: further experience with radical wide excision and selective inguinal lymphadenectomy. *Gynecol Oncol* 1995;57:215–220.

49. Podczaski E, Sexton M, Kaminski P, et al. Recurrent carcinoma of the vulva after conservative treatment for "microinvasive" disease. *Gynecol Oncol* 1990;39:65–68.

50. Stehman FB, Bundy BN, Dvoretsky PM, Creasman WT. Early stage I carcinoma of the vulva treated with ipsilateral superficial inguinal lymphadenectomy and modified radical hemivulvectomy. A prospective study of the Gynecologic Oncology Group. *Obstet Gynecol* 1992; 79:490–497.

51. Levenbeck C, Burke TW, Gershenson DM, et al. Intraoperative lymphatic mapping for vulvar cancer. *Obstet Gynecol* 1994;84:163–167.

52. Binder SW, Huang I, Fu YS, et al. Risk factors in the development of lymph metastasis in vulvar squamous carcinoma. *Gynecol Oncol* 1990;37:9–16.

53. Figge DC, Tamimi HK, Greer BE. Lymphatic spread in carcinoma of the vulva. *Am J Obstet Gynecol* 1985;152:387–394.

54. Boyce J, Fruchter RG, Kasambilides E, et al. Prognostic factors in carcinoma of the vulva. *Gynecol Oncol* 1985;20:364–377.

55. Abrao FS, Baracat EC, Marques AF, et al. Carcinoma of the vulva. Clinico-pathologic factors involved in inguinal and pelvic lymph node metastasis. *J Reprod Med* 1990;35:1113–1116.

56. Shimm DS, Fuller AF, Orlow BS, et al. Prognostic variables in the treatment of squamous cell carcinoma of the vulva. *Gynecol Oncol* 1986; 24:243–258.

57. Sedlis A, Homesley H, Bundy BN, et al. Positive groin lymph nodes in superficial squamous cell vulvar cancer. *Am J Obstet Gynecol* 1987;156: 1159–1164.

58. Gomez Rueda N, Vighi S, Garcia A, et al. Histologic predictive factors: therapeutic impact in vulvar cancer. *J Reprod Med* 1994;39:71–76.

59. Krupp PJ Jr. Invasive tumors of vulva: clinical features, staging and management. In: Coppleson M, ed. *Gynecologic oncology*, vol. 1. 2nd ed. Edinburgh: Churchill Livingstone, 1992:479–492.

60. Hacker NF, Van der Velden J. Conservative management of early vulvar cancer. *Cancer* 1993;71:4:1673–1677.

61. Morris JMcL. A formula for selective lymphadenectomy, its application to cancer of the vulva. *Obstet Gynecol* 1977;50:2:152–158.

62. Hoffman MS, Roberts WS, LaPolla JP, Cavanagh D. Recent modifications in the treatment of invasive squamous carcinoma of the vulva. *Obstet Gynecol Surv* 1989;44:227–233.

63. Trelford JD, Deer DA, Ordorica E, et al. Ten-year prospective study in a management change of vulvar carcinoma. *Am J Obstet Gynecol* 1984;150:288–296.

64. Siller BS, Alvarez RD, Conner WD, et al. Vulva cancer: a case-control study of triple incision versus en bloc radical vulvectomy and inguinal lymphadenectomy. *Gynecol Oncol* 1995;57: 335–339.

65. Ross MJ, Ehrmann RL. Histologic prognosticators in stage I squamosquamous cell carcinoma of the vulva. *Obstet Gynecol* 1987;70:774–784.

66. Heaps JM, Fu YS, Montz FJ, et al. Surgical-pathologic variables predictive of local recurrence in squamous cell carcinoma of the vulva. *Gynecol Oncol* 1990;38:309–314.

67. Berman ML, Soper JT, Creasman WT, et al. Conservative surgical management of superficially invasive stage 1 vulvar carcinoma. *Gynecol Oncol* 1989;35:352–357.

68. Hacker NF, Berek JS, Lagasse LD, et al. Individualization of treatment for stage I squamous cell vulvar carcinoma. *Obstet Gynecol* 1984;63: 155–162.

69. Rowley KC, Gallion HH, Donaldson ES, et al. Prognostic factors in cancer. *Gynecol Oncol* 1988;31:43–49.

70. Di Saia PJ, Creasman WT, Rich WM. An alternate approach to early cancer of the vulva. *Am J Obstet Gynecol* 1979;133:825–830.

71. Homesley HD. Management of vulvar cancer. *Cancer* 1995;76:2159–2170.

72. Wilkinson EJ, Rico MJ, Pierson KK. Microinvasive carcinoma of the vulva. *Int J Gynecol Pathol* 1982;1:29–39.

73. Hoffman JS, Kumar NB, Morley GW. Prognostic significance of groin lymph node metastases in squamous carcinoma of the vulva. *Obstet Gynecol* 1985;66:402–405.

74. Magrina JF, Webb MJ, Gaffey TA, Symmonds RE. Stage I squamous cell cancer of the vulva. *Am J Obstet Gynecol* 1979;134:453–457.

75. Van der Velden J, Kooyman CD, Van Lindert AC, Heintz APM. A stage Ia vulvar carcinoma with an inguinal lymph node recurrence after local excision. A case report and literature review. *Int J Gynecol Cancer* 1992;2:157–159.

76. Iversen T, Abeler VC, Aalders J. Individualized treatment of stage I carcinoma of the vulva. *Obstet Gynecol* 1981;57:85–89.

77. Piura B, Masotina A, Murdoch J, et al. Recurrent squamous cell carcinoma of the vulva: a study of 73 cases. *Gynecol Oncol* 1993;48:189–195.

78. Hopkins MP, Reid GC, Morley GW. The surgical management of recurrent squamous cell carcinoma of the vulva. *Obstet Gynecol* 1990;75:1001–1005.

79. Hoffman MS, Mark JE, Cavanagh D. A management scheme for postoperative groin lymphocysts. *Gynecol Oncol* 1995;56:262–265.

80. Barnhill DR, Hoskins WJ, Metz P. Use of the rhomboid flap after partial vulvectomy. *Obstet Gynecol* 1983;62:444–447.

81. Ballon SC, Donaldson RC, Roberts JA. Reconstruction of the vulva using a myocutaneous graft. *Gynecol Oncol* 1979;7:123–127.

82. Burke TW, Morris M, Roh MS, et al. Using single gracilis myocutaneous flaps. *Gynecol Oncol* 1995;57:221–225.

83. Knapstein PG, Friedberg V. Reconstructive operations of the vulva and vagina. In: Knapstein PG, Friedberg V, Sevom BU, eds. *Reconstructive surgery in gynecology.* New York: Thieme Medical, 1990:11–70.

84. International Federation of Gynecology and Obstetrics. 21st annual report on the results of treatment of gynecological cancer. *Int J Gynecol Obstet* 1991;36(suppl):1–315.

85. Iversen T, Aalders JG, Christensen A, Kolstadt P. Squamous cell carcinoma of the vulva. A review of 424 patients, 1956–1974. *Gynecol Oncol* 1980;9:271–279.

86. Grimshaw RN, Ghazal Aswad S, Monaghan JM. The role of ano-vulvectomy in locally advanced carcinoma of the vulva. *Int J Gynecol Cancer* 1991;1:15–18.

87. Hoffman MS, Cavanagh D, Roberts WS, et al. Ultraradical surgery for advanced carcinoma of the vulva. An update. *Int J Gynecol Cancer* 1993; 3:369–372.

88. Cavanagh D, Shepherd JH. Pelvic exenteration for advanced carcinoma of the vulva. *Gynecol Oncol* 1982;13:318–322.

89. Thornton WN, Flanagan WC. Pelvic exenteration in the treatment of advanced malignancy of the vulva. *Am J Obstet Gynecol* 1973;117:774–781.

90. Morley GW, Hopkins MP, Lindenauer SM, Roberts JA. Pelvic exenteration, University of Michigan: 100 patients at 5 years. *Obstet Gynecol* 1989;74:934–942.

91. Boronow RC. Therapeutic alternative to primary exenteration for advanced vulvo-vaginal cancer. *Gynecol Oncol* 1973;1:233–255.

92. Boronow RC, Hickman BT, Reagan MT, et al. Combined therapy as an alternative to exenteration for locally advanced vulvovaginal cancer. II. Results, complications, and dosimetric and surgical considerations. *Am J Clin Oncol* 1987; 10:171–181.

93. Boronow RC. Combined therapy as an alternative to exenteration for locally advanced vulvo-vaginal cancer. Rationale and results. *Cancer* 1982;49:1085–1091.

94. Hacker NF, Berek JS, Juillard GJF, Lagasse LD. Preoperative radiation therapy for locally advanced vulvar cancer. *Cancer* 1984;54:2056–2061.

95. Papillon J, Montbarbon J. Epidermoid carcinoma of the anal canal. A series of 276 cases. *Dis Colon Rectum* 1987;30:324–333.

96. Nigro ND, Vaitevicius VK, Considine B. Combined therapy for cancer of the anal canal. A preliminary report. *Dis Colon Rectum* 1974; 17:354–356.

97. Hacker NF, Berek JS, Lagasse LD, et al. Management of regional lymph nodes and their prognostic influence in vulvar cancer. *Obstet Gynecol* 1983;61:408–412.

98. Thomas G, Dembo A, DePetrillo A, et al. Concurrent radiation and chemotherapy in vulva cancer. *Gynecol Oncol* 1989;34:263–267.

99. Sebag-Montefiore DJ, McLean C, Arnott SJ, et al. Treatment of advanced carcinoma of the

vulva with chemoradiotherapy—can exenterative surgery be avoided? *Int J Gynecol Cancer* 1994;4:150–155.

100. Carson LF, Twiggs LB, Adcock LL, et al. Multimodality therapy for advanced and recurrent vulvar squamous cell carcinoma. A pilot project. *J Reprod Med* 1990;35:1029–1032.

101. Burger PM, Hollema H, Emmanuels AG, et al. The importance of the groin node status for the survival of T1 and T2 vulval carcinoma patients. *Gynecol Oncol* 1995;57:327–334.

102. Homesley HD, Bundy BN, Sedlis A, Adcock L. Radiation therapy versus pelvic node resection for carcinoma of the vulva with positive groin nodes. *Obstet Gynecol* 1986;68:733–738.

103. Van der Velden J, Van Lindert ACM, Lammes FB, et al. Extracapsular growth of lymph node metastases in squamous cell carcinoma of the vulva. *Cancer* 1995;75:2885–2890.

104. Henderson RH, Parsons JT, Morgan L, Million RR. Elective ilioinguinal lymph node irradiation. *Int J Radiat Oncol Biol Phys* 1984;10:811–815.

105. Stehman F, Bundy B, Bell J, et al. Groin dissection versus groin radiation in carcinoma of the vulva: a Gynecologic Oncology Group study. *Int J Radiat Oncol Biol Phys* 1992;24:389–396.

106. McCall AR, Olson MC, Potkul RK. The variation of inguinal lymph node depth in adult women and its importance in planning elective irradiation for vulvar cancer. *Cancer* 1995;75:2286–2288.

107. Miller B, Morris M, Levenback C, et al. Pelvic exenteration for primary and recurrent vulvar cancer. *Gynecol Oncol* 1995;58:202–205.

108. Schulz MJ, Penalver M. Recurrent vulvar carcinoma in the intervening tissue bridge in early invasive stage I disease treated by bilateral groin dissection through separate incisions. *Gynecol Oncol* 1989;35:383–386.

109. Ndubisi B, Kaminski PF, Olt G, et al. Staging and recurrence of disease in squamous cell carcinoma of the vulva. *Gynecol Oncol* 1995;59:34–37.

110. Kirschner CV, Yordan EL, De Geest K, Wilbanks GD. Smoking, obesity and survival in squamous cell carcinoma of the vulva. *Gynecol Oncol* 1995;56:79–84.

111. Microinvasive cancer of the vulva: report of the ISSVD task force. *J Reprod Med* 1984;29:454–457.

112. Hacker NF. Vulvar cancer. In: Berek JS, Hacker NF, eds. *Practical gynecologic oncology.* Baltimore: Williams & Williams, 1994:403–440.

113. Origoni M, Sideri M, Garsia S, et al. Prognostic value of pathological patterns of lymph node positivity in squamous cell carcinoma of the vulva. Stage III and IVA FIGO. *Gynecol Oncol* 1992;45:313–316.

114. Brand E, Fu YS, Lagasse LD, Berek JS. Vulvovaginal melanoma. Report of seven cases and literature review. *Gynecol Oncol* 1989;33:54–60.

115. Beller V, Demopolous RI, Beckman EM. Vulvovaginal melanoma: a clinicopathologic study. *J Reprod Med* 1986;31:315–319.

116. Blessing K, Kernohan NM, Miller ID, Al Nafussi AI. Malignant melanoma of the vulva. Clinicopathological features. *Int J Gynecol Oncol* 1991;1:81–87.

117. Phillips GL, Twiggs LB, Okagaki T. Vulvar melanoma. A microstaging study. *Gynecol Oncol* 1982;14:80–88.

118. Clark WH Jr, From L, Bernadino EA, Mihm MC. Histogenesis and biologic behavior of primary human malignant melanoma of the skin. *Cancer Res* 1969;29:705–726.

119. Breslow A. Thickness of cross-sectional areas and depth of invasion in the prognosis of cutaneous melanoma. *Ann Surg* 1970;172:902–908.

120. Look KY, Roth LM, Sutton GP. Vulvar melanoma reconsidered. *Cancer* 1993;72:143–146.

121. Rose PG, Piver MS, Tsukada Y, Lou T. Conservative therapy for melanoma of the vulva. *Am J Obstet Gynecol* 1988;159:52–55.

122. Davidson T, Kissin M, Wesbury G. Vulvovaginal melanoma—should radical surgery be abandoned? *Br J Obstet Gynaecol* 1987;94:473–476.

123. Phillips GL, Bundy BN, Okagaki T, et al. Malignant melanoma of the vulva treated by radical hemivulvectomy. *Cancer* 1994;73:2626–2632.

124. Veronesi U, Adamus J, Bandiera DC, et al. Delayed regional lymph node dissection in stage I melanoma of the skin of the lower extremities. *Cancer* 1982;49:2420–2430.

125. Slingluff CL Jr, Stidham KR, Ricci WM, et al. Surgical management of regional lymph nodes in patients with melanoma. Experience with 4682 patients. *Ann Surg* 1994;219:120–130.

126. Copeland LJ, Sneige N, Gershenson DM, et al. Bartholin gland carcinoma. *Obstet Gynecol* 1986;67:794–801.

127. Copeland LJ, Sneige N, Gershenson DM, et al. Adenoid cystic carcinoma of Bartholin gland. *Obstet Gynecol* 1986;67:115–120.

128. Leuchter RS, Hacker NF, Voet RL, et al. Primary carcinoma of Bartholin gland. A report of 14 cases and review of the literature. *Obstet Gynecol* 1982;60:361–365.

129. Hoffman MS, Roberts WS, Ruffolo EH. Basal cell carcinoma of the vulva with inguinal lymph node metastases. *Gynecol Oncol* 1988;29:113–119.

130. Gallousis S. Verrucous carcinoma. Report of three vulvar cases and a review of the literature. *Obstet Gynecol* 1972;40:502–507.

131. Crowther ME, Lowe DG, Shepherd JH. Verrucous carcinoma of the female genital tract: a review. *Obstet Gynecol Surv* 1988;43:263–280.

132. Isaacs HJ. Verrucous carcinoma of the female genital tract. *Gynecol Oncol* 1976;4:259–269.

133. Japaze H, van Dinh T, Woodruff JD. Verrucous carcinoma of the vulva. Study of 24 cases. *Obstet Gynecol* 1982;60:462–466.

134. Hays DM, Shimada H, Raney RB, et al. Clinical staging and treatment results in rhabdomyosarcoma of the female genital tract among children and adolescents. *Cancer* 1988;61:1893–1903.

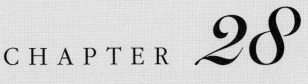

CHAPTER 28

Gynecologic Melanoma

MOLLY A. BREWER
DIANE C. BODURKA
CREIGHTON L. EDWARDS

Malignant melanomas of gynecologic origin are rare, accounting for less than 1% of all gynecologic cancers and only 2% to 3% of all melanomas. Due to the relative rarity of gynecologic melanomas, the literature is scant, with the vast majority of studies having too few numbers for accurate conclusions to be drawn. Most cutaneous melanomas are linked to sun exposure, but it is unclear if this holds true for those of gynecologic origin. In addition, gynecologic melanomas occur in areas that are poorly visualized and therefore are diagnosed later than the more accessible cutaneous melanomas, which may partially account for their relatively poorer prognosis. With such few numbers available, there is a paucity of data supporting different methods of treatment. The trend over the last 20 years, however, has been toward less radical surgery, without an apparent decline in survival.

Epidemiology

Cutaneous melanomas are more prevalent in people with greater exposure to ultraviolet light. In addition, changes in lifestyle and clothing habits have been linked to the current trend of an increasing incidence of cutaneous melanoma. Melanomas may occur in non-sun-exposed areas in Caucasians with a history of excessive sun exposure, although it is unclear whether there is a concomitant increase in incidence in perineal melanomas. The mechanism may be related to elevated sun-induced circu-

latory melanocyte-stimulating factors such as melanocyte-stimulating hormone (MSH).

Most cutaneous melanomas arise in pre-existing nevi that undergo a malignant transformation. However, the vulvar skin is obscured in hair and folds so nevi may be difficult to see prior to a lesion becoming larger (1). Vaginal melanomas are also thought to arise from nevi and occasionally from areas of benign melanosis, which are areas of benign melanocytes in the basal layer of the vagina found in 3% of women (2).

Vulvar melanoma is a disease that affects older women (3). It is rarely seen in individuals younger than 50 years. A large study in Sweden, with 245 cases collected over 24 years, described a range of ages from 15 to more than 75 years, but the majority of women were at least 60 years old. This same study showed a decrease in vulvar melanoma, in contrast to cutaneous melanoma, from an age-standardized incidence of 0.27 in 1960 to 1964 to 0.14 in 1980 to 1984 (4).

Vulvar melanoma affects Caucasians two to four times more frequently than other races. In a classic paper by Morrow and Rutledge (5), which evaluated 30 women with vulvar melanoma, 23 (78%) of the women were white, 2 (6.7%) were black, and 2 (6.7%) were Latin American. Four of the 30 patients had been treated for other malignancies, and 2 of the 30 had a family member with a history of melanoma. Fourteen of the patients had a family history of other nonmelanoma cancers (5). In a study of 44 patients from Memorial Sloan Kettering Cancer Center, only 1 patient gave a family history of melanoma. It is therefore difficult to draw conclusions regarding the significance of family history.

Vaginal cancer is a rare disease, comprising only 1% of all gynecologic malignancies. Poronas first reported vaginal melanoma in 1887 (6), and only 140 cases have been documented in the literature to date. Primary vaginal melanoma accounts for less than 1% of all melanomas and less than 5% of malignant vaginal neoplasms (7). The mean age at the time of diagnosis of vaginal melanoma is 57 years, with a range of 22 to 83 years (8). A disproportionately large number of vaginal melanomas have been reported in Japanese women, with white and then black women following in frequency (7–9).

Biology

Melanocytes originate in neural crest cells that migrate early during fetal development and reside in the basal layer of the epidermis. These cells synthesize melanin, which helps protect the skin against ultraviolet damage. MSH is secreted by the pituitary gland and acts by both stimulating melanin production from melanocytes and supporting their growth. Melanocytes are also regulated by melatonin, a molecule that arises in the pineal gland and suppresses melanocyte function when ambient light is decreased.

Malignant melanocyes may also produce growth factors that upregulate melanoma growth. Interestingly, cases of spontaneous remission have been documented, suggesting that the immune system plays an important role in melanoma biology. A defect in natural killer (NK) cells has been associated with metastatic melanoma, along with a lack of human leukocyte antigen (HLA) expression, which is associated with a lack of recognition by lymphocytes (10).

Types

Four subtypes of cutaneous melanoma have been described: superficial spreading, nodular, lentigo maligna, and acral-lentiginous. These subtypes each have a somewhat different prognosis. Seventy percent of nongynecologic melanomas are superficial spreading and 15% to 30% are nodular. The lentigo maligna and acral-lentiginous types account for the remaining cases. Superficial spreading and lentigo maligna melanomas have the best prognosis, while nodular melanoma has the poorest prognosis. An attempt has been made to correlate these cell types with vulvar melanoma and, in a classic study by Podratz et al (11), histologic cell type had a significant effect on both long- and short-term survival. The majority of patients in Podratz's study had superficial spreading or nodular melanoma. As with the nongynecologic melanomas, superficial spreading had the best prognosis, with a 71% five-year survival rate, while nodular melanoma had the worst prognosis, with a 38% five-year survival rate. Ten-year survival data revealed a similar disparity, 66% and 25% survival rates, respectively. However, only 45 patients were evaluated for histologic classification and such small numbers lack statistical significance.

Even less is known about primary malignant melanoma of the vagina, although the majority of lesions are nodular. An epithelioid histologic pattern is most commonly seen; spindle cell (sarcomatous) and mixed patterns may also be identified. Vaginal melanomas do not have a distinctive microscopic pattern. Immunohistochemical studies that demonstrate the presence of protein S-100 and antigen HMB-45 are useful to identify melanoma. Staining for keratin and desmin will be negative. The prognosis of patients with any histologic type of vaginal melanoma is uniformly poor.

Diagnosis

Cutaneous malignant melanoma is thought to arise from a preexisting nevus that has undergone malignant transformation. It should be suspected in any pigmented lesion or mucosal lesion that changes in size or color, begins to itch, or bleeds spontaneously (12). Morrow and Rutledge (5) described a patient who had such intense pruritis that she cut off her lesion with a razor blade! In the vulvar area, it is unclear whether melanomas arise in nevi, as they are hidden by skinfolds and hair. In most reports, the most common presenting complaint is a lump either on the vulva or in the groin, followed by pruritis and bleeding (5,10,13–17). Occasionally, melanoma is found on routine examination. The majority of patients have presented historically with advanced disease and consequently a poor prognosis, making early diagnosis even more desirable. Vaginal melanomas may present as fungating, nodular, or polypoid gray or black soft masses. Lesions can vary from 0.5 to 8.0 cm in diameter (6,7). The overlying epithelium is frequently ulcerated. Vaginal bleeding is the most frequent clinical presentation, followed by vaginal discharge and the presence of a mass (18). Tumors are most commonly located in the lower third of the vagina. Six percent of vaginal melanomas are amelanotic, and can easily be mistaken for epithelial lesions (12).

Staging

Staging of melanoma is highly controversial. Podratz et al (11) found a significant difference in survival when Clark's levels I to IV (see Addendum) were compared to level V. Patients with level I or II had a survival rate of 100%; with level III, 83%; with level IV, 81%; and with level V, 28%. There was no statistical difference in survival when they were analyzed using Breslow's staging system (see Addendum) except for Breslow level V (disease reached 3.0 mm), for which the survival rate was significantly less at 23%. However, Bradgate et al (16) found statistically different survival rates when they analyzed stages with both methods, again emphasizing the controversy regarding how best to develop a method to predict prognosis.

Cutaneous melanomas are staged by both methods, but some authors found Breslow's classification to be more accurate and more reproducible in terms of predicting lymph node metastases (12). Most authors think that Breslow's classification fails to predict survival for patients with vulvar melanoma (15,16) and believe Chung's method is more predictive (13,15,16). There have been difficulties in identifying a well-defined papillary dermis in the vulva; Johnson et al (1) were only able to stage 50% of their patients with either method. Chung et al (13) defined a modification which determined depth of invasion by measuring depth with a micrometer in relation to the epidermis. Some authors (13,15,16) had difficulty quantifying depth of invasion with Clark's method because of the lack of a well-defined papillary dermis in vulvar skin and mucous membranes of the labia, and proposed use of Chung's modification.

In 1964, Das Gupta and D'Urso (19) proposed that treatment of gynecologic melanomas

be based on the principles of cutaneous melanoma treatment. Lesion thickness (Breslow's classification) and level of invasion (Clark's levels) are the most important variables in predicting the survival of patients with cutaneous melanomas (20). Jaramillo et al (21) reported that tumor thickness and Clark's level correlated best with survival in patients with vulvar melanoma. It is difficult, however, to apply Clark's levels to vaginal melanoma, since there is no papillary or reticular dermis in the vagina. Although lesion thickness is thought to be a prognostic factor for survival, the majority of studies on vaginal melanoma did not quantify this value, making lesion thickness difficult to document as a prognostic factor.

Treatment

The most controversial topic associated with vulvar melanoma is treatment. The two classic papers by Morrow and Rutledge (5) and Podratz et al (11) strongly recommend radical surgery as the most appropriate procedure. However, over the last 20 years, radical surgery has been increasingly criticized because of its failure to improve survival and its high morbidity.

In Morrow and Rutledge's retrospective study (5) at the M. D. Anderson Cancer Center of 30 patients with primary vulvar melanoma, 21 patients were treated with radical vulvectomy and node dissection, either groin alone or groin combined with pelvic node dissection; 1 was treated with anterior exenteration; 3 patients were treated conservatively; and 2 palliatively. The overall 5-year survival rate was 50%. Eleven of the 27 patients treated with curative intent had a recurrence. Three of these 11 patients had distant metastases, while 7 had a recurrence in the operative field. There was no information available regarding the eleventh patient. The authors concluded that radical surgery was the preferred treatment for melanoma.

Podratz and his group (11) at the Mayo Clinic reviewed 30 years of cases of primary vulvar melanoma; 48 patients were identified. Forty of the 48 patients were treated with radical en bloc resection. The 5-year survival rate was 54%; 16 patients (41%) survived 10 years. In almost half of the patients with recurrent disease, the recurrence was outside of the pelvis. This group of patients clearly would not have benefited from more aggressive surgery.

All of these patients with distal recurrence had invasion into the subcutaneous tissue at the time of initial surgery. The authors concluded that en bloc inguinal lymph node dissection prevented groin recurrence, as only 1 patient had a recurrence in the groin; however, it is questionable whether a lack of recurrence in the groin supports radical lymph node dissection, as there was no randomization. The authors attributed the 32% local recurrence rate to inadequate margins. However, these recurrences were probably more of a function of tumor biology rather than of inadequate surgical resection. One trial on cutaneous melanoma concluded that a 2-cm margin is probably adequate (22).

A 1975 retrospective study from Memorial Sloan Kettering Cancer Center (13) included 44 patients with vulvar melanoma. Although data at that time suggested that a superficial lesion (Clark's level II) might be adequately treated with a less radical excision, radical dissection remained the standard treatment approach. Despite radical surgery, the 5-year survival rate remained a dismal 30%.

Radical surgery is associated with multiple complications. Early problems include wound breakdown, lymphocyst formation, thrombophlebitis, and hemorrhage. Late complications, which carry significant long-term morbidity, include lymphedema, lymphangitis, urinary incontinence, genital prolapse, and sexual dysfunction. Eighty-five percent of patients undergoing radical surgery have wound breakdown, 30% to 70% have chronic leg edema, and 15% require reoperation for complications. Edwards and Stringer (23) identified complications in 41 patients who underwent a modified procedure and 163 who underwent the standard radical procedure. Sixty-three percent of patients treated with radical vulvar surgery had early complications, versus 19% of those who had modified surgery. Fifty-eight percent had late complications, versus 21% of those treated more conservatively.

Burke et al (24) reviewed 32 patients with T1 and T2 vulvar tumors treated with wide radical excision rather than radical surgery. They showed that only 10 (31%) had early complications and only 5 (15%) had delayed complications.

Newer studies failed to show increased survival rates with radical surgery (22,25–28). Davidson et al (25) reviewed 32 patients with vulvovaginal melanoma and suggested that there was no statistically significant difference in survival between treatment with local excision, simple vulvectomy, or radical vulvectomy. Bradgate et al (16) reviewed 50 patients with vulvar melanoma and found only a slightly improved survival with radical surgery compared to local excision, but this finding was not statistically significant. Rose et al (26) compared patients with similar lesions; 12 patients were treated with local therapy and 13 patients were treated with radical therapy. The authors found no significant difference in survival between the two groups. Depth of invasion and younger patient age were associated with increased survival. Adequacy of margin may be an important prognosticator of survival, as 6 of the 12 patients who had local resection had an inadequate margin (<2 cm). Three of the four recurrences occurred in this group. The numbers are too small to draw significant conclusions and the study was retrospective without any randomization. However, this is the only study that addressed depth of invasion and survival in a group of patients with vulvar melanoma treated with conservative therapy or with radical therapy.

The treatment of primary vaginal melanoma remains controversial. Despite multiple treatment regimens, the overall 5-year survival rate ranges from 5% to approximately 20% (12). Chung et al (7) retrospectively reviewed 19 patients with primary vaginal melanoma treated with either radical surgery or radiotherapy. The overall 5-year survival rate was 21% (7).

Bonner et al (29) evaluated 10 patients with vaginal melanoma treated at the University of Michigan Hospital between 1964 and 1987. Of the 5 patients who underwent radical surgery and had adequate information regarding the first site of relapse, 4 had a relapse in the pelvis or in local or regional lymph nodes. Three patients were treated with local resection, and all had locoregional recurrences. The authors suggested that preoperative whole-pelvic radiotherapy might improve the local control rate when surgery alone is utilized as the primary treatment modality (29).

Van Nostrand et al (30) reviewed 119 patients with vaginal melanoma reported prior to 1994, and added 8 additional patients treated at the University of California at Irvine from 1972 to 1992. Patients were divided into two treatment groups according to the primary therapy, radical versus conservative treatment. Of the 8 patients treated, 4 received radical treatment and 4 received conservative treatment. The average lesion size was 6.4 cm² for the radical group and 16 cm² for the conservative group; however, the size difference was not statistically significant (30). Seventy-five percent of the patients treated radically survived 2 years; none of the patients treated conservatively survived 2 years. By reviewing all reported cases, the authors felt they had validated an improvement in 2-year survival in patients with lesions smaller than 10 cm² and treated radically. This survival benefit did not extend to 5 years (30).

Two separate studies analyzed clinicopathologic findings. Borazjani et al (18) examined depth of invasion, presence of melanin pigment, vascular invasion, junctional activity, mitotic count, and histologic cell type in 10 patients with primary vaginal malignant melanoma. The mean survival time was significantly correlated to mitotic count, and the authors concluded that patients with mitotic counts of less than 6/10 high-power fields had a better survival time (21 months) when compared to those with mitotic counts higher than 6/10 high-power field (mean survival time of only 7 months).

In an analysis of 15 patients treated at the University of Michigan Medical Center and Bowman Gray School of Medicine, Reid et al (31) demonstrated a cumulative 5-year survival rate of 17.4%. Their data were incorporated into a meta-analysis, which demonstrated several conclusions. Tumor thickness (≤6 mm) significantly affected the disease-free interval. Lesion size (<3 cm) significantly influenced survival, while stage, age, tumor location, and tumor thickness did not. Treatment modality and radicality of surgery did not significantly affect survival (31).

Discussion

Melanoma behaves much more aggressively than squamous cell cancer of the vulva, and unfortunately, is commonly diagnosed in an advanced state. There is clear evidence that the size and depth of invasion correlate significantly with patient survival, so early diagnosis is linked to better survival. Although earlier studies suggested that patients with melanoma need radical surgery, it is less clear that this will provide better survival than local excision will. It is difficult to tolerate the substantial complications associated with radical surgery when an uncertain improval in survival exists. Most studies utilizing surgical therapy demonstrated survival rates of 30% to 50%, depending on the size of the lesion. More advanced disease is associated with a poorer outcome. It is evident that a 30% to 50% survival rate, irrespective of radical or conservative surgery, is poor and fails to support radical surgery, especially given its inherent complication rate. Chemoimmunotherapy shows promising response rates, especially when compared to the poor responses of traditional chemotherapy, radiation therapy, and surgical therapy.

Pigmented lesions are not always associated with melanoma; in fact, they are more likely to be a nevus. However, because the survival rate for patients with larger lesions is so poor, biopsy of the pigmented lesions seen on the vulva and vagina should always be performed. If a small melanoma is present, the patient is an ideal candidate for surgical management, as early, superficial lesions are clearly associated with a significantly improved outcome.

REFERENCES

1. Johnson A, Mathai G, Robinson W. Malignant melanoma of the perineum. *J Surg Oncol* 1993; 54:185–189.

2. Nigogosyan G, De La Pava S, Pickren JW. Melanoblasts in vaginal mucosa. *Cancer* 1964; 17:912.

3. Dunton C, Kautsky M, Hanau C. Malignant melanoma of the vulva: a review. *Obstet Gynecol Surv* 1995;50:739–746.

4. Olding B, Johansson H, Rutqvist L, Ringborg U. Malignant melanoma of the vulva and vagina. *Cancer* 1993;71:1893–1897.

5. Morrow C, Rutledge F. Melanoma of the vulva. *Obstet Gynecol* 1972;39:745–752.

6. Liu L-Y, Hou Y-J, Li J-Z. Primary malignant melanoma of the vagina: a report of seven cases. *Obstet Gynecol* 1987;70:569.

7. Chung AF, Casey MJ, Flannery JT, et al. Malignant melanoma of the vagina—report of 19 cases. *Obstet Gynecol* 1980;55:720.

8. Levitan Z, Gordon AN, Kaplan AL, Kaufman RH. Primary malignant melanoma of the vagina: report of four cases and review of the literature. *Gynecol Oncol* 1989;33:85.

9. Hasumi K, Sakamoto G, Sugano H. Primary melanoma of the vagina. Study of four autopsy

cases with ultrastructural findings. *Cancer* 1978; 42:2675.

10. Anderson C, Tabacof J, Legha S. Malignant melanoma: biology, diagnosis and management. In: *Medical oncology: a comprehensive review.* Huntington, NY: PRR 1995:493–509.

11. Podratz K, Gaffey T, Symmonds R, et al. Melanoma of the vulva: an update. *Gynecol Oncol* 1983;16:153–168.

12. Ariel IM. Malignant melanoma of the female genital system: a report of 48 patients and review of the literature. *J Surg Oncol* 1981;15:371.

13. Chung A, Woodruff J, Lewis J. Malignant melanoma of the vulva. *Obstet Gynecol* 1975;45: 638–646.

14. Fenn M, Abell M. Melanoma of vulva and vagina. *Obstet Gynecol* 1973;41:902–911.

15. Piura B, Egan M, Lopes A, Monaghan J. Malignant melanoma of the vulva: a clinicopathologic study of 18 cases. *J Surg Oncol* 1992;50:234–240.

16. Bradgate M, Rollason T, McConkey C, Powell J. Malignant melanoma of the vulva: a clinico-pathologic study of 50 women. *Br J Obstet Gynaecol* 1990;97:124–133.

17. Trimble E, Lewis J, Williams L, et al. Management of vulvar melanoma. *Gynecol Oncol* 1992; 45:254–258.

18. Borazjani G, Prem KA, Okagaki T, et al. Primary malignant melanoma of the vagina: a clinico-pathologic analysis of 10 cases. *Gynecol Oncol* 1990;37:264.

19. Das Gupta T, D'Urso J. Melanoma of the female genitalia. *Surg Obstet Gynecol* 1964;119:1074.

20. Chanda JJ. Clinical recognition of primary cutaneous malignant melanoma. *Med Clin North Am* 1986;70:39.

21. Jaramillo BA, Ganjei P, Averette HE, et al. Malignant melanoma of the vulva. *Obstet Gynecol* 1985;66:398.

22. Balch C, Urist M, Karakousis C. Efficacy of 2 cm surgical margins for intermediate-thickness melanomas: results of a multi-institutional randomized trial. *Ann Surg* 1993;218:262–267.

23. Edwards C, Stringer C. Management of early stage carcinoma of the vulva. *Ann Cl Conf Cancer* 1987;29:285–290.

24. Burke T, Stringer C, Gershenson D, et al. Radical wide excision and selective inguinal node dissection for squamous cell carcinoma of the vulva. *Gynecol Oncol* 1992;38:328–332.

25. Davidson T, Kissin M, Westbury G. Vulvo-vaginal melanoma—should radical surgery be abandoned? *Br J Obstet Gynaecol* 1987;94:473–476.

26. Rose P, Piver S, Tsukada Y, Lau T. Conservative therapy for melanoma of the vulva. *Am J Obstet Gynecol* 1988;159:52–55.

27. Thomas G, Dembo A, Bryson S, et al. Changing concepts in the management of vulvar cancer. *Gynecol Oncol* 1991;42:9–21.

28. Tasseron EW, Esch E, Hart A, et al. A clinico-pathologic study of 30 melanomas of the vulva. *Gynecol Oncol* 1992;46:170–175.

29. Bonner JA, Perez-Tamayo C, Reid GC, et al. The management of vaginal melanoma. *Cancer* 1988; 62:2066.

30. Van Nostrand KM, Lucci JA III, Schell M, et al. Primary vaginal melanoma: improved survival with radical pelvic surgery. *Gynecol Oncol* 1994; 55:243.

31. Reid GC, Schmidt RW, Roberts JA, et al. Primary melanoma of the vagina: a clinicopathologic analysis. *Obstet Gynecol* 1989;74:190.

Addendum: Staging System for Melanoma

WHO Stage	Extent of Disease	
I	Limited to skin	
II	Regional lymph node	
III	Distant metastases	

Stage	Extent of Disease	10-Year Survival Rates
American Joint Commission on Cancer		
Stage I	Localized, 0.76–1.50-mm involvement	85%
Stage Ia	Localized, <0.75 mm	
Stage IIa	Localized, 1.6–4.0 mm	60%
Stage IIb	Localized, >4.0 mm	
Stage III	Involved regional node or in transit metastasis	20%
Stage IV	Distant metastasis	<5%
Breslow's Staging		
Level I	<0.75 mm	100%
Level II	0.76–1.50 mm	100%
Level III	1.51–2.26 mm	89%
Level IV	2.26–3.00 mm	72%
Level V	>3.00 mm	22%
Clark's Levels		
Level I	In situ lesion	100%
Level II	Lesion penetrates basement membrane,	100%

	extends into loose papillary dermis	
Level III	Melanoma invades and fills papillary dermis, involves reticular dermis	74%
Level IV	Invasion of deep reticular dermis	50%
Level V	Melanoma invades subcutaneous adipose tissue	30%

Chung's Levels

Level I	Tumor confined to epithelium
Level II	Lesion penetrates basement membrane, extends into dermis/lamina propria, to 1 mm or less from granular layer, its estimated position in the epidermis, or from the outermost epithelial layer
Level III	Melanoma penetrates 1–2 mm into subepithelial tissue
Level IV	Invasion beyond 2 mm but not into underlying fat
Level V	Melanoma invades subcutaneous adipose tissue

Ovary
and
Fallopian
Tube

CHAPTER 29

Origins of Ovarian Cancer

HAROLD FOX

The term *ovarian cancer* embraces three broad groups of neoplasms, the epithelial tumors, tumors of sex cord–stromal origin, and germ cell neoplasms. These three broad groups of neoplasms differ markedly from each other in terms of their histogenesis, etiology, and clinical features and any discussion of the origin of ovarian cancer will have to consider these three groups separately.

Malignant Epithelial Tumors

Epithelial neoplasms account for 75% of all ovarian tumors. They can exist in a benign form, can grow as noninvasive tumors of borderline malignancy, or form malignant neoplasms. The malignant epithelial tumors are adenocarcinomas and these account for 90% of all malignant disease of the ovary. Indeed, the term *ovarian cancer*, when used without any qualification, usually refers to ovarian adenocarcinoma. There are five main forms of ovarian adenocarcinoma: 1) the serous adenocarcinomas, which resemble carcinomas of the fallopian tube; 2) mucinous carcinomas, which are histologically similar to endocervical carcinomas; 3) endometrioid carcinomas, which do not differ in any way from endometrial adenocarcinomas; 4) transitional cell carcinomas, which are identical to transitional cell neoplasms of the urinary tract; and 5) clear-cell adenocarcinomas, which are histologically identical to the clear-cell carcinomas of the vagina seen in girls who have been exposed prenatally to diethylstilbestrol.

Histogenesis

The generally accepted view is that most epithelial neoplasms arise, either directly or indirectly, from the surface epithelium, or serosa, of the ovary (1), though it is recognized that this unitary theory is too all embracing and a proportion have a quite different origin.

The ovarian serosa is the direct descendant, and exact postnatal equivalent, of the coelomic epithelium, which during embryogenesis overlies the parent structure of the ovary, the nephrogenital ridge. As the embryo develops, the coelomic epithelium of the nephrogenital ridge gives rise, by a process of evagination, to the müllerian ducts from which the endocervical epithelium, the endometrium, and the epithelium of the fallopian tube develop. The wolffian ducts, from which parts of the urinary system develop, also arise from the coelomic epithelium of the nephrogenital ridge. It is a basic histogenetic concept in ovarian neoplasia that tumors are derived from undifferentiated cells that have the same potential for differentiation as do the embryonic cells from which the adult tissue was derived. Hence, undifferentiated cells in the ovarian serosa can undergo a neoplastic change while retaining their embryonic potential to differentiate along various müllerian pathways. Thus, differentiation of neoplastic cells along a tubal pathway produces the serous group of neoplasms, differentiation along an endocervical route results in mucinous neoplasms, and differentiation along endometrial lines yields the endometrioid tumors. The transitional cell carcinomas (and their benign counterparts, the Brenner tumors) are formed of urinary tract–type epithelium and appear to arise from the surface epithelium by a process of wolffian, rather than müllerian, differentiation. It is not surprising that there is a residual capacity for wolffian differentiation in undifferentiated ovarian serosal cells in view of the origin of the wolffian ducts from the coelomic epithelium of the nephrogenital ridge. The clear-cell carcinomas are of müllerian nature and are best considered as a variant of an endometrioid tumor.

This concept of the epithelial tumors of the ovary having a common origin from the surface epithelium but showing different patterns of differentiation has been supported by tissue culture experiments which showed that the ovarian surface epithelium, unlike most other adult epithelia, appears relatively uncommitted and retains a considerable phenotypic plasticity (2). There are, however, exceptions to this general rule. Thus, some endometrioid and clear-cell carcinomas arise in and from foci of ovarian endometriosis. It is difficult to assess the proportion of ovarian adenocarcinomas that develop in this manner, for a neoplasm, as it grows, may obliterate any residual evidence of a preceding endometriotic focus, but circumstantial evidence suggests that about 30% of endometrial carcinomas and 50% of clear-cell carcinomas arise in this manner (3).

It is also possible that not all mucinous carcinomas develop from the ovarian serosa, for some, indeed many, are formed not of endocervical-type epithelium but of gastrointestinal-type epithelium: Neoplasms of this type may arise from the ovarian serosa via a process of gastrointestinal metaplasia, a change now known to occur with some frequency in müllerian tissues (1), but there is a possibility that some are monophyletic teratomas.

An actual origin directly from the ovarian serosa is very difficult to prove in most ovarian adenocarcinomas, for these usually have attained a large size by the time of the initial diagnosis and no site of origin can be determined. A small number of very early ovarian adenocarcinomas have, however, been described and did appear to involve the surface epithelium (4,5), while changes such as nuclear pleomorphism, irregularity of nuclear chromatin, stratification, and loss of nuclear polarity, thought to represent intraepithelial neoplasia, have been observed in the surface epithelium adjacent to ovarian adenocarcinomas (6,7). Expression of the p53 protein, indicative of a mutation in the tumor suppressor gene p53, is also frequently detectable in the serosa adjacent to an adenocarcinoma (8). It is probable that some ovarian adenocarcinomas do not arise directly from the serosa but from inclusion cysts that result from invagination of the serosa. Credence has been lent to this view by reports that the contralateral ovaries from women with unilateral ovarian adenocarcinoma contain an increased number of inclusion cysts (9), that inclusion cysts associated with ovarian adenocarcinoma have a high incidence of metaplastic changes (10) and cytologic atypia (8), and that the epithelium in these cysts may show overexpression of the oncogene c-*erb* B-2 and expression of the protein p53 (8). It must be noted, however, that an increased incidence of inclusion cysts in association with adenocarcinoma has not been confirmed in all studies (8,11).

Etiology

It is now known that a proportion of ovarian adenocarcinomas, probably no more than 5%, are genetically determined. However, any etiologic theory for sporadic ovarian epithelial neoplasia has to take into account the fact that epithelial neoplasms, relatively common in the human ovary, occur very rarely in the testes and are rather infrequent in animals (12,13). This suggests that the human ovary is exposed to carcinogenic stimuli from which both the testes and the animal ovary are shielded. Attempts to define the nature of such stimuli have rested largely on epidemiologic studies, for there has been a failure of experimental techniques to provide a suitable animal model for ovarian epithelial neoplasia (14).

Reproductive Factors

It has emerged from epidemiologic studies with considerable clarity that population groups with a high incidence of ovarian cancer are those that, on average, have small families (15) and that within any given population nulliparity is an important risk factor (16,17). It could be, and indeed has been, argued that nulliparity is not the real risk factor, but that the apparent relationship between the nulliparous state and ovarian cancer simply reflects a tendency for infertile women with ovarian malfunction to develop this form of neoplasia. Ovarian cancer is, however, unduly common in nuns (18), and nulliparous women who have never been married have the same risk as do married nulliparous women. These facts suggest not only that infertility per se is not an independent risk factor but also that the elevated risk in nulliparous women is attributable to deprivation of a direct protective effect conferred by pregnancy (17). That this is the case is shown by the fact that the more pregnancies a woman has, the less is her chance of developing ovarian adenocarcinoma (16,17,19,20). It is of note, however, that the first pregnancy has a greater protective effect than later pregnancies and that the pregnancy need not be complete, for failed gestations (e.g., ectopic pregnancies and abortions) also reduce the risk of ovarian cancer, though the magnitude of protection is less than that obtained from a full-term pregnancy (16,17,19,21). In some studies the age at which the first pregnancy occurs did not appear to be of any significance (16,17), though one recent population-based case-control study demonstrated that the older the woman at the time of her first gestation, the greater the degree of protection (20).

Breast-feeding also decreases the risk of ovarian cancer and the measure of protection increases with the length of the breast-feeding period (17,22,23). Studies of the effects of age at menarche and at menopause on the risk of ovarian cancer have not yielded any consistent pattern (17,23,24) but there has been general agreement, in a very large number of studies, that the use of combined oral contraceptives diminishes the risk of ovarian carcinoma, the magnitude of the risk reduction increasing with lengthening duration of usage (16,17,25–27). The protective effect of oral contraception usage is most marked in older women (28) and this may indicate that the early high-potency contraceptives were more protective than those in current use.

As discussed already, fertility per se does not appear to be a risk factor for ovarian cancer but it has been suggested that there is a subset of infertile women, those who have received drug therapy, who are at increased risk of developing ovarian adenocarcinoma (17). One later study found that only the use of clomiphene citrate was associated with an increased risk of ovarian cancer (29) while another found no association between the use of fertility drugs and ovarian cancer (30).

Both hysterectomy and tubal ligation reduce the risk for ovarian adenocarcinoma (17,31) and there is some evidence that hysterectomy before the age of 40 confers greater protection than does a similar operation after this age (17).

Genetic Factors

Since the early reports of familial ovarian cancer (32,33), it has become clear that hereditary forms of ovarian adenocarcinoma are far from rare (34). There are three different forms of familial ovarian adenocarcinoma: site-specific ovarian cancer, ovarian carcinoma associated with the Lynch II syndrome, and the breast/ovarian cancer syndrome. The latter syndrome is due largely to mutations in the *BRCA1* gene on chromosome 17q (35,36), which is probably a tumor suppressor gene, and, to a lesser extent mutations in the *BRCA2* locus on chromosome 13q (37). Many cases of site-specific ovarian cancer also seem to be related to *BRCA1* (38). The increased risk of ovarian cancer associated with *BRCA1* is considerable but difficult to quantify exactly, largely because there are possibly two alleles of *BRCA1* (39) and therefore significant heterogeneity of risk between different ovarian cancer families (40). The least common form of familial ovarian cancer is that associated with the Lynch II syndrome, which consists of hereditary nonpolyposis colorectal cancer together with a number of other carcinomas including ovarian cancer. This syndrome is associated with hereditary defects in mismatch repair genes, particularly on chromosomes 2p and 3p21 (41). The actual proportion of cases of ovarian cancer that have a genetic familial basis is also difficult to quantitate, for it is very dependent on what exactly is defined as a family history, and while estimates range from 3% (42) to 17% (43), a balanced view would be that approximately 5% of cases of ovarian cancer have a familial basis (41).

The genetic factors involved in sporadic ovarian cancer are still far from being fully understood, but they include abnormalities of growth factors (transforming growth factor-β, macrophage colony-stimulating factor), growth factor receptors (c-*fos*, epidermal growth factor receptor, c-*erb* B-2), genes involved in signal transduction (Ki-*ras*), genes involved in transcriptional regulation (c-*myc*, p53), and loss of heterozygosity at various chromosomal loci (41). These changes form a complex interlocking mosaic that is still in the process of elucidation.

Other Factors

The protective effect of hysterectomy has led some to suggest that an ascending carcinogen is involved in ovarian neoplasia and the finger of guilt has been pointed at talc (44,45), but overall the evidence in favor of a causal connection between talc and ovarian cancer is not convincing (46).

There have been repetitive claims that dietary factors play a role in ovarian carcinogenesis, dietary fat intake being particularly implicated in this respect (23,47,48). However, the evidence for this is far from convincing (49). It has also been maintained that milk consumption and lactose intake are related to the risk for ovarian cancer (50,51), but two recent studies (52,53) did not confirm this. Cigarette smoking has no effect on the risk for ovarian cancer while alcohol ingestion may have a protective effect (54).

Pathogenesis

Consideration of all the factors known either to increase or to decrease the risk of ovarian adenocarcinoma allows for the formulation of two etiologic hypotheses. The first of these is the "incessant ovulation" hypothesis, which argues that any factor that reduces the number of ovulations during a woman's reproductive life will decrease the risk of ovarian epithelial neoplasia (55). The possible mechanisms by which repetitive ovulation could influence the development of ovarian adenocarcinoma include an increased formation of inclusion cysts (56), repeated bathing of the surface epithelium by estrogen-rich follicular fluid (57), excess production of growth factors or cytokines (58), or an aberration of the repeated repair process that follows the trauma to the surface epithelium consequent to ovulation (59). This last suggestion has some experimental support, for repeated subculture in vitro of rat ovarian surface epithelial cells leads to their spontaneous transformation with acquisition of tumorigenicity (60), possibly because of mutations that result in somatic activation of oncogenes and tumor suppressor genes (41). Most

of the data with regard to reproductive factors are in accord with the incessant ovulation hypothesis, in particular the protective effects of pregnancy, oral contraception, and breast-feeding, all of which inhibit ovulation. The protective effects of hysterectomy and tubal ligation can also be explained in these terms, for there is a tendency for anovulatory cycles to occur after both procedures (61,62). Arguments against the excessive ovulation hypothesis include the weak, if any, influences of age at menarche and menopause, the greater risk reduction offered by pregnancy compared to a similar period of oral contraception, and the differential protective effect of first and subsequent pregnancies.

The alternative hypothesis is that raised gonadotropin levels play an etiologic role in the development of ovarian adenocarcinoma and that any factor reducing the levels of these hormones would protect against ovarian cancer (63). The hypergonadotropic hypothesis does not accord, however, with the protective effects of breast-feeding, hysterectomy, or tubal ligation, or with the lack of any reduction in risk with estrogen replacement therapy (17).

It is clear that neither of the two etiologic theories would explain all the known epidemiologic data and it is perhaps a little oversimplistic to seek a unitary theory of ovarian carcinogenesis. Possibly both incessant ovulation and high gonadotropin levels contribute, almost certainly together with other currently unidentified factors, to the development of ovarian adenocarcinoma, but neither is, in itself, *the* cause of the disease. The molecular genetics of ovarian carcinoma are complex (41) and it would be unduly simplistic to believe that any single factor can be held responsible for this disease.

Sex Cord–Stromal Tumors

Histogenesis

The only malignant neoplasm in this group that is encountered with any frequency is the granulosa cell tumor. A relatively simple, and widely held, view is that these neoplasms originate from undifferentiated cells that are ultimately derived from the sex cords of the early gonad (1). However, convincing evidence that granulosa cell tumors originate in this way is lacking and the results of experimental studies suggest a quite different histogenesis. In such studies granulosa cell neoplasms only developed when the oocytes were destroyed or genetically deleted. The oocytes appeared to be the organizers of the granulosa cells (64) and their loss led to disorganization or atresia of the follicles, circumstances under which a granulosa cell tumor was induced. This supports the suggestion that granulosa cell neoplasms arise from persisting granulosa cells in atretic follicles (65). In some animal studies granulosa cell tumors arose from stromal cells after follicular destruction (12) or from the surface epithelium (66). Nevertheless, oocyte depletion appears to be a key factor in the histogenesis of granulosa cell tumors, though this concept is unlikely to be applicable to the tumors of this type, about 5%, that occur in prepubertal girls.

Etiology

There are numerous experimental techniques for the induction of granulosa cell tumors in animals (12) and they have in common the facts that these neoplasms only develop when the pituitary gland is functioning normally and when there is depletion of ovarian oocytes. A spontaneously occurring animal model for ovarian granulosa cell tumors that bears a considerable resemblance to the experimental models is the F1 hybrid W^w/W^v mouse in which there is a genetic deletion of oocytes and a high incidence of granulosa cell neoplasia (67).

The sequence of events in experimentally induced granulosa cell tumors, and in some genetically determined spontaneous mouse tumors, appears to be oocyte destruction or loss, subsequent disorganization of follicular granulosa cells, a compensatory increase in pituitary gonadotropin output and resulting irregular proliferation, and eventually neoplasia, of the granulosa cells. These models reflect reasonably accurately the granulosa cell tumors found in many humans, for a significant proportion of these neoplasms occur at or soon after the menopause when oocytes are depleted and gonadotropin levels are high. It is therefore possible that an excessive gonadotropin response at the time of the menopause is an important factor in the etiology of at least some granulosa cell tumors.

Clearly, however, this etiologic theory will not account for the granulosa cell tumors that develop well before the menopause, sometimes before the menarche. A model for such neoplasms exists in SWR/J mice. In these animals ovarian granulosa cell tumors develop at an early age but there is no loss of oocytes and gonadotropin levels are normal (68). This model suggests that genetic factors may be implicated in the premenopausal development of granulosa cell tumors.

The sparse information about the epidemiology of human sex cord–stromal tumors has been collected and analyzed (69). Having had one full-term pregnancy appears to increase slightly the risk of developing a sex cord–stromal tumor but this risk is not further increased by subsequent pregnancies. The later the age at which the first pregnancy occurs, the greater the risk of neoplasia. A history of ever having used oral contraceptives is associated with a decreased risk of developing a sex cord–stromal tumor, as is estrogen replacement therapy after the age of 40. No change in risk is associated with breast-feeding, age at menarche, age at menopause, hysterectomy, or tubal ligation. These findings present difficulties in interpretation but they do offer some qualified support for the view that high gonadotropin levels play a role in the etiology of these neoplasms.

The study of genetic alterations in sex cord–stromal tumors is still in a rudimentary stage but there does seem to be a definite relationship between granulosa cell neoplasms and trisomy 12 (70).

Germ Cell Tumors

Histogenesis

There are three broad groups of germ cell neoplasms of the ovary, the dysgerminomas, those (such as the yolk sac tumors) that show differentiation into extraembryonic tissues, and tumors formed of tissues normally found in the embryo or adult, namely, the teratomas. All these neoplasms can occur together in various combinations and all have a similar distribution in gonadal and extragonadal sites, facts suggesting that they all have a common parentage. The most commonly occurring germ cell tumor is the teratoma and the histogenesis of all these allied neoplasms is best considered in the light of our knowledge of the origin of teratomas.

Numerous studies, detailed elsewhere (1,71), of spontaneously occurring and experimentally induced teratomas in mice showed that although teratomas are ultimately derived from primordial germ cells, these must first undergo parthenogenetic embryonic development (72) and that the stem cell of a mouse teratoma is an embryonal cell. Chromosomal and genetic studies of human teratomas confirmed the germ cell origins of these neoplasms and showed that teratoma formation is related to a meiotic defect in these cells (73–76). Further, studies of cell lines derived from immature, and hence malignant, human teratomas showed that their stem cells are very similar to those of mouse teratomas (77) and correspond to a cell in the early cleavage-stage embryo.

Hence, human teratomas arise from primordial germ cells as a result of a meiotic error and the germ cell must then undergo abortive parthenogenetic embryogenesis to give rise to the embryo-derived teratoma stem cell.

Etiology

The quite profound understanding of germ cell neoplasms arrived at by research studies is far from being matched by our knowledge of etiologic factors in human germ cell neoplasia.

There is evidence that prenatal exposure of male fetuses to excess estrogens increases the postnatal risk of developing an immature testicular teratoma (78,79) but there have been conflicting reports about any association between ovarian teratomas and maternal use of exogenous estrogens during pregnancy, one study finding such an association (80) and one not (81). Women with mature ovarian teratomas have some epidemiologic characteristics in common with men who have testicular immature teratomas, namely, high social class, high educational status, and a history either of being unmarried or of having married late in life (81). Unexplained, and indeed inexplicable, associations between ovarian mature teratomas and a history of exercise or alcohol ingestion have also been noted (81).

An analysis of reproductive factors associated with ovarian teratomas of all types found a slightly decreased risk in women who have had one to three full-term pregnancies, an increased risk in women who have had an abortion, and an increased risk with oral contraceptive usage (69). In a study confined to mature ovarian teratomas these neoplasms were associated with a history of infertility but there

was no relationship to parity, abortion history, or oral contraceptive usage (82).

Interpretation of these findings is difficult, especially when they are set in the context of our knowledge of the histogenesis of germ cell neoplasms.

REFERENCES

1. Langley FA, Fox H. Ovarian tumours: classification, histogenesis and aetiology. In: Fox H, ed. *Haines and Taylor: obstetrical and gynaecological pathology.* 4th ed. New York: Churchill Livingstone, 1995:727–742.

2. Auersperg N, Mainees-Bandiera SL, Dyck HG. Phenotypic plasticity of ovarian surface epithelium: implications for ovarian carcinogenesis. In: Sharp F, Blackett T, Leake R, Berek J, eds. *Ovarian cancer 4.* London: Chapman & Hall, 1996:3–17.

3. Toki T, Fujii S, Silverberg SG. A clinicopathologic study on the association of endometriosis and carcinoma of the ovary using a scoring system. *Int J Gynecol Cancer* 1996;6:68–75.

4. Scully RE. Early ovarian cancer. In: Sharp F, Mason WP, Creasman W, eds. *Ovarian cancer 2: biology, diagnosis and management.* London: Chapman & Hall, 1992:199–205.

5. Bell DA, Scully RE. Early de novo ovarian carcinoma: a study of fourteen cases. *Cancer* 1994;73:1859–1864.

6. Deligdisch L, Gill J. Characterization of ovarian dysplasia by interactive morphometry. *Cancer* 1989;63:748–755.

7. Plaxe SC, Deligdisch L, Dottino PR, Cohen CJ. Ovarian intraepithelial neoplasia demonstrated in patients with stage I ovarian carcinoma. *Gynecol Oncol* 1990;38:367–372.

8. Hutson R, Ramsdale J, Wells M. p53 Protein expression in putative precursor lesions of epithelial ovarian cancer. *Histopathology* 1995; 27:367–371.

9. Mittal KR, Zeleniuch-Jacquotte A, Cooper R, Demopoulos RI. Contralateral ovary in unilateral ovarian carcinoma: a search for preneoplastic lesions. *Int J Gynecol Pathol* 1993;12:59–63.

10. Resta L, Russo S, Colucci GA, Prat J. Morphologic precursors of ovarian epithelial tumors. *Obstet Gynecol* 1993;82:181–186.

11. Westhoff C, Murphy C, Heller D, Halim A. Is ovarian cancer associated with an increased fre-

quency of germinal inclusion cysts? *Am J Epidemiol* 1993;138:90–93.

12. Marchant J. Animal models for tumours of the ovary. In: Murphy ED, Beamer WG, eds. *Biology of ovarian neoplasia.* Geneva: UICC, 1980: 50–65.

13. Damjanov I. Ovarian tumors in laboratory and domestic animals. *Curr Top Pathol* 1989;78:1–10.

14. Fox H. Human ovarian tumours: classification, histogenesis and criteria for animal models. In: Murphy ED, Beamer WG, eds. *Biology of ovarian neoplasia.* Geneva: UICC, 1980:22–55.

15. Beral V. The epidemiology of ovarian cancer. In: Newman CE, Ford CMJ, Jordan JA, eds. *Ovarian cancer.* Oxford: Pergamon, 1980:29–36.

16. Parazzini F, Franceschi S, La Vecchia C, Fasoli M. The epidemiology of ovarian cancer. *Gynecol Oncol* 1991;42:9–23.

17. Whittemore AS, Harris R, Imyre J. Characteristics relating to ovarian cancer risk: collaborative analysis of 12 US case control studies. *Am J Epidemiol* 1992;136:1184–1203.

18. Fraumeni JF, Lloyd JW, Smith EM, Wagoner JK. Cancer mortality amongst nuns: role of marital status in etiology of neoplastic disease in women. *J Natl Cancer Inst* 1969;42:455–468.

19. Negri E, Franceschi S, Tzonou A, et al. Pooled analysis of 3 European case-control studies. I. Reproductive factors and risk of epithelial ovarian cancer. *Int J Cancer* 1991;49:50–56.

20. Adami H-O, Hsieh CC, Lambe M, et al. Parity, age at first childbirth, and risk of ovarian cancer. *Lancet* 1994;344:1250–1254.

21. Mori M, Harabuchi I, Miyake H, et al. Reproductive, genetic, and dietary risk factors for ovarian cancer. *Am J Epidemiol* 1988;128:771–777.

22. Rosenblatt KA, Thomas DB. Lactation and the risk of epithelial ovarian cancer. *Int J Epidemiol* 1993;22:192–197.

23. Shoham Z. Epidemiology, etiology, and fertility drugs in ovarian epithelial carcinomas: where are we today? *Fertil Steril* 1994;62:433–448.

24. Franceschi S, La Vecchia C, Booth M, et al. Pooled analysis of 3 European case-control studies of epithelial ovarian cancer. II. Age at menarche and at menopause. *Int J Cancer* 1991; 49:57–60.

25. Vessey M, Metcalfe A, Wells C, et al. Ovarian neoplasms, functional ovarian cysts, and oral contraceptives. *BMJ* 1987;294:1518–1520.

26. Beral V, Hannaford P, Kay C. Oral contraceptive use and malignancies of the genital tract. *Lancet* 1988;2:1331–1334.

27. Franseschi S, Parazzini F, Negri E, et al. Pooled analysis of 3 European case-control studies of epithelial ovarian cancer. III. Oral contraceptive use. *Int J Cancer* 1991;49:61–65.

28. Whittemore A. Personal characteristics relating to risk of invasive epithelial ovarian cancer in older women in the United States. *Cancer* 1993;71(2 suppl):558–565.

29. Rossing MA, Daling JR, Weiss NS, et al. Ovarian tumors in a cohort of infertile women. *N Engl J Med* 1994;331:771–776.

30. Franceschi S, La Vecchia C, Negri E, et al. Fertility drugs and risk of epithelial ovarian cancer in Italy. *Hum Reprod* 1994;9:1673–1675.

31. Parazzini F, Negri E, La Vecchia C, et al. Hysterectomy, oophorectomy, and subsequent ovarian cancer risk. *Obstet Gynecol* 1993;81:363–366.

32. Franceschi S, La Vecchia C, Mangioni C. Familial ovarian cancer: eight more families. *Gynecol Oncol* 1982;13:31–36.

33. Piver MS, Barlow J, Sawler DM. Familial ovarian cancer: increasing in frequency? *Obstet Gynecol* 1982;60:397–399.

34. Piver MS, Baker TR, Piedmonte M, Sandecki AM. Familial ovarian cancer: a report of 658 families from the Gilda Radner Familial Ovarian Cancer Registry 1981–1991. *Cancer* 1993;71(2 suppl):582–588.

35. Miki Y, Swensen J, Shattuck-Eidenes D, et al. A strong candidate for the breast and ovarian cancer susceptibility gene BRCA1. *Science* 1994; 266:66–71.

36. Futreal PA, Liu Q, Shattuck-Eidenes D, et al. BRCA1 mutations in primary breast and ovarian carcinomas. *Science* 1994;266:120–122.

37. Wooster R, Neuhausen SL, Mangion J, et al. Localization of a breast cancer susceptibility gene, BRCA2, to chromosome 13q12-13. *Science* 1994;265:2088–2090.

38. Steichen Gersdorf E, Gallion HH, Ford D, et al. Familial site specific ovarian cancer is linked to BRCA1 on 17q12-21. *Am J Hum Genet* 1994;55: 870–875.

39. Narod SA, Ford D, Devilee P, et al. An evaluation of genetic heterogeneity in 145 breast-ovarian cancer families: Breast Cancer Linkage Consortium. *Am J Hum Genet* 1995;56:254–264.

40. Easton DF, Ford D, Bishop DT. Breast and ovarian cancer incidence in BRCA1-mutation carriers. Breast Cancer Linkage Consortium. *Am J Hum Genet* 1995;56:265–271.

41. Jacobs I, Lancaster J. The molecular genetics of sporadic and familial epithelial ovarian cancer. *Int J Gynecol Cancer* 1996;6:337–355.

42. Webb MJ. Screening for ovarian cancer. *BMJ* 1993;306:1015–1016.

43. Houlston RS, Collins A, Slack J, et al. Genetic epidemiology of ovarian cancer: segregation analysis. *Ann Hum Genet* 1991;55:291–299.

44. Cramer DW, Welch WR, Scully RE, Wojoeckowski RN. Ovarian cancer and talc: a case control study. *Cancer* 1982;50:372–376.

45. Harlow BL, Cramer DW, Bell DA, Welch WR. Perineal exposure to talc and ovarian cancer risk. *Obstet Gynecol* 1992;80:19–23.

46. Wehner AP. Biologic effects of cosmetic talc. *Food Chem Toxicol* 1994;32:1173–1184.

47. La Vecchia C, Decarli A, Negri E, et al. Dietary factors and the risk of epithelial ovarian cancer. *J Natl Cancer Inst* 1987;79:663–669.

48. Prentice RL, Sheppard L. Dietary fat and cancer: consistency of the epidemiologic data and disease prevention that may follow from a practical reduction in fat consumption. *Cancer Causes Control* 1990;1:81–97.

49. Doyle P, dos Santos Silva I. Pathogenesis and epidemiology of ovarian cancer. In: Shingleton HM, Fowler WC Jr, Jordan JA, Lawrence WD, eds. *Gynecologic oncology: current diagnosis and treatment.* London: Saunders, 1996:165–173.

50. Cramer DW, Harlow BL, Willett WC, et al. Galactose consumption and metabolism in relation to the risk of ovarian cancer. *Lancet* 1989;2:66–71.

51. Cramer DW. Lactase persistence and milk consumption as determinants of ovarian cancer risk. *Am J Epidemiol* 1989;130:904–910.

52. Risch HA, Jain M, Marrett LD, Howe GR. Dietary lactose intake, lactose intolerance and the risk of epithelial ovarian cancer in southern Ontario (Canada). *Cancer Causes Control* 1994;5:540–548.

53. Herrington LJ, Weiss NS, Beresford SA, et al. Lactose and galactose intake and metabolism in relation to the risk of epithelial ovarian cancer. *Am J Epidemiol* 1995;141:407–416.

54. Kato I, Tominaga S, Terao C. Alcohol consumption and cancers of hormone-related organs in women. *Jpn J Clin Oncol* 1989;19:202–207.

55. Fathalla MF. Incessant ovulation—a factor in ovarian neoplasia? *Lancet* 1971;2:163.

56. Zajicek J. Ovarian cystomas and ovulation: a histogenetic concept. *Tumori* 1977;63:429–435.

57. Venter PF. Ovarian epithelial cancer and chemical carcinogenesis. *Gynecol Oncol* 1981;12:281–285.

58. Berek JS, Martinez-Maza O. Molecular and biologic factors in the pathogenesis of ovarian cancer. *J Reprod Med* 1994;39:241–248.

59. Casagrande JT, Louie EW, Pike MC, et al. "Incessant ovulation" and ovarian cancer. *Lancet* 1979; 2:170–173.

60. Godwin AK, Testa JR, Handel LM, et al. Spontaneous transformation of rat ovarian surface epithelial cells: association with cytogenetic changes and implications of repeated ovulation in the etiology of ovarian cancer. *J Natl Cancer Inst* 1992;84:592–601.

61. Cattanach J. Oestrogen deficiency after tubal ligation. *Lancet* 1985;1:847–849.

62. Destefano F, Perlman JA, Peterson HB, et al. Long-term risk of menstrual disturbances after tubal sterilization. *Am J Obstet Gynecol* 1985;152: 835–841.

63. Stadel BV. The etiology and prevention of ovarian cancer. *Am J Obstet Gynecol* 1975;123: 772–774.

64. Gospadarowicz D. Growth and differentiation factors for cell populations in the normal ovary. In: Murphy ED, Beamer WG, eds. *Biology of ovarian neoplasia.* Geneva: UICC, 1980:2–21.

65. McKay DG, Hertig AT, Hickey WI. The histogenesis of granulosa and thecal cell tumors of the ovary. *Obstet Gynecol* 1953;1:125–136.

66. Gardner WH. Development of tumors in ovaries transplanted into the spleen. *Cancer Res* 1955;13:109–117.

67. Murphy ED. Major experimental models of ovarian tumors: histogenesis and evaluation. In: Murphy ED, Beamer WG, eds. *Biology of ovarian neoplasia.* Geneva: UICC, 1980:66–73.

68. Beamer WG. Endocrinology of human tumors. In: Murphy ED, Beamer WG, eds. *Biology of ovarian neoplasia.* Geneva: UICC, 1980:82–97.

69. Horn-Ross PL, Whittemore AS, Harris R, Itnyre J. Characteristics relating to ovarian cancer risk: collaborative analysis of 12 US case-control studies. VI. Non-epithelial cancers among adults. *Epidemiology* 1992;3:490–495.

70. Fletcher JA, Gibas Z, Donovan K, et al. Ovarian granulosa-stromal cell tumors are characterized by trisomy 12. *Am J Pathol* 1991;138:515–520.

71. Fox H. Biology of teratomas. In: Anthony P, MacSween RNM, eds. *Recent advances in histopathology 13.* Edinburgh: Churchill Livingstone, 1987:33–43.

72. Solter D. Experimental mouse teratocarcinoma: a model for human teratocarcinoma? In: Damjanov I, Knowles BB, Solter D, eds. *The human teratomas: experimental and clinical biology.* Clifton, NJ: Humana, 1983:323–356.

73. Carritt B, Partington J, Welch H, Povey S. Diverse origins of multiple ovarian teratomas in a single individual. *Proc Natl Acad Sci USA* 1982;79:7400–7404.

74. Partington J, West I, Povey S. The origin of ovarian teratomas. *J Med Genet* 1984;21:4–12.

75. Ohama K, Nomura K, Okamoto E, et al. Origin of immature teratomas of the ovary. *Am J Obstet Gynecol* 1985;152:869–890.

76. Surti U, Hoffner L, Chakravarti A, Ferrel RE. Genetics and biology of human ovarian teratomas. I. Cytogenetic analysis and mechanism of origin. *Am J Hum Genet* 1990;47:635–643.

77. Andrews PW, Goodfellow PN, Damjanov I. Human teratocarcinoma cells in culture. *Cancer Surv* 1983;2:41–73.

78. Schottenfeld D, Warshauer M, Sherlock S, et al. The epidemiology of testicular cancer in young adults. *Am J Epidemiol* 1980;112:232–246.

79. Depue R, Pike M, Henderson B. Estrogen exposure during gestation and risk of testicular cancer. *J Natl Cancer Inst* 1983;71:1151–1155.

80. Walker AH, Ross RK, Haile RWC, Henderson BE. Hormonal factors and risk of ovarian germ cell cancer in young women. *Br J Cancer* 1988;57:418–422.

81. Westhoff C, Pike M, Vessey M. Benign ovarian teratomas: a population-based case-control study. *Br J Cancer* 1988;58:93–98.

82. Parazzini F, La Veccia C, Negri E, et al. Risk factors for benign ovarian teratomas. *Br J Cancer* 1995;71:644–646.

CHAPTER 30

Pathology of Ovarian Cancer

HAROLD FOX

The term *ovarian cancer* is used here to include not only the malignant primary epithelial tumors of the ovary but also the various malignant sex cord–stromal and germ cell neoplasms.

Epithelial Tumors

As discussed in a previous chapter, these neoplasms are, for the most part, derived from the surface epithelium of the ovary. They comprise 60% to 65% of all ovarian neoplasms and about 90% of those that are malignant. Those that are frankly malignant are collectively classed as *ovarian adenocarcinoma*, this portmanteau term encompassing several histologic subsets, namely, serous, mucinous, endometrioid, and clear-cell adenocarcinomas and malignant Brenner tumors (transitional cell carcinomas). Some epithelial ovarian neoplasms show the cytologic features of malignancy but are noninvasive and these are classed as tumors of borderline malignancy.

Adenocarcinoma

Among malignant epithelial ovarian tumors, serous adenocarcinomas are the most common form, accounting for between 40% and 50% of these tumors. Endometrioid and mucinous adenocarcinomas form about 20% and 10% of the total, respectively, whereas clear-cell carcinomas account for between 5% and 10% of adenocarcinomas. Malignant Brenner tumors are uncommon, though in the past their infrequency has been markedly overestimated.

Some carcinomas are so poorly differentiated that no diagnosis more specific than undifferentiated adenocarcinoma can be made whereas a significant proportion of epithelial neoplasms contain more than one type of epithelium, it being not uncommon, for instance, to encounter a mixture of serous carcinoma and mucinous carcinoma within a given tumor: These latter neoplasms are classified in terms of the predominant type of epithelium and are only diagnosed as "mixed" if the second epithelial component is a prominent feature of the tumor.

Gross Appearances

There is little point to describing the gross appearance of each individual type of ovarian adenocarcinoma, for specific features are generally absent. The tumors are usually bulky, typically measuring between 15 and 30 cm in diameter, and may have a smooth or bosselated outer surface that can be studded with papillae. On section the neoplasm may appear cystic, partially cystic, or solid throughout. Cystic areas may be unilocular or, more commonly, multiloculated and can contain either serous or mucinous fluid that may be turbid, blood stained, or frankly hemorrhagic. Fleshy or firm mural nodules often protrude into cystic spaces while, particularly but not specifically in serous adenocarcinomas, the cyst cavities may be partly or wholly filled with soft friable villi. Solid areas may be crumbly, soft, fleshy, firm, or rubbery and are commonly white, whitish-yellow, or gray. Foci of hemorrhage and necrosis, often extensive, are a characteristic feature.

Histologic Appearances

Well-differentiated serous adenocarcinomas have a predominantly papillary pattern (Fig. 30-1). The papillae tend to be fine, often branching, and not infrequently fused at their tips. They have a delicate connective tissue support and a covering but invading epithelium in which the constituent cells bear an anarchic resemblance to those normally found in the tubal epithelium. A purely papillary pattern is, however, relatively uncommon and there are often a few areas showing an irregular acinar pattern, the acini tending to have slitlike lumens. Poorly differentiated serous adenocarcinomas have a predominantly solid histologic appearance with sheets of small, relatively uniform cells, sometimes showing a syncytial-like pattern, admixed with poorly formed glandular acini or abortive papillae. Serous tumors of moderate differentiation occupy an intermediate position, often containing a melange of papillary, acinar, and solid areas. Psammoma bodies, which are small laminated calcospherites, are a characteristic but not a specific feature of serous adenocarcinomas and are seen most commonly, and most conspicuously, in well-differentiated neoplasms.

Well-differentiated mucinous adenocarcinomas (Fig. 30-2) tend to show a locular and acinar pattern, the lining epithelium being recognizably formed of columnar mucus-secreting cells that show varying degrees of multilayering, mitotic activity, and atypia. Goblet cells are commonly seen. Stromal invasion is evident but it is not uncommon for well-differentiated tumors, if extensively sampled, to also contain

F I G U R E **30-1**

A well-differentiated serous adenocarcinoma.

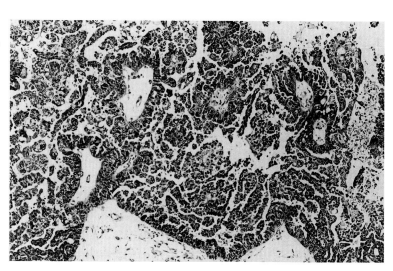

F I G U R E **30-2**

A well-differentiated mucinous adenocarcinoma.

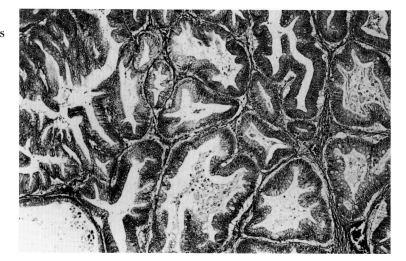

areas having the appearance of a benign mucinous cystadenoma or areas showing the appearance of a tumor of borderline malignancy. Poorly differentiated mucinous adenocarcinomas may be formed largely of solid sheets of anaplastic cells interspersed with poorly formed glandular acini. There may be clusters or single infiltrating cells while signet-ring cells may be a noticeable feature. In all grades of mucinous carcinoma there may be extrusion of mucus into the stroma. This is sometimes extensive, with the formation of large pools of mucus in which tumor cells appear to be floating (pseudomyxoma ovarii).

Endometrioid adenocarcinomas have a histologic appearance that is very similar to, indeed virtually identical with, that of endometrioid adenocarcinomas of the endometrium (Fig. 30-3). It is of interest that despite the histologic similarity between the endometrial and ovarian neoplasms, they differ markedly from each other in genetic terms (1). Most endometrioid adenocarcinomas are well differentiated and have a well-formed acinar pattern, with the cells lining the acini often showing multilayering and irregular budding. The cells resemble those of the glandular epithelium of a proliferative-phase endometrium but show a greater degree of pleomorphism and atypia. The stroma of the tumor resembles that of the ovary rather than that of the endometrium and stromal invasion is usually readily apparent. A papillary pattern may be present in some areas and may even predominate. However, the papillae are blunter and broader than those in a serous adenocarcinoma. Squamous metaplasia is a common occurrence while a clear-cell pattern is often

focally present. Moderately differentiated adenocarcinomas show a more complex microglandular pattern with a greater degree of pleomorphism whereas poorly differentiated endometrioid tumors have a predominantly solid growth pattern with residual microglandular areas. Some endometrioid tumors adopt a pattern resembling a Sertoli cell neoplasm (2,3) but in such tumors there is usually a transition, in at least some areas, to a more conventional endometrioid appearance. It should be noted that the term *malignant endometrioid tumor of the ovary* encompasses all the various neoplasms that can also occur in the endometrium, such as carcinosarcomas, adenosarcomas, adenosquamous carcinomas, and endometrioid stromal sarcomas.

Malignant Brenner tumors have generally been regarded as rare neoplasms but it is probable that their apparent infrequency has been overemphasized by an insistence on unnecessarily rigid and restrictive diagnostic criteria. In essence, a malignant Brenner tumor is a transitional cell carcinoma that resembles neoplasms of similar type found in the bladder (Fig. 30-4). The tumor may grow in a solid fashion but papillary areas may also be present. Areas of squamous differentiation are common whereas foci of adenocarcinomatous differentiation are sometimes apparent. It has traditionally been insisted that a malignant Brenner tumor can only be diagnosed if there is an observable transition from benign Brenner elements, but this implies that a malignant Brenner tumor invariably originates from a previously present benign neoplasm, a view not held for any other form of ovarian carcinoma. However, a distinc-

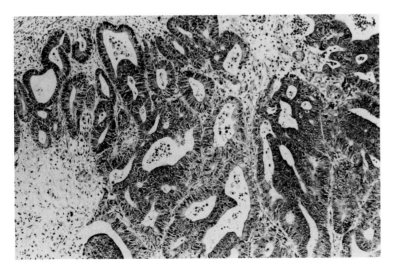

FIGURE **30-3**

A well-differentiated endometrioid adenocarcinoma.

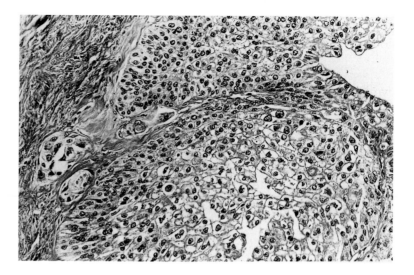

F I G U R E **30-4**

A malignant Brenner tumor.

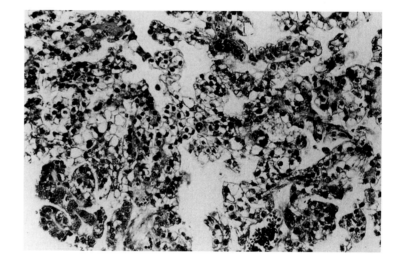

F I G U R E **30-5**

A clear-cell adenocarcinoma.

tion has been drawn between malignant Brenner tumors, which are associated with benign Brenner elements, and pure transitional cell carcinomas (4), a distinction that appears to be valid for while the latter behave in a more malignant fashion, they appear to be unusually sensitive to radiotherapy (5,6).

Clear-cell adenocarcinomas show a variety of architectural patterns that may occur singly or in any combination within an individual neoplasm (7–9). In clear-cell adenocarcinomas with the diffuse pattern there are sheets of polyhedral cells with distinct boundaries, abundant clear cytoplasm, and eccentric, angular nuclei. The tubulocystic pattern is characterized by tubules and cysts that may be lined by flattened, cuboidal, or columnar clear cells or by hobnail-shaped cells (Fig. 30-5), the latter having prominent nuclei that occupy the bulbous tips of the cells and protrude into the lumen. In the pap-

illary pattern the papillae may be simple or complex and have delicate mesenchymal cores that often show hyalinization. The papillae are covered by clear, hobnail-shaped, or nondescript cuboidal cells. Oxyphilic cells, with abundant eosinophilic cytoplasm, are often present in clear-cell adenocarcinomas and sometimes predominate (10).

Spread

Bilateral involvement of the ovaries by adenocarcinoma is common and it is often far from clear whether this is due to metastatic spread or to a multicentric origin. It appears highly probable, however, that spread to the contralateral ovary contributes substantially to the incidence of bilaterality, for the frequency of bilateral involvement increases progressively with advancing clinical stage. Possible routes of spread to the opposite ovary include transperitoneal seeding, cell migration through the tubes and endometrial cavity, and lymphatic spread via anastomoses between ovarian and uterine lymphatic vessels. The uterus is frequently involved by tumor, either because of direct extension or because of retrograde lymphatic spread, whereas extension to the endometrium may be either via the lymphatics or by luminal migration of tumor cells through the tube.

Transperitoneal spread is very common and is not limited to neoplasms with external tumor excrescences, occurring with almost equal frequency in tumors with an apparently intact capsule. Direct seeding leads to implants on the pelvic peritoneum, in the pouch of Douglas, and in the omentum. Deposits in the pouch of Douglas may grow through to the vagina but those in the pelvic peritoneum tend to spread over the surface, leading to widespread adhesions. Tumor cells also seed directly into the small amount of normally present peritoneal fluid and are carried by this fluid to be deposited in the paracolic gutters (11) and on the undersurface of the right leaf of the diaphragm (spread to the left diaphragm not occurring because the phrenicocolic ligament blocks the upward movement of the fluid on this side) (12). Tumor cells also seed to involve the gastrointestinal tract, often to form multiple small superficial nodules on the peritoneum of the small bowel. Involvement of large areas of the wall of the sigmoid colon or rectum is common whereas less frequently there is diffuse infiltration of the mesentery (13).

Lymphatic spread is a common feature of ovarian carcinoma. Six to eight lymphatic channels accompany the ovarian blood vessels to the para-aortic nodes but lymphatic vessels also run via the broad ligament to the obturator nodes. As there are numerous anastomoses between the obturator nodes and the iliac and para-aortic nodes, the retroperitoneal nodes that drain the ovary are interconnected to the level of the aortic bifurcation (14). Autopsy studies found metastases in the pelvic lymph nodes in between 48% and 80% of ovarian carcinoma patients and metastases in the para-aortic nodes in between 58% and 78% of patients (15,16). However, nodal metastasis is not a late event, for it is found in between 14% and 24% of women with apparent stage I disease (17,18). The incidence of nodal metastasis doubles in patients with apparent stage II disease and exceeds 70% in those in stage III (12,14,17–20).

The topographic distribution of nodes involved by ovarian carcinoma is unpredictable, but metastases confined to the pelvic nodes are somewhat more common than are metastases confined to the para-aortic nodes whereas in 44% of patients both sets of nodes are involved (18).

Hematogenous spread of ovarian carcinoma is uncommon but does occur, usually late in the course of the disease, to sites such as the liver, spleen, lungs, brain, and bones.

Prognostic Pathologic Factors

The overall 5-year survival rate for women with ovarian carcinoma is in the region of 30% and the most important prognostic factor is the surgicopathologic stage at the time of initial diagnosis. Staging is, however, not of absolute prognostic value to the individual patient, for some women with stage I or II disease die quite quickly whereas others with stage III or IV disease survive for surprisingly long periods.

Many clinicians believe the histologic type of ovarian carcinoma is of prognostic importance, the claim often being that endometrioid and mucinous adenocarcinomas have a relatively good prognosis, that serous carcinomas have an unusually poor prognosis, and that the outlook for women with clear-cell adenocarcinomas lies somewhere between these two extremes (21–23). When considering the significance of histologic type, one must keep in mind that many pathologists tend to diagnose endometrioid adenocarcinomas as such only if they are well differentiated, and often relegate all poorly differentiated neoplasms into the serous category; this partially, though not completely, accounts for the very considerable interobserver variation in the histologic typing of ovarian adenocarcinomas (24,25). Equally, or perhaps more importantly, evidence for the prognostic value of histologic type has usually been based on univariate analysis, and multivariate analysis has generally shown that, stage for stage and grade for grade, the histologic type of an ovarian adenocarcinoma is of little or no prognostic significance (26–31). However, this conclusion applies largely to serous, mucinous, and endometrioid adenocarcinomas and there is still some dispute about the prognostic significance of a clear-cell and a transitional cell pattern. Thus, debate continues as to whether early-stage clear-cell carcinomas have an unusually poor prognosis or not (32) and as to whether the histologic pattern within such tumors is of prognostic significance (33–36). The transitional cell carcinomas were originally thought to have a poor prognosis (4) but more recent reports claimed that these neoplasms are associated with a relatively good outlook, even when at an advanced stage, and respond unusually well to chemotherapy (5,37,38).

The prognostic value of histologic grading of ovarian carcinoma has been widely accepted (26,30,39,40), but it is far from clear how these neoplasms should be graded. Some clinicians find Broders' system, in which the percentage of undifferentiated cells is assessed, useful but it is highly subjective and difficult to apply in a consistent pattern. Most commonly, therefore, ovarian carcinomas are graded in architectural terms as well, moderately, or poorly differentiated. This system works to the extent that pathologists can easily recognize very well and very poorly differentiated tumors but the borderlines between "well" and "moderately" differentiated neoplasms and between "moderately" and "poorly" differentiated tumors have never been defined and are interpreted in an inconsistent and subjective fashion. Therefore, it is not surprising that there are very high interobserver and intraobserver differences in the assessment of ovarian carcinoma grades (41–43).

In the last few decades the introduction of quantitative techniques has allowed for a more objective and consistent approach to the grading of ovarian carcinomas. Tumor aneuploidy, demonstrated by DNA flow cytometry, is an important independent adverse prognostic factor in both early- and late-stage ovarian epithelial cancer according to the results of most studies (44–51), though admittedly there have been some dissenters from this view (52–54).

Quantitative morphometric and stereologic analysis of tumors using automated image analysis systems provides information that is both objective and reproducible. Measurements that can be made in such systems include mean nuclear area, volume, longest axis, and shortest axis, and parameters such as the volume percentage epithelium (i.e., the percentage of the volume of a tumor that is formed of epithelium) and the mitotic activity index can also be quantitatively assessed. Techniques such as these have been applied to ovarian adenocarcinomas. It has been shown that the estimation of the mitotic activity index and the volume percentage epithelium allows for stratification of tumors

into "high-risk" and "low-risk" groups (55–61) whereas the addition of the mean nuclear area to these variables adds a further element of prognostic precision, this latter measurement probably being the single best indicator of clinical outcome in ovarian cancer (61–65).

Estrogen and progesterone receptors are present in a high proportion of ovarian adenocarcinomas (66) and there have been both claims and denials that expression of these receptors is associated with a relatively good prognosis (67–72), but no clear agreement has been attained.

Within the past few years the search for prognostic factors in ovarian carcinomas has widened to include studies of cell proliferation markers, expression of proto-oncogenes and their products, and mutations within tumor suppression genes. Two cell proliferation markers have been studied, proliferating cell nuclear antigen (PCNA) and Ki-67. Staining for the cell proliferation marker PCNA has yielded conflicting results about the prognostic value of this marker in ovarian adenocarcinoma (73–77), and while the range of Ki-67–positive cells in ovarian carcinomas is variable, high values correlated with poor patient survival in some studies (78–81) but not in others (77,82).

Mutation of the tumor suppressor gene p53 with positive immunostaining for p53 protein is common in ovarian carcinomas (83–91) and has been related to poor tumor differentiation and an adverse clinical outcome in patients with stage I ovarian carcinomas (92,93). Some studies found that, overall, detectable p53 in ovarian carcinomas is associated with poor tumor differentiation and with decreased survival (89,93–97) but others were unable to show any correlation between p53 expression and either tumor-related features or an adverse clinical outcome (83,86,90). In a carefully studied and well-analyzed series of ovarian carcinomas, p53 expression was associated with poor tumor differentiation, advanced stage, and bulky residual disease but did not, on multivariate analysis, have a significant independent effect on patient survival or disease-free interval (98).

In ovarian neoplasms, p62c-*myc*, which is the product of the c-*myc* oncogene, has been detected in serous tumors, both frank adenocarcinomas and tumors of borderline malignancy to much the same extent and degree (99,100), and in mucinous adenocarcinomas (101). It has been suggested that c-*myc* overexpression is associated with unusually aggressive tumor behavior (102). K-*ras* point mutations occur in 20% to 40% of ovarian carcinomas (103,104) and the *ras* oncogene product p21 is often detectable in ovarian neoplasms (105,106) but this has not been shown to have any correlation with tumor characteristics or clinical outcome. Overexpression of the c-*erb* B-2 oncogene is found in 20% of early-stage ovarian adenocarcinomas (107) and more commonly in advanced-stage disease (108) but there has been considerable disagreement about the prognostic significance of this finding, some noting that c-*erb* B-2 expression is associated with a poor prognosis (108–112) and others finding it to have no prognostic significance (107,113–120).

Epithelial Tumors of Borderline Malignancy

To some gynecologists a histopathologic diagnosis of ovarian epithelial tumor of borderline malignancy indicates indecision on the part of the pathologist as to whether a tumor is benign or malignant, an attitude that led to the view that "there are no borderline tumors, only borderline pathologists." If this were indeed the case, then the gynecologist would have legitimate grounds for complaint, for there is little point to elevating pathologic uncertainty into a nosologic entity. Ovarian tumors of borderline malignancy are, however, a well-delineated and clearly defined group, the diagnosis of which is a positive one based on specific histologic findings. It is true that the term *borderline malignancy* hints at uncertainty and irresolution but it is marginally less objectionable than any of the other suggested forms of nomenclature (121).

Only mucinous and serous tumors of borderline malignancy have been clearly defined in clinicopathologic terms. Endometrioid, clear-cell, and Brenner tumors of borderline malignancy have been described but the status of these neoplasms remains uncertain and their clinical course is ill defined.

Many reports of the behavior and management of ovarian tumors of borderline malignancy consider the serous and mucinous types together as if they were a single homogeneous group with respect to pathology, clinical course, and management. This approach is increasingly seen to be invalid and, apart from considerations of nomenclature and definition, the mucinous and serous tumors require separate consideration.

Definition

The currently employed World Health Organization (WHO) definition of a tumor of borderline malignancy (122) is woefully imprecise and that of the Ovarian Tumour Panel of the Royal College of Obstetricians and Gynaecologists (123) is much preferred (and will be the definition of choice in the new WHO classification). The panel defined a borderline tumor as one in which the epithelial component shows some, or all, of the characteristics of malignancy but in which there is no stromal invasion. It should be recognized that this definition takes no account of the degree of epithelial abnormality and employs lack of stromal invasion as the cardinal defining feature of these neoplasms. It should also be noted that the presence or absence of apparent extraovarian spread plays no role in the definition of a neoplasm of borderline malignancy, and that even if extensive extraovarian lesions are present, the ovarian tumor will still be placed in the borderline category if it fulfills the histologic criteria for that diagnosis.

Insistence on the prime diagnostic importance of a lack of stromal invasion, though undoubtedly the correct approach, has nevertheless led to some conceptual and practical problems. Thus, because difficulties may be encountered in deciding whether stromal invasion is present or not, there has been an increasing tendency to insist on a lack of "destructive" invasion (124). Unfortunately, the term *destructive* has not been defined in this context and hence its recognition may be highly subjective. Identification of stromal invasion may be particularly difficult in mucinous tumors of borderline malignancy that have a complex glandular pattern with many epithelial outpouchings. This has led to the proposal that such neoplasms showing a marked overgrowth of atypical epithelial cells with cellular stratification of four or more cell layers in thickness should be classed as mucinous carcinomas even in the absence of overt stromal invasion (125–127). This concept has won some support (124,128–130) but others have not found it to confer any added prognostic precision and have argued against its use (131–136).

Although evidence of stromal invasion negates a diagnosis of borderline malignancy, there have been several reports of "microinvasion" of the stroma of both serous and mucinous tumors that otherwise showed the typical features of a neoplasm of borderline malignancy (136–138). Such neoplasms followed the same clinical course and had the same prognosis as did borderline tumors without microinvasion. Conceptually, neoplasms with microinvasion are not of borderline malignancy but clinically they are not adenocarcinomas.

Serous Tumors of Borderline Malignancy

These are usually cystic and differ from a benign papillary serous cystadenoma only by an unusually luxuriant proliferation of fine papillae on their inner surface and by the presence of exophytic papillary excrescences on their outer surface. A proportion resemble a benign serous surface papillary tumor but tend to have a rather more complex and dense papillary pattern. Histologically, these neoplasms are formed of rather fine branching papillae (Fig. 30-6). In the neoplasms with only minimal epithelial atypia, the cellular mantle of the papillae can be clearly recognized as being tubal in type but in tumors with marked epithelial abnormalities this resemblance tends to be lost and the cells become predominantly round or cuboidal. The epithelial component of the tumor shows a variable degree of multilayering and has a marked tendency to form cellular buds or tufts. These buds may break off to float freely within the cyst whereas fusion of the tips of adjacent epithelial buds may result in a honeycomb pattern. Nuclear crowding, atypia, and hyperchromatism are of variable degree but mitotic figures are uncommon. Psammoma

bodies are frequently present. In most of these neoplasms there is a very sharp interface between epithelium and stroma and the possibility of stromal invasion can be excluded with relative ease. Furthermore, the borderline pattern tends to be consistent throughout, it being rather unusual to encounter an intermingling with areas showing a benign appearance or with areas showing a focal evolution into a frank adenocarcinoma.

There is a very high incidence of bilaterality in serous tumors of borderline malignancy, the reported frequency in different series ranging from 26% to 66% (131,139–149). The variation in the reported incidence of bilaterality probably reflects the fact that involvement of the contralateral ovary to that containing an obvious neoplasm may not be apparent to the naked eye, being recognized only on histologic examination. It is virtually certain that the presence of bilateral tumors represents the synchronous development of two primary neoplasms rather than spread of one tumor to the contralateral side.

A further and often disconcerting feature of serous borderline tumors is that in a significant proportion of patients, variously reported as being between 16% and 48%, but averaging at about 35%, there is at the time of initial diagnosis apparent extraovarian spread in the form of tumor implants in the pelvic peritoneum and infracolic omentum (131,139–141,143–149,150–154). Histologically the extraovarian lesions may be plastered onto the surface of the peritoneum or lie in the subperitoneal connective tissue and show a variety of patterns (155–157). Some have a fully benign appearance and

F I G U R E **30-6**

A papillary serous tumor of borderline malignancy.

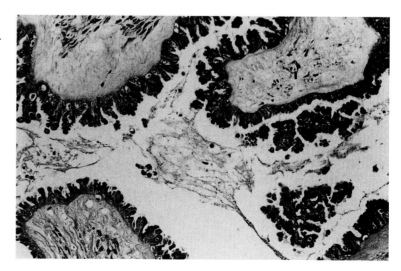

consist of simple tubules lined by tubal-type epithelium or indifferent cuboidal cells; psammoma bodies may be present. Others consist of papillae lying within mesothelial-lined spaces; there is some degree of epithelial atypia and multilayering but no invasion and the appearances closely resemble those seen in a serous tumor of borderline malignancy. In a small minority of patients the subserosal "implants" are invasive with infiltrating epithelial cells that have the appearances of an adenocarcinoma. In any given patient there may be an admixture of different patterns, with some lesions having a benign appearance, others resembling a borderline tumor, and rarely, yet others resembling an adenocarcinoma (156).

Over the years, there has been much argument as to whether the extraovarian lesions represent true implantation metastases or whether they are independent of the ovarian neoplasm and develop in situ within the secondary müllerian system, that is, the submesothelial connective tissues (158,159). It is probable that the superficial lesions are true seeding deposits from serous tumors of borderline malignancy that show an exophytic growth pattern (160) but there is strong evidence that the subserosal lesions are independent of the ovarian tumor and develop in situ. Thus, those with a fully benign appearance clearly correspond to the well-recognized condition of endosalpingiosis (161,162), which can occur in the absence of an ovarian neoplasm and can also be found in association with a benign ovarian tumor (163). Those showing some degree of atypia but no evidence of invasion are sometimes categorized as *atypical endosalpingiosis* (164) and can also occur in the absence of any ovarian tumor, often being classed as primary serous borderline tumors of the peritoneum (165,166). The frequently found admixture of atypical and typical endosalpingiosis indicates a common derivation. Finally, the invasive lesions can similarly occur independently of an ovarian tumor as primary peritoneal adenocarcinomas (163), which are also thought to be derived from foci of endosalpingiosis (167).

In recent studies, in which a full staging procedure had been performed, the long-term survival rate (excluding deaths from other causes) for patients with stage I serous tumors of borderline malignancy has been virtually 100% (147–149,168–177), the few deaths that did occur being due to the subsequent development of a frank ovarian adenocarcinoma. The

long-term survival rate for women with extra-ovarian disease has been reported as between 75% and 79% (173,174). It is widely thought that the prognosis in such patients depends on the nature of the peritoneal lesions, those patients in whom the peritoneal lesions have a non-invasive pattern having an excellent prognosis and those with invasive implants tending to develop progressive peritoneal disease that takes the form of a low-grade peritoneal serous adenocarcinoma (155,157,174,178,179), though it has not been everyone's experience that invasive implants are necessarily associated with a poor prognosis (149,153,156,173,180). It has been suggested that invasive implants are true metastases from a subgroup of noninvasive ovarian tumors characterized by a complex papillary architecture with fibrous stalks covered by proliferating rounded cells showing a filigree pattern, and that these should be regarded as low-grade adenocarcinomas (micropapillary serous adenocarcinomas) (178,179). However, this is still a matter for debate.

Mucinous Tumors of Borderline Malignancy

There are two quite different types of ovarian mucinous tumors of borderline malignancy. In most such neoplasms the mucinous epithelium is of intestinal type but in a minority it is of endocervical type (181). These two forms differ significantly from each other, both pathologically and clinically, but virtually the entire literature on mucinous borderline tumors relates solely to the intestinal type.

Intestinal Type The intestinal-type mucinous tumors of borderline malignancy usually present as large multilocular cysts. The cyst lining is generally smooth but there may be focal areas of thickening or nodularity. The epithelial component may show a complex glandular pattern but is often characterized by short papillary infoldings that give the epithelium a serrated appearance (Fig. 30-7). There are varying degrees of multilayering, loss of nuclear polarity, and cytologic atypia whereas mitotic figures are quite frequently seen. The outpouching of the epithelium and the formation of secondary glands in many borderline mucinous tumors of intestinal type make the assessment of stromal invasion more difficult than is the case with serous tumors, but this is not usually an impossible task. Many of these

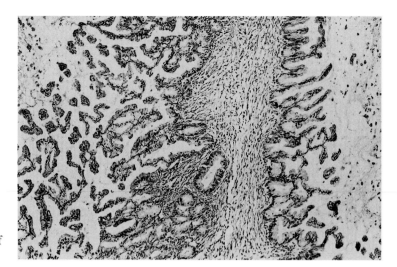

F I G U R E **30-7**
An enteric-type mucinous tumor of
borderline malignancy.

neoplasms, like their serous counterparts, show
a stereotyped pattern of noninvasive epithelial
atypia throughout, but in a proportion there is
a variety of patterns. Some show an admixture
of benign and borderline areas, others borderline areas with foci of frankly invasive carcinoma, and yet others demonstrate the complete
range of appearances, containing benign epithelium, areas of borderline malignancy, and
focal adenocarcinoma. Therefore, these neoplasms require extensive sampling.

Bilaterality of intestinal-type mucinous borderline tumors is uncommon and it has become
increasingly evident that the long-term survival
rate for women with stage I enteric-type mucinous ovarian tumors of borderline malignancy
is extremely good; indeed it is probable that
the survival rate for thoroughly sampled and
adequately staged tumors approaches 100%
(125,128,129,143,148,149,170,182–187).

While the outlook for patients with stage I
intestinal-type mucinous ovarian tumors of borderline malignancy is excellent, that for the
rather small minority of women having such
neoplasms but with apparent extraovarian
spread is poor, largely because this takes the
form of pseudomyxoma peritonei. The traditional view of the pathogenesis of this condition is that the accumulation of thick gelatinous
mucoid material within the peritoneal cavity is
due either to leakage of mucin or to seeding of
mucin-secreting cells from the ovarian tumor.
However, most mucinous ovarian tumors associated with pseudomyxoma peritonei are not
overtly ruptured and it is now becoming apparent that pseudomyxoma peritonei rarely, if ever,

occurs in the absence of a synchronous appen-
dicular or, much less commonly, an intestinal
neoplasm of low-grade malignancy (188–190).
It is currently still a matter for debate but the
balance of evidence favors the view that
pseudomyxoma peritonei is usually, perhaps
invariably, secondary to a gastrointestinal neoplasm and that the associated ovarian tumors
are metastatic in origin despite their usually
having an appearance of only borderline malignancy; thus, it is not surprising that they are
associated with a poor prognosis.

Müllerian (Endocervical) Type Mucinous
tumors of borderline malignancy of müllerian
(endocervical) type are architecturally very
similar to serous borderline tumors, the only difference being that the papillae are covered by
endocervical-type columnar epithelial cells and
that the tumor stroma almost invariably contains
an acute inflammatory infiltrate (181).

The müllerian type of borderline mucinous
neoplasm has more in common with borderline
serous tumors than it does with enteric-type
mucinous borderline neoplasms. Thus, bilaterality is quite common, there is no association
with pseudomyxoma peritonei, and although
apparent extraovarian spread does occur, this
takes the form of endocervicosis, that is, mucinous glands set in a fibrous stroma, which is
considered to be analogous to endosalpingiosis
and similarly arise in situ within the secondary
müllerian system. Too little information is currently available about the natural history of this
type of mucinous neoplasm to allow for any
firm statement about the long-term prognosis,

but so far all reported patients have remained well and symptom free after removal of the ovarian neoplasm (136,181).

Prognostic Features

In ovarian epithelial tumors of borderline malignancy, the most important, perhaps the only, prognostic factor is the nature of the extraovarian lesions. Nevertheless there have been many attempts to determine prognostic factors within the ovarian neoplasm. Some investigators suggested that histologic grading, in terms of the degree of budding, multilayering, and atypia, is of prognostic value (129,182), but others failed to confirm that such grading is of any predictive value (141,191). Morphometric analysis appears to be of value in identifying those borderline tumors likely to pursue an unfavorable course (192) but there has been quite marked disagreement about the prognostic value of flow cytometry. Some studies (193,194) found tumor aneuploidy to be a highly significant prognostic indicator of a poor clinical outcome but others did not (149,195–197).

Sex Cord–Stromal Tumors

This group of neoplasms includes all those containing granulosa cells, Sertoli cells, thecal cells, Leydig cells, or fibroblasts of specialized gonadal stromal origin, or the precursors of these cells, either singly or in any combination. Many sex cord–stromal tumors are benign and only the malignant forms are considered here.

Adult-Type Granulosa Cell Tumors

These neoplasms, which are usually estrogenic, differ both clinically and morphologically from juvenile granulosa cell tumors, and whereas they occur most commonly in perimenopausal and postmenopausal women, they can, despite their name, develop at any age, 5% occurring in premenarchal girls.

The tumors are usually unilateral, solid, and hard or rubbery. They have a smooth outer surface, commonly measure about 12 cm in diameter, and have a white, yellow, or gray cut surface. A very small minority of adult-type granulosa cell tumors are cystic and resemble a cystadenoma. Such neoplasms often exert an

androgenic rather than an estrogenic effect (198,199).

Histologically, the cells in an adult-type granulosa cell tumor are smooth, round or polygonal, and have little cytoplasm and indistinct cell margins. Their large round or ovoid nuclei characteristically show longitudinal grooving. The cells are arranged in a variety of patterns and although in any individual neoplasm a particular pattern may predominate, there is usually an admixture of cellular arrangements. In the insular pattern the cells are arranged in compact masses or islands whereas in the trabecular pattern the cells form anastomosing ribbons or cords. Alternatively the cells may be arranged in sheets to give a diffuse pattern (sometimes misleadingly classed as a "sarcomatoid" pattern). In the microfollicular pattern (Fig. 30-8), granulosa cells are arranged around small spaces containing nuclear debris (Call-Exner bodies) while a macrofollicular pattern with large follicles, resembling follicular cysts, is sometimes seen. The cystic granulosa cell tumors have a lining which resembles that of a graafian follicle but which contains microfollicles.

There is usually little pleomorphism but about 2% of these neoplasms contain a population of cells with large, bizarre, hyperchromatic nuclei (200). Mitotic figures are characteristically scanty. The stromal component of a granulosa cell tumor is variable in amount and may have a fibromatous or thecomatous appearance.

All adult-type granulosa cell tumors should be regarded as malignant, though the degree of malignancy is often very low and the course pursued by the tumor is frequently extremely indolent. Recurrences or metastases tend to occur late, commonly after 5 years, not infrequently after 10 years, and sometimes after 20 years. The long-term survival rate is only in the region of 50% (23,201,202) and the only absolute indication of a poor short-term prognosis is the presence of extraovarian spread at the time of initial diagnosis. Prognostic factors for tumors confined to the ovary are very difficult to define (201–204). The histologic pattern is of no prognostic importance but it is possible that large size (>10 cm in diameter) and an abundance of mitotic figures may indicate a relatively poor outlook. There have been conflicting reports about the prognostic significance of aneuploidy (205,206).

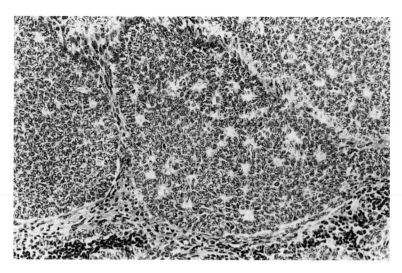

FIGURE **30-8**

An adult-type granulosa cell tumor.

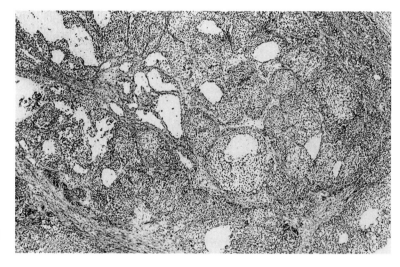

FIGURE **30-9**

A juvenile-type granulosa cell tumor.

Juvenile Granulosa Cell Tumor

Neoplasms of this type, which are also estrogenic, occur most commonly in, but are not confined to, the first two decades of life. About 3% arise after the age of 30 years (207).

The tumors are usually unilateral and largely solid, though cystic forms are occasionally encountered. Histologically (Fig. 30-9) there is a nodular or, less commonly, a diffuse pattern of tumor cells set in a loose edematous stroma. The nodules may be solid but usually contain a number of sharply etched, round, or irregular follicles that are lined by one or more layers of granulosa cells. Thecal cells may lie adjacent to the granulosa cell nodules but the two cell types may be intermingled. Luteinization is often a striking feature of these neoplasms and the granulosa cell nuclei tend to be hyperchromatic and lack the typical longitudinal groove seen in adult-type granulosa cell tumors. A degree of cytologic atypia is not unusual and mitotic figures are plentiful in many tumors.

Juvenile granulosa cell tumors behave in a fashion quite unlike that of adult-type granulosa cell neoplasms. The vast majority are confined to the ovary at the time of the initial diagnosis and only about 5% of these will behave in a malignant fashion, with recurrence and wide dissemination throughout the abdominal cavity occurring within 2 years of the time of the initial diagnosis (207). The prognosis for patients with extraovarian spread is poor (208).

Cellular Fibroma and Fibrosarcoma

Fibromatous ovarian tumors that are unusually cellular but contain fewer than 4 mitotic figures per 10 high-power fields are classed as *cellular fibromas* (209). These neoplasms will recur if surgical removal is incomplete. Ovarian fibrosarcomas are bulky, soft, lobulated neoplasms that are densely cellular and contain more than 4 mitotic figures per 10 high-power fields; these aggressive neoplasms pursue a highly malignant course (209).

Androblastoma

Androblastomas are neoplasms composed of Sertoli cells, Leydig cells, or a combination of the two cell types.

Pure Sertoli cell neoplasms, which are commonly estrogenic, are rare and occur as small, solid, yellowish masses. Histologically the tumors show highly differentiated tubules lined by a single layer of radially orientated Sertoli cells. These neoplasms are usually benign but there has been one instance, in a young girl, of such a tumor evolving into a fatal carcinoma (210).

Pure Leydig cell neoplasms may arise either from stromal cells or from preexisting hilar cells (211–214). They are usually androgenic and occur as small, unilateral, well-circumscribed, solid, brown, yellow, or orange masses. Histologically they consist of rounded or polygonal Leydig cells with abundant eosinophilic cytoplasm that are arranged in sheets, nests, and cords. Leydig cell tumors are usually androgenic but a small minority are estrogenic. They are nearly always benign but occasionally these neoplasms pursue a malignant course despite the absence of any histologic features to indicate their aggressive nature.

Sertoli-Leydig cell tumors are rare, occur most commonly in relatively young women, and are usually androgenic, though occasional well-differentiated neoplasms are estrogenic (215). The tumors, which are usually solid, firm, and yellowish, show a wide range of histologic differentiation. Well-differentiated neoplasms (Fig. 30-10) are formed by well-defined tubules lined by Sertoli cells that are set in a fibrous stroma containing a variable number of Leydig cells. In less well-differentiated tumors the Sertoli cells are arranged in cords, sheets, islands, or trabeculae; solid or hollow tubules are occasionally seen. The Sertoli cell component is set in a mesenchymal stroma in which Leydig cells are present singly, in clumps, or as sheets. Poorly differentiated Sertoli-Leydig cell tumors are formed largely of sheets of spindle-shaped cells in which occasional poorly formed tubules or irregular cordlike structures are present together with small clusters of Leydig cells.

About 10% of Sertoli-Leydig cell neoplasms contain, at least in part, a pattern resembling that of the rete testis (216–218) and this retiform pattern can sometimes be a predominant, even exclusive, feature. Heterologous elements are present in about 20% of Sertoli-Leydig cell tumors and are thought to arise by a process of neometaplasia: Most commonly gastrointestinal epithelium is present but muscle, cartilage, and hepatocytes can also be seen (219,220).

Well-differentiated Sertoli-Leydig cell tumors are always benign (221) as are the vast majority of those of intermediate differentiation (222,223). About 40% of poorly differentiated neoplasms pursue a malignant course, these

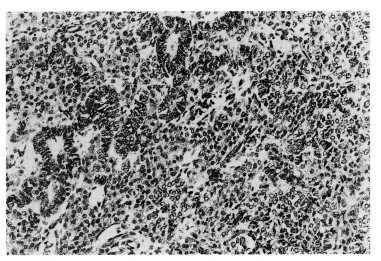

F I G U R E **30-10**

A well-differentiated Sertoli-Leydig cell tumor.

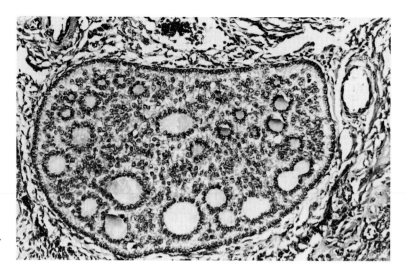

F I G U R E **30-11**
A sex cord tumor with annular tubules.

most commonly being those with high mitotic counts, with a predominant retiform pattern, or with heterologous cartilage or muscle (224). Recurrence or metastases usually appear within a year of the time of the initial diagnosis and metastases are found most commonly in the omentum, abdominal lymph nodes, or liver.

Sex Cord Tumor with Annular Tubules

This uncommon, but histologically distinctive (Fig. 30-11) neoplasm contains rounded nests in which immature sex cord cells are palisaded along the periphery of the cell nests and around hyaline bodies that are formed of basement membrane protein (225–227). About one third of these tumors are associated with the Peutz-Jeghers syndrome and under these circumstances are usually bilateral, commonly of microscopic size only, frequently calcified, and invariably benign (228). The tumors unassociated with the Peutz-Jeghers syndrome are unilateral, large, and uncalcified and may show an overgrowth of granulosa or Sertoli cells (229,230). About 20% of these behave in a malignant fashion (228).

Germ Cell Tumors

Tumors derived from germ cells may show no evidence of differentiation into either embryonic or extraembryonic tissues (dysgerminomas), can differentiate into embryonic tissues (teratomas), or may differentiate along extraembryonic pathways into trophoblast (choriocarcinoma) or yolk sac structures (yolk sac

neoplasms). Not infrequently there may be an admixture of different germ cell tumor patterns within a single neoplasm. Germ cell neoplasms account for about 30% of primary ovarian tumors, largely in the form of mature cystic teratomas, and only about 5% are malignant. They account for 1% to 3% of malignant ovarian tumors in Western countries but account for two thirds of ovarian cancers in children and adolescents (231).

Dysgerminoma

Dysgerminomas commonly arise in patients between 10 and 30 years old and, although they have a particular tendency to develop in individuals with abnormal gonads, they usually occur in otherwise fully normal females.

The tumors are bilateral in 15% of patients, usually measure about 15 cm in diameter, have a smooth or bosselated outer surface, are solid, and appear firm or rubbery and pinkish-gray on section. Histologically (Fig. 30-12) the neoplastic cells resemble primordial germ cells and are large, uniform, round, oval, or polyhedral with well-defined limiting membranes, abundant cytoplasm, and large vesicular nuclei. The cells are commonly arranged in solid nests separated by delicate fibrous septa but may form cords or strands embedded in a fibrous stroma. A lymphatic infiltration of the stroma, sometimes aggregated into follicles with germinal centers, and small stromal granulomas are characteristic features. About 3% of dysgerminomas contain multinucleated syncytiotrophoblast-like cells that stain positively for β-human chorionic

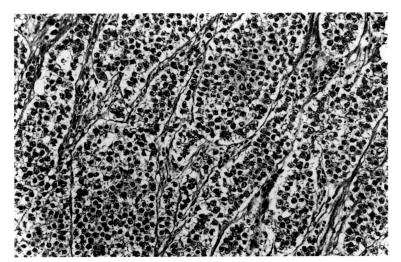

F I G U R E **30-12**
A dysgerminoma.

gonadotropin (hCG) (232,233). A few dysgerminomas are of the "anaplastic" variety and show marked pleomorphism and mitotic activity (234) but these features are not of prognostic significance (231).

Dysgerminomas are malignant: rupture of their capsule may lead to direct implantation of tumor onto the pelvic peritoneum and omentum while lymphatic spread to para-aortic, retroperitoneal, and mediastinal nodes occurs relatively early. Hematogenous spread to the liver, lungs, kidneys, and bones occurs at a late stage. They are, however, highly sensitive to both radiotherapy and chemotherapy and the 5-year survival rate is virtually 100% for patients with stage I disease and 80% to 90% for those with higher-stage or recurrent disease (231). The only definite prognostic factor is stage.

Choriocarcinoma

These germ cell tumors show trophoblastic differentiation. They are often combined with other germ cell elements but pure ovarian choriocarcinomas are sometimes encountered (235,237). In women of reproductive age it is usually impossible to tell, unless one resorts to genetic analysis, whether such a neoplasm is a germ cell tumor, a metastasis from a regressed uterine choriocarcinoma, or a tumor arising from the placental tissue of an ectopic ovarian pregnancy. It is therefore only in premenarchal girls that a diagnosis of a pure choriocarcinoma of germ cell origin can be accepted.

The tumors form large hemorrhagic masses and their histologic appearances are identical to those of a gestational uterine choriocarcinoma, with both cytotrophoblast and syncytiotrophoblast being present. Ovarian choriocarcinomas respond poorly to the therapeutic regime, which is so successful for gestational choriocarcinoma, and are associated with a poor prognosis (235).

Yolk Sac Tumors

Yolk sac tumors are rare, occur predominantly in girls between 4 and 20 years old, represent neoplastic germ cell differentiation into extraembryonic mesoblast and yolk sac endoderm, and share with yolk sac structures the ability to secrete α-fetoprotein (AFP).

Yolk sac tumors form unilateral, large, smooth or nodular, soft masses showing conspicuous hemorrhage, necrosis, and microcystic change. Their histologic appearances are very complex (231,236,237) but there is characteristically a loose vacuolated labyrinthine network containing microcysts lined by flattened cells together with Schiller-Duval bodies, these having a mesenchymal core containing a central capillary and an epithelial investment of cuboidal or columnar cells (Fig. 30-13). A glandular pattern, sometimes resembling an endometrioid adenocarcinoma (238), is often seen while there may be hepatoid or endodermal differentiation (239–241); hematopoietic foci are occasionally seen (242). Eosinophilic hyaline droplets are almost invariably present and consist predominantly of AFP. A polyvesicular-vitelline pattern is seen in many yolk sac tumors and sometimes predominates: This is characterized by the presence of cysts lined by flattened or cuboidal cells and having an eccen-

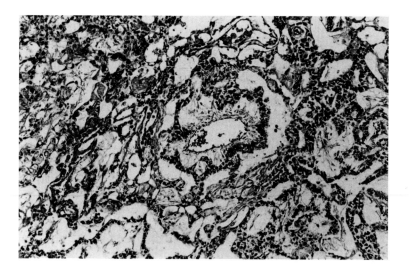

F I G U R E **30-13**

A yolk sac tumor.

tric constriction, simulating the conversion of the primary to the secondary yolk sac (243).

Yolk sac tumors are highly malignant and spread rapidly within the abdomen and to distant sites. Their previously appalling prognosis has, however, been transformed by the introduction of effective chemotherapy, with survival rates of 70% to 90% for patients with stage I disease and 30% to 50% for those with tumors of higher stage (231).

Embryonal Carcinoma

Ovarian tumors of this type are extremely rare (244,245). They occur at a median age of 12 years, form large masses, and are characterized histologically by the presence of sheets and nests of large primitive cells admixed with syncytiotrophoblast-like giant cells that stain positively for hCG. Hyaline bodies staining positively for AFP are almost invariably present. These are aggressive tumors but some do respond well to chemotherapy.

Teratomas

These germ cell neoplasms show differentiation along embryonic lines. In most there is a melange of tissues, but in some, known as *monodermal teratomas*, there is differentiation along only a single tissue pathway, for example, solely into thyroid tissue. The terms *benign* and *malignant* are not truly applicable to teratomas, for the prognosis of any given neoplasm is determined not by the usual criteria of malignancy but by the degree of maturity of its constituent tissues: Those in which all the tissue

components are fully mature behave in a benign fashion, and increasing degrees of tissue immaturity are associated with a progressive tendency for the neoplasm to pursue a malignant course. Hence, teratomas are classed as either "mature" or "immature," the term *malignant* being reserved for mature teratomas in which a conventional malignant change has occurred, for instance, when a squamous cell carcinoma develops in a mature cystic teratoma.

The vast majority of ovarian teratomas are mature and cystic. Malignant change occurs in about 1% to 2% of mature cystic teratomas, usually in women between 40 and 60 years old. The vast majority (85%) of these are squamous cell carcinomas whereas most of the remainder are adenocarcinomas (246,247).

A small proportion of mature teratomas are solid rather than cystic, but most solid teratomas are of the immature variety. These latter occur predominantly during the first two decades of life as unilateral, large (averaging about 18 cm in diameter) masses, with a smooth glistening outer surface and a predominantly solid appearance on cut section. Histologically these neoplasms contain an admixture of both mature and immature tissue, though immature mesenchyme or neuroepithelium (Fig. 30-14) is often a salient feature. The immature tissues resemble those of the normal embryo. The amount of such tissue varies from small foci to a predominant component and these neoplasms are graded in term of their content of immature neuroectodermal tissue (248).

Immature teratomas behave in a malignant fashion, implanting onto the peritoneum, metastasizing to retroperitoneal and para-aortic

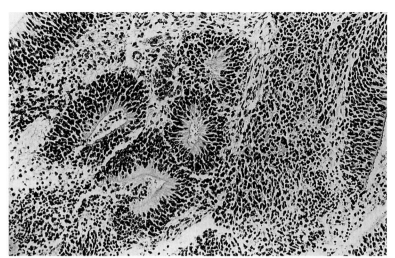

F I G U R E **30-14**
An immature teratoma.

nodes, and being disseminated via the blood-stream to the lungs and liver. The previously dismal prognosis for patients with high-grade immature teratomas has, however, been transformed by chemotherapy, with sustained remissions now being obtained in virtually all patients (249).

Monodermal teratomas (250), in which differentiation is into only one tissue, are typified by the struma ovarii, which consists predominantly or solely of tissue that is histologically, physiologically, and pharmacologically identical to normal cervical thyroid tissue. This ovarian thyroid tissue sometimes undergoes malignant change, with a resulting thyroid adenocarcinoma that metastasizes, albeit in a very indolent manner, to lymph nodes, liver, and spleen (251,252).

Many carcinoid tumors of the ovary occur in a mature cystic teratoma, in association with gastrointestinal or respiratory epithelium, but a few are pure and not admixed with any other tissues, these being regarded as *monodermal teratomas*. Ovarian carcinoid tumors are similar to those that occur in the gastrointestinal tract but are associated with a high incidence of a typical carcinoid syndrome (250,253), this reflecting the ability of these neoplasms to secrete products directly into the systemic, rather than the portal, circulation. The usual thinking has been that about 5% of ovarian carcinoid tumors behave in a malignant fashion (253), but in a recent series of 17 patients, 6 had stage III or IV disease at the time of the original diagnosis, and only 1 of them survived (254).

A strumal carcinoid is a rare neoplasm that combines the features of a struma ovarii and a carcinoid tumor (255–257). It is thought that the carcinoid component of these neoplasms is derived from the parafollicular cells of the thyroid tissue and that it is thus homologous with the medullary carcinoma of the thyroid gland.

Other rare monodermal teratomas of the ovary include neuroectodermal tumors, malignant melanoma, and retinal anlage tumor (250).

Tumors of Uncertain Cell Type

Not all malignant neoplasms of the ovary can be fitted into a specific category, such as "epithelial" or "germ cell," and can hence only be classed as *tumors of uncertain cell type*.

Small-cell carcinomas of the hypercalcemic type are highly aggressive neoplasms that occur in young women (mean age, 22 years) (258–260). Despite their name they are not carcinomas and hypercalcemia is only present in about half the patients. These tumors occur as unilateral, large, solid masses showing extensive hemorrhage and necrosis and are formed by sheets, islands, and cords of small cells with scanty cytoplasm and hyperchromatic nuclei. These tumors spread quickly, respond poorly to chemotherapy, and usually prove rapidly fatal, though some patients with stage Ia neoplasms have survived.

The small-cell carcinoma of the pulmonary type is probably of neuroendocrine origin and histologically resembles a small-cell carcinoma of the bronchus (261). These neoplasms occur at a much later age than do the small-cell carcinomas of hypercalcemic type and are often bilateral. They are highly aggressive and have an extremely poor prognosis.

Hepatoid carcinomas occur in relatively elderly women. They bear a very close histologic similarity to a hepatocellular carcinoma and are highly malignant (262,263).

REFERENCES

1. Yonescu R, Currie JL, Hedrick L, et al. Chromosome abnormalities in primary endometrioid ovarian carcinoma. *Cancer Genet Cytogenet* 1996;87:167–171.

2. Young RH, Prat J, Scully RE. Ovarian endometrioid carcinomas resembling sex cord-stromal tumors: a clinicopathologic analysis of 13 cases. *Am J Surg Pathol* 1982;5:513–522.

3. Remadi S, Ismail A, Tawil A, MacGee W. Ovarian sertoliform endometrioid carcinoma. *Virchows Arch* 1995;426:533–536.

4. Austin RM, Norris HJ. Malignant Brenner tumors and transitional cell carcinoma of the ovary. *Int J Gynecol Pathol* 1987;6:29–39.

5. Robey SS, Silva EG, Gershenson DM, et al. Transitional cell carcinoma in high-grade high-stage ovarian carcinoma: an indicator of favorable response to chemotherapy. *Cancer* 1989; 63:839–847.

6. Silva EG, Robey-Cafferty SS, Gershenson DM, et al. Ovarian carcinoma with transitional cell carcinoma pattern. *Am J Clin Pathol* 1990;93: 457–465.

7. Scully RE, Barlow JF. "Mesonephroma" of the ovary: tumor of müllerian nature related to the endometrioid carcinoma. *Cancer* 1967;20:1405–1417.

8. Eastwood J. Mesonephroid (clear cell) carcinoma of the ovary and endometrium: a comparative prospective clinicopathological study and review of the literature. *Cancer* 1978;41: 1911–1928.

9. Shevchuk MM, Winkler-Monsanto B, Fenoglio CM, Richart RM. Clear cell carcinoma of the ovary: a clinicopathologic study with review of the literature. *Cancer* 1981;47:1244–1251.

10. Young RH, Scully RE. Oxyphilic clear cell carcinoma of the ovary: a report of nine cases. *Am J Surg Pathol* 1987;11:661–667.

11. Meleka F, Rafla S. Variation of spread of ovarian malignancy according to site of origin. *Gynecol Oncol* 1975;3:108–113.

12. Fuks Z. Patterns of spread of ovarian carcinoma: relation to therapeutic strategies. In: Newman CE, Ford CHJ, Jordan JE, eds. *Ovarian cancer*. Oxford: Pergamon, 1980:39–51.

13. Wu P-C, Lang J-H, Huang R-L, et al. Intestinal metastasis and operation in ovarian cancer: a report on 62 cases. *Ballieres Clin Obstet Gynaecol* 1989;3:95–108.

14. Pickel H, Lhousen M, Stetner H, Girardi F. The spread of ovarian cancer. *Ballieres Clin Obstet Gynaecol* 1989;3:3–12.

15. Bergman F. Carcinoma of the ovary: a clinical-pathological study of 86 autopsied cases with special reference to mode of spread. *Acta Obstet Gynecol Scand* 1966;45:211–231.

16. Rose PG, Piver MS, Tsukada Y, Lau T. Metastatic patterns in histologic variants of ovarian cancer: an autopsy study. *Cancer* 1989;64:1508–1513.

17. Wu P-C, Lang J-H, Huang R-L, et al. Lymph node metastasis and retroperitoneal lymphadenectomy in ovarian cancer. *Ballieres Clin Obstet Gynaecol* 1989;3:143–155.

18. Burghardt E, Girardi F, Lahousen M, et al. Patterns of pelvic and paraaortic lymph node involvement in ovarian cancer. *Gynecol Oncol* 1991;40:103–106.

19. Knapp RC, Friedman EA. Aortic lymph node metastases in early ovarian cancer. *Am J Obstet Gynecol* 1974;119:1013–1017.

20. Burghardt E, Lahousen M, Stettner H. Die operative Behandlung des Ovarialkarzinoms. *Geburtshilfe Frauenheilkd* 1990;50:670–677.

21. Kottmeier HL. Surgical management—conservative indications according to the type of the tumour. In: Gentil F, Junquiera AC, eds. *Ovarian cancer*. UICC monograph series, vol. 11. Berlin: Springer, 1968:257–266.

22. Bjorkholm E, Pettersson F, Einhorn N, et al. Long-term follow up and prognostic factors in ovarian carcinoma: the Radiumhemmet series 1958–1973. *Acta Radiol Oncol* 1982;21:413–419.

23. Kolstad P. *Clinical gynecologic oncology: the Norwegian experience*. Oslo: Norwegian University Press, 1986.

24. Cramer SF, Roth LM, Ulbright TM, et al. Evaluation of the reproducibility of the World Health Organization classification of common ovarian

cancers. *Arch Pathol Lab Med* 1987;111:819–829.

25. Lund B, Thomsen HK, Olsen J. Reproducibility of histopathological evaluation in epithelial ovarian carcinoma. *APMIS* 1991;99:353–358.

26. Sorbe B, Frankendal BO, Veress B. Importance of histologic grading in the prognosis of epithelial ovarian carcinoma. *Obstet Gynecol* 1982;59:576–582.

27. Sigurdsson K, Alm P, Gullberg P. Prognostic factors in malignant epithelial ovarian tumors. *Gynecol Oncol* 1983;15:370–380.

28. Malkasian GD, Melton LJ, O'Brien PC, Greene MH. Prognostic significance of histologic classification and grading of epithelial malignancies of the ovary. *Am J Obstet Gynecol* 1984;149:274–284.

29. Einhorn N, Nilsson BO, Sjovall K. Factors influencing survival in carcinoma of the ovary: study from a well-defined Swedish population. *Cancer* 1985;55:2019–2025.

30. Swenerton KD, Hislop TG, Spinelli J, et al. Ovarian carcinoma: a multivariate analysis of prognostic factors. *Obstet Gynecol* 1985;65:264–270.

31. Miller DS, Ballon SC, Teng NNH, et al. A critical reassessment of second-look laparotomy in epithelial ovarian carcinoma. *Cancer* 1986;57:530–535.

32. O'Brien MER, Schofield JB, Tan S, et al. Clear cell epithelial ovarian cancer (mesonephroid): bad prognosis only in early stages. *Gynecol Oncol* 1993;49:250–254.

33. Kennedy AW, Biscotti CV, Hart WR, Webster KD. Ovarian clear cell adenocarcinoma. *Gynecol Oncol* 1989;32:342–349.

34. Crozier MA, Copeland CJ, Silva EG, et al. Clear cell carcinoma of the ovary: a study of 59 cases. *Gynecol Oncol* 1989;35:199–203.

35. Montag AG, Jenison EL, Griffiths CT, et al. Ovarian clear cell carcinoma: a clinicopathologic analysis of 44 cases. *Int J Gynecol Pathol* 1989;8:85–96.

36. Imachi M, Tsukamoto N, Shimamoto T, et al. Clear cell carcinoma of the ovary: a clinicopathologic analysis of 34 cases. *Int J Gynecol Cancer* 1991;1:113–120.

37. Gersall DJ. Primary ovarian transitional cell carcinoma: diagnostic and prognostic considerations. *Am J Clin Pathol* 1990;93:586–588.

38. Gershenson DM, Silva EG, Mitchell MF, et al. Transitional cell carcinoma of the ovary: a

matched controlled study of advanced-stage patients treated with cisplatin-based chemotherapy. *Am J Obstet Gynecol* 1993;168:1178–1187.

39. Decker DG. Epithelial ovarian cancer. In: Bender HG, Beck L, eds. *Carcinoma of the ovary.* Stuttgart: Gustav Fischer Verlag, 1983:137–141.

40. Hogberg T, Carstensen J, Simonsen E. Treatment results and prognostic factors in a population-based study of epithelial ovarian cancer. *Gynecol Oncol* 1993;48:38–49.

41. Baak JPA, Langley FA, Talerman A, Delemarre JFM. Interpathologist and intrapathologist disagreement in ovarian tumor grading and typing. *Anal Quant Cytol Histol* 1986;8:354–357.

42. Baak JPA, Langley FA, Talerman A, Delemarre JFM. The prognostic variability of ovarian tumor grading by different pathologists. *Gynecol Oncol* 1987;27:166–172.

43. Bertelsen K, Holund B, Andersen E. Reproducibility and prognostic value of histologic type and grade in early epithelial ovarian cancer. *Int J Gynecol Cancer* 1993;3:72–79.

44. Rodenberg CJ, Cornelisse CJ, Heintz PA, et al. Tumor ploidy as a major prognostic factor in advanced ovarian cancer. *Cancer* 1987;59:317–323.

45. Volm M, Kleine W, Pfleiderer A. Flow cytometric prognostic factors for the survival of patients with ovarian carcinoma: a 5 year follow-up study. *Gynecol Oncol* 1989;35:84–89.

46. Klemi PJ, Joensuu H, Naenpaa J, Kiiholma P. Influence of cellular DNA content on survival in ovarian carcinoma. *Obstet Gynecol* 1989;74:200–204.

47. Khoo SK, Hurst T, Kearsley GD, et al. Prognostic significance of tumor ploidy in patients with advanced ovarian cancer. *Gynecol Oncol* 1990;139:284–288.

48. Jakobsen A, Bichel P, Stornes I. Prognostic significance of DNA index in advanced ovarian cancer. *Int J Gynecol Cancer* 1991;1:195–197.

49. Vergote IB, Kaern J, Abeler VM, et al. Analysis of prognostic factors in stage I epithelial ovarian carcinoma: importance of degree of differentiation and DNA ploidy in predicting relapse. *Am J Obstet Gynecol* 1993;169:40–52.

50. Gajewski WH, Fuller AF, Pastel-Ley C, et al. Prognostic significance of DNA content in epithelial ovarian cancer. *Gynecol Oncol* 1994;53:5–12.

51. Kaern J, Trope CG, Kristensen CB, et al. Evaluation of DNA ploidy and S-phase fraction as prognostic parameters in advanced epithelial ovarian carcinoma. *Am J Obstet Gynecol* 1994; 170:479–487.

52. Kigawa J, Minagawa Y, Ishihara H, et al. Tumor DNA ploidy and prognosis of patients with serous cystadenocarcinoma of the ovary. *Cancer* 1993;72:804–808.

53. Pfisterer J, Kommoss F, Sauerbrei A, et al. Cellular DNA content and survival in advanced ovarian cancer. *Cancer* 1994;74:2509–2515.

54. Rice LW, Mark SD, Berkowitz RS, et al. Clinicopathologic variables, operative characteristics, and DNA ploidy in predicting outcome in ovarian epithelial carcinoma. *Obstet Gynecol* 1995;86:379–385.

55. Baak JPA, Langley FA, Talerman A, Delemarre JFM. Morphometric data in the prognosis of ovarian tumors in addition to FIGO stage, histologic type and grade. *J Clin Pathol* 1986;39: 1340–1346.

56. Baak JPA, Wisse-Brekelmans ECM, Uyterlinde AM, Schipper NW. Evaluation of the prognostic value of morphometric features and cellular DNA content in FIGO 1 ovarian cancer patients. *Anal Quant Cytol Histol* 1987;9:287–290.

57. Baak JPA, Schipper NW, Wisse-Brekelmans ECM, et al. The prognostic value of morphometrical features and cellular DNA content in cisplatin treated late ovarian cancer patients. *Br J Cancer* 1988;57:503–508.

58. Haapasalo H, Collan Y, Atkin NB, et al. Prognosis of ovarian carcinomas: prediction by histoquantitative methods. *Histopathology* 1989;15: 167–178.

59. Schipper NW, Smeulders AWM, Baak JPA. Evaluation of automated estimation of epithelial volume and its prognostic value in ovarian tumors. *Lab Invest* 1989;61:228–234.

60. Haapasalo H, Collan Y, Seppa A, et al. Prognostic value of ovarian carcinoma grading methods: a method comparison study. *Histopathology* 1990;16:1–7.

61. van Diest PJ, Baak JPA, Brugghe J, et al. Quantitative prognostic features as predictors of long-term survival in patients with advanced ovarian cancer treated with cisplatin. *Int J Gynecol Cancer* 1994;3:174–180.

62. Ludescher C, Weger AR, Lindholm J, et al. Prognostic significance of tumor cell morphometry, histopathology, and clinical parameters in advanced ovarian carcinoma. *Int J Gynecol Pathol* 1990;9:343–351.

63. Hogberg T, Wang G, Risberg B, et al. Nuclear morphometry: a strong prognostic factor for survival after secondary surgery in advanced ovarian cancer. *Int J Gynecol Cancer* 1992;2: 198–206.

64. Brinkhuis M, Baak JPA, van Diest PA, et al. In Dutch and Danish patients with FIGO III ovarian carcinoma, geographic survival differences are associated with differences in quantitative pathologic features. *Int J Gynecol Cancer* 1996;6: 108–114.

65. Brinkhuis M, Lund B, Meijer GA, Bak JPA. Quantitative pathologic variables as prognostic factors for overall survival in Danish patients with FIGO stage III ovarian cancer. *Int J Gynecol Cancer* 1996;6:168–174.

66. Bizzi A, Codegoni AM, Landoni F, et al. Steroid receptors in epithelial ovarian carcinoma: relation to clinical parameters and survival. *Cancer Res* 1988;48:6222–6226.

67. Rose PJ, Reale FR, Longcope C, Hunter RE. Prognostic significance of estrogen and progesterone receptors in ovarian epithelial cancer. *Obstet Gynecol* 1990;76:258–263.

68. Sevelda P, Denison U, Schemper M, et al. Oestrogen and progesterone receptor content as a prognostic factor in advanced epithelial ovarian carcinoma. *Br J Obstet Gynaecol* 1990; 97:706–712.

69. Slotman BJ, Narta JJP, Rao BR. Survival of patients with ovarian cancer: apart from stage and grade, tumor progesterone receptor content is a prognostic indicator. *Cancer* 1990;66: 740–744.

70. Leake RE, Owens O. The prognostic value of steroid receptors, growth factors and growth factor receptors in ovarian cancer. In: Sharp F, Mason WP, Leake RE, eds. *Ovarian cancer: biological and therapeutic challenges.* London: Chapman & Hall, 1990:69–75.

71. Scambia G, Benedetti-Panici P, Ferrandina G, et al. Epidermal growth factor, oestrogen and progesterone receptor expression in primary ovarian cancer: correlation with clinical outcome and response to chemotherapy. *Br J Cancer* 1995;72: 361–365.

72. Kieback DG, Press MF, McCamant SK, et al. Die prognostische Differenzierung von Ovarialkarzinomen durch immunohistochemische Analyse

der Ostrogenrezeptorexpression. *Geburtshilfe Frauenheilkd* 1995;55:189–194.

73. Hartmann LC, Sebo TJ, Kamel NA, et al. Proliferating cell nuclear antigen in epithelial ovarian cancer: relation to results at second-look laparotomy and survival. *Gynecol Oncol* 1992;47: 191–195.

74. Guo L-N, Wilkinson N, Buckley CH, et al. Proliferating cell nuclear antigen (PCNA) immunoreactivity in ovarian serous and mucinous neoplasms: diagnostic and prognostic value. *Int J Gynecol Cancer* 1993;3:391–394.

75. Nakopoulou L, Janinis J, Panagos G, et al. The immunohistochemical expression of proliferating cell nuclear antigen (PCNA/cyclin) in malignant and benign epithelial ovarian neoplasms and correlation with prognosis. *Eur J Cancer* 1993;29A:1599–1601.

76. Thomas H, Nasim MM, Sarraf CE, et al. Proliferating cell nuclear antigen (PCNA) immunostaining—a prognostic factor in ovarian cancer? *Br J Cancer* 1995;71:357–362.

77. Khalifa MA, Chase GA, Lage JM, et al. Ki-67 and proliferating cell nuclear antigen (PCNA) staining in ovarian adenocarcinoma using MIB-1 and PC 10 monoclonal antibodies: correlation with prognostic factors. *Int J Gynecol Cancer* (in press).

78. Isola J, Kallioniemi O-P, Korte J-M, et al. Steroid receptors and Ki-67 reactivity in ovarian cancer and in normal ovary: correlation with DNA flow cytometry, biochemical receptor assay, and patient survival. *J Pathol* 1990;162:295–301.

79. Kerns BM, Jordan PA, Faerman LL, et al. Determination of proliferation index with MIB-1 in advanced ovarian cancer using quantitative image analysis. *Am J Clin Pathol* 1994;101: 192–197.

80. Hendriksen R. Ovarian carcinogenesis: a study of markers for growth regulatory mechanisms in epithelial ovarian tumors. Dissertation, University of Uppsala, 1994.

81. Garzetti GG, Ciavattini A, Goteri G, et al. Ki67 antigen immunostaining (MIB 1 monoclonal antibody) in serous ovarian tumors: index of proliferative activity with prognostic significance. *Gynecol Oncol* 1995;56:169–174.

82. de Nictolis M, Garbisa S, Lucarini G, et al. 72 Kilodalton type IV collagenase, type IV collagen, and Ki67 in serous tumors of the ovary: a clinicopathologic, immunohistochemical, and serological study. *Int J Gynecol Pathol* 1996;15: 102–109.

83. Marks JR, Davidoff AM, Kerns BJ, et al. Overexpression and mutation of p53 in epithelial ovarian cancer. *Cancer Res* 1991;51:2979–2984.

84. Eccles DM, Brett L, Lessells A, et al. Overexpression of the p53 protein and allelic loss of 17p13 in ovarian carcinoma. *Br J Cancer* 1992; 65:40–44.

85. Kupryjanczyk J, Thor AD, Beauchamp R, et al. p53 Gene mutations and protein accumulation in human ovarian cancer. *Proc Natl Acad Sci USA* 1993;90:4961–4965.

86. Kohler MF, Marks JR, Wiseman RW, et al. Spectrum of mutation and frequency of allelic deletion of the p53 gene in ovarian cancer. *J Natl Cancer Inst* 1993;85:1513–1519.

87. Milner BJ, Allan LA, Eccles DM, et al. p53 Mutation is a common genetic event in ovarian carcinoma. *Cancer Res* 1993;53:2128–2132.

88. Kiyokawa T. Alteration of p53 in ovarian cancer: its occurrence and maintenance in tumor progression. *Int J Gynecol Pathol* 1994;13: 311–318.

89. Henriksen R, Strang P, Wilander E, et al. p53 expression in epithelial ovarian neoplasms: relationship to clinical and pathological parameters, Ki-67 expression and flow cytometry. *Gynecol Oncol* 1994;53:301–306.

90. Niwa K, Itoh M, Murase T, et al. Alteration of p53 gene in ovarian carcinoma: clinicopathological correlation and prognostic significance. *Br J Cancer* 1994;70:1191–1197.

91. McManus DT, Yep EPH, Maxwell P, et al. p53 expression, mutation and allelic deletion in ovarian cancer. *J Pathol* 1994;174:159–168.

92. Kupryjanczyk J, Bell DA, Yandell DW, et al. p53 expression in ovarian borderline tumors and stage 1 carcinomas. *Am J Clin Pathol* 1994;102: 671–676.

93. Levesque MA, Katsaros D, Yu H, et al. Mutant p53 protein overexpression is associated with poor outcome in patients with well or moderately differentiated ovarian carcinoma. *Cancer* 1995;75:1327–1338.

94. Klemi PJ, Takahashi S, Joensuu H, et al. Immunohistochemical detection of p53 protein in borderline and malignant serous ovarian tumors. *Int J Gynecol Pathol* 1994;13:228–233.

95. Hartmann LC, Podratz KC, Keeney GL, et al. Prognostic significance of p53 immunostaining in epithelial ovarian cancer. *J Clin Oncol* 1994; 12:64–69.

96. Herod JJ, Eliopoulos AG, Warwick J, et al. The prognostic significance of Bcl-2 and p53 expression in ovarian carcinoma. *Cancer Res* 1996;56:2178–2184.

97. Diebold J, Baretton G, Felchner M, et al. bcl-2 Expression, p53 accumulation and apoptosis in ovarian carcinomas. *Am J Clin Pathol* 1996;105:341–349.

98. Allan LA, Campbell MK, Eccles RCF, et al. The significance of p53 mutation and over-expression in ovarian cancer prognosis. *Int J Gynecol Cancer* 1996;6:483–490.

99. Watson JV, Curling OM, Hudson CN. Flow cytometric quantitation of p62myc and DNA in serous papillary ovarian cancer. In: Sharp F, Mason WP, Leake RE, eds. *Ovarian cancer: biological and therapeutic challenges.* London: Chapman & Hall, 1990:123–138.

100. Sasano H, Nagura H, Silverberg SG. Immunolocalization of c-myc oncoprotein in mucinous and serous adenocarcinomas of the ovary. *Hum Pathol* 1992;23:491–495.

101. Polocarz SV, Hey NA, Stephenson TJ, Hill AS. c-myc oncogene product P62c-myc in ovarian mucinous neoplasms: immunohistochemical study correlated with malignancy. *J Clin Pathol* 1990;42:896–899.

102. Bauknecht T, Bermelin G, Kommoss F. Clinical significance of oncogenes and growth factors in ovarian carcinoma. *J Steroid Biochem Med Biol* 1990;37:855–862.

103. van Dam PA, Vergote IB, Lowe DG, et al. Expression of c-erbB-2, c-myc, and c-ras oncoproteins, insulin-like growth factor receptor I, and epidermal growth factor receptor in ovarian carcinoma. *J Clin Pathol* 1944;47:914–919.

104. Park JS, Kim HK, Han SK, et al. Detection of c-K-ras point mutation in ovarian cancer. *Int J Gynecol Cancer* 1995;5:107–111.

105. Yaginuma Y, Yamashita K, Kuzumaki N, et al. ras oncogene product p21 expression and prognosis of human ovarian tumors. *Gynecol Oncol* 1992;46:45–50.

106. Scambia G, Catozzi L, Panici PB, et al. Expression of ras p21 protein in normal and neoplastic ovarian tissues: correlation with histopathologic features and receptors for estrogen, progesterone, and epidermal growth factor. *Am J Obstet Gynecol* 1993;168:71–78.

107. Leeson SC, Morphopoulos G, Buckley CH, Hale RJ. c-erbB2 oncogene expression in stage 1 epithelial ovarian cancer. *Br J Obstet Gynaecol* 1995;102:65–67.

108. Felip E, Del Campo JM, Rubio D, et al. Over-expression of c-erbB-2 in epithelial ovarian cancer. *Cancer* 1995;75:2147–2152.

109. Berchuck A, Kamel A, Whitaker R, et al. Over-expression of HER-2/neu is associated with poor survival in advanced epithelial ovarian cancer. *Cancer Res* 1990;50:4087–4091.

110. Meden H, Marx D, Rath W, et al. Overexpression of the oncogene c-erbB-2 in primary ovarian cancer: evaluation of the prognostic value in a Cox proportional hazards multiple regression. *Int J Gynecol Pathol* 1994;13:45–53.

111. Meden H, Marx D, Rab T, et al. EGF-R and overexpression of the oncogene c-erbB-2 in ovarian cancer: immunohistochemical findings and prognostic value. *J Obstet Gynaecol* 1995;21:167–178.

112. Wong YF, Cheung TH, Lam SK, et al. Prevalence and significance of HER-2/neu amplification in epithelial ovarian cancer. *Gynecol Obstet Invest* 1995;40:209–212.

113. Haldane JS, Hird V, Hughes CM, Gullick WJ. c-erbB-2 oncogene expression in ovarian cancer. *J Pathol* 1990;162:231–237.

114. Wilkinson N, Todd N, Buckley CH, et al. An immunohistochemical study of the incidence and significance of c-erbB-2 oncoprotein overexpression in ovarian neoplasia. *Int J Gynecol Cancer* 1991;1:285–289.

115. Rubin SC, Finstad CL, Wong GY, et al. Prognostic significance of HER-2/neu expression in advanced epithelial ovarian cancer: a multivariate analysis. *Am J Obstet Gynecol* 1993;168:162–169.

116. Rubin SC, Finstad CL, Federici MG, et al. Prevalence and significance of HER-2/neu expression in early epithelial ovarian cancer. *Cancer* 1994;73:1456–1459.

117. Singleton TP, Perrone T, Oakley G, et al. Activation of c-erbB-2 and prognosis in ovarian carcinoma. *Cancer* 1994;73:1460–1466.

118. Makar AP, Holm R, Kristensen GB, et al. The expression of c-erbB-2 (HER-2/neu) oncogene in invasive ovarian malignancies. *Int J Gynecol Cancer* 1994;4:194–199.

119. Fajac A, Bernard J, Lhomme C, et al. c-erbB-2 Gene amplification and protein expression in ovarian epithelial tumors: evaluation of their respective prognostic significance by multivariate analysis. *Int J Cancer* 1995;64:146–151.

120. Medl M, Sevelda P, Czerwenka K, et al. DNA amplification of HER-2/neu and INT-2 oncogenes in epithelial ovarian cancer. *Gynecol Oncol* 1995;59:321–326.

121. Fox H. Ovarian tumours of borderline malignancy: time for a reappraisal? *Curr Diagn Pathol* 1996;3:143–151.

122. Serov SF, Scully RE, Sobin LH. *International histological classification of tumours. No 9. Histological typing of ovarian tumours.* Geneva: World Health Organization, 1973.

123. Ovarian Tumour Panel of the Royal College of Obstetricians and Gynaecologists. Ovarian epithelial tumours of borderline malignancy: pathological features and current status. *Br J Obstet Gynaecol* 1983;90:743–750.

124. Bell DA, Rutgers JL, Scully RE. Ovarian epithelial tumors of borderline malignancy. In: Damjanov I, Cohen A, Mills SE, Young RH, eds. *Progress in reproductive and urinary tract pathology,* vol. 1. Philadelphia: Field and Wood, 1989:1–30.

125. Hart WR, Norris HJ. Borderline and malignant mucinous tumors of the ovary. *Cancer* 1973;31:1031–1045.

126. Hart WR. Ovarian epithelial tumors of borderline malignancy (carcinomas of low malignant potential). *Hum Pathol* 1977;8:541–549.

127. Hart WR. Pathology of malignant and borderline (low malignant potential) epithelial tumors of the ovary. In: Coppleson M, Monaghan J, Morrow CP, Tattersall MRN, eds. *Gynecologic oncology.* 2nd ed. Edinburgh: Churchill Livingstone, 1992:863–887.

128. Chaitin BA, Gershenson DM, Evans HL. Mucinous tumors of the ovary: a clinicopathologic study of 70 cases. *Cancer* 1985;55:1958–1962.

129. Sumithran E, Susil BJ, Looi L. The prognostic significance of grading in borderline mucinous tumors of the ovary. *Hum Pathol* 1988;19:15–18.

130. Watkin W, Silva EG, Gershenson DM. Mucinous carcinoma of the ovary: pathologic prognostic factors. *Cancer* 1992;69:208–212.

131. Russell P. The pathological assessment of ovarian neoplasms. II. The proliferating epithelial tumors. *Pathology* 1979;11:251–282.

132. Fox H. The concept of borderline malignancy in ovarian tumors. *Curr Top Pathol* 1989;78:111–134.

133. Russell P. Ovarian epithelial tumours with atypical proliferation. In: Lowe D, Fox H, eds. *Advances in gynaecological pathology.* Edinburgh: Churchill Livingstone, 1992:299–320.

134. Fox H. Ovarian tumours of borderline malignancy. In: Ratnam SS, Sen DK, Arulkumaran S, eds. *Contributions to obstetrics and gynaecology,* vol. 3. Singapore: Churchill Livingstone, 1994:327–341.

135. Russell P. Surface epithelial-stromal tumours of the ovary. In: Fox H, ed. *Haines and Taylor: textbook of obstetrical and gynaecological pathology.* 4th ed. New York: Churchill Livingstone, 1995:743–821.

136. Siriaunkgul S, Robbins KM, McGowan L, Silverberg SG. Ovarian mucinous tumors of low malignant potential: a clinicopathologic study of 54 tumors of intestinal and müllerian type. *Int J Gynecol Pathol* 1995;14:198–208.

137. Tavassoli FA. Serous tumor of low malignant potential with early stromal invasion (serous LMP with microinvasion). *Mod Pathol* 1988;1:407–414.

138. Bell DA, Scully RE. Ovarian serous borderline tumors with stromal microinvasion: a report of 21 cases. *Hum Pathol* 1990;21:397–403.

139. Purola E. Serous papillary ovarian tumours: a study of 233 cases with special reference to the histological type of tumour and its influence on prognosis. *Acta Obstet Gynaecol Scand Suppl* 1963;3:1–77.

140. Julian CG, Woodruff JD. The biologic behavior of low grade papillary serous carcinoma of the ovary. *Obstet Gynecol* 1972;40:360–368.

141. Katzenstein AA, Mazur MT, Morgan TE, Kao GF. Proliferative serous tumors of the ovary: histologic features and prognosis. *Am J Surg Pathol* 1978;2:339–355.

142. Tang M, Lian L, Liu T. The characteristics of ovarian serous tumors of borderline malignancy. *Chin Med J* 1980;92:459–464.

143. Tasker M, Langley FA. The outlook for women with borderline epithelial tumours of the ovary. *Br J Obstet Gynaecol* 1985;92:969–973.

144. Tazelaar HD, Bostwick DG, Ballon SC, et al. Conservative treatment of borderline ovarian tumors. *Obstet Gynecol* 1985;66:417–422.

145. Kliman L, Rome RM, Fortune DW. Low malignant potential tumors of the ovary: a study of 76 cases. *Obstet Gynecol* 1986;68:338–344.

146. Nakashima N, Nagasaka T, Oiwa N, et al. Ovarian epithelial tumors of borderline malignancy in Japan. *Gynecol Oncol* 1990;38:90–98.

147. Massad LS, Hunter VJ, Szpakca CA, et al. Epithelial ovarian tumors of low malignant potential. *Obstet Gynecol* 1991;78:1027–1032.

148. Kaern J, Trope CG, Abeler VM. A retrospective study of 370 ovarian borderline tumors treated at the Norwegian Radium Hospital from 1970 to 1982: a clinical and histopathological review. *Cancer* 1993;71:1810–1820.

149. Sykes P, Quinn M, Rome R. Ovarian tumors of low malignant potential: a retrospective study of 234 patients. *Int J Gynecol Cancer* 1997;7: 218–226.

150. Aure JC, Hoeg K, Kolstad P. Clinical and histologic studies of ovarian carcinoma: long term follow-up of 990 cases. *Obstet Gynecol* 1971;37: 1–9.

151. Nikrui N. Survey of clinical behavior of patients with borderline epithelial tumors of the ovary. *Gynecol Oncol* 1981;12:107–119.

152. Russell P. Borderline epithelial tumors of the ovary: a conceptual dilemma. *Clin Obstet Gynecol* 1984;11:259–277.

153. Gershenson DM, Silva EG. Serous ovarian tumors of low malignant potential with peritoneal implants. *Cancer* 1990;65:578–585.

154. Trimble CL, Trimble EL. Management of epithelial ovarian tumors of low malignant potential. *Gynecol Oncol* 1994;55:552–561.

155. McCaughey WTE, Kirk ME, Lester W, Dardick I. Peritoneal epithelial lesions associated with proliferative serous tumors of the ovary. *Histopathology* 1984;8:195–208.

156. Michael H, Roth LM. Invasive and non-invasive implants in ovarian serous tumors of low malignant potential. *Cancer* 1986;57:1240–1247.

157. Bell DA, Weinstock MA, Scully RE. Peritoneal implants of ovarian serous borderline tumors: histologic features and prognosis. *Cancer* 1988;62:2212–2222.

158. Lauchlan SC. The secondary müllerian system. *Obstet Gynecol Surv* 1972;27:133–146.

159. Lauchlan SC. The secondary müllerian system revisited. *Int J Gynecol Pathol* 1994;13:73–79.

160. Segal GH, Hart WR. Ovarian serous tumors of low malignant potential (serous borderline tumors): the relationship of exophytic surface tumor to peritoneal "implants." *Am J Surg Pathol* 1992;16:577–583.

161. Tutschka BG, Lauchlan SC. Endosalpingiosis. *Obstet Gynecol* 1980;55:57s–60s.

162. Zinser KR, Wheeler JE. Endosalpingiosis in the omentum: a study of autopsy and surgical material. *Am J Surg Pathol* 1982;6:109–117.

163. Bell DA. Pathology of the peritoneum and secondary müllerian system. In: Fox H, ed. *Haines and Taylor: obstetrical and gynaecological pathology.* 4th ed. New York: Churchill Livingstone, 1995:997–1014.

164. Dallenbach-Hellweg G. Atypical endosalpingiosis: a case report with consideration of the differential diagnosis of glandular subperitoneal inclusions. *Pathol Res Pract* 1987;182:180–182.

165. Bell DA, Scully RE. Serous borderline tumors of the peritoneum. *Am J Surg Pathol* 1990;14:230–239.

166. Biscotti CV, Hart WR. Peritoneal serous micropapillomatosis of low malignant potential (serous borderline tumors of the peritoneum): a clinicopathologic study of 17 cases. *Am J Surg Pathol* 1992;16:467–475.

167. Farnsworth H, Russell P. Extraovarian tumours of müllerian type. In: Lowe D, Fox H, eds. *Advances in gynaecological pathology.* Edinburgh: Churchill Livingstone, 1992:321–341.

168. Lim-Tan SK, Cagigas HA, Scully RE. Ovarian cystectomy for serous borderline tumors: a follow-up study of 35 cases. *Obstet Gynecol* 1988;72:775–781.

169. Dgani R, Blickstein I, Stroham Z, et al. Clinical aspects of ovarian tumors of low malignant potential. *Eur J Obstet Gynecol Reprod Biol* 1990; 35:251–258.

170. Rice LW, Berkowitz RS, Mark SD, et al. Ovarian epithelial tumors of borderline malignancy. *Gynecol Oncol* 1990;39:195–198.

171. Ayhan A, Atakin R, Develioglu O, et al. Borderline epithelial tumours. *Aust N Z J Obstet Gynaecol* 1991;31:174–176.

172. Sawada M, Yamasaki M, Urabe T, et al. Stage I epithelial ovarian tumors of low malignant potential. *Jpn J Clin Oncol* 1991;21:30–34.

173. Manchul LA, Simm J, Levin W, et al. Borderline epithelial ovarian tumors: a review of 81 cases with an assessment of the impact of treatment. *Int J Radiat Oncol Biol Phys* 1992;22:867–874.

174. de Nictolis M, Montironi R, Tommasoni S, et al. Serous borderline tumors of the ovary: a clinicopathologic, immunohistochemical, and quantitative study of 44 cases. *Cancer* 1992;70: 152–160.

175. Piura B, Dgani R, Blickstein I, et al. Epithelial ovarian tumors of borderline malignancy: a study of 50 cases. *Int J Gynecol Cancer* 1992;2: 189–197.

176. Kurman RJ, Trimble CL. The behaviour of serous tumors of low malignant potential: are they ever malignant? *Int J Gynecol Pathol* 1993; 12:120–127.

177. Barnhill DR, Kurman RJ, Brady MF, et al. Preliminary analysis of the behavior of stage I ovarian serous tumors of low malignant potential: a Gynecologic Oncology Group study. *J Clin Oncol* 1995;13:2752–2756.

178. Burks RT, Sherman ME, Kurman RJ. Micropapillary serous carcinoma of the ovary and peritoneum: a distinctive low grade carcinoma related to serous borderline tumors. *Am J Surg Pathol* (in press).

179. Seidman JD, Kurman RJ. Subclassification of serous borderline tumors of the ovary into benign and malignant types: a clinicopathologic study of 65 advanced stage cases. *Hum Pathol* (in press).

180. Padberg BC, Stegner HE, von Sengbusch S, et al. DNA cytophotometry and immunocytochemistry in ovarian tumours of borderline malignancy and related peritoneal lesions. *Virchows Arch A Pathol Anat Histopathol* 1992;421: 497–503.

181. Rutgers JL, Scully RE. Ovarian müllerian mucinous papillary cystadenomas of borderline malignancy: a clinicopathologic analysis of 30 cases. *Cancer* 1988;61:340–348.

182. Russell P, Merkur H. Proliferating ovarian "epithelial" tumours: a clinicopathologic analysis of 144 cases. *Aust N Z J Obstet Gynaecol* 1979;19:45–51.

183. Barnhill D, Heller P, Brzozowski P, et al. Epithelial ovarian carcinoma of low malignant potential. *Obstet Gynecol* 1985;65:53–58.

184. Bostwick DG, Tazelaar HD, Ballon SC, et al. Ovarian epithelial tumors of borderline malignancy: a clinical and pathologic study of 109 cases. *Cancer* 1986;58:2052–2065.

185. Nation JG, Krepart GV. Ovarian carcinoma of low malignant potential: staging and treatment. *Am J Obstet Gynecol* 1986;154:290–293.

186. de Nictolis M, Montironi R, Tommasoni S, et al. Benign, borderline, and well differentiated malignant intestinal mucinous tumors of the ovary: a clinicopathologic, immunohistochemi-cal, and nuclear quantitative study of 57 cases. *Int J Gynecol Pathol* 1994;13:10–21.

187. Guerriere C, Hogberg T, Wingren S, et al. Mucinous borderline and malignant tumors of the ovary. *Cancer* 1994;74:2329–2335.

188. Young RH, Gilks SB, Scully RE. Mucinous tumors of the appendix associated with mucinous tumors of the ovary and pseudomyxoma peritonei: a clinicopathological analysis of 22 cases. *Am J Surg Pathol* 1991;15:415–429.

189. Ronnett BM, Kurman RJ, Zahn CM, et al. Pseudomyxoma peritonei in women: a clinicopathologic analysis of 30 cases with emphasis on site of origin, prognosis, and relationship to ovarian mucinous tumors of low malignant potential. *Hum Pathol* 1995;26:509–524.

190. Ronnett BM, Zahn CM, Kurman RJ, et al. Disseminated peritoneal adenomucinosis and peritoneal carcinomatosis. *Am J Surg Pathol* 1995; 19:1390–1408.

191. Fox H. Ovarian tumors of borderline malignancy. In: Morrow CP, Bonnar J, O'Brien TJ, Gibbons WE, eds. *Recent clinical developments in gynecologic oncology.* New York: Raven, 1983:137–150.

192. Baak J, Fox H, Langley FA, Buckley CH. The prognostic value of morphometry in ovarian epithelial tumors of borderline malignancy. *Int J Gynecol Pathol* 1985;4:186–191.

193. Padberg P-C, Arps H, Franke U, et al. DNA cytophotometry and prognosis in ovarian tumors of borderline malignancy: a clinicopathological study of 80 cases. *Cancer* 1992;69:2510–2514.

194. Kaern J, Trope CG, Kristensen GB, et al. DNA ploidy: the most important prognostic factor in patients with borderline tumors of the ovary. *Int J Gynecol Cancer* 1993;3:349–358.

195. Harlow BL, Fuhr JE, McDonald TW, et al. Flow cytometry as a prognostic indicator in women with borderline epithelial ovarian tumors. *Gynecol Oncol* 1995;50:305–309.

196. Kuoppala T, Heinola M, Aine R, et al. Serous and mucinous borderline tumors of the ovary: a clinicopathologic and DNA-ploidy study of 102 cases. *Int J Gynecol Cancer* 1996;6:302–308.

197. Demirel D, Laucirica R, Fishman A, et al. Ovarian tumors of low malignant potential: correlation of DNA index and S-phase fraction with histopathologic grade and clinical outcome. *Cancer* 1996;77:1494–1500.

198. Norris HJ, Taylor HB. Virilization associated with cystic granulosa cell tumors. *Obstet Gynecol* 1969;34:629–635.

199. Nakashima N, Young RH, Scully RE. Androgenic granulosa cell tumors of the ovary: a clinicopathologic analysis of 17 cases and review of the literature. *Arch Pathol Lab Med* 1984; 108:786–791.

200. Young RH, Scully RE. Ovarian sex cord–stromal tumors with bizarre nuclei: a clinicopathologic analysis of 17 cases. *Int J Gynecol Pathol* 1983; 1:325–335.

201. Fox H, Agrawal, K, Langley FA. A clinicopathological study of 92 cases of granulosa cell tumor of the ovary with special reference to the factors influencing prognosis. *Cancer* 1975;35: 231–241.

202. Pautier P, Lhomme C, Culine S, et al. Adult granulosa cell tumor of the ovary: a retrospective study of 45 cases. *Int J Gynecol Cancer* 1997;7:58–65.

203. Malmstrom H, Hogberg T, Risberg B, Simonsen E. Granulosa cell tumor of the ovary prognostic factors and outcome. *Gynecol Oncol* 1994; 52:50–55.

204. King LA, Okagaki T, Gallup DH, et al. Mitotic count, nuclear atypia, and immmunohistochemical determination of Ki-67, c-myc, p21-ras, c-erbB2, and p53 expression in granulosa cell tumors of the ovary: mitotic count and Ki-67 are indicators of poor prognosis. *Gynecol Oncol* 1996;61:227–232.

205. Holland DR, Le Riche J, Swenerton KD, et al. Flow cytometric assessment of DNA ploidy is a useful prognostic factor for patients with granulosa cell ovarian tumors. *Int J Gynecol Cancer* 1991;1:227–232.

206. Palmquist-Evans M, Webb MJ, Gaffey TA, et al. DNA ploidy of ovarian granulosa cell tumors: lack of correlation between DNA index or proliferative index and outcome in 40 patients. *Cancer* 1995;75:2295–2298.

207. Young RH, Dickersin GR, Scully RE. Juvenile granulosa cell tumor of the ovary: a clinicopathologic analysis of 125 cases. *Am J Surg Pathol* 1984;8:575–596.

208. Powell JL, Johnson NA, Bailey CL, Otis CN. Management of advanced juvenile granulosa cell tumor of the ovary. *Gynecol Oncol* 1993; 48:119–123.

209. Prat J, Scully RE. Cellular fibromas and fibrosarcomas of the ovary: a comparative clinico-pathologic analysis of seventeen cases. *Cancer* 1981;47:2663–2670.

210. Young RH, Scully RE. Ovarian Sertoli cell tumors: a report of ten cases. *Int J Gynecol Pathol* 1984;2:349–363.

211. Sternberg WH, Roth LM. Ovarian stromal tumors containing Leydig cells: I. Stromal Leydig cell tumor and non-neoplastic transformation of ovarian stroma to Leydig cells. *Cancer* 1973;32:940–951.

212. Sternberg WH, Roth LM. Ovarian stromal tumors containing Leydig cells. II. Pure Leydig cell tumor, non-hilar type. *Cancer* 1973;32:952–960.

213. Salm R. Ovarian hilus-cell tumors: their varying presentations. *J Pathol* 1974;113:117–127.

214. Paraskevas M, Scully RE. Hilus cell tumor of the ovary: a clinicopathological analysis of 12 Reinke-crystal-positive and 9 crystal-negative cases. *Int J Gynecol Pathol* 1989;8:299–310.

215. Young RH. Sertoli-Leydig cell tumors of the ovary: a review with emphasis on historical aspects and unusual variants. *Int J Gynecol Pathol* 1993;12:141–147.

216. Young RH, Scully RE. Ovarian Sertoli-Leydig cell tumors with a retiform pattern: a problem in histopathologic diagnosis; a report of 25 cases. *Am J Surg Pathol* 1983;7:755–771.

217. Roth LM, Slayton RE, Brady LW, et al. Retiform differentiation in ovarian Sertoli-Leydig cell tumors: a clinicopathologic study of six cases from a Gynecologic Oncology Group study. *Cancer* 1985;55:1093–1098.

218. Talerman A. Ovarian Sertoli-Leydig cell tumor (androblastoma) with retiform pattern. *Cancer* 1987;60:3056–3064.

219. Young RH, Prat J, Scully RE. Ovarian Sertoli-Leydig cell tumors with heterologous elements. (i) Gastrointestinal epithelium and carcinoid: a clinicopathologic analysis of thirty six cases. *Cancer* 1982;50:2448–2456.

220. Prat J, Young RH, Scully RE. Ovarian Sertoli-Leydig cell tumors with heterologous elements. (ii) Cartilage and skeletal muscle: a clinicopathological analysis of twelve cases. *Cancer* 1982;50:2465–2475.

221. Young RH, Scully RE. Well differentiated ovarian Sertoli-Leydig cell tumors: a clinicopathological analysis of twenty five cases. *Int J Gynecol Pathol* 1984;3:277–290.

222. Roth LM, Anderson MC, Govan ADT, et al. Sertoli-Leydig cell tumors: a clinicopathol-

ogic study of 34 cases. *Cancer* 1981;48:187–197.

223. Zaloudek C, Norris HJ. Sertoli-Leydig cell tumors of the ovary: a clinicopathologic study of 64 intermediate and poorly differentiated neoplasms. *Am J Surg Pathol* 1984;8:405–418.

224. Young RH, Scully RE. Ovarian Sertoli-Leydig cell tumors: a clinicopathologic analysis of 207 cases. *Am J Surg Pathol* 1985;9:543–569.

225. Scully RE. Sex cord tumor with annular tubules: a distinctive ovarian tumor of the Peutz-Jeghers syndrome. *Cancer* 1970;25:1107–1121.

226. Anderson MC, Govan ADT, Langley FA, et al. Ovarian sex cord tumors with annular tubules. *Histopathology* 1980;4:135–145.

227. Shen K, Wu PC, Lang JH, et al. Ovarian sex cord tumor with annular tubules: a report of six cases. *Gynecol Oncol* 1993;48:180–184.

228. Young RH, Welch WR, Dickersin GR, Scully RE. Ovarian sex cord tumor with annular tubules: review of 74 cases including 27 with Peutz-Jeghers syndrome and four with adenoma malignum. *Cancer* 1982;50:1384–1402.

229. Hart WR, Kumar N, Crissman JD. Ovarian neoplasms resembling sex cord tumors with annular tubules. *Cancer* 1980;45:2252–2263.

230. Ahn HG, Chi JG, Lee SK. Ovarian sex cord tumor with annular tubules. *Cancer* 1986;57:1066–1077.

231. Clement PB, Young RH. Non-teratomatous germ cell tumors. *Curr Diagn Pathol* 1995;2:199–207.

232. Zaloudek C, Tavassoli CA, Norris HJ. Dysgerminoma with syncytiotrophoblastic giant cells: a histologically and clinically distinctive subtype of dysgerminoma. *Am J Surg Pathol* 1981;5:361–367.

233. Kaplan C, Hawley R. Dysgerminoma with giant cells: a case report with immunoperoxidase. *Diagn Gynecol Obstet* 1981;3:325–329.

234. Gillespie JJ, Arnold LK. Anaplastic dysgerminoma. *Cancer* 1978;42:1886–1889.

235. Jacobs AJ, Newland ER, Green RK. Primary choriocarcinoma of the ovary. *Obstet Gynecol Surv* 1982;37:603–609.

236. Axe SR, Klein VR, Woodruff JD. Choriocarcinoma of the ovary. *Obstet Gynecol* 1985;66:111–114.

237. Grover V, Grover RK, Usha R, Logami KB. Pure primary choriocarcinoma of the ovary. *Gynecol Obstet Invest* 1990;30:61–63.

238. Clement PB, Toung RH, Scully RE. Endometrioid-like yolk sac tumor of the ovary: a clinicopathological analysis of eight cases. *Am J Surg Pathol* 1987;11:767–778.

239. Prat J, Bhart AK, Dickersin GR, et al. Hepatoid yolk sac tumor of the ovary (endodermal sinus tumor with hepatoid differentiation): a light microscopic, ultrastructural and immunohistochemical study of seven cases. *Cancer* 1982;50:2355–2368.

240. Cohen MB, Mulchahey KM, Molnar JJ. Ovarian endodermal sinus tumor with intestinal differentiation. *Cancer* 1986;57:1580–1583.

241. Nakashima N, Fukatsu T, Nagasaki T, et al. The frequency and histology of hepatic tissue in germ cell tumors. *Am J Surg Pathol* 1987;11:682–692.

242. Nogales FF. Germ cell tumours of the ovary. In: Fox H, ed. *Haines and Taylor: obstetrical and gynaecological pathology.* 4th ed. New York: Churchill Livingstone, 1995:847–896.

243. Nogales FF, Matilla A, Nogales-Ortiz F, Galera-Davidson HL. Yolk sac tumors with pure and mixed polyvesicular vitelline patterns. *Hum Pathol* 1978;9:553–566.

244. Kurman RJ, Norris HJ. Embryonal carcinoma of the ovary: a clinicopathologic entity distinct from endodermal sinus tumor resembling embryonal carcinoma of the adult testis. *Cancer* 1976;38:2420–2433.

245. Ueda G, Abe Y, Yoshida M, Fujiwara T. Embryonal carcinoma of the ovary: a six year survival. *Int J Gynecol Obstet* 1990;31:287–292.

246. Peterson WF. Malignant degeneration of benign cystic teratomas of the ovary: a collective review of the literature. *Obstet Gynecol Surv* 1957;12:793–830.

247. Hirakawa T, Tsuneyoshi M, Enjoji M. Squamous cell carcinoma arising in mature cystic teratoma of the ovary: clinicopathologic and topographic analysis. *Am J Surg Pathol* 1989;13:397–405.

248. Norris HJ, Zirkin HJ, Benson WL. Immature (malignant) teratoma of the ovary: a clinical and pathologic study of 58 cases. *Cancer* 1976;37:2359–2372.

249. Clement PB, Young RH. Teratomas excluding monodermal teratomas. *Curr Diagn Pathol* 1995;2:208–213.

250. Clement PB, Young RH. Monodermal teratomas. *Curr Diagn Pathol* 1995;2:214–221.

251. Hasleton PS, Kelehan P, Whittaker JS, et al. Benign and malignant struma ovarii. *Arch Pathol Lab Med* 1978;102:180–184.

252. Devaney K, Snyder R, Norris HJ, Tavassoli FA. Proliferative struma ovarii and histologically malignant struma ovarii. *Int J Gynecol Pathol* 1993;12:333–343.

253. Robboy SJ, Norris HJ, Scully RE. Insular carcinoid primary in the ovary: a clinicopathologic analysis of 48 cases. *Cancer* 1975;36:404–418.

254. Davis KP, Hartmann LK, Keeney GL, Shapiro H. Primary ovarian carcinoid tumors. *Gynecol Oncol* 1996;61:608–615.

255. Robboy SK, Scully RE. Strumal carcinoid of the ovary: an analysis of 50 cases of a distinctive tumor composed of thyroid tissue and carcinoid. *Cancer* 1980;46:2019–2034.

256. Snyder RR, Tavassoli FA. Ovarian strumal carcinoid: immunohistochemical, ultrastructural, and clinicopathologic observations. *Int J Gynecol Pathol* 1986;5:187–201.

257. Stagno PA, Petras RE, Hart WR. Strumal carcinoids of the ovary: an immunohistologic and ultrastructural study. *Arch Pathol Lab Med* 1987;111:440–446.

258. Dickersin GR, Kline EW, Scully RE. Small cell carcinoma of the ovary with hypercalcemia: a report of 11 cases. *Cancer* 1982;49:188–197.

259. Scully RE. Small cell carcinoma of hypercalcemic type. *Int J Gynecol Pathol* 1993;12:148–152.

260. Young RH, Oliva E, Scully RE. Small cell carcinoma of the ovary, hypercalcemic type: a clinicopathological analysis of 150 cases. *Am J Surg Pathol* 1994;18:1039–1047.

261. Eichhorn JH, Young RH, Scully RE. Primary ovarian small cell carcinoma of pulmonary type: a clinicopathologic, immunohistologic and flow cytometric analysis of eleven cases. *Am J Surg Pathol* 1992;18:926–938.

262. Ishikura H, Scully RE. Hepatoid carcinoma of the ovary: a newly described tumor. *Cancer* 1987;60:2775–2784.

263. Matsuta M, Ishikura H, Murakami K, et al. Hepatoid carcinoma of the ovary: a case report. *Int J Gynecol Pathol* 1991;10:302–310.

CHAPTER 31

Early-Stage Ovarian Carcinoma

AKIRA SUGIMOTO
GILLIAN THOMAS

Introduction

Epithelial ovarian carcinoma presents with disease limited to the pelvis in up to one-third of cases (1). The overall prognosis of this group is good; however, a significant proportion of patients will still suffer recurrence and die of disease. The risk of recurrence for the individual patient can vary from as low as 2% to nearly 50%. There are no universally accepted criteria for identifying patients who are at high enough risk that adjuvant therapy should be offered. There is even more uncertainty about the benefit of adjuvant therapy in those patients at risk for recurrence. Current practice ranges from no further treatment to adjuvant radiotherapy, chemotherapy, intraperitoneal agents, or combinations of both. The two fundamental issues with early-stage ovarian carcinoma are identification of patients at significant risk of recurrence and development and administration of effective treatment to improve their survival. Limitations in our understanding of the behavior of this disease and its treatment underscore the difficulty in achieving these objectives.

Defining Early-Stage Disease

The concept of early-stage disease arose from historical observations that patients with overt abdominal metastases did not survive, while those with disease limited to the pelvis often fared better. Cure was possible with surgical removal of the entire tumor in early-stage disease. A significant number of patients still developed recurrent disease and, interestingly, these failures were often in the upper abdomen. Mechanisms for abdominal dissemination of disease have been elucidated by in vivo studies of the flow of radioactive labels through the peritoneal cavity and anatomical studies of the lymphatic drainage of the ovaries into the para-aortic and pelvic lymph nodes. Hence, disease that is apparently in its early stage appeared to have the potential for occult metastases in the lymph nodes and/or the peritoneal cavity. This observation led to surgically staging ovarian carcinoma by biopsy of the upper abdomen and the retroperitoneal lymph nodes. Further studies showed that even in the absence of overt abdominal disease, the presence of ascites or positive cytology in the abdominal cavity, surface involvement of the ovary with tumor, and disruption of the tumor capsule were often associated with disease recurrence (2). These conclusions were based on univariate analysis of a limited number of surgicopathologic factors without taking other prognostic variables into consideration. Nonetheless, they formed the basis of the surgical staging system put forth by the International Federation of Gynecology and Obstetrics (FIGO) in 1988 (Table 31-1) (3). FIGO staging is currently the most standardized tool for estimating prognosis. Several clinicopathologic studies demonstrate that the 5-year survival rate is 5% to 15% for advanced-stage disease compared with 40% to 90% for stage I and II disease (4). The parameters of FIGO staging may be best thought of as "first-generation" prognostic

T A B L E **31-1**

FIGO Staging of Early-stage Ovarian Carcinoma

FIGO Stage	Description
I	Disease limited to the ovaries
Ia	Disease limited to one ovary, no ascites, no surface involvement, capsule intact
Ib	Disease limited to both ovaries, no ascites, no surface involvement, capsule intact
Ic	Either stage Ia or stage Ib with ascites containing malignant cells or positive peritoneal cytology, capsule ruptured, or surface involvement
II	Disease involving one or both ovaries with pelvic extension
IIa	Extension and/or metastases to the fallopian tube or uterus
IIb	Disease spread to other pelvic organs including the pelvic sidewall
IIc	Either stage IIa or stage IIb with ascites containing malignant cells or positive peritoneal cytology, capsule ruptured, or surface involvement

factors that are capable of broadly defining patients with advanced disease and poor prognosis from those with early disease and better prognosis.

Limitations of FIGO Staging

Stage I disease is substaged depending on whether disease is found to be unilateral (Ia), bilateral (Ib), or associated with positive peritoneal cytology or capsular rupture (Ic).

Stage II disease is substaged based on the finding of spread to the fallopian tubes or uterus (stage IIa), to other pelvic organs including the sidewall (stage IIb), or to either location in association with positive peritoneal cytology or capsular rupture (stage IIc). Notably, while disease can extend to the pelvis either by transcoelomic transfer or by direct extension, FIGO does not acknowledge a difference in these two entities.

It is implied by FIGO substages that progressive substages are associated with progressively worsening prognosis. However, careful interpretation of the literature demonstrates little conclusive evidence that bilaterality, ovarian excrescences, and peritoneal cytology are independent adverse prognostic factors.

Webb et al retrospectively studied 271 cases of stage I ovarian carcinoma to determine the prognostic significance of the FIGO parameters in stage I disease. The treatments were mixed and not controlled for, and univariate rather than multivariate analysis was used to assess the impact of each FIGO variable. Recognizing these limitations, the study was unable to

T A B L E **31-2**

5-Year Survival in Individual FIGO Substages

FIGO Stage	No.	Treatment	% Year Survival
Ia	81	None/XRT/Chemo	84
Ib	22	None/XRT/Chemo	68
Ic	14	None/XRT/Chemo	86
IIa	16	None/XRT/Chemo	81
IIb	55	None/XRT/Chemo	40
IIc	13	None/XRT/Chemo	62

demonstrate that FIGO parameters in stage I disease, namely bilaterality and positive washings, carry any prognostic significance (5).

Sigurdsson et al retrospectively studied 117 stage I and 84 stage II patients, examining the prognosis in FIGO substages. Table 31-2 illustrates again that indeed, these substages have little direct correlation with prognosis (6).

Thus, while FIGO staging as a historical "first-generation" staging system can broadly identify those patients with advanced-stage disease destined to do poorly, in early-stage disease one cannot rely on FIGO staging alone to estimate prognosis. Other prognostic factors must be operational.

"Second-Generation" Prognostic Factors

Recognizing that the prognosis for stage I disease can vary widely from 40% to 90% (7), in the mid-1980s several investigators began studying other surgicopathologic tumor factors that would better predict outcome in early-stage disease.

The impact of individual prognostic factors on the natural history of early-stage disease is difficult to study for two reasons: the incidence of early-stage disease is low and the event rate for recurrence is relatively low. Furthermore, many studies in the literature do not correctly identify patients with only early-stage invasive disease. Surgical staging data are often limited and histologic interpretation may not discriminate between patients who may have unrecognized borderline tumors. Many patients included in "natural history" studies have actually received treatment. Finally, there are likely to be several important prognostic factors that interact with each other, but individual studies usually assess one at a time in univariate analysis. Table 31-3 illustrates the surgicopathologic parameters that have been studied. Using Cox multivariate analysis, it has been shown that age, FIGO stage, integrity of the capsule, and histologic type have no bearing on prognosis whereas histologic grade does (6,8,9). Although generally assumed to be an adverse prognostic factor, the significance of positive peritoneal cytology is questionable. Small comparative case series have demonstrated that the 5-year survival rate is similar in stage I and II disease whether washings are positive or not (10).

In 1990, Dembo et al studied several surgicopathologic variables concomitantly using multivariate analysis in order to determine which tumor characteristics are truly important in predicting outcome, and which are confounders (11). A single pathologist in each center was used to determine histologic subtype and grade, and borderline tumors were excluded. In the analysis, tumor grade, the presence of dense tumor-associated adhesions, and large-volume ascites (irrespective of cytology)

were the only three significant independent prognostic factors.

Baak et al point out that when relying upon tumor grade as a prognostic factor, one must be aware of the potential for a significant degree of variability in pathologic interpretation of tumor grade (12). According to Dembo, once grade, adherence, and large-volume ascites are controlled for, the traditional prognostic parameters of bilaterality, positive washings, capsular invasion, tumor size, patient age, and histologic subtype could not be shown to have any independent prognostic significance. In order to validate these findings, the same multivariate analysis was carried out on a database of patients from the Norwegian Radium Hospital by Carey, and the results were nearly the same: tumor grade and dense tumor adherence remained independent factors; however, large-volume ascites was not in the second database (13). By comparing the prognosis of individual subgroups based on these new prognostic factors, Carey and Dembo suggested three groupings of patients based on 5-year survival. "Low risk" was defined as stage I, grade 1 disease; "intermediate risk" as stage I, grade 2/3 disease or stage II tumors with no residuum; and "high risk" consisted of stage II disease with residuum of less than 2 cm (Table 31-4). Again, that the prognosis of those patients with stage I, grade 2/3 disease was similar to that of patients with optimally debulked stage III disease highlights the fact that early FIGO stage does not always correlate with good prognosis. Using these "second-generation" prognostic factors, the outcome of patients with early-stage disease can be predicted to a much more narrow range than with FIGO staging.

Surgical Staging

Identifying cases of early-stage ovarian carcinoma involves meticulous surgical staging for three metastatic processes: direct extension, transperitoneal, and lymphatic spread. The standard procedure consists of peritoneal washings, bilateral salpingo-oophorectomy, total abdominal hysterectomy, omentectomy, random peritoneal biopsies, and pelvic and para-aortic lymph node biopsies. On occasion, the initial operation for early-stage disease will not have included complete surgical staging. In this instance the value of a second procedure must

T A B L E **31-3**

Surgicopathologic Variables in Early Ovarian Cancer

Tumor size
Presence of dense tumor adhesions
Capsular rupture
Presence of surface excrescences
Presence of ascites
Bilaterality
Presence of positive peritoneal cytology
Patient age

T A B L E   **31-4**

Defining High-, Intermediate-, and Low-risk Early-stage Disease

Stage	Grade 1 (All Histologic Subtypes)	Grade 2/3 (Mucin./Endomet.) Grade 2 Serous	Grade 2/3 (Clear Cell or Grade 3 Serous)
I	96 ± 2% (*n* = 80)	75 ± 5% (*n* = 79)	66 ± 9% (*n* = 31)
II No Residuum	91 ± 4% (*n* = 45)	74 ± 14% (*n* = 60)	40 ± 9% (*n* = 33)
II <2 cm Residuum	100 % (*n* = 5)	78 ± 14% (*n* = 9)	21 ± 11% (*n* = 14)

Figures represent 5-year relapse-free rates ± standard deviation.

be assessed on the basis of the likelihood of detecting occult disease, the risks of the procedure, and the ability to make a treatment decision that will alter outcome.

When hysterectomy and bilateral salpingo-oophorectomy alone have been carried out, the likelihood of finding occult advanced disease at a second laparotomy has been shown to be 31% for patients with apparent stage I disease, and 41% for patients with apparent stage II disease (14,15). What is unclear from these studies is the degree of simple inspection and palpation of the abdomen at the initial operation. It is possible that many of these cases of presumed early-stage disease could have been upstaged by careful palpation and inspection alone (16).

Estimates from the literature suggest that if cases with presumed early-stage disease are restaged, roughly 10% to 24% of stage I and 20% of stage II patients will have para-aortic nodal metastases (17–24). Again, in many of these studies the quality and reporting of intraperitoneal staging and associated disease in the peritoneal cavity are not well described. Therefore, the true incidence of para-aortic node metastases where adequate intraperitoneal staging is negative is likely to be lower, although this situation is known to occur (22,25). In an analogous fashion, it is estimated that approximately 8% of patients with early-stage disease will have pelvic node metastases (18–21).

With respect to the value of intraperitoneal staging, approximately 3% of patients with presumed stage I disease will have occult omental metastases at omentectomy (10,28) and in patients of all stages where the pretest likelihood of occult disease is higher, the presence of occult disease in an otherwise normal-appearing omentum is as high as 22% (21,26).

Roughly one-third of patients with apparent stage I disease will have malignant cells identified in peritoneal washings; however, as mentioned previously, the prognostic significance of this finding is not clear (27,28).

Laparoscopic staging provides a safe and less morbid approach to surgical staging while being technically more challenging, time consuming, and technology dependent than laparotomy (29,30). There has been literature to suggest that peritoneoscopy is in fact more sensitive than laparotomy at detecting occult diaphragmatic disease (30). Conversely, there is also the suggestion that negative staging laparoscopy may miss disease in up to 50% of a small number of patients (30).

While laparoscopy has played a tremendous role in the advancement of surgical technique in gynecology, one must exercise caution in assessing and removing a pelvic mass through the laparoscope (31). Metastatic deposits of tumor within the trochar sites have been reported (32). It is controversial as to whether a laparoscopic approach to the patient highly suspected to have early-stage ovarian carcinoma is appropriate. Careful preoperative assessment of the patient and the use of ultrasound and CA-125 are useful in assessing the likelihood of malignancy before proceeding to laparoscopy.

When to Restage

The preoperative likelihood of finding more advanced disease upon restaging is related to the presence of associated surgicopathologic prognostic factors, notably histologic grade, presence of dense tumor adhesions, and large-volume ascites. There are no standardized recommendations as to when to reoperate on the patient who has been incompletely staged. In favor of restaging is the argument that the patient with presumed early-stage disease may have treatment decisions altered on the basis of finding advanced disease. On the other hand, if low- or intermediate-risk prognostic factors are present, the preoperative likelihood of there being disease is only 4% and 28%, respectively, as judged by 5-year survival statistics (11). Furthermore, one must assume that the yield of restaging as mentioned earlier may be as low as 50%, thereby reducing the yield in populations of low- and intermediate-risk patients to as low as 2% and 14%. Finally, adjuvant therapy administered in the setting of these 2% and 14% with presumably optimally debulked stage III disease (0 or <2 cm residuum) is roughly 40% (13). In other words, if all patients with low- or intermediate-risk disease are restaged, the highest possible survival benefit attributable to restaging may be as low as 1% to 6%. Roughly 90% of all stage I and II patients will fit into this category (13). The most dogmatic solution to this dilemma is to reoperate on every case of incompletely staged early ovarian carcinoma. This approach will yield the highest number of cases of occult advanced disease, but at the expense of up to 95% of the procedures leading to no improvement in survival. Individualized decisions about restaging that consider prognostic factors, patient tolerance, and efficacy of available treatment are most likely to reduce the number of unnecessary procedures.

The sensitivity of "thorough" staging laparotomy is difficult to measure directly as there is presently no biochemical or imaging technique that can act as a better "gold standard" for occult disease. An approximation of the false-negative rate of a staging laparotomy is the number of patients who develop recurrent disease after negative second-look staging procedure. The sensitivity of the staging procedure will be directly correlated with the thoroughness of surgery, including sampling the peritoneal cavity for cytology, the peritoneum itself, and the pelvic lymph nodes. When patients following treatment have laparotomy, peritoneal cytology, random peritoneal biopsies, and pelvic and para-aortic lymph node sampling performed following treatment, and all biopsies are negative, up to 54% of patients will still develop recurrent disease, indicating that the falsenegative rate of staging laparotomy may be

similarly high (33). On the other hand, there are other possible explanations for false-negative second-look procedures. Post-treatment adhesions may form a sanctuary for persistent disease. Abdominal recurrence could theoretically occur after true-negative staging from malignant cells in the peritoneal fluid that do not implant until after the staging procedure is performed. Furthermore, abdominal "recurrence" may be the result of a field process in the peritoneal cavity and the development of new primary peritoneal tumors.

Although abdominal hysterectomy and bilateral salpingo-oophorectomy are considered standard parts of surgery, younger patients with stage I disease who wish to preserve childbearing raise the issue of conservative surgery. Some studies have suggested that patients with apparent "stage I" disease treated by unilateral salpingo-oophorectomy alone have worse prognosis than those after abdominal hysterectomy, bilateral salpingo-oophorectomy, and omentectomy (62% vs. 84%) (8). Unfortunately, many of the patients treated did not undergo thorough abdominal staging. It is thus possible that the difference in survival is attributable to occult advanced disease rather than an effect of hysterectomy and contralateral salpingo-oophorectomy.

Proper assessment for planned conservative surgery should include an estimation of the risk of contralateral occult disease in a grossly normal ovary. In all stages combined, the incidence of bilaterality is up to 50% of serous tumors, 5% of mucinous tumors, and 35% of endometrioid tumors. There are two theoretical risks to leaving a normal-appearing contralateral ovary, namely the risk of leaving existing occult disease in that ovary and the risk of developing contralateral ovarian disease as a second primary. Whether to biopsy a normal-appearing ovary is controversial. The risk is of adhesion formation to the fallopian tube, compromising fertility. Furthermore, the true prevalence of occult microscopic disease in a normal-appearing contralateral ovary is unknown.

Having estimated the risk to the patient of leaving occult disease in the contralateral ovary and counseled the patient thoroughly with respect to this risk, it would appear reasonable to consider unilateral salpingo-oophorectomy for selected patients where preservation of fertility is appropriate, thorough inspection of the contralateral ovary and uterus is negative, and comprehensive surgical staging of the abdomen is performed. If conservative surgery is performed, close follow-up of patients with serial ultrasound and CA-125 treatment is prudent, although the value of such follow-up in this setting has not been confirmed. In every case, the patient must be prepared to accept a small risk of occult disease and the possibility of reduced survival in that event.

Adjuvant Therapy

The recurrence rate for all patients with early-stage disease after surgery and adjuvant therapy is on the order of 70%. Unfortunately, most studies of adjuvant therapy have not compared treated patients with those not receiving adjuvant therapy and it is not known whether there is actually an incremental benefit from the adjuvant treatment. Despite this fact, the apparent efficacy of adjuvant chemotherapy in advanced-stage disease, combined with ethical and medicolegal influences, has made adjuvant therapy common practice in North American centers.

Several epidemiologic factors make it difficult to determine whether adjuvant therapy improves survival. Because there are differing rates of relapse among patients with early-stage disease, substantial numbers of patients are required to study the effect of therapy in individual risk groups. In fact for most patients with early-stage disease, the incidence of relapse is very low even without treatment and it is very difficult to detect any reduction attributable to treatment.

Adjuvant therapies that have been described for early-stage disease include systemic chemotherapy, intraperitoneal chemotherapy, intraperitoneal radiocolloid treatment, external beam radiation therapy, or combinations of these.

Systemic Chemotherapy

In theory, occult residual cells in early-stage disease should be more sensitive than in advanced disease because of fewer clonogenic cells, fewer chemoresistant cell lines, distribution of drug to a higher percentage of tumor, and fewer areas of tumor hypoxia. Unfortunately, even unrecognized "microscopic residuum" in apparent early-stage disease can consist of 10^8 to 10^{10} cells. Since any reduction

in clonogenic cells with systemic chemotherapy is limited to only 3 to 4 logs, it is not surprising that adjuvant chemotherapy does not cure all patients with apparent early-stage disease (34). Nonetheless, agents that have been studied include single-agent cisplatin, cisplatin-cyclophosphamide, oral melphalan (35), and currently cisplatin-paclitaxel (Taxol).

When low-risk disease is defined as stage Ia or Ib, grade 1 or 2, the recurrence rate without treatment appears to be less than 10%. Detecting an improvement in survival with such a low natural recurrence rate would require extremely large numbers of patients and it is not surprising that a randomized controlled trial failed to show an improvement in survival with adjuvant oral melphalan (36). In patients with well-differentiated stage Ia, Ib, and Ic, a "wait-and-see" approach appears to be appropriate and has been advocated by Trimbos et al, who reported a 94% to 100% survival rate (37).

For those patients considered to have high-risk disease (stage I, grade 3 disease, or stage II disease), studies to date have compared systemic chemotherapy to whole abdominal radiotherapy (38), intraperitoneal chromic phosphate (36,38,39), or no further therapy (39).

Young et al found that high-risk patients treated with oral melphalan had a 5-year survival rate of 80% and there was no statistically significant difference when compared to intraperitoneal chromic phosphate (36).

Klassen et al compared pelvic radiation plus oral melphalan to pelvic radiotherapy plus whole abdominal radiotherapy, or intraperitoneal chromic phosphate. There was no statistically significant difference in 5-year survival between all three groups (61%, 62%, and 66%, respectively). Notably, 4% of patients receiving melphalan developed either myelodysplasia or acute leukemia (38).

Until recently, few studies have compared adjuvant treatment to a no-treatment arm, and none had conclusively shown any benefit to survival or recurrence rates. In 1995, Bolis et al published the results of two randomized trials of adjuvant cisplatin versus no further therapy. The results are noteworthy. In 85 patients with stage Ia/Ib, grade 2–3 disease randomized to receive cisplatin versus no further therapy, there was a statistically significant reduction in risk of relapse for those patients treated with cisplatin (83% disease free at 5 years vs. 63%). However, the 5-year survival was no different despite the higher recurrence rate in the nontreated group (39). The authors conclude that it is possible that longer follow-up and a larger population of patients may eventually reveal a survival benefit. However, the lack of demonstration of a survival benefit in a such a well-designed study suggests an alternative approach to the management of early-stage disease. It is possible that "high-risk" early-stage patients could be observed, with treatment being reserved for those patients who relapse. If this is implemented, it could result in a marked reduction in the number of patients who require treatment with no compromise in ultimate survival (39). Longer follow-up and more studies are necessary.

Intraperitoneal Chemotherapy

Intraperitoneal chemotherapy has theoretical appeal in the management of ovarian cancer by maximizing the tumor/host drug concentration gradient. There have been no trials that have specifically addressed the value of intraperitoneal chemotherapy in early-stage disease. In advanced-stage disease, intraperitoneal chemotherapy appears to have a complete response rate of approximtely 30% (40). There are preliminary data to suggest that in more advanced disease intraperitoneal chemotherapy may be superior to systemic chemotherapy in terms of prolongation of survival. The Gynecologic Oncology Group is currently studying the difference in survival between intraperitoneal chemotherapy and systemic therapy in advanced-stage disease.

Intraperitoneal Radiocolloids

The use of radiocolloids in the treatment of ovarian cancer has been thoroughly reviewed by Rosenshein (41). ^{63}Zn, ^{198}Au, and ^{32}P have all been used in ovarian cancer. Both ^{63}Zn and ^{198}Au were described early and then abandoned because of excessive toxicity related to the emission of both beta and gamma rays. On the other hand, ^{32}P is a pure beta emitter, has a favorable therapeutic index, and therefore has been more extensively studied. Theoretical problems with using intraperitoneal ^{32}P are nonuniform distribution throughout the peritoneal cavity and the rapid decline in radiation dose after only a few cell layers. Most reports of intraperitoneal ^{32}P are small case series of

adjuvant intraperitoneal ^{32}P in patients with combined high- and low-risk early-stage disease, and surgical staging is sometimes not complete (42,43); however, several clinical trials have been performed. Intraperitoneal ^{32}P in high-risk early-stage patients has been compared to three cycles of cisplatin-cyclophosphamide single-agent cisplatin (39), external beam pelvic radiotherapy, and oral melphalan plus whole abdominopelvic radiotherapy (36). It appears from these studies that the 5-year survival rate in patients with grade 3 or stage II disease receiving intraperitoneal ^{32}P is approximately 66% to 78%. It has not been demonstrated that there is a statistically significant difference in survival between intraperitoneal ^{32}P and any of the other treatments, although six cycles of cisplatin have been shown to reduce recurrence rate.

In only one of the studies was ^{32}P compared to a no-treatment arm to separate the effect of treatment from natural history of disease, and, although the scope of this study was limited, no difference in survival occurred when adjuvant treatment was used. Despite lack of positive studies, it is still possible that adjuvant intraperitoneal ^{32}P after surgery in early-stage disease does improve survival, but the overall benefit is likely to be small and limited to a select number of patients where all tumor is within the peritoneal cavity, no tumor is more than a few cells in thickness, and the distribution and dose of radiation are adequate.

Radiotherapy

As a treatment modality the therapeutic index of radiation is extremely dependent on dose, fraction, treatment time, and technique, which can vary greatly and in general have improved over time. Unfortunately, studies on the use of radiotherapy rarely report on these parameters. Early work on the use of radiotherapy in epithelial tumors of the head and neck suggested that a dose of 45 to 50 Gy is required to gain 98% control over microscopic disease in cervical lymph nodes. These data formed the basis for the traditional assumption that a similar dose is required to achieve control in epithelial ovarian cancer. Studies that have applied this dose to the pelvis alone found that survival was not improved, as patients would relapse in the upper abdomen. The proportion of pelvic relapses was reduced, however, confirming that ovarian cancer is a radiosensitive disease. The problem is that when 45 to 50 Gy are administered to the entire abdominal cavity, the enteric complications became unacceptable. It was believed initially that a tolerable dose of 25 Gy would not significantly impact on survival. However, in the past 5 years the application of radiation in ovarian cancer has been revisited. For patients with apparent early-stage disease, the degree of malignant cellular burden within the abdominal cavity at the time of adjuvant treatment will be determined by three factors: 1) the ability of the malignant cells to spread, 2) the net growth rate of these cells, and 3) the time from surgery to adjuvant treatment. As these three parameters vary, the magnitude of the disease burden will form a spectrum from no disease to small-volume burden to large, unmanageable amounts of burden. Recognizing that a dose of 45 to 50 Gy is required to attain 98% control, it has been found that a smaller dose of 25 to 28 Gy will reduce recurrence rates by 3% to 35%. In properly selected populations this treatment could result in significant improvement in survival. Furthermore, it has been suggested that the addition of chemotherapy to radiation may futher improve survival.

To Treat or Not to Treat?

To date, no study has conclusively demonstrated an improvement in survival with any form of adjuvant therapy for early-stage disease. In recognition of methodologic difficulties, however, it is still quite possible that an undetected benefit does exist for some selected patients. Whether or not to treat then becomes predicated on philosophy.

One approach is to treat patients at high risk on the assumption that there is a survival benefit. There are several arguments in defense of this approach. Recurrences in advanced-stage disease are incurable and since the risk of recurrence in selected patients with early-stage disease is high, attempts to lower the risk with adjuvant therapy are appropriate. Furthermore, as mentioned above, there are theoretical reasons as to why systemic therapy that is effective in advanced-stage disease might be even more effective in early-stage disease.

A fundamentally different approach to adjuvant treatment is to rely on the existing evidence that despite an apparent reduction in relapse rate there does not appear to be any improvement in survival. With this approach, therapy could be withheld until relapse occurs without compromising survival.

The Future: "Third-Generation" Prognostic Factors

To be sure, if ovarian carcinoma were truly limited to the ovary in stage I disease then recurrences would not develop. In order for recurrence to develop, there must be occult disease that is not detected at surgical staging, and furthermore the occult malignant cells must be biologically capable of invasion and the host must be susceptible to invasion. To what extent these factors determine whether an individual develops recurrence of early-stage disease is as yet unknown, but forms the concept of "third-generation" prognostic factors.

Evidence is now pointing toward the presence of determinants of recurrence that are operating at the molecular level, and many of these biomolecular prognostic factors may be determined genetically (44,45). The factors that have been studied include DNA flow cytometry for tumor ploidy (46–48), S-phase fraction (49), *Her-2/neu* oncogene expression (50), and steroid receptor content (51). These studies are too preliminary to draw any useful conclusions. It is clear that our understanding of this disease is rapidly changing. Rather than trying to predict outcome by relying on static parameters such as histologic grade, adherence, and presence of gross metastases, we will soon be able to assess the behavior of a particular tumor by examining its biomolecular activity. The number of important factors may eventually be vast; however, these determinants will revolutionize the clinical management of ovarian cancer, leading to an abandonment of the concept of "early-stage" disease in favor of "high risk" for death and "low risk" for death, irrespective of the actual FIGO stage.

Summary

"Early-stage" ovarian cancer is a heterogeneous disease with widely divergent prognoses from as high as 98% expected survival to as low as 50%. The evidence to date suggests that histologic grade, dense adherence, and possibly large-volume ascites are the most important predictors of outcome. Tumor size, bilaterality, ascites, and positive peritoneal cytology appear to predict for survival independently despite strong historical inferences to the contrary. Advanced-stage disease confers a poor prognosis and thorough abdominal staging for its detection is paramount. The impact on survival of repeated laparotomy for staging purposes in patients with apparent early-stage disease may be limited. Although many patients in certain "high-risk" groups are destined to develop recurrent disease, there is no convincing evidence that the use of adjuvant treatment is of benefit to survival. The use of adjuvant treatment is becoming polarized between a North American tendency to treat all at risk upfront and a European propensity to observe and treat at the time of recurrence. Further study is required to clarify which is the best approach.

Our knowledge of the behavior of ovarian carcinoma has extended from gross observations to histologic correlates and is rapidly progressing to biomolecular and genetic factors that can predict behavior. In consort with the better prediction of outcome, our ability to impact on the survival of patients with early-stage carcinoma still hinges on the development of more effective treatment.

REFERENCES

1. Young RC. Initial therapy of early stage ovarian cancer. *Cancer* 1987;60:2042–2049.

2. Creasman WT, Rutledge F. The prognostic significance of peritoneal cytology in gynaecologic malignant disease. *Am J Obstet Gynecol* 1971;110:773–781.

3. Pettersson F, ed. *Annual report on the results of treatment on gynaecological cancer.* International Federation of Gynecology and Obstetrics, vol 20, Stockholm, Sweden, 1988.

4. Friedlander ML, Dembo AJ. Prognostic factors in epithelial ovarian cancer. *Semin Oncol* 1991;18:205–212.

5. Webb MJ, Decker DG, Mussey E, Williams T. Factors influencing survival in stage I ovarian cancer. *Am J Obstet Gynecol* 1973;116:222–228.

6. Sigurdsson K, Alm P, Gullberg B. Prognostic factors in malignant epithelial ovarian tumours. *Gynecol Oncol* 1983;15:370–380.

7. Swenerton KD, Hislop TG, Spinelli J, et al. Ovarian carcinoma: a multivariate analysis of prognostic factors. *Obstet Gynecol* 1985;65:264–269.

8. Sevelda P, Vavra N, Schemper M, Salzer H. Prognostic factors for survival in stage I epithelial ovarian carcinoma. *Cancer* 1990;65:2349–2352.

9. Malkasian GD, Melton LJ, O'Brien PC, Greene MH. Prognostic significance of histological classification and grading of epithelial malignancies of the ovary. *Am J Obstet Gynecol* 1984;149:274–284.

10. Yoshimura S, Scully, RE, Taft PD, Herrington JB. Peritoneal fluid cytology in patients with ovarian cancer. *Gynecol Oncol* 1984;17:161–167.

11. Dembo A, Davy M, Stenwig AE, et al. Prognostic factors in patients with stage I epithelial ovarian cancer. *Obstet Gynecol* 1990;75:263–273.

12. Baak JP, Langley FA, Talerman A, Delemarre JF. The prognostic variability of ovarian tumor grading by different pathologists. *Gynecol Oncol* 1987;27:166–172.

13. Carey MS, Dembo AJ, Simm JE, et al. Testing the validity of a prognostic classification in patients with surgically optimal ovarian carcinoma: a 15-year review. *Int J Gynecol Cancer* 1993;3:24–35.

14. Young RC, Decker DG, Wharton JT, et al. Staging laparotomy in early ovarian cancer. *JAMA* 1983;250:3072–3073.

15. Helewa ME, Krepart GV, Lotocki R. Staging laparotomy in early epithelial ovarian carcinoma. *Am J Obstet Gynecol* 1986;154:282–286.

16. Bagley CM, Young RC, Scein PS, et al. Ovarian carcinoma metastatic to the diaphragm frequently undiagnosed at laparotomy. *Am J Obstet Gynecol* 1973;116:397–400.

17. Chen SS, Lee L. Incidence of paraaortic and pelvic lymph node metastases in epithelial carcinoma of the ovary. *Gynecol Oncol* 1983;16:95–100.

18. Musumeci R, Banfi A, Bolis G, et al. Lymphangiography in patients with ovarian epithelial cancer. *Cancer* 1977;40:1444–1449.

19. Musumeci R, et al. *Proceedings of the Sixth International Congress on Lymphology.* Prague, Czechoslovakia, 1977.

20. Knapp RC, Friedman EA. Aortic lymph node metastases in early ovarian cancer. *Am J Obstet Gynecol* 1974;119:1013–1017.

21. Delgado G, Chun B, Caglar H, Bepko F. Paraaortic lymphadenectomy in patients with gynaecologic malignancies confined to the pelvis. *Obstet Gynecol* 1977;50:418–423.

22. Burghardt E, Girardu F, Lahousen M, et al. Patterns of pelvic and paraaortic lymph node

involvement in ovarian cancer. *Gynecol Oncol* 1991;40:103–106.

23. Benedetti-Panici P, Greggi S, Maneschi F, et al. Anatomical and pathological study of retroperitoneal nodes in epithelial ovarian cancer. *Gynecol Oncol* 1993;51:150–154.

24. Petru E, Lahousen M, Tanussino K, et al. Lymphadenectomy in stage I ovarian cancer. *Am J Obstet Gynecol* 1994;70:656–662.

25. Creasman WT, Abu-Ghazaleh S, Schmidt HJ. Retroperitoneal metastatic spread of ovarian cancer. *Gynecol Oncol* 1978;6:447–450.

26. Steinberg JJ, Demopoulos RI, Bigelow B. The evaluation of the omentum in ovarian cancer. *Gynecol Oncol* 1986;24:327–330.

27. Piver MS, Barlow JJ, Lele SB. Incidence of subclinical metastases in stage I and II ovarian carcinoma. *Obstet Gynecol* 1978;52:100–104.

28. Keetel WC, Pixley EE, Buschbaum HJ. Experience with peritoneal cytology in the management of gynaecologic malignancies. *Am J Obstet Gynecol* 1974;120:174–182.

29. Pomel C, Provencher D, Dauplat J, et al. Laparoscopic staging of early ovarian cancer. *Gynecol Oncol* 1995;58:301–306.

30. Rossenoff SH, DeVita VT, Hubbard S, Young RC. Peritoneoscopy in the staging and follow-up of ovarian cancer. *Semin Oncol* 1975;2:223–228.

31. Maiman M, Seltzer V, Botce J. Laparoscopic excision of ovarian neoplasms subsequently found to be malignant. *Obstet Gynecol* 1991;77:563–565.

32. Gleeson NC, Nicosia SV, Mark JE, et al. Abdominal wall metastases from ovarian cancer after laparoscopy. *Am J Obstet Gynecol* 1993;169:522–533.

33. Rubin SC, Hoskins WJ, Saigo PE. Prognostic factors for recurrence following negative second-look laparotomy in ovarian cancer patients treated with platinum-based chemotherapy. *Gynecol Oncol* 1991;42:137–141.

34. Thomas GM. Radiotherapy in early ovarian cancer. *Gynecol Oncol* 1994;S73–S79.

35. Gallion HH, van Nagell JR, Donaldson ES, et al. Adjuvant oral alkylating agent in patients with stage I epithelial ovarian cancer. *Cancer* 1989;63:1070–1073.

36. Young RC, Walton LA, Ellenberg SS, et al. Adjuvant therapy in stage I and stage II epithelial ovarian cancer. *N Engl J Med* 1990;322:1021–1027.

37. Trimbos JB, Schueler JA, van der Burg M, et al. Watch and wait after careful surgical treatment and staging in well-differentiated early ovarian cancer. *Cancer* 1991;67:597–602.

38. Klassen D, Starreveld SA, Kirk ME, et al. Early stage ovarian cancer: a randomized clinical trial comparing whole abdominal radiotherapy, melphalan, and intraperitoneal chromic phosphate: a National Cancer Institute of Canada clinical trials group report. *J Clin Oncol* 1988;6:1254–1263.

39. Bolis G, Colombo N, Pecorelli S, et al. Adjuvant treatment for early epithelial ovarian cancer: results of two randomized trials comparing cisplatin to no further treatment or chromic phosphate (32P). *Ann Oncol* 1995;6:887–893.

40. ten Bokkel Huinink WW, Dubbleman R, Aarsten E, et al. Experimental and clinical results with intraperitoneal cisplatin. *Semin Oncol* 1985;12:43.

41. Rosenshein NB. Radioisotopes in the treatment of ovarian cancer. *Clin Obstet Gynecol* 1983;10:279–295.

42. Soper JT, Berchuck A, Clarke-Pearson DL. Adjuvant intraperitoneal chronic phosphate therapy for women with apparent early ovarian carcinoma who have not undergone comprehensive surgical staging. *Cancer* 1991;68:725–729.

43. Soper JT, Berchuck A, Dodge R, Clarke-Pearson DL. Adjuvant intraperitoneal chronic phosphate (32P) therapy for women with apparent early ovarian carcinoma after comprehensive surgical staging. *Obstet Gynecol* 1992;79:993–997.

44. Watson JD, Hopkins NH, Roberts JW, et al. The origins of human cancer. In: Gillen JR, ed. *Molecular biology of the gene.* Redwood City, CA: Benjamin/Cummings, 1987;1058–1096.

45. Miki Y, Swenson J, Lynch HT. A strong candidate for the breast and ovarian cancer susceptibility gene BRCA 1. *Science* 1994;226:66–71.

46. Punnonen R, Kallioniemi OP, Mattila J, et al. Prognostic assessment in stage I ovarian cancer using a discriminate analysis with clinicopathological and flow cytometric data. *Gynecol Obstet Invest* 1989;27:213–216.

47. Freidlander ML, Taylor IW, Russel P, et al. Ploidy as a prognostic factor in ovarian carcinoma. *Int J Gynecol Pathol* 1983;1:55–62.

48. Hedley DW, Freidlander ML, Taylor IN. Application of DNA flow cytometry to paraffin-embedded archival material for the study of aneuploidy and its clinical significance. *Cytometry* 1985;6:327–333.

49. Freidlander ML, Taylor IN, Russel P, et al. Cellular DNA content-A stable feature in epithelial ovarian cancer. *Br J Cancer* 1984;49:173–179.

50. Slamon DJ, Godolphin W, Jones LA, et al. Studies of the Her-2/Neu protooncogene in human breast and ovarian cancer. *Science* 1989;244:707–712.

51. Bizzi A, Codegoni AM, Landoni F, et al. Steroid receptors in epithelial ovarian carcinoma. Relation to clinical parameters and survival. *Cancer Res* 1988;48:6222–6226.

CHAPTER *32*

Management of Advanced Ovarian Cancer: Surgical Aspects

A. PETER M. HEINTZ

The treatment of ovarian cancer patients remains one of the biggest challenges in gynecologic oncology. Because the disease has a long asymptomatic phase, many patients have advanced disease at the time of presentation. Advanced disease is defined as the spread of disease outside the ovaries and the uterus, that is, stages IIb to IIc, III, and IV. The first consideration in the treatment of these patients is surgical. Surgery is important to establish the diagnosis, to stage the disease, and to appropriately reduce the tumor volume. The surgical findings also define the need for and the type of adjuvant therapy. The standard adjuvant treatment after cytoreduction is cisplatin- and cyclophosphamide-based chemotherapy. The results of recent studies suggest further improvement of survival by combining cisplatin with paclitaxel (Taxol). In spite of all these efforts, the overall survival rate for patients with advanced ovarian cancer remains poor: 25%. In this chapter the principles of surgical treatment, including its limitations, are discussed.

History and Definitions

The role of surgery in advanced ovarian cancer has been discussed since Meigs (1) suggested that the removal of as much tumor as possible followed by radiation treatment improved the survival of patients, as compared to those who were treated by surgery alone. In spite of this suggestion, extensive surgery for advanced epithelial ovarian cancer remained unpopular because of the generally poor prognosis, the 5-year survival rate being less than 10% (2). In 1968 Munnell (3) introduced the concept of "maximum surgical effort." This concept included a total abdominal hysterectomy and bilateral oophorectomy, partial omentectomy, and resection of local metastases. Meigs (4) and Pemberton (5) had already advocated omentectomy because of the frequent occurrence of omental metastases. These metastases together can far exceed the volume of the primary tumor. Removal of this "omental cake" should decrease the production of ascites and contribute to better personal relief. Munnell (3) reported that a successful maximum surgical effort should result in a 5-year survival rate of 40%. However, he did not exclude borderline and nonepithelial ovarian malignancies. Terms such as *maximum surgical effort* do not define an objective for the procedure nor do they give detailed guidelines for an effective operation. In 1975 Griffiths (6) introduced the concept of cytoreductive surgery. He defined quantitatively the goal of surgery, from a vague exhortation to remove as much as possible to a well-defined objective being a residual tumor smaller than 1.5 cm in diameter. If this objective goal was achieved, median survival time was 17 months better than that in patients with larger residual tumors, irrespective of the total tumor volume. Griffiths and Fuller (7), Wharton and Herson (8), and Hacker et al (9) provided general guidelines on how to reach this objective. In fact, the technique is a combination of the retroperitoneal approach to a pelvic mass, as described by Hudson and Chir (10), and upper abdominal tumor resections. The feasibility of achieving the objective is about 70% to 90% for experienced physicians, but in general practice the success rate is reported to be much lower: 30% to 40% (11). Subsequently, others (12) reported improved survival when no residual disease was left behind. In this subset of patients, 5-year survival rates higher than 50% were reported (12). In this chapter I consider three different types of cytoreductive surgery:

1. Primary cytoreductive surgery: The cytoreduction is performed before the start of chemotherapy.
2. Intervention cytoreductive surgery: The cytoreductive surgery is performed during first-line chemotherapy treatment but before completion of the primary course.
3. Secondary cytoreductive surgery: The cytoreduction is performed after the completion of the primary treatment.

Rationale for Cytoreductive Surgery

Cytoreductive surgery is only effective for ovarian carcinoma and Burkitt's lymphoma. This makes the procedure controversial. The arguments for cytoreductive surgery are mainly based on three different considerations (13,14):

1. The physiologic benefits of tumor mass excision
2. Perfusion and cell kinetics
3. Immunology

Physiologic Benefits

The intra-abdominal spread of ovarian carcinoma causes extensive involvement of all serosal surfaces. This can result in an omental cake and a jeopardized gastrointestinal function. Together with the catabolic effect of the tumor itself, this results in inanition and finally in death. Adequate tumor resection can restore gastrointestinal function and interrupt this catabolic process.

Tumor Perfusion and Cell Kinetics

The observation that cytoreductive surgery is not effective in all tumors might be related to the degree of chemosensitivity of these tumors. If the tumor is 100% chemosensitive, any surgical attempt to remove it is useless because the outcome of treatment will be excellent regard-

less of the amount of residual disease. If a tumor is resistant to chemotherapy, the outcome of treatment will be dismal even when the smallest amount of tumor cells is left behind. Perhaps ovarian cancer involves an intermediate chemosensitivity. In this particular disease, resection might help to optimize the effect of chemotherapy, by removing poorly perfused bulky tumor masses that are characterized by decreased oxygenation and a decreased growth fraction and that, as a result, are less sensitive to chemotherapy or radiotherapy (15). The main obstacle to this way of thinking is the development of permanent drug resistance. This resistance may be a result of prior exposure to chemotherapeutic agents, but is mainly caused by spontaneous mutation to phenotypic drug resistance. This mutation occurs as an intrinsic property of genetically unstable malignant cells (16). The development of a resistant clone is a random event, dependent on the growth curve of the tumor and the mutation rate. This event cannot be altered surgically and limits the value of surgery in metastasized disease.

Immunology

The definite role of the immune system in the defense against cancer is unknown. However, there is some evidence that the patient's immune competence is enhanced by the removal of large tumor masses (17–19).

Limitations of Cytoreductive Surgery

Limitations

The work of Griffiths (6) provided major impetus for the use of radical resection of disease. Since then, many others showed a strong correlation between postoperative residuum and survival data (Fig. 32-1) (8,9, 12,14,20–24). However, it should be stated that most patients with advanced ovarian cancer will die of their disease. Therefore, 5-year survival rates are not the standard by which the value of cytoreduction should be measured. Rather, the two most important parameters are the quantity of the patient's life (progression-free interval, median survival time) and the quality of her life (symptom-free survival). Currently it is still accepted that if all the tumor and metas-

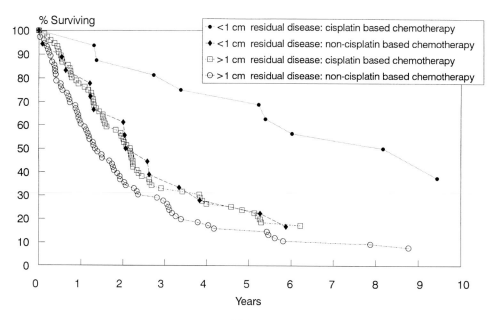

Survival in relation to tumor diameter and treatment in 106 patients with advanced ovarian cancer. (Reproduced by permission from Lawton FG, Neijt JP, Swenerton KD, eds. *Epithelial cancer of the ovary*. London: BMJ Publishing Group, 1995.)

tases cannot be removed, the maximum diameter of the largest tumor mass remaining should optimally not exceed 1.0 to 1.5 cm because of its influence on survival. Other factors, such as type of chemotherapy, intrinsic chemosensitivity, and the presence of other biologic variables, however, may be as or more important to outcome as the extent of surgery (25) (see Fig. 32-1). For example, colleagues and I (20) found that the factors that influence the ability to perform optimal cytoreductive surgery are the same as those influencing disease-free and overall survival. Optimal cytoreduction was easier to achieve in young patients with low-grade tumors, small metastases, and no ascites or peritoneal carcinomatosis (Table 32-1). Patients with tumor nodules smaller than 20 mm after the operation had the best disease-free interval and overall survival rate. Analysis of the influence of pretreatment factors on survival showed only the diameter of the largest metastases, the presence of ascites, and the existence of peritoneal carcinomatosis to have a significant effect (20) (Table 32-1). Eisner et al (22) recently confirmed the negative effect of the number of residual masses on survival, even when all the masses had a small diameter. Their finding also underlines the importance of the

initial tumor load for survival (22), and is also in agreement with Goldie and Goldman's model of developing drug resistance (16). Studying the joint influence of these factors using the Cox regression model, only the presence of ascites and performance proved to be independent factors (Table 32-2), which reflects the strong interrelationship between most prognostic factors. This also means that these factors have to be looked at as a whole, representing the disease status of the patient and reflecting prognosis.

Feasibility and Morbidity

The main reasons for nonoptimal tumor resection are the presence of an unresectable abdominal mass and the poor general condition of the patient. Disease is usually considered unresectable when it involves the base of the small-bowel mesentery, the liver parenchyma, particularly multiple such lesions, the hepato-duodenal ligament, the lesser sac, or retroperitoneal lymph nodes above the renal vessels, or when there are multiple large metastases on the peritoneal surfaces. In experienced hands the feasibility of the procedure is reported to be 70% to 90% (11).

T A B L E   **32-1**

Pretreatment Factors Influencing Resectability at the First Operation
and Survival

	Resectability to Optimal Status, p^*	Disease-Free Survival, p^*	Overall Survival, p^*
Age	0.05	NS	NS
Performance	NS	NS	0.03
Stage	0.03	NS	0.05
Histologic type	NS	NS	NS
Grade	0.03	0.03	0.05
Diameter of primary tumor	NS	NS	NS
Diameter of largest metastasis before cytoreduction	0.0001	0.2	0.03
Ascites	0.008	0.008	0.005
Peritoneal carcinomatosis	0.001	0.003	0.005

$^*p$ based on χ^2 test.

NS = not significant.

Source: Heintz APM, van Oostrom AT, Trimbos JBMC, et al. The treatment of advanced ovarian carcinoma (I): clinical variables associated with prognosis. *Gynecol Oncol* 1988;30:348–358.

T A B L E   **32-2**

Cox Regression Model Studying the Joint Influence on Overall Survival and Disease-Free Interval

	Overall Survival	Disease-Free Interval
Performance	0.003	0.05
Stage	NS	NS
Grade	NS	NS
Diameter of largest metastasis ≤15 mm	NS	NS
Ascites	0.005	0.03
Peritoneal carcinomatosis	NS	NS
Diameter of residual disease <15 mm	NS	NS
$+\chi^2$	27.2	25.3

$^*\chi^2$ = values for the model; NS = not significant.

Source: Heintz APM, van Oostrom AT, Trimbos JBMC, et al. The treatment of advanced ovarian carcinoma (I): clinical variables associated with prognosis. *Gynecol Oncol* 1988;30:348–358.

The mean hospital stay after cytoreductive surgery is 10 to 14 days. The mean operating time is $2^1/_2$ hours and the mean blood loss 1200 mL. In general, postoperative complications do not differ from those encountered after major abdominal surgery (26).

Who Should Undergo Cytoreductive Surgery When and Where?

Primary Cytoreductive Surgery

The size of the residual mass in itself does not indicate anything about the operation, because by the nature of the disease one third of patients have tumor diameters smaller than 1 cm at the time of the first operation. In the group with initially small tumors the operation is usually not more than a total abdominal hysterectomy with bilateral salpingo-oophorectomy, an infracolic omentectomy, and resection of isolated metastases. This operation requires no special technical skills and can be performed by every gynecologist. As stated before, the feasibility of optimal cytoreduction is reported to be at least 70% in experienced hands. This means that in about 40% of patients with large metastatic disease, the tumor can be optimally reduced. Recently, Guidozzi and Ball (27) reported their experience with extensive primary surgery in patients with significantly advanced peritoneal metastatic disease (>10 cm in diameter). In their selected group of 30 patients, the authors achieved the optimal status in 76%, which is nearly twice as high as the usually reported rate, except by experienced gynecologic oncologists. However, the rate of serious morbidity was very high, 43%, and 2 patients died within 48 hours. The conclusion is that ultraradicality has its limits and its price. Many reports confirmed the observation that optimal cytoreductive surgery influences the survival following platinum-based combination chemotherapy (8,9,12–14, 20,21,24–31). Only a few studies of ovarian cancer reported survival data based on the amount of residual disease according to the International Federation of Gynecology and Obstetrics (FIGO) stages of disease (24). Recently Allen et al (24) performed a review analysis of residual disease and survival for stage III and IV carcinoma of the ovary. They showed clearly for stage III as well as stage IV that survival at 2 and 5 years was better for patients with no residual disease than for patients with macroscopic residual disease of more than 2 cm or less (odds ratios, 3.37 and 4.35), and that this latter group survived better than did patients with residual disease of more than 2 cm (odds ratios, 3.43 and 4.55). Within our group of patients with residual disease of less than 15 mm, the patients with extensive initial disease had a tendency toward shorter survival times compared with those who had limited disease from the beginning: 35 months compared with longer than 5 years (20). However, the median survival time for patients

in whom the cytoreduction was not successful was only 23 months. Thus, the best result that might be expected from more radical surgery in patients with extensive initial disease is lengthening of the median survival time from 23 to 35 months. In the study of Hoskins et al (28) on cytoreduction, the probable survival benefit in the nonoptimal group would be 9 months. Therefore, retrospectively, the effect of cytoreductive surgery seems to be an additional 9 to 12 months of life. Another question that has to be answered is what amount of residual disease, as measured by diameter, should be classified as optimal. In the literature a variety of diameters from 0 to 20 mm are reported to be significant cutoff points for survival. However, all these results are influenced by patient selection, sample size, and the chemotherapy administered. From a theoretical point of view, it seems unlikely that a difference of a few millimeters in diameter of the largest residual nodule will alter the prognosis dramatically. As already shown several times and recently again by Potter et al (29), improved survival is gradual, is related to the volume of residual disease, and does not increase by leaps and bounds, and there is no magic volume of residual disease that portends a better prognosis (Fig. 32-2). These authors also showed that extensive debulking procedures such as peritoneal stripping techniques or bowel resections demonstrate no improvement in survival. Despite extensive debulking efforts, patients who had bowel resection(s) to achieve "no residual disease" did not fare better than

F I G U R E **32-2**

Relation between the diameter of residual disease in millimeters and survival in years according to Potter et al (29).

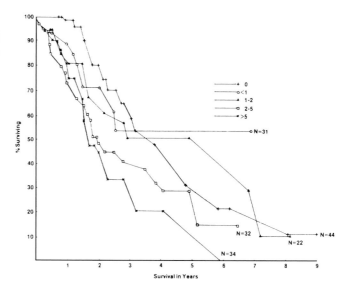

patients who still had residual disease at the completion of surgery. This observation is in agreement with our observation that both the initial tumor burden and the tumor residue influence prognosis (20). This again indicates the limited value of cytoreductive surgery in patients with extensive peritoneal spread and large extrapelvic metastases.

Recently Eisenkop et al (30) showed in a small group of patients that removal of all small metastases can improve survival. They succeeded in removing all peritoneal implants from 21 patients. Their survival rates were compared with the survival rates of 30 patients who had macroscopic residual disease of less than 1 cm left behind on the peritoneal surfaces, and with the survival rates of 7 patients who did not have any peritoneal implants after removal of the primary tumor. The group with peritoneal implants left behind had worse survival rates than did the other two groups: a 4-year survival rate of 18%, versus 53% and 60% for the group that underwent excision and the group without peritoneal metastases, respectively. Although the results of this study were strongly influenced by patient selection, they also show the strong influence of total tumor volume on survival, irrespective of individual tumor size. In this respect, the study results are in agreement with those of the other studies mentioned.

Intervention Cytoreductive Surgery

Several authors advocated a second attempt of cytoreductive surgery in patients who respond to chemotherapy. Others who used cisplatin-based chemotherapy as first-line treatment could not confirm the benefit of these second surgical attempts.

In 1987 the European Organization for Research and Treatment of Cancer Gynaecological Cancer Cooperative Group started a randomized study in patients with tumor residues of more than 1 cm after primary debulking surgery (31). Patients with a response or stable disease after three courses of cyclophosphamide with cisplatin were randomized to undergo intervention tumor debulking or no tumor debulking. Three hundred and nineteen patients were randomized and 278 patients were evaluable: 140 in the surgical group and 138 in the nonsurgical group. Surgical data were available on 127 patients. All patients received at least six cycles of combination chemother-

apy. In the surgical group, 83 patients (65%) had lesions of more than 1 cm in diameter. The surgeons succeeded in reducing the size of the tumors in 37 patients (45%) to diameters less than 1 cm. The survival time in this intervention surgery group was significantly longer than that in the nonsurgical group ($p = 0.01$). The difference in median survival time was 6 months. The 2-year survival rate in the surgical group was 56% and in the nonsurgical group was 46%. A multivariate analysis revealed successful cytoreduction to be an independent prognostic factor ($p = 0.012$). Statistical analysis showed that a successful operation helped to decrease the risk of dying by 33% ($p = 0.008$). There was no postoperative mortality and no serious morbidity. This study (31) was the first randomized trial to demonstrate the value of cytoreductive surgery.

In this study (31) a second operation was not necessary for 44 of the patients (35%) because the largest tumor residual after chemotherapy was smaller than 1 cm in diameter. The operation was successful for 37 patients (45%) of the 83 patients (65%) with residual masses larger than 1 cm, that is, 29% of the entire group. This also means that for 71% of the patients the second operation was useless. This rate is acceptable in a prospective study, but underlines the necessity to perform an adequate operation during the first laparotomy if possible. These findings also indicate that the team that performs the surgery must feel confident with the principles of the procedure. In experienced hands, the success rate of cytoreductive surgery must be at least 70%, which is higher than the 45% found in this and many other multicenter studies. The conclusion is that these patients should be referred to gynecologic oncologists, or an experienced gynecologic oncologist should be invited to assist the less experienced colleague with the procedure.

The Timing of Cytoreductive Surgery

As stated before, the group with unresectable large disease, mostly in the upper abdomen, will not benefit at all from cytoreductive surgery. The first laparotomy will only help to make a diagnosis and to stage the disease properly. An attempt to perform extensive cytoreductive surgery will only delay the start of chemotherapy. For this reason, patients with an unresectable large tumor should undergo intervention cytoreductive surgery after they have had at least three courses of chemotherapy and demonstrated a partial response. Hence, real primary cytoreductive surgery will only make sense in 30% to 40% of all patients with advanced disease. It is important that an experienced gynecologist who is familiar with all aspects of abdominal and retroperitoneal surgery operate on these patients. In most instances, this experienced gynecologist is a gynecologic oncologist. Based on the data reported in the literature, most of these patients do not get optimal primary surgical treatment, as indicated by the percentage (almost always <50%) of patients in multicenter trials with postoperative residual disease smaller than 1.5 cm in diameter.

It is important that all patients with ovarian cancer be operated on and nursed by well-trained personnel familiar with the disease. Because gastrointestinal and urologic procedures might be necessary, the gynecologist and his or her team should know how to deal with them. In many patients the diagnosis of ovarian cancer is not definite preoperatively. Therefore, for these patients it is advisable to invite a gynecologic oncologist to assist with the procedure. This is especially the case for patients with a mobile pelvic mass, no ascites, no signs of upper abdominal disease, or raised CA-125 levels. In patients with ascites or an upper abdominal mass and a raised CA-125 level, the physician must decide whether to perform primary or intervention cytoreductive surgery. If the histologic diagnosis is already made based on cytology or biopsy results, the indication to delay the operation is the presence of stage IV disease. Indications to restrict the operation to a diagnostic laparotomy include the presence of large metastases in the liver hilus, retroperitoneal metastases above the level of the renal vein, or large metastases in the mesentery of the small bowel. For many patients this decision can only be made during laparotomy. When during laparotomy it is clear that successful cytoreductive surgery is not possible, the gynecologist should only sample the tumor and restrict himself or herself to those procedures that provide personal relief for the patient. Chemotherapy should be started as soon as possible after the operation and intervention cytoreductive surgery is indicated after three courses of chemotherapy have been given and a response has been demonstrated.

The Operation

Perioperative Management

Cytoreductive surgery is a major abdominal operation. For this reason, a general physical check-up must be performed. Laboratory tests should include full blood cell count; measurement of serum creatinine levels, electrolyte concentrations, and CA-125 levels; liver function tests; and blood typing. Especially in women with advanced ovarian cancer, it is necessary to correct hemoglobin and electrolyte levels. If the patient has lost more than 10% of her body weight, preoperative parenteral nutrition for 10 days is necessary to correct the catabolic state of her metabolism. A chest x-ray study is necessary to evaluate the pulmonary status (effusions, metastases?) and ultrasonography is necessary for evaluation of the kidneys (hydronephrosis?) and the liver (metastases?). Computed tomography (CT) and magnetic resonance imaging (MRI) do not add essential information and do not influence the indication for the surgical procedure. CT or MRI should only be performed in patients in whom a laparotomy is not performed. Mammography should be done if any suspicious lump is found in the breast. A barium enema is indicated only in patients with changed bowel habits. Bowel preparation is necessary because of the possibility of performing a bowel resection. Prophylactic antibiotics are indicated and should be given at the start of anesthesia. Subcutaneous heparin is started the evening before the operation to prevent deep venous thrombosis.

If food intake is not expected to be possible within 5 days after the operation, total parenteral nutrition is started the first postoperative day.

Surgical Technique

The operation is performed with the patient in the low lithotomy position to facilitate bowel reanastomosis, if necessary. A midline abdominal incision is made, extending from the symphysis pubis up to at least 10 cm above the umbilicus; it can be extended to the processus xiphoideus if extensive upper abdominal resection is required. After the peritoneum is opened, ascites is suctioned away after a sample is obtained for cytology. Care must be taken not to remove the ascitic fluid too rapidly because of the hemodynamic consequence—a rapid drop in blood pressure and shock. If there is no ascites, or after the ascites has been removed, careful inspection and palpation of all intra-abdominal organs is carried out. The localization and diameter of the primary tumor and its extension into surrounding organs are described as are the metastatic pattern throughout the whole abdominal cavity and the diameter of the largest metastases outside the ovaries. The presence of an omental cake is noted. The bowel and its mesentery are inspected for tumor ingrowth. Special attention has to be paid to the existence of possible metastases in the right and left hemodiaphragms and the existence of peritoneal carcinomatosis. The diameter of the largest peritoneal carcinomatosis nodule is noted. After this, the pelvic and periaortic lymph nodes are palpated if possible. Sometimes these regions cannot be inspected before the large tumor masses are removed. After this general inspection, the decision as to whether cytoreductive surgery is possible has to be made. Optimal cytoreduction is considered to be impossible if there are areas where tumor masses of more than 15 mm cannot be removed. This is usually the case if masses of this size are located near the base of the small-bowel mesentery, close to the origin of the superior mesenteric artery, in para-aortic nodes above the renal artery, in the porta hepatis, in the liver parenchyma, or in the lungs (11).

Omentectomy

Often in advanced epithelial ovarian cancer the omentum is totally replaced by carcinoma and adheres to the parietal peritoneum of the anterior abdominal wall, making entry into the peritoneal cavity difficult. A dissection plane between the peritoneum and omental cake can be developed and extended caudally and laterally to the paracolic gutters. Often the omental cake is adherent to or confluent with the pelvic tumor mass. Small-bowel involvement with the undersurface of the omentum can vary but is usually restricted to adherent planes that are easy to separate. After the edges of the omentum are mobilized, the pelvic attachments can be separated. The next step is to separate the infracolic omentum from the transverse colon. Since the attachment between the transverse colon to the omentum is avascular, this

separation is done by lifting the omentum and pulling it gently in the cranial direction. A dissection plane is then easily discovered and the separation can be performed by sharp dissection along the serosa of the transverse colon. Small vessels close to the dissection plane can be ligated with hemoclips or coagulated with electrocautery. The omentum can be separated from the stomach by ligating the right and left gastroepiploic arteries and individually ligating their gastric branches (Figs. 32-3 and 32-4). This phase of the procedure can be facilitated by traction downward and medially on the omental cake. During the mobilization of the omental cake one has to take into account that the blood supply to the omentum is still intact and is often more intensive than usual. Dissection with the use of electrocautery can be of help in preventing extensive blood loss. In patients with only limited metastases to the omentum, an infracolic omentectomy is usually sufficient to obtain the optimal status. This can be achieved by transecting the infracolic omentum along the transverse colon.

Since epithelial ovarian tumors tend to spread via the gastrocolic ligament to the hilus of the spleen, special attention has to be paid

FIGURE 32-3

The anatomic relation between the omentum, transverse colon, and stomach.

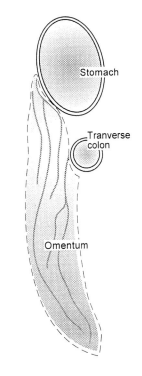

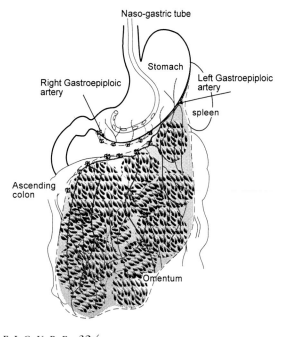

F I G U R E 32-4

Total omentectomy.

to this region. Splenectomy seldom needs to be performed because epithelial ovarian cancer usually grows around and not into the spleen. Splenectomy is only indicated if it results in optimal cytoreduction.

Total Abdominal Hysterectomy and Bilateral Salpingo-oophorectomy

The next step is to remove the primary tumor together with the other adnexa and the uterus. If the primary tumor is limited to the ovaries and the uterus, without extension to other organs and metastasis to the pelvic peritoneum, total abdominal hysterectomy and bilateral salpingo-oophorectomy can be performed in the routine way. However, advanced ovarian cancer often results in a tumor mass involving both adnexa and the uterus. Often the bladder or rectum and cecum are also involved in the pelvic mass and metastasis to the pelvic peritoneum causes an intensive nodularity in the cul-de-sac. In these patients total abdominal hysterectomy and bilateral salpingo-oophorectomy together with resection of the local pelvic tumor mass can be achieved by the retroperitoneal approach as first described by Hudson and Chir (10). The rationale for this approach is that even large bulky epithelial ovarian car-

cinomas usually do not infiltrate deeply in the peritoneum of the pelvic wall or into the walls of the rectum and bladder. This means that the iliac vessels, ureter, and pelvic muscles are rarely directly invaded by tumor. Retroperitoneal mobilization of the pelvic peritoneum allows use of this as a pseudocapsule that surrounds the pelvic mass. The mobilization of this pelvic mass can be accomplished further by mobilization of the rectum via exploration of the avascular space behind the rectum and in front of the fascia of Waldeyer and by retrograde resection of the uterus. The pelvic tumor can then be dissected from the rectum under direct vision. The end result will be a cul-de-sac and rectum denuded of peritoneum. The peritoneum of the pelvis is incised as shown in Figures 32-5 and 32-6. The exact plane of the incision depends on the extent of tumor involvement of the pelvic peritoneum. After the incision is made, the mesentery of the sigmoid is mobilized and the left ovarian vessels and ureter are identified. Both ureters are freed from the posterior peritoneum as far as possible. The ovarian vessels are double ligated above the pelvic brim. To prevent unnecessary blood loss, the uterine artery is now identified, isolated, and ligated. In the same way, the ovarian vessels and uterine artery are ligated on the right side. Sometimes the volume and immobility of the pelvic mass makes ligation of the uterine arteries in this phase of the operation impossible. In that case the ligation has to be performed as soon as possible. Next, both round ligaments are divided. The anterior leaf of the ligamentum latum on both sides is incised toward the bladder. If there are tumor metastases on the bladder dome, the incision has to continue proximally from them, and the bladder dome has to be denuded of peritoneum. Then the bladder can be sharply dissected from the cervix. On the left side, the retrorectal space is entered. This has to be done with special care to prevent damaging the fascia of Waldeyer, which can result in serious bleeding from presacral veins. Next, the presacral space on the right side is explored and connected to the retrorectal space, resulting in one big retroperitoneal space. In this phase of the operation the mobility of the tumor mass has strongly increased (Fig. 32-7). Both ureters are freed from the posterior leaf of the broad ligament. The vagina is opened and cut round without opening the cul-de-sac. A tenaculum is placed on the posterior part of the cervix, allowing it

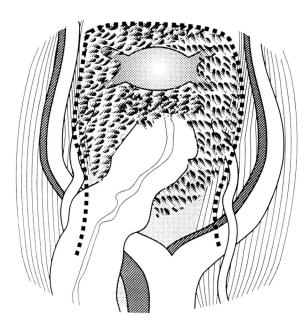

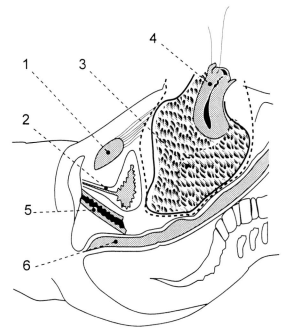

F I G U R E   **32-5**

Incision of the pelvic peritoneum.

F I G U R E   **32-7**

The retroperitoneal approach to a fixed pelvic tumor mass: the retrograde hysterectomy: sagittal view. 1 = symphysis; 2 = bladder; 3 = tumor; 4 = uterus; 5 = vagina; 6 = rectum.

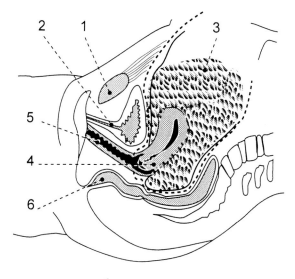

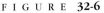

F I G U R E   **32-6**

The retroperitoneal approach to a fixed pelvic tumor mass: sagittal view. 1 = symphysis; 2 = bladder; 3 = tumor; 4 = uterus; 5 = vagina; 6 = rectum.

rectal wall is involved, a segment of the wall must be excised or a part of the rectum must be removed together with the uterus. If not all of the tumor can be removed from the pelvis, a subtotal hysterectomy can be performed.

Large-Bowel Resection

If the tumor infiltrates into the muscularis of the rectum, a resection with reanastomosis has to be performed. In this situation it is desirable to transect the sigmoid colon early in the dissection with the gastrointestinal anastomosis (GIA) stapler, and then to ligate and divide the vessels in the sigmoid mesentery, in order to gain access to the presacral space. As much distal rectum as possible should be spared to facilitate primary reanastomosis with the end-to-end anastomosis (EEA) stapler. A protecting colostomy is required only if the patient has received previous pelvic radiation.

Small-Bowel Resection

The tumor usually implants on the serosa but does not invade the muscularis. This fa-

to be pulled upward. The peritoneum over the posterior fornix is dissected as far as the attachment of the rectum. On both sides the ureter is dissected from the specimen. Both parametria are clamped and divided. Next, the serosa of the rectum is incised just above the tumor and the tumor is removed from the rectal wall by resecting the serosa. If the muscularis of the cilitates local excision of nodules larger than 15 mm in diameter. If there are multiple nodules in a limited area of bowel, resection is indicated if it will ensure an optimal dissection. The GIA stapler facilitates this procedure and saves time.

Urinary Tract Resection

Occasionally the tumor will invade the bladder or distal end of the ureter. If the bladder is invaded, partial cystectomy with primary repair can be performed. If the distal part of the ureter is involved in the mass, primary resection of the ureter in continuity with the mass and primary reconstruction have to be considered. Depending on the extent of ureter dissection, an end-to-end reanastomosis, a ureteroneocystostomy, or a transureteroureterostomy might be required. These resections are only indicated when the optimal status can be achieved.

Resection of Other Metastases

If possible, all metastases larger than 15 mm in diameter are removed from the parietal peritoneum. If larger metastases are located on the liver serosa or diaphragm, removal is not advised because it is technically difficult and associated with high morbidity (blood loss). Large pelvic and para-aortic nodes are only removed if removal contributes to the optimal status.

The Role of Lymphadenectomy

One of the main reasons for the bad prognosis of ovarian cancer is its early retroperitoneal spread (32,33). Therefore, several oncologists addressed the importance of systematic resection of pelvic and para-aortic nodes (34–39). The reasoning for this approach is the reported beneficial effect on survival: This is explained by the hypothesis that retroperitoneal nodes are a pharmacologic sanctuary that makes cisplatin less effective in the retroperitoneal area (34,37,39), or by the "hypothetical development of a network of subperitoneal lymphangiosis" that is also less accessible for chemotherapy (38).

Severe criticisms of these viewpoints include the following:

1. None of the studies was prospective.
2. None of them was randomized.

3. The experience with cisplatin-based chemotherapy in patients with germ cell tumors on the ovary and testis, with lymph node metastases, is excellent. Therefore, less chemosensitivity of tumor metastases in lymph nodes reflects the development of drug resistance that is related to the age of the tumor and is also present in other metastases which are a result of the same number of cell doublings.

Di Re et al (39) recently showed in his analysis of 488 ovarian cancer patients that the lymph node status, together with FIGO stage and residual disease, had a significant influence on survival. However, in the multivariate analysis, FIGO stage was the strongest covariate. Unfortunately these investigators did not add lymphadenectomy to the multivariate analysis. According to their univariate analysis the performance of a lymphadenectomy in this highly selected group of patients resulted in a survival benefit in the short term. However, stage II, IIIa, and borderline tumors were included in their analysis and accounted for 19.9% of the tumors. Only 50.8% of the patients underwent a total lymphadenectomy. In fact the patients with the worst prognostic factors had the highest incidence of positive nodes, which suggests that looking at the lymph node status is just another way of looking to the biology of the tumor, which cannot be changed by surgery.

For this reason we do not advise performing a total lymphadenectomy routinely in patients with advanced ovarian cancer, but rather performing resection of just the enlarged nodes. A complete lymphadenectomy is only justified as a part of a research protocol after informed consent has been obtained.

Closure of the Wound

Patients with advanced ovarian carcinoma are at high risk for dehiscence of the wound. We advise mass closure using the Smead-Jones closure technique or the continuous Polydioxanone suture (PDS) or a similar monofilament suture to prevent this complication.

Postoperative Care

Since many patients with advanced ovarian carcinoma are very ill, postoperative intensive care nursing is mandatory. All patients need careful monitoring of their fluid balance by a central venous pressure catheter and an indwelling bladder catheter for at least 72 hours. Urine output per catheter should be at least 30 mL/hr. Prophylactic minidose heparin is continued for at least 1 week. Oral fluids are withheld until bowel movements are clearly heard or gas is passed. Early ambulation is encouraged.

A nasogastric tube is desirable to prevent patients from vomiting and aspirating. Such a tube is mandatory in patients who underwent bowel surgery, because they are not able to cope with the production of their own gastric juices. If prolonged gastric suction is expected, a gastrostomy can be desirable to increase postoperative comfort. When oral fluid intake can be started, the nasogastric or gastrostomy tube is changed, to see if it is tolerated. The tube can be removed if the result is satisfactory.

If a small-bowel resection was performed, the patient should have nil by mouth for at least 4 days. Oral fluid intake may commence after passage of flatus. If the fluid is tolerated well, a low-residue diet can be started 1 day later. If a large-bowel resection was performed, the patient should have no oral intake for 7 days.

Perioperative antibiotics are required during 24 hours, starting at the beginning of anesthesia. The drugs chosen have to cover aerobic as well as anaerobic microorganisms. If a large-bowel resection has to be performed in the absence of preoperative bowel preparation, broad-spectrum antibiotics should be given for at least 1 week.

Surgical Assessment of Response

All patients with low-stage ovarian cancer (stages I–IIa, IIc) and most patients with advanced-stage disease (IIb, III, IV) who have had optimal cytoreductive surgery and subsequent cytotoxic treatment will have no evidence of disease after treatment has been stopped. Unfortunately, there is no reliable laboratory test or radiologic technique to diagnose subclinical disease. For this reason second-look operations (laparoscopy and laparotomy) have been advocated for formal reassessment.

Wangensteen et al (40) first introduced the term *second-look operation* in 1951 and applied it to the re-exploration of the abdomen of patients with colonic cancer while they remained clinically free of disease after primary treatment. The idea was that if recurrences were

discovered, they might be treated in the preclinical stage. Rutledge and Burns (41) introduced the concept into the planned treatment of ovarian carcinoma and used the operation to evaluate the need for continuation of chemotherapy in patients with asymptomatic disease.

The term *second-look operation* should be used only for the first surgical evaluation in patients who are clinically free of disease after adequate first-line treatment. The benefit of this approach has always been earlier discontinuation of chemotherapy in patients with pathologically confirmed complete remission, or a change to a more effective treatment in patients in the asymptomatic phase.

Because it is known that the number of patients with a complete response will not increase after six courses of platinum-based combination chemotherapy and because there is no effective second-line treatment available, second-look operations have ceased to be of importance for patients who have completed their first-line treatment. For this reason, these reassessment operations should be done only in the interest of research when second-line treatments are being studied and after informed consent is obtained from the patient. Three types of procedures are advocated as reassessment operations: laparoscopy, laparotomy, and a combination of the two.

Second-Look Laparoscopy

The laparoscope has been advocated for the inspection of the peritoneal cavity after treatment. Because second-look laparoscopy is always done for patients with a history of surgery or radiotherapy, or both, it is not surprising that the procedure is often inadequate or unsuccessful. When adequate visualization is defined as the ability of the surgeon to visualize the entire peritoneal cavity from the cul-de-sac to the diaphragm including the paracolic gutters, adequate laparoscopy is reported to be successful in 50% to 72% of the procedures (42,43).

The incidence of persistent disease ranges from 20% to 50% based on peritoneal washings taken during laparoscopy (42–46), but a second-look laparoscopy that fails to show disease does not correlate with complete pathologic response, as the incidence of persistent disease at laparotomy after a laparoscopy failed to show disease is reported to be 30% to 50%

T A B L E   **32-3**

Incidence of Persistent Disease at Second-Look Laparotomy after Laparoscopy Failed to Show Evidence of Disease in Patients with Ovarian Carcinoma

First Author	Reference No.	Total No. of Patients	No. (%) with Tumor at Second-Look Laparotomy
Mangioni	43	11	6 (54)
Heintz	46	15	8 (53)
Rosenoff	47	4	2 (50)
Smith	48	11	5 (45)

(Table 32-3) (43,46–48). These reports clearly indicate that second-look laparoscopy is of limited value in assessing extent of disease in the follow-up of a patient with ovarian carcinoma.

In addition, laparoscopy after one or more previous laparotomies carries a certain morbidity. The reported incidence of serious complications ranges between 1% and 10%, with bowel injury being most common (43,48,49). Puncture of the pneumoperitoneum with a thin needle on a syringe filled half with sterile water is an easy test to locate bowel loops adherent to the abdominal wall at the puncture site. Aspiration of air indicates that there is no bowel loop fixed to the wall at this site. Aspiration of green or brown fluid is suspicious for bowel fluid and one should not puncture the abdominal wall at this site. I advise doing two tests per puncture site, 1 cm from each other. In selected patients, open laparoscopy is indicated.

Second-Look Laparotomy

The diagnostic value of a second-look laparotomy is illustrated by the reported incidence of persistent disease (50%–75%) in patients diagnosed with advanced disease who are clinically free of disease (46,50–62). However, the value of a pathologically confirmed complete response is also questionable, as 13% to 50% of patients with such a response have been reported to develop recurrences sooner or later (46,50–53,55–61,63–74). The technique of the second-look laparotomy is similar to the technique and guidelines used for a staging laparotomy.

Second-Look Laparoscopy Before Second-Look Laparotomy

It is frustrating to find disease during a second-look laparotomy in a patient without clinical evidence of residuum because this means an unnecessary laparotomy, since the laparotomy itself does not contribute to the survival of the patient but is purely a diagnostic procedure. Because of the inaccuracy of the laparoscope alone, a few authors mentioned the possibility of combining laparoscopy and laparotomy for second-look procedures, which allows only those patients in whom no tumor is detected by laparoscopy to be selected for laparotomy (42,43,46). In our experience this combination prevents half of the second-look laparotomies (46).

In conclusion, second-look procedures are very accurate in evaluating the degree of cancer in patients who are clinically free of disease after an adequate number of courses of chemotherapy (75). In this respect, the combination of laparoscopy and laparotomy can prevent unnecessary laparotomies, but the benefits of second-look procedures for individual patients have undoubtedly contributed to our understanding of the biologic behavior of the disease, and continue to contribute to our understanding of the value of new treatment strategies. This conclusion also clearly underlines the limited value of the procedure for individual patients who are not treated in a research setting.

Secondary Cytoreductive Surgery

The term *secondary cytoreductive surgery* is used for operations on patients with persistent disease after they completed first-line treatment or on patients who develop recurrent disease after a disease-free interval.

Benefits from this operation have especially been noted in patients who did not receive cisplatin-based chemotherapy as first-line treatment (76). Without any doubt the tumor status of the patient after completed first-line treatment and secondary cytoreductive surgery is related to survival time (77,78). However, it has never been proved that secondary cytoreduction itself has influenced that outcome.

Several groups (77–80) studied second cytoreductive surgery in patients who were clinically free of disease for some time. Survival was better especially in patients who had a disease-free interval of more than 12 months and a successful second cytoreductive procedure.

Conclusions

From a theoretical point of view, cytoreductive surgery can be of value in the treatment of a malignant solid tumor like ovarian carcinoma. However, the availability of effective chemotherapy with high fractional cell kill is of major importance in this concept. A result of the same theoretical concept is that cytoreductive surgery might become less important if more effective drugs or combinations of drugs are developed. An important limitation of the value of cytoreductive surgery in this concept is the development of clones of cells resistant to available chemotherapy.

The surgical technique that has to be employed concerns the entire abdominal cavity and requires knowledge of gynecologic as well as gastrointestinal and urologic surgery. Intensive care is mandatory after this type of surgery. All patients with advanced ovarian cancer should have a laparotomy to establish the diagnosis. If cytoreduction is not possible, the abdomen is closed and a second attempt is made after three courses of chemotherapy. If possible, cytoreduction is completed at the time of the first operation. The objective of the procedure should be to remove all visible tumor.

If the gynecologist is not familiar with the principles and techniques of ovarian cancer surgery, the patient should be referred to a gynecologic oncologist for further treatment. To date there are no data that justify replacing all primary cytoreductive surgery with intervention cytoreductive surgery.

Surgical assessment of response (second-look) is only justified in a research setting after informed consent is obtained.

Secondary cytoreduction seems to be of benefit, especially to those women who had a clinically complete response for more than 12 months and for those who were not treated with cisplatin-based combination chemotherapy.

REFERENCES

1. Meigs JV. *Tumors of the female pelvic organs.* New York: Macmillan, 1934.
2. Henderson DN, Bean JL. Results of treatment of primary ovarian malignancy. *Am J Obstet Gynecol* 1957;74:1187.
3. Munnell EW. The changing prognosis and treatment in cancer of the ovary. *Am J Obstet Gynecol* 1968;100:790.
4. Meigs JV. Cancer of the ovary. *Surg Gynecol Obstet* 1940;71:44.
5. Pemberton FA. Carcinoma of the ovary. *Am J Obstet Gynecol* 1940;40:751.
6. Griffiths CTH. Surgical resection of tumor bulk in the primary treatment of ovarian carcinoma. Symposium on ovarian cancer. *Natl Cancer Inst Monogr* 1975;42:101.
7. Griffiths CTH, Fuller AF. Intensive surgical and chemotherapeutic management of advanced ovarian cancer. *Surg Clin North Am* 1978;58:131.
8. Wharton JT, Herson J. Surgery for common epithelial tumors of the ovary. *Cancer* 1981;48:582.
9. Hacker NF, Berek JS, Alberts D, Surwit EA, eds. *Cytoreductive surgery in ovarian cancer. Gynecologic oncology II: ovarian cancer.* The Hague: Martinus Nijhoff, 1984.
10. Hudson CN, Chir M. Surgical treatment of ovarian cancer. *Gynecol Oncol* 1973;1:370.
11. Heintz APM, Hacker NF, Berek JS, et al. Cytoreductive surgery in ovarian carcinoma: feasibility and morbidity. *Obstet Gynecol* 1986;67:783–788.
12. Hacker NF, Wain GV, Trimbos JB. Management and outcome of stage III epithelial ovarian cancer. In: Sharp F, Mason WP, Creasman W, eds. *Ovarian cancer.* New York: Chapman & Hall Medical, 1992:351–356.
13. Heintz APM. Surgery in ovarian cancer: the concept of cytoreductive surgery. *Curr Opin Obstet Gynecol* 1996;8:8–11.
14. Heintz APM. Advanced ovarian carcinoma: surgical treatment and prognosis. Academic thesis, Leiden University, Netherlands, 1985.
15. Bruchovsky N, Goldie JH. Drug and hormone resistance in neoplasia. Boca Raton, FL: CRC, 1982:22–53.
16. Goldie JH, Goldman AJ. A mathematical model for relating the drug sensitivity of tumors to their spontaneous mutation rate. *Cancer Treat Rep* 1979;63:1727–1732.

17. Morton DC. Changing concepts in cancer surgery; surgery as immunotherapy. *Am J Surg* 1978;135:367–372.

18. Khoo SK, Tillack SV, Mackay EV. Cell-mediated immunity: effects of female genital tract cancer, pregnancy and immunosuppressive drugs. *Aust N Z Obstet Gynaecol* 1975;15:156–161.

19. Patillo RA, Rackert ACF, Story MT, et al. Immunodiagnosis in ovarian cancer: blocking factor activity. *Am J Obstet Gynecol* 1979;133:791–797.

20. Heintz APM, van Oostrom AT, Trimbos JBMC, et al. The treatment of advanced ovarian carcinoma (I): clinical variables associated with prognosis. *Gynecol Oncol* 1988;30:348–358.

21. Neijt JP, ten Bokkel Huinink WW, van den Burg MEL, et al. Randomized trial comparing two combination chemotherapy regimens (CHAP-5 vs CP) in advanced ovarian carcinoma. *Clin Oncol* 1987;5:1157–1162.

22. Farias-Eisner R, Oliveira M, Teng F, et al. The influence of tumor distribution, number and size after optimal primary cytoreductive surgery for epithelial ovarian cancer. *Gynecol Oncol* 1992; 46:267.

23. Hunter RW, Alexander NDE, Soutter WP. Management of surgery in advanced ovarian carcinoma: is maximum cytoreductive surgery an independent determinant of prognosis? *Am J Obstet Gynecol* 1992;166:504–511.

24. Allen DG, Heintz APM, Touw FWMM. A meta-analysis of residual disease and survival in stage III and IV carcinoma of the ovary. *Eur J Gynecol Oncol* 1995;16:349–356.

25. Levin L, Lund B, Heintz APM. An overview of multi-variate analysis of prognostic variables with special reference to the role of cytoreductive surgery. *Ann Oncol* 1993;4:23–24.

26. Hacker NF. Surgical management of advanced ovarian cancer. In: Lawton FG, Neijt JP, Swenerton KD, eds. *Epithelial cancer of the ovary.* London: BMJ Publishing Group, 1995:144–171.

27. Guidozzi F, Ball JHS. Extensive primary cytoreductive surgery for advanced epithelial cancer. *Gynecol Oncol* 1994;53:326–330.

28. Hoskins WJ, Bundy BN, Thigpen JT, Omura GA. The influence of cytoreductive surgery on recurrence-free interval and survival in small-volume stage III epithelial ovarian cancer: a Gynecologic Oncology Group study. *Gynecol Oncol* 1992;47:159–166.

29. Potter ME, Partridge EE, Hatch KD, et al. Primary surgical therapy of ovarian cancer. How much and when? *Gynecol Oncol* 1991;40: 195–200.

30. Eisenkop S, Nalick R, Teng N. Peritoneal implant excision or ablation during cytoreductive surgery. The impact on survival. *Gynecol Oncol* 1992;45:97.

31. Van den Burg MEL, van Lent M, Buyse M, et al. The effect of debulking surgery after induction chemotherapy on the prognosis in advanced epithelial ovarian cancer. *N Engl J Med* 1995; 332:629–634.

32. Bergman F. Carcinoma of the ovary: a clinico-pathological study of 86 autopsied cases with special reference to node of spread. *Acta Obstet Gynecol Scand* 1966;45:211–231.

33. Chen SS, Lee L. Incidence of para-aortic and pelvic node metastases in epithelial carcinoma of the ovary. *Gynecol Oncol* 1983;16:95–100.

34. Burghardt E, Pickel H, Lahousen M, Stettner H. Pelvic lymphadenectomy in operative treatment of ovarian cancer. *Am J Obstet Gynecol* 1986; 155:315–319.

35. Wu PC, Qu JY, Lang JH, et al. Lymph node metastases of ovarian cancer. A preliminary survey of 74 cases of lymphadenectomy. *Am J Obstet Gynecol* 1986;155:1103–1108.

36. Benedetti-Panici P, Scambia G, Baiocchi G, et al. Technique and feasibility of systemic para-aortic lymphadenectomy for gynecological malignancies. *Int J Gynecol Cancer* 1991;1:133–140.

37. Spirtos NM, Gross GM, Freddo JL, Ballon SC. Cytoreductive surgery in advanced epithelial cancer of the ovary: the impact of aortic and pelvic lymphadenectomy. *Gynecol Oncol* 1995; 56:345–352.

38. Scarabelli C, Gallo A, Zarrelli A, et al. Systemic pelvic and para-aortic lymphadenectomy during cytoreductive surgery in advanced ovarian cancer. Potential benefit on survival. *Gynecol Oncol* 1995;56:328–337.

39. Di Re F, Baiocchi G, Fontanelli R, et al. Systemic pelvic and para-aortic lymphadenectomy for advanced ovarian cancer. Prognostic significance of node metastases. *Gynecol Oncol* 1996; 62:360–365.

40. Wangensteen OH, Lewis FJ, Tongen LA. The "second look" in cancer surgery. *Cancer* 1951; 71:303.

41. Rutledge F, Burns BC. Chemotherapy of advanced ovarian cancer. *Am J Obstet Gynecol* 1966;96:761–772.

42. Berek JS, Griffiths CT, Leventhal JM. Laparoscopy for second-look evaluation in ovarian cancer. *Obstet Gynecol* 1981;58:192–198.

43. Mangioni C, Bolis G, Molteni P, et al. Indications, advantages and limits of laparoscopy in ovarian cancer. *Gynecol Oncol* 1979;7:47.

44. Quinn MA, Bischop GJ, Campbell JJ, et al. Laparoscopic follow-up of patients with ovarian carcinoma. *Br J Obstet Gynaecol* 1980;87:1132.

45. Ozols RF, Fisher RI, Anderson T, et al. Peritoneoscopy in the management of ovarian cancer. *Am J Obstet Gynecol* 1981;140:1611.

46. Heintz APM, van Oosterom AT, Trimbos JBMC, et al. The treatment of advanced ovarian carcinoma (II): interval reassessment operations during chemotherapy. *Gynecol Oncol* 1988;30:359–371.

47. Rosenoff SH, de Vita VT, Hubbard S, et al. Peritoneoscopy in the staging and follow-up of ovarian carcinoma. *Semin Oncol* 1975;2:223.

48. Smith GW, Day TG, Smith JP. The use of laparoscopy to determine the results of chemotherapy for ovarian cancer. *J Reprod Med* 1977;18:257.

49. Lacey CG. Laparoscopy in gynecologic oncology. In: Morrow CP, Bonnar J, O'Brien TG, Gibbons WE, eds. *Recent clinical developments in gynecologic oncology*. New York: Raven, 1983:181–189.

50. Webb MJ, Snijder JA, Williams TJ, et al. Second-look laparotomy in ovarian cancer. *Gynecol Oncol* 1982;14:285.

51. Raju KS, McKinna JA, Barker GH, et al. Second-look operations in the planned management of advanced ovarian carcinoma. *Am J Obstet Gynecol* 1982;144:650.

52. Roberts WS, Hodel K, Rich WM. Second-look laparotomy in the management of gynecologic malignancy. *Gynecol Oncol* 1982;13:345.

53. Phibbs GD, Smith JP, Stanhoper CR. Analysis of sites of persistent cancer at "second-look" laparotomy in patients with ovarian cancer. *Am J Obstet Gynecol* 1983;147:611.

54. Berek JS, Hacker NF, Lagasse LD, et al. Second-look laparotomy in stage 3 epithelial ovarian cancer. Clinical variables associated with disease status. *Obstet Gynecol* 1984;64:207.

55. Barnhill DR, Hoskins WJ, Heller PB, et al. The second look surgical reassessment for epithelial ovarian carcinoma. *Gynecol Oncol* 1984;19:148.

56. Gershenson DM, Copeland LJ, Wharton JT, et al. Prognosis of surgically determined complete

57. Podratz KC, Malkasian G Jr, Hilton JF, et al. Second-look laparotomy in ovarian cancer: evaluation of pathologic variables. *Am J Obstet Gynecol* 1985;152:230–238.

58. Cain J, Saigo P, Pierce V, et al. A review of second-look laparotomy for ovarian cancer. *Gynecol Oncol* 1986;23:14.

59. Carmichael JA, Shelly WE, Brown LB, et al. A predictive index of cure versus no cure in advanced ovarian carcinoma patients—replacement of second-look laparotomy as a diagnostic test. *Gynecol Oncol* 1987;27:269–281.

60. Podczaski ES, Stevens CJ, Manetta A, et al. Use of second-look laparotomy in the management of patients with ovarian epithelial malignancies. *Gynecol Oncol* 1987;28:205–214.

61. Ghatage P, Krepart GV, Lotocki R. Factor analysis of false negative second-look laparotomy. *Gynecol Oncol* 1990;36:172–175.

62. Lund B, Williamson P. Prognostic factors for outcome of and survival after second-look laparotomy in patients with advanced ovarian carcinoma. *Obstet Gynecol* 1990;76:617–622.

63. Curry SL, Zembomm, Nahhas WA, et al. Second-look laparotomy for ovarian cancer. *Gynecol Oncol* 1981;11:114.

64. Schwartz PE, Smith JP. Second-look operations in ovarian cancer. *Am J Obstet Gynecol* 1980;138:1124–1130.

65. Smirz LR, Stehman FB, Ulbright TM, et al. Second-look laparotomy after chemotherapy in the management of ovarian malignancy. *Am J Obstet Gynecol* 1985;152:661–668.

66. Copeland LJ, Gershenson DM. Ovarian cancer recurrences in patients with no macroscopic tumor at second-look laparotomy. *Obstet Gynecol* 1986;86:873–874.

67. Miller DS, Ballon SC, Teng NN, et al. A critical reassessment of second-look laparotomy in epithelial ovarian carcinoma. *Cancer* 1986;57:530–535.

68. Gallup DG, Talledo OE, Dudzinski MR, Brown KW. Another look at the second assessment procedure for ovarian epithelial carcinoma. *Am J Obstet Gynecol* 1987;157:590–596.

69. McCusker MC, Hoffman JS, Curry SL, et al. The role of second-look laparotomy in treatment of epithelial ovarian cancer. *Gynecol Oncol* 1987;28:83–88.

70. Lippman SM, Alberts DS, Slijmen DJ, et al.

Second-look laparotomy in epithelial ovarian carcinoma. Prognostic factors associated with survival duration. *Cancer* 1988;61:2571–2577.

71. Podratz KC, Malkasian GJ, Wieand HS, et al. Recurrent disease after negative second-look laparotomy in stages III-IV ovarian carcinoma. *Gynecol Oncol* 1988;29:274–282.

72. Rubin SC, Hoskins WJ, Hakes TB, et al. Recurrence after second look laparotomy for ovarian cancer: analysis of risk factors. *Am J Obstet Gynecol* 1988;159:1094–1098.

73. Sonnendecker EW. Is routine second-look laparotomy for ovarian cancer justified? *Gynecol Oncol* 1988;31:249–255.

74. Luesley DM, Chan KK, Lawton FG, et al. Survival after negative second-look laparotomy. *Eur J Surg Oncol* 1989;15:205–210.

75. Rubin SC, Hoskins WJ, Saigo PE, et al. Prognostic factors for recurrence following negative second-look laparotomy in ovarian cancer patients treated with platinum-based chemotherapy. *Gynecol Oncol* 1991;42:137–141.

76. Berek JS, Hacker NF, Lagasse LD, et al. Survival of patients following secondary cytoreductive surgery in ovarian cancer. *Obstet Gynecol* 1983; 61:189–194.

77. Creasman WT. Evaluation of debulking surgery at second-look laparotomy. In: Sharp F, Mason WP, Creasman W, eds. *Ovarian cancer.* New York: Chapman & Hall Medical, 1992:375–383.

78. Hoskins WJ, Rubin SC, Dulamey E, et al. Influence of secondary cytoreduction at the time of second-look laparotomy on the survival of patients with epithelial ovarian cancer. *Gynecol Oncol* 1989;34:365–371.

79. Janicke F, Holscher M, Kuhn W, et al. Radical surgical procedure improves survival time in patients with recurrent ovarian cancer. *Cancer* 1992;70:2129–2136.

80. Segna RA, Dottino PR, Mandeli JP, et al. Secondary cytoreduction for ovarian cancer following cisplatin therapy. *J Clin Oncol* 1993;11: 434–439.

CHAPTER *33*

Chemotherapy in Advanced Ovarian Cancer

JOHN J. KAVANAGH

A majority of patients present with advanced disease (stage III or IV). Standard treatment for advanced ovarian cancer patients has been cytoreductive surgery (or debulking surgery) to remove as much as possible of the primary tumor and the associated metastatic disease and to determine accurately the extent of disease, followed by combination chemotherapy. Among the advanced-disease patients, the volume of residual disease is predictive of the patient's response to chemotherapy as well as survival (1). Systemic chemotherapy is the standard treatment for advanced epithelial ovarian cancer (2). Oral single-agent alkylating therapy had been used for many years (3), but the introduction of cisplatin in the latter half of the 1970s changed the therapeutic approach in the United States. Recently, paclitaxel has become available, and its combination with platinum is often used as initial treatment. The use of single-agent chemotherapy for metastatic epithelial ovarian cancer is generally reserved for patients whose overall physical condition precludes the use of more toxic therapy such as the elderly or debilitated patients.

Combination Chemotherapy

The relatively large number of active drugs available for the treatment of epithelial ovarian cancer points to the potential for the development of effective combination therapy. Combination chemotherapy may be superior to single-agent therapy in patients with advanced ovarian cancer (4). The first study to show the benefit of combination therapy compared the hexamethylmelamine, cyclophosphamide (Cytoxan), methotrexate, and 5-fluorouracil (5-FU) regimen (Hexa-CAF) with melphalan and showed that the response rate and the median survival time with the combination regimen were better than with the single drug (5). The Hexa-CAF regimen produced a complete response rate of 33% with a median survival time of 29 months, compared with 16% and 17 months, respectively, for melphalan. A variety of combination chemotherapeutic regimens have been studied in the treatment of advanced epithelial ovarian cancer (Table 33-1).

Platinum-Based Combination Chemotherapy

Since they were first introduced into the clinic in the late 1970s, the platinum compounds have remained some of the most active drugs in epithelial ovarian cancer (6). Cisplatin, the most extensively studied platinum compound, has clear-cut activity in patients with no prior chemotherapy as well as in those who received prior alkylating agent therapy (7,8). Subsequently, platinum compounds were incorporated into combination chemotherapeutic regimens with other active drugs, like cyclophosphamide, hexamethylmelamine, and doxorubicin. One such regimen, cyclophosphamide, hexamethylmelamine, doxorubicin (Adriamycin), and cisplatin (CHAP), was shown to be active and generally tolerable (9). Because of

T A B L E **33-1**

Chemotherapeutic Regimens for Advanced Ovarian Cancer

Regimen		Interval
PC	Cisplatin (75–100 mg/m²) Cyclophosphamide (650–1000 mg/m²)	q 3 wk
CC	Cisplatin (75–100 mg/m²) Cyclophosphamide (650–1000 mg/m²)	q 4 wk
PAC	Cisplatin (75–100 mg/m²) Doxorubicin (Adriamycin) (50 mg/m²) Cyclophosphamide (650–1000 mg/m²)	q 3–4 wk
CHAP	Hexamethylmelamine (150 mg/m² orally days 1–14) Cyclophosphamide (350 mg/m² IV day 1 and day 8) Doxorubicin (Adriamycin) (20 mg/m² IV day 1 and day 8) Cisplatin (60 mg/m² IV day 1)	q 3–4 wk
PT	Cisplatin (75–100 mg/m²) Taxol (135–210 mg/m²)	q 3 wk
CT	Carboplatin (starting dose, AUC = 5 mg·min/mL) Taxol (135–175 mg/m²)	q 3–4 wk

AUC = area under the curve.

the toxicity of hexamethylmelamine, particularly the depression that some patients experience with the drug, many oncologists omitted that agent.

In a meta-analysis performed on studies of patients with advanced-stage disease, those given cisplatin-containing combination chemotherapy were compared with those treated with regimens that did not include cisplatin (4). Survival differences between the groups were seen at 2 to 5 years, with the cisplatin group having a slight survival advantage, but the difference disappeared by 8 years (4). At a consensus meeting on the treatment of advanced ovarian cancer, there was agreement that after appropriate cytoreductive surgery, platinum-based chemotherapy yields superior response rates, progression-free survival, and superior overall survival (10).

The addition of doxorubicin to cisplatin and cyclophosphamide regimens is another controversial issue. The recent consensus (11) is that either cyclophosphamide (750 mg/m²) plus cisplatin (75 mg/m²) every 3 weeks or cyclophosphamide (500 mg/m²) plus doxorubicin (50 mg/m²) plus cisplatin (50 mg/m²) (CAP) every 3 weeks is acceptable standard therapy. However, four prospective randomized trials (12–15) comparing cisplatin and cyclophosphamide with the CAP regimen failed to show statistically significant differences in the overall survival. The largest of the above-mentioned trials was from the Italian Cooperative Gynecologic Oncology Group (GICOG), which randomized

529 patients to receive CAP, cisplatin with cyclophosphamide (PC), or cisplatin alone (12). No statistical difference was seen in overall survival (minimum follow-up, 5 years) among the three groups. Meta-analysis of these four trials (16) revealed a 6-year survival advantage of 7% in patients receiving the doxorubicin-containing regimen, but it remains unclear whether the benefit was a result of the addition of doxorubicin or the greater dose intensity achieved by its addition. Gadducci et al (17) reported their update data, which revealed no significant difference in progression-free survival between PC and CAP regimens. However, there is a trend in favor of the CAP regimen among patients with residual disease more than 2 cm in diameter (17). Because of the cardiotoxicity of doxorubicin, it would be desirable to omit the drug if overall response or survival rates were not significantly changed. A large prospective randomized Dutch study of CHAP versus PC showed that response rates and median survival times were almost identical (18). Because the toxicity of PC was significantly less than that of the four-drug regimen, it was concluded that PC should be considered the preferred treatment.

Another controversial issue is the number of cycles of chemotherapy to be given. Most studies reported six to eight courses of treatment, and it is generally agreed that most responses occur within four courses of chemotherapy. Two prospective randomized trials failed to demonstrate any significant benefit of the more prolonged treatment (18,19). The current recommendation is to give six to eight courses of treatment. There is no evidence so far to show that additional treatment produces any further benefit in an unselected population of patients.

Cisplatin Dose Intensity

Several investigators analyzed the importance of dose intensity (mg/m^2/time period) in relation to clinical outcome in ovarian cancer (Table 33-2) (12,20–23). At present the published data from randomized trials of dose intensity in ovarian cancer failed to confirm a benefit in favor of the dose-intense approach (20–28). A large Scottish trial (20) showed a difference in survival but included in its population patients with stage Ic to IV disease whose tumors had been optimally debulked. Recently, the mature results of this group showed the overall survival rates for the high-dose- and low-dose-intensity treatment arms to be 32.4% and 26.6%, respectively, and the overall relative death rate 0.68 ($p = 0.043$) (24). This represents a reduction in overall benefit with longer follow-up compared with the first 2 years of study (relative death rate of 0.52). Toxicity, particularly neurotoxicity, was

still evident in the fourth year (10/31 on high-dose- compared with 1/24 on low-dose-intensity treatment). The Hong Kong trial included stage III to IV patients who showed improved survival with high-dose regimens, but the patient population was small (24).

The Gynecologic Oncology Group (GOG) trial of patients with suboptimally debulked stage III or IV disease failed to demonstrate survival advantage for the high-dose-intensity chemotherapy arm (22). However, it is important to note that the final assessment of clinical response was based on a relatively small subset of patients with measurable disease (34%), and that in this study the high-intensity treatment arm consisted of only four courses of chemotherapy (12,19–27). It is possible that a greater increase in dose intensity is required to produce clinically meaningful improvement in patients with advanced disease. A critical problem, however, with evaluation of dose intensity in ovarian cancer is that multiple chemotherapy-related toxicities preclude marked increases in dose intensity for prolonged periods.

Studies that focused on patients with suboptimally debulked disease consistently found no statistically significant improvement in response rates and overall survival. However, studies focusing on patients with optimally

T A B L E   **33-2**

Randomized Trials of Cisplatin Plus Cyclophosphamide (CTX) Dose Intensity

Group	Disease Stage	No. of Patients	Drug Regimens	Dose Intensity	Cumulative Dose	Assigned Increase in Dose-Intensified Arm	Results
Hong Kong (22)	Stage III/IV	60	Cisplatin 100 mg/m^2 + CTX 1000 mg/m^2 vs cisplatin 50 mg/m^2 + CTX 1000 mg/m^2 × 6 cycles	+	+	×2	3-yr survival rates: higher dose = 60%, lower dose = 30%
Gynecology Oncology Group (23)	Untreated, suboptimal stage III/IV	458	Cisplatin 100 mg/m^2 + CTX 1000 mg/m^2 × 4 vs cisplatin 50 mg/m^2 + CTX 500 mg/m^2 × 8	+	−	×2	Median survival duration: higher dose = 21.9 mo, lower dose = 18.9 mo.
Scottish (21)	Stage I–IV	165	Cisplatin 100 mg/m^2 + CTX 750 mg/m^2 vs cisplatin 50 mg/m^2 + CTX 750 mg/m^2 × 6 cycles	+	−	×2	Median survival duration: higher dose = 28.5 mo, lower dose = 17.2 mo.
Italian (12)	Stage III/IV	296	Cisplatin 75 mg/m^2 every 3 wk × 6 vs cisplatin 50 mg/m^2 every wk × 9 cycles	+	−	×2	Median survival duration: higher dose = 36 mo, lower dose = 33 mo.
Danish (20)	Stage II–IV	78	AUC escalation from: 3–8 mg/mL/min	+	+	AUC × 4 vs AUC × 8	Higher PCR survival too early for analysis

AUC = area under the curve; PCR = pathologic complete response.

debulked disease reported improvement in response rates and overall survival. Increased dose intensity may be more likely to enhance survival of patients with small-volume disease.

Carboplatin Versus Cisplatin

Carboplatin, a second-generation platinum analogue, was introduced in the hope that it had less toxicity and broader activity than its parent compound, cisplatin. Carboplatin does have lower toxicity with fewer gastrointestinal sick effects, especially nausea and vomiting, less neurotoxicity, less nephrotoxicity, and less ototoxicity but more thrombocytopenia than cisplatin (29–32).

Several studies comparing carboplatin with cisplatin in treating ovarian cancer have been performed (Table 33-3) (30,32–37). The Advanced Ovarian Cancer Trialist Group (AOCTG) (4) conducted a meta-analysis that incorporated data from more than 2000 patients and compared carboplatin and cisplatin treatment. It failed to demonstrate any significant differences in overall survival between the two drugs. A similar conclusion came from two large North American trials: a trial by the Southwest Oncology Group (SWOG) (32) (342 patients with stage III or IV disease randomized to

receive cisplatin, $100 \, \text{mg/m}^2$, plus cyclophosphamide, $600 \, \text{mg/m}^2$, or carboplatin, $300 \, \text{mg/m}^2$, plus cyclophosphamide, $600 \, \text{mg/m}^2$) and a trial by the National Cancer Institute of Canada (33) (447 patients randomized to receive cisplatin, $75 \, \text{mg/m}^2$, plus cyclophosphamide versus carboplatin and cyclophosphamide). All three of these studies failed to demonstrate a significant difference in overall survival. However, the carboplatin regimen had a better therapeutic index and produced a better quality of life (32,33). In contrast, a recent French trial (34) involving 144 patients with stage III or IV disease who received either cisplatin or carboplatin together with cyclophosphamide and doxorubicin demonstrated different results, as seen in Table 33-3 (29,33–38). The planned doses of cyclophosphamide ($500 \, \text{mg/m}^2$) and doxorubicin ($40 \, \text{mg/m}^2$) were the same in both groups. The pathologic complete remission and overall response rates were significantly higher in the cisplatin treatment arm than in the carboplatin arm (33% versus 15% and 73% versus 47%, respectively). The median survival time was 27.9 months for the cisplatin arm and 20.6 months for the carboplatin arm. However, the actual delivered dose intensity for the two arms of the study was not reported (35).

At the recent National Institutes of Health

T A B L E   **33-3**

Carboplatin Versus Cisplatin (Carb/Cis) in Combination Chemotherapy for Advanced Ovarian Cancer: Treatment Results

Group	No. of Patients	Carb/Cis Dose (mg/m²)	Carb/Cis PDI (mg/m²/wk)	Combine w/Drug	SOD (%)	Carb/Cis PCR	Carb/Cis Median PFS (mo)	Carb/Cis Median Survival Time (mo)
National Cancer Institute of Canada (33)	417	300/75	75/18.75	CTX	59[a]	11/15	13.4/12.9	25.8/23.8
EORTC (30)	342	350/100	70/20	DOX CTX HMM	63[b]	23/27	13.1/16.8	22.7/24.6
Southwest Oncology Group (32)	291	300/100	75/25	CTX	100[a]	8/7	N/A	19.8/17.4
GONO (35)	164	200/50	50/12.5	DOX CTX	66[b]	14/20	15.5/13.2	23.1/22.6
ARTAC (34)	144	300/75	75/18.75	DOX CTX	N/A	10/25	N/A	20.6/27.9
NCCTG/Mayo (36)	103	150/60	37.5/15	CTX	35[a]	N/A	12.0/17.0	20.0/27.0
United Kingdom (37)	56	300/100	75/25	CTX	77[b]	N/A	24.0/13.0	24.0/19.0

PDI = planned dose intensity, $20 \, \text{mg/m}^2/\text{day} * 5$; DOX = doxorubicin; CTX = cyclophosphamide; HMM = hexamethylmelamine; SOD = suboptimally debulked; PCR = pathologic complete response; PFS = progression-free survival; N/A = not available.

[a] Lesions > 2 cm.

[b] Lesions > 1 cm.

Consensus Conference on Ovarian Cancer (39), it was concluded that data from mature randomized clinical trials indicate that the combination of carboplatin and cyclophosphamide is effective therapy and the substitution of carboplatin for cisplatin leads to a more acceptable toxicity profile.

In summary, carboplatin appears to be equivalent to cisplatin in terms of overall antitumor activity in the treatment of ovarian cancer (6,39–41). Platinum-based chemotherapy with the two-drug combination of cyclophosphamide and cisplatin or carboplatin remains the standard treatment, with 60% to 80% overall response rates and 40% to 50% clinical complete response rates.

Paclitaxel and Docetaxel

The taxanes, paclitaxel and docetaxel, represent a novel class of antineoplastic drugs. They share similar mechanisms of action, that is, the promotion of microtubule assembly and the inhibition of microtubule disassembly (41–43). Paclitaxel (Taxol) is a taxane alkaloid extracted from the bark of the Pacific yew, *Taxus brevifolia*. Docetaxel (Taxotere) is a semisynthetic taxane synthesized from a precursor alkaloid derived from the needles of the European yew, *Taxus baccata*. Although the molecular structures are similar, the toxicities are somewhat different. Docetaxel causes cumulative edema but less neuropathy (44). Premedication to prevent an anaphylactoid reaction is recommended with both taxanes. For paclitaxel, premedication consists of oral steroids and parenteral diphenhydramine plus cimetidine prior to drug administration. With docetaxel, oral steroids are started 24 hours before treatment and continued for a total of 5 days. Taxanes must be administered through tubes and bags that are not made of polyvinyl chloride. Both compounds have significant clinical activity in platinum-resistant ovarian cancer (Tables 33-4 and 33-5) (45–57).

Paclitaxel as a Single Agent in Previously Treated Patients

In platinum-refractory ovarian cancer, paclitaxel has a consistent activity, with response rates ranging from 15% to 50% (see Table 33-4). The activity of paclitaxel seems to depend on dose and schedule. The doses most commonly reported in trials range from 135 to 250 mg/m^2 with an infusion duration of 3 to 24 hours. Three phase II trials included 111 patients with prior platinum-based combination chemotherapy (46–48). The paclitaxel dose ranged from

T A B L E   **33-4**

Studies of Paclitaxel in Refractory and Advanced Ovarian Cancer

Institution		No. of Patients	Dose (mg/m²)	Overall Response (%)	% with CR (No.)	Median Survival (mo)
Single agent						
JHOC	(45)	40	135 (110–170)	30	2.5 (1)	8.2
Gynecology Oncology Group	(46)	41	170	37	12 (5)	15.9
Einstein	(47)	30	180–250	20	3 (1)	6.5
National Cancer Institute Treatment Referral Center	(48)	619	135	22	3	9
European-Canadian	(49)	195	135	15	1 (2)	11.0
		187	135	20	2 (4)	11.5
High dose (with G-CSF)						
National Cancer Institute	(50,51)	44	250	48	14	11.5
M. D. Anderson	(52)	48	250	48	4	12.0
United Kingdom	(53)	155	135–175	16	1.3 (2)	8.1

G-CSF = granulocyte colony-stimulating factor; CR = complete remission.

Source: Holmes FA, Kudelka AP, Kavanagh JJ, et al. Current status of clinical trials with paclitaxel and docetaxel. In: George GI, Chen TT, Ojima I, Vyas DM, eds. *ACS symposium series. Taxane anticancer agents. Basic science and current status. 207th national meeting of American Chemical Society, San Diego, CA.* 1994;3:31–57.

T A B L E   **33-5**

Docetaxel Phase II Trials in Advanced Ovarian Cancer

Study	No. of Patients	No. with CR (%)	Total Response (CR + PR)
EORTC (54)	97	4 (4)	23 (24)
EORTC (55)	76	3 (4)	26 (34)
MSKCC (56)	23	—	8 (35)
MDACC (57)	55	3 (6)	22 (40)

CR = complete remission; PR = partial remission; MDACC = M. D. Anderson Cancer Center; MSKCC = Memorial Sloan-Kettering Cancer Center; EORTC = European Organization for Research and Treatment of Cancer.

110 to 250 mg/m^2 infused over 24 hours every 3 weeks. Overall, 20% to 37% of the patients achieved a partial response and 7 patients (67%) achieved a complete response. Response rates were 40% to 50% for platinum-sensitive tumors and 24% to 30% for platinum-resistant tumors. The median duration of response was 6 months. The overall median survival time was 11 months (17 months in patients with platinum-sensitive tumors and 9 months in those with platinum-resistant tumors) (51). The National Cancer Institute (NCI)–designated Comprehensive Centers Care provided paclitaxel, 135 mg/m^2, in a 24-hour infusion to patients with platinum-refractory ovarian cancer and demonstrated a 22% response rate (4% complete response, 18% partial response) (48). The median survival time was 9 months.

Several studies in ovarian cancer suggested an effect of dose intensification of paclitaxel on outcome. Nonrandomized studies were performed to better define dose intensification with paclitaxel in this disease (52,53). Paclitaxel was given as a single agent at 250 mg/m^2 over 24 hours to patients with platinum-resistant ovarian cancer. Granulocyte colony-stimulating factor (G-CSF) was also administered starting 24 hours after completion of the paclitaxel infusion. Objective tumor response was seen in 48% of the patients. The duration of response was 6 months and the median survival time was 12 months.

In an attempt to define the optimal dose and duration of paclitaxel infusion, a joint European and Canadian trial coordinated by the National Cancer Institute of Canada prospectively randomized patients to receive one of two dose levels of paclitaxel (135 or 175 mg/m^2) and two different infusion schedules (3 or 24 hours) (49).

Responses were more frequent at the larger dose (20% versus 15%) and with the longer infusion duration (19% versus 16%). Although neither of these differences in response was statistically significant, the study authors recommended paclitaxel at 175 mg/m^2 given over 3 hours. The recommendation was based on the higher response rate, the lesser hematopoietic toxicity, more convenience, and the lower cost of the 3-hour infusion. A recent multigroup study involving the GOG, SWOG, National Canadian Clinical Trials Group (NCCTG), and Eastern Cooperative Oncology Group (ECOG) (protocol 134) compared a paclitaxel dose of 175 mg/m^2 with 250 mg/m^2 infused over 24 hours with G-CSF support administered every 3 weeks (58). The authors concluded that there is a dose-response effect in response rates but more toxicity and no prolongation of survival for the dose 250 mg/m^2 versus 175 mg/m^2 as a second-line therapy (objective response rates of 27.5% for 175 mg/m^2 versus 36% for 250 mg/m^2; survival times of 12.5 versus 11.9 months, respectively). Kudelka et al (59) reported similar results from two nonrandomized studies performed in a single institution. The median survival time was comparable, 10 to 12 months, in the two dose groups despite the difference in response rates (objective response rates of 21% for 135 mg/m^2 versus 48% for 250 mg/m^2) (59). The role of high-dose paclitaxel remains to be elucidated. Perhaps it will prove to be most beneficial in patients with significant symptomatology from their cancer.

Interestingly, patients with at least a 6-month paclitaxel-free interval and previously treated with low-dose paclitaxel (135 mg/m^2), or who achieved a complete response with high-dose paclitaxel (250 mg/m^2) may respond to high-dose paclitaxel retreatment of 250 mg/m^2 over 24 hours (60,61).

Paclitaxel-Based Regimens in Newly Diagnosed Patients

Paclitaxel Plus Cisplatin

McGuire et al (62) reported the final result of the GOG 111 study that compared cisplatin plus cyclophosphamide and cisplatin plus paclitaxel as first-line therapy in patients with suboptimally debulked (residual mass >1 cm in diameter) refractory ovarian cancer (62). Patients were randomized to receive either 750 mg/m^2 of cyclophosphamide and 75 mg/m^2 of cisplatin or 135 mg/m^2 of paclitaxel and 75 mg/m^2 of cisplatin. They reported an objective response rate of 73% and a median survival time of 38 months in the paclitaxel plus cisplatin arm and an objective response rate of 60% and median survival time of 24 months in the cisplatin plus cyclophosphamide arm, respectively. The progression-free survival times for each treatment arm were 18 and 13 months, respectively. The toxicity of the paclitaxel-cisplatin combination was considered to be clinically manageable. However, some doubts exist about the reproducibility of this result (63–66). Moreover, the overall survival data on the patients in the cyclophosphamide arm who were later rescued with paclitaxel have not been reported. The use of salvage paclitaxel may result in an overall survival rate that is comparable to that when platinum is used as primary therapy. The dose schedule of paclitaxel used in this study may not have been optimal, as that remains to be defined. Confirmatory trials are underway.

Paclitaxel Plus Carboplatin

The rationale for the substitution of carboplatin for cisplatin is that carboplatin is as effective as cisplatin with less toxicity, especially neurotoxicity. Based on early clinical data, carboplatin (like cisplatin) should be administered after the paclitaxel infusion (67). Currently, carboplatin is infused after the completion of paclitaxel infusion. Interestingly, thrombocytopenia appears to be less severe than expected, leading to the suggestion that paclitaxel provides some protection against carboplatin-induced thrombocytopenia (68). A phase I study by the GOG of this combination reported an overall response rate of 75% (complete response 67%) and a median progression-free survival time of 15 months (69). Accordingly, the combination of paclitaxel, 175 mg/m^2 infused over 3 hours, followed by carboplatin dosed with a target area under the curve (AUC) of 7.5 mg·min/mL every 3 weeks was recommended for a phase III GOG trial (70). Meerpohl et al (71) recommended similar doses for a phase III trial: paclitaxel dose of 185 mg/m^2 and carboplatin dose of AUC 6 mg·min/mL (71).

Paclitaxel-Based Combination Regimens in Pretreated Patients

Guastella et al (72) performed a study of paclitaxel, 175 mg/m^2 infusion over 3 hours, with carboplatin, AUC of 5 mg·min/mL infusion over 30 minutes, administered every 3 weeks in pretreated, advanced ovarian cancer patients (72). They reported an overall response rate of 41% (complete response 12%) with a median duration of response of 8 months. They concluded that this regimen is effective, safe, and convenient for outpatient administration.

Docetaxel

Docetaxel has significant activity in the treatment of many malignancies such as breast, lung, gastric, pancreatic, and ovarian cancer (see Table 33-5). For ovarian cancer, it achieves response rates of 17% to 37% (73–75). Kaye et al (75) reported the results of an EORTC study; in 200 patients previously treated with platinum, an overall response rate of 31.5% was noted after treatment with docetaxel at a dose of 100 mg/m^2 as a 1-hour intravenous infusion every 3 weeks. Similarly, Piccart et al (54), in their study using docetaxel at the same dose and schedule in 97 patients with platinum-refractory ovarian cancer, found an overall response rate of 23.5% with a median overall survival time of 8.4 months. A study from the M. D. Anderson Cancer Center evaluated docetaxel, 100 mg/m^2 given as a 1-hour infusion every 3 weeks, in 55 platinum-refractory patients. A response rate of 40% and median overall survival time of 10 months were noted (57). Premedications to prevent an anaphylactoid reaction were used with this drug. The main nonhematologic total dose-limiting toxicity associated with docetaxel use is the development of fluid retention, including pleural effusions and ascites. The frequency and severity increase with the total dose of this drug. This side effect becomes problematic as the cumulative dose exceeds 400 mg/m^2. It has been ameliorated with systemic steroids and with early diuretic use on evidence of fluid retention.

Second-Line Chemotherapy for Refractory Ovarian Cancer: Platinum Reinduction

Retreatment with platinum in patients with relapsing disease that previously responded to this agent resulted in response rates of 30% to 100% with a platinum-free interval of 6 months to over 2 years (76–79). The likelihood of achieving a response in patients with initially platinum-sensitive tumors increases when the interval from the last cycle of initial platinum-based treatment is longer than 12 months. That time interval may allow for the regrowth of platinum-sensitive cells or for resistant cells to lose their resistance to the cytotoxic drugs. However, the response rate in patients whose disease failed to achieve a complete response or recurred within 6 months of platinum treatment is less than 20% (79,80).

At the M. D. Anderson Cancer Center, 33 patients with ovarian cancers refractory to platinum and taxane therapy were treated with single-agent carboplatin reinduction once the disease progressed with a taxane (81). The starting dose of carboplatin was 300 mg/m² at 28-day intervals. The objective response rate was 21% and the proportion of patients whose disease ceased to progress was 39% (13/33), which is clinically significant in these prognostically highly unfavorable patients with bulky disease. The use of targeted AUC concentration as a function of time and renal clearance (i.e., glomerular filtration rate) to determine the carboplatin dose may reduce the toxicity and augment activity of this treatment (30). Accordingly, carboplatin retreatment has clinical benefit in patients with platinum- and taxane-refractory disease and represents a viable option for this group of patients for whom the number of effective agents is severely limited.

Ifosfamide

Ifosfamide is an analogue of cyclophosphamide that appears to be more active than its chemical cousin. The drug has clear-cut activity in ovarian carcinoma with responses noted in patients who were clinically refractory to platinum-cyclophosphamide combinations (82, 83). The overall response rates for platinum-refractory ovarian cancer to ifosfamide are 13% to 20% (82–86). The major toxicity other than myelosuppression is hemorrhagic cystitis, which is prevented by the use of mesna (2-mercaptoethanesulfonate), a specific antidote to the urothelial effects. With the use of mesna, other toxicities, typically hematologic toxicity, become dose limiting. Ifosfamide is commonly administered daily for 5 days as a bolus schedule of 1.2 to 1.8 g/m² with 300 to 400 mg/m² of mesna given 0, 4, and 8 hours after each ifosfamide dose. An alternative is ifosfamide, 5 to 8 g/m² as a continuous 24-hour infusion, with an overlapping continuous infusion of mesna

(administered for at least 12 hours after completion of ifosfamide infusion). Other significant toxicities include renal tubular abnormalities and toxic encephalopathy. The toxic encephalopathy is probably underreported and appears to be more common with high-dose schedules, although there is controversy over the relationship between central nervous system toxicity and the dose of ifosfamide, peak plasma levels, or the AUC concentration as a function of time (87,88). Neurotoxicity may be more common in older patients and also patients with renal dysfunction or hypoalbuminemia. In this regard, neurotoxicity may be more common in the patient who has received prior cisplatin therapy, secondary to subclinical renal impairment, but no publication to date has prospectively evaluated the effect of prior cisplatin therapy on ifosfamide-induced neurotoxicity.

Ifosfamide has also been used in combination therapy for advanced ovarian cancer. Of interest is the regimen of ifosfamide, carboplatin, and etoposide (ICE) in platinum-refractory patients (89). The response rate was 52% (13/25 patients) with 7 (28%) complete responses.

Topoisomerase I Inhibitors

Topoisomerase I is an enzyme necessary for DNA replication and RNA transcription (90). It mediated the relaxation of supercoiled DNA by binding to specific regions of DNA, inducing single-strand breaks, and then resealing the DNA breaks after it has uncoiled the DNA. The intracellular level of topoisomerase I is higher in malignant than in normal cells (91). The main topoisomerase inhibitors are analogues of camptothecin. Camptothecins bind to the topoisomerase I–DNA complex and prevent resealing of the DNA single-strand breaks. As a result, the DNA fragments during its synthesis.

Topotecan

Topotecan (Hycamptin) is a semisynthetic water-soluble camptothecin analogue that is a specific and potent inhibitor of topoisomerase I. It has demonstrated antitumor activity in preclinical and phase I studies (92–95). In a recent phase II study at the M. D. Anderson Cancer Center, topotecan was administered by a daily intravenous infusion over 30 minutes each day for 5 days every 3 weeks. Objective partial responses were observed in 4 (14%) of 28 patients with measurable disease. Most of the patients (61%) achieved clinical stabilization of previously progressive disease (96). Topotecan's major toxic effect was myelosuppression (neutropenia and thrombocytopenia) and its sequelae. There was no significant neurologic, cardiovascular, or renal toxicity in this study. Optimization of dose schedules and incorporation of multilineage hematopoietins are being studied. Other groups also demonstrated 13.0% to 16.3% response rates for platinum- and platinum-paclitaxel–refractory ovarian cancer (97). Currently, studies of topotecan in combination with cisplatin are ongoing (98). In summary, topotecan has definite activity in patients with platinum-refractory ovarian cancer with a manageable toxicity profile.

Irinotecan

Irinotecan (CPT-11) is a water-soluble semisynthetic derivative of camptothecin. Irinotecan is a pro-drug that undergoes de-esterification to produce SN-38, a metabolite that is 1000-fold more potent than the parent compound (99). Irinotecan is a potent topoisomerase I inhibitor with a broad spectrum of experimental antitumor activity. Objective response rates of 18% to 28% are seen with this compound in recurrent or refractory ovarian cancers. A 23% response rate was observed in patients who had prior platinum therapy. The dose-limiting toxicity was diarrhea or myelosuppression, depending on the dose schedule (100–103). Puzzling cholinergic symptoms were observed with irinotecan (104). In a recent study of irinotecan combined with cisplatin in 18 patients with relapsed ovarian cancer, there were 2 complete responses, 4 partial responses, and 4 with stable disease (105).

9-Nitrocamptothecin

9-Nitrocamptothecin (9-NC) is a water-insoluble derivative of camptothecin that is administered orally 4 or 5 days a week on a continuous schedule. It is metabolized to 9-aminocamptothecin, a topoisomerase I inhibitor with broad activity in refractory human tumors (106). A recent phase I study at the Stehlin Foundation and M. D. Anderson Cancer Center demonstrated a 20% overall response rate in 27 patients, including 8 patients with refractory ovarian cancer. At $2 mg/m^2$, the dose-limiting toxicity was hematologic, with 25%, 17%, and 29% of patients manifesting grade 4 neutropenia, thrombocytopenia, and anemia, respectively. Significant gastrointestinal side effects were noted, with 48% of the patients experiencing nausea and vomiting and 33% diarrhea. These preliminary data showed that 9-NC may have significant antitumor activity, although the overall toxicity is substantial (106).

Gemcitabine

Gemcitabine (2′,2′-difluorodeoxycytidine) was developed as a new deoxycytidine analogue (108). Gemcitabine inhibits DNA synthesis. It was originally synthesized as an antiviral agent but was found to have excellent in vivo activity against a variety of animal tumors. In a phase II study, gemcitabine was given intravenously at a dose of 800 to $1250 mg/m^2$ once a week for 3 consecutive weeks, followed by 1 week of rest, in patients with platinum-refractory ovarian cancer (107–111). A partial response of 15% to 19% was demonstrated, with a median response duration of 8.1 months. Leukopenia and thrombocytopenia were the main toxic effects. Based on the evidence of activity in platinum-refractory ovarian cancer at a dose of 800 to $1250 mg/m^2$ and the apparently higher tolerated dose demonstrated in later phase I studies, a phase II study in refractory ovarian cancer at a higher dose ($2000 mg/m^2$) is being performed. Gemcitabine is a well-tolerated drug with activity in platinum-resistant ovarian cancer patients (112).

Acknowledgments

The author wishes to thank Andrzej P. Kudelka and Wichai Termrungruanglert for their contributions.

REFERENCES

1. Thigpen JT. Chemotherapy in the management of celomic epithelial carcinoma of the ovary. In: Markman M, Hoskins WJ, eds. *Cancer of the ovary.* New York: Raven, 1993:277–286.

2. Berek JS. Epithelial ovarian cancer. In: Berek JS, Hacker NF, eds. *Practical gynecologic oncology.* 2nd ed. Baltimore: William & Wilkins, 1994: 327–375.

3. Smith JP, Day TG. Review of ovarian cancer at the University of Texas System Cancer Center,

M.D. Anderson Hospital and Tumor Institute. *Am J Obstet Gynecol* 1979;135:984–993.

4. Advanced Ovarian Cancer Trialists Group. Chemotherapy in advanced ovarian cancer: an overview of randomized clinical trials. *BMJ* 1991;303:884–893.

5. Young RC, Chabner BA, Hubbard SP, et al. Advanced ovarian adenocarcinoma: a prospective clinical trial of melphalan (L-PAM) versus combination chemotherapy. *N Engl J Med* 1978; 299:1261–1266.

6. Ozols RF. Current status of chemotherapy for ovarian cancer. *Semin Oncol* 1995;5(suppl 12): 61–66.

7. Wiltshaw E, Kroner T. Phase II trial of platinum (II) (NSC-119875) in advanced adenocarcinoma of the ovary. *Cancer Treat Rep* 1976;60:55–60.

8. Thigpen T, Blessing JA, Homesley H, et al. Cisplatinum in the treatment of advanced or recurrent adenocarcinoma of the ovary: a phase II study of the Gynecologic Oncology Group. *Am J Clin Oncol* 1983;6:431–435.

9. Greco FA, Julian CG, Richardson RL. Advanced ovarian cancer: brief intensive combination chemotherapy and second-look laparotomy. *Obstet Gynecol* 1981;58:199–205.

10. Allen DG, Baak J, Belpomme D, et al. Consensus group on advanced epithelial ovarian cancer: 1993 consensus statement. *Ann Oncol* 1993;4(suppl):83–89.

11. Ozols RF. Ovarian cancer: part II. Treatment. *Curr Probl Cancer* 1992;16:63–126.

12. GICOG (Gruppo Interregionale Cooperativo Oncologico Gynecologica). Randomized comparison of cisplatin with cyclophosphamide/cisplatin and with cyclophosphamide/doxorubicin/cisplatin in advanced ovarian cancer. *Lancet* 1989;2:355–359.

13. Omura GA, Bundy BN, Berek JS, et al. Randomized trial of cyclophosphamide plus cisplatin with or without doxorubicin in ovarian carcinoma: a GOG study. *J Clin Oncol* 1989;7: 457–465.

14. Bertelsen K, Jacobsen A, Andersen JE, et al. A randomized study of cyclophosphamide and cisplatin with or without doxorubicin in advanced ovarian cancer. *Gynecol Oncol* 1987;26:161–169.

15. Conte PF, Bruzzone M, Chiara S, et al. A randomized trial comparing cisplatin plus cyclophosphamide vs. cisplatin, doxorubicin, and cyclophosphamide in advanced ovarian cancer. *J Clin Oncol* 1986;4:965–971.

16. The Ovarian Cancer Meta-analysis Group. Cyclophosphamide plus cisplatin versus cyclophosphamide, doxorubicin, and cisplatin chemotherapy of ovarian carcinoma: a meta-analysis. *J Clin Oncol* 1991;9:1668–1674.

17. Gadducci A, Bruzzone M, Carnino F, et al. Twelve-year follow-up of a randomized trial comparing cisplatin and cyclophosphamide with cisplatin, doxorubicin and cyclophosphamide in patients with advanced epithelial ovarian cancer. *Int J Gynecol Cancer* 1996;6: 286–290.

18. Neijt JP, ten Bokkel Huinink WW, van der Burg ME, et al. Randomized trial comparing two combination chemotherapy regimens (CHAP-5 versus CP) in advanced ovarian carcinoma: a randomized trial of the Netherlands joint study group for ovarian cancer. *J Clin Oncol* 1987;5: 1157–1168.

19. Hakes TB, Cholas E, Hoskins WJ, et al. Randomized prospective trial of 5 vs. 10 cycles of cyclophosphamide, doxorubicin, and cisplatin in advanced ovarian carcinoma. *Gynecol Oncol* 1992;45:284–289.

20. Bertelsen IF, Jacobsen A, Hansen MK, et al. A randomized trial of six vs. twelve cycles of cyclophosphamide, Adriamycin, in advanced ovarian cancer. *Proc Am Soc Clin Oncol* 1989;8: 15. Abstract.

21. Kaye SB, Lewis CR, Paul JP, et al. Randomized study of two doses of cisplatin with cyclophosphamide in epithelial ovarian cancer. *Lancet* 1992;340:329–333.

22. Ngan HY, Choo YC, Cheung M, et al. A randomized study of high-dose versus low-dose cisplatinum combined with cyclophosphamide in the treatment of advanced ovarian cancer. *Chemotherapy* 1989;35:221–227.

23. Kaye SB, Cassidy JP, Lewis CR, et al. Mature results of a randomized trial of two doses of cisplatin for the treatment of ovarian cancer. *J Clin Oncol* 1996;14:2113–2119.

24. McGuire WP, Hoskins WJ, Brady MF, et al. A phase III trial of dose intense (DI) versus standard dose (DS) cisplatin (CDDP) and Cytoxan (CTX) in advanced ovarian cancer. *Br J Cancer* 1992;11:226.

25. Bella M, Cocconi G, Lotticci R, et al. Conventional versus high dose intensity regimen of cis-

platin in advanced ovarian carcinoma. A prospective randomized study. *Proc Am Soc Clin Oncol* 1992;11:223.

26. Ehrlich CE, Einhorn L, Stehman FB, et al. Treatment of advanced epithelial ovarian cancer using cisplatin, Adriamycin and Cytoxan, the Indiana University experience. *Clin Obstet Gynecol* 1983;10:325–335.

27. Colombo N, Pittelli MR, Parma G, et al. Cisplatin dose-intensity in advanced ovarian cancer: a randomized study of dose-intensity versus standard dose cisplatin monochemotherapy. *Proc Am Soc Clin Oncol* 1993;12:255.

28. Conte PF, Bruzzone M, Carnino F, et al. High-dose versus low-dose cisplatin in combination with cyclophosphamide and epidoxorubicin in suboptimal ovarian cancer: a randomized study of the Gruppo Oncologico Nord-Ovest. *J Clin Oncol* 1996;14:351–356.

29. Fennelly D. Dose intensity in advanced ovarian cancer: have we answered the question? *Clin Cancer Res* 1995;1:575–582.

30. ten Bokkel Huinink WW, van der Burg MET, van Oosterom AT, et al. Carboplatin in combination therapy for ovarian cancer. *Cancer Treat Rev* 1988;15:9–15.

31. Calvert AH, Newell DR, Gumbrell LA, et al. Carboplatin dosage prospective evaluation of a simple formula based on renal function. *J Clin Oncol* 1989;7:1748–1756.

32. Alberts DS, Green S, Hannigan EV, et al. Improved therapeutic index of carboplatin plus cyclophosphamide versus cisplatin plus cyclophosphamide: final report by the Southwest Oncology Group of a phase III randomized trial in stages III (suboptimal) and IV ovarian cancer. *J Clin Oncol* 1992;10:706–717.

33. Swenerton K, Jefffrey J, Stuart G, et al. Cisplatin-cyclophosphamide versus carboplatin-cyclophosphamide in advanced ovarian cancer: a randomized phase III study of the National Cancer Institute of Canada Clinical Trials Group. *J Clin Oncol* 1992;10:718–726.

34. Belpomme D, Bugat R, Rives M, et al. Carboplatin vs. cisplatin in association with cyclophosphamide and doxorubicin as first line therapy in stage III–IV ovarian carcinoma: results of an ARTAC phase III trial. *Proc Am Soc Clin Oncol* 1992;11:227.

35. Conte PF, Bruzzone M, Caruino F, et al. Carboplatin, doxorubicin, and cyclophosphamide vs. cisplatin, doxorubicin, and cyclophosphamide. A randomized trial in stage III-IV epithelial ovarian carcinoma. *J Clin Oncol* 1991;9:658–663.

36. Edmondson JH, McCormack GM, Wieand HS, et al. Cyclophosphamide-cisplatin vs cyclophosphamide-carboplatin in stage III–IV ovarian carcinoma: a comparison of equally myelosuppressive regimens. *J Natl Cancer Inst* 1989; 81:1500–1504.

37. Gurney H, Crowther D, Anderson H, et al. Five-year follow up and dose delivery analysis of cisplatin, iproplatin, or carboplatin in combination with cyclophosphamide in advanced ovarian carcinoma. *Ann Oncol* 1990;1:427–433.

38. NIH Consensus Conference. Ovarian cancer screening, treatment, and follow up *JAMA* 1995; 273:491–497.

39. Alberts DS. Carboplatin versus cisplatin in ovarian cancer. *Semin Oncol* 1995;22(suppl 12): 88–90.

40. Mainwaring PN, Gore ME. The importance of dose and schedule in cancer chemotherapy: epithelial ovarian cancer. *Anticancer Drugs* 1995;6(suppl 5):29–41.

41. Pazdur R, Kudelda AP, Kavanagh JJ, et al. The taxoids: paclitaxel (Taxol) and docetaxel (Taxotere). *Cancer Treat Rev* 1993;19:351–386.

42. Holmes FA, Kudelka AP, Kavanagh JJ, et al. Current status of clinical trials with paclitaxel and docetaxel. In: George GI, Chen TT, Ojima I, Vyas DM, eds. *Taxane anticancer agents: basic science and current status.* Washington, DC: American Chemical Society, 1995:31–57.

43. Rowinsky EK, Donehower RC. Paclitaxel (Taxol). *N Engl J Med* 1995;322:1004–1014.

44. van Oosterom AT, Schriivers D. Docetaxel (Taxotere), a review of preclinical and clinical experience. Part II: clinical experience. *Anticancer Drugs* 1995;6:356–368.

45. McGuire WP, Rovinsky EK, Rosenshein NB, et al. Taxol: a unique antineoplastic agent with significant activity in advanced ovarian epithelial neoplasms. *Ann Intern Med* 1989;111: 273–279.

46. Thigpen JT, Blessing JA, Ball H, et al. Phase II trial of paclitaxel in patients with progressive ovarian carcinoma after platinum-based chemotherapy: a Gynecologic Oncology Group study. *J Clin Oncol* 1994;12:1748–1753.

47. Einzig AI, Wiernik P, Sasloff J, et al. Phase II study and long term follow-up of patients

treated with Taxol for advanced ovarian adenocarcinoma. *J Clin Oncol* 1992;10:1748–1753.

48. Timble E, Adams J, Vena D, et al. Paclitaxel for platinum refractory ovarian cancer: results from the first 1,000 patients registered to National Cancer Institute Treatment Referral Center 9103. *J Clin Oncol* 1993;11:2405–2410.

49. Eisenhauer EA, ten Bokkel Huinink WW, Swenerton KD. European-Canadian randomized trial of paclitaxel in relapsed ovarian cancer: high-dose versus low-dose and long versus short infusion. *J Clin Oncol* 1994;12:2654–2666.

50. McGuire WP. Paclitaxel in the treatment of ovarian cancer. In: *American Society of Clinical Oncology educational book*. PP 204–213, 3014 Annual Meeting, Dallas Texas, 1994.

51. Sarosy G, Kohn E, Stowe A, et al. Phase I study of Taxol and granulocyte colony-stimulating factor in patients with refractory ovarian cancer. *J Clin Oncol* 1992;10:1165–1170.

52. Kavanagh JJ, Kudelka AP, Edwards CL, et al. A randomized crossover trial of parenteral hydroxyurea vs. high-dose Taxol in cisplatin/carboplatin-resistant epithelial ovarian cancer. *Proc Am Soc Clin Oncol* 1993;13:259.

53. Gore ME, Levy V, Rustin G, et al. Paclitaxel (taxol) in relapsed and refractory ovarian cancer: the UK and Eire experience. *Br J Cancer* 1995;72:1016–1019.

54. Piccart MJ, Gore M, ten Bokkel Huinink WW, et al. Docetaxel: an active new drug for treatment of advanced epithelial ovarian cancer. *J Natl Cancer Inst* 1995;87:676–681.

55. Aapro M, Pujade-Lauraine E, Lhomme C, et al. EORTC clinical screening group: phase II study of Taxotere in ovarian cancer. *Ann Oncol* 1994;5:202.

56. Francis P, Schneider J, Hann L, et al. Phase II trial of docetaxel in patients with platinum-refractory advanced ovarian cancer. *J Clin Oncol* 1994;12:2301–2308.

57. Kavanagh JJ, Kudelka AP, Gonzalez de Leon C, et al. Phase II study of docetaxel in patients with epithelial ovarian carcinoma refractory to platinum. *Clin Cancer Res* 1996;2:837–842.

58. Omura GA, Brady MF, Delmore JE, et al. A randomized trial of paclitaxel at 2 dose levels and filgrastim (G-CSF) at 2 doses in platinum pretreated epithelial ovarian cancer: a Gynecologic Oncology Group, SWOG, NCCTG and ECOG study. *Proc Am Soc Clin Oncol* 1996;15:A755.

59. Kudelka AP, Tresukosol D, Gonzalez de Leon C, et al. Paclitaxel in patients with platinum-resistant ovarian cancer: a selected review of literature and clinical experience. *J Med Assoc Thai* 1996;79:240–244.

60. Tresukosol D, Kudelka AP, Gonzales de Leon C, et al. Paclitaxel retreatment in patients with platinum and paclitaxel resistant ovarian cancer. *Eur J Gynaecol Oncol* 1996;17:188–191.

61. Aghajanian C, Gogas H, Fennelly D, et al. Second-line paclitaxel therapy in patients with ovarian cancer previously treated with a taxane. *Proc Am Soc Clin Oncol* 1996;15:A776.

62. McGuire WP, Hoskins WJ, Brady MF, et al. Cyclophosphamide and cisplatin compared with paclitaxel and cisplatin in patients with stage III and stage IV ovarian cancer. *N Engl J Med* 1996;334:1–6.

63. Parmar MKB, Sandercock J. Letter to editor. *N Engl J Med* 1996;334:1268–1269.

64. Cvitkovic E, Misset JL. Letter to editor. *N Engl J Med* 1996;334:1269.

65. Lacave AJ, Pelaez I, Palacio I. Letter to editor. *N Engl J Med* 1996;334:1269–1270.

66. Seetalarom K, Kudelka AP, Verschraegen CF, Kavanagh JJ. Taxanes in ovarian cancer treatment. *Curr Opin Obstet Gynecol* 1997;9:14–20.

67. Clark JW, Santos-Moore AS, Choy H. Sequencing of taxol and carboplatinum therapy. *Proc Am Assoc Cancer Res* 1995;36:A1772.

68. Calvert AH, Boddy A, Bailey NP, et al. Carboplatin in combination with paclitaxel in advanced ovarian cancer: dose determination and pharmacokinetics and pharmacodynamic interactions. *Semin Oncol* 1995;22(suppl 12):91–98.

69. Bookman MA, McGuire WP, Kilpatrick D, et al. Carboplatin and paclitaxel in ovarian carcinoma: a phase I study of the Gynecologic Oncology Group. *J Clin Oncol* 1996;14:1895–1902.

70. Reszka R, du Bois A, Luck HJ, et al. Clinical pharmacokinetics of paclitaxel and carboplatin in combination therapy. *Proc Am Assoc Cancer Res* 1996;37:A1245.

71. Meerpohl HG, du Bois A, Kuhnle H, et al. Paclitaxel combined with carboplatin in the first-line treatment of advanced ovarian cancer. *Semin Oncol* 1995;22(suppl 15):7–12.

72. Guastella JP, Pujade Lauraine E, Orfeuvre H, et al. Efficacy and safety of carboplatin-paclitaxel

CHAPTER 33 **Chemotherapy in Advanced Ovarian Cancer**   **483**

association in pretreated ovarian cancer patients. *Proc Am Soc Clin Oncol* 1996;15:A746.

73. Kaye SB. Docetaxel (Taxotere) in the treatment of solid tumors other than breast and lung cancer. *Semin Oncol* 1995;22(suppl 4):30–35.

74. Cortes JE, Pazdur R. Docetaxel. *J Clin Oncol* 1995;13:2643–2655.

75. Kaye SB, Piccart M, Aapro M, Kavanagh J. Docetaxel in advanced ovarian cancer: preliminary results from three phase II trials. EORTC Early Clinical Trials Group and Clinical Screening Group, and the M.D. Anderson Cancer Center. *Eur J Cancer* 1995;31(suppl 4):14–17.

76. Gershenson DM, Kavanagh JJ, Copeland LJ, et al. Re-treatment of patients with recurrent epithelial ovarian cancer with platin based chemotherapy. *Obstet Gynecol* 1989;73:798–802.

77. Blackledge G, Lawton F, Redman C, et al. Response of patients in phase II studies of chemotherapy in ovarian cancer: implications for patient treatment and the design of phase II trials. *Br J Cancer* 1989;59:650–653.

78. Gore ME, Fryatt I, Wiltshaw E, et al. Treatment of relapses of carcinoma of the ovary with cisplatin or carboplatin following initial treatment with these compounds. *Gynecol Oncol* 1990;36:207–211.

79. Markman M, Rothman R, Hakes T, et al. Second-line platinum therapy in patients with ovarian cancer previously treated with cisplatin. *J Clin Oncol* 1991;9:389–393.

80. Kavanagh JJ, Nicaise C. Carboplatin in refractory epithelial ovarian cancer. *Semin Oncol* 1989;2(suppl 5):45–48.

81. Kavanagh JJ, Tresukosol D, Edwards CL, et al. Carboplatin reinduction after taxane in patients with platinum-refractory epithelial ovarian cancer. *J Clin Oncol* 1995;13:1584–1588.

82. Sutton GP, Blessing JA, Homesley HD, et al. Phase II trial of ifosfamide and mesna in advanced ovarian carcinoma: a Gynecologic Oncology Group trial. *J Clin Oncol* 1989;7:1672–1676.

83. Thigpen T, Lambuth B, Vance R. Ifosfamide in the management of gynecologic cancers. *Semin Oncol* 1990;17(suppl 4):11–18.

84. Hakes T, Markman M, Reichman B, et al. Ifosfamide therapy of ovarian cancer previously treated with cisplatin and Cytoxan. *Proc Am Soc Clin Oncol* 1991;10:A603.

85. Sutton G. Ifosfamide and mesna in epithelial ovarian cancer. *Gynecol Oncol* 1993;51:104–108.

86. Srensen P, Pfeiffer P, Bertelsen K. A phase II trial of ifosfamide/mesna as salvage therapy in patients with ovarian cancer refractory to or relapsing after prior platinum-containing chemotherapy. *Gynecol Oncol* 1995;56:75–78.

87. Meanwell CA, Blake AC, Kelly KA, et al. Prediction of ifosfamide/mesna associated encephalopathy. *Eur J Cancer Clin Oncol* 1986;22:815–819.

88. Perren TJ, Turner RC, Smith IE. Encephalopathy with rapid infusion ifosfamide/mesna. *Lancet* 1987;1:390–391.

89. Fanning J, Hilgers RD, Hutson E. Carboplatin, etoposide, and ifosfamide as second-line treatment for ovarian cancer. *Am J Clin Oncol* 1994;17:335–337.

90. Balat O, Mohammed E, Kudelka AP, et al. Frontiers of ovarian cancer therapy. *Cancer Control* 1996;3:137–144.

91. Liu LF. DNA topoisomerase poisons as antitumor drugs. *Annu Rev Biochem* 1989;58:351–375.

92. Chabner BA. Camptothecins. *J Clin Oncol* 1992;10:3–4.

93. Burris HA, Rothenberg ML, Kuhn JG, et al. Clinical trials with the topoisomerase I inhibitors. *Semin Oncol* 1992;19:663–669.

94. Slichenmyer WJ, Rowinsky EK, Donehower RC, et al. The current status of camptothecin analogues as antitumor agents. *J Natl Cancer Inst* 1993;85:271–291.

95. Rowinsky EK, Grochow LB, Hendricks CB, et al. Phase I and pharmacologic study of topotecan: a novel topoisomerase I inhibitor. *J Clin Oncol* 1992;10:647–656.

96. Kudelka AP, Tresukosol D, Edwards CL, et al. Phase II study of intravenous topotecan as a 5-day infusion for refractory epithelial ovarian carcinoma. *J Clin Oncol* 1996;14:1552–1557.

97. Gordon A, Bookman M, Malmstrom H, et al. Efficacy of topotecan in advanced epithelial ovarian cancer after failure of platinum and paclitaxel: International Topotecan Study Group Trial. *Proc Am Soc Clin Oncol* 1996;15:A763.

98. ten Bokkel Huinink W, Gore M, Bolis G, et al. A phase II trial of topotecan for the treatment of relapsed advanced ovarian carcinoma: European

Topotecan Oncology Group. *Proc Am Soc Clin Oncol* 1996;15:A768.

99. Lilenbaum RC, Miller AA, Batist G, et al. Phase I study of continuous IV infusion topotecan (TT) in combination with cisplatin (C) in patients with advanced cancer (CALGB 9462). *Proc Am Soc Clin Oncol* 1996;15:A1543.

100. Furue H. Irinotecan hydrochloride (CPT-11). *Jpn J Cancer Chemother* 1994;21:709–717.

101. Mori H, Itoh N, Kondoh H, et al. Treatment of recurrent gynaecologic malignancies with a new camptothecin derivative. *Eur J Cancer* 1992;28:613.

102. Takeuchi S, Takamizawa H, Takeda Y, et al. Clinical study of CPT-11, camptothecin derivative, on gynecological malignancy. *Proc Am Soc Clin Oncol* 1991;10:A617.

103. Noda K, et al. Late phase II study of CPT-11, new camptothecin derivative, in cervical and ovarian carcinoma. *Proceedings of the 13th World Congress of Gynecology and Obstetrics (FIGO)* 1991;271:A936.

104. Takeuchi S, Dobashi I, Fujimoto S, et al. A late phase II study of CPT-11 on uterine cervical cancer and ovarian cancer. *Jpn J Cancer Chemother* 1991;18:1681–1689.

105. Gandia D, Abigerges D, Armand JP, et al. CPT-11 induced cholinergic effects in cancer patients. *J Clin Oncol* 1993;11:196–197.

106. Sugiyama T, Nishida T, Ushijima K, et al. Irinotecan hydrochloride (CPT-11) combined with cisplatin (CDDP) in patients with relapsed or metastatic ovarian cancer. *Proc Am Soc Clin Oncol* 1996;15:A796.

107. Verschraegen CF, Natelson E, Giovanella B, et al. Phase I study of oral 9-nitrocamptothecin (9NC). *Proc Am Soc Clin Oncol* 1996;15:A1532.

108. Lund B, Kristjansen PE, Hansen HH. Clinical and preclinical activity of 2′,2′-difluorodeoxycytidine (gemcitabine). *Cancer Treat Rev* 1993;19:45–55.

109. Lund B, Hansen OP, Theilade K, et al. Phase II study of gemcitabine (2′,2′-difluorodeoxycytidine) in previously treated ovarian cancer patients. *J Natl Cancer Inst* 1994;86:1530–1533.

110. Lund B, Hansen OP, Neijt JP, et al. Phase II study of gemcitabine in previously platinum treated ovarian cancer patients. *Anticancer Drugs* 1995;6(suppl 6):61–62.

111. Millward MJ, Rischin D, Toner GC, et al. Activity of gemcitabine in ovarian cancer patients resistant to paclitaxel. *Proc Am Soc Clin Oncol* 1995;14:A776.

112. Martin C, Lund B, Anderson H, et al. Gemcitabine: once-weekly schedule active and better tolerated than twice-weekly schedule. *Anticancer Drugs* 1996;7:351–357.

CHAPTER 34

Rare Malignant Tumors of the Ovary

DAMRONG TRESUKOSOL
HAROLD FOX

*I*n this chapter the clinical and therapeutic aspects of nonepithelial tumors of the ovary are discussed, albeit only briefly and in very general outline form. Because of their relative rarity, diagnosis of these neoplasms is rarely made preoperatively and, in most instances, the tumor is only correctly identified on histopathologic examination of the resected specimen. Hence, primary intraoperative evaluation of the extent and spread of the disease is often inadequate.

The pathogenesis and pathology of those nonepithelial tumors of specifically gonadal type are discussed in Chapters 29 and 30 and are not reiterated here.

Malignant Sex Cord–Stromal Tumors

Granulosa Cell Tumors

Granulosa cell tumors account for a majority of malignant sex cord–stromal tumors but are rare in absolute terms and comprise only 1% to 3% of all ovarian neoplasms (1–3). They occur over a wide age range, from newborns to old age, but approximately 40% of granulosa cell tumors occur after the menopause, with only a very small proportion occurring before puberty (4). It should be noted that although granulosa cell tumors may be of either adult or childhood type, this distinction is made, as discussed in Chapter 30, on the basis of their histologic features and not on the age at which they occur. In this account the term *granulosa cell tumor*,

unless otherwise specified, applies solely to the adult type.

Diagnosis

Most patients present either with nonspecific tumor symptoms such as awareness of an abdominal mass, abdominal pain, abdominal distension, or bloating or with symptoms related to the endocrine activity of the functioning ovarian tumor, or both (1,3,4). Occasionally, granulosa cell tumors present as an acute abdomen due to internal tumor hemorrhage or rupture of a cystic neoplasm.

Granulosa cell tumors are usually estrogenic and their most striking symptoms in premenopausal women are menstrual disorders such as menometrorrhagia, oligomenorrhea, or secondary amenorrhea. Under these circumstances the ovarian tumors are often missed at the initial presentation (1,3), though this problem will diminish as transvaginal sonography, which can detect nonpalpable adnexal masses, is progressively incorporated into the routine investigation of aberrant bleeding patterns. When granulosa cell tumors occur in prepubertal girls, about 75% of them experience isosexual precocious puberty with the development of secondary sex characteristics. In postmenopausal patients vaginal bleeding is common and is due to estrogenic stimulation of the endometrium, stimulation that can result in endometrial hyperplasia or carcinoma. The reported frequency of associated endometrial hyperplasia has ranged from 32% to 85% (4–10), while that of accompanying endometrial carcinoma has varied from 3% to 22% with an average of about 10% (1,4,5,7–12). The endocrine-related endometrial carcinomas are usually well differentiated, are often confined to the endometrium, and have little potential for causing death. It is of interest that patients in Thailand with granulosa cell tumors have a much lower incidence of associated endometrial hyperplasia and adenocarcinoma than do similar women in Western countries. This may be related to the slender body configuration among Asian women who, as a group, have a strikingly low incidence of endometrial carcinoma.

Although the vast majority of granulosa cell neoplasms are estrogenic, a small minority are androgenic (13,14) and patients with such neoplasms will present with symptoms and signs related to masculinization and defeminization.

An elevated serum level of inhibin, a nonsteroidal polypeptide hormone secreted by most granulosa cell tumors, has been proposed as a diagnostic tumor marker for these neoplasms (15–18) but there have been reports denying the specificity of this substance, which, it is claimed, is also secreted by many other ovarian neoplasms (19,20). Nevertheless, even if such claims are confirmed, serum inhibin levels will retain their important role as a marker for detection of tumor recurrence, though more information will probably have to be acquired before the determination of inhibin levels becomes a routine part of clinical practice.

Principles of Treatment

Early Disease Most granulosa cell tumors are diagnosed at an early stage because their presence is heralded by the development of hormonally induced symptoms (1,3,4,9,10,21–24) and surgery is, in such cases, the mainstay of treatment. Many patients present with unilateral tumors confined to the ovary, and in these patients surgical excision as a sole treatment seems to be adequate; there is no compelling necessity for, or proven benefit of, adjuvant therapy (9,24–26). Young patients with stage Ia tumors who wish to retain their fertility and have been adequately staged may be treated by unilateral salpingo-oophorectomy (10) but in all other patients a hysterectomy and bilateral salpingo-oophorectomy is the procedure of

choice. Because of the relative rarity of this type of tumor, however, data concerning the natural pattern of spread or sites and frequency of occult metastasis are not available (24,25). A complete staging procedure is therefore warranted if only to serve as a basis for better defining the natural history of these tumors and the value of surgical staging.

All granulosa cell tumors should be regarded as having a potential for recurrence or metastasis, but attempts have been made to define prognostic factors that could identify the stage I neoplasms that pose the highest risk of recurrence. Adverse prognostic factors that have been defined include large tumor size, bilateral involvement, intra-abdominal rupture of cyst wall, nuclear atypia, and a high mitotic rate (4,8,24,27–29). The prognostic significance of aneuploidy has been disputed (30–33) but there has been wide agreement that the histologic pattern of the neoplasm is of no predictive value (34). The delineation of these risk factors has been largely based on retrospective studies with a multitude of confounding factors and their validity as independent indicators of a poor prognosis has not been firmly established (24). Nevertheless, postoperative adjuvant treatment has been advocated for patients with one or more of the risk factors mentioned, even though it is not known with any degree of certainty whether any form of postoperative treatment results in improvement in disease-free interval or overall survival (26). Both platinum-based chemotherapy (3,35) and anticancer hormonal therapy (36) have had their proponents as adjuvant therapy in patients with multiple risk factors for tumor recurrence but radiation is considered less attractive because there is no good evidence that it conveys any benefit (8,37). Long-term surveillance is necessary after primary treatment is completed, for the natural history of granulosa cell tumors is a prolonged and indolent one with recurrences occurring late, many more than 10 years and some more than 20 years after the initial treatment (4,24,25,38).

Advanced and Recurrent Disease In patients with advanced or recurrent disease it is generally recommended that initial debulking surgery should be done to remove, if feasible, the primary tumor and its metastatic deposits, although there are no supporting data that identify the volume of residual tumor as an adverse prognostic factor. Platinum-based chemotherapy is currently widely used (39–41) and the highest response rates have been reported using a vinblastine, bleomycin, and cisplatin combination (42,43). Unfortunately, the reported chemotherapeutic trials recruited only a small number of patients and follow-up time was too short to be able to draw any conclusions regarding any improvement of long-term survival. Further, any responses obtained usually were of short duration and most patients with advanced or recurrent disease eventually died. Responses have been obtained with both paclitaxel and a gonadotropin-releasing hormone agonist in patients with metastatic or recurrent granulosa cell tumor (44,45) but too few patients have been studied for any clear-cut role for these agents to be defined.

Juvenile Granulosa Cell Tumor

Only about 5% of granulosa cell tumors are of this type, which occurs predominantly, but not solely, in the first two decades of life (46). The vast majority of tumors are in stage I at the time of the initial diagnosis and require treatment only by salpingo-oophorectomy (7). Only a small proportion of juvenile granulosa cell tumors metastasize (47) and those that do behave in a malignant fashion either are at an advanced stage at the time of diagnosis or recur within 2 years of the original treatment, the protracted course of adult-type granulosa tumors not being a feature of these neoplasms. Too few patients with recurrent or advanced disease have been treated to give any data about the type or value of chemotherapy in these circumstances, but the prognosis is generally poor (45).

Sertoli-Leydig Cell Tumors

Sertoli-Leydig cell tumors are rare and occur most frequently between the ages of 20 and 30 years, with fewer than 5% occurring in prepubertal girls (48). They are usually androgenic and patients commonly present with evidence of progressive masculinization such as hirsutism, temporal balding, deepening of the voice, and enlargement of the clitoris. Secondary amenorrhea and breast atrophy are manifestations of defeminization (49).

However, occasional Sertoli-Leydig cell tumors are estrogenic and some are endocrinologically inert.

Principles of Treatment

Sertoli-Leydig cell tumors are, for the most part, considered to be neoplasms of only low malignancy and treatment generally follows the same guidelines as described for granulosa cell tumors. Surgery seems to be adequate treatment and removal of the tumor will halt, but not fully reverse, the masculinizing process (26,50). Since most Sertoli-Leydig tumors occur in women of reproductive age, conservation with unilateral salpingo-oophorectomy is justified. Adjuvant chemotherapy is clearly indicated if there is evidence of extraovarian extension, whereas a case can be made for considering such treatment for stage I tumors thought to be at increased risk of recurrence, namely, those that are poorly differentiated, show extensive areas of a retiform pattern, or contain heterologous muscle or cartilage (51). There are, however, no data to suggest that adjuvant therapy is of any value in preventing recurrence in stage I patients and the rarity of advanced or recurrent disease makes it impossible to have sufficient data to propose any chemotherapeutic regimen of choice.

Sertoli Cell Tumor

Pure Sertoli cell tumors of the ovary are extremely rare; they tend to occur in young patients and are commonly estrogenic, though about 20% are either androgenic or endocrinologically inactive. They are almost invariably benign but there has been one reported example of a neoplasm of this type that evolved into a fatal adenocarcinoma (52). Conservative fertility-sparing surgery is adequate treatment and adjuvant therapy is not indicated in the absence of any histologic evidence of frank malignant change (50).

Hilus Cell Tumors

Hilus cell tumors are rare virilizing ovarian neoplasms usually found in perimenopausal or postmenopausal women. Most of the tumors are unilateral and often of insufficient size to present as a palpable mass. The presence of symptoms or signs of a virilization syndrome usually initiates a thorough endocrinologic investigation, though measurement of circulating hormones may provide only evidence of testosterone overproduction. In the absence of a palpable mass the detection and localization of a hormone-producing tumor of this type often depends on the use of magnetic resonance or computed tomography. Even these imaging techniques are not always successful if the neoplasm is extremely small and in some patients a blind exploratory laparotomy has to be undertaken (53). Venous sampling of both the ovarian vein and adrenal vein for hormonal profile measurement may be helpful for disclosing tumor location (54), but if all else fails, surgical removal of both apparently normal ovaries may have to be considered. These neoplasms are usually benign and only exceptional ones have pursued a malignant course. Surgery alone is, therefore, the treatment of choice and adjuvant therapy is not indicated.

Malignant Germ Cell Tumors

Despite their varied nature, malignant ovarian germ cell neoplasms can be considered a single entity in clinical terms. They occur predominantly in the first three decades of life and patients usually present with nonspecific tumor symptoms, such as abdominal pain or awareness of a pelvic mass (55); tumors that contain trophoblastic elements, such as choriocarcinomas and some dysgerminomas, may, depending on the age of the patient, cause precocious isosexual puberty, breast enlargement, or menstrual irregularities.

Patients with germ cell neoplasms can be monitored for a number of tumor markers, including α-fetoprotein (AFP), human chorionic gonadotropin (hCG), and lactic acid dehydrogenase (LDH) isoenzymes. These not only are of diagnostic value but also will, in many cases, serve to monitor the response to treatment and aid in the detection of subclinical recurrence.

About 60% to 70% of germ cell tumors will be stage I at the time of initial diagnosis, most of the remainder being stage III (55). In the past most of these neoplasms proved to be highly malignant and were associated with very high death rates, but with current therapeutic techniques excellent long-term survival rates are now being obtained (56).

Principles of Treatment

Stage I Disease

It is generally agreed that unilateral salpingo-oophorectomy with adequate staging is the correct initial treatment for patients with early-stage disease (55–57). It has also been widely accepted that postoperative adjuvant therapy is not indicated for patients with a completely resected grade 1 malignant teratoma and that it is safe for these patients to be carefully followed by clinical assessment, radiology, and measurement of tumor markers (58). There has been considerable debate as to whether a similar approach should be adopted for stage I dysgerminomas (26,59) but it has been usual to use adjuvant therapy for all other stage I malignant germ cell neoplasms (60,61). However, this policy was recently questioned, and excellent results have been achieved by following a surveillance policy for all patients with resected stage I malignant germ cell tumors, chemotherapy only being given when evidence of recurrent or metastatic disease emerges (62).

Advanced or Recurrent Disease

The role of surgery in advanced or recurrent disease is questionable, for there is no clear-cut evidence that debulking improves the prognosis, there being only a suggestion that such surgery, if successful, is associated with a higher response rate to chemotherapy (26). In the past radiotherapy was the treatment of choice for patients with advanced-stage or recurrent dysgerminoma whereas chemotherapy was administered for all other malignant germ cell neoplasms that were at a high stage or had recurred. There is now, however, an increasing tendency for all patients to be treated by chemotherapy irrespective of tumor type. Dysgerminoma is usually treated with the same chemotherapeutic regime as that used for testicular seminoma, namely, etoposide and cisplatin (63), though single-agent carboplatin has also been recommended (64,65). Other malignant germ cell neoplasms are currently treated with bleomycin, etoposide, and cisplatin (BEP) (56,61,66) or with a POMB/ACE regimen (67). The value of second-look laparotomy in the management of recurrent or high-stage malignant germ cell tumors is controversial and remains a subject for debate (56,68).

Ovarian Sarcoma

The term *sarcoma* is used here to denote an ovarian tumor that is formed either wholly or partially of malignant cells of mesenchymal origin, these constituting less than 3% of all ovarian neoplasms (69). Their rarity and heterogeneity make diagnosis and treatment difficult whereas their inherent complexity has been compounded by complex classifications. It is probably simplest to consider ovarian sarcomas as being either müllerian or nonmüllerian in nature. In many patients the müllerian sarcomas, which comprise endometrioid stromal sarcoma (70,71) and carcinosarcoma (72–75) (the latter often misleadingly known as *mixed mesodermal sarcoma* or *malignant mixed mesenchymal tumor*), probably arise from foci of ovarian endometriosis, though the carcinosarcomas, which occur predominantly in elderly women, may also be considered a form of endometrioid neoplasia, a view strengthened by the increasing evidence that they are metaplastic carcinomas rather than true sarcomas (76–78). Nonmüllerian sarcomas, such as chondrosarcoma, fibrosarcoma, rhabdomyosarcoma, liposarcoma, and leiomyosarcoma (79–84), all of which are very rare, are usually derived from mesenchymal components of the ovary that are not committed to the specific gonadal function of the organ. However, occasional cases arise in teratomas, in the heterologous components of a Sertoli-Leydig cell tumor, or in the wall of a cystic epithelial neoplasm (81,85–88).

Principles of Treatment

Many nonmüllerian sarcomas of the ovary form a discrete mass that, in contrast to soft tissue sarcomas arising in sites elsewhere, allows for a possible complete tumor resection. Hence, the initial treatment of these neoplasms is radical surgery. Adjuvant radiation or combined chemotherapy, or both, are generally recommended for stage I tumors and are mandatory for those patients with extraovarian spread of the disease. However, the prognosis is generally very poor.

The primary approach to primary endometrioid stromal sarcomas of the ovary is also surgical. If the patient is menopausal or postmenopausal, a hysterectomy with bilateral salpingo-oophorectomy is the treatment of choice and, because of the high frequency of bilateral ovarian involvement and the possibility of synchronous or subsequent uterine endometrial stromal sarcoma, a similar approach may be optimal even for younger women (89). Both progesterone and radiation therapy have been used for residual or recurrent disease but it is extremely difficult to assess the value of such treatment insofar as these tumors are of low-grade malignancy and typically run a very indolent course; patients with untreated residual disease may remain well for many years and in some the extraovarian lesions appear to regress spontaneously.

Carcinosarcomas have, in general, an extremely poor prognosis and most have spread beyond the ovary at the time of initial diagnosis. Aggressive surgery is generally recommended as the most appropriate treatment (1,69,90) and postoperative adjunctive combined chemotherapy, using varied regimens, has achieved objective responses (72,90–92). Recently, carcinosarcomas were shown to respond to platinum-based regimens in a manner similar to high-grade epithelial ovarian carcinoma (93,94). The overall response rate to this form of therapy has been impressive but the impact on survival is still doubtful. Prognostic factors, apart from stage, have not been specifically defined for ovarian carcinosarcomas but a relatively prolonged survival time has been noted in patients with completely resected tumors that were positive for estrogen receptors (95). It is probable, however, that prognostic factors defined for uterine carcinosarcomas also apply to those occurring in an ovarian site. Predominant among these, again apart from stage, are the grade and histologic type of the epithelial component (96).

Malignant Lymphoma

A lymphoma is one of the rarest tumors of the ovary. Most examples of ovarian lymphoma, which is nearly always of the non-Hodgkin's type, represent ovarian involvement in overt or covert systemic disease (97,98) but there has been considerable debate as to whether a lymphoma can arise as a primary tumor of the ovary. The theoretical possibility of such a neoplasm arising de novo in the ovary certainly exists, for it was recently shown that, contrary to previously held views, lymphoid aggregates are not uncommon in otherwise normal ovaries (98). The minimal criteria, which are rarely if ever met, for the recognition of a primary lymphoma of the ovary include extensive search for systemic disease and a disease-free interval of at least 5 years following treatment of the ovarian lesion by surgery alone (97–100).

Patients with lymphomas localized mainly, or apparently solely, to one ovary may experience abdominal symptoms but the neoplasms are often discovered incidentally on clinical examination or during surgery for unrelated conditions. A correct diagnosis is usually only attained by histopathologic examination and the tumor should then be staged, preferably using the Ann Arbor, rather than the International Federation of Gynecology and Obstetrics (FIGO), staging system (97,101). Unilateral surgical resection is considered the correct approach for tumors apparently localized to the ovary (99), and because ovarian lymphoma should always be considered for therapeutic purposes as a localized manifestation of a systemic disease, surgery should be followed by systemic chemotherapy of a type appropriate to the form of lymphoma. With this treatment patients with lymphoma of this type have an appreciable survival advantage when compared to those with obvious systemic lymphoma (98). In the more common situation in which ovarian involvement is clearly a component of a systemic lymphoma, surgical removal of the pelvic mass seems to have little impact on subsequent treatment. In this form of the disease the prognosis is based on the cell type and the stage of the disease (98,101).

REFERENCES

1. DiSaia PJ, Creasman WT. *Clinical gynecologic oncology.* 4th ed. St Louis: Mosby Year Book, 1994:445–457.

2. Jones HW III. Sex cord-stromal tumors of the ovary. In: Jones HW III, Wentz AC, Burnett LS, eds. *Novak's textbook of gynecology.* 11th ed. Baltimore: Williams & Wilkins, 1988:849–862.

3. Segal R, DePetrillo AD, Thomas G. Clinical review of adult granulosa cell tumors of the ovary. *Gynecol Oncol* 1995;56:338–344.

4. Fox H, Agrawal K, Langley FA. A clinicopathologic study of 92 cases of granulosa cell tumor of the ovary with special reference to the factors influencing prognosis. *Cancer* 1975;35:231–241.

5. Busby T, Anderson GA. Feminizing mesenchymomas of the ovary: includes 107 cases of granulosa-, granulosa-theca-, and theca-cell tumors. *Am J Obstet Gynecol* 1954;68:1391–1417.

6. Salerno IJ. Feminizing mesenchymomas of the ovary: an analysis of 28 granulosa-thecal cell tumors and their relationship to co-existent carcinoma. *Am J Obstet Gynecol* 1962;84:731–737.

7. Norris HJ, Taylor HB. Prognosis of granulosa-theca cell tumors of the ovary. *Cancer* 1968;21:255–263.

8. Stenwig JT, Hazekamp JT, Beechman JB. Granulosa cell tumors of the ovary: a clinicopathological study of 118 cases with long term follow-up. *Gynecol Oncol* 1979;7:136–152.

9. Evans AT, Gaffey TA, Malkasian GD, Annegers JF. Clinicopathologic review of 118 granulosa and theca cell tumors. *Obstet Gynecol* 1980;55:231–238.

10. Pautier P, Lhomme C, Culine S, et al. Adult granulosa cell tumor of the ovary: a retrospective study of 45 cases. *Int J Gynecol Cancer* 1997;7:58–65.

11. Greene JW Jr. Feminizing mesenchymomas (granulosa and theca cell tumors) with associated endometrial carcinoma: review of the literature and a study of the material of the Ovarian Tumor Registry. *Am J Obstet Gynecol* 1957;74:31–41.

12. Gusberg SB, Kardon P. Proliferative endometrial response to theca-granulosa cell tumors. *Am J Obstet Gynecol* 1971;111:633–643.

13. Norris HJ, Taylor HB. Virilization associated with cystic granulosa cell tumors. *Obstet Gynecol* 1969;34:629–635.

14. Nakashima N, Young RH, Scully RE. Androgenic granulosa cell tumors of the ovary. A clinicopathologic analysis of 17 cases and review of the literature. *Arch Pathol Lab Med* 1984;108:786–791.

15. Lappohn RE, Burger HG, Bouma J, et al. Inhibin as a marker for granulosa cell tumor. *Acta Obstet Gynecol Scand Suppl* 1992;155:61–65.

16. Jobling T, Mamers P, Healy DL, et al. A prospective study of inhibin in granulosa cell tumors of the ovary. *Gynecol Oncol* 1994;55:285–289.

17. Flemming P, Wellmann A, Maschek H, et al. Monoclonal antibodies against inhibin represent key markers of adult granulosa cell tumors of the ovary even in their metastases. A report of three cases with late metastasis, being previously

misinterpreted as hemangiopericytoma. *Am J Surg Pathol* 1995;19:927–933.

18. Cook I, O'Brien M, Charnock M, et al. Inhibin as a marker for ovarian cancer. *Br J Cancer* 1995; 71:1046–1050.

19. Bremmer WJ. Inhibin: from hypothesis to clinical application. *N Engl J Med* 1989;321:790–793.

20. Healy DL, Burger HG, Manners P, et al. Elevated serum inhibin concentrations in postmenopausal women with ovarian tumors. *N Engl J Med* 1993;329:1539–1542.

21. Schweppe K-W, Beller FK. Clinical data on granulosa cell tumors. *J Cancer Res Clin Oncol* 1982;104:161–169.

22. Scharl A, Vierbuchen M, Kusche M, Bolte A. Zur Klinik und Prognose von Granulosazelltumoren des Ovars. *Geburtshilfe Frauenheilk* 1988;48: 567–573.

23. Petru E, Pickel H, Heydarfadal M, et al. Experience with stromal tumors and germ-cell tumors of the ovary. *Int J Gynecol Cancer* 1991;1:9–14.

24. Malmstrom H, Hogberg T, Risberg B, Simonsen E. Granulosa cell tumors of the ovary: prognostic factors and outcome. *Gynecol Oncol* 1994;52:50–55.

25. Kietlinska Z, Pietrzak K, Drabik M. The management of granulosa-cell tumors of the ovary based on long term follow up. *Eur J Gynecol Oncol* 1993;14:118–127.

26. Williams SD, Sutton GP. Non-epithelial ovarian cancer. In: Shingleton HM, Fowler WC Jr, Jordan JA, Lawrence WD, eds. *Gynecologic oncology: current diagnosis and treatment*. London: Saunders, 1996:224–233.

27. Bjorkholm E, Silfversward C. Prognostic factors in granulosa-cell tumors. *Gynecol Oncol* 1981; 11:261–274.

28. Suh KS, Silverberg SG, Rhame JG, Wilkinson DS. Granulosa cell tumor of the ovary. *Arch Pathol Lab Med* 1990;114:496–501.

29. King LA, Okagaki T, Gallup DH, et al. Mitotic count, nuclear atypia, and immunohistochemical determination of Ki-67, c-myc, p21-ras, c-erbB2, and p53 expression in granulosa cell tumors of the ovary: mitotic count and Ki-67 are indicators of poor prognosis. *Gynecol Oncol* 1996;61: 227–232.

30. Klemi PJ, Joensuu H, Salmi T. Prognostic value of flow cytometric DNA content analysis in granulosa cell tumor of the ovary. *Cancer* 1990;65: 1189–1193.

31. Suh K-S, Silverberg SG, Rhame JG, Wilkinson DS. Granulosa cell tumor of the ovary: histopathologic and flow cytometric analysis with clinical correlation. *Arch Pathol Lab Med* 1990; 114:496–501.

32. Holland DR, Le Riche J, Swenerton KD, et al. Flow cytometric assessment of DNA ploidy is a useful prognostic factor for patients with granulosa cell ovarian tumors. *Int J Gynecol Cancer* 1991;1:227–232.

33. Palmquist-Evans M, Webb MJ, Gaffey TA, et al. DNA ploidy of ovarian granulosa cell tumors: lack of correlation between DNA index or proliferative index and outcome in 40 patients. *Cancer* 1995;75:2295–2298.

34. Fox H, Buckley CH. Pathology of malignant gonadal stromal tumors of ovary. In: Coppleson M, ed. *Gynecologic oncology*. 2nd ed. Edinburgh: Churchill Livingstone, 1992:947–959.

35. Gershenson DM. Management of early ovarian cancer: germ cell and sex cord-stromal tumors. *Gynecol Oncol* 1994;55:S62–S72.

36. Kauppila A, Bangah M, Burger H, Martikainen H. GnRH agonist analog therapy in advanced/recurrent granulosa cell tumors: further evidence of a role of inhibin in monitoring response to treatment. *Gynecol Endocrinol* 1992;6:271–274.

37. Pankratz E, Boyes DA, White GW, et al. Granulosa cell tumors: a clinical review of 61 cases. *Am J Obstet Gynecol* 1978;52:718–723.

38. Kohlstad P. *Clinical gynecologic oncology: the Norwegian experience*. Oslo: Norwegian University Press, 1986.

39. Gershenson DM, Copeland LJ, Kavanagh JJ, et al. Treatment of metastatic stromal tumors of the ovary with cisplatin, doxorubicin, and cyclophosphamide. *Obstet Gynecol* 1987;70:765–768.

40. Muntz HG, Goff BA, Fuller AF. Recurrent ovarian granulosa cell tumor: role of combination chemotherapy with report of a long term response to a cyclophosphamide, doxorubicin and cisplatin regimen. *Eur J Gynecol Oncol* 1990;11:263–268.

41. Pectasides D, Alevizakos N, Athanassiou AE. Cisplatin-containing regimen in advanced or recurrent granulosa cell tumours of the ovary. *Ann Oncol* 1992;3:316–318.

42. Colombo N, Sessa C, Landoni F, et al. Cisplatin, vinblastine, and bleomycin combination chemotherapy in metastatic granulosa cell tumor

of the ovary. *Obstet Gynecol* 1986;67:265–268.

43. Zambetti M, Escoebedo A, Pilotti S, De Palo G. Cisplatinum/vinblastine/bleomycin combination chemotherapy in advanced or recurrent granulosa cell tumors of the ovary. *Gynecol Oncol* 1990;36:317–320.

44. Tresukosol D, Kudelka AP, Edwards CL, et al. Recurrent ovarian granulosa cell tumor: a case report of a dramatic response to taxol. *Int J Gynecol Cancer* 1995;5:156–159.

45. Martikainen H, Penttinen J, Huhtaniemi I, Kauppila A. Gonadotropin-releasing hormone agonist analog therapy effective in ovarian granulosa cell malignancy. *Gynecol Oncol* 1988;35:406–408.

46. Young RH, Dickersin RG, Scully RE. Juvenile granulosa cell tumor of the ovary. A clinicopathological analysis of 125 cases. *Am J Surg Pathol* 1984;8:575–596.

47. Powell JL, Johnson NA, Bailey CL, Otis CN. Management of advanced juvenile granulosa cell tumor of the ovary. *Gynecol Oncol* 1993;48:119–123.

48. Jones W. Sex cord-stromal tumors of the ovary. In: Markman M, Hoskins WJ, eds. *Cancer of the ovary.* New York: Raven, 1993:385–405.

49. Larsen WG, Felmar EA, Wallace ME, Frieder R. Sertoli-Leydig cell tumor of the ovary: a rare cause of amenorrhea. *Obstet Gynecol* 1992;79:831–833.

50. Hoskins WJ, Rubin SC. Malignant gonadal stromal tumors of ovary: clinical features and management. In: Coppleson M, ed. *Gynecologic oncology.* 2nd ed. Edinburgh: Churchill Livingstone, 1992:961–970.

51. Young RH, Scully RE. Ovarian Sertoli-Leydig cell tumors: a clinicopathologic analysis of 207 cases. *Am J Surg Pathol* 1985;9:543–569.

52. Young RH, Scully RE. Ovarian Sertoli cell tumors: a report of 10 cases. *Int J Gynecol Pathol* 1984;2:349–463.

53. Dunn S. Bilateral virilizing hilus (Leydig) cell tumors of the ovary. *Acta Obstet Gynecol Scand* 1994;73:76–77.

54. Surrey ES, Ziegler D, Gambone JC, Judd HL. Preoperative localization of androgen-secreting tumors: clinical, endocrinologic, and radiologic evaluation of ten patients. *Am J Obstet Gynecol* 1988;158:1313–1322.

55. Gershenson DM. Malignant germ cell tumors of ovary: clinical features and management. In: Coppleson M, ed. *Gynecologic oncology.* 2nd ed. Edinburgh: Churchill Livingstone, 1992:935–945.

56. Curtin JP, Morrow CP, D'Ablaing G, Schlaerth JB. Malignant germ cell tumors of the ovary: 20 year report of LAC-USC Womens Hospital. *Int J Gynecol Cancer* 1994;4:29–35.

57. Peccatori F, Bonazzi C, Chiari S, et al. Surgical management of malignant ovarian germ cell tumors: 10 years' experience of 129 patients. *Obstet Gynecol* 1995;86:367–372.

58. Gershenson DM. Management of early ovarian cancer: germ cell and sex cord-stromal tumors. *Gynecol Oncol* 1994;55:S62–S72.

59. Thomas GM, Dembo AJ, Hacker NF, Depetrillo AD. Current therapy for dysgerminoma of the ovary. *Obstet Gynecol* 1987;70:268–275.

60. Williams SD. Chemotherapy of ovarian germ cell tumors. *Hematol Oncol Clin North Am* 1991;5:1261–1269.

61. Williams SD, Blessing JA, Liao S-Y, et al. Adjuvant therapy of ovarian germ cell tumors with cisplatin, etoposide, and bleomycin: a trial of the Gynecologic Oncology Group. *J Clin Oncol* 1994;12:701–706.

62. Dark GG, Bower M, Newlands ES, et al. Surveillance policy for stage 1 ovarian germ cell tumours. *J Clin Oncol* 1997;15:620–624.

63. Mencel PJ, Motzer RJ, Mazumdar M, et al. Advanced seminoma: treatment results, survival and prognostic factors in 142 patients. *J Clin Oncol* 1994;12:120–126.

64. Oliver RTD, Edmonds PM, Ong JYH, et al. Pilot studies of 2 and 1 course carboplatin as adjuvant for stage I seminoma: should it be tested in a randomized trial against radiotherapy? *Int J Radiat Oncol Biol Phys* 1994;29:3–8.

65. Horwich A, Dearnaley DP, Duchesne GM, et al. Simple non-toxic treatment of advanced metastatic seminoma with carboplatin. *J Clin Oncol* 1989;7:1150–1156.

66. Segelov E, Campbell J, Ng M, et al. Cisplatin-based chemotherapy for ovarian germ cell malignancies: the Australian experience. *J Clin Oncol* 1994;12:378–384.

67. Bower M, Fife K, Holden L, et al. Chemotherapy for ovarian germ cell tumours. *Eur J Cancer* 1996;32a:593–597.

68. Gershenson DM, Copeland LJ, Del Junco G, et al. Second look laparotomy in the management of malignant germ cell tumors of the ovary. *Obstet Gynecol* 1986;67:789–793.

69. Disaia PJ, Pecorelli S. Gynecological sarcomas. *Semin Surg Oncol* 1994;10:369–373.

70. Silverberg SG, Nogales F. Endolymphatic stromal myosis of the ovary: a report of three cases and literature review. *Gynecol Oncol* 1981; 12:129–138.

71. Young RH, Prat J, Scully RE. Endometrioid stromal sarcomas of the ovary: a clinicopathologic analysis of 23 cases. *Cancer* 1984;53: 1143–1155.

72. Hanjani P, Petersen RO, Lipton SE, Nolte SA. Malignant mixed mesodermal tumors and carcinosarcoma of the ovary: report of eight cases and review of the literature. *Obstet Gynecol Surv* 1983;38:537–545.

73. Dictor M. Malignant mixed mesodermal tumor of the ovary: a report of 22 cases. *Obstet Gynecol* 1985;65:720–724.

74. Dinh TV, Slavin RE, Bhagavan BS, et al. Mixed mesodermal tumors of the ovary: a clinicopathologic study of 14 cases. *Obstet Gynecol* 1988;72:409–412.

75. Pfeiffer P, Hardt-Madsen M, Rex S, et al. Malignant mixed müllerian tumors of the ovary: report of 13 cases. *Acta Obstet Gynecol Scand* 1991;70:79–84.

76. George E, Manivel JC, Dehner LP, Wick MR. Malignant mixed müllerian tumors: an immunohistochemical study of 47 cases, with histogenetic considerations and clinical correlation. *Hum Pathol* 1991;22:215–223.

77. de Brito PA, Silverberg SG, Orenstein JM. Carcinosarcoma (malignant mixed müllerian (mesodermal) tumor) of the female genital tract: immunohistochemical and ultrastructural analysis of 28 cases. *Hum Pathol* 1993;24:132–142.

78. Emeto M, Iwasaki H, Kikuchi M, Shirakawa K. Characteristics of cloned cells of mixed müllerian tumors of the uterus: carcinoma cells showing myogenic differentiation in vitro. *Cancer* 1993;71:3065–3075.

79. Prat J, Scully RE. Cellular fibromas and fibrosarcomas of the ovary: a comparative clinicopathologic analysis of seventeen cases. *Cancer* 1981;47:2663–2670.

80. Guerard MJ, Arguelles MA, Ferenczy A. Rhabdomyosarcoma of the ovary: ultrastructural study of a case and review of the literature. *Gynecol Oncol* 1983;15:325–339.

81. Shafeh SM, Woodruff JD. Primary ovarian sarcomas: report of 46 cases and review of the literature. *Obstet Gynecol Surv* 1984;42:331–349.

82. Friedman HD, Mazur MT. Primary ovarian leiomyosarcoma: an immunohistochemical and ultrastructural study. *Arch Pathol Lab Med* 1991; 115:941–945.

83. Monk BJ, Nieberg R, Berek JS. Primary leiomyosarcoma of the ovary in a perimenarchal female. *Gynecol Oncol* 1993;48:389–393.

84. Stellato G, Bonito MD, Tramontana S. Primary fibrosarcoma of the ovary. *Acta Obstet Gynecol Scand* 1995;74:649–652.

85. Prat J, Scully RE. Sarcomas in ovarian mucinous tumors: a report of two cases. *Cancer* 1979; 44:1327–1331.

86. De Nictolis M, di Loreto C, Clinti S, Prat J. Fibrosarcomatous mural nodule in an ovarian mucinous cystadenoma. *Surg Pathol* 1990;3: 309–315.

87. Tsujimura T, Kawano K. Rhabdomyosarcoma coexistent with ovarian mucinous cystadenocarcinoma: a case report. *Int J Gynecol Pathol* 1992;11:58–62.

88. Rahilly MA, Candlish W, Al-Nafussi A. Fibrosarcoma arising in an ovarian mucinous tumor: a case report. *Int J Gynecol Cancer* 1994;4: 211–214.

89. Russell P, Bannatyne P, Solomon HJ. Malignant müllerian and miscellaneous mesenchymal tumors of ovary ("ovarian sarcomas"). In: Coppleson M, ed. *Gynecologic oncology.* 2nd ed. Edinburgh: Churchill Livingstone, 1992:971–986.

90. Prendiville J, Murphy D, Renninson J, et al. Carcinosarcoma of the ovary treated over a 10-year period at the Christie Hospital. *Int J Gynecol Cancer* 1994;4:200–205.

91. Lele SB, Piver MS, Barlow JJ. Chemotherapy in management of mixed mesodermal tumors of the ovary. *Gynecol Oncol* 1980;10:298–302.

92. Morrow CP, D'Ablaing G, Brady LW, et al. A clinical and pathological study of 30 cases of malignant müllerian epithelial and mesenchymal ovarian tumors: a Gynecologic Oncology Group study. *Gynecol Oncol* 1984;18:278–292.

93. Anderson WA, Young DE, Peters WA, et al. Platinum-based combination chemotherapy for malignant mixed mesodermal tumors of the ovary. *Gynecol Oncol* 1989;32:319–322.

94. Bicher A, Levenback C, Silva EG, et al. Ovarian malignant mixed müllerian tumors treated with platinum-based chemotherapy. *Obstet Gynecol* 1995;85:735–739.

95. Geisler JP, Wiemann MC, Miller GA, et al. Estrogen and progesterone receptors in malignant mixed mesodermal tumors of the ovary. *J Surg Oncol* 1995;59:45–47.

96. Silverberg SG, Major FJ, Blessing JA, et al. Carcinosarcoma (malignant mixed mesodermal tumor) of the uterus: a Gynecologic Oncology Group pathologic study of 203 cases. *Int J Gynecol Pathol* 1990;9:1–19.

97. Fox H, Langley FA, Govan ADT, et al. Malignant lymphoma presenting as ovarian tumor: a clinicopathologic analysis of 34 cases. *Br J Obstet Gynaecol* 1988;95:386–390.

98. Monterroso V, Jaffe ES, Merino MJ, Medeiros LJ. Malignant lymphomas involving the ovary. A clinicopathologic analysis of 39 cases. *Am J Surg Pathol* 1993;17:154–170.

99. Paladugu RR, Bearman RM, Rappaport H. Malignant lymphoma with primary manifestation in the gonad: a clinicopathologic study of 38 patients. *Cancer* 1980;45:561–571.

100. Skrodras G, Field V, Kragel PJ. Ovarian lymphoma and serous carcinoma of low malignant potential arising in the same ovary. A case report with literature review of 14 primary ovarian lymphomas. *Arch Pathol Lab Med* 1994;118:647–650.

101. Osborne BM, Robboy SJ. Lymphomas or leukemias presenting as ovarian tumors: analysis of 42 cases. *Cancer* 1983;52:1933–1943.

CHAPTER 35

Primary Fallopian Tube Carcinoma

APICHAI VASURATNA

JOHN J. KAVANAGH

*P*rimary fallopian tube carcinoma (PFTC) is one of the rarest gynecologic malignancies. Its incidence ranges from 0.1% to 1.8% of all female reproductive cancers (1–3). In the United States, the annual incidence is only 3.6 cases/million population/yr (4) and the incidence does not appear to have changed much over time. Due to its rarity, most of the data are derived from retrospective studies. There is a belief that this type of malignancy behaves like epithelial ovarian cancer. Although PFTC shares many features with ovarian cancer, it also expresses many of its own characteristics. Since more than a century ago, when the first case was reported by Ranaud (5), the natural history of PFTC and its treatment has remained unclear.

PFTC usually occurs in the fifth or sixth decade of life (6). The age of patients ranges from 14 to 88 years (3,7), with a mean age of 56.7 years (3). Two thirds of the patients are postmenopausal; only four cases in adolescents have been reported (3). The average parity is 1.7. Nulliparity was found in 27.5% to 34.4% of patients (3). One report did show a high infertility rate of up to 71% in patients with the disease (8). Given the age group, parity, and infertility status, it is believed that PFTC possibly shares the same etiologic factors as endometrial and ovarian cancers. Recent studies demonstrated a high proportion of genetic abnormalities—c-*erb* B-2, p53, and K-*ras* mutations—that are similar to those seen with ovarian and endometrial cancer (9–11). Many studies revealed a high incidence of second primary malignancies, that is, of the breast, endometrium, and ovary, in PFTC patients (6,12). It is unclear whether this suggests similar genetic or environmental factors. Previously, endometriosis and salpingitis were suspected to be the etiologic factors. Now most authors disagree (3,4,6).

Clinical Features

PFTC is more likely to have symptoms earlier than ovarian cancer. The most common presentation is vaginal bleeding, occurring in more than half of patients (11–19). The literature reports abdominal or pelvic pain as the most common presenting symptom, occurring in 31% to 51% of patients (20–22). The pain is secondary to tubal distention. There has been one report of acute abdominal pain due to torsion of a distended tube (3). Abnormal vaginal discharge, either watery or serosanguineous, is also a common symptom, found in 30% to 58% of patients (13,23,24). The classic presentation, "hydrops tubae profluens," occurs in less than 10% of patients (3,22). It has been described as intermittent, colicky lower abdominal pain relieved by a profuse, serous watery or yellow vaginal discharge. These symptoms are neither early nor specific for PFTC (5,6); they can also mimic vesicovaginal fistula, as reported in two patients (3).

On physical examination, two thirds of patients have a pelvic mass (2,3,19). Typically, this mass is sausage like. The triad of Latzko, consisting of abdominal pain, a pelvic mass, and abnormal vaginal discharge, is uncommon in most series (5). Ascites is found in 6% to 20% of patients (2,3) and it reflects an earlier stage of disease, whereas with ovarian cancer the presentation of ascites reflects an advanced stage.

Although Sedlis (25) reported a high rate (60%) of abnormal Pap smears, in most series the rate was less than 20% (3,6,11). This may be due to variations in sample collection. The diagnosis of PFTC should always be kept in mind whenever there is a discrepancy between an abnormal Pap smear and negative findings on colposcopy, cervical biopsy, or endometrial curettage in a patient with recurrent postmenopausal bleeding (2,17).

The introduction and use of high-frequency transvaginal ultrasonography have led to an increasing number of reports of preoperative diagnosis of PFTC (26,27). The characteristic findings are a cystic, fusiform, or sausage-shaped mass with inner papillary projection (26,28). One report noted a change in shape and size accompanied by passage of free fluid through the uterine cavity during transvaginal ultrasonographic examination (26). However, ultrasonographic findings are not specific and can be seen with other abnormalities of the tube such as hydrosalpinx, hematosalpinx, and pyosalpinx (28). The new transvaginal color Doppler imaging technique may help to distinguish PFTC from the benign conditions (29,30).

Computed tomography (CT) and magnetic resonance imaging (MRI) are other noninvasive investigations. However, the accuracy of these modalities over transvaginal ultrasonography is still controversial (29). There have been some reports that CT and MRI may be superior in distinguishing between benign and malignant adnexal masses (29).

As with nonmucinous epithelial ovarian cancer, CA-125 is a useful tumor marker for PFTC. Abnormally elevated levels of CA-125 are found in 78% to 100% of patients with PFTC (31–33). The marker may be used to monitor the results of treatment or the progression of disease. The markers carcinoembryonic antigen (CEA) and CA19-9 are of limited use for detecting PFTC (3).

PFTC can be diagnosed by hysteroscopy although there are no specific findings. Hysteroscopy can be used to obtain fallopian tubal fluid for cytologic study. Laparoscopy might be the only diagnostic tool in an equivocal case. Some clinicians suggest early laparoscopy when PFTC is suspected. Hysterosalpingography can aid in the diagnosis of PFTC (18); however, its usage is not common.

By using monoclonal antibody techniques in combination with immunolymphoscintigraphy or immunoscintigraphy, Lehtovirta et al (34) demonstrated improvement in the detection of retroperitoneal node metastasis of ovarian cancer and PFTC. This technique may aid in the preoperative evaluation or staging of PFTC patients (34). Even with the modern techniques available, the number of accurate preoperative diagnoses of PFTC remains the same. It is common to misdiagnose the lesion before surgery (1,3,6,13,19,21–23,28,33), owing to the rarity of the tumor and the common clinical features with other upper genital tract malignancies. Misdiagnosis also reflects a low index of suspicion.

Spread Pattern

The pattern of spread is similar to that for ovarian carcinoma, with intraperitoneal metastases being the most frequent route. However, Tamimi and Figge (35) reported more lymphatic spread than what they found with ovarian cancer. The fallopian tubes are rich in their lymphatic supplies, and there is evidence showing retroperitoneal node involvement in early-stage disease (35–37). These observations are further supported by the observation that lymph nodes are the common site of recurrence. The overall incidence of retroperitoneal node involvement ranges from 35% to 59% (35,37–39). When lymph nodes are involved, the para-aortic group is dominant (35,38). Many authors suggested routine retroperitoneal node sampling even in patients with early-stage disease (6,36,37). Basically, there are three lymphatic channels in the fallopian tube: 1) The proximal portion of the tube drains into the para-aortic nodes; 2) the distal portion drains into the pelvic nodes; and 3) there is the unusual route to the round ligament of the uterus, which drains into the inguinal nodes. Inguinal node metastasis of PFTC has been reported (40). Another venue of spreading is direct extension to adjacent organs, which creates the problem of diagnosis of PFTC in patients with advanced disease. Hematogenous metastasis is not uncommon (41).

Staging

Staging presents a perplexing problem in relation to the management of PFTC. Numerous staging classifications have been used and confused the treatment. Due to the rarity of PFTC, many retrospective studies were conducted prior to the development of staging systems. Increasing stage is reported with more recent publications. This tendency may be attributed to more complete staging procedures or investigations in recent years; earlier patients may have been understaged (1,11,42).

Staging systems used ovarian cancer as a model and have been endorsed by Erez et al (43), Dodson et al (44), and the American College of Obstetrics and Gynecology (ACOG) (45). In 1971 Schiller and Silverberg (46) proposed a different concept. They considered the fallopian tube as a hollow viscus and suggested a staging classification like Duke's staging system for rectal cancer. Several authors emphasized the importance of depth of tubal wall invasion (1,12,46,47). In 1992, the International Federation of Gynecology and Obstetrics (FIGO) published the first official fallopian tube cancer staging classification (Table 35-1) (48).

This has been proposed as the standard system in the care of PFTC patients.

About half of PFTCs are classified as early stage (2). However, many publications (6,20,24) revealed a delayed diagnosis. The resulting short interval of recurrence and high incidence of lymph node metastasis suggest the disease may have been understaged (6,13,16,23,37). Another possibility that explains the high proportion of early-stage cancer is the misdiagnosis of advanced PFTC as ovarian or endometrial cancer.

Pathology

On gross examination, the affected tube is usually diffused and enlarged, a sausage-shaped mass. The fimbrial ends are occluded in half of the patients. When the neoplasm is found in an early stage, only a localized nodular enlargement at the involved area may be noted. The tubal wall itself may be normal in thickness or

T A B L E **35-1**
FIGO Fallopian Tube Staging, 1992 (48)

Stage 0	Carcinoma in situ (limited to tubal mucosa).
Stage I	Growth limited to the fallopian tubes.
Stage IA	Growth is limited to one tube with extension into the submucosa and/or muscularis but not penetrating the serosal surface; no ascites.
Stage IB	Growth is limited to both tubes with extension into the submucosa and/or muscularis but not penetrating the serosal surface; no ascites.
Stage IC	Tumor either stage IA or IB with tumor extension through or onto the tubal serosa; or with ascites present containing malignant cells or with positive peritoneal washings.
Stage II	Growth involving one or both fallopian tubes with pelvic extension.
Stage IIA	Extension and/or metastasis to the uterus and/or ovaries.
Stage IIB	Extension to other pelvic tissues.
Stage IIC	Tumor either stage IIA or IIB and with ascites present containing malignant cells or with positive peritoneal washings.
Stage III	Tumor involves one or both fallopian tubes with peritoneal implants outside of the pelvis and/or positive retroperitoneal or inguinal nodes. Superficial liver metastases equals stage III. Tumor appears limited to the true pelvis but with histologically proven malignant extension to the small bowel or omentum.
Stage IIIA	Tumor is grossly limited to the true pelvis, with negative nodes but with histologically confirmed microscopic seeding of abdominal peritoneal surfaces.
Stage IIIB	Tumor involving one or both tubes with histologically confirmed implants of abdominal peritoneal surfaces, none exceeding 2 cm in diameter. Lymph nodes are negative.
Stage IIIC	Abdominal implants greater than 2 cm in diameter and/or positive retroperitoneal or inguinal nodes.
Stage IV	Growth involving one or both fallopian tubes with distant metastases. If pleural effusion is present, there must be positive cytology to be stage IV. Parenchymal liver metastases equals stage IV.

Note: Staging for fallopian tube is by the surgical pathologic system. Operative findings designating stage are determined prior to tumor debulking.

Source: Petersson F. Staging rules for gestational trophoblastic tumors and fallopian tube cancer. *Acta Obstet Gynecol Scand* 1992;71:224–225.

thinner than normal, even in the presence of large lesions. Its consistency may be soft so that it mimics benign lesions such as a hydrosalpinx, hematosalpinx, or pyosalpinx. It is not surprising that intraoperative diagnosis may be in error 50% of the time (19). Another study reported PFTC as an incidental finding from pathologic review in 12% of patients (20). These results emphasize the necessity to open every specimen containing an abnormal fallopian tube (2,6). Most tumors arise in the distal two thirds of the tube. The tumor usually causes distal obstruction rather than proximal obstruction, one reason why many patients present with abnormal vaginal discharge. Bilaterality is found in 10% to 26% of patients (2,3). Several authors believed that the bilaterality represents a multifocal origin rather than metastasis (3,46,49,50). This evidence does not support a conservative approach such as unilateral salpingectomy.

More than 90% of PFTCs are papillary serous adenocarcinomas. The microscopic findings resemble epithelial ovarian cancer of the same cell type. The plicae, treelike papillary projections of the tubal wall, are covered with multiple layers of atypical columnar or cuboidal epithelium. Frequent mitotic figures are encountered. The fusion of plicae results in a papillary alveolar pattern, similar to a glandular structure. When the tumor enlarges, necrosis becomes a common feature. Sometimes tuberous salpingitis may produce a prominent adenomatous change that can be mistaken as PFTC.

Because of the similarity in clinical features and microscopic appearances between PFTC and ovarian cancer, it is difficult to distinguish PFTC from ovarian cancer, especially when the disease is advanced. Finn and Javert, in 1949, first proposed the diagnostic criteria differentiating primary from metastatic cancer involving

the fallopian tubes (51). These criteria were modified in 1950 by Hu et al (Table 35-2) (5) and later in 1978 by Sedlis (52). The latter are generally accepted worldwide as the principal diagnostic criteria (Table 35-3).

These criteria are helpful to identify PFTC; nevertheless, some authors questioned that PFTC might be misdiagnosed as ovarian cancer or endometrial cancer instead of advanced PFTC (13,19).

Immunohistochemical staining for CA-125 is positive in 87% of PFTC patients (31,32). This technique may predict which patients will benefit most from serial antigen determination (31). As part of the müllerian system, the fallopian tubal epithelium also expresses estrogen receptor.

Hu et al (5) classified PFTC into three grades:

Grade I: Papillary. The pure papillary growth is confined to the lumen of the tube and the transition between normal and malignant epithelium is clearly seen. The high-power view shows the cells to be fairly well differentiated and to be columnar in shape, and mitotic figures are scanty.

Grade II: Papillary-alveolar. There is a beginning of glandular formation with invasion of the tubal wall. The individual cells are undifferentiated and there is a moderate number of mitotic figures.

Grade III: Alveolar-medullary. The growth is more solid with a lack of papillary projections, and the cells are arranged in a medullary or glandular pattern. There is definite invasion in the lymphatic vessels of the tubal wall. Under higher power, the cells appear poorly differentiated, show vacuolization, and have abundant atypical mitoses.

T A B L E 35-2

Pathologic Criteria for Diagnosis of Primary Fallopian Tube Malignancy

1. Grossly, the main tumor is in the tube.
2. Microscopically, chiefly the mucosa should be involved, and should show a papillary pattern.
3. If the tubal wall is found to be involved to great extent, the transition between benign and malignant epithelium should be demonstrated.

Source: Hu CY, Taymor ML, Hertig AT. Primary carcinoma of the fallopian tube. *Am J Obstet Gynecol* 1950; 59:58–67.

T A B L E 35-3

Pathologic Criteria for Diagnosis of Primary Fallopian Tube Malignancy (52)

1. The tumor arises from the endosalpinx.
2. The histologic pattern reproduces the epithelium of tubal mucosa.
3. Transition from benign to malignant epithelium is found.
4. The ovaries and endometrium are either normal or with a tumor smaller than the tumor in the tube.

Source: Sedlis A. Carcinoma of the fallopian tube. *Surg Clin North Am* 1978;58:121–129.

This system of grading has been generally accepted. Whether these criteria assist in determining the prognosis of disease is controversial.

Treatment

Surgery

Surgery is the cornerstone of the initial treatment for PFTC and usually follows the practices for epithelial ovarian cancer. The procedure involves not only removing as much tumor burden as possible but also properly staging the disease. The operative approach to PFTC should include the following:

Collection of ascitic fluid or peritoneal fluid for cytology

Careful evaluation of the extent of disease

Total abdominal hysterectomy

Bilateral salpingo-oophorectomy

Infracolic omentectomy

Sampling of pelvic and/or para-aortic lymph nodes

Appendectomy

Abdominal and/or pelvic peritoneal biopsies

The role of cytoreductive surgery in PFTC is not clear. Based on extrapolated experiences with epithelial ovarian cancer, most authors suggested a similar procedure (10,19).

As mentioned, the rate of lymphatic metastasis is high despite diagnosis at an early stage, and several authors (2,3,6,7,11) stressed the importance of retroperitoneal lymph node sampling.

Conservative surgery may be considered in a young patient desiring future pregnancy. However, some authors (1,2,6,21) disagreed with this practice because there is a high percentage of bilateral involvement.

Adjuvant Therapy

There is no consensus about what the treatment should be after surgery. Except for stage IA disease, adjuvant therapy of some type is recommended. Either radiation or chemotherapy has been used. There are increasing data concerning platinum based chemotherapy in treat-

ing PFTC and they mimic the results of chemotherapeutic management of ovarian cancer (6,7,11,23,49,53–57). For stage IA disease, most authors suggest surgery to be adequate therapy. However, one should note reports of poor survival for patients with early disease (11,16,40), possibly reflecting understaging or an aggressive behavior of early-stage PFTC.

Chemotherapy

Boronow (53), in 1973, first reported the activity of a single alkylating agent in PFTC. Since then, there have been many publications concerning chemotherapy for this kind of tumor. Chemotherapeutic agents that have shown some activity include alkylating agents such as melphalan, cyclophosphamide, doxorubicin, and platinum compounds. Experience with single-agent chemotherapy in advanced PFTC has been discouraging. In the series of Peters et al (54), the response rate to therapy with a single alkylating agent for advanced or recurrent disease was only 9%. This may be an underestimation because patients not receiving cisplatin were more likely to be treated for a recurrence and to have previously received irradiation therapy.

Parallel to the management of ovarian cancer, cisplatin-based regimens were introduced into the treatment of PFTC. Deppe et al (55), in 1980, first reported use of a cisplatin combination chemotherapy. The combination of cisplatin and cyclophosphamide or these two drugs and doxorubicin was frequently investigated. Although most studies were retrospective and not randomized, combination chemotherapy with platinum compounds seemed to demonstrate higher response rates. The activity ranged from 53% to 92% (7,54,56,57). As expected, there was a close parallel to epithelial ovarian cancer. One report demonstrated similar activity of paclitaxel against platinum-resistant PFTC (58).

Radiotherapy

Radiotherapy was previously the traditional adjuvant treatment for PFTC. With the customary use of chemotherapy for ovarian cancer, the question of using radiotherapy for tubal cancer became controversial. Several studies advocated the usefulness of radiotherapy, especially for stage I and II PFTC. Others (59,60) did not find an apparent difference in survival between surgical treatment alone or with adjuvant radiotherapy.

Second-Look Laparotomy

Until now, about a hundred patients with PFTC reported in the literature have undergone second-look laparotomy (SLL) (61–63). As with ovarian cancer, SLL was applied to the management of PFTC. It was defined as exploratory laparotomy performed after completion of therapy in patients without clinical evidence of disease. The objectives of SLL are first, to determine the effectiveness of therapy; second, to provide prognostic information; and third, to allow further treatment. SLL appeared to serve the first two purposes. Based on the study of Barakat et al (61), the recurrence rate after negative findings on SLL was 19%, which compared to 31% in the study by Frigerio et al (63). Those who had negative SLL findings seemed to live longer. However, the role of SLL for secondary cytoreduction is undefined.

Hormonal Treatment

There is sparse literature on hormonal treatment for PFTC. Usually progestins were combined with chemotherapy or radiotherapy. Even though there is evidence of estrogen receptors in normal fallopian tubes, there are no solid data to confirm the effectiveness of hormonal treatment in PFTC.

Prognosis

The overall 5-year survival rate for patients with PFTC ranges from approximately 30% to 40% in most series. Because these rates have been accumulated over long periods of time during which staging systems and treatments varied, the accuracy of the survival data is difficult to assess. Survival data from several series are shown in Table 35-4 (11–13,15,17,21–23,62,63). Overall the median survival time was approximately 23 to 28 months (1,20,49). Recurrence most likely occurred within 2 to 3 years after treatment (6).

Studies often found that extraperitoneal disease was a common pattern of recurrence. The median time to relapse ranged from 9.0 to 13.5 months (1,11). Late recurrence was not uncommon in many series (6,11,24,58).

In patients with disease limited to the fallopian tube, depth of tubal wall invasion is a significant prognostic factor (12,47). For those who had extratubal extension, the stage of disease and the amount of residual tumor after cytoreduction appeared to correlate with survival (12). Podratz et al (11) found the result of peritoneal cytologic study to have significant prognostic value. Histologic grading, bilaterality, tubal end occlusion, and lymph-vascular invasion are controversial issues. Although Rosen et al (64) detected positive staining for estrogen receptor in 26% and for progesterone receptor in 42% of patients, they observed no prognostic influence. DNA ploidy and abnormal expression of oncogene are under investigation for their prognostic value.

TABLE   **35-4**

Five-Year Survival (%) per Stage

Author	Years	No.	Staging	I	II	III	IV	Overall
Benedet et al (17)	1946–1976	32	Schiller	88	20	3	0	34.4
Roberts and Lifshitz (22)	1938–1979	102	Dodson	77	42	6*	—	42.3
Eddy et al (62)	1948–1981	71	Dodson	71	40	40	0	22
Denham and MacLennon (21)	1951–1981	40	ACOG	69	39	21	0	—
McMurray et al (13)	1951–1981	30	Dodson	56	27	14	0	—
Podratz et al (11)	1964–1983	47	Dodson	64	60	18	25	41
Peters et al (12)	1928–1987	115	Dodson	61	29	17	—	—
Pfeiffer et al (23)	1978–1983	52	Dodson	64	40	6*	—	37.4
Muntz et al (15)	1960–1980	19	Dodson	100	63	0	0	—
Frigerio et al (63)	1970–1988	29	Dodson	48	48	25*	—	41.3

*Stages III and IV considered together.

Other Fallopian Tubal Malignancies

Malignant mixed müllerian tumors of the fallopian tube are exceedingly rare (3,65,66). To date, fewer than 60 cases have been reported in the literature. The clinical picture resembles that of adenocarcinoma. However, survival is generally poor. A 2-year survival rate of only 40% was observed. Surgical removal with adjuvant therapy is considered for all stages. As part of the müllerian tumor, gestational choriocarcinoma after ectopic pregnancy has been reported. Its behavior and treatment were suggested to be like uterine choriocarcinoma.

Other histologic cell types including clear-cell carcinoma, squamous cell carcinoma, endometrioid carcinoma, pure sarcoma, and immature teratoma have been reported.

REFERENCES

1. Jereczek B, Jaseem J, Kobierska A. Primary cancer of the fallopian tube: report of 26 patients. *Acta Obstet Gynecol Scand* 1996;75: 281–286.

2. Morrow CP, Curtin JP. Tumors of the vagina broad ligament and fallopian tube. In: *Gynecologic cancer surgery.* New York: Churchill Livingstone, 1996:717–743.

3. Nordin AJ. Primary carcinoma of the fallopian tube: a 20-year literature review. *Obstet Gynecol Surv* 1994;49:349–361.

4. Rosenblatt KA, Weiss NS, Schwartz SM. Incidence of malignant fallopian tube tumors. *Gynecol Oncol* 1989;35:236–239.

5. Hu CY, Taymor ML, Hertig AT. Primary carcinoma of the fallopian tube. *Am J Obstet Gynecol* 1950;59:58–67.

6. Baekelandt M, Kockx M, Wesling F, Gerris J. Primary adenocarcinoma of the fallopian tube: review of the literature. *Int J Gynecol Cancer* 1993;3:65–71.

7. Maxson WZ, Stehman FB, Ulbright TM, et al. Primary carcinoma of the fallopian tube: evidence for activity of cisplatin combination therapy. *Gynecol Oncol* 1987;26:305–313.

8. Boutselis JG. Clinical aspects of primary carcinoma of the fallopian tube: a clinical study of 14 cases. *Am J Obstet Gynecol* 1971;111:98–101.

9. Mizuuchi H, Mori Y, Sato K, et al. High incidence of point mutation in K-*ras* codon 12 in

carcinoma of the fallopian tube. *Cancer* 1995;76:86–90.

10. Bardi G, Sukhikh T, Pandis N, et al. Complex karyotypic abnormalities in a primary carcinoma of the fallopian tube. *Genes Chromosomes Cancer* 1994;10:207–209.

11. Podratz KC, Podczaski E, Gaffey TA, et al. Primary carcinoma of the fallopian tube. *Am J Obstet Gynecol* 1986;154:1319–1326.

12. Peters WA, Andersen WA, Hopkins MP, et al. Prognostic features of carcinoma of the fallopian tube. *Obstet Gynecol* 1988;71:757–762.

13. McMurray EH, Jacobs AJ, Perez CA, et al. Carcinoma of the fallopian tube: management and sites of failure. *Cancer* 1986;58:2070–2075.

14. Calero F, Armas A, Abarca L, et al. Primary tubal carcinoma. *Eur J Gynaecol Oncol* 1994;15:288–294.

15. Muntz HG, Tarraza HM, Granai CO, Fuller AF. Primary adenocarcinoma of the fallopian tube. *Eur J Gynaecol Oncol* 1989;10:239–249.

16. Asmussen M, Kaern J, Kjoerstad K, et al. Primary adenocarcinoma localized to the fallopian tubes: report on 33 cases. *Gynecol Oncol* 1988;30:183–186.

17. Benedet JL, White GW, Fairey RN, Boyes DA. Adenocarcinoma of the fallopian tube: experience with 41 patients. *Obstet Gynecol* 1977;50:654–657.

18. Hirai Y, Kaku S, Teshima H, et al. Clinical study of primary carcinoma of the fallopian tube: experience with 15 cases. *Gynecol Oncol* 1989;34:20–26.

19. King A, Seraj IM, Thrasher T, et al. Fallopian tube carcinoma: a clinicopathological study of 17 cases. *Gynecol Oncol* 1989;33:351–355.

20. Eddy GL, Copeland LJ, Gershenson DM, et al. Fallopian tube carcinoma. *Obstet Gynecol* 1984;64:546–552.

21. Denham JW, MacLennan KA. The management of primary carcinoma of the fallopian tube: experience of 40 cases. *Cancer* 1984;53:166–172.

22. Roberts JA, Lifshitz S. Primary adenocarcinoma of the fallopian tube. *Gynecol Oncol* 1982;13:301–308.

23. Pfeiffer P, Mogensen H, Amtrup F, Honore E. Primary carcinoma of the fallopian tube: retrospective study of patients reported to the Danish Cancer Registry in a five-year period. *Acta Oncol* 1989;28:7–11.

24. Semrad N, Watring W, Fu Y, et al. Fallopian tube adenocarcinoma: common extraperitoneal recurrence. *Gynecol Oncol* 1986;24:230–235.

25. Sedlis A. Primary carcinoma of the fallopian tube. *Obstet Gynecol Surv* 1961;16:209–226.

26. Ajjimakorn S, Bhamarapravati Y. Transvaginal ultrasound and the diagnosis of fallopian tubal carcinoma. *J Clin Ultrasound* 1991;19:116–119.

27. Kol S, Gal D, Friedman M, Paldi E. Preoperative diagnosis of fallopian tube carcinoma by transvaginal sonography and CA125. *Gynecol Oncol* 1990;37:129–131.

28. Yamamoto K, Katoh S, Nakayama S, et al. Ultrasonic evaluation of fallopian tube carcinoma. *Gynecol Obstet Invest* 1988;25:202–208.

29. Yamashita Y, Torashima M, Hatanaka Y, et al. Adnexal masses: accuracy of characterization with transvaginal US and precontrast and post-contrast MR imaging. *Radiology* 1995;194: 557–565.

30. Fleischer AC, Rogers WH, Rao BK, et al. Transvaginal color Doppler sonography of ovarian masses with pathological correlation. *Ultrasound Obstet Gynecol* 1991;1:275–278.

31. Puls LE, Davey DD, DePriest PD, et al. Immunohistochemical staining for CA-125 in fallopian tube carcinomas. *Gynecol Oncol* 1993;48: 360– 363.

32. Tokunaka T, Miyazaki K, Matsuyama S, Okamura H. Serial measurement of CA 125 in patients with primary carcinoma of the fallopian tube. *Gynecol Oncol* 1990;36:335–337.

33. Makar AP, Kristensen GB, Nesland J, et al. Serum CA125 as a tumor marker and the expression of c-erbB-2 oncogene in tubal malignancies. *Int J Gynecol Cancer* 1993;3:116–121.

34. Lehtovirta P, Kairemo KJ, Liewendahl K, Seppala M. Immunolymphoscintigraphy and immunoscintigraphy of ovarian and fallopian tube cancer using F(ab')₂ fragments of monoclonal antibody OC125. *Cancer Res* 1990; 50(suppl):937s–940s.

35. Tamimi HK, Figge DC. Adenocarcinoma of the uterine tube: potential for lymph node metastases. *Am J Obstet Gynecol* 1981;141:132–137.

36. Yoonessi M, Leberer JP, Crickard K. Primary fallopian tube carcinoma: treatment and spread pattern. *J Surg Oncol* 1988;38:97–100.

37. Di Re E, Grosso G, Raspagliesi F, Baiocchi G. Fallopian tube cancer: incidence and role of lymphatic spread. *Gynecol Oncol* 1996;62: 199–202.

38. Schray MF, Podratz KC, Malkasian GD. Fallopian tube cancer: the role of radiation therapy. *Radiother Oncol* 1987;10:267–275.

39. Klein M, Rosen A, Lahousen M, et al. Lymphogenous metastasis in the primary carcinoma of the fallopian tube. *Gynecol Oncol* 1994;55: 336–338.

40. Harrison CR, Averette HE, Jarrell MA, et al. Carcinoma of the fallopian tube: clinical management. *Gynecol Oncol* 1989;32:357–359.

41. Southwood WF. Carcinoma of the fallopian tube. A review and a description of a case with unusual clinical features, presenting as an acute abdominal surgery. *Br J Surg* 1956;44:487.

42. Gurney H, Murphy D, Crowther D. The management of primary fallopian tube carcinoma. *Br J Obstet Gynaecol* 1990;97:822–826.

43. Erez S, Kapland AL, Well JA. Clinical staging of carcinoma of the uterine tube. *Obstet Gynecol* 1967;30:547–550.

44. Dodson MG, Ford JH, Averette HE. Clinical aspects of fallopian tube carcinoma. *Obstet Gynecol* 1970;36:935–939.

45. *Classification and staging of malignant tumors of the female pelvis.* American College of Obstetrics and Gynecology technical bulletin no. 12. American College of Obstetrics and Gynecology, May 1969.

46. Schiller HM, Silverberg SG. Staging and prognosis in primary carcinoma of the fallopian tube. *Cancer* 1971;28:389–395.

47. Klein M, Rosen A, Lahousen M, et al. Evaluation of adjuvant therapy afer surgery for primary carcinoma of the fallopian tube. *Arch Gynecol Obstet* 1994;225:19–24.

48. Pettersson F. Staging rules for gestational trophoblastic tumors and fallopian tube cancer. *Acta Obstet Gynecol Scand* 1992;71: 224–225.

49. Rose PG, Piver MS, Tsukada Y. Fallopian tube cancer: the Roswell Park experience. *Cancer* 1990;66:2661–2667.

50. Woodruff JD, Solomon D, Sullivant H. Multifocal disease in the upper genital canal. *Obstet Gynecol* 1985;65:695–698.

51. Finn WF, Javert CT. Primary and metastatic cancer of the fallopian tube. *Cancer* 1949;2:803–814.

52. Sedlis A. Carcinoma of the fallopian tube. *Surg Clin North Am* 1978;58:121–129.

53. Boronow RC. Chemotherapy for disseminated tubal cancer. *Obstet Gynecol* 1973;42:62–66.

54. Peters WA, Andersen WA, Hopkins MP. Results of chemotherapy in advanced carcinoma of the fallopian tube. *Cancer* 1989;63:836–838.

55. Deppe G, Bruckner HW, Cohen CJ. Combination chemotherapy for advanced carcinoma of the fallopian tube. *Obstet Gynecol* 1980;56:530–532.

56. Pectasides D, Barbounis V, Sintila A, et al. Treatment of primary fallopian tube carcinoma with cisplatin-containing chemotherapy. *Am J Clin Oncol* 1994;17:68–71.

57. Morris M, Gershenson DM, Burke TW, et al. Treatment of fallopian tube carcinoma with cisplatin, doxorubicin, and cyclophosphamide. *Obstet Gynecol* 1990;76:1020–1023.

58. Tresukosol D, Kudelka AP, Edwards CL, et al. Primary fallopian tube adenocarcinoma: clinical complete response after salvage treatment with high dose paclitaxel. *Gynecol Oncol* 1995;58: 258–261.

59. Pakisch B, Poschauko J, Stucklschweiger G, et al. Die Behandlung des primaren Karzinomas der Ruba Fallopii. *Geburtshilfe Frauenheilkd* 1990;50:593–596.

60. Klein M, Rosen A, Lahousen M, et al. Evaluation of adjuvant therapy after surgery for primary carcinoma of the fallopian tube. *Arch Gynecol Obstet* 1994;225:19–24.

61. Barakat RR, Rubin SC, Saigo PE, et al. Second-look laparotomy in carcinoma of the fallopian tube. *Obstet Gynecol* 1993;82:748–751.

62. Eddy GL, Copeland LJ, Gershenson DM. Second-look laparotomy in fallopian tube carcinoma. *Gynecol Oncol* 1984;19:182–186.

63. Frigerio L, Pirondini A, Pileri M, et al. Primary carcinoma of the fallopian tube. *Tumori* 1993;79: 40–44.

64. Rosen AC, Reiner A, Klein M, et al. Prognostic factors in primary fallopian tube carcinoma. *Gynecol Oncol* 1994;53:307–313.

65. Hellstrom AC, Auer G, Silfversward C, Petersson F. Prognostic factors in malignant mixed müllerian tumor of the fallopian tube: the Radiumhemmet series 1923-1994. *Int J Gynecol Cancer* 1996;6:467–472.

66. Patton GW, Goldstein DP. Gestational choriocarcinoma of the tube and ovary. *Surg Gynecol Obstet* 1973;137:608–612.

$\mathcal{S}$ECTION 6

Special Topics

CHAPTER *36*

Cancer Prevention in Women: Clues from Epidemiology

PETER BOYLE
PATRICK MAISONNEUVE

Cancer Burden in Women

It has been estimated that in 1985 there were approximately 7.6 million new cases of cancer diagnosed throughout the world (1). This figure, as with others presented below, omits nonmelanoma skin cancers from the calculations. Of this total, there were 3,774,200 new cases of cancer in women. The most frequent form in women was breast cancer, with 719,000 new cases annually (Table 36-1) (1–3). To many observers in Western countries, it is somewhat surprising to see that there were 437,000 cases of cervical cancer each year and that this was the second most common form of cancer in women worldwide. The entity of colon and rectum cancer was third most common, followed by stomach cancer. In contrast, the most common cancer in men (lung cancer, with 676,000 victims annually) is the fifth most common form of cancer in women.

In the European Community, the incidence of cancer was estimated for the single year 1980 (4). In women, the most common form of cancer was breast cancer, with 135,000 new cases and an annual incidence rate of 56.8 cases/100,000 population/annum (Table 36-2). Breast cancer was nearly four times more frequent than the second most common form of cancer observed in women (colon cancer) and nearly six times as frequent as the third most common form (stomach cancer). Cancers of the ovary, cervix, and endometrium were, respectively, the fourth, fifth, and sixth most common forms of cancer found.

It is also useful to consider the mortality rate from specific cancers as well as the incidence rates. In women in Canada in 1992, breast cancer was the most common form of cancer (28% of all new cases) and also the most common cause of cancer death (20%). It is of major importance to note that while lung cancer is only the third most frequent incident cancer in women (12%) and much less frequent than breast cancer, lung cancer approaches breast cancer as a cause of cancer death in women, being responsible for 19% of cancer deaths in women in Canada (5).

Causes of Cancer in Men and Women

The best estimates of the proportion of cancer deaths attributable to various factors remain those based on the initial work of Richard Doll and Richard Peto (6). However, the estimates are not made for each gender group separately because it is very difficult to imagine that the effect of a human carcinogen at the same dose and in the same circumstances would produce a different effect in men and women.

Tobacco smoking remains the most important, best-understood human carcinogenic factor and it is estimated that 30% of cancer deaths (in a population with a cancer pattern such as in the United Kingdom or the United States) can be attributable to this factor (6). The evidence of the carcinogenic effect of tobacco smoking is so overwhelming (7) that the range of the size of the effect (25%–40%) is so relatively small (Table 36-3). Diet is widely re-

	1975	1980	1985
Mouth and pharynx	105,600 (6)	121,200 (8)	143,000 (7)
Esophagus	102,300 (7)	108,200 (9)	108,000 (10)
Stomach	260,600 (3)	260,600 (4)	282,000 (4)
Colorectal	255,600 (4)	285,900 (3)	346,000 (3)
Liver	76,700 (9)	79,500 (−)	101,000 (11)
Lung	126,700 (5)	146,900 (6)	219,000 (5)
Breast	541,200 (1)	572,100 (1)	719,000 (1)
Cervix	459,400 (2)	465,600 (2)	437,000 (2)
Lymphoma	91,300 (8)	98,000 (10)	135,000 (9)
Leukemia	75,400 (10)	81,300 (−)	96,000 (12)
All sites	2,901,800	3,100,000 (10)	3,774,200

T A B L E   36-1

Estimated Annual Cancer Incidence Burden Worldwide in Women in 1975, 1980, and 1985*

*Estimates of the global cancer burden have been made for 1975 (2), 1980 (3), and 1985 (1). These estimates are for all forms of cancer excluding nonmelanoma skin cancers. Numbers in parentheses indicate order from highest incidence to lowest.

T A B L E   36-2

Cancer Incidence Estimates in Women in European Community Around 1980

Site	No. of Cases	Rate/100,000
1. Breast	135,000	56.8
2. Colon	51,000	15.8
3. Stomach	38,000	11.1
4. Ovary	26,000	11.0
5. Cervix uteri	22,000	10.4
6. Corpus uteri	24,000	9.7
7. Liver	27,000	8.5
8. Lung	23,000	8.2
9. Brain	17,000	8.0
10. Rectum	20,000	6.6

Source: Jensen OM, Esteve J, Moller H, Renard H. Cancer in the European Community and its member states. *Eur J Cancer* 1990;24:1167–1256.

T A B L E   36-3

Estimate of the Proportion of Cancer Deaths That Will Be Found to Be Attributable to Various Factors*

	Best Estimate	Range
Tobacco	30	25–40
Alcohol	3	2–4
Diet	35	10–70
Food additives	<1	5–2
Sexual behavior	1	1
Yet to be discovered hormonal analogies of reproductive factors	Up to 6	0–12
Occupation	4	2–8
Pollution	2	1–5
Industrial products	<1	<1–2
Medicines and procedures	1	0.5–3
Geographic factors	3	2–4
Infective processes	10	1–?

*Refers to United Kingdom or United States cancer pattern.
Source: Peto 1985.

cognized as an important cause of cancer, with approximately 35% of cancer deaths attributable to this factor. However, the epidemiologic data available regarding all aspects of this complex exposure are not as conclusive as for tobacco smoking and this is reflected in the wide limits quoted for the magnitude of the effect (between 10% and 70%) (see Table 36-3).

Recent research involving successful collaboration between epidemiologists and basic scientists identified clear associations between cancer risk and certain infective processes. The associations between hepatitis viruses and liver cancer are important to women, as are the striking associations demonstrated between Epstein-Barr virus (EBV) and nasopharyngeal cancer risk in Southeast Asia and also between EBV

and Hodgkin's disease. However, in view of the fact that cervical cancer is the second most frequent cancer in women worldwide, the recent demonstration of a strong association between exposure to human papillomavirus (HPV) and an increased risk of cervical cancer is of considerable importance to women. It is now thought that at least 10% of human cancers may be the result of infective processes. As more and more evidence emerges, it is believed that this proportion could be even higher.

Most other identified causes of cancer account for smaller proportions of cancer deaths (see Table 36-3). Alcohol drinking accounts for around 3% of human cancer although the greatest effect of alcohol drinking comes via its inter-action with the effect of cigarette smoking on increasing the risk of cancers of the oral cavity, larynx, and esophagus (8). Occupational exposures to carcinogens account for a small proportion of the total cancer burden, with an independent contribution to the statistics for occupation coming from working in occupa-tions of a sedentary nature: The risk associated with such exposures and increased colorectal cancer risk is increasing. Pollution accounts for a small proportion of cancer overall and the effect of air pollution on cancer risk is greatest among, if not confined to, smokers (9).

Industrial products, food additives, medi-cines and procedures, and geographic factors account for small proportions of the total cancer burden. It is clearly recognized that some aspects of reproductive habits influence the risk of cancer in women, notably breast cancer risk (10). However, these are merely surrogate mea-sures of some hormonal imbalance or change that alter cancer risk. These have not been clearly identified although they could account for a total of about 6% of cancer deaths (see Table 36-3).

It is clear that the major causes of cancer are tobacco smoking, diet, and infective pro-cesses and that while tobacco smoking and diet are important causes of cancer in men and in women, there may be a separate gender effect of certain infective processes.

Tobacco Smoking and Cancer Risk

Current low levels of smoking among physi-cians and research scientists, in many countries, have led them unconsciously to overlook tobacco smoking as an important cause of cancer (11). However, there is a very substan-tial body of evidence from many sources in-cluding epidemiology and toxicology data that indicates the carcinogenicity of tobacco smoking (7). Not only does cigarette smoking greatly increase the risk of lung cancer in smokers, but also the risks of oral cavity cancer, larynx cancer, esophageal cancer, bladder can-cer, pancreas cancer, and kidney cancer are increased. The risk of cancer of the cervix and stomach may also be increased, although the evidence of this is much less consistent (9).

There is at present a worldwide epidemic of tobacco-related disease: Not only does

smoking cause increased levels of many dif-ferent common forms of cancer, but also it increases the risk of cardiovascular disease. Deaths from cancer of the lung, the cancer site most strongly linked to cigarette smoking, have increased in Japan by a factor of 10 in men and 8 in women since 1950. In central and eastern Europe, more than 400,000 premature deaths are currently caused each year by tobacco smoking (12). In young men in all countries of central and eastern Europe, there are levels of lung cancer that are greater than anything seen before in Western countries and these rates are still rising (13). In Poland, a country severely hit by the tobacco epidemic, the life expectancy of a 45-year-old man has been falling for over a decade now due to the increasing pre-mature death rates from tobacco-related cancers and cardiovascular disease. Tragically, cigarette smoking is still increasing in central and eastern Europe and also in China, where an epidemic of tobacco-related deaths is building up quickly.

The situation in women worldwide is alarm-ing, with the number of women smokers climb-ing and with the incidence and mortality of lung cancer in many countries increasing rapidly (14). In the past, it was thought that women have a different reaction to tobacco than men do, owing to the wide disparity between tobacco-cancer rates in men and women. However, the effect on cancer rates only man-ifests itself beginning 20 years after the expo-sure to tobacco smoke first commences. Thus, there is a period of longer than 20 years, prob-ably 30 or even 40 years, when the effects of smoking do not make an impression on national cancer mortality rates. Therefore, when one sees a large proportion of women and par-ticularly young women smoking, and no real impression on the rates of lung cancer, it is important to bear in mind that the real effect of the current tobacco-smoking habits in younger women will not manifest themselves into cancer rates for at least 30 or 40 years. The current low levels of lung cancer and many other smoking-related cancers are falsely reassuring: Women are not immune to the adverse health conse-quences of smoking tobacco, as future cancer rates will clearly reflect.

The effects of smoking tobacco and the dif-ference in the patterns between men and women are clear, based on lung cancer rates in several countries. Lung cancer mortality data for each sex were abstracted from the World Health

Organization database for the years 1950 to 1989. Data were available as annual numbers of deaths presented by sex and 5-year age groups. The data were analyzed by age-period-cohort modeling and the results presented as time period–specific relative risks (the referent time period is 1950–1954) and birth cohort–specific relative risks (the referent birth cohort is that born in the period around 1910) (15). The methodology was implemented as described in more detail elsewhere (16).

In the United Kingdom, the cohort-specific relative risks in men increased until the cohort born around 1910 and subsequently stabilized and declined. In women, the risk rose until the cohort born around 1930 and also subsequently declined. In Italy, the cohort-specific risks rose in each sex until the cohort born around 1930 and then stabilized. In the Netherlands, the cohort-specific risk in men increased until the 1910 cohort and subsequently stabilized and decreased. However, in women in the Netherlands, the cohort-specific relative risk continued to rise without any decline in evidence.

These data clearly illustrate a number of points. Firstly, men appear to have heeded the health education messages earlier than women. Secondly, there are indications that in several countries lung cancer rates in women will continue to increase for the foreseeable future. Thirdly, the recent increase in smoking in younger women in several countries has not yet manifested itself as a lung cancer hazard, although based on current knowledge and past experience, this will happen.

Obviously, the problem of women smoking tobacco is a current research and public health priority.

Diet and Cancer Risk

The second major cause of cancer is the complex exposures occurring through diet, nutrition, and dietary practices (17). At the present time, it is very difficult to quantify the exact mechanisms of carcinogenesis of human dietary exposures, but as epidemiologic studies of diet and cancer become more sophisticated and exposure assessment more reliable, associations will become clearer and mechanisms more obvious. Current evidence suggests that 35% of human cancers may be associated with

dietary practices, although there are broad limits on this estimation (6), with associations already described with many different sites of cancer (18).

Diet is a very complicated field of research, with the concept of "diet" being so difficult to define clearly. There is evidence that the effects of certain aspects of diet are associated with cancer risk. For example, obesity is one consequence of a number of factors including diet that is associated with an increased risk of a number of cancers including endometrial cancer, breast cancer, and colorectal cancer, all of which are common in women (9). Similarly, being underweight during adolescence has been associated with a reduced risk of subsequent breast cancer (10).

The focus of research on specific dietary intakes and patterns and cancer risk has centered on the role of the dietary intake of fats and vitamins. There is now good evidence that the risk for colorectal cancer is increased by total fat intake, that there is an additional contribution from saturated fat over and above its contribution to total fat intake, and that there is also a separate contribution from meat intake (9). Despite much conflicting evidence and many different arguments, the time may have come to accept that the available evidence in humans does not support an association between adult intake of total fat or saturated fat and the risk of breast cancer. There is little substantive and no conclusive evidence of a link between fat intake and the risk of other forms of cancer at the present time. Clearly more research is needed on dietary fat intake and cancer risk before definite conclusions in this area can be made, but the current evidence is clearly pointing in certain directions.

At the same time that the association with fat intake and the risk of certain forms of cancer has been moving to-and-fro, there has been an impressive build-up of evidence linking the consumption of fruits and vegetables with reduced risks of certain cancers (19). There is strong and consistent evidence for protective effects of increased consumption of fruits and vegetables against cancers of the lung, larynx, stomach, colorectum, esophagus, bladder, oral cavity, and pancreas (9). Unfortunately, there is little consistent evidence of any major effect of fruit and vegetable consumption on the risk of hormone-related cancers such as those of the endometrium, cervix, ovary, and prostate. Until recently, the evidence relating to breast cancer had been very weak but there has been an important recent development. Using the data collected in the prospective study of U.S. nurses, Hunter et al (20) showed an apparent protective effect of an index of vitamin A intake on breast cancer risk that had a significant dose-response relationship. Furthermore, there was a demonstrable effect of protection offered by the use of vitamin A supplements in the fifth of women in the study who had the lowest intake levels of vitamin A. Thus, this issue is not yet resolved and the possibility remains that there may be some protection against breast cancer offered by increased intake of foods rich in vitamin A.

What is clear, however, is that there is good evidence that an increased consumption of fruits and vegetables can lead to a reduction in the risk of certain forms of cancer that are common in women (as well as men). At the present time, more evidence is needed regarding the effect of dietary intake on the risk of hormonally related cancers.

Infective Processes and Cancer Risk

Infection, viruses, and infective processes are increasingly recognized as one of the three major groups of cancer causes.

A large number of ecologic studies suggested an association between elevated nasopharyngeal cancer risk and EBV infection. Clinical progression of the disease is accompanied by increases in the antiviral antibody; nucleic acid hybridization has shown the presence of EBV DNA in squamous epithelial cells, indicating the strong probability that the virus is not simply a passenger in the process of carcinogenesis. The "late host response" model for Hodgkin's disease (21) was developed in response to a number of observations including the similarity of the age distribution of Hodgkin's disease with that of EBV infections. Prospective studies demonstrated higher antibody titers to EBV (22), an increased incidence of infectious mononucleosis, and a later incidence of childhood infections (23) in patients with young-onset Hodgkin's disease. Furthermore, EBV genomes have been found within Reed-Sternberg cells (24), although they do not appear to have been isolated from lymphoid cells. Although the "late host response" model does not require evidence for social contact

between patients, numerous studies addressed this issue, presumably motivated by anecdotal reports (25). Studies of space-time clustering generally produced inconsistent results but recent investigations of purely spatial clustering were somewhat consistent in showing weak evidence of clustering (26). It appears that shared social experience during childhood and adolescence may be a feature of subsequent Hodgkin's disease.

It is well established that there is a strong and specific association between infection with hepatitis B virus (HBV) and the risk of hepatocellular carcinoma (27). The association appears to be restricted to chronically active forms of HBV infection, which are characterized by the presence in serum of hepatitis B surface antigen (HBsAg), commonly referred to as *carrier status*. The association is strong: In a cohort study from Taiwan based on 22,000 subjects, of whom 345 were HBsAg positive, the relative risk for hepatocellular carcinoma was found to be 104 [95% confidence interval (CI): 51, 212] and the calculated attributable risk was nearly 94% (27). This relative risk is one whole order of magnitude greater than that commonly reported from case-control studies from Europe; this may be related to the influence of some cofactor (such as poorer diet in East Asia) or a different duration of exposure to the virus (which is generally transmitted perinatally in East Asia but which in North America and Europe is contracted later in life).

Epidemiologic studies demonstrated a clear association between a woman's risk of developing cervical cancer and the number of sex partners she, or her current partner, have had: This strongly suggests that a sexually transmitted agent is involved in the etiology of cervical cancer, and a number of candidate viruses including herpes simplex virus type 2 and HPV have been identified as possible carcinogenic agents. Most studies of herpes simplex type 2 failed to find any difference in the prevalence of these antibodies between women who developed cervix cancer and women who did not (9). A major difficulty in studying the role of HPV is that it cannot be grown in vitro and it has only recently been possible to clone the DNA of HPV in bacteria. However, there is now evidence from first-class epidemiologic studies demonstrating that among the more than 60 different types of HPV, HPV-16 and, to a lesser extent, HPV-18 are associated with advanced cervical intraepithelial neoplasia (CIN) whereas

HPV-6 and HPV-11 are found more often in association with lower-grade CIN and condylomata (28). This is an important advance in a cancer that is second on the list of the most frequent forms of cancer in women.

Again, it is clear that infective processes are important determinants of some common forms of cancer in women.

Cancers Specific to Women

Cancer of the Breast

Globally, breast cancer is the most frequent malignancy among women, with an estimated 422,000 new cases occurring in developed countries around 1985. In developing countries breast cancer, with an estimated 298,000 new cases, follows cancer of the cervix uteri in frequency (344,000). The disease is rare in males.

The highest incidence rates of breast cancer in women are exclusively in the United States (Table 36-4); the highest rate outside the United States is from Porto Alegre, Brazil, which has the fifteenth highest incidence rate (78.5). Incidence rates exceeding 100 cases/100,000 population are reported for the white population of the San Francisco Bay area (104.2) and the Hawaiian population of Hawaii (100.2). Rates in western Europe are much lower, with the highest recorded incidence rate in Geneva, Switzerland (73.5/100,000).

The highest incidence rate in central and eastern Europe was reported from the former German Democratic Republic (46.3). Low rates are reported from other central and eastern European countries, Asia, and Africa (see Table 36-4).

In Singapore, the incidence in Hokkien and Cantonese females is some 30% greater than that in Teochew, Hainanese, and Hakka females. An urban-rural gradient is generally found, with the incidence higher in urban than in rural areas (29).

Although the breast, rather than the cervix uteri, is the most common female cancer site in a large number of Muslim countries (Egypt,

T A B L E **36-4**

Cancer of the Breast (ICD9 175): 10 Highest and 10 Lowest Incidence Rates per 100,000 Person-Years

Male Registry	No. of Cases	Rate	Female Registry	No. of Cases	Rate
Kuwait: non-Kuwaitis	10	2.2	U.S., Bay area: white	9,736	104.20
France, Tarn	21	1.5	U.S., Hawaii: Hawaiian	351	100.2
Italy, Trieste	7	1.4	U.S., Hawaii: white	735	99.3
Bermuda: black	1	1.3	U.S., Alameda: white	2,864	99.2
Switzerland, Neuchâtel	7	1.1	U.S., Seattle	8,976	94.2
Israel: born Europe, America	59	1.1	U.S., Detroit: white	9,779	91.4
U.S., New York City	237	1.0	U.S., Atlanta: white	3,748	91.0
Philippines, Manila	42	1.0	U.S., Connecticut: white	10,155	88.9
France, Calvados	17	1.0	U.S., Los Angeles: O. white	16,057	88.5
Portugal, V N de Gaia	5	1.0	U.S., Alameda: black	541	83.8
U.S., Los Angeles: Chinese	0	—	Japan, Yamagata	647	17.6
Singapore: Malay	0	—	Kuwait: Kuwaitis	141	17.2
Bermuda: white and other	0	—	Israel: non-Jews	172	17.0
The Gambia	0	—	U.S., Los Angeles: Korean	48	16.9
U.S., Los Angeles: Filipino	0	—	Thailand, Chiang Mai	308	13.7
Peru, Trujillo	0	—	Mali, Bamako	44	10.2
Kuwait: Kuwaitis	0	—	Thailand, Khon Kaen	111	9.9
Canada, Northwest Territory and Yukon	0	—	China, Qidong	265	9.5
U.S., Hawaii: Chinese	0	—	Algeria, Sétif	85	6.4
U.S., Los Angeles: Korean	0	—	The Gambia	22	3.4

Source: Parkin DM, Pisani P, Ferlay J. Estimates of the worldwide frequency of sixteen major cancers in 1985. *Int J Cancer* 1993;54:594–606.

Tunisia, Sudan, Iran, Kuwait, and Pakistan), the high relative frequencies in these countries do not necessarily mean that the incidence will be high. For example, although the relative frequency in Kuwaiti females is 22%, the incidence is 15.9, whereas in Maoris a relative frequency of 20% is associated with an incidence of 59.9.

The continued rise in the age-specific incidence of female breast cancer, following Clemmesen's hook, is particularly marked in the highest incidence areas, whereas in several Asian countries a plateau or even a slight decline is observed after the menopause. Intermediate age-incidence curves are seen for eastern European countries.

Muir et al (30) drew attention to similarities of the cross-sectional age-incidence curves for breast cancer at various times in the past in Iceland, with current cross-sectional curves in regions of contrasting incidence, namely, Connecticut, Finland, and Miyagi Prefecture, Japan, suggesting that these represented birth cohort effects reflecting differing times of entry of risk factors into the environment. Thus, the risk in Iceland in 1911 to 1929, 1930 to 1949, and 1950 to 1972 was the same as in Japan in 1959 to 1960, Finland in 1959 to 1961, and Connecticut in 1960 to 1962, respectively.

The change in risk of breast cancer in migrants from low-incidence to high-incidence areas, and in their descendants, argues strongly for environmental influences. The incidence in Hawaiian and San Francisco Bay area Japanese women is now double that in Japan, although the difference is less in Los Angeles (1.4-fold). A similar phenomenon is observable for Chinese: The incidence in Singapore and Hong Kong Chinese women is about 50% higher than that in Shanghai and Tianjin, but well below that in U.S. Chinese women. In Singapore, the incidence in the Singapore-born Chinese women in 1968 to 1982 was 29.5, whereas that for those born elsewhere, mainly in China, was 18.2, a difference significant for all dialect groups (31).

The incidence of breast cancer is increasing slowly in most countries, with the rate of increase tending to be greatest where rates were the lowest (e.g., 3.2% per annum in Singapore Chinese women, an increase most noticeable in the 0–49-year age group). Mortality rates have also been increasing in, for example, Japan and Hong Kong, but have had a tendency to remain stationary in Western countries. In the United States, mortality in white women less than 50 years old has fallen, and overall mortality was remarkably stable between 1950 and 1982 (32).

Temporal trends in mortality from female breast cancer are interesting because incidence rates are subject to "artificial" influences such as the introduction and widespread use of screening programs. While these may also affect mortality, this is the aim of such programs and mortality is an important end point. It is difficult to summarize the worldwide trends in breast cancer mortality easily (9,33). The risk seems to have stabilized among younger birth cohorts in countries such as the United Kingdom, Denmark, Australia, Canada, and Italy but still appears to be rising in Germany. The risk is rising among younger cohorts in central European countries such as Poland and Czechoslovakia and also in Japan, although the acceleration expected from the westernization of the diet has not yet materialized (34).

Etiology of Breast Cancer and Risk Factors

Despite many detailed epidemiologic studies, including a large number with biologic measurements, the etiology of breast cancer remains unclear (10). The breast cancer incidence in urban population groups is about 30% higher than that in rural groups, and is similarly elevated among black compared with white members of the same community (9). These observations, together with the international patterns of both geographic and temporal variation and findings of alterations to incidence and mortality rates in migrant groups (35–37), lead us to believe that a large proportion of breast cancer is related to environmental or lifestyle factors and therefore is theoretically avoidable. However, it is not yet clear what these factors are.

Hormonal and Reproductive Factors

The risk of breast cancer is increased by about 50% in nulliparous compared with parous women. Risk increases with age at first birth until the age at first birth is older than (approximately) 35, which carries a higher risk than nulliparity, indicating that first childbirth after this age no longer confers protection against breast cancer (38,39). Trichopoulos et al (40) estimated that age at any birth after the first was an independent risk factor. The association with parity is more complex, owing to the relationship between age at first birth and parity, particularly high parity, but it still appears that there may be some independent contribution of high parity to reducing breast cancer risk (41).

La Vecchia et al (42) tried to clarify these associations by conducting a meta-analysis of 26 published studies of parity, age at first birth, and breast cancer risk. Among these studies, 1 found no significant association with either age at first birth or parity, 7 found an association with age at first birth but not parity, 6 found an association with parity but not with age at first birth, and 12 found associations with both age at first birth and parity. Age at first birth appeared to be more important, with a trend of increasing risk with older age evident across all stratification levels, while the protection of parity, even in those studies where the association was evident, seemed to be quantitatively relevant only for women with four or more births. Another meta-analysis from the Nordic countries found a risk with both age at first birth and parity (43).

Thompson and Janerich (44) recently reported that among parous women, a 15-year increase of maternal age at birth is associated with a 25% increase in the risk of breast cancer in the daughters. This finding was examined in a prospective study which found a weak and nonsignificant trend in risk of breast cancer with increasing maternal age at birth but there was no relation with paternal age (45). Daughters born to mothers 30 to 34 years old had an age-adjusted relative risk of breast cancer of 1.11 (95% CI: 0.89, 1.37) compared with daughters born to mothers younger than 20 years. If this association is true, Trichopoulos (46) raised the intriguing possibility that breast cancer may be initiated in utero, noting that serum levels of total estrogens during pregnancy are substantially higher among older as opposed to younger women (47).

Risk is increased by a late age at menopause (48,49); an early menopause, whether natural or artificial (50,51), contributes to reducing risk. The association posited between an early age at menarche and increased breast cancer risk is not supported by all studies of the issue and can be best described as "weak" (10). Breast-feeding was initially thought to be an important breast cancer risk determinant but subsequently fell from favor. However, it has made a comeback in recent years with strength-

ening evidence of a protective effect in premenopausal women (52). However, the recent prospective U.S. Nurses Health Study (53) found no association between lactation and breast cancer risk.

The association between breast cancer risk and spontaneous and induced abortions remains difficult to interpret. For example, Pike et al (54) reported a relative risk of 2.4 among women under the age of 33 who had a first-trimester abortion, either spontaneous or induced, before their first full-term pregnancy. Subsequently, several studies failed to confirm this association although a number of further studies found elevated risks in subsets of their data. Howe et al (55) reported a 70% excess of interrupted pregnancies among breast cancer patients in New York State; the excess occurred regardless of prior pregnancy history.

In a large study conducted in Greece, the risk of breast cancer was not increased for women who had a history of abortion compared to nulliparous women with no history of abortion. When the analysis was restricted to parous women, using parous women with no history of abortion as the baseline, the risk of breast cancer associated with an induced abortion before first-term pregnancy was 2.06 (95% CI: 1.45, 2.90), for an induced abortion after first full-term pregnancy it was 1.59 (1.24, 2.04), and for a spontaneous abortion the risk was 1.10 (0.82, 1.40) (56).

In an equally large study, but with a younger age limitation, conducted in Seattle, Washington, the risk of breast cancer among women who had been pregnant at least once, the risk of breast cancer in those who had experienced an induced abortion was 50% higher than among other women (95% CI: 1.2, 1.9). The highest risks were seen in women who had an abortion before the age of 18 and those who had an abortion after 8 weeks' gestation (57). The authors concluded that their data support the hypothesis that an induced abortion can adversely affect a woman's subsequent risk of breast cancer (57). Lipworth et al (56) concluded that an interrupted pregnancy does not impart the long-term protective effect of a full-term pregnancy against breast cancer.

The potential association of an induced abortion and subsequent breast cancer risk remains an open question in cancer epidemiology at the present time. Given the large numbers of abortions induced worldwide and the common nature of breast cancer, it is important to resolve this issue as soon as possible.

Ionizing Radiation

Radiation to the breast in high doses increases the risk of breast cancer, whether the radiation was from exploding nuclear devices (58), from treatment of acute postpartum mastitis (59), or as a result of fluoroscopy (60). Exposure of the breast to radiation around menarche is associated with a particularly high risk of breast cancer (61), indicating that breast tissue may be particularly vulnerable at this time either because the breasts are developing rapidly or because most women have not given birth. Modan et al (62) reported an increased risk of breast cancer among a cohort of children subjected to scalp irradiation when they immigrated to Israel; risk was only elevated among those irradiated between the ages of 5 and 9. These results are very similar to those of cohorts exposed to much larger doses of radiation, although they are based on small numbers of patients.

Dietary and Nutritional Factors

The risk of breast cancer appears to increase with increasing body mass index among postmenopausal women (63), and a number of studies suggested that the same risk factor reduces the risk of breast cancer at premenopausal ages, although a number of biases, including the increased likelihood of finding a lump in thinner women, complicate the interpretation of these findings (64). Former college athletes have a reduced risk of breast cancer compared with nonathletes (65), as do ballet dancers (66). This may be associated with physical activity or reduced body weight around the time of menarche, during early adolescence, or throughout life.

The association with diet, particularly dietary fat intake, remains the subject of a great deal of controversy (67). Theoretical considerations of biologic processes lead to the conclusion that an increased risk of breast cancer with increasing saturated fat intake in postmenopausal women is plausible (68). However, the evidence from studies of human subjects with breast cancer is unclear. Case-control studies provided minimal support for this association, but no such association was found in the prospective studies reported to date. In fact,

these studies could be interpreted as supporting an inverse (protective) association between fat and breast cancer. Boyd et al (69) conducted a meta-analysis of 23 studies that examined fat as a nutrient and calculated the summary odds ratio to be 1.12 (95% CI: 1.04, 1.21) comparing women in the highest fifth of daily intakes with women in the lowest fifth. The finding was driven by results from case-control studies (overall risk: 1.21; 95% CI: 1.10, 1.34), particularly those conducted in Europe, and the authors reasoned that this was because of the greater heterogeneity in the European diet (69). Interpretation of these findings is still not altogether straightforward. Meta-analysis is a technique that needs more thought when applied to observational studies than to randomized trials, and many issues remain unresolved (70). It is also somewhat discomforting that the positive association between breast cancer risk and fat intake is based on findings from case-control studies, which are perceived to have a "weaker" design than the prospective design of the cohort studies for the analysis of dietary associations (10).

Most prospective studies of diet and breast cancer demonstrated a lack of association between intake of dietary fat and risk of breast cancer. They each have been criticized for involving a small number of subjects, homogeneous fat intake, and measurement errors in estimates of fat intake. A pooled analysis of all existing, good-quality data was conducted to clarify the nature of the association between fat intake and breast cancer risk. Seven prospective studies, conducted in Canada, the United States, Sweden, and the Netherlands, satisfied the criteria for inclusion in this pooled analysis. There were at total of 4980 cases of breast cancer among 337,819 women included in this study (71).

When women in the highest quintile of energy-adjusted total fat intake were compared to women in the lowest quintile, the multivariate, pooled relative risk (RR) of breast cancer was 1.05 (95% CI: 0.94, 1.16). Relative risks for saturated, monounsaturated, and polyunsaturated fat and for cholesterol, considered individually, were close to unity. There was little overall association between the percentage of energy intake from fat and the risk of breast cancer, even among women whose energy intake from fat was less than 20%. This analysis revealed no evidence of a positive association between total dietary fat intake and the risk of breast cancer. There was no reduction in risk even among women whose energy intake from fat was less than 20% of total energy intake. In the context of the Western lifestyle, lowering the total intake of fat in midlife is unlikely to reduce the risk of breast cancer substantially.

Early investigational studies of the association between diet and breast cancer were essentially retrospective (case-control) studies with conflicting findings. In the 1980s, belief in the association between breast cancer risk and dietary fat intake was a matter of faith in the epidemiologic community. Like many issues of faith, schisms developed and positions became entrenched and dogmatic while the community awaited findings from the prospective studies. For a variety of putative reasons, some sects failed to believe the early cohort studies, but the findings reported here are quite convincing. Prospective studies showed no evidence of an association between adult fat intake and the risk of developing breast cancer.

Can we now dismiss the hypothesis that associates breast cancer risk and fat intake? It is impossible to rule out dietary fat intake in early childhood as being important in the subsequent development of breast cancer. It probably always will be because it is very difficult to imagine how to study such an association (in the absence of reliable biologic markers of breast cancer risk). It is also useful to examine the possible different effects of fat at different periods before breast cancer develops. Cohort studies frequently have gaps of 8 to 15 years between the exposure assessment at the cancer diagnosis, whereas case-control studies are restricted to very recent diet. This is a lesser issue and should be resolved in the near future.

The findings from this study have implications in two other areas. From a scientific viewpoint, they raise real questions about the utility of conducting intervention studies aimed at reducing breast cancer risk by altering dietary fat intakes in women in middle life. There do not appear to be data to support the conduction of such studies at present. Much more importantly, the findings do not provide carte blanche for women to eat as much fatty foods as they wish: High-fat diets are still associated with an increased risk of several common serious diseases.

Martin-Moreno et al (72) reported from a large case-control study in Spain that higher consumption of olive oil is significantly related to a lower risk of breast cancer. For highest to

lowest quartile of consumption, the odds ratio was 0.66 (95% CI: 0.46, 0.97). A large case-control study in Greece confirmed this finding: A higher consumption of olive oil was significantly associated with a reduced risk of breast cancer (73). A case-control study conducted in Italy (74) further supported the finding.

The association between breast cancer risk and dietary intake of nutrients was investigated in a prospective study of 85,000 U.S. nurses followed for 8 years (20). When the highest quintile of intake was compared to the lowest (the referent category with an odds ratio of 1), the odds ratios for vitamin C was 1.03 (95% CI: 0.87, 1.21); for vitamin E, 0.99 (0.83, 1.19); and for vitamin A, 0.84 (0.70, 0.98). Furthermore, when the effect of vitamin supplementation was investigated, a protective effect of vitamin A supplementation was identified but only among women in the lowest fifth of the daily intake of this vitamin. This is a particularly interesting finding whose true significance will become apparent as the results of other ongoing epidemiologic studies become available (18). In Greece, vegetable and fruit consumption were independently associated with statistically significant reductions of breast cancer risk by 12% and 8%, respectively, per quintile increase of consumption (73).

The results of these and other studies (72,75) suggest that consumption of green vegetables is an indicator of a low-risk dietary pattern. This may simply reflect low intake of fat or calories, or suggest that some constituent of green vegetables may be protective (76). However, this was not a consistent finding in studies of the association between fruit and vegetable consumption and cancer risk (19).

Alcohol Drinking

A large number of studies consistently observed a modest increase in the risk of breast cancer with increased alcohol intake (77,78), although no satisfactory biologic explanation has been proposed. In their overview Longnecker et al (78) concluded the following: 1) At intakes of 24g/day (two drinks/day) the published data are strongly supportive of an association between alcohol consumption and an increased risk of breast cancer; 2) at lower levels of intake, weaker or modest associations are found, although the CI generally includes 1.0; 3) evidence in favor of a dose-response relationship is strong; and 4) the pooled RR of 1.1 for ever-versus never-drinkers does not alter the conclusions since most women are light or moderate drinkers. Longnecker et al did not interpret their findings as proof of causality but as being strongly supportive of an association between alcohol consumption and an increased risk of breast cancer.

Oral Contraceptives

A large number of studies investigated the role of oral contraceptive use in breast cancer risk (79). Initially, there appeared to be consistent evidence supporting an increased risk of breast cancer in "young" women associated with current prolonged use (>5 years) of oral contraceptives; "young" is certainly less than 35 years old and perhaps less than 45 years old (79). The risk appears to level off after use of oral contraceptives has stopped. An important meta-analysis was undertaken recently to help clarify this situation. All available epidemiologic data collected on this association were analyzed by the ICRF Cancer Epidemiology Group at Oxford, United Kingdom. The Collaborative Group on Hormonal Factors in Breast Cancer (80) brought together and reanalyzed the entire epidemiologic database available regarding the relationship between breast cancer risk and use of hormonal contraceptives. The objective was to obtain a clearer picture of the quantitative nature of the putative relationship between patterns of use of hormonal contraceptives and the subsequent risk of breast cancer in users.

Individual data on 53,297 women with breast cancer and 100,239 women without breast cancer from 54 studies conducted in 25 countries were collected in a central database. After the data were checked, a central analysis was performed. Estimates of the relative risk for breast cancer were determined using a modification of the Mantel-Haenszel procedure. All analyses were stratified by study, age at diagnosis, parity, and, where appropriate, the age a woman was when her first child was born and the age she was when her risk of conception ceased.

Data regarding risk factors were obtained from individual epidemiologic studies which differed in their basic design, some studies being retrospective (case-control studies) while others were prospective in design (cohort studies).

The findings from this analysis provide strong support for two main conclusions. First, while women are taking combined oral contraceptives and in the 10 years after stopping, there is a small increase in the relative risk of having breast cancer diagnosed (RR in current users: 1.24; 95% CI: 1.15, 1.33; 1–4 years after stopping use RR: 1.16; 95% CI: 1.08, 1.23; 5–9 years after stopping use RR: 1.07; 95% CI: 1.02, 1.13).

Second, there is no significant excess risk of having breast cancer diagnosed 10 or more years after stopping oral contraceptive use (RR: 1.01; 95% CI: 0.96, 1.05). Breast cancers diagnosed in women who had used combined oral contraceptives were less advanced clinically than those diagnosed in women who had never used these contraceptives. For ever-users compared to never-users the RR for tumors that had spread beyond the breast compared to localized tumors was 0.88 (0.81, 0.95). The analysis demonstrated no obvious association for recency of use between women with different background risks of breast cancer, including women from different countries and ethnic groups, women with different reproductive histories, and those with or without a family history of breast cancer. Other features of hormonal contraceptive use such as duration of use, age at first use, and the dose and type of the hormone within the contraceptives had little additional effect on breast cancer risk once recency of use had been taken into account.

The relationship between breast cancer risk and hormonal contraceptive use is unusual and it is not possible to infer from these data whether it is due to an earlier diagnosis of breast cancer in ever-users, the biologic effects of breast cancer in ever-users, or a combination of reasons. Women who are currently using combined oral contraceptives or who have used them in the past 10 years are at a slightly increased risk of having breast cancer diagnosed, although the additional cancers diagnosed tend to be localized to the breast. There is no evidence of an increase in the risk of having breast cancer diagnosed 10 years or later after cessation of use, and the cancers diagnosed then appear to be less advanced clinically than the breast cancers diagnosed in never-users.

Further reassuring news is that the relative risks are small and the *period-at-risk* appears confined to times of life when the incidence of breast cancer, although not negligible, has not reached the highest levels attained in the latter part of the sixth and seventh decades of life.

Hormonal Replacement Therapy

The other important, and increasingly common, source of exogenous hormones is hormonal replacement therapy (HRT). There have been several important recent studies of breast cancer risk and HRT. To quantify the relationship between the use of hormones in postmenopausal women and the risk of breast cancer, the follow-up in the Nurses Health Study was extended to 1992. There were 1935 cases of invasive breast cancer recorded during 725,550 woman-years of follow-up among the postmenopausal women (81). The risk of breast cancer was significantly increased among women who were currently using estrogen alone (RR: 1.32; 95% CI: 1.14, 1.54) compared to postmenopausal women who had never used hormones. The risk of breast cancer was also significantly increased among women who were currently using estrogen plus progestin (RR: 1.41; 95% CI: 1.15, 1.74) (81).

Women currently taking hormones and who had used such therapy for 5 to 9 years had an adjusted RR of breast cancer of 1.46 (95% CI: 1.22, 1.74). Women currently taking hormones and who had used such therapy for 10 years or longer had an adjusted RR of breast cancer of 1.46 (95% CI: 1.20, 1.76) (81). Breast cancer incidence associated with postmenopausal hormone therapy for 5 years or longer was greater among older women (RR for women aged 60–64 years: 1.71; 95% CI: 1.34, 2.18). The RR of death from breast cancer was 1.45 (1.01, 2.09) among women who had taken estrogen for 5 years or longer (81).

Recent meta-analyses of the available studies on HRT use and breast cancer agree that little excess risk is associated with ever-use or short-term use of estrogen replacement therapy. A small increase in relative risk has a large impact on the number of women developing breast cancer because of the high baseline rates. For women in the United States aged 65, the baseline rate is 210 new cases/100,000 women/yr. An RR as small as 1.2 increases a woman's chances of developing breast cancer each year from 1 in 250 to 1 in 200 (82).

There is some evidence of an association between use of HRT and an increased risk of breast cancer. The risk appears to increase with duration of use and there does not appear to be a beneficial effect of progestin use. There also seems to be a suggestion of an association with recent use. The absolute effect could be quite large due to the common nature of breast cancer and HRT use.

Other Risk Factors

Although there is an antiestrogenic effect of cigarettes (83), which theoretically should lead to an apparent protective effect of cigarette smoking in breast cancer risk, the majority of published studies have not demonstrated this (7).

Of the other factors for breast cancer that have been studied, a positive family history has the effect of increasing the risk of breast cancer (84), with the maximum effect apparent in premenopausal women who have a first-degree relative with breast cancer at premenopausal ages. Genetics are discussed in more detail later in this volume. Women with primary biliary cirrhosis appear to have an increased risk of breast cancer (85). A number of other risk factors have been identified, albeit inconsistently, and are reviewed elsewhere (10), although their effect is thought to be limited.

Summary

In summary, there are one million reasons why breast cancer is and will remain an important public health problem. Between 1950 and 1979 one million women in the United States died from breast cancer. In the year 2000, more than one million women worldwide are expected to be diagnosed for the first time as having breast cancer.

Mortality is generally the first important thought when one considers the impact of breast cancer. The social dimension to the effects of breast cancer is not fully appreciated. Breast cancer robs families of their mother frequently at times of life when social dependence is maximum. During childhood a child is much more likely to lose his or her mother to breast cancer than the mother is to lose the child to cancer of any form. Breast cancer mortality will not be eliminated by a single approach but will only be reduced by a series of coordinated actions.

The underlying concept of breast cancer control is to specify a series of actions that will bring about a reduction in breast cancer mortality: *primary prevention*, by identification of risk determinants and their alteration; *secondary prevention*, by earlier diagnosis and increased survival over and above lead time; and *tertiary prevention*, by improving treatment outcome.

The classic approach to prevention is through the identification of risk factors and their alteration in a population. A risk factor is an exposure or habit that is associated with the occurrence of a disease. A litany of risk factors for breast cancer have been identified. A risk determinant is a member of a subset of risk factors whose alteration would lead directly to an alteration in the risk of a disease. For breast cancer, two, and possibly three, risk determinants have been identified: exposure to ionizing radiation around the time of puberty and long-term use of HRT (86). The third possibility is alcohol consumption.

Thus, there is little hope at the present time for greatly altering the risk of an individual woman developing breast cancer in her lifetime given the current state of knowledge derived from classic epidemiology. However, as discussed below, there may be possibilities arising from less-classic approaches to prevention.

Cancer of the Uterus

Cancer of the cervix, choriocarcinoma, and cancer of the corpus uteri are generally well separated in incidence statistics and analytical studies. However, there is some difficulty in obtaining a clear interpretation of mortality statistics. Cancer of the cervix uteri is the second most common cancer among women worldwide. Some 80% of these cancers occur in developing countries.

Descriptive Epidemiology of Cancer of the Cervix Uteri (ICD9 180)

Cancer of the cervix is the second most common form of cancer in women worldwide and the leading female cancer in sub-Saharan Africa, Central and South America, and Southeast Asia. The highest incidence rate is recorded in Trujillo in Peru (54.6 cases/100,000 population). High incidence rates are also recorded in regions of South America and India (Table 36-5). Low incidence rates of cervical cancer are found in a variety of population settings, with the lowest rates recorded in two population groups of Israel, non-Jews (2.6) and Jews born in Israel (3.4). However, there is no region of

T A B L E 36-5

Cancer of the Cervix Uteri (ICD9 180): 10 Highest and 10 Lowest Incidence Rates per 100,000 Person-Years

Registry	No. of Cases	Rate
Peru, Trujillo	312	54.6
Brazil, Goiânia	290	48.9
India, Madras	2878	47.2
Paraguay, Asunción	626	47.1
Colombia, Cali	1017	42.2
Ecuador, Quito	357	34.0
Brazil, Pôrto Alegre	209	31.2
India, Bangalore	1526	31.1
New Zealand: Maori	153	29.9
Thailand, Chiang Mai	691	29.2
Finland	875	4.4
China, Shanghai	986	4.3
Israel: all Jews	384	4.2
Kuwait: Kuwaitis	32	4.1
Israel: born Europe, America	168	4.0
U.S., Hawaii: Chinese	8	3.8
China, Qidong	108	3.7
U.S., Hawaii: Japanese	43	3.6
Israel: born Israel	74	3.4
Israel: non-Jews	27	2.6

Source: Parkin DM, Pisani P, Ferlay J. Estimates of the worldwide frequency of sixteen major cancers in 1985. *Int J Cancer* 1993;54:594–606.

the world with truly low rates of cancer of the cervix; this is perhaps the only form of cancer to exhibit this phenomenon.

The highest incidence rates recorded previously were in Recife in Brazil (83.2) and in the Pacific Polynesian Islanders (64.4); these rates are somewhat higher than the current highest rates. High incidence rates are seen in several large Indian cities. The rates are intermediate in eastern Europe, but much lower in North America, Australasia, and northern and western Europe. The lowest rates are seen in Israel and in Kuwait. In Europe, very low rates are noted in Finland, Spain, and southern Ireland.

In the United States large differences are seen between ethnic groups, with a twofold difference between the black and white populations. The incidence is also lower in Japanese populations, but is higher in Hispanics and American Indians. Ethnic differences are also seen in New Zealand between the Maoris, the non-Maoris, and the Pacific Polynesian Islanders. Urban populations frequently show higher rates than rural populations.

A decline in the incidence and mortality rates for cervical cancer has been observed virtually everywhere. Where effective national screening programs have been introduced, as in Finland, mortality has fallen substantially (87). However, rises in mortality rates for women born around 1930 were recently observed in New Zealand, Australia, and the United Kingdom (88), suggesting greater exposure to risk factors, whether new or preexisting, in the more recent birth cohorts in these countries.

Descriptive Epidemiology of Choriocarcinoma (ICD9 181)

Choriocarcinoma is a rare disease of the trophoblast, the incidence of which seems to be much higher in Asian countries than elsewhere (89). Incidence rates are very low and exceed 1 per 100,000 in only two populations, in each of which the number of cases is very low. There are also many regions where no cases were recorded in a 5-year period. The etiology of these cancers is very poorly understood and researched, undoubtedly on grounds related to the rare nature of the condition. Maternal age and history of a prior hydatidiform mole seem to be the only two established risk factors for the disease (90). There is a suggestion that choriocarcinoma is declining in incidence, but this is difficult to prove given the rarity of the condition.

Descriptive Epidemiology of Cancer of the Corpus Uteri (ICD9 182)

The highest rates of cancer of the corpus uteri are reported from the United States and Canada, specifically from populations that are white or mainly white. The highest incidence rate (22.3 cases/100,000 population) is from the white population of the San Francisco Bay area. Low incidence rates are reported from populations of India, Southeast Asia, and Africa (Table 36-6).

In Israel, the incidence in Jews born in Europe or America is higher than in those born in Africa, Asia, or Israel. The Chinese and Japanese in the United States experience rates that are more than four times those in China and Japan.

Leiomyosarcoma of the uterus accounts for 6.8% of these cancers in black American women compared with 2.2% in white women (91). In

T A B L E   36-6

Cancer of the Corpus Uteri (ICD9 182): 10 Highest and 10 Lowest Incidence Rates per 100,000 Person-Years

Registry	No. of Cases	Rate
U.S., Bay area: white	2186	22.3
U.S., Alameda: white	659	22.1
U.S., Seattle	2101	21.8
U.S., Detroit: white	2306	21.2
U.S., Los Angeles: O. white	3714	19.0
U.S., Hawaii: white	141	18.9
U.S., Iowa	2029	18.4
U.S., Hawaii: Hawaiian	64	18.3
Canada, Manitoba	679	18.0
U.S., Utah	720	17.7
U.S., Los Angeles: Korean	4	2.0
Bermuda: white and other	3	1.9
Brazil, Goiânia	12	1.8
India, Madras	91	1.7
India, Ahmadabad	74	1.7
India, Bangalore	73	1.6
The Gambia	8	1.2
Algeria, Sétif	12	1.1
Mali, Bamako	4	0.8
China, Qidong	14	0.5

Source: Parkin DM, Pisani P, Ferlay J. Estimates of the worldwide frequency of sixteen major cancers in 1985. *Int J Cancer* 1993;54:594–606.

Singapore in 1968 to 1982, the proportion was 11.6% (31).

Whereas mortality rates from cancer of the corpus uteri largely declined, incidence trends are more variable. In the United States a substantial increase in incidence, more marked in the age group 55 to 64 years old and ascribed to the use of postmenopausal estrogens, occurred in the 1970s. Incidence rates have now declined to, or below, previous levels after use of these drugs ceased (92). Increases in Europe were much smaller.

Individual mortality statistics for cancer of the cervix and endometrium are unreliable (93). Thus, it is necessary to consider uterine cancer as a single entity when one discusses mortality data and investigates temporal trends. Of course, this is a major problem on account of the differences in the epidemiology of the two sites. However, the mortality rate appears to be falling in most countries (9,33), although it is difficult to say whether this is due to changing patterns of cervical or endometrial cancer.

Etiology of Cancer of the Cervix

Epidemiologic studies of cervical cancer demonstrated a clear association between a woman's risk of developing this cancer and the number of sexual partners she, or her partner, have had. This association strongly suggests that a sexually transmitted agent is involved in the etiology of cervical cancer, and viruses, particularly herpes simplex virus type 2, HPV, and cytomegalovirus, have been considered among the candidates. A simple interpretation of the results of many studies is limited by problems with the lack of specificity of the laboratory techniques employed to conduct the biologic measurements.

A cohort study of 10,000 women in which a technique to detect herpes simplex virus type 2 antibodies was used failed to find any difference in the prevalence of these antibodies between women who developed cervical cancer and those who did not (94); however, the number of cases arising in this cohort was probably too small to allow definitive conclusions. Further studies did not support the existence of an association with herpes simplex virus type 2, and molecular, immunologic, and other experimental studies failed to provide clear evidence that herpes simplex virus type 2 has oncogenic potential (95).

HPV also may have a role in the causation of cervical cancer. A major difficulty in the study of this virus is that it cannot be grown in vitro, which has made the development of laboratory tests to detect markers of HPV in human tissues difficult. However, the DNA of HPV can now be cloned in bacteria, and more than 60 types have been identified. Results suggest that HPV-16 and, to a lesser extent, HPV-18 are associated with advanced CIN or invasive cervical carcinoma, whereas HPV-6 and HPV-11 are more often associated with lower-grade CIN and condylomata. The strength of the association is now becoming very much clearer and stronger, and can almost be accepted as causal (28).

Cervical cancer resembles a sexually transmitted disease in several aspects (96): It is related inversely to age at the time of first intercourse and directly to the number of sexual partners (97), and is apparently independently related to multiparity (98). Moreover, epidemiologic data indicate that the risk is elevated in lower social classes, long-term oral contraceptive users (99,100), and cigarette smokers (101).

Pre–vitamin A (carotenoids) or other aspects of a vegetable-rich diet may be protective, although it is not clear whether this merely indicates a more health-conscious lifestyle (102). In terms of prevention, rational use of cytologic screening services is undoubtedly the key to reducing rates of invasive cervical cancer. It has been estimated that screening at 3-year intervals for women aged 35 to 64 can reduce the incidence of invasive cervical cancer by over 90% (7).

Etiology of Endometrial Cancer

The descriptive epidemiology of endometrial cancer is similar to that of breast cancer in several aspects. High incidence rates are reported in developed countries of North America and Europe (except the United Kingdom), and low rates in Japan and other cancer registration areas in Asia. Although endometrial cancer is a disease of older women, its age-incidence curve shows a flattening of the slope around the time of menopause.

In terms of hormonal correlates, endometrial cancer is the best-understood gynecologic malignancy. It is strongly related to elevated levels or availability of exogenous or endogenous estrogens, and correspondingly low levels of progestogens. Thus, it is related to anovularity in many women, estrogen replacement treatment during the menopause, and obesity, which increases endogenous estrogen levels. The RRs for long-term use and severe obesity are of the order of 5 to 10 in various populations investigated (103). However, in terms of attributable risk, menopausal replacement treatment was the major determinant of the epidemic of endometrial cancer observed in the United States during the 1970s (104), whereas obesity is the major established risk determinant of endometrial cancer in Europe (105) where menopausal HRT has not been so widely used. The situation in the 1990s may not be so clear.

While HRT has been widely shown to be beneficial against the symptoms of the menopause, there is a long history of an association with an increased risk of endometrial cancer. Thirty epidemiologic studies were available to conduct a meta-analysis to assess the association of unopposed estrogen or estrogen plus progestin and the risk of developing endometrial cancer or of dying from that disease (106). The summary RR was 2.3 (95%

CI: 2.1, 2.5) for estrogen users compared to nonusers. The RR was much higher for long-term use, being 9.5 for those who took estrogen for 10 years or longer, compared to nonusers.

The relative risk remained elevated 5 years or more after discontinuation of unopposed estrogen therapy (RR: 2.3). Interrupting estrogen for 5 to 7 days per month was not associated with a lower risk of endometrial cancer compared to using estrogens every day. Users of unopposed conjugated estrogen had a greater increase in relative risk of developing endometrial cancer than did users of synthetic estrogens.

The risk of endometrial cancer death was also elevated among unopposed estrogen users (RR: 2.7; CI: 0.9, 8.0). Among users of estrogen plus progestin, cohort studies showed a decreased risk of endometrial cancer (RR: 0.4) whereas case-control studies showed an increased risk (RR: 1.8).

These data are limited and conflicting and difficult to interpret at the present time (106). The Postmenopausal Estrogen/Progestin Interventions (PEPI) trial was a 3-year randomized trial of placebo, unopposed estrogen, or three estrogen-progestin combinations in 875 women. The risk of adenomatous or atypical endometrial hyperplasia was about 1% in women allocated to the placebo arm or to any of the estrogen-progestin combinations, but was 34% in women assigned to treatment with estrogen alone (107).

There is convincing evidence that use of unopposed estrogens leads to a risk of endometrial cancer that is higher than that in women who do not use such HRT. The risk of endometrial cancer increases with long-term use of unopposed estrogens and remains elevated for at least 5 years after discontinuation. The overall evidence concerning estrogen plus progestin on the risk of endometrial cancer cannot yet be properly evaluated but initial findings look promising.

Recent analysis of incidence data from Sweden reveals patterns of cohort-specific risk that are compatible with the effect of estrogen-only HRT (as prescribed in the 1960s) in increasing risk, while the addition of progestins approximately 10 years later was not so obviously associated with an increased risk (108). This is compatible with the results from case-control and cohort studies (109). Further simultaneous examination of mortality data revealed a discrepancy between incidence and mortality data, which the authors suggest is partly due to improved survival but also supports the hypothesis that endometrial cancers associated with exogenous estrogens may be associated with a favorable clinical course (108).

Use of combined oral contraceptives, and the consequent relative progestin excess, considerably decrease the risk of the endometrial cancer (110). The combined evidence from studies showed a very consistent protection (approximately 50%) in ever-users compared with never-users, and the risk is inversely related to duration of use. However, endometrial cancer is rare in younger women, and the ultimate evaluation of the public health impact of this protection is related to the observation of much reduced risks at older ages (111).

Other determinants of endometrial cancer include nulliparity, late menopause and perhaps early menarche, diabetes, and hypertension (112), although it is not known whether these risk factors are partly mediated through a mutual association with being overweight.

All these established and potential risk factors explain only a fraction of endometrial cancers (approximately 50% in Europe and perhaps two thirds in the United States), but cannot account for the 30-fold worldwide variation in the disease incidence. There is some suggestion that not only nutritional status but also diet composition are related to endometrial cancer. Ecologic studies found positive correlations with consumption of meat, eggs, milk, proteins, fats, and total calorie intake. The few analytical studies available suggested positive associations with total calorie intake, carbohydrates, fats, and oils, and protection by green vegetables (19). Methodologically sound studies, with adequate allowance for total energy intake, are even more important for endometrial cancer than for other cancers that are less strongly related to obesity (113).

Cancer of the Ovary

Ovarian cancer is a moderately frequent disease representing the most frequent cause of death from gynecologic malignancies in the Western world. It is the sixth most frequent form of cancer worldwide, with an estimated 162,000 incident cases in 1985 (1). Epithelial cystadenocarcinomas constitute the large majority of ovarian malignancies. The less-frequent germ cell tumors have a younger age distribution. The range of geographic variation for this disease is rather small.

Descriptive Epidemiology

The highest incidence rate of cancer of the ovary is reported from St. Gallen in Switzerland (17.0 cases/100,000 population). High rates are also recorded from four Scandinavian countries: Iceland (16.6/100,000), Denmark (14.9), Sweden (14.6), and Norway (14.6) [Finland has the eighty-second highest rate (9.9)]. There is little geographic pattern to the regions with the lowest rates (Table 36-7).

Hawaiians and Pacific Polynesian Islanders have higher rates than Maoris, in whom the incidence is similar to that of non-Maoris in New Zealand. The highest rates reported from Europe are 17.3 in Ardèche in France (114) and around 15 in Norway, Sweden, and Israel (for women born in Europe or America). Most rates in Europe and North America range between 8

T A B L E   **36-7**

Cancer of the Ovary (ICD9 183): 10 Highest and 10 Lowest Incidence Rates per 100,000 Person-Years

Registry	No. of Cases	Rate
Switzerland, St. Gallen	307	17.0
Iceland	118	16.6
Israel: born Europe, America	742	15.2
Denmark	3058	14.9
Canada, Northwest Territory and Yukon	15	14.7
U.K., N.E. Scotland	300	14.6
Sweden	5097	14.6
Norway	2300	14.6
U.K., S.E. Scotland	680	14.0
Czechoslovakia, Boh. and Moravia	5195	13.6
Italy, Latina	38	4.3
U.S., Los Angeles: Korean	10	4.1
India, Ahmadabad	190	4.0
Kuwait: Kuwaitis	28	3.7
France, Martinique	30	3.2
Israel: non-Jews	27	2.4
Algeria, Sétif	22	1.6
China, Qidong	45	1.5
The Gambia	7	1.4
Mali, Bamako	7	1.0

Source: Parkin DM, Pisani P, Ferlay J. Estimates of the worldwide frequency of sixteen major cancers in 1985. *Int J Cancer* 1993;54:594–606.

and 12. Rates for black American women are about two thirds those for white women. Although women in Asia have a relatively low incidence of ovarian tumors (in the range of 5–7), Chinese and Japanese women who reside in the United States tend to have slightly higher rates although they are less than those in the white population.

Little change has been observed in the incidence of the disease in most registries. The rise in incidence has been slightly greater in Japan than elsewhere. There is great variation in the cohort-specific patterns of ovarian cancer mortality worldwide (9,33). Risk appears to be falling in younger cohorts in countries such as Canada, Germany, Denmark, and Australia but rising in Japan, Czechoslovakia, and Italy.

Etiology

Epithelial ovarian cancer is the most common type of ovarian neoplasia and the leading cause of death from gynecologic neoplasms in most Western countries. This term represents a very wide and diverse range of pathologic entities. As for other female hormone–related neoplasms, its age curve tends to flatten off around the time of menopause (115).

The risk of ovarian cancer is increased approximately twofold in nulliparous women compared with parous women. An increased risk has been suggested for late age at first birth, early menarche, and late menopause, but the evidence is inconsistent.

Results of more than a dozen studies uniformly indicate that oral contraceptive use is protective against ovarian carcinogenesis, with the incidence of epithelial invasive cancer being reduced by approximately 40% in ever-users of oral contraceptives, and to a greater extent in long-term users (116–119). Thus, on a population scale, combined oral contraceptives have probably been the major determinant of the (favorable) decrease in ovarian cancer rates observed in several Western countries (120).

As for breast and endometrial cancers, nutrition and diet are the major open questions in ovarian cancer epidemiology. The American Cancer Society One Million Study showed an elevated risk of ovarian cancer among obese women (103), but the evidence from case-control studies is largely negative, possibly because of loss of weight secondary to the neoplastic process. Ecologic studies found positive correlations with fats, proteins, and calories, although these are less strong than those for endometrial cancer. Case-control studies showed a possible association with total fat intake and some protection by consumption of green vegetables (19), but further research is required in the area, particularly because diet may be more amenable to intervention than reproductive or menstrual history.

Prospects for Cancer Prevention in Women

There are several enigmas in the descriptive epidemiology of cancer in women whose detailed study may shed important etiologic clues. These include the higher incidence rates in many countries of malignant melanomas in women, the higher incidence rates of thyroid cancer in women, and the consistent finding of lower levels of gastric cancer in women than in men. The latter is most surprising given our belief that diet is such an overwhelming risk factor for this condition.

There is increasing evidence supporting an unexpected association between HRT use and a reduced risk of colorectal cancer. Colorectal cancer is the fourth most common form of cancer. In 1985, there were 678,000 incident cases, representing 8.9% of all new cancers (1). In men, colorectal cancer is the third most common form of cancer (331,000 cases, 8.6%). In women, it also is the third most common cancer (346,000 cases, 9.2%).

A MEDLINE search was used to identify observational studies published between January 1974 and December 1993 for a meta-analysis (121). The overall risk for colorectal cancer and estrogen replacement therapy was 0.92 (95% CI: 0.74, 1.5). There was not a separate effect when colon and rectal cancers were considered separate entities (121). Subsequent to this report further studies have been published.

A case-control study from Seattle of 193 women aged 30 to 62 years with colon cancer and an equal number of control subjects was conducted to examine the relationship between colon cancer and female hormone use (122). Use of noncontraceptive hormones after age 40 was associated with a reduced risk of colon cancer (odds ratio: 0.60; 95% CI: 0.35, 1.01). The risk among women taking noncontraceptive hormones for 5 years or more was 0.47 (0.24, 0.91) (122).

The American Cancer Society Prospective Study examined in some detail colorectal cancer mortality. With the risk set to 1.0 among women who reported to be never-users of HRT (the referent group), the risk associated with ever-use was 0.69 (95% CI: 0.60, 0.79) (123). Relative to the risk in never-users, the risk associated with use for less than 1 year was 0.81 (0.63, 1.03), that associated with use for 2 to 5 years was 0.76 (0.61, 0.95), with use for 6 to 10 years the risk was 0.55 (0.39, 0.77), and with use of HRT for 11 years or longer it was 0.54 (0.39, 0.76).

Of 19 published studies of HRT and colorectal cancer risk, 10 supported an inverse association and the remaining 5 showed a significant reduction in risk. The risk seems lowest among long-term users. Although there are still some contradictions in the available literature, it appears likely that use of HRT reduces the risk of colorectal cancer in women. The risk appears to be decreased in half with such use for 5 to 10 years. The role of unopposed as compared to combination HRT is an open issue for colorectal cancer.

Thus, there is a complicated pattern of cancers potentially increased by HRT use (endometrium and breast cancers) and potentially reduced by its use (at least colorectal cancer), as well as beneficial effects of HRT use against heart disease and osteoporosis. Decision analysis has been used to assess the relative risks and benefits of estrogen replacement therapy in a hypothetical cohort of women assumed to be 50 years old. Health outcomes were extrapolated to age 75 and risks were based on accepted values from the literature (124). On balance, 25 years of estrogen replacement therapy would prevent 574 deaths and these 10,000 women would gain 3951 quality-adjusted life years. Sensitivity analysis revealed that the benefits of estrogen replacement therapy outweigh the risks under most assumptions (124).

HRT can be effective in reducing the symptoms frequently associated with the menopause. Increasingly HRT is being prescribed to women on a long-term basis in the hope that it will reduce the incidence and mortality from heart disease and osteoporosis. From the findings of the observational studies available, the net effect of long-term HRT use in a large group of women *appears* to be of benefit at the present time. This net benefit is the result of the overall trade-offs between reduced risks of cardiovascular disease and osteoporosis (and probably also colorectal cancer) and the increased risks of endometrial cancer and breast cancer: It will depend to some extent on the background rates of these conditions in the population of interest. However, there is as yet no confirmation of this effect from large-scale randomized trials, although these are now under way.

An approach to health that focuses on a single cause or preventive strategy is severely limited. The decision to prescribe HRT to a woman must always be made on an individual basis with a careful assessment of all possible risks and benefits. So should the management scheme available for women who are using HRT.

Another essential issue surrounds the advice given to a woman taking oral contraceptives or HRT, particularly with regard to breast cancer. Advice should be constrained. Participation in organized mammographic screening programs has been demonstrated unequivocally to reduce the mortality rate from breast cancer among women over the age of 50 (125). However, there is no evidence of a statistically significant reduction in breast cancer mortality among women younger than 50 years. Thus, with regards to reducing breast cancer mortality, at present there is little to offer women at the ages frequently associated with maximum social responsibility and at the ages when they are frequently exposed to exogenous hormonal therapy.

The physician, in discussing with a woman contemplating to undertake long-term HRT, is likely to be influenced by the potential large reductions in the mortality of heart disease, which is a more important cause of death than breast cancer in women. However, Stampfer (126) made the very shrewd observation that we know of several alternative ways to reduce the risk of heart disease (through changes in lifestyle) but that very little can be done at present to lower the risk of breast cancer.

The situation regarding the effects on mortality of long-term HRT will remain unclear for at least several more years until the results of randomized trials become available. This difficult situation will be compounded if recent findings from a large U.S. study are validated in other clinical situations. Laya et al (127) recently demonstrated that women currently taking HRT had an increased mammographic breast density that led to a lower specificity and lower sensitivity of screening mammography. Lower specificity could increase the cost of breast cancer screening and the lower sensitivity may decrease its effectiveness: There would be an increase in the number of recalls and an increase in the number of biopsies required. This further confuses an already difficult situation, particularly in women using such exogenous hormones and who are younger than 50 years.

These findings need to be verified urgently before an evidence-based position can be taken (128), and in the immediate short term, studies must be undertaken to investigate whether the stopping of HRT for short periods before mammography is performed can avoid this loss of effectiveness of screening mammography. The best advice at the present time for a woman taking HRT is to continue to participate in organized mammographic screening programs, but careful attention needs to be paid by the organizers of such programs to the status of the women with respect to current HRT use. The publication of further studies of this issue will allow a more quantified measured response to be made.

While this association remains without the formal proof of an intervention trial, there is enough information already available to indicate important prospects for cancer prevention in women, two of which are within our ability to influence, one of which is beyond it at present, and a further is an empirical observation.

1. Elimination of tobacco smoking or at the very least its reduction in women should be a cornerstone of any cancer control policy in women (and in men also). Cigarettes are the only product ever marketed that cause significant morbidity and premature mortality among those who use the product as the manufacturer intended (11). It is clear that women are not immune to the adverse effects of smoking and that this is a major international public health problem (14).

2. Increasing daily consumption of vegetables and fruits would serve to reduce the incidence of a number of common forms of cancer. No one type of vegetable or fruit appears to be more closely involved with this protective effect than any other and there is no indication as to what molecule in fruits and vegetables is necessary to confer this protection.

These two actions are clearly possible and should be pursued aggressively. There could also be important contributions to the reduction in cancer risk from a variety of other actions including reducing consumption of alcoholic beverages to 2 units/day, avoiding obesity, taking part in physical exercise, and reducing intake of fatty foods, as well as observing safety regulations at work and taking care in the sun (9). Paying attention to the early warning signs of cancer would also pay off in reducing mortality from cancer and participation of women in organized screening programs for cervical (Pap smear) and breast cancer (mammography), where quality-control standards are high at all steps of the process, would serve to contribute to cancer control in women (9).

In the future it might be possible to develop vaccines that have an important effect on reducing cancer risk in women. The development of a vaccine against EBV would reduce the incidence of nasopharyngeal cancer in Southeast Asia in men and women. The development of a vaccine against HPV types responsible for the increased risk of cervical cancer would reduce the risk of a cancer that is very common and responsible for 500,000 new cases of cancer each year around the world. Similarly, vaccination against hepatitis B could also lead to a reduction in primary liver cancer. In parts of Asia and Africa, liver and nasopharyngeal cancers are important forms of cancer in women.

There might also be some opportunity to alter cancer risk in women, since in recent decades it has become common for many women to use exogenous estrogens and progestins for purposes such as contraception and treatment of menopausal symptoms. The use of such substances regularly and for long periods could serve as one possible mechanism to alter the cancer risk in women. There is already evidence that exogenous hormone intake can alter cancer risk, both in increasing cancer risk (HRT and breast and endometrial cancers, oral contraceptives and breast cancer) and in reducing cancer risk (oral contraceptives and ovarian and endometrial cancers, probably HRT and colorectal cancer, tamoxifen and contralateral breast cancer). It seems theoretically attractive to pursue research to identify the *correct* ingredients of exogenous hormonal therapy that have a beneficial effect on a number of important cancers in women. If the goal is to reduce the global cancer burden in women, it makes greater sense at the present time to invest resources in cigarette avoidance and dietary modification.

Acknowledgments

This work was conducted within the framework of support from the Associazione Italiana per la Ricerca sul Cancro (Italian Association for Cancer Research) and the Consiglio Nazionale per la Ricerca (Italian Medical Research Council).

REFERENCES

1. Parkin DM, Pisani P, Ferlay J. Estimates of the worldwide frequency of sixteen major cancers in 1985. *Int J Cancer* 1993;54:594–606.

2. Parkin DM, Stjernsward J, Muir CS. Estimates of the worldwide frequency of twelve major cancers. *Bull World Health Organ* 1984;62:163–182.

3. Parkin DM, Laara E, Muir CS. Estimates of the worldwide frequency of sixteen major cancers in 1980. *Int J Cancer* 1988;41:184–197.

4. Jensen OM, Esteve J, Moller H, Renard H. Cancer in the European Community and its member states. *Eur J Cancer* 1990;26:1167–1256.

5. Illing EM, Gaudette LA, McLaughlin J, McBride M. Canadian Cancer Statistics, 1992. *Health Rep* 1992;4:161–174.

6. Doll R, Peto R. The causes of cancer: quantitative estimates of avoidable risks of cancer in the United States today. *J Natl Cancer Inst* 1981;66:1191–1308.

7. International Agency for Research on Cancer (IARC). Tobacco smoking. *Monogr Eval Carcinog Risk Hum* 1986;38.

8. International Agency for Research on Cancer (IARC). Alcohol drinking. *Monogr Eval Carcinog Risk Hum* 1988;44.

9. Boyle P, La Vecchia C, Maisonneuve P, et al. Cancer epidemiology and prevention. In: Peckam MJ, Pinedo H, Veronesi U, eds. *Oxford textbook of oncology.* Oxford: Oxford Medical, 1995:199–273.

10. Boyle P. Epidemiology of breast cancer. *Baillieres Clin Oncol* 1988;2:1–59.

11. Boyle P. The hazards of passive and active smoking. *N Engl J Med* 1993;328:1708–1709.

12. Peto R, Lopez AD, Boreham J, et al. Mortality from tobacco in developed countries: indirect

estimation from national vital statistics. *Lancet* 1992;39:1268–1278.

13. Boyle P, Maisonneuve P. Lung cancer and tobacco smoking. *Lung Cancer* 1995;12:167–181.

14. Chollat-Traquet C. *Women and tobacco.* Geneva: World Health Organization, 1992.

15. Decarli A, La Vecchia C. Cancer mortality in Italy, 1980. *Tumori* 1986;72:31–240.

16. Macfarlane GJ, Boyle P, Evstifeeva TV, et al. Rising trends of oral cancer mortality among males worldwide: the return of an old public health problem. *Cancer Causes Control* 1994; 5:259–265.

17. Peto R. The preventability of cancer. In: Vessey MP, Gray M, eds. *Cancer risks and prevention.* Oxford: Oxford University Press, 1985:1–15.

18. Boyle P. Dietary factors in the aetiology of cancer. *Oncol Haematol Lit Serv* 1994;1(2):7–8. Editorial.

19. Steinmetz KA, Potter JD. Vegetable, fruit, and cancer. I. Epidemiology. *Cancer Causes Control* 1991;2:325–358.

20. Hunter DJ, Manson J, Colditz GA, et al. A prospective study of the intake of vitamins C, E, and A and the risk of breast cancer. *N Engl J Med* 1993;329:234–240.

21. Gutensohn N, Cole P. Epidemiology of Hodgkin's disease. *Semin Oncol* 1980;7:92–102.

22. Mueller N, Evans A, Harris NL, et al. Hodgkin's disease and Epstein-Barr virus. Altered antibody pattern before diagnosis. *N Engl J Med* 1989; 320:689–695.

23. Paffenbarger RS, Wing AL, Hyde RT. Characteristics in youth indicative of adult-onset Hodgkin's disease. *J Natl Cancer Inst* 1977; 58:1489–1491.

24. Boiocchi M, Carbone A, DeRe V, Dolcetti R. Is the Epstein-Barr virus involved in Hodgkin's disease? *Tumori* 1989;75:345–350.

25. Alexander FE, Williams J, McKinney PA, et al. A specialist leukaemia/lymphoma registry in the UK. Part 2. Clustering of Hodgkin's disease. *Br J Cancer* 1989;60:948–952.

26. Boyle P, Walker AM, Alexander FE. Historical aspects of investigation of disease clusters. In: Alexander FE, Boyle P, eds. *Statistical investigation of disease clustering.* Lyon: IARC Scientific, 1996.

27. Beasley RP, Lin C, Hwang LY, Chien CS. Hepatocellular carcinoma and hepatitis B virus. A prospective study of 22,707 men in Taiwan. *Lancet* 1981;2:1129–1133.

28. Munoz N, Bosch FX. HPV and cervical neoplasia: review of case-control and cohort studies. *IARC Sci Publ* 1992;119:251–261.

29. Boyle P, Hsieh C-C, Maisonneuve P. Descriptive epidemiology of breast cancer. In: Zatonski W, Boyle P, Tzyznski J, eds. *Cancer epidemiology: vital statistics to prevention.* Warsaw: Interpresse, 1990.

30. Muir CS, Choi NW, Schifflers E. Time trends in cancer mortality in some countries—their possible causes and significance. In: *Proceedings of the Skandia international symposium, Stockholm.* Copenhagen: Munksgaard, 1990: 269–309.

31. Lee HP, Day NE, Shanmugaratnam K, eds. Trends in cancer incidence in Singapore 1968–1982. *IARC Sci Publ* 1988;91.

32. Devesa SS, Silverman DT, Young JL, et al. Cancer incidence and mortality among whites in the United States, 1974–1984. *J Natl Cancer Inst* 1987;79:701–770.

33. La Vecchia C, Lucchini F, Negri E, et al. Trends of cancer mortality in Europe, 1955–89. III. Breast and genital sites. *Eur J Cancer* 1992;28: 927–998.

34. Boyle P, La Vecchia C, Negri E, et al. Trends in diet-related cancers in Japan: a conundrum? *Lancet* 1993;342:752. Letter.

35. Haenszel W, Kurihara M. Studies of Japanese migrants. I. Mortality from cancer and other diseases among Japanese in the United States. *J Natl Cancer Inst* 1968;40:43–68.

36. Armstrong BK, Woodings TL, Stenhouse NS, et al. Mortality from cancer in migrants to Australia 1962–1971. NH & MRSC Research Unit in Epidemiology and Preventive Medicine, University of Western Australia, 1983.

37. McCredie M, Coates M. Cancer incidence in migrants to New South Wales. *Int J Cancer* 1990;46:228–232.

38. MacMahon B, Cole P, Lin TM, et al. Age at first birth and cancer of the breast. A summary of an international study. *Bull World Health Organ* 1970;43:209–221.

39. Ewertz M, Duffy SW, Adami HO, et al. Age at first birth, parity and risk of breast cancer: a meta-analysis of 8 studies from the Nordic Countries. *Int J Cancer* 1990;46:597–603.

40. Trichopoulos D, Hsieh CC, MacMahon B, et al. Age at any birth and breast cancer risk. *Int J Cancer* 1983;31:701–709.

41. Kvale G, Heuch I, Eide GE. A prospective study of reproductive factors and breast cancer. I: parity. *Am J Epidemiol* 1987;126:831–841.

42. La Vecchia C, Negri E, Boyle P. Reproductive factors and breast cancer: an overview. *Soz Praventivmed* 1989;34:101–107.

43. Ewertz M, Duffy SW, Adami HO, et al. Age at first birth, parity and risk of breast cancer: a meta-analysis of 8 studies from the Nordic countries. *Int J Cancer* 1990;46:597–603.

44. Thompson WD, Janerich DT. Maternal age at birth and risk of breast cancer in daughters. *Epidemiology* 1990;1:101–106.

45. Colditz GA, Willett WC, Stampfer MJ, et al. Parental age at birth and risk of breast cancer in daughters: a prospective study among US women. *Cancer Causes Control* 1990;1:31–36.

46. Trichopoulos D. Is breast cancer initiated in utero? *Epidemiology* 1990;1:95–96.

47. Panagiotopolou K, Katsouyani K, Petridou E, et al. Maternal age, parity and pregnancy estrogens. *Cancer Causes Control* 1990;1:119–124.

48. Bucallosi P, Veronesi U. Researches on the etiological factors in human breast cancer. *Acta Union Int Contre Cancer* 1959;15:1056–1060.

49. Ewertz M, Duffy SW. Risk of breast cancer in relation to reproductive factors in Denmark. *Br J Cancer* 1988;58:99–104.

50. Herity BA, O'Halloran MJ, Bourke GJ, Wilson-Davies K. A study of breast cancer in Irish women. *Br J Prev Soc Med* 1975;29:178–181.

51. Trichopoulos D, MacMahon B, Cole P. Menopause and breast cancer risk. *J Natl Cancer Inst* 1972;48:605–613.

52. Skegg DCG. Alcohol, coffee, fat and breast cancer. *BMJ* 1987;295:1011–1012. Editorial.

53. London SJ, Colditz GA, Stampfer MJ, et al. Lactation and risk of breast cancer in a cohort of US women. *Am J Epidemiol* 1990;132:17–26.

54. Pike MC, Henderson BE, Casagrande JT, et al. Oral contraceptive use and early abortion as risk factors for breast cancer in young women. *Br J Cancer* 1981;43:72–79.

55. Howe HL, Senie RT, Bzduch H, Herzfeld P. Early abortion and breast cancer risk among women under age 40. *Int J Epidemiol* 1989;18:300–304.

56. Lipworth L, Katsouyanni K, Ekbom A, et al. Abortion and the risk of breast cancer: a case-control study in Greece. *Int J Cancer* 1995;61:181–184.

57. Daling JR, Malone KF, Voigt LF, et al. Risk of breast cancer among young women: relationship to induced abortion. *J Natl Cancer Inst* 1994;86:1584–1592.

58. McGregor DH, Land CE, Choi K, et al. Breast cancer incidence among atomic bomb survivors, Hiroshima and Nagasaki, 1950–1969. *J Natl Cancer Inst* 1977;59:799–811.

59. Shore RE, Hempelmann LH, Kowaluk E, et al. Breast neoplasms in women treated with X-rays for acute postpartum mastitis. *J Natl Cancer Inst* 1977;59:813–822.

60. Boice JD, Monson RR. Breast cancer in women after repeated fluoroscopic examinations of the chest. *J Natl Cancer Inst* 1977;59:823–832.

61. Boice JD. Cancer following medical irradiation. Cancer 1981;47(suppl):1081–1090.

62. Modan B, Chetrit A, Alfandary E, Katz L. Increased risk of breast cancer after low-dose irradiation. *Lancet* 1989;1:629–631.

63. de Waard F, Baanders-van Halewijn EA, Huizinga J. The bimodal age distribution of patients with mammary carcinoma. *Cancer* 1964;17:141–151.

64. Swanson CA, Jones DY, Schatzkin A, et al. Breast cancer risk assessed by anthropometry in NHANES 1 epidemiological follow-up study. *Cancer Res* 1988;48:5363–5367.

65. Frisch RE, Wyshak G, Albright NL, et al. Lower prevalence of breast cancer and cancers of the reproductive system among former college athletes compared to non-athletes. *Br J Cancer* 1985;52:885–891.

66. Warren MP. The effects of exercise on pubertal progression and reproduction function in girls. *J Clin Endocrinol Metab* 1980;51:1150–1157.

67. Willett WC. The search for the causes of breast and colon cancer. *Nature* 1989;338:389–394.

68. Boyle P, Leake RE. Progress in understanding breast cancer: epidemiologic and biologic interactions. *Breast Cancer Res Treat* 1986;11:91–112.

69. Boyd NF, Martin LJ, Noffel M, et al. A meta-analysis of studies of dietary fat and breast cancer risk. *Br J Cancer* 1993;68:627–636.

70. Spitzer WO. Meta-meta analysis: unanswered questions about aggregating data. *J Clin Epidemiol* 1991;44:103–107.

71. Hunter DJ, Spiegelman D, Adami H-O, et al. Cohort studies of fat intake and the risk of breast cancer—a pooled analysis. *N Engl J Med* 1996;334:356–361.

72. Martin-Moreno JM, Boyle P, Gorgojo L, et al. Dietary fat, olive oil intake and breast cancer risk. *Int J Cancer* 1994;58:774–780.

73. Trichopolou A, Katsouyanni K, Stuver S, et al. Consumption of olive oil and specific food

groups in relation to breast cancer risk in Greece. *J Natl Cancer Inst* 1995;87:110–116.

74. La Vecchia C, Negri E, Franceschi S, et al. Olive oil, other dietary fats and the risk of breast cancer (Italy). *Cancer Causes Control* 1995;6: 545–550.

75. La Vecchia C, Decarli A, Parazzini F, et al. General epidemiology of breast cancer in northern Italy. *Int J Epidemiol* 1987;16:347–355.

76. Minchovicz JJ, Bradlow HL. Induction of estradiol metabolism by dietary indole-3-carbinol in humans. *J Natl Cancer Inst* 1990;82:947–949.

77. Willett WC, Stampfer MJ, Colditz GA, et al. Moderate alcohol consumption and risk of breast cancer. *N Engl J Med* 1987;316:1174–1180.

78. Longnecker MP. Alcoholic beverage consumption in relation to risk of breast cancer: meta-analysis and review. *Cancer Causes Control* 1994;5:73–82.

79. Prentice RL, Thomas DB. On the epidemiology of oral contraceptives and diseases. *Adv Cancer Res* 1987;49:285–401.

80. Collaborative Group on Hormonal Factors in Breast Cancer. Breast cancer and hormonal contraceptives: collaborative reanalysis of individual data on 53,297 women with breast cancer and 100,239 women without breast cancer from 54 epidemiological studies. *Lancet* 1966;347: 1713–1727.

81. Colditz GA, Hankinson SE, Hunter DJ, et al. The use of estrogens and progestins and the risk of breast cancer in post-menopausal women. *N Engl J Med* 1995;332:1589–1593.

82. Hulka BS, Liu ET, Lininger RA. Steroid hormones and risk of breast cancer. *Cancer* 1994; 74:1111–1124.

83. Baron JA. Smoking and estrogen-related disease. *Am J Epidemiol* 1984;119:9–22.

84. Macklin MT. Comparison of the number of breast cancer deaths observed in the relatives of breast cancer patients, and the number expected on the basis of mortality rates. *J Natl Cancer Inst* 1959;22:927–951.

85. Goudie BM, Burt AD, Boyle P, et al. Breast cancer in women with primary biliary cirrhosis. *BMJ* 1985;291:1597–1598.

86. Bergkvist L, Adami HO, Persson I, et al. The risk of breast cancer after estrogen and estrogen-progestin replacement. *N Engl J Med* 1989; 321:293–297.

87. Hakama M, Magnus K, Petterson F, et al. Effect of organised screening on the risk of cervix cancer in the Nordic countries. In: Miller AB, Chamberlain J, Day NE, et al, eds. *Cancer screening.* Geneva: International Union Against Cancer, 1991.

88. Muñoz N, Bosch FX. Epidemiology of cervical cancer. *IARC Sci Publ* 1989;94:9–39.

89. Shanmugaratnam K, Muir CS, Tow SH, et al. Rates per 100,000 births and incidence of choriocarcinoma and malignant mole in Singapore Chinese and Malays. Comparison with Connecticut, Norway and Sweden. *Int J Cancer* 1971;8:165–175.

90. Bracken MB, Brinton LA, Hayashi K. Epidemiology of hydatidiform mole and choriocarcinoma. *Epidemiol Rev* 1984;6:52–75.

91. Young JL, Percy CL, Asire AJ, eds. *Surveillance, epidemiology and end results. Incidence and mortality data 1973–77.* NCI Monograph 57. NIH publication no. 81-2330. Bethesda: National Cancer Institute, 1981.

92. Austin DF, Roe KM. The decreasing incidence of endometrial cancer: public health implications. *Am J Public Health* 1982;72:65–68.

93. Cuzick J, Boyle P. Trends in cervix cancer mortality. *Cancer Surv* 1988;7:417–439.

94. Vonka V, Kanka J, Jelinek I, et al. Prospective study on the relationship between cervical neoplasia and herpes-simplex type-2 virus. I. Epidemiological characteristics. *Int J Cancer* 1984; 33:49–60.

95. Vonka V, Kanka J, Roth Z. Herpes simplex type 2 virus and cervical neoplasia. *Adv Cancer Res* 1987;48:149–191.

96. Brinton LA, Fraumeni JF Jr. Epidemiology of uterine cervical cancer. *J Chron Dis* 1986;39: 1051–1065.

97. Brinton LA, Hamman RF, Huggins GR, et al. Sexual and reproductive risk factors for invasive squamous cell cervical cancer. *J Natl Cancer Inst* 1987;79:23–30.

98. Brinton LA, Reeves WC, Brenes MM, et al. Parity as a risk factor for cervical cancer. *Am J Epidemiol* 1989;130:486–496.

99. WHO Collaborative Study of Neoplasia and Steroid Contraceptives. Invasive cervical cancer and combined oral contraceptives. *BMJ* 1985; 290:961–965.

100. Brinton LA, Huggins GR, Lehmann HF, et al. Long-term use of oral contraceptives and risk of invasive cervical cancer. *Int J Cancer* 1986;38: 339–344.

101. La Vecchia C, Franceschi S, Decarli A, et al. Cigarette smoking and the risk of cervical neoplasia. *Am J Epidemiol* 1986;123:22–29.

102. La Vecchia C, Decarli A, Fasoli M, et al. Dietary vitamin A and the risk of intraepithelial and invasive cervical neoplasia. *Gynecol Oncol* 1988;30:187–195.

103. Lew EA, Garfinkel L. Variations in mortality by weight among 750,000 men and women. *J Chron Dis* 1979;32:563–576.

104. Ziel HK, Finkle WD. Increased risk of endometrial carcinoma among users of conjugated estrogens. *N Engl J Med* 1975;293:1167–1170.

105. Parazzini F, Negri E, La Vecchia C, et al. Population attributable risk for endometrial cancer in northern Italy. *Eur J Cancer Clin Oncol* 1989;25:1451–1456.

106. Grady D, Gebretsadik T, Kerlikowske K, et al. Hormone replacement therapy and endometrial cancer risk: a meta-analysis. *Obstet Gynecol* 1995;85:304–314.

107. The Postmenopausal Estrogen/Progestin Interventions (PEPI) trial. The Writing Committee for the PEPI trial. Effects of hormone replacement therapy on endometrial histology in postmenopausal women. *JAMA* 1996;275:370–375.

108. Persson I, Schmidt M, Adami H-O, et al. Trends in endometrial cancer incidence and mortality in Sweden, 1960–1984. *Cancer Causes Control* 1990;1:201–208.

109. Persson I, Adami H-O, Bergkvist L. Risk of endometrial cancer after treatment with oestrogens alone or in conjunction with progestogens: results of a prospective study. *BMJ* 1989;298:147–151.

110. Schlesselman JJ. Oral contraceptives and neoplasia of the uterine corpus. *Contraception* 1991;43:557–579.

111. Key TJA, Pike MC. The dose-effect relationship between unopposed oestrogens and endometrial mitotic rate: its central role in explaining and predicting endometrial cancer risk. *Br J Cancer* 1988;57:205–212.

112. Wynder EL, Escher GC, Mantel N. An epidemiological investigation of cancer of the endometrium. *Cancer* 1966;19:489–520.

113. Shu XO, Gao YT, Yuan JM, et al. Dietary factors and epithelial ovarian cancer. *Br J Cancer* 1989;59:92–96.

114. Olaya F, Nectoux J. Le cancer en Ardèche du Nord, incidence 1983–86. Registre des Tumeurs de l'Ardèche du Nord. Annonay, 1987.

115. Pike MC. Age-related factors in cancers of the breast, ovary, and endometrium. *J Chron Dis* 1987;40(suppl 2):595–695.

116. Rosenberg L, Shapiro S, Slone D, et al. Epithelial ovarian cancer and combination oral contraceptives. *JAMA* 1982;247:3210–3212.

117. La Vecchia C, Franceschi S, Decarli A. Oral contraceptive use and the risk of epithelial ovarian cancer. *Br J Cancer* 1984;50:31–34.

118. CASH (Cancer and Steroid Hormone) Study of the Centers for Disease Control and the National Institute of Child Health and Human Development. The reduction in risk of ovarian cancer associated with oral-contraceptive use. *N Engl J Med* 1987;316:650–655.

119. WHO Collaborative Study of Neoplasia and Steroid Contraceptives. Epithelial ovarian cancer and combined oral contraceptives. *Int J Epidemiol* 1989;18:538–545.

120. Adami HO, Bergstrom R, Persson I, Sparen P. The incidence of ovarian cancer in Sweden, 1960–1984. *Am J Epidemiol* 1990;132:446–452.

121. MacLennan SC, MacLennan AH, Ryan P. Colorectal cancer and oestrogen replacement therapy: a meta-analysis of epidemiological studies. *Med J Aust* 1995;162:491–493.

122. Jacobs EJ, White E, Weiss NS. Exogenous hormones, reproductive history and colon cancer. *Cancer Causes Control* 1994;5:359–366.

123. Calle EE, Miracle-McMahill HL, Thun MJ, Heath CW. Estrogen replacement therapy and risk of fatal colon cancer in a prospective cohort of postmenopausal women. *J Natl Cancer Inst* 1995;87:517–523.

124. Gorsky RD, Koplan JB, Peterson HB, Thacker SB. Relative risks and benefits of long-term estrogen replacement therapy: a decision analysis. *Obstet Gynecol* 1994;83:161–166.

125. Wald NJ, Chamberlain J, Hackshaw A, et al. Report of the European Society of Mastology (EUSOMA) Breast Cancer Screening Evaluation Committee. *Breast* 1993;2:209–216.

126. Stampfer MJ. Hormone replacement grows: some experts worried. *J Natl Cancer Inst* 1996;88:637–639.

127. Laya MB, Larson EB, Taplin SH, White E. Effect of estrogen replacement therapy on the sensitivity and specificity of screening mammography. *J Natl Cancer Inst* 1996;88:643–649.

128. Black WC, Fletcher SW. Effects of estrogen on screening mammography: another complexity. *J Natl Cancer Inst* 1996;88:627–628.

CHAPTER 37

Laparoscopy for Diagnosis and Staging of Gynecologic Cancer

DANIEL DARGENT

*L*aparoscopy plays three roles in gynecologic oncology: diagnosis, staging, and assistance to extirpative surgery. Use of laparoscopy for diagnosis began with Raoul Palmer, Michel Mintz, and Jean de Brux (1) who demonstrated that it was possible to detect some early ovarian cancers during puncture of ovarian cysts under guidance of the "celioscope." Nowadays, despite controversies that persist about techniques and strategy, diagnosis of early ovarian cancer remains the most consensual justification of laparoscopy in gynecologic oncology. The second use, staging of disease, started when laparoscopic assessment of the retroperitoneal space became possible. I demonstrated such an assessment in 1987 (2) while devising "panoramic retroperitoneal pelviscopy" (PRPP). Denis Querleu et al (3) expanded its use for staging in 1989 (3) when they described transumbilical transperitoneal laparoscopic pelvic lymphadenectomy. More recently, the concept of laparoscopic assistance to extirpative surgery emerged with the description in 1990 (4) of the so-called laparoscopic radical hysterectomy. Since then, laparoscopy has played a more or less important role in radical surgery and cytoreductive surgery.

Diagnosis of Early Ovarian Cancer

In two of every three patients, the diagnosis of ovarian cancer is made as the disease reaches stages III and IV. Only in one of three patients is the clinical presentation a "pelvic mass." In most instances, the true nature of this pelvic mass is malignant, as assessed by palpation, ultrasound, and measurements of biologic markers. However, early ovarian cancer can appear as a trivial ovarian cyst, and when discovered at this stage, the chance of cure is high. A lot of such cysts are borderline tumors or low-grade infiltrative adenocarcinomas. It is important not to miss or mismanage such tumors.

Since the time when puncture of the cyst and cytologic assessment of the fluid were the only means to establish the diagnosis of early ovarian cancer, much progress has been made, leading to a precise operative strategy.

Operative Strategy

For assessing an ovarian cyst, laparoscopy is generally performed using the standard technique. Because each ovarian cyst has the potential to be an early ovarian cancer, I use the gasless technique rather than classic laparoscopy, which is performed under permanent insufflation with CO_2. Actually, insufflation of CO_2 is likely to be the cause of the tumoral graft one can observe after laparoscopic surgery for intraperitoneal tumors. The more suspicious the cyst is, the more the gasless technique is indicated.

Once the peritoneal cavity has been entered, peritoneal fluid is collected or, if no fluid is present, peritoneal washing is carried out. This has to be done before any manipulation of the lesion.

In order to see the lesions and their peritoneal environment, two ancillary trocars are introduced at the very beginning; these enable the physician to work with two forceps and to perform palpation and mobilization at the same time as inspection. The features to look for are very well known: irregular papillary growths implanted on the cystic wall, unequal thickness of the cystic wall, and atypical vessels. Since these features can be seen either on the prominent aspect or on the hidden aspect of the cyst, mobilization of the tissues is mandatory. This mobilization can be difficult or even impossible to perform, in most cases because of the volume of the lesions or the presence of inflammatory of endometriotic adhesions; such findings may be the only indication of malignancy.

In the absence of suspicious laparoscopic findings, the diagnosis of malignancy cannot be entirely withdrawn and the possibility of endocystic malignant growth has to be entertained. If the cyst is less than 6 cm in diameter, it can be dissected en bloc, put into an endoscopic bag, and punctured inside the bag before it is extracted and assessed outside the abdomen. If the cyst is more than 6 cm in diameter, one has to perform cystoscopy before deciding to extract the cyst. Ideally, cystoscopy is done using as cystoscope, a 1.2-, 5.0-, or 10.0-mm endoscope introduced through the sheath of an appropriate trocar. Practically, it is difficult to avoid the spillage of fluid during cystoscopy. Finally, the simplest procedure is the best: Open the cyst with scissors, wash and aspirate the cyst, then observe directly the inner aspect of the cyst, dissect the wall of the cyst, and extract it.

When the findings of the first step of the operation (extracystic assessment) or the second one (endocystic assessment) are suspicious, I generally recommend an examination of frozen sections. If the diagnosis of infiltrative malignant disease is made, I recommend opening the abdomen and treating the patient in the usual manner. If the diagnosis of noninfiltrative malignant disease is made, the definitive decision has to be delayed until the results of the assessment of the embedded specimen are known. The worst-appearing papillary growth can be benign (cystadenofibroma). The apparently smooth surface of a perfectly free and poorly vascularized cystic wall can be affected by an infiltrative carcinomatous proliferation.

Ovarian Cancer "Discovered" in a Laparoscopic Cystectomy Specimen

Most of the ovarian cancers mimicking trivial ovarian cysts after the preoperative workup are identified during the multistep laparoscopic procedure. However, some of them are evidenced only at the time of pathologic assessment of the specimen. Maiman et al (5) reported a series of 42 patients in whom cancer was diagnosed at pathologic examination. The survey by Maiman et al (5) demonstrates some important points.

First, the rate of borderline malignant lesions in these patients was higher than that currently found: 12 of 36 epithelial tumors (the other 6 tumors comprised 4 ovarian germ cell tumors and 2 stromal tumors).

The second point concerns the delay that elapsed between the time of the laparoscopy and the definitive treatment. The laparotomy was performed immediately in 7 patients, within 2 weeks in 16 patients, between 2 and 4 weeks in 8 patients, and later than 4 weeks in 6 patients (laparotomy was not performed in 5 patients).

At the time of definitive treatment, 20 (50%) of the 40 staged lesions were classified as stage II, III, or IV (6%, 11%, and 3%, respectively). On the other hand, the treatment outcome was considered poor: At the end of the follow-up [<1 year in 26 (62%) of the patients], 1 patient was dead and 7 were alive with disease (remember that 1 of every 3 epithelial tumors was a borderline tumor).

Discussions persist about the facilitation of tumor recurrences after laparoscopic surgery (see later). However, no doubt exists about the responsibility of the laparoscopic tool, when a metastasis develops at a trocar site on the abdominal wall. This complication was mentioned for the first time in 1978 (6). Since then, a lot of case reports have been published (7–13) and a Dutch team (14) demonstrated that such metastases impair the chances of survival independent of other prognostic factors.

In summary regarding "missed ovarian cancer," the negative impact of the laparoscopic tool is not attributable to the rationale of its use but rather to the conditions in which it is used. The surgical rules of laparoscopic ovarian surgery obviously were not respected in most of the published disasters. If a correct laparoscopic technique is followed, the discovery later of an ovarian cancer in a laparoscopic cystectomy specimen will be a rare event.

Prelaparoscopic Workup

An analysis of the literature demonstrates that a lot of the cancers found unexpectedly during examination of cystectomy specimens were in patients in whom a prelaparoscopic workup either was not carried out or was not taken into account. Now ultrasonography and measurement of biologic markers are able to detect most of the malignancies or at least to indicate patients in need of special attention.

Concerning ultrasound, several scoring systems for interpreting the images have been proposed. The system devised by Timor-Tritsch et al (15) in 1993 is a good model (Table 37-1). With this system the average score is 1.8 for benign lesions and 5.6 for malignant lesions. If the cutoff is put at 3.0, the sensitivity is 96.8% and the specificity 77.4% in detecting malignancies. These data are very close to the data published in 1990 by Granberg et al (16) who used another scoring system: 96.8% and 78.8%, respectively. However, the positive (PPV) and negative predictive values (NPV) were quite different in the two surveys: 32.6% versus 86.8% for the PPV and 99.6% versus 93.4% for the NPV. The values indicate that all the scoring systems are equally good (without being perfect) but the results of their practical use depend on the population to which they are applied. In the Timor-Tritsch series the prevalence of malignancy was low (31/350): The PPV is low and the NPV is high. In the Granberg series the prevalence of malignancy was high (178/289): The PPV is higher and the NPV is lower. These mathematical data are very important in interpreting the results of prelaparoscopic ultrasonography; familial history, age, and reproductive background interfere a lot in the decision-making process.

Assessment of biologic markers (CA-125, CA 19-9) is the second tool to use before performing laparoscopy for a pelvic mass. Based on a lot of surveys (17), the sensitivity of measuring CA-125 to detect ovarian cancer does not exceed 80%. For stage I ovarian cancer, the sensitivity drops to 50% and the specificity is very low, especially in young women. The causes of the false-positive findings are well known (e.g., endometriosis, inflammatory disease). The false-negative findings are linked with an absence of synthesis of the CA-125 oncoprotein by some ovarian cancers. Some of them do produce other oncoproteins. From a practical point of view, only the marker CA 19-9, which is mainly produced by mucinous adenocarcinoma, has to be measured during prelaparoscopic workup, but it has to be measured systematically in the presence of a pelvic mass. Last but not least, the results of the two assessments (CA-125 and CA 19-9) have to be interpreted while taking the risk factors into account.

The best accuracy in the prelaparoscopic workup is obviously based on both ultrasound and biologic marker measurement. The Italian multicenter study (18) demonstrated, for example, that in a population of 290 postmenopausal patients operated on for pelvic masses (166 were benign and 132 were malignant), the values for specificity, sensitivity, and accuracy, respectively, were 77.6%, 84.9%, and 80.3% for ultrasound; 82.0%, 78.3%, and 80.4% for CA-125 (cutoff 35 IU/mL); and 86.1%, 91.7%, and 94.3% for ultrasound combined with CA-125. More interesting is the NPV of the combined approach: 100% if the class II ultrasonograms ("equivocal") are combined with the class III ultrasonograms ("possibly malignant"). Hence, one virtually can reduce to nil the rate of "unexpected ovarian cancers" by interpreting the results of the preoperative workup with the highest rigor. However, this rigor leads to an excessive rate of laparotomies. Based on

T A B L E **37-1** **Scoring System for Interpreting** **Ultrasound Images**		0	1	2	3
	Wall structure	Smooth	—	Solid	Papillae >3 mm
	Shadowing	Yes	No	—	—
	Septa	<3 mm	>3 mm	—	—
	Echogenicity	Low	—	—	High

Source: Timor-Tritsch IE, Lerner JP, Monteagudo A, Santos R. Transvaginal ultrasonographic characterization of ovarian masses by means of color flow directed measurements and a morphologic scoring system. *Am J Obstet Gynecol* 1993;168:909–913.

the results of the Italian study, reserving laparoscopy for the patients who show both a class I ultrasonogram ("probably benign") and a CA-125 level lower than 35IU/mL leads to laparotomy being performed in half of the patients with a benign pelvic mass (NPV of the combined approach: 56.4%). The rate of useless laparotomy may be even higher in premenopausal patients. I advocate a more sensible interpretation of the preoperative workup.

Comprehensive Management of the Pelvic Masses

The management of pelvic masses is a multistep procedure in which laparoscopy is certainly not the alpha and the omega: Initial workup, laparoscopy, and definitive treatment are the three main stages of the global approach. Using laparoscopy without careful preoperative assessment, or with the aim of treating the patient without laparotomy whatever the endoscopic symptoms are, surely is an error. However, making the decision to treat the patient either by laparoscopy or by laparotomy on the basis of only the clinical, ultrasonographic, and biologic data is harmful to the patient as well. In my opinion, laparoscopy has to be undertaken in all patients but a correct technique must be used and the final decision made while not forgetting the results of the prelaparoscopic workup. Under these circumstances, laparoscopy, instead of appearing as a danger, can be the best ally of the gynecologic oncologist in the fight against ovarian cancer, as shown in most of the well-documented series (19–21). In my opinion, three situations have to be distinguished regarding use of laparoscopy in the management of pelvic masses.

The first situation is when the ultrasonographic score is low, the levels of CA-125 and CA 19-9 are in the normal range, and risk factors are absent. In this situation, the standard laparoscopic technique can be used (CO_2 insufflation). The endoscopic assessment generally confirms the findings of the prelaparoscopic workup. The lesion can be removed laparoscopically: cystectomy if the patient is young, bilateral annexectomy if the patient is more than 45 years old (40 for some authors). But even if suspicious endoscopic symptoms are totally absent, all precautions have to be taken during the assessment of the inner surface of the cystic wall and during the dissection and extraction of

the lesions (see above). Pathologic assessment of the embedded specimen is mandatory and the patient has to be followed. Moreover, the patient must be aware of a potential reoperation.

The second situation is when the ultrasonographic score is high. The likelihood of malignancy is high, especially if the level of CA-125 or CA 19-9 is high and the patient is menopausal or postmenopausal or at risk. In such patients the gasless open laparoscopy is a good choice. If the endoscopic assessment reveals a dermoid cyst, endometrioma, or even bleeding into a luteal cyst, I operate as in the previously described situation. When the presumption of malignancy is confirmed, biopsies are performed and frozen sections required. If the results confirm the malignancy and demonstrate the infiltrative nature of it, a laparotomy has to be performed and the treatment is undertaken following the usual rules.

The third situation is when the ultrasonographic scores are intermediate. The results of laparoscopic assessment can be entirely negative or frankly positive: such patients should be managed as previously described. However, for some patients laparoscopy does not resolve the diagnosis: A moderate amount of unclear ascites, papillary growth of undetermined nature, or vessels of ambiguous significance may be found. Obviously, this can occur in the first two situations, but for didactic reasons I separated them from the third one. Fast cytologic assessment of the peritoneal fluid and examination of frozen sections must be done. If the results are positive, I treat the case as an infiltrative cancer: False-positive results are rare. However, if the laboratory findings are negative or uncertain (an answer that becomes more frequent as the pathologist is more scrupulous), the management is hard to decide. Especially in young patients, I treat the case as a benign or borderline lesion. All precautions have to be taken during dissection and extraction of the specimen, but it is better to await the results of the assessment of the embedded specimen before making the definitive decision. The discovery of a truly infiltrative ovarian cancer on a cystectomy specimen can be raised to the level of good clinical practice assuming that management is carried out properly.

There are three possible final results of the pathologic assessment. The first is the one where benignity is asserted: This represents no problem. The second is the one where a malignant borderline lesion is evidenced. If the cystectomy was performed correctly, no further treatment is needed, except maybe for the mucinous borderline cystadenocarcinoma where a complementary appendectomy can be recommended. The third situation is the most embarrassing: infiltrative ovarian cancer. In such a situation laparotomy is considered mandatory in order to complete the peritoneal inspection (and palpation), perform the complementary omentectomy (and ipsilateral and/or contralateral adnexectomy plus appendectomy), and perform the pelvic and lumboaortic lymphadenectomy (or lymph node sampling). This laparotomy has to be done as soon as possible and must be followed by appropriate chemotherapy, the necessity and protocol of which depend on the final diagnosis. The post-laparoscopic laparotomy is finished after the scars of the trocar wounds are dissected to prevent abdominal recurrence.

Systematic progression to laparotomy after discovery of an infiltrative ovarian cancer in a laparoscopic cystectomy specimen may be bypassed if there is certainty that the initial laparoscopy was performed under good conditions: no extraovarian extension, correct dissection, and riskless extraction of the specimen. I do not agree with deliberate laparoscopic treatment of early ovarian cancer. However, in the very particular situation of a cancer mimicking a benign or borderline lesion at laparoscopy, a second laparoscopy is allowed. The treatment has been made at the time of the first laparoscopy. What is required is a complete staging and it is important not to lose more time with laparotomy than with laparoscopy. As a matter of fact, the use of laparoscopy for extirpative surgery may be criticized but it appears as a good tool for staging (or restaging) surgery.

Staging of Uterine Carcinomas

The concept of staging surgery began when Nelson et al (22) published data concerning para-aortic lymph node metastases in late invasive carcinoma of the cervix and proposed to assess these lymph nodes before radiotherapy is started. The concept was adopted (23) and then extended to early disease (24,25), with a double goal: 1) selecting among the early-disease patients those who could be treated by surgery only (stage IB and IIA with no lymph node involvement), and 2) selecting among the patients who should be treated using radiation those who should be treated using extended-field radiotherapy (positive para-aortic lymph node involvement) rather than classic pelvic radiotherapy.

Such a strategy led to a significant improvement in the outcome of radical hysterectomy; however, this improvement was totally artificial because patients with a poor prognosis were not operated on. The overall results did not show improvement at all. Moreover, for the patients submitted to radiotherapy, the rate of complications significantly increased, owing to the postoperative adhesions which were the consequence of the extensive dissections that preceded the irradiation. Using an extraperitoneal approach instead of transperitoneal laparotomy led to a significant decrease in some of the complications (26). Nevertheless, the complications rate remained too high in relation to the expected benefits and the concept of staging surgery was progressively dropped. Laparoscopy can breathe a second life into this concept while enabling physicians to perform the pretherapeutic staging with the same accuracy but without the drawbacks of laparotomy.

Techniques of Laparoscopic Staging

The idea of assessing endoscopically the retroperitoneal lymph nodes was launched by Bartel (27) who was the first to do it in the aortic area using the mediastinoscope. Ten years later Hald and Rasmussen (28) used the same instrument for assessing the pelvic lymph nodes as well. Wurst and Luck (29) first described the use of the technique in gynecologic oncology. The aortic assessment was performed through a minilaparotomy and the pelvic assessment through a mini-inguinotomy. Not having a mediastinoscope and not being convinced that the direct approach obtained with this instrument is accurate enough, in December 1986 I started assessing the pelvic lymph nodes using the laparoscopic tool. Hence was born the PRPP I described with Salvat in a monograph published in 1989 (30). Two years later Querleu et al (3) wrote about pelvic lymphadenectomy under guidance of a transumbilical laparoscope. Subsequently it was demonstrated that assessment of the aortic lymph nodes was possible under laparoscopic guidance as well (31–33). Nowadays staging laparoscopy can mimic completely the former staging laparotomy.

The Transumbilical Transperitoneal Approach

The transumbilical transperitoneal approach can be used in all circumstances; the preperitoneal route is reserved for selected patients (see later).

The setting used for laparoscopic lymphadenectomy does not differ from the one used for the trivial laparoscopic surgery except one has to avoid putting a stent into the uterus. Two ancillary trocars are put on the interiliac line lateral to the epigastric vessels. A third ancillary trocar is put on the median line at the same level or a little more caudally. After careful evaluation of the peritoneal cavity, the pelvic peritoneum is opened and the retroperitoneal space is developed.

For the pelvic lymphadenectomy, the landmarks of the operative field are the superior vesical artery and the iliac vessels on which contours can be easily observed in the ventral part of the sphere of vision. The incision of the peritoneum is made between the two landmarks and then is extended dorsally along the infundibulopelvic ligament. With the broad ligament opened, the dorsal fold of it is pushed medially and maintained in this medial position: This puts the ureter, which is attached to the deep surface of the peritoneum, out of danger. The dissection of the lymph nodes starts at the level where the iliac vessels cross Cooper's ligament and is continued from front to back until arriving at the level of the bifurcation of the common iliac artery: All the lymph nodes along the lateral and caudal surfaces of the external vein are prepared and then removed. After the medial (or prevascular) lymph nodes are removed, the lateral (or retrovascular) lymph nodes are prepared. For this preparation, the external iliac vein is detached from the external iliac artery and then from the pelvic wall. Removal of the lymph nodes located between the external iliac artery and the psoas muscle is not useful in the situations one usually faces. This point is discussed later.

Before proceeding further in the description of the laparoscopic lymphadenectomy, I have to make two points concerning the removal of the lymph nodes. First, when the lymph nodes appear obviously metastatic (enlarged, infiltrated, and adherent), I do not remove them. As explained later, the laparoscopic tool is not made for debulking surgery. However, I do puncture the nodes to obtain a specimen for documenting the metastatic involvement by cytologic examination. The second point is based on the same rationale. It concerns the lymph nodes that appear normal but may actually be involved. Be careful not to morcellate the glands and not to contaminate the abdominal wall while removing them; that is, use the Coelioextractor (Lépine, Lyon) for the normal-size glands and use laparoscopic bags for the enlarged ones.

When the lymph node assessment has to be extended to the common iliac and the aortic areas either as continuation of the pelvic assessment or as a separate evaluation, one of two techniques can be used. Childers et al (33) proposed the first one. The surgeon stands on the left side of the patient. The video camera is turned clockwise 90 degrees. The intestinal loops are driven back into the diaphragmatic domes. The peritoneum is opened along the aorta (the vertical incision appears horizontal on the video monitor). The right ureter and gonadic vessels are identified and pushed upward, then the preparation and removal of the right aortic lymph nodes are carried out. The same is done on the left side. In the technique devised by Querleu (32), the surgeon stays between the legs of the patient and watches upwardly with the laparoscope (the video monitor has to be placed at the head of the bed). The peritoneum is opened transversly along the last ileal loop. The right common iliac artery is identified. Then the surgeon proceeds along the vascular axis while the assistant lifts the peritoneum, making a sort of tent under the cover of which the surgeon can work without being disturbed by the intestinal loops. Whatever the technique used, the lymph node assessment and removal can be pushed up to the level of the left renal vein.

The Preperitoneal Approach

At the very beginning of my experience, the route I used for assessing the pelvic lymph nodes was the inguinal one. The main advantage of this approach was direct access to the iliac vessels. The drawbacks were a lack of distance and difficulty in introducing ancillary instruments of performing a true lymphadenectomy. I moved quickly to the suprapubic median approach and devised the PRPP.

The PRPP is performed using a microlaparotomy on the median line 3 cm above the pubic bone. The cutaneous incision is transversal. The aponeurotic incision is vertical. As soon as it is opened, the preperitoneal space is entered with the forefinger and developed with the same "instrument," moving along the pubic bone toward the iliac vessels. Then the peritoneum is separated from the posterior surface of the rectus abdominis muscle. Once the suprapubic preperitoneal space (cranial extension of the Retzius space) is developed, the laparoscopic trocar is introduced into it. The CO_2 insufflation is given through the sheath of the trocar, the "pneumostasis" being obtained by placement of a circular suture around the cutaneous incision (use of an autostatic trocar—Blunt Tip Origin—highly facilitates the progress of the surgery). The laparoscope is introduced, with the surgeon staying lateral to the patient on the side opposite to the pelvic wall he or she intends to assess. Cooper's ligament is visualized. A first ancillary trocar is pushed level with the pubic bone, and then a second one symmetric to the first. With the instruments introduced through the two ancillary doors, the peritoneal sac is developed along the axis of the iliac vessels up to the level of the bifurcation. The lymph nodes are separated, then delivered: All the interiliac lymph nodes including the retrovascular ones can be removed.

Recent improvements in the instrumentation enable the performance of PRPP while avoiding the microlaparotomy. A simple 10-mm cutaneous incision is made. The Optiview trocar Ethicon (or the Visiport Autosuture) is introduced. The subcutaneous fat and the aponeurosis are opened using the cutting tip of the trocar, the penetration of which can be watched endoscopically (the tip of the trocar is transparent). As soon as the preperitoneal space is entered, the trocar is removed while leaving in place its sheath through which the insufflation of CO_2 will be done at the same time the preperitoneal space is developed using the laparoscope as a blunt dissector. The continuation of the surgery is the same as previously described.

For the assessment of the pelvic lymph nodes, the extraperitoneal approach can be started from the infraumbilical area rather than the suprapubic one. The 10-mm incision is made at the inferior margin of the umbilicus and the preperitoneal space is entered using, as previously described, the Optiview trocar. The preperitoneal space is developed around

the median line. A first ancillary trocar is introduced on the median line in the suprapubic area, then the dissection of the posterior surface of the abdominal wall, which is pushed laterally under direct laparoscopic guidance. Scissors are used after introduction on the median line. After passing the level of the epigastric vessels, one can open two more lateral ancillary doors (one on each side) close to the point of McBurney. With dissection one gets a view into the pelvic cavity that is identical to the one obtained by transumbilical transperitoneal laparoscopy. The interiliac lymphadenectomy is performed in the same manner. If the common iliac lymph nodes are to be assessed, one can push more dorsally the mobilization of the peritoneal sac while cutting the round ligaments at the level of their penetration into the inguinal rings. For the aortic lymph nodes one can use the ipsilateral iliac door for the laparoscope and the contralateral iliac door for an endoretractor with which one pushes medially the peritoneal bag. For the first dissecting forceps, one uses the umbilical door. For the second dissecting forceps, one opens a new door located cranially and laterally to the ipsilateral iliac door.

When I intend to assess only the common iliac and aortic lymph nodes (see later), I use the procedure just described. Nevertheless, arriving directly in the preperitoneal space is not easy in the iliac area, owing to the local reinforcement of the fascia parietalis. I recommend performing first transumbilical transperitoneal laparoscopy and entering the preperitoneal space while watching the progression from inside. Moreover I think that making a true microlaparotomy at McBurney's point is better than using the Optiview system.

Results of Laparoscopic Staging

Ten years after its first use, the feasibility, cost-effectiveness, and accuracy of laparoscopic staging are still questioned.

Concerning the feasibility, the only problem is the risk of vascular injuries. This risk concerns the aortic assessment more than the pelvic one. The risk is not greater than it is during open surgery. The injuries, in most instances, can be treated laparoscopically using compression, bipolar cauterization, or clips. In case of failure, the conversion to laparotomy has to be decided without delay. It is of paramount importance that the laparoscopic surgeon be trained both in laparoscopic surgery and in oncologic surgery.

The cost of laparoscopic staging surgery may be less than the cost of open surgery but there are several confounding factors. The time elapsed in the operation room is longer, especially if there is a complication and even more so if a conversion to laparotomy is needed. A lot of money can be spent on the instrumentation if disposable instruments are used (a practice that can be avoided). However, the hospital stay and the recovery time are much shorter and the benefit is huge, especially for aortic assessment, which can be done as a 1-day procedure.

The feasibility and cost-effectiveness of laparoscopic staging surgery to a certain extent depend on the route followed for performing the lymph node assessment. The preperitoneal route has, for the gynecologist, the drawback of being less familiar. This difficulty can be overcome after appropriate training. In the same manner, the excess of CO_2 transfer can be compensated while adapting the artificial ventilation (34). From all other points of view the direct route appears superior: no trouble with the guts, which remain in their natural bag; no trouble with the ureters, which remain attached to the inner aspect of the peritoneum; no hemodynamic problem, then absence of compression of the vena cava (except during the right para-aortic lymph node assessment). For these reasons the direct approach is, for me as for many urologists (35–37), the approach of choice with two limits. In endometrial cancer where the assessment of the peritoneal cavity is as important as the assessment of the retroperitoneal space, the transumbilical route has to be preferred. On the other hand, in cervical cancer, glancing into the peritoneal cavity has a certain importance, especially in patients with late disease: Use the preperitoneal approach but do a peritoneotomy either at the beginning or at the end of the procedure. Last but not least, the preperitoneal approach can be hard to perform in patients previously operated on by a suprapubic laparotomy, either transversal or vertical: The transumbilical route should be used.

The accuracy of laparoscopic staging is often considered inferior to the accuracy of laparotomic staging. Actually the removal of the adventitia of the blood vessels on which the lymph nodes are dependent can be performed in the same manner if not better (Fig. 37-1). However, the number of lymph nodes delivered after laparoscopy (3,38) is generally inferior to the number of lymph nodes delivered after systematic lymphadenectomy (39). The difference is not due to technical differences but to strategy. During systematic lymphadenectomy, which is done with a therapeutic perspective, one tries to remove all the lymph nodes that potentially could be involved by the disease's spread; for laparoscopic staging lymphadenectomy, one aims only to do a "targeted lymphadenectomy" or a "panoramic lymph node sampling." These two operations, which are completely different from a conceptual point of view, are similar in terms of quantitative results, and inferior to systematic lymphadenectomy.

Indications of Laparoscopic Staging

Before elaborating about each of the indications of laparoscopic staging, I have to say one last

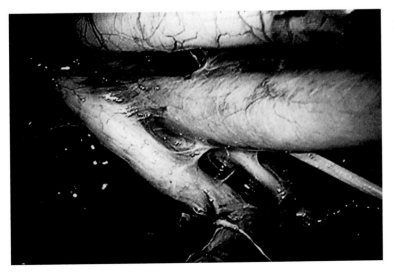

F I G U R E **37-1**

The bifurcation of the left common artery as it is seen after interiliac lymphadenectomy performed laparoscopically using the preperitoneal suprapubic route.

word about technique and define the concept of "targeted lymphadenectomy" and "panoramic lymph node sampling." In the targeted lymphadenectomy the goal is cleaning out perfectly an anatomic area where one knows that the sentinel lymph nodes lie, that is, the nodes of which uninvolvement enables one to assert, with a risk of error less than 2%, that no metastases exist anywhere else. The rationale for panoramic lymph node sampling is based on the same data but interpreted the opposite way. Even if a very small (<2%) risk of lymph node "skipping" during the process of extension does exist, it is better to perform panoramic lymph node sampling. Both practices leave an open door to fate but the role of fate is less (and better documented) with the first strategy (targeted lymphadenectomy). That is why I choose this strategy. But I have another motivation that is of a technical nature: The area where I do lymph node dissection becomes, from the surgical point of view, a prohibited zone, that is, a zone where a second dissection is impossible or at least difficult and dangerous. For this reason I perform a complete lymphadenectomy, and the benefit of systematic lymphadenectomy not being worth the risk, I limit this lymphadenectomy to the sentinel area.

Early Cervical Cancer

Numerous surgicopathologic surveys showed that the volume of the tumor is the first discriminant in the prognosis of cancer of the cervix. If the maximal tumor diameter is less than 4 cm, the chances of cure after radical hysterectomy are around 85% (40). One can obtain the same results using radiation therapy but at a much higher price. Therefore, radical hysterectomy appears to be the treatment of choice. However, a subpopulation does exist in which the chances are less: patients with lymph node involvement. Among this subpopulation, which accounts for 15% of patients, two groups have to be considered: Patients with involvement of one or two lymph nodes (2/3 patients) have 60% chance of survival after radical hysterectomy and patients with involvement of three lymph nodes or more have a very low chance of survival after radical hysterectomy, even if followed by adjuvant radiotherapy (41).

These findings are the bases of the algorithm presented in Figure 37-2, which shows the role of laparoscopic staging surgery in the management of stage IB1 and small (<4cm in diam-

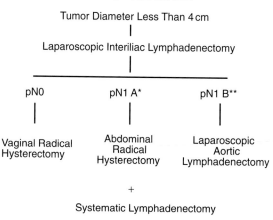

CANCER OF THE CERVIX

Tumor Diameter Less Than 4 cm

Laparoscopic Interiliac Lymphadenectomy

pN0 — pN1 A* — pN1 B**

Vaginal Radical Hysterectomy — Abdominal Radical Hysterectomy — Laparoscopic Aortic Lymphadenectomy

+

Systematic Lymphadenectomy

*pN1A = 1 or 2 positive lymph nodes
**pN1B = 3 or more positive lymph nodes

F I G U R E **37-2**

Algorithm for the treatment of early forms of cervical cancer.

eter) stage II disease. Three subpopulations can be defined:

Patients with no lymph node involvement: Treatment is radical hysterectomy, which can be done through the vaginal route with minimal surgical stress and a 90% chance of cure.

Patients with involvement of one or two lymph nodes: Treatment is radical hysterectomy with systematic lymphadenectomy, which is performed more quickly and safely by laparotomy than the laparoscopic vaginal approach. There is a 60% chance of cure. Postoperative radiotherapy is optional.

Patients with involvement of three or more lymph nodes: Radiotherapy affords very few chances of survival but the chances are better after a simple laparoscopic staging than after a radical hysterectomy. The radiation schedule is adapted to the result of the comprehensive laparoscopic lymph node assessment. Adjuvant radical hysterectomy is optional (use laparotomy and complete the lymphadenectomy).

Advanced Cervical Cancer

As soon as the maximal diameter of the tumor exceeds 4 cm, the chances of cure after radical hysterectomy drop to less than 60%. It is not absolutely proved that radiotherapy offers better chances. However, there is general agreement about the preference for radiotherapy, if only based on the risk-benefit ratio.

Laparoscopic staging with its high accuracy (more than imaging) and low risk (less than laparotomic staging) can play a very important role in selecting pelvic radiotherapy or extended-field radiotherapy. One can start the lymph node assessment in the pelvic area and proceed further only in patients with pelvic lymph node involvement. It is better to go directly to aortic assessment, which provides the key to the radiation schedule. Moreover, by not manipulating the pelvic area during the pretherapeutic assessment, one does not impair the radical surgery that can be added to the radiation therapy. This is the rationale of the algorithm presented in Figure 37-3.

Endometrial Carcinoma

In stage I endometrial carcinoma (80% of the patients) extrafascial hysterectomy is the treatment of choice. Bilateral salpingo-oophorectomy is mandatory. Lymphadenectomy is reserved for grade 2 or 3 stage IB or C cancers: It is not mandatory for stage IA, grade 1 disease in which the rate of lymph node involvement is less than 2%. Tumor grade is known at the time of the inaugural curettage. Stage (myometrial infiltration) can be assessed by ultrasound or magnetic resonance imaging with great accuracy.

Starting from these bases, one can select a subpopulation for which hysterectomy can be carried out using the vaginal approach. In this subpopulation, there is no need for laparoscopic staging. For the other patients laparoscopic staging appears as highly interesting. This is the rationale of the algorithm presented in Figure 37-4.

When laparoscopy, which has to be performed through the transumbilical transperitoneal route, reveals peritoneal or salpingo-ovarian involvement, the patient has to be treated as an ovarian cancer patient, that is, by laparotomy and with integrated therapies. In the other patients a laparoscopic lymphadenectomy has to be undertaken, leading either to vaginal hysterectomy or to laparotomy (as for the modalities of the lymph node dissection I think that targeted pelvic lymphadenectomy is better than panoramic lymph node sampling).

The algorithm shown in Figure 36-4 is not applicable to everybody. Obesity is considered a contraindication to the minimally invasive approach. Such a view is unfair and a laparoscopic vaginal approach is generally less difficult and dangerous than laparotomy. An excessive uterine volume does represent a contraindication: Before undertaking a vaginal hysterectomy for endometrial cancer, one has to be sure not to morcellate the uterus. A second contraindication involves the deep infiltration of the myometrium. If this infiltration reaches the subserous layer, laparoscopic preparation and vaginal extirpation are dangerous.

Laparoscopic Assistance to Extirpative Surgery

Extirpative surgery, whatever the progress of the nonsurgical therapies, remains the "queen of the battles" in the fight against cancer. It survived radiotherapy and chemotherapy as well and it probably will survive gene therapy because it is the most cost-effective treatment in a lot of situations. Two types of surgery have to be considered: radical surgery and cytoreductive or debulking surgery. What is the place for laparoscopy in surgery?

Before answering in detail about each of the situations encountered in gynecologic oncology, I have to say straight away that the role of the laparoscopic approach is limited by the doubts one has about the safety of laparoscopic manipulations in organs affected by malignant tumors. These doubts come from the experience of general surgeons treating colorectal cancer: The

F I G U R E **37-3**

Algorithm for the treatment of late forms of cancer of the cervix.

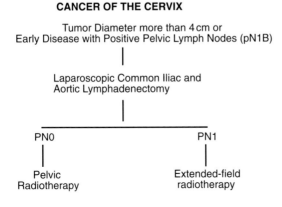

CANCER OF THE CERVIX

Tumor Diameter more than 4 cm or
Early Disease with Positive Pelvic Lymph Nodes (pN1B)

Laparoscopic Common Iliac and
Aortic Lymphadenectomy

PN0 — Pelvic Radiotherapy

PN1 — Extended-field radiotherapy

ENDOMETRIAL CARCINOMA

Ultrasound ± MRI

Stages IA, IB   Stage IC   Stages II & III

Grade 1   Grades 2 & 3

Laparoscopy

Stage IC   Stage III

Lymphadenectomy

N–   N+

Vag. hyst.   Integrated therapies

Laparoscopic complement
— If BSO impossible to perform transvaginally
— If stage IC on frozen sections

Laparotomic conversion if hysteroscopy impossible to
perform transvaginally

F I G U R E **37-4**

Algorithm for the treatment of endometrial carcinoma. MRI = magnetic resonance imaging; N = node; BSO = bilateral salpingo-oophorectomy.

rate of abdominal recurrences, which was 1.5% after classic surgery (42), is more than twice that rate after laparoscopic surgery (43). At the moment there is no biologic explanation for this phenomenon. The modifications of the peritoneal milieu that inhibit the natural reaction to the mechanical traumatism of surgery (no postoperative adhesions) probably facilitate the seeding of tumoral deposits and the growth of them, as demonstrated in an experimental assay (44). From a practical point of view, it is very important to know that the increased risk of abdominal recurrences is observed only in Dukes B and C cancers as it remains nil in Dukes A cancer, that is, cancer not involving the muscular layer of the colic wall. Hence, the only cancers that can be treated using a laparoscopic approach are the ones in which invasion is at a distance from the peritoneum.

In the field of gynecologic oncology the situations where laparoscopic assistance to extirpative surgery is both useful and safe are few. Endometrial carcinoma is the first of them if the tumoral infiltration is confined to the uterus and

does not reach the subserosal layer of it. Cervical carcinoma equally fulfills the conditions for making laparoscopic assistance possible at least in patients with early disease, who anyway are the only ones treated electively by radical surgery. On the contrary, ovarian carcinoma, especially in the early stage, is a contraindication. However, in the late stages, one can make a case for laparoscopic surgery, as it is made by general surgeons for metastatic colorectal carcinoma.

Uterine Cancer

Even if the surgeries performed for the treatment of endometrial cancer and for the treatment of early cervical cancer are very different, some common rules do exist as far as laparoscopic assistance is concerned.

The first rule is to avoid use of a uterine stent. This use is considered mandatory for trivial laparoscopic surgery. Experienced gynecologic oncologists can perform the most sophisticated operations without using this stent, the handling of which leads to a risk of perforation or tumoral dissemination.

The second rule of safety is to try to make as short as possible the time devoted to the preparation in the laparoscopic atmosphere and to move as quickly as possible to the removal of the operative specimen, which has to be performed without friction. Concerning uterine cancer such a conversion is easy: The vaginal route can be used but has to be taken as soon as possible.

The third rule is linked to the second one. Actually moving to the vaginal approach, in the same time as reducing the length of the laparoscopic step of the operation (and the total length of the surgery as well), enables one to prevent contamination of the vaginal wall and surrounding cellular tissue. The first thing I do at the beginning of the vaginal part of the operation is make a vaginal cuff and close the uterine cervix.

Endometrial Carcinoma

Laparoscopy can be used in the management of endometrial carcinoma, enabling one to select the definitive treatment (see Fig. 36-2). It can be used for assistance in extirpative surgery as well. The laparoscopically assisted vaginal hysterectomy (LAVH) could be the best approach for the treatment of endometrial cancer. In this operation the round and infundibulopelvic ligaments are divided under laparoscopic guidance, then the vesicouterine fold is opened and the bladder mobilized, the uterine arteries and paracervical ligaments are cut, and the vagina finally opened through which the uterus is delivered.

Manipulating in the laparoscopic atmosphere for too long is dangerous and increases the total length of the surgery. For this reason I think one does well to use the laparoscopic approach for only those things that cannot be done through the vaginal approach: assessing the peritoneum and the ovaries and tubes and performing the lymph node assessment. As for the hysterectomy and even bilateral salpingo-oophorectomy, the vaginal approach is quicker and safer. Accordingly my recommendation is to move to the vaginal approach as soon as the lymph node dissection is carried out, while leaving in place the laparoscopic instrumentation, which can be used again in case difficulties occur during the vaginal operation, especially during bilateral salpingo-oophorectomy.

As said before, the laparoscopic vaginal approach, while having all the advantages of minimally invasive surgery, cannot be used in all circumstances. Laparoscopy is useless in stage IA, grade 1 tumor. Vaginal hysterectomy is contraindicated for stage IC cancer and in patients with a big uterus as well. However, when it can be used, there is no doubt that this approach is the best one. The data published in recent literature are more than encouraging (45–47).

Early Cervical Cancer

The most important contribution of laparoscopy to the treatment of early cervical carcinoma is that it enables us to select the indications to vaginal radical hysterectomy (VRH), an operation that was completely withdrawn in spite of its obvious advantages. This operation can be made easier with laparoscopic assistance: One can move from VRH to radical LAVH (48–51).

Laparoscopic assistance to VRH can be pushed very far: One can, mimicking the successive stages of the abdominal radical hysterectomy, perform a purely laparoscopic radical hysterectomy (52,53). Actually some stages are easy to accomplish under laparoscopic guidance and others are not. Opening and developing completely the paravesical and pararectal spaces is very easy. Dividing the paracervical ligaments at the very level of their pelvic insertion is very easy as well (especially if endoscopic staplers are used). Opening the rectovaginal fold and dividing the sacrouterine ligaments is not difficult. Opening the vesicouterine fold and mobilizing the bladder is easy, but dividing the vesicouterine ligaments and deroofing the ureter is not that simple. Moreover, separating the elements inside the paracervix that depend on the vaginal cuff (paracervix stricto sensu) and those that depend on the vaginal sheath (para colpos) is very difficult, bloody, and time-consuming. For these reasons, added to the ones previously set out, I think the role of laparoscopic assistance has to be limited to the really useful components.

Radical hysterectomy can be tailored depending on the volume of the tumor. Rather than the classic Piver and Rutledge five classes, I use a two-class classification: the "proximal radical hysterectomy" and the "distal radical hysterectomy." In the first operation the paracervix is divided midway; it is divided at the very level of its pelvic insertion in the second one. The first operation is for tumors less than 2 cm in diameter (the "free interval" will surely be more than 2 cm). The second operation is indicated for the tumors 2 to 4 cm in diameter (the only way to be sure the free interval will be more than 2 cm). Regarding the laparoscopic vaginal approach, the two operations are different: Dividing the paracervix midway is easier to do transvaginally; dividing it at the very level of its origin is easier to do laparoscopically.

My recommendation, after the points made previously, is finally to adapt the blend of laparoscopic and transvaginal surgeries to tumoral volume. For tumors less than 2 cm in diameter, I advocate the "proximal radical LAVH" (or proximal Coelio-Schauta): opening the paravesical and the pararectal spaces and cutting the uterine arteries under laparoscopic guidance, then moving to the vaginal route for performing a Schauta Stoeckel operation, which ends with clamping and cutting the paracervical ligaments midway. For tumors 2 to 4 cm in diameter, I advocate the distal radical LAVH or distal Coelio-Schauta: developing completely

paravesical and pararectal spaces and cutting the paracervical ligaments at the level of their pelvic insertion (endostapler) under laparoscopic guidance, then moving to the vaginal route for performing a Schauta Amreich operation, achievement of which is highly facilitated by the laparoscopic preparation (no bleeding, easy treatment of the bladder pillar, no need for the paravaginal incision or Schuchardt's incision, which is mandatory for the classic Schauta Amreich operation).

Contrary to LAVH in endometrial carcinoma, radical LAVH can be used in all cases of early cervical carcinoma. There are no contraindications linked with the tumor itself. Neither are there contraindications linked with the morphology of the patient. The laparoscopic preparation makes easy the most difficult-appearing VRH.

As for the curative value of the laparoscopic vaginal approach, I can assert, based on my personal experience (54) with 98 patients (December 1986–June 1992), that the rate of failures is not higher than expected (12% at 3 years). The

FIGURE 37-5

Algorithm for treatment of stage III ovarian carcinoma. CR = complete response; PR = partial response; NR = no response.

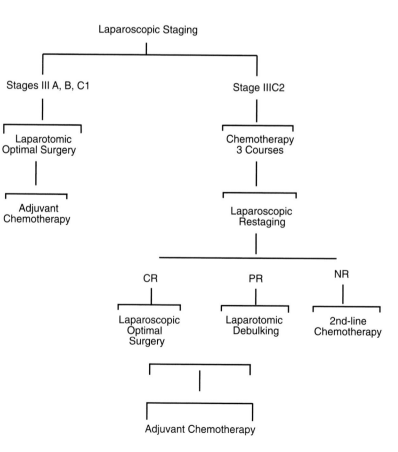

OVARIAN PERITONEAL CARCINOSIS

rate of primary complications is low (no postoperative fistula, one ureteral stenosis). The recovery time is short. The patient is cured without a scar, a point that may seem unimportant to the gynecologic oncologist but is of seminal importance for women. These data concern the time I used laparoscopy only for lymphadenectomy and then did the classic Schauta operation. There are not enough data for assessing the benefit of the introduction of laparoscopic assistance to the Schauta operation (55). I can assert that the laparoscopic vaginal approach surely overtakes the purely laparoscopic approach regarding operative time and primary complications.

Ovarian Cancer

As previously said, operating laparoscopically on early ovarian cancer is strictly forbidden. It is the best way to make a stage I tumor into stage III. As for stage III and IV disease a new trend does exist now favoring the so-called intervention surgery, that is, surgery undertaken after three courses of chemotherapy. The European Organization for Research and Treatment of Cancer (EORTC) study (56) demonstrated that such a strategy can improve the overall results. Laparoscopy may have a role in such a strategy, in the way schematized by the algorithm shown as Figure 37-5. Laparoscopy could be a tool for triage of stage III disease, to differentiate the patients in whom an immediate debulking has to be attempted (optimal debulking appearing as possible) and those in whom it does not. Such a laparoscopic assessment is not dangerous; it is immediately followed either by laparotomy or by a first course of chemotherapy, which has to be scheduled in the 24 hours following surgery.

The second role of laparoscopy is in the evaluation of the response to chemotherapy. The information provided is better than that provided by imaging or biologic surveillance. Such a laparoscopic re-evaluation can lead to laparotomic debulking or to second-line chemotherapy, two situations where the risk of dissemination is controlled. It can lead to purely laparoscopic extirpative surgery as well. The risk of such surgery is nil if we limit its indications to only those patients with a true complete response.

The algorithm presented in Figure 37-5 far from enjoys a general consensus. The Tucson team (Surwit E, personal communication, 1996)

is studying this closely. The Heidelberg team (Walweiner D, personal communication, 1996) is launching a phase-one study regarding whether we can rely on laparoscopy for identifying the "primary, not optimally debulkable cancers." However, no data are available for backing the concept of laparoscopic triage before neoadjuvant chemotherapy. On the contrary, the role of laparoscopy in the evaluation of responses to chemotherapy is well documented (57,58). This practice can be, inside or outside the global program I propose, recommended, as laparoscopic restaging was recommended for "missed ovarian cancer" at the beginning of this chapter. In gynecologic cancer laparoscopy is a tool that certainly is promised a great future (it may be that endoscopic surgery is the only sort of surgery that will survive the progress to conservative approaches), but needs to be thoroughly evaluated in most of the fields in which it is already applied.

REFERENCES

1. De Brux J, Palmer R, Mintz M. Cytology of parauterine tumors punctured under coelioscopy. *J Int Fed Gynaecol Obstet* 1967;5:247–254.

2. Dargent D. A new future for Schauta's operation through presurgical retroperitoneal pelviscopy. *Eur J Gynaecol Oncol* 1987;8:292–296.

3. Querleu D, LeBlanc E, Castelain B. Laparoscopic pelvic lymphadenectomy. *Am J Obstet Gynecol* 1991;164:579–581.

4. Canis M, Mage G, Wattiez A, et al. La chirurgie coelioscopique a-t-elle une place dans la chirurgie radicale du cancer du col utérin? *J Gynecol Obstet Biol Reprod* 1990;19:921.

5. Maiman M, Seltzer W, Boyce J. Laparoscopic excision of ovarian neoplasms subsequently found to be malignant. *Obstet Gynecol* 1991; 77:563–565.

6. Dobronte Z, Wittmann T, Karacsony G. Rapid development of malignant metastases in the abdominal wall after laparoscopy. *Endoscopy* 1978;10:127–130.

7. Stockdale AD, Pocok TJ. Abdominal wall metastasis following laparoscopy: a case report. *Eur J Surg Oncol* 1985;11:373–375.

8. Hsiu JG, Given FT, Kemp GM. Tumor implantation after diagnostic laparoscopic biopsy of serous ovarian tumors of low malignant potential. *Obstet Gynecol* 1986;68S:90–93.

9. Miralles RM, Petit J, Gine L, Balaguero L. Metastatic cancer spread at the laparoscopic puncture site: report of a case in a patient with carcinoma of the ovary. *Eur J Gynaecol Oncol* 1989;10:442–444.

10. Crouet H, Heron JF. Dissemination du cancer de l'ovaire lors de la chirurgie coelioscopique: un danger réel. *Presse Med* 1991;20:1738–1739.

11. Benifla JL, Hauuy JP, Guglielmina JN, et al. Kystectomie per coelioscopique: découverte fortuite d'un carcinome ovarien. *J Gynecol Obstet Biol Reprod* 1992;21:45–49.

12. Gleeson NC, Nicosia SV, Mark JE, et al. Abdominal wall metastases from ovarian cancer after laparoscopy. *Am J Obstet Gynecol* 1993;169: 522–533.

13. Canis M, Wattiez A, Pouly JL, et al. Dissemination tumorale après traitement par kystectomie coelioscopique d'un cancer de Stade IA1. La prise en charge coelioscopique des kystes annexiels est-elle justifiable? *Ref Gynecol Obstet* 1993;1:41–49.

14. Kruitwagen RFPM, Swinkels BM, Keyser KG, et al. Incidence and effect on survival of abdominal wall metastases at trocar or puncture sites following laparoscopy or paracentesis in women with ovarian cancer. *Gynecol Oncol* 1996;60: 233–237.

15. Timor-Tritsch IE, Lerner JP, Monteagudo A, Santos R. Transvaginal ultrasonographic characterization of ovarian masses by means of color flow directed measurements and a morphologic scoring system. *Am J Obstet Gynecol* 1993;168: 909–913.

16. Granberg S, Nostrom A, Wikland M. Tumors in the lower pelvis as imaged by vaginal sonography. *Gynecol Oncol* 1990;37:224–229.

17. Jacobs E, Bast R. The CA125 tumor associated antigen: a review of the literature. *Hum Reprod* 1989;4:1–12.

18. Maggino T, Gaducci A, D'Addario V, et al. Prospective multicenter study on CA 125 in post menopausal pelvic masses. *Gynecol Oncol* 1994; 54:117–123.

19. Canis M, Mage G, Wattiez A, et al. Kyste de l'annexe: place de la coelioscopie en 1991. *Contracept Fertil Sex* 1992;20:345–352.

20. Nezhat F, Nezhat C, Welander LE, Benigno B. Four ovarian cancers diagnosed during laparoscopic management of 1011 women's adnexal masses. *Am J Obstet Gynecol* 1992;167:790–796.

21. Mettler L, Caesar G, Neunzling S, Semm K. Stellenwert der endoskopischen Ovar-chirurgie— kritische Analyse von 626 pelviskopisch operierten Ovarialzysten an der Universitäts-Frauenklinik Kiel 1990–1991. *Geburtshilfe Frauenheilk* 1993;53:253–257.

22. Nelson JH, Macasaet MA, et al. The incidence and significance of para-aortic lymph node metastases in late invasive carcinoma of the cervix. *Am J Obstet Gynecol* 1974;118:749–756.

23. Piver MS, Barlow JJ. Para-aortic lymphadenectomy in staging patients with advanced local cervical carcinoma. *Obstet Gynecol* 1974;43:544–548.

24. Lagasse LD, Creasman WT, Shingleton HM, et al. Results and complication of operative staging in cervical cancer: experience of the GOG. *Gynecol Oncol* 1980;9:90–98.

25. Averette HE, Doinato DM, Lovecchio JL. Sevin BU. Surgical staging of gynecologic malignancies. *Cancer* 1987;60:2010–2020.

26. Weiser EB, Bundy BN, Hoskins WT, et al. Extraperitoneal vs transperitoneal selective para-aortic lymphadenectomy in the pretreatment surgical staging of advanced cervical carcinoma (a GOG study). *Gynecol Oncol* 1989;33:283–289.

27. Bartel M. Die Retroperitoneoskopie. Eine endoskopische Method zur Inspektion und bioptischen Untersuchung des retroperitonealen Raumes. *Zentralbl Chir* 1969;94:377–383.

28. Hald T, Rasmussen F. Extraperitoneal pelviscopy, new aid in staging of lower urinary tract tumors: a preliminary report. *J Urol* 1980; 124:245–248.

29. Wurtz H, Luck H. Réflexion à propos de la retroperitonéoscopie "opératoire" en gynécologie. *Presse Med* 1987;16:1865.

30. Dargent D, Salvat J. *Envahissement ganglionnaire pelvien. Place de la pelviscopie retroperitoneale.* Paris: Medsi McGraw Hill, 1989.

31. Nezhat CR, Burrell MO, Nezhat FR, et al. Laparoscopic radical hysterectomy with para-aortic and pelvic node dissection. *Am J Obstet Gynecol* 1992;166:864–865.

32. Querleu D. Laparoscopic para-aortic lymphadenectomy: a preliminary experience. *Gynecol Oncol* 1993;68:90–93.

33. Childers JM, Hatch KD, Tran AN, Surwit EA. Laparoscopic para-aortic lymphadenectomy in gynecologic malignancy. *Obstet Gynecol* 1993; 82:741–747.

34. Mullet Ch, Vialle JP, Sagnard PE, et al. Pulmonary CO_2 elimination during surgical procedures using intra or extraperitoneal CO_2 insufflation. *Anesth Anal* 1993;76:622–626.

35. Ferzli G, Raboy A, Kleinerman D, Albert P. Extraperitoneal endoscopic pelvic lymph node dissection vs. laparoscopic lymph node dissection in the staging of prostatic and bladder carcinoma. *J Laparoendosc Surg* 1992;2:219–222.

36. Das S, Tashima M. Extraperitoneal laparoscopic staging pelvic lymph node dissection. *J Urol* 1994;151:1321–1323.

37. Etwaru D, Raboy A, Ferzli G, Albert P. Extraperitoneal endoscopic gasless pelvic lymph node dissection. *J Laparoendosc Surg* 1994;4: 113–116.

38. Dargent D, Arnould P. Percutaneous pelvic lymphadenectomy under laparoscopic guidance. In: Nichols D, ed. *Gynecologic and obstetric surgery.* St Louis: Mosby, 1993:583–605.

39. Winter R. Lymphadenectomy. In: Burghardt E, ed. *Surgical gynecologic oncology.* New York: Thieme, 1993:281.

40. Dargent D, Keita N, Mathevet P, et al. Histoire naturelle du cancer du col: confrontation entre les données morphologiques et les chances de survie *Ref Gynecol Obstet* 1993;1:548–549.

41. Fuller A, Elliot N, Kosloff C, Lewis T. Lymph node metastasis from carcinoma of the cervix stage IB and IIA: implications for prognosis and treatment. *Gynecol Oncol* 1982;13:165–175.

42. Hughes FSR, MacDermott FT, Polglase AL, Johnson WR. Tumor recurrence in the abdominal wall scar tissue after large bowel cancer surgery. *Dis Colon Rectum* 1983;26:571–572.

43. Boulez J. Chirurgie du cancer colo-rectal par voie coelioscopique. *Annal Chir* 1996;50:219–230.

44. Volz J, Koster S, Weiss M, et al. *Gynecol Endosc* 1996 (in press).

45. Childers JM, Brzechffa PR, Hatch K, Surwit E. Laparoscopically assisted surgical staging of endometrial carcinoma. *Gynecol Oncol* 1993;51: 33–38.

46. Mage G, Bournazeau JA, Canis M. Le traitement des adénocarcinomes de l'endomètre Stade I clinique par coelio chirurgie à propos de 17 cas. *J Gynecol Obstet Biol Reprod* 1995;24: 485–490.

47. Boike GM, Sciarra JJ. Le traitement laparoscopique des cancers utérins. *Gynecol Int* 1996;5: 108–112.

48. Querleu D. Hystérectomies élargies de Schauta Amreich et Schauta Stoeckel assistées par coelioscopie. *J Gynecol Obstet Biol Reprod* 1991;20: 747–748.

49. Dargent D, Mathevet P. Hystérectomie élargie laparoscopico-vaginale. *J Gynecol Obstet Biol Reprod* 1992;21:709–710.

50. Querleu D. Case report: laparoscopically assisted radical vaginal hysterectomy. *Gynecol Oncol* 1993;51:248–254.

51. Kadar N, Reich H. Laparoscopically assisted radical Schauta hysterectomy and bilateral laparoscopic pelvic lymphadenectomy for the treatment of bulky stage IB carcinoma of the cervix. *Gynecol Endosc* 1993;2:135–142.

52. Canis M, Mage G, Wattiez A, et al. Vaginally assisted laparoscopic radical hysterectomy. *J Gynecol Surg* 1992;8:103–106.

53. Sedlacek TV, Campion MJ, Reich H, Sedlacek T. Laparoscopic radical hysterectomy: a feasibility study. *Gynecol Oncol* 1995;56:126. Abstract.

54. Dargent D. Laparoscopic surgery and gynecologic cancer. *Curr Opin Obstet Gynecol* 1993;5: 294–300.

55. Dargent D. Schauta's vaginal hysterectomy combined with laparoscopic lymphadenectomy. *Baillieres Clin Obstet Gynaecol* 1995;9:691–705.

56. Van der Burg MEL, Van Lent M. To evaluate the benefits and risks of intervention surgery: phase III study for the treatment of ovarian cancer FIGO stage II b and c, III and IV. Presented at the ASCO meeting, 1993.

57. Canis M, Chapron C, Mage G. Technique et résultats préliminaires du second look coelioscopique dans les tumeurs épithéliales malignes de l'ovaire. *J Gyn Obstet Biol Rep* 1992;21: 655–663.

58. Shinozuka T, Miyamoto T, Hirazono K, et al. Follow up laparoscopy in patients with ovarian cancer. *Tohai J Exp Clin Med* 1994;19:53–59.

ᏢART **III**

Psychosocial and Genetic Aspects

CHAPTER 38

Psychosocial Considerations for Breast Cancer Patients and Their Families

BETH E. MEYEROWITZ
BETH LEEDHAM
STACEY HART

The psychosocial aspects of breast cancer have received considerable attention in the research literature, far more than cancer at any other site (1). Initially this attention was in response to a perceived lack of sensitivity on the part of the medical community to the tremendous disruption that breast cancer can cause in a woman's life. Psychosocial researchers speculated that breast cancer and mastectomy would have a uniquely devastating impact because of the central role that the breasts play in defining body image and femininity. However, research conducted for more than 20 years documented that breast cancer, while certainly distressing and disruptive, is no more likely than other cancers to result in serious psychological difficulties. Nonetheless, this extensive body of research provides invaluable information on the psychosocial aspects of breast cancer for patients and their families. In this chapter we review key findings, using representative research from a large and growing literature. We emphasize information that may be useful to clinicians working with breast cancer patients and survivors.

Adjustment to the Diagnosis

Immediate Reactions

Receiving any diagnosis of cancer is a terrifying experience that changes the lives of patients and their families forever. Since most breast cancer patients begin treatment shortly after receiving the diagnosis, it is difficult to separate reactions to diagnosis from reactions to treatments. The few studies that obtained information from patients during the pretreatment phase identified reactions in the emotional, cognitive, and social domains.

Anxiety, typically at moderate levels, is an almost universal reaction to receiving a breast cancer diagnosis (2). Women diagnosed with malignant disease report significantly higher levels of psychological distress—including tension, depression, and anger—than do women who receive benign diagnoses (3–5). In fact, evidence suggests that during the period between diagnosis and treatment, patients with early-stage disease may reach their highest levels of distress and uncertainty (4,6). In one study, more than two thirds of breast cancer patients described the diagnostic phase prior to surgery as the most stressful (7).

In addition to causing discomfort, this anxiety can impede cognitive functioning (8). Cancer-related fears can interfere with the ability to process and remember information about cancer (9). Research also suggests that recently diagnosed breast cancer patients are likely to experience high levels of confusion (4). Such confusion can impair the patient's ability to participate in important treatment-related decisions soon after receiving the cancer diagnosis. Cognitive difficulties, however, do not mean that patients should be excluded from the decision-making process. Several studies confirmed that having the opportunity to make treatment-related choices predicts better psychological adjustment for breast cancer patients and their partners (10,11), as we discuss later in this chapter. Providing patients with tape recordings of consultations to review at home and including companions in discussions of treatment options can aid patients as they consider difficult decisions (12,13).

The literature suggests that certain coping strategies may be more or less helpful to patients adjusting to a cancer diagnosis. Stanton and Snider (4) found that attempts to cope with cancer during the prebiopsy period through cognitive avoidance were associated with greater distress both prior to and following surgery. These efforts to escape thinking about cancer should not be confused with efforts to maintain a positive and hopeful outlook, which were associated with less distress prior to biopsy.

Family members, as well as patients, are affected by a diagnosis of breast cancer. The diagnostic phase can be one of the most stressful periods for partners of cancer patients, marked by depression and fear (7,14). Many partners appear to have needs for information and for involvement in decision-making similar to those of the patient (11,12,14).

Long-Term Adjustment

The distress and disruption associated with breast cancer continue long after the immediate postdiagnostic period. In some patients, ongoing difficulties are associated with specific treatments for breast cancer or with spread of the disease, and these specific problems are discussed in subsequent sections. Here we focus on those aspects of long-term adjustment that appear to be general reactions common to many breast cancer patients, regardless of treatment or disease progression.

Emotional Distress

Researchers have consistently found that breast cancer patients experience mild to moderate levels of anxiety and depression for several months following surgery. Breast cancer patients report greater emotional distress than do healthy women, women undergoing cholecystectomy, and patients undergoing biopsy for benign breast disease (3,5,15), and psychological symptoms requiring some intervention are found in a sizeable minority of patients (16). Severe psychopathologic symptoms and serious psychological maladjustment, however, are rare (15,17,18).

It is not unusual for breast cancer survivors to continue to report being upset for more than a year following the termination of treatment (5). However, most women who remain disease free experience a gradual reduction in emotional distress following treatment and, by 2 years after treatment, no longer report elevated levels of distress (3,19,20). A minority of disease-free women, ranging from approximately 10% to 25% depending on the study, do not return to preoperative levels of emotional functioning (17,19). These women may experience consistently high levels of distress or increasing distress during the posttreatment period (21).

Although elevated mood disturbance abates for most patients during the first 2 years following treatment, some fears and concerns continue. For most people, having cancer is a transition point in their lives (22). Even years after remission, patients may experience an ongoing sense of increased vulnerability and decreased control over life. Although patients are usually able to avoid thinking about cancer, periodic reminders such as routine medical examinations or minor aches and pains can provoke fear (20).

Social Interactions

The vast majority of breast cancer patients, from 70% to 95% in most studies, report that they receive excellent support from their family and friends (23–25). In fact, levels of support appear to be higher for breast cancer patients than for women who have not had cancer (18). Despite these high levels of support, temporary impairments in social functioning appear to be common. In one study, for example, researchers measured the levels of distress associated with social and interpersonal relationships that mastectomy patients reported as compared to healthy women, female cholecystectomy patients, and women who underwent biopsy for benign breast disease (15). They found elevated social distress among the cancer patients during the first few months following surgery; however, the four groups reported equivalent levels of interpersonal distress by 1 year.

High levels of support coupled with interpersonal difficulties create an apparent paradox that some researchers have sought to understand by identifying specific areas of interpersonal difficulty. Approximately 25% of patients have specific interpersonal problems and a larger proportion describe isolated cases of hurtful interactions (23,24). In addition to overt rejection and withdrawal, patients find comments that minimize their problems or suggest that they should not worry to be particularly unhelpful. Even when friends intend to be supportive, they may misperceive the patient's concerns. For example, people who have not had breast cancer, particularly men, often overestimate the extent to which breast cancer patients are bothered by breast disfigurement relative to survival concerns (26). It is also common for friends and family to assume that the impact of breast cancer ends shortly after the termination of treatment. They can become impatient when survivors continue to be upset about having had cancer, leaving survivors to feel that they must keep their concerns to themselves. In addition, some issues—such as discussing fears about cancer, asking for help, and beginning new dating relationships—can be difficult even within a supportive environment (20).

Social interactions are complicated by the fact that family and friends are dealing with their own reactions to breast cancer. Most of the research on reactions to breast cancer in significant others focuses on husbands and confirms that they experience many of the same reactions that patients do. For both partners, survival concerns are paramount (7,27). Husbands also have concerns about communicating about cancer and their wives' emotional needs (28). In addition to specific concerns, most husbands report high levels of emotional distress during their wives' hospitalization (29), and a substantial minority experience high

levels of distress which may increase throughout at least the first year following treatment (30). In fact, in many cases husbands appear to experience levels of distress equivalent to the patients' (31). While both patients and partners tend to report high levels of marital satisfaction (24,29,32), husbands perceive less support from friends and the medical team than do patients (7).

Attending more closely to the partner's needs may benefit both the partner and the patient, in that patient's and partner's levels of anxiety and depression tend to be highly correlated (31). Negative mood in the couple, in turn, leads to marital maladjustment which has a negative impact on coping for the entire family (33). While most good marriages remain strong, troubled relationships can worsen, and for a minority of couples the illness can cause ongoing serious conflict (24,29,32). Although little has been written about the reactions of children when their mother is diagnosed with breast cancer, there is evidence that some daughters may be particularly distressed (33, 34).

Job Discrimination

In addition to personal relationships, breast cancer can have a long-term impact on a patient's work relationships and employment. Hoffman (35) estimated that approximately 25% of cancer patients experience some form of job discrimination due to their illness. Despite the fact that work performance and productivity are not decreased by cancer (35), there appears to be discrimination against patients in hiring, promotion, and workplace atmosphere (36,37). These problems are most common and severe for women with blue-collar jobs (37). Problems at work can be exacerbated by fears that losing or changing employment may result in loss of both medical insurance and income. Nevertheless, although there are often problems, most patients report that their coworkers have generally positive and supportive attitudes (37,38).

Body Image and Sexuality

In two areas of psychosocial functioning—body image and sexuality—problems do not appear to abate over time, even for disease-free patients who are well adjusted in other domains (20). In fact, there is some evidence that sexual functioning may actually worsen (39). Sexual difficulties are among the most common, severe, and persistent problems reported by breast cancer patients (17,25). Women with breast cancer report significantly more sexual problems than do healthy outpatients (40), and in retrospective reports, husbands describe sexual satisfaction as decreasing for both themselves and their partners (29). Commonly reported problems include decreased sense of physical and sexual attractiveness, discomfort being seen naked, difficulty becoming sexually aroused and reaching orgasm, decreased libido, and less frequent kissing and intercourse (19,20,25,40).

Sexual difficulties may result from disfiguring surgery, breast cancer–related weight gain, premature menopause caused by chemotherapy and hormonal therapy, withdrawal from hormone replacement therapy necessitated by the cancer diagnosis, reactions of partners, difficulty in relaxing and being vulnerable, or many other concerns faced by breast cancer survivors. Consequently, clinicians should assess for sexual and body image problems with all breast cancer patients (41).

Positive Changes

Despite the distress and disruption associated with receiving a cancer diagnosis, most cancer survivors report that their lives were improved in some respects by the experience. Zemore and Shepel (18), for example, found that 73% of breast cancer patients reported positive consequences, such as having a more positive outlook on life and closer family ties. Many cancer survivors report that they are more aware of what is important in life and no longer allow trivial matters to bother them.

Predictors of Adjustment

A major focus of research on adjusting to cancer has been on identifying characteristics of the patient and her experience that are associated with optimal psychosocial adjustment. Understanding how some breast cancer patients adjust to their illness and treatments can provide critical information on how to help other patients learn to adjust more effectively. Researchers found that it is possible to identify patients who adjust well and those who are likely to fall into the minority who experience serious psychopathology or who do not fully recover psychologically from breast cancer (20). The

most promising predictors of adjustment are described below.

Patient Characteristics That Predate Cancer

A history of prior psychiatric problems, depression, anxiety, or stressful life events has been consistently associated with poorer adjustment among breast cancer patients and their families (3,29,30,42–44). Similarly, marital relationships that are most seriously stressed following breast cancer are likely to be those that had more problems before cancer (24,29).

Social Support

A variety of aspects of social support for breast cancer patients—including family cohesion, marital support, emotional support, social contacts, and practical help—has been associated with better adjustment (7,23,33,45,46). Moreover, there is some evidence to suggest that social support may lead to increased natural killer cell activity and improved chances of survival among breast cancer patients (46,47).

Coping

Psychological research suggests that a pattern of passive coping and emotional withdrawal predicts worse outcomes in cancer patients (48). On the other hand, good adjustment may be most likely in cancer patients who hold optimistic beliefs (49,50), seek social support (51), and engage in active problem solving (49). This pattern of positive, active coping may predict better physical health and longer survival as well, although these data are limited and preliminary (48).

Communication with the Medical Team

From the time that a patient contacts a physician, her relationship with the medical team will play a central role in her psychosocial well-being. Unfortunately, this relationship often takes place in the context of a confusing and bureaucratic medical system that is not well structured to be supportive to patients and their families (52). Moreover, medical examinations and treatment are highly stressful for breast cancer patients and survivors (20), heightening the need for the medical team to provide information and a supportive milieu.

Providing Information and Involvement in Decision Making

When patients are asked to describe their interactions with physicians, they consistently list providing information as one of the most helpful things that physicians can do (53–56). Good communication with the medical team is an important component of patients' and families' satisfaction with medical care, whereas communication problems are associated with distress (53,57–59). Unfortunately, many patients do experience difficulty communicating with their medical caregivers (56,58). The most commonly reported communication problems include finding it difficult to understand physicians and to express feelings to them (20,58). On the other hand, when information is provided clearly and in a way that patients can understand, even distressing information appears not to be detrimental to patients (59,60). Nonetheless, physicians and nurses should be careful to consider patients' individual needs and cultural backgrounds when deciding how best to convey information (61).

Information can be essential for early-stage breast cancer patients, to allow them to be involved in making decisions about treatment options. Physicians and patients agree that the physician should play the dominant role in decision making (62). Nonetheless, patients benefit psychologically when they are consulted about the decision-making process, even if they choose to turn over all decisions to their medical team. For example, Fallowfield et al (63) found that patients who were offered a choice about surgery, regardless of whether they had mastectomy or conservative treatment, were less likely to be depressed than women who were not offered a choice. Differences in anxiety and depression were maintained at a 3-year follow-up, despite the fact that, when consulted, the majority of patients had requested that the surgeon make the decision rather than making the decision themselves (64). Increased psychological morbidity was not found, however, when no involvement in decision making was offered because of medical constraints that determined treatment (64). These data do not suggest that patients should be pressured to play a role in making decisions, but that they benefit from being given the option to participate if they so choose. Involvement in decision making also may reduce anxiety and depression among partners (11).

Providing Emotional Support

Although patients expect and prefer their family and friends to be the primary providers of emotional support (23,54), a caring and understanding attitude on the part of the physician is very important as well (43,56). Patients who perceive better emotional support, empathy, and interpersonal skill on the part of the physician report greater satisfaction with their care and better psychological adjustment overall (43,53,57). Since patients differ in their preferences and needs (60), it is difficult for the medical team to know what will be helpful to a given patient or her family. Research has documented that, without direct consultation with the patient, physicians are at high risk of making inaccurate judgments about patients' concerns and needs (65). In addition, most patients have difficulty asking their physicians questions (58), leaving the medical team with the responsibility for initiating discussion. When physicians encourage questions, patients ask more questions and express greater satisfaction with their care (66).

The way in which physicians express support, as well as the specific information that they provide, can be of great importance to patients. Simple interpersonal behaviors, such as sitting down when talking and not interrupting, are appreciated by patients (67). Reassuring the patient that she will not be abandoned and not appearing overly worried may also be important (60,68). While most research focuses on the patient-physician relationship, patients may rely on nurses for expressing concern and empathy and being available to answer questions (54,69).

Psychological Impact of Treatment

Surgery

Breast-Conserving Surgeries

Prior to the availability of breast-conserving surgeries, it was widely believed that the disfigurement caused by mastectomy was the primary cause of distress and disruption for breast cancer patients. This belief led to the expectation that breast-conserving surgeries would prevent most of the problems experienced by patients. However, evidence from over 25 studies comparing the psychological reactions of patients who received mastectomy versus breast-conserving surgeries does not support the belief that breast-conserving surgeries protect women from the distress and difficulties associated with breast cancer (65, 70,71).

In most areas of adjustment, there do not appear to be differences between mastectomy and breast-conserving surgery. Researchers failed to find differences on a variety of psychological variables, including self-concept, mood, overall quality of life, and social adjustment, for either patients or their partners (5,6,72–75). Functional status also is equivalent between the two group of patients (6). Any breast surgery can result in difficulties in performing daily activities (25) and in persistent symptoms such as numbness, pain, and skin sensitivity for some women (39). Women who experience lymphedema, a common side effect of both surgeries with nodal dissection, have greater psychological and physical impairment than do women without arm swelling (76,77). In addition, patients report decreases in their capacity to concentrate in the days following either of the two surgeries (78). Early concerns that conservative surgery might foster greater fears of recurrence among patients have not been substantiated (79,80). The psychological outcomes of these surgeries may have as much to do with whether the patient was allowed to be involved in the decision making than with the extent of surgery, as discussed previously.

Despite the similarities between the surgeries in psychological adjustment and quality of life, differences in some discrete domains have been found reliably. Patients who have had conservative surgeries consistently report better body image (65,71); these women feel more comfortable with their appearance and have fewer concerns about finding attractive clothes (73,80). Some studies (5), but not others (80), demonstrated that women who have had conservative surgeries also show advantages in terms of sexual satisfaction and functioning. On the other hand, patients who have had conservative surgery with radiation treatment report greater difficulties in some areas (73),

as we discuss in the section on radiation therapy.

Breast Reconstruction

Approximately 10% of mastectomized women have reconstructive surgery (81). The primary reason why most women have reconstruction is to avoid the discomfort of external prostheses (81,82). A substantial majority of women, approximately 80% in most studies, report being satisfied with the cosmetic results of surgery (81,83). Some patients also experience positive effects in other domains, such as body image and psychological adjustment (83,84). Women who seek reconstruction in hopes of improving their marital or sexual relationships, on the other hand, are typically disappointed (81,82).

While most women who choose reconstruction seem to benefit from it, they do not appear to experience psychological advantages relative to other breast cancer patients. Women who have had breast reconstruction do not report better psychological adjustment, body image satisfaction, or sexual functioning compared to women who did not have breast reconstruction (81,85). Moreover, in comparison to women who have breast-conserving surgeries, women who undergo immediate reconstruction report worse body image and less patient satisfaction (74,80). In addition, removal of tissue from the abdomen or back to reconstruct the breast leaves some patients with concerns about scarring and pain (80).

Radiation Therapy

Radiotherapy, whether administered as adjuvant treatment following surgery or as a primary treatment, can have negative effects on patients' lives. Many patients experience disturbingly high levels of fatigue, which can increase during the first few weeks of treatment (86). Disruptions in daily activities are common (87), especially in recreational and social domains (73). Women also are likely to have breast soreness and skin changes (76,88). Research findings are inconsistent regarding the extent to which emotional distress is increased during radiation.

Most women who remain disease free recover from the negative impact of radiation. Fatigue typically begins to diminish approximately 3 weeks after the completion of treatment (86), whereas decreases in activity level seem to persist for several months. In one study cosmetic results declined for as long as 3 years following treatment, although 85% of patients were rated as having excellent or good cosmetic results eventually (88). Almost all of the lingering cosmetic problems were found in patients who had a radiation boost dose. To the extent that there is mood disturbance, it also appears to diminish after treatment.

Chemotherapy

Patients receiving chemotherapy are likely to experience greater psychological distress, worse body image, and more sexual dysfunction than other patients with treatable breast cancer (75,89). Almost all patients experience high levels of fatigue and many have weight gain, hair loss, and other side effects (90). Premenopausal women also are likely to go through an abrupt and premature menopause (76). Menopausal symptoms, without the option of hormone replacement, can be very distressing to these young women.

The period immediately prior to the beginning of chemotherapy is particularly distressing for many patients. Clinically elevated levels of depression and anxiety can be present in up to 40% of patients beginning chemotherapy (91,92). Distress is typically most intense at the initiation of treatment and subsides gradually over the treatment period (91–93). However, a substantial proportion of patients experience a resurgence of distress at the end of chemotherapy, possibly because the completion of treatments signifies the loss of a "safety net" (93).

Whereas depression typically decreases across the treatment period, physical side effects such as nausea, fatigue, and hair loss intensify. Somatic side effects and physical impairment due to chemotherapy impede work and social functioning and predict psychological distress (94,95). In addition, some patients undergoing chemotherapy experience measurable cognitive impairment (96). Unfortunately, many cancer patients underestimate how difficult side effects are going to be (94), and many report that they either were not adequately prepared by their medical caregivers for the range and possible intensity of negative side effects or were not taught how to cope with them (94,97).

Many patients also experience negative physical side effects in anticipation of chemotherapy treatments. In the most clinically well-known example, patients feel nauseated or vomit simply at the sight, sound, or smell of things associated with their chemotherapy, such as the sight of their oncology nurse, or the smell of disinfectant (98). Anticipatory nausea and vomiting appear to be learned behaviors acquired through a process of classical conditioning, and are worse in highly anxious patients (99).

Other negative effects of chemotherapy are also acquired through classical conditioning. Up to half of patients develop conditioned food aversions, which may occur even in patients who do not experience nausea and vomiting with chemotherapy treatments (100). Such acquired aversions are typically transient, and do not appear to have a significant negative impact on quality of life or nutritional status (101). There is also growing evidence that patients can experience elevated distress (98,102) and conditioned immune suppression (103,104) when exposed to cues associated with chemotherapy treatments.

The side effects of chemotherapy can cause impairment in quality of life to such a great extent that 45% of patients consider prematurely ending their treatments (94), although few in fact do. Most patients report a substantial decrease in their daily activities due to the effects of the chemotherapy, and over a third report negative changes in their family or sexual lives (90). Despite these difficulties, however, most patients state they would definitely recommend chemotherapy treatments to a friend in a similar situation (90). Fortunately, by 2 years after adjuvant chemotherapy is concluded, most patients' quality of life in most areas is restored to pretreatment levels (105), although some patients continue to experience physical problems due to their treatments, such as weight gain or persistent fatigue (105). For patients undergoing palliative chemotherapy, however, the end of treatments can represent the beginning of the final stage of their disease with the attendant deterioration in most aspects of quality of life.

Most of the literature on quality of life in breast cancer patients receiving chemotherapy focuses on patients receiving adjuvant treatment. Patients undergoing chemotherapy as a primary or palliative treatment are likely to experience even greater psychological and physical difficulties, both because of the greatly increased stress of having advanced disease and the likelihood that the chemotherapy will be more toxic.

Recurrence and Advanced Disease

The diagnosis of cancer recurrence is devastating to patients and their families. The news of a recurrence can be substantially more upsetting than the initial cancer diagnosis (25,106), with high levels of anxiety and depressive symptoms being common among both patients and family members (107,108). Many patients with newly diagnosed recurrence report that their medical caregivers give them less attention and information than they received after their initial diagnosis with cancer, and a substantial majority feel that their physicians and nurses incorrectly assumed that they are coping well and that they have adequate social support (106). Some patients may be less active in seeking social support for fear of burdening their families with the demands of caring for them (106).

Advanced disease, for both patients who experienced a period of remission and patients who present with advanced cancer, is associated with anxiety, depression, lower self-esteem, and feelings of hopelessness (109–111). Although some patients are able to maintain a good quality of life even through the terminal phase of cancer (112), substantial impairment in quality of life is typical. Symptoms of fatigue (113) and anorexia (114) are common among advanced breast cancer patients, and can significantly impair quality of life. Patients also report needing considerable help with activities of daily living (115). These physical and functional symptoms can stem from a variety of causes and may have a reciprocal relationship with pain and mood disturbance (114).

Lack of adequate social support can also become a major problem for patients during the terminal stages of cancer. Patients with advanced disease report more interpersonal problems and family discord (23,116), and many experience an erosion of social support in general as their disease progresses and they become less able to engage in rewarding social activities (117). Family members also report increased emotional distress (109) and inadequate social support (118). A particular area of difficulty is coping with the physical care of the patient (118). For example, problems with

feeding can cause significant distress in patients' family members, whereas patients are less likely to experience these problems as distressing (119). This discrepancy can result in considerable stress for the patient, with about three fourths of patients in one study wishing their caregivers would refrain from pressuring them to eat (119). Communication with the medical team can be difficult as well, especially for patients who are unaccustomed to dealing with a hospital environment and who may have views of illness and death that differ from those of the medical team (61,120).

One of the most serious problems for the advanced cancer patient is poorly controlled pain. Up to three fourths of advanced cancer patients have pain sufficiently intense to interfere severely with daily living (121,122). Patients with undercontrolled pain are more likely to experience depression and anxiety (121–124), and pain can severely interfere with daily activities and social functioning (125). Medical caregivers are often poor judges of a patient's pain and may fail to provide adequate analgesia because of discrepancies between their perceptions of the patient's pain and the patient's own subjective experience (125). The medical team needs to conduct a careful pain assessment, as many patients may be reluctant to complain. The patients least likely to be adequately treated for their cancer pain are minority patients, women, and the elderly (125), placing breast cancer patients at high risk.

Women at Risk for Breast Cancer

Because of the prevalence of breast cancer and the multiple biologic and behavioral risk factors for the disease, clinicians routinely encounter patients presenting with elevated breast cancer risk. Given the rapid recent progress in genetic research, the number of such high-risk patients seeking medical counseling is likely to increase dramatically. For example, as many as 1 in 200 women may carry the *BRCA1* gene (126), and the majority of women from high-risk families intend to seek genetic testing when it becomes available (127). Psychological research on high-risk women can inform efforts to provide clinical care to this growing patient group.

Women at high risk for breast cancer are in an unfortunate psychological predicament for at least two reasons. First, high-risk women tend to have inaccurate perceptions about their true susceptibility to breast cancer (128,129). Most women at high risk tend to have exaggerated perceptions of their susceptibility to the disease (130), probably because they make the common cognitive error of overestimating the role of genetics in cancer etiology and underestimating the importance of other risk factors. Second, many high-risk women have had frightening firsthand experiences with breast cancer and its sometimes-difficult treatments. These women may have cared for relatives suffering through very difficult treatments, and may have lost their mothers or other relatives to the disease.

The combination of overestimated susceptibility and very salient negative cancer experiences can create high levels of cancer anxiety. Although some at-risk women may experience little anxiety about cancer, up to one third of women at risk for breast cancer have clinically elevated anxiety levels (131) that can impair mood and general functioning (132,133). Moreover, women with high cancer anxiety are less likely than those with moderate anxiety to perform breast self-examinations (131,132), seek clinical breast examinations (131), and obtain mammograms (133). Educational programs are least effective among women with high cancer anxiety (130), probably because high anxiety can impair learning and memory about cancer (9). Obviously, to be effective, consultation with high-risk women must address explicitly the patient's level of anxiety and fear related to cancer. Researchers at the University of Michigan published a useful detailed protocol for risk counseling that includes intensive education and anxiety management components (126). Because patients tend to overestimate the importance of genetics in cancer development, it is essential with patients testing negative for breast cancer mutations to examine carefully what other risk factors may be present.

Women at greatly elevated risk for breast cancer face a choice between increased medical surveillance, prophylactic mastectomy with or without oophorectomy, and tamoxifen therapy (134). For certain patients, surgery may be preferable to the waiting and wondering of surveillance or tamoxifen therapy. Some patients may in fact feel relief at finally being free of a body part about which they have come to feel resentful and suspicious (135). However, little is known about the quality of life in women

opting for preventive surgery. Anecdotal reports provide no evidence for major psychological disturbance in patients opting for prophylactic surgery, even when they undergo prophylaxis and later learn they are likely negative for breast cancer mutations (129). Nevertheless, caution is obviously required in counseling the at-risk woman considering surgery, as the impact of removing healthy tissue for cancer prevention remains unclear. In addition to the dearth of research on quality of life in patients at genetic risk for breast cancer, the social and ethical ramifications of genetic testing remain unclear. Women contemplating genetic testing face financial and insurance concerns: Prophylaxis is costly, and insurance companies may wish to drop patients testing positive or may fail to reimburse for preventive measures or increased early-detection efforts. In addition, medical ethicists will have to grapple with difficult questions about confidentiality of results, prenatal testing, and testing of patients who are minors.

Referrals for Mental Health Consultation

Although it is beyond the scope of this chapter to provide a comprehensive review of research on the treatment of the psychological and behavioral problems associated with breast cancer, it is important that the people treating patients be aware that effective interventions are available (136). As described earlier, a minority of breast cancer patients and survivors are at risk for ongoing or worsening psychosocial problems, and these problems can be prevented or minimized through timely intervention. Other breast cancer patients may experience a range of less-severe difficulties that require appropriate assessment and intervention, including treatment side effects, sexual dysfunction, anxiety, and relationship difficulties. Even women who recover psychologically from cancer may benefit from interventions that speed their recovery or that address circumscribed areas of continuing difficulties. Many patients can benefit from referral to a mental health clinician who has experience working with cancer patients.

Interventions for Psychiatric Disorders

As among women in general (137), depressive disorders are the most common type of disturbance found among breast cancer patients (138). Moderate distress and anxiety are normative reactions to a breast cancer diagnosis. However, patients require assessment and treatment when these symptoms become severe and interfere significantly with daily activity and enjoyment of life (16). Differentiating between stress reactions and depression can be difficult in the cancer patient, because cancer treatments may cause depressive somatic symptoms such as fatigue and insomnia. Additionally, because pain can cause psychiatric symptoms, depression is not diagnosable in the context of untreated cancer pain. For breast cancer patients, diagnosis of depression relies more on psychological symptoms such as sadness, hopelessness, guilt, worthlessness, anhedonia and apathy, tearfulness, and suicidal thoughts. Such disturbance may be underdiagnosed because of the myth that depression is an appropriate and unavoidable reaction to cancer; in fact, depression is highly treatable through psychotherapy (139), psychopharmacology (16), or a combination.

Social Support Interventions

As discussed earlier, abundant correlational research links social support to better psychological adjustment in cancer patients. In addition, randomized controlled-outcome intervention studies showed that increasing social support through support groups has benefits for patients' emotional adjustment (140). Research on social support groups demonstrates that the best group interventions for cancer patients are structured and time limited (136). Effective groups include emotional support, information and education, and coping skills–training components. For patients with advanced or terminal disease, the groups that are most beneficial also include discussion of death and dying, as well as behavioral training for management of pain and disability (136).

Some research suggests that social support groups may improve the physical health in cancer patients as well (141). In the work of Spiegel et al (141), for example, advanced breast cancer patients were randomized to a no-treatment condition or a structured group intervention that included emotional support, coping skills training, and relaxation for pain management. Patients receiving the intervention experienced significantly less pain than did

control patients, and also survived longer (124,141). Some preliminary evidence suggests that social support may exert its beneficial effects on the physical health of cancer patients by stimulating immune functioning (47,142).

Psychological and Behavioral Interventions

A wide range of time-limited, empirically supported, and targeted interventions are available that can be helpful for patients who have not recovered psychologically from cancer and for patients who are recovering but have concerns in specific areas. In some cases, programs can be integrated into ongoing medical care, without special mental health expertise. For example, preparatory patient education prior to treatment can decrease distress and improve coping among patients (143,144). In other cases, referral to mental health professionals who are expert in working with cancer patients may be optimal. Behavioral interventions have been developed that prevent or reduce the anticipatory nausea and vomiting, pain, and insomnia associated with cancer treatments (99). Behavioral, cognitive behavioral, and counseling approaches can be highly effective in stress management, treatment of depression, problem-solving skills training, treatment of sexual dysfunction, and a variety of other issues with special relevance to cancer patients (139).

Conclusions

In this chapter we summarized the extensive literature on the psychosocial aspects of breast cancer for patients and their families. Although we did not provide a comprehensive review of all of the hundreds of papers that have been published on this topic, the findings cited here are representative and consistent with the larger literature. This literature is limited in several respects. Almost all of the patients and survivors studied are middle-class, non-Hispanic white women in heterosexual relationships, and most were being treated at teaching hospitals for early-stage disease. We know much less about the reactions of women and families from ethnic minority backgrounds, about lesbian breast cancer patients and their partners, and about women who present with advanced disease. Also, we made no attempt to review the literature on psychosocial aspects of compliance with medical recommendations or on psychosocial predictors of disease onset and prognosis.

Despite these drawbacks, the literature provides a great deal of information that may be of use to patients, their families, and their medical teams. The medical team can use this information to make judgments about when a woman's reactions are within normal limits and when a mental health referral might be beneficial. Moreover, by including this information in discussions with patients and their families, they can be fully informed and, in most cases, reassured that their reactions are normal. In the treatment of early-stage breast cancer, in particular, physicians and patients often make decisions—for example, between mastectomy and conservative surgeries and about breast reconstruction—on the basis of psychosocial outcomes, in part. To make these decisions in a fully informed manner, patients should be provided with information on both the medical and psychosocial consequences of these treatment decisions.

Acknowledgments

The writing of this manuscript was supported in part by a grant from the National Cancer Institute (CA63028).

R E F E R E N C E S

1. Meyerowitz BE, Hart S. Women and cancer: have assumptions about women limited our research agenda? In: Stanton AL, Gallant SJ, eds. *The psychology of women's health: progress and challenges in research and application.* Washington, DC: American Psychological Association, 1995:51–84.

2. Hughes J. Emotional reactions to the diagnosis and treatment of early breast cancer. *J Psychosom Res* 1982;26:277–283.

3. Morris T, Greer HS, White P. Psychological and social adjustment to mastectomy: a two-year follow-up study. *Cancer* 1977;40:2381–2387.

4. Stanton AL, Snider PR. Coping with a breast cancer diagnosis: a prospective study. *Health Psychol* 1993;12:16–23.

5. Wolberg WH, Romsaas EP, Tanner MA, Malec JF. Psychosexual adaptation to breast cancer surgery. *Cancer* 1989;63:1645–1655.

6. Hughes KK. Psychosocial and functional status of breast cancer patients: the influence of diagnosis and treatment choice. *Cancer Nurs* 1993;16:222–229.

7. Northouse LL. The impact of breast cancer on patients and husbands. *Cancer Nurs* 1989;12:276–284.

8. Scott DW. Anxiety, critical thinking and information processing during and after breast biopsy. *Nurs Res* 1983;32:24–28.

9. Jepson C, Chaiken S. Chronic issue-specific fear inhibits systematic processing of persuasive communications. *J Soc Behav Pers* 1990;5:61–84.

10. Morris J, Ingham R. Choice of surgery for early breast cancer: psychosocial considerations. *Soc Sci Med* 1988;27:1257–1262.

11. Morris J, Royle GT. Offering patients a choice of surgery for early breast cancer: a reduction in anxiety and depression in patients and their husbands. *Soc Sci Med* 1988;26:583–585.

12. Beisecker AE, Moore WP. Oncologists' perceptions of the effects of cancer patients' companions on physician-patient interactions. *J Psychosoc Oncol* 1994;12:23–39.

13. Hogbin B, Fallowfield L. Getting it taped: the "bad news" consultation with cancer patients. *Br J Hosp Med* 1989;41:330–333.

14. Lewis FM. Strengthening family supports: cancer and the family. *Cancer* 1990;65:158–165.

15. Psychological Aspects of Breast Cancer Study Group. Psychological responses to mastectomy: a prospective comparison study. *Cancer* 1987;59:189–196.

16. Massie MJ, Holland JC. Depression and the cancer patient. *J Clin Psychiatry* 1990;51(suppl):12–17.

17. Hughson AVM, Cooper AF, McArdle CS, Smith DC. Psychosocial consequences of mastectomy: levels of morbidity and associated factors. *J Psychosom Res* 1988;32:383–391.

18. Zemore R, Shepel LF. Effects of breast cancer and mastectomy on emotional support and adjustment. *Soc Sci Med* 1989;28:19–27.

19. Omne-Ponten M, Holmberg L, Sjoden PO. Psychosocial adjustment among women with breast cancer stages I and II: six-year follow-up of consecutive patients. *J Clin Oncol* 1994;12:1778–1782.

20. Schag CAC, Ganz PA, Polinsky ML, et al. Characteristics of women at risk for psychosocial distress in the year after breast cancer. *J Clin Oncol* 1993;11:783–793.

21. Ell K, Nishimoto R, Morvay T, et al. A longitudinal analysis of psychological adaptation among survivors of cancer. *Cancer* 1989;63: 406–413.

22. Mages NL, Mendelsohn GA. Effects of cancer on patients' lives: a personological approach. In: Stone GC, Cohen F, Adler NE, eds. *Health psychology—a handbook: theories, applications, and challenges of a psychological approach to the health care system.* San Francisco: Jossey-Bass, 1979:255–284.

23. Dunkel-Schetter C. Social support and cancer: findings based on patient interviews and their implications. *J Soc Issues* 1984;40:77–98.

24. Lichtman RR, Taylor SE, Wood JV. Social support and marital adjustment after breast cancer. *J Psychosoc Oncol* 1987;5:47–74.

25. Silberfarb PM, Maurer H, Crouthamel CS. Psychosocial aspects of neoplastic disease: I. Functional status of breast cancer patients during different treatment regimens. *Am J Psychiatry* 1980;137:450–455.

26. Peters-Golden H. Breast cancer: varied perceptions of social support in the illness experience. *Soc Sci Med* 1982;16:483–491.

27. Gotay CC. The experience of cancer during early and advanced stages: the views of patients and their mates. *Soc Sci Med* 1984;18:605–613.

28. Zahlis EH, Shands ME. Breast cancer: demands of the illness on the patient's partner. *J Psychosoc Oncol* 1991;9:75–93.

29. Wellisch DK, Jamison KR, Pasnau RO. Psychological aspects of mastectomy: II. The man's perspective. *Am J Psychiatry* 1978;135:543–546.

30. Ell K, Nishimoto R, Mantell J, Hamovitch M. Longitudinal analysis of psychological adaptation among family members of patients with cancer. *J Psychosom Res* 1988;32:429–438.

31. Baider L, De-Nour AK. Adjustment to cancer: who is the patient—the husband or the wife? *Isr J Med Sci* 1988;24:631–636.

32. Lewis FM, Hammond MA. Psychosocial adjustment of the family to breast cancer: a longitudinal analysis. *J Am Med Wom Assoc* 1992;47: 194–200.

33. Lewis FM, Hammond MA, Woods NF. The family's functioning with newly diagnosed breast cancer in the mother: the development of an explanatory model. *J Behav Med* 1993;16: 351–370.

34. Lichtman RR, Taylor SE, Wood J, et al. Relations with children after breast cancer: the mother-daughter relationship at risk. *J Psychosoc Oncol* 1984;2:1–19.

35. Hoffman B. Cancer survivors at work: job problems and illegal discrimination. *Oncol Nurs Forum* 1989;16:39–43.

36. Bordieri JE, Drehmer DE, Taricone PF. Personnel selection bias for job applicants with cancer. *J Appl Soc Psychol* 1990;20:244–253.

37. Feldman FL. Female cancer patients and caregivers: experiences in the workplace. *Women Health* 1987;11:137–153.

38. Staley JC, Kagle JD, Hatfield AK. Cancer patients and their co-workers: a study. *Soc Work Health Care* 1987;13:101–112.

39. Ganz PA, Coscarelli A, Fred C, et al. Breast cancer survivors: psychosocial concerns and quality of life. *Breast Cancer Res Treat* 1996;38: 183–199.

40. Andersen BL, Jochimsen PR. Sexual functioning among breast cancer, gynecologic cancer, and healthy women. *J Consult Clin Psychol* 1985;53: 25–32.

41. Kaplan HS. A neglected issue: the sexual side effects of current treatments for breast cancer. *J Sex Marital Ther* 1992;18:3–19.

42. Maunsell E, Brisson J, Deschenes L. Psychological distress after initial treatment of breast cancer. *Cancer* 1992;70:120–125.

43. Roberts CS, Cox CE, Reintgen DS, et al. Influence of physician communication on newly diagnosed breast patients' psychologic adjustment and decision-making. *Cancer* 1994;74: 336–341.

44. Weisman AD, Worden JW. The existential plight in cancer: significance of the first 100 days. *Int J Psychiatry Med* 1976–77;7:1–15.

45. Friedman LC, Baer PE, Nelson DV, et al. Women with breast cancer: perception of family functioning and adjustment to illness. *Psychosom Med* 1988;50:529–540.

46. Waxler-Morrison N, Hislop TG, Mears B, Kan L. Effects of social relationships on survival for women with breast cancer: a prospective study. *Soc Sci Med* 1991;33:177–183.

47. Levy SM, Herberman RB, Whiteside T, et al. Perceived social support and tumor estrogen/progesterone receptor status as predictors of natural killer cell activity in breast cancer patients. *Psychosom Med* 1990;52:73–85.

48. Leedham B, Meyerowitz BE. The mind and breast cancer risk. In: Stoll BA, ed. *Reducing*

breast cancer risk in women. Amsterdam: Kluwer, 1995:223–229.

49. Carver CS, Pozo C, Harris SD, et al. How coping mediates the effect of optimism on distress: a study of women with early stage breast cancer. *J Pers Soc Psychol* 1993;65:375–390.

50. Carver CS, Pozo-Kaderman C, Harris SD, et al. Optimism versus pessimism predicts the quality of women's adjustment to early stage breast disease. *Cancer* 1994;73:1213–1220.

51. Taylor SE, Lichtman RR, Wood J, et al. Illness-related and treatment-related factors in psychological adjustment to breast cancer. *Cancer* 1985;55:2506–2513.

52. Taylor SE. Hospital patient behavior: reactance, helplessness, or control? *J Soc Issues* 1979;35:156–184.

53. Burton MV, Parker RW. Satisfaction of breast cancer patients with their medical and psychological care. *J Psychosoc Oncol* 1994;12:41–63.

54. Dakof GA, Taylor SE. Victims' perceptions of social support: what is helpful from whom? *J Pers Soc Psychol* 1990;58:80–89.

55. Sutherland HJ, Llewellyn-Thomas HA, Lockwood GA, et al. Cancer patients: their desire for information and participation in treatment decisions. *J R Soc Med* 1989;82:260–263.

56. Wiggers JG, Donovan KO, Redman S, Sanson-Fisher RW. Cancer patient satisfaction with care. *Cancer* 1990;66:610–616.

57. Blanchard CG, Ruckdeschel JC, Fletcher BA, Blanchard EB. The impact of oncologists' behaviors on patient satisfaction with morning rounds. *Cancer* 1986;58:387–393.

58. Lerman C, Daly M, Walsh WP, et al. Communication between patients with breast cancer and health care providers. *Cancer* 1993;72:2612–2620.

59. Mosconi P, Meyerowitz BE, Liberati MC, Liberati A. Disclosure of breast cancer diagnosis: patient and physician reports. *Ann Oncol* 1991;2:273–280.

60. Sardell AN, Trierweiler SJ. Disclosing the cancer diagnosis: procedures that influence patient hopefulness. *Cancer* 1993;72:3355–3365.

61. Trill MD, Holland JH. Cross-cultural differences in the care of patients with cancer: a review. *Gen Hosp Psychiatry* 1993;15:21–30.

62. Beisecker AE, Helmig L, Graham D, Moore WP. Attitudes of oncologists, oncology nurses, and patients from a women's clinic regarding medical decision making for older and younger

breast cancer patients. *Gerontologist* 1994;34:505–512.

63. Fallowfield LJ, Hall A, Maguire GP, Baum M. Psychological outcomes of different treatment policies in women with early breast cancer outside a clinical trial. *BMJ* 1990;301:575–580.

64. Fallowfield LJ, Hall A, Maguire P, et al. Psychological effects of being offered choice of surgery for breast cancer. *BMJ* 1994;309:448.

65. Meyerowitz BE. Quality of life in breast cancer patients: the contribution of data to the care of patients. *Eur J Cancer* 1993;29A:S59–S62.

66. Thompson SC, Nanni C, Schwankovsky L. Patient-oriented interventions to improve communication in a medical office visit. *Health Psychol* 1990;9:390–404.

67. Blanchard CG, Labrecque MS, Ruckdeschel JC, Blanchard EB. Physician behaviors, patient perceptions, and patient characteristics as predictors of satisfaction of hospitalized adult cancer patients. *Cancer* 1990;65:186–192.

68. Shapiro DE, Boggs SR, Melamed BG, Graham-Pole J. The effect of varied physician affect on recall, anxiety, and perceptions in women at risk for breast cancer: an analogue study. *Health Psychol* 1992;11:61–66.

69. Northouse LL. Psychological impact of the diagnosis of breast cancer on the patient and her family. *J Am Med Wom Assoc* 1992;47:161–164.

70. Glanz K, Lerman C. Psychosocial impact of breast cancer: a critical review. *Ann Behav Med* 1992;14:204–212.

71. Hall A, Fallowfield L. Psychological outcome of treatment for early breast cancer: a review. *Stress Med* 1989;5:167–175.

72. Baider L, Rizel S, De-Nour AK. Comparison of couples' adjustment to lumpectomy and mastectomy. *Gen Hosp Psychiatry* 1986;8:251–257.

73. Ganz PA, Schag AC, Lee JJ, et al. Breast conservation versus mastectomy: is there a difference in psychological adjustment or quality of life in the year after surgery? *Cancer* 1992;69:1729–1738.

74. Mock V. Body image in women treated for breast cancer. *Nurs Res* 1993;42:153–157.

75. Schover LR, Yetman RJ, Tuason LJ, et al. Partial mastectomy and breast reconstruction: a comparison of their effects on psychosocial adjustment, body image, and sexuality. *Cancer* 1995;75:54–64.

76. Knobf MT. Symptoms and rehabilitation needs of patients with early stage breast cancer during primary therapy. *Cancer* 1990;66:1392–1401.

77. Tobin MB, Lacey HJ, Meyer L, Mortimer PS. The psychological morbidity of breast cancer-related arm swelling: psychological morbidity of lymphoedema. *Cancer* 1993;72:3248–3252.

78. Cimprich B. Attentional fatigue following breast cancer surgery. *Res Nurs Health* 1992;15:199–207.

79. Lasry JM, Margolese RG. Fear of recurrence, breast-conserving surgery, and the trade-off hypothesis. *Cancer* 1992;69:2111–2115.

80. Noguchi M, Kitagawa H, Kinoshita K, et al. Psychologic and cosmetic self-assessments of breast conserving therapy compared with mastectomy and immediate breast reconstruction. *J Surg Oncol* 1993;54:260–266.

81. Rowland JH, Holland JC. Breast cancer. In: Holland JC, Rowland JH, eds. *Handbook of psychooncology.* New York: Oxford University Press, 1989:188–207.

82. Schain WS, Wellisch DK, Pasnau RO, Landsverk J. The sooner the better: a study of psychological factors in women undergoing immediate versus delayed breast reconstruction. *Am J Psychiatry* 1985;142:40–46.

83. Schain WS. Breast reconstruction: update of psychosocial and pragmatic concerns. *Cancer* 1991;68:1170–1175.

84. Rowland JH, Holland JC, Chaglassian T, Kinne D. Psychological response to breast reconstruction: expectations for and impact on postmastectomy functioning. *Psychosomatics* 1993;34:241–250.

85. Reaby LL, Hort LK. Postmastectomy attitudes in women who wear external breast prostheses compared to those who have undergone breast reconstructions. *J Behav Med* 1995;18:55–67.

86. Greenberg DB, Sawicka J, Eisenthal S, Ross D. Fatigue syndrome due to localized radiation. *J Pain Symptom Manage* 1992;7:38–45.

87. Johnson JE, Lauver DR, Nail LM. Process of coping with radiation therapy. *J Consult Clin Psychol* 1989;57:358–364.

88. Beadle GF, Silver B, Botnick L, et al. Cosmetic results following primary radiation therapy for early breast cancer. *Cancer* 1984;54:2911–2918.

89. Hughson AVM, Cooper AF, McArdle CS, Smith DC. Psychological impact of adjuvant chemotherapy in the first two years after mastectomy. *BMJ* 1986;293:1268–1271.

90. Meyerowitz BE, Sparks FC, Spears IK. Adjuvant chemotherapy for breast carcinoma: psychosocial implications. *Cancer* 1979;43:1613–1618.

91. Jacobsen PB, Bovbjerg DH, Redd WH. Anticipatory anxiety in women receiving chemotherapy for breast cancer. *Health Psychol* 1993;12:469–475.

92. Middelboe T, Ovesen L, Mortensen EL, Bech P. Depressive symptoms in cancer patients undergoing chemotherapy: a psychometric analysis. *Psychother Psychosom* 1994;61:171–177.

93. Ward SE, Viergutz G, Tormey D, et al. Patients' reactions to completion of adjuvant breast cancer therapy. *Nurs Res* 1992;41:362–365.

94. Love RR, Leventhal H, Easterling DV, Nerenz DR. Side effects and emotional distress during cancer chemotherapy. *Cancer* 1989;63:604–612.

95. Given CW, Stommel M, Given B, et al. The influence of cancer patients' symptoms and functional states on patients' depression and family caregivers' reaction and depression. *Health Psychol* 1993;12:277–285.

96. Silberfarb PM, Philibert D, Levine PM. Psychosocial aspects of neoplastic disease: II. Affective and cognitive effects of chemotherapy in cancer patients. *Am J Psychiatry* 1980;137:597–601.

97. Tierney AJ, Leonard RCF, Taylor J, et al. Side effects expected and experienced by women receiving chemotherapy for breast cancer. *BMJ* 1991;302:272.

98. Sabbioni MEE, Bovbjerg DH, Jacobsen PB, et al. Treatment related psychological distress during adjuvant chemotherapy as a conditioned response. *Ann Oncol* 1992;3:393–398.

99. Carey MP, Burish TG. Etiology and treatment of the psychological side effects associated with cancer chemotherapy: a critical review and discussion. *Psychol Bull* 1988;104:307–325.

100. Bernstein IL, Borson S. Learned food aversion: a component of anorexia syndromes. *Psychol Rev* 1986;93:462–472.

101. Mattes RD, Curran WJ, Alavi J, et al. Clinical implications of learned food aversions in patients with cancer treated with chemotherapy or radiation therapy. *Cancer* 1992;70:192–200.

102. Jacobsen PB, Bovbjerg DH, Schwartz MD, et al. Conditioned emotional distress in women receiving chemotherapy for breast cancer. *J Consult Clin Psychol* 1995;63:108–114.

103. Bovbjerg DH, Redd WH, Maier LA, et al. Anticipatory immune suppression and nausea in

women receiving cyclic chemotherapy for ovarian cancer. *J Consult Clin Psychol* 1990;58: 153–157.

104. Fredrikson M, Furst CJ, Lekander M, et al. Trait anxiety and anticipatory immune reactions in women receiving adjuvant chemotherapy for breast cancer. *Brain Behav Immun* 1993;7: 79–90.

105. Meyerowitz BE, Watkins IK, Sparks FC. Psychosocial implications of adjuvant chemotherapy: a two-year follow-up. *Cancer* 1983;52: 1541–1545.

106. Cella DF, Mahon SM, Donovan MI. Cancer recurrence as a traumatic event. *Behav Med* 1990;16:15–22.

107. Jenkins PL, May VE, Hughes LE. Psychological morbidity associated with local recurrence of breast cancer. *Int J Psychiatry Med* 1991;21: 149–155.

108. Wright K, Dyck S. Expressed concerns of adult cancer patients' family members. *Cancer Nurs* 1984;7:371–374.

109. Cassileth BR, Lusk EJ, Strouse TB, et al. A psychological analysis of cancer patients and their next-of-kin. *Cancer* 1985;55:72–76.

110. Lewis FM. Experienced personal control and quality of life in late-stage cancer patients. *Nurs Res* 1982;31:113–119.

111. Wellisch D, Landsverk J, Guidera K, et al. Evaluation of psychosocial problems of the homebound cancer patient: I. Methodology and problem frequencies. *Psychosom Med* 1983;45: 11–21.

112. Morris JN, Suissa S, Sherwood S, et al. Last days: a study of the quality of life of terminally ill cancer patients. *J Chron Dis* 1986;39:47–62.

113. Bruera E. Asthenia in patients with advanced cancer: a review and update of our experience. *J Pain Symptom Manage* 1988;3:1–19.

114. Nelson KA, Walsh, D, Sheehan, FA. The cancer anorexia-cachexia syndrome. *J Clin Oncol* 1994; 12:213–225.

115. Houts PS, Yasko JM, Harvey HA, et al. Unmet needs of persons with cancer in Pennsylvania during the period of terminal care. *Cancer* 1988;62:627–634.

116. Wellisch DK, Wolcott DL, Pasnau RO, et al. An evaluation of the psychosocial problems of the homebound cancer patient: relationship of patient adjustment to family problems. *J Psychosoc Oncol* 1989;7:55–76.

117. Bloom JR, Spiegel D. The relationship of two dimensions of social support to the psychological well-being and social functioning of women with advanced breast cancer. *Soc Sci Med* 1984; 19:831–837.

118. Hinds C. The needs of families who care for patients with cancer at home: are we meeting them? *J Adv Nurs* 1985;10:575–581.

119. Holden C. Anorexia in the terminally ill cancer patient: the emotional impact on the patient and the family. *Hospice J* 1991;7:73–84.

120. Mathews HF, Lannin DR, Mitchell JP. Coming to terms with advanced breast cancer: black women's narratives from eastern North Carolina. *Soc Sci Med* 1994;38:789–800.

121. Arathuzik MD. The appraisal of pain and coping in cancer patients. *West J Nurs Res* 1991; 13:714–731.

122. Rankin MA. Use of drugs for pain with cancer patients. *Cancer Nurs* 1982;5:181–190.

123. Cleeland CS. The impact of pain on the patient with cancer. *Cancer* 1984;54:2635–2641.

124. Spiegel D, Bloom JR. Pain in metastatic breast cancer. *Cancer* 1983;52:341–345.

125. Cleeland CS, Gonin R, Hatfield AK, et al. Pain and its treatment in outpatients with metastatic cancer. *N Engl J Med* 1994;330:592–596.

126. Biesecker B, Boehnke M, Calzone K, et al. Genetic counseling for families with inherited susceptibility to breast and ovarian cancer. *JAMA* 1993;269:1970–1974.

127. Lerman C, Daly M, Masny A, Balshem A. Attitudes about genetic testing for breast-ovarian cancer susceptibility. *J Clin Oncol* 1994;12: 843–850.

128. Evans DGR, Burnell LD, Hopwood P, Howell A. Perception of risk in women with a family history of breast cancer. *Br J Cancer* 1993;67: 612–614.

129. Lynch HT, Watson P, Conway TA, et al. DNA screening for breast/ovarian susceptibility based on linked markers. *Arch Intern Med* 1993;153: 1979–1987.

130. Lerman C, Lustbader E, Rimer B, et al. Effects of individualized breast cancer risk counseling: a randomized trial. *J Natl Cancer Inst* 1995;87: 286–292.

131. Kash KM, Holland JC, Halper MS, Miller G. Psychological distress and surveillance behaviors of women with a family history of breast cancer. *J Natl Cancer Inst* 1992;84:24–30.

132. Lerman C, Trock B, Rimer BK, et al. Psychological side effects of breast cancer screening. *Health Psychol* 1991;10:259–267.

133. Lerman C, Daly M, Sands C, et al. Mammography adherence and psychological distress among women at risk for breast cancer. *J Natl Cancer Inst* 1993;85:1074–1080.

134. King M, Rowell S, Love S. Inherited breast and ovarian cancer: what are the risks? What are the choices? *JAMA* 1993;269:1975–1980.

135. Breo DL. Altered fates—counseling families with inherited breast cancer. *JAMA* 1993;269: 2017–2022.

136. Andersen BL. Psychological interventions for cancer patients to enhance quality of life. *J Consult Clin Psychol* 1992;60:552–568.

137. American Psychiatric Association. *Diagnostic and statistical manual of mental disorders.* 4th ed. Washington, DC: American Psychiatric Association, 1994.

138. Derogatis LR, Morrow GR, Fetting J, et al. The prevalence of psychiatric disorders among cancer patients. *JAMA* 1983;249:751–757.

139. Task Force on Promotion and Dissemination of Psychological Procedures, Division of Clinical Psychology, American Psychological Association. Training in and dissemination of empirically-validated psychological treatments: report and recommendations. *Clin Psychol* 1995;48:3–23.

140. Meyer TJ, Mark MM. Effects of psychosocial interventions with adult cancer patients: a meta-analysis of randomized experiments. *Health Psychol* 1995;14:101–108.

141. Spiegel D, Bloom JR, Kraemer HC, Gottheil E. Effect of psychosocial treatment on survival of patients with metastatic breast cancer. *Lancet* 1989;2:888–891.

142. Fawzy FI, Cousins N, Fawzy NW, et al. A structured psychiatric intervention for cancer patients: I. Changes over time in immunological measures. *Arch Gen Psychiatry* 1990;47:729–735.

143. Burish TG, Snyder SL, Jenkins RA. Preparing patients for cancer chemotherapy: effects on coping preparation and relaxation interventions. *J Consult Clin Psychol* 1991;59:518–525.

144. Rainey LC. Effects of preparatory patient education for radiation oncology patients. *Cancer* 1985;56:1056–1061.

CHAPTER *39*

Familial Ovarian Cancer

DAVID E. C. COLE
WINSTON TAM
K. JOAN MURPHY
BARRY ROSEN

The Biologic Basis of Hereditary Cancers

The central role of genetic mutation in the development of cancer is now widely accepted. Knudson first elaborated the paradigm as the "two-hit hypothesis" for retinoblastoma (1,2). Then Vogelstein and others (3–5) modified it to embrace the multiple genetic events underlying common cancers. Thus, ovarian cancer can be considered to arise by a series of deleterious mutations in genes that regulate cell proliferation and differentiation (6). In inherited ovarian cancer, the first genetic mutation occurs in cells that transmit genetic information to the next generation (Fig. 39-1). Called *germline mutations*, these changes are passed on through egg(s) or sperm in an autosomal dominant fashion to all cells in half of the children. Therefore, the affected offspring are at increased risk of cancer. The subsequent mutagenic steps of the ovarian cancer sequence are more likely to lead to an earlier cancer because the germline mutation is present from birth, but the mutational events themselves still follow a probabilistic time line. Thus, carriers of a germline mutation may go an entire lifetime without cancer if later mutational events in the multistep process do *not* occur. Carriers who remain asymptomatic for an entire lifetime are said to be nonpenetrant. Nonpenetrance is not just a random process though, and the factors that contribute to nonpenetrance in some families or

individuals, but not others, are not understood. These uncertainties are crucial considerations for the families that harbor a predisposing mutation and the health-care workers who offer them clinical advice on the risk of cancer.

Epidemiology and Definition

Ovarian cancer is the most common lethal gynecologic cancer in North America. In Canada, there are 2100 new cases and 1300 deaths each year (7), and the numbers are more than 10 times higher in the United States. The disease is difficult to detect in its earliest stages and is resistant to therapy later in its course. The population lifetime risk for ovarian cancer is approximately 1 in 70. Familial clustering of ovarian cancer has been recognized for decades. For those with one affected first-degree relative, the estimated lifetime risk increases 1.5-fold to 3.6-fold and the risks rise steeply with additional affected family members (8). The increased risk is not uniformly distributed, as epidemiologic surveys tend to suggest. Rather, most of the cancer risk in women with one affected first-degree relative resides in the small fraction whose family carries a single gene mutation that greatly enhances predisposition to cancer.

We use the term *familial ovarian cancer* to denote families or individuals with a positive family history (9) and reserve the term *hereditary ovarian cancer syndrome* for those in

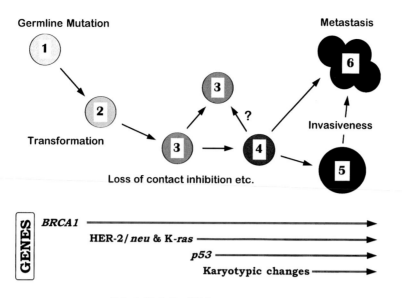

F I G U R E 39-1

Postulated genetic events in familial ovarian cancer. Cells already carrying a germline mutation such as *BRCA1* (No. 1) may be more susceptible to further mutations resulting in earlier and more frequent transformation (No. 2), dedifferentiation, loss of contact inhibition (No. 3), and deregulation of cell cycling, resulting in ovarian epithelial clones with recognizable premalignant changes, such as papillary cystadenomatosis and epithelial inclusion cysts (No. 4). Both HER-2/*neu* overexpression and K-*ras* mutations (164) have been implicated in the transformation process (165), as have mutations of the *p53* gene (62). Mutations of *p53* may also be late events (65) and tissue localization has been used to identify clonal reversions of neoplastic cells with loss of transforming mutations and resumption of a benign cellular phenotype (166,167). Healthy women with germline mutations appear to have increased risks for microinvasive and borderline ovarian cancer and for a variety of premalignant changes (145), which has been taken as evidence supporting this model of inherited ovarian cancer (168). In the final stages of the carcinogenesis sequence, a variety of chromosomal deletions and karyotypic rearrangements (169) and loss of heterozygosity (169,170) are observed frequently and are a common feature of cell types demonstrating invasiveness (No. 5) and the potential for metastasis (No. 6).

whom there are clear indications of a genetic etiology. Narod et al (10) examined family history patterns in 450 of 631 ovarian cancers reported to a Canadian registry over a 3-year period. Of the 71 patients with a positive family history (familial ovarian cancer), 18 had multiple relatives with breast or ovarian cancer, which suggested a hereditary ovarian cancer syndrome. In the 18 families, there were 81 asymptomatic women whose age and relationship to the ovarian cancer case placed them at 50% risk of carrying the gene themselves. Overall, the proportion of ovarian cancer that could be considered hereditary from detailed

family history alone was estimated to be between 2.9% and 6.9% (10). Accordingly, for every 20 women with ovarian cancer, one would potentially benefit from detailed genetic counseling and pass on information to an average of four asymptomatic relatives at high risk for ovarian and other cancers.

Syndromes Associated with Hereditary Ovarian Cancer

There are at least three different classes of genes that confer increased risk for ovarian cancer and several patterns of clinical presentation (Table 39-1). The class of syndrome designated *BRCA* is typified by mutations of *BRCA1*, a gene that codes for a protein expressed in a wide variety of tissues (Table 39-2). Germline mutations in this gene, localized to chromosome 17q12-21, have been identified in more than 400 different families (Narod S, personal communication, 1997) with multiple breast or ovarian cancer occurrences. At the time of writing, 70% of the reported mutations are small deletions or insertions or nonsense mutations, so-called because they introduce a stop codon that prematurely truncates the BRCA1 protein (11–30). However, despite careful searches, mutations have not been found in several families with strong *BRCA1* linkage (31). To complicate matters, there are numerous benign polymorphisms scattered throughout the gene. Validation of conservative missense mutations as causative is still dependent on linkage and accurate histologic diagnosis in multiple affected family members. One notable exception is the frequency of recurrent mutations in individuals of Ashkenazi Jewish background. First identified through a common haplotype of closely linked polymorphic flanking markers (32), the exon 2 truncating mutation—185delAG—is found in about 1% of the Ashkenazi Jewish population (33,34). The 185delAG mutation is also recurrent in two British families with a distinctly different haplotype background and no known Jewish ancestry, and so probably represents a separate mutational event (35). Another recur-

rent mutation of *BRCA1*, the 5382insC mutation, is found in 0.1% of the Jewish population (34), but it is also recurrent in many families without Jewish ancestry (35). As expected, Jewish women with a positive family history for breast and ovarian cancer have a significantly higher risk of having these specific mutations, and this is a key point for genetic counseling of these women (36).

For *BRCA*, there are four clinical patterns (see Table 39-1). One is the so-called site-specific ovarian cancer syndrome. These families are now known to be genetically linked to the *BRCA1* locus (37) while at the other end of the spectrum, many breast-only cancer families also have mutations of the *BRCA1* gene (38). In between are families with both cancers (39) which divide epidemiologically into two types (Table 39-3). In type 1 (breast predominant), the lifetime risk of breast cancer may be very high (91% by age 70) and there is an increased relative risk for colon cancer in male or female family members. In type 2 (ovarian predominant), the risk for breast cancer is lower (70% by age 70), while the risk for ovarian cancer is higher (84% by age 70). Recent studies of consecutive case series (40,41) indicate that the risks may be lower for many families. Both types confer increased relative risk for prostate cancer. A gene that appears to be involved in the expression of the CA-125 tumor marker for ovarian cancer (the *1A1-3B* gene) has been found in immediate physical juxtaposition to the *BRCA1* gene (42–44), in a duplicated region of

T A B L E   **39-1**

Hereditary Ovarian Cancer Syndromes

Syndrome	Risk of Ovarian Cancer in Gene Carriers	Gene(s)	Genetic Locus (Reference)
1. *Breast/ovarian syndromes* (111)			
a. Site-specific ovarian cancer (37)	↑↑		
b. Breast/ovarian—type 1 or "breast predominant" (112)	≤32%	*BRCA1*	17q12–21 (9)
c. Breast/ovarian—type 2 or "ovarian predominant" (112)	≤84%	*BRCA2*	13q12–13 (46)
d. Site-specific breast cancer	↑		
2. *Hereditary nonpolyposis colorectal cancer (HNPCC)*	8%*	*hMSH2*	2p16 (113)
		hMLH1	3p21 (114)
		hPMS1	2q31–33 (115)
		hPMS2	7p22 (115)
3. *p53 Familial cancer syndrome (rare)*	Slight ↑	*p53*	17p13 (68)

*Much of the increase may be specifically associated with *hMSH2* mutations (116).

↑↑ ≡ greatly increased; ↑ ≡ increased, in comparison to the population risk.

T A B L E   **39-2**

Characteristics of the *BRCA1* Gene and
Its Protein Product

- Single-copy gene of >70 kb in size localized to 17q12–21 (38).
- Full-length mRNA transcript (7.8 kb) composed of 24 exons, 22 encoding the protein (38).
- At least 2 transcription start sites, with 2 mRNA species (117).
- Predicted protein of 1863 amino acids, but multiple transcript lengths (38).
- Zinc finger (118) of the RING type (119), binds RING-containing ligand, *BARD1* (120).
- C-terminus functions as a transcriptional activation factor (121,122).
- Functional splice variants expressed in nonmalignant and tumor cells (123).
- Antibody epitopes shared with epidermal growth factor receptor (124,125).
- 220-kd *BRCA1* peptide expressed in the nucleus and phosphorylated in a cell cycle–dependent manner (126).
- Granin motif (amino acids 1214–1223) (127,128) of disputed functional significance (129).
- Component of RNA polymerase II holoenzyme (130).
- Mutations of the 5′ end lose their growth repression (tumor suppressor) properties (131).
- Expressed in adult ovary (132).
- Mutations clustered at sites of homonucleotide tracts, repeats, and methylation sites (26).
- Protein detected in the nucleus (125,133) and cytoplasm (134).
- Germline but not somatic mutations of *BRCA1* are found in sporadic ovarian cancer (19,135).
- Loss of heterozygosity (LOH) for *BRCA1* in familial ovarian tumors is *not* uncommon (136–138).
- *BRCA1* LOH in sporadic ovarian tumors is infrequent (135,139,140).
- 17q11–21 LOH in sporadic tumors suggests a nearby tumor suppressor locus (140–142).
- Founder effect and increased carrier frequency of 185delAG in affected and asymptomatic women of (Ashkenazi) Jewish background (15,32–34,36,45,143–145).
- Recurrent *BRCA1* mutations associated with founder effects in French Canada (11), Sweden (27), Norway (146), Austria (147), and Tuscany (29).

the gene. The sequence data suggest that the two genes lie head to head and that the *BRCA1* 5′ region may share one or more overlapping promoter properties with the *1A1-3B* gene complex and another pseudogene (encoding a ribonucleoprotein, *ARPP*) in the flanking region (43). This finding may be relevant to the clinical observation (18,45) of a stronger association

between ovarian cancer with mutations lying in the 5′ region of *BRCA1* (Table 39-4). Other characteristics of *BRCA1*-related ovarian tumors have been reported (see Table 39-4), but so far they appear sufficiently nonspecific that they offer only suggestive indications in the context of a clinical evaluation. Perhaps the most tantalizing recent finding is the evidence for prolonged survival of *BRCA1* carriers with ovarian cancer (46), but this may not be true for all groups (Narod S, personal communication, 1997).

Most of the families without linkage to the chromosome 17 locus are linked to the second locus, designated *BRCA2* (47) and found on chromosome 13q12-13 (48). The gene product has structural similarities to the BRCA1 protein, but there is little genetic homology (Table 39-5). Like *BRCA1*, *BRCA2* is infrequently found in sporadic tumors and therefore does not likely play a classic tumor suppressor role in the majority of ovarian cancers (49). A recurrent identified *BRCA2* mutation—6174delT—that is seen recurrently in Ashkenazi Jews (34,50), confers a much lower risk of ovarian cancer (36). Families carrying *BRCA2* mutations are also likely to have risks for a different spectrum of associated cancers—particularly breast cancer in males (51,52), pancreatic cancer (36,47,53), and perhaps laryngeal cancer (47) and colorectal cancer (54). Whether there are other *BRCA* loci with associated increased risks for ovarian cancer is not known.

The second group of mutations associated with a predisposition to ovarian cancer are those affecting DNA mismatch repair genes (55,56). At least four of these genes have been described (see Table 39-1), although two (*hMSH2* and *hMLH1*) account for the majority of known families (57). The associated clinical syndrome is hereditary nonpolyposis colon cancer, or HNPCC (58,59). The absolute lifetime and relative risks for colorectal and endometrial cancer are much higher overall in affected families, and there appears to be a significantly increased risk for ovarian cancer also (60) (see Table 39-1). However, the risk for breast cancer is not markedly increased.

A third candidate gene that may confer risk for ovarian cancer—*p53*—is better known as the cause of Li-Fraumeni syndrome (61). Somatic mutations of this tumor suppressor gene are frequently seen in the ovarian carcinogenic process (62–66). However, at least two studies suggested that germline *p53* mutations can be

T A B L E   **39-3**

Estimated Risks of Cancer in *BRCA1* Carriers*

	Type 1 (Breast Predominant)	Type 2 (Ovarian Predominant)
Risk for breast cancer by age 70	91%	70%
Risk for ovarian cancer by age 70	32%	84%
Relative risk for colon cancer (95% CI)[a]	6.40[b] (3.59–11.40)	1.11 (0.19–6.40)
Relative risk for prostate cancer (95% CI)	3.33[b] (1.78–6.20)	

*Studies of consecutive case series suggest the risks may be lower in many families (40,41).

[a] Risks are relative to national incidence rates and given with the 95% confidence interval (CI).

[b] Statistically increased risk ($p < 0.01$).

Source: Data abstracted from Ford D, Easton DF, Bishop DT, et al. Risks of cancer in BRCA-1 mutation carriers. *Lancet* 1994;343:692–695.

T A B L E   **39-4**

Characteristics of Ovarian Cancer in *BRCA1* Carriers

- Decreased age at diagnosis (16,46,89,148,149)
- No strong association with stage or grade (46)
- Positive association with premalignant changes and microinvasive tumors in asymptomatic carriers (150)
- Negative association with borderline malignancies (142,143,151)
- Negative association with mucinous tumors (149,152)
- Positive association with papillary serous histopathology (46,149)
- Positive association (compared to breast cancer) with 5′ *BRCA1* mutations (18)*
- Positive association with decreased age at last childbirth (153)
- Positive association with rare *hRas1* alleles (154)
- Possible association with prolonged survival (46)

*A similar positive association exists between the predominance of ovarian cancer and *BRCA2* mutations, giving rise to an "ovarian cancer cluster region" (OCCR) in exon 11 of that gene (155).

T A B L E   **39-5**

Characteristics of the *BRCA2* Gene and Its Protein Product

- Single-copy gene >70 kb in size localized to 13q12–13 (156).
- Full-length mRNA transcript (11–12 kb) composed of 27 exons (47,156).
- Predicted acidic, highly charged protein 3418 amino acids in length (156) and 380 kd in molecular mass (127).
- Interacts with the Rad51 DNA-repair protein (157).
- Expressed in adult human ovary (156).
- Increased prevalence (1.36%) of 6187delT mutation with Jewish ancestry (34,36,50,158), but is recurrent in those without known Jewish background (158).
- Founder *BRCA2* mutation in Iceland (159).
- Somatic mutations are no more frequent than germline mutations in sporadic ovarian tumors (160,161).
- Coordinately regulated with *BRCA1* in mammary epithelial cells (162).

observed in familial cancer clusters that could be clinically indistinguishable from the hereditary *BRCA* syndromes (67,68). Nevertheless, *p53* mutations are rare causes of familial ovarian cancer (69) and the risk in known *p53* mutation families is at most modestly increased.

Finally, it should be mentioned that epithelial ovarian cancer with small-cell histopathology may show familial clustering. Seen in younger women (mean age, 23.9 years), this rare but highly malignant type of tumor has been identified in a mother-daughter pair (70)

and a review of 150 cases refers to clusters of three sisters, of two cousins, and of another potential mother-daughter pair (71). Whether these clusters are due to chance, to one of the *BRCA* predispositions, or to a different type of syndrome is not known.

Assessing Genetic Risk

Individuals often make critical decisions about health and reproduction without the benefit of genetic information that should underlie a truly "informed" decision. Genetic counselors recognize this fact and consider it their task as healthcare professionals to help verify a genetic diagnosis or refute it (72). Where possible, they also provide more accurate estimation of risk to the family and marshal the appropriate support—clinical, psychological, and social (73–75). A well-informed clinical diagnosis starts with a detailed interview that includes questions about second- and third-degree relatives, followed by construction of a family pedigree (19,73,76–78). From such a pedigree, it may be relatively easy to recognize an affected family because there are multiple same-site cancers over several generations, all of early onset. On the other hand, some individuals have only one affected family member, so the risks appear much smaller. From the family history alone, it is possible to estimate the likelihood of a *BRCA1* mutation (Fig. 39-2). Other important factors include reliability of the history, evidence for tumor bilaterality or multiple primary lesions (e.g., ovarian *and* colorectal cancer), recognition of sex-specific expression (e.g., ovary, breast, and prostate), and prior surgery (bilateral oophorectomy). Any high-risk clinic should consider documentation of pathologic diagnoses in affected family members as an essential part of clinical care. This often requires a combination of patience, determination, and tact on the part of the clinical personnel requesting the information. However, a well-documented family is one in which screening and genetic testing will be most beneficial. For the asymptomatic woman at age 44 (individual III:4 in Fig. 39-3), confirmation of pathology in her deceased mother (II:6) and affected sister (III:3) is clear indication for extended pedigree analysis. Additional information of early-onset metachronous bilateral breast cancer in a cousin (III:2—left-sided breast cancer at age 31 and independent right-sided breast cancer at age 34) increases the likelihood of a genetic etiology substantially, even though the intermediate relative (the maternal aunt, II:4) is unaffected. Review of this pedigree with the family members can be the most direct demonstration to them that there is reduced penetrance [i.e., "the gene (mutation) is *not* the cancer") and requires careful counseling if the genetic risks are to be fully understood.

The presence of a living first cousin with later-onset unilateral breast cancer (III:1) might be considered further support for a hereditary

FIGURE **39-2**

Probability of carrying a *BRCA1* mutation. The estimated prior probability of a particular cluster of cases being due to a *BRCA1* mutation is taken from that reported by Shattuck-Eidens et al (14). Br = breast cancer; Ov = ovarian cancer; Dx = diagnosis; Br < 30 = individual with breast cancer before the age of 30; Br < 40 and Br < 40 = two sisters, both with breast cancer before the age of 40; 3+ Br with Dx < 50 = a family cluster of at least three members with breast cancer all under the age of 50; 2+ Br & 2+ Ov = a family cluster of two or more members with breast cancer and two or more with ovarian cancer, without regard for age at diagnosis.

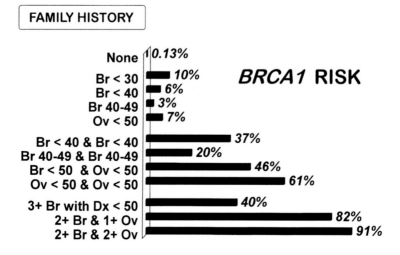

breast/ovarian cancer syndrome. However, there is a significant possibility that she is sporadically affected, so the pedigree symbol is shaded (see Fig. 39-3). Genetic testing of the unaffected living aunt (II:4) is actually more likely to reveal that she is an asymptomatic carrier of the gene—given her daughter's early bilateral breast disease. If both the aunt (II:4) as "obligate" carrier and the affected sister (III:3) bear the same deleterious *BRCA1* mutation, the proband's risk of carrier status is 50% and the associated lifetime risk of ovarian cancer may be upwards of 16% (half of 32%, see Table 39-3).

It may seem trivial to add that the contribution of affected relatives must be evaluated according to which parent they are related to. However, all too frequently, the various affected "high-risk" relatives are scattered among genetically unrelated branches of the family. For the asymptomatic women in these families, pedigree analysis will seem imprecise or inconclusive. These women can be reassured that the risk contributions of different family branches are more likely to be additive than multiplicative, but extensive counseling may be required to fully explain this critical difference.

At-risk individuals should be given an age-specific, limited-period risk figure for a genetic cancer, relative to their risk for sporadic cancer. Thus, an asymptomatic 50-year-old woman with a sister affected by ovarian cancer has a *higher risk of nongenetic breast cancer than of either genetic or nongenetic ovarian cancer*. It is important, therefore, that she be advised of the potentially greater benefits of mammography and breast screening, at least until genetic testing can identify her real risk of a hereditary breast/ovarian cancer syndrome with its altered risks for these two cancers.

Management of Asymptomatic Women at Risk for Hereditary Ovarian Cancer

Transvaginal ultrasound, particularly with Doppler flow studies (79), can be a useful diagnostic tool for the early identification of epithe-

F I G U R E **39-3**

An example of a pedigree for a family with hereditary breast/ovarian cancer syndrome. The woman who is the source of the family history (III:4) is denoted by the arrow. Very often one can only guess that women in previous generations (I:2, shaded circle) had ovarian cancer. Family members may describe typical signs, such as loss of weight and a swollen, fluid-filled abdomen, but the diagnosis known to the family may be "stomach cancer." The presence of asymptomatic carriers (II:4) may also be confusing, and transmission through males may not be recognized. Abbreviations: R br = cancer of the right breast (with age at diagnosis); ov = ovarian cancer; diagonal slash = deceased; black filled circle = affected female; square with question mark = male, possibly affected.

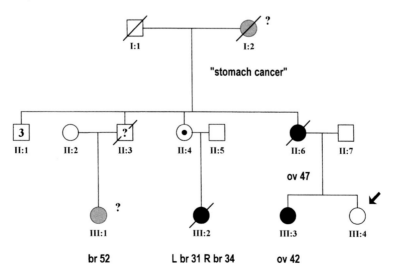

lial ovarian cancer (80), but it remains an operator-dependent screening procedure with a significant number of false-positive and -negative results (81). Measurement of the serum marker CA-125 is also a valid screening test, but even in combination, these tests do not have sufficient predictive value to be recommended for asymptomatic women (82). Prevalence estimates and results of preliminary studies (83) suggest some benefit for periodic screening of high-risk women. Combined ultrasonography and CA-125 measurement have been recommended for at-risk individuals in a breast/ovarian cancer family (84), but their true predictive value is not known.

Similarly, bilateral oophorectomy may benefit women with a strong family history but prophylactic surgery is not 100% protective. It is still unclear whether bilateral oophorectomy should be accompanied by total abdominal hysterectomy, as there is some suggestion that fallopian tube carcinoma may be an associated risk. Either way, there is a significant residual risk for peritoneal carcinomatosis, presumably on the basis of a common embryologic origin for peritoneal and ovarian epithelial tissues (85,86). Thus, women who choose surgery may still need routine screening and follow-up. Women considering prophylactic surgery should be advised of the other medical issues that arise from bilateral oophorectomy, such as premature menopause and an end to normal childbearing options (87). In premenopausal women, the family history should be reviewed for a history of early atherosclerotic disease and osteoporosis, as the risks of death from these disorders may outweigh the benefits associated with ovarian surgery, particularly if hormone replacement therapy (HRT) is contraindicated (88). One concern is whether there are substantially increased risks associated with prolonged HRT in *BRCA1/2* carriers; unfortunately, it may be some time before data are available to resolve this issue completely.

Not so uncertain is the increased risk of ovarian cancer in gene carriers who already have breast cancer. For *BRCA1* carriers, Ford et al (89) estimated that the risks of contralateral breast cancer were 48% by age 50 and 64% by age 70, and the risks of ovarian cancer, 24% by age 50 and 44% by age 70. The options may be clear for breast cancer survivors with a family history of ovarian cancer, but for women without any experience with familial ovarian cancer, other criteria (age, completion of family,

concomitant pelvic surgery such as hysterectomy) may dominate their perception of relative risks. Whether the increasingly accepted view that there are benefits to ovarian ablation in breast cancer (90) will alter these women's view of bilateral oophorectomy remains to be seen. Clearly, carriers surviving their first cancer should be fully informed of these risks and benefits in comparison to those associated with screening and surgical prophylaxis.

Genetic Testing

Who should receive genetic testing now? Among those most eligible are families that meet research-defined criteria for a hereditary cancer syndrome (91,92). Narod (93,94) argued that we are ready to test *and* to provide genetic information to some breast/ovarian cancer families. This has been echoed by more recent statements (95), including an official recommendation of the American Society of Clinical Oncology (92). Similar arguments have been made for HNPCC families. However, there is an

T A B L E   39-6

Procedures Used in Mutational Analysis of *BRCA1* and *BRCA2*

Mutational screening
- Direct sequencing* (38,47,102)
- Chemical cleavage mismatch (163)
- Single-strand conformation polymorphism (SSCP) analysis (54,102,163)
- Conformation-sensitive gel electrophoresis (CSGE) (51)
- RNA SSCP for loss of heterozygosity (22)
- High-density oligonucleotide arrays with fluorescence detection (164)
- Protein truncation test (PTT) (20,165–167)
- Multiplex heteroduplex (HDX) analysis (168)
- Polymerase chain reaction (PCR)-SSCP-HDX analysis (169)

Direct mutation detection
- Heteroduplex analysis (del185AG) (167)
- Restriction fragment length polymorphism (RFLP) analysis (38)
- Acrylamide gel electrophoresis (50)
- Allele-specific oligonucleotide (ASO) hybridization (15,34,38)
- Allele-specific PCR (158)
- PCR-mediated site-directed mutagenesis (170)

*Only the primary references are cited here. For most laboratories, other detection methods are validated or confirmed by direct sequencing.

understandable reluctance to accept the same arguments even for well-defined *p53* familial cancer families, because of the extensive variation in tumor type and presentation (61). Once patients are told they are at increased risk, even without testing, they will expect professional health-care givers to provide expert advice about benefits and risks of all possible preventive options (96). Health-care authorities generally recognize that people at high risk of familial cancer require preventive care guidelines that differ from those for the population at large (97). However, recommendations for high-risk individuals are more likely to be based on theoretical modeling than on real data used to analyze and establish guidelines for application to the general population (98). Clearly, some form of outcome analysis is needed for women who are tested, but such studies await the kind of case definition that can only come with widespread genetic testing. To this end, various institutions and funding agencies are sponsoring the establishment of multidisciplinary teams (consisting of gynecologists, oncologists, geneticists, ethicists, and sociologists, among others) to address the whole spectrum of outcome issues (99–102).

The transformation of laboratory research data into clinically reliable laboratory services introduces another set of problems that requires specialized laboratory expertise (103). Consistent testing procedures and risk estimation algorithms are needed, particularly given the wide number of molecular protocols being reported (Table 39-6). The fact that there is a subset of recurrent mutations, some of which are much more common in certain ethnic backgrounds, has led to the development of simple mutation screens (Fig. 39-4). Yet even where the family mutation is known, the possibility, albeit quite small, of an undetected predisposing mutation, either cosegregated with the known mutation or being transmitted from another branch of the family, cannot be altogether ignored (104,105). These and other limitations and pitfalls inherent in any molecular study should be well understood by the health-care providers involved (106) so that they can provide clear and concise information for their patients.

Molecular diagnosis is usually achieved by mutational assay or by indirect linkage analysis. In the best of all possible worlds, there would be a small subset of known mutations for each syndrome, easily testable in a one-shot approach. However, this is not the case.

Rather, testing in many families may require a protracted search for the mutation or involve detailed linkage studies that call for extensive collaboration among members of a committed family. In some searches, the laboratory will be faced with the need to distinguish a disabling mutation from a benign genetic variant or a mild functional polymorphism (107), or to decide if there should be a search for another mutation.

Technical matters are equally important for laboratories carrying out genetic studies. Each laboratory must develop protocols to ensure that the proffered molecular tests are as accurate as possible. At the same time, reports to clinicians should explicitly state the small probability of error that is inherent in any genetic testing methodology, so that neither clinician nor patient remains uninformed about these irreducible residual error rates when they come to make major health-care decisions. To maintain quality assurance in this area, a program of surveillance and a set of standards are essential, and proposals for such programs are just now emerging.

Conclusions

Genetic counseling for familial ovarian cancer should include a careful pedigree analysis with provisional assignment of genetic risk and approximate assessment of common cancer risks. This should be accompanied by provision of information regarding the spectrum of screening and surgical options along with a clear statement of their relative benefits and risks. Genetic testing should be introduced in this context, along with its attendant risks and benefits. At present, this testing should be directed toward the families with a more than 90% risk of harboring a *BRCA1* mutation (see Figs. 39-2 and 39-3), but it should be gradually introduced for the patients and close relatives of those 15% of all ovarian cancer patients with a positive family history. Counseling those who test negative will require care to ensure that they appreciate the continued risk for sporadic cancers as well as the potential of a false-negative test result. Conversely, those who test positive and are therefore genetically affected will need a comprehensive surveillance system for effective prevention (105). Some genetically affected individuals will remain asymptomatic, and it may be possible to identify in them the

A

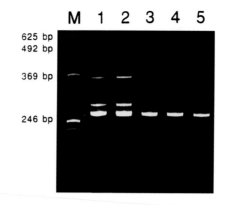

B

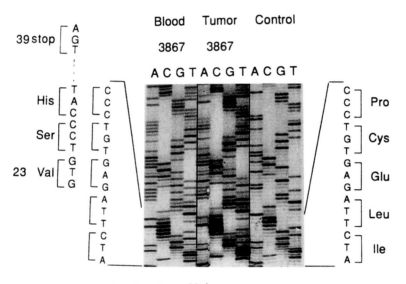

FIGURE 39-4

Diagnosis of the 185delAG mutation (160). The most common recurrent mutation can be simply detected by heteroduplex analysis (A). In this example, primers specific to intronic sequences around exon 2 were used to amplify DNA from the patient's blood (lane 1), the patient's tumor (lane 2), and three control cell lines (lanes 3-5). The amplified products were held at denaturing conditions and allowed to reanneal and the products separated on 12% polyacrylamide gels and stained with ethidium bromide. Because the mutant DNA copy in the patient's lymphocytes and tumor differs from the normal copy by the loss of two nucleotides, the duplex DNA formed from mixed mutant and normal single DNA strands is mismatched, producing "kinked" heteroduplexes that migrate more slowly in the gel (upper bands in lanes 1 and 2). This rapid polymerase chain reaction (PCR)-based diagnosis is confirmed by direct sequencing (B). A partial nucleotide sequence is shown for the blood and tumor for the patient (No. 3867), and a control subject. The resultant normal amino acid sequence (right) is disrupted after Leu-22 by the deletion of the A and G residues at position 186 and all subsequent amino acids in the mutated DNA (left) are abnormal until a stop signal is reached at amino acid 39. Thus, instead of the normal 1863-amino acid BRCA1 protein, only a small 39-amino acid peptide is coded for and the patient essentially has only one functional BRCA1 gene.

protective effects of genetic variation at sites other than the primary susceptibility gene. In the end, genetic counseling and testing will not provide the kind of certainty that patients or practitioners may expect or desire (106,107), but it can substantially improve risk estimates for the many families afflicted with an increased predisposition for this disease.

Acknowledgments

We wish to acknowledge the central role that our counselors, Linda Bradley, Michelle Phillips, and Laura Brown, have played in the provision of care through the Familial Ovarian Cancer Clinic at the Toronto Hospital. We also thank Karen Gronau for proofreading the manuscript and Steven Narod (Department of Preventive Medicine and Epidemiology, University of Toronto) for helpful comments and suggestions.

REFERENCES

1. Knudson AG. Mutation and cancer: statistical study for retinoblastoma. *Proc Natl Acad Sci USA* 1971;68:820–823.

2. Knudson AG. Hereditary cancer: two hits revisited. *J Cancer Res Clin Oncol* 1996;122:135–140.

3. Vogelstein B, Fearon ER, Hamilton SR, et al. Genetic alterations during colorectal-tumor development. *N Engl J Med* 1988;319:525–532.

4. Renan MJ. How many mutations are required for tumorigenesis? Implications from human cancer data. *Mol Carcinog* 1993;7:139–146.

5. Goddard AD, Solomon E. Genetic aspects of cancer. *Adv Hum Genet* 1993; 21:321–376.

6. Hartwell LH, Kastan MB. Cell cycle control and cancer. *Science* 1994;266:1821–1828.

7. National Cancer Institute of Canada. Probability of developing/dying from cancer. In: Gaudette LA, Lee J, eds. *Canadian cancer statistics 1995.* Toronto: National Cancer Institute of Canada, 1995:1–87.

8. Amos CI, Struewing JP. Genetic epidemiology of epithelial ovarian cancer. *Cancer* 1993;71: 566–572.

9. Narod SA. Genetics of breast and ovarian cancer. *Br Med Bull* 1994;50:656–676.

10. Narod SA, Madlensky L, Bradley L, et al. Hereditary and familial ovarian cancer in southern Ontario. *Cancer* 1994;74:2341–2346.

11. Simard J, Tonin P, Durocher F, et al. Common origins of BRCA1 mutations in Canadian breast and ovarian cancer families. *Nat Genet* 1994; 8:392–398.

12. Castilla LH, Couch FJ, Erdos MR, et al. Mutations in the BRCA1 gene in families with early-onset breast and ovarian cancer. *Nat Genet* 1994; 8:387–391.

13. Friedman LS, Ostermeyer EA, Szabo CI, et al. Confirmation of BRCA1 by analysis of germline mutations linked to breast and ovarian cancer in ten families. *Nat Genet* 1994;8:399–404.

14. Shattuck-Eidens D, McClure M, Simard J, et al. A collaborative survey of 80 mutations in the BRCA1 breast and ovarian cancer susceptibility gene: implications for presymptomatic testing and screening. *JAMA* 1995;273:535–541.

15. Friedman LS, Szabo CI, Ostermeyer EA, et al. Novel inherited mutations and variable expressivity of BRCA1 alleles, including the founder mutation 185delAG in Ashkenazi Jewish families. *Am J Hum Genet* 1995;57:1284–1297.

16. Inoue R, Fukutomi T, Ushijima T, et al. Germline mutation of BRCA1 in Japanese breast cancer families. *Cancer Res* 1995;55:3521–3524.

17. Struewing JP, Brody LC, Erdos MR, et al. Detection of eight BRCA1 mutations in 10 breast/ovarian cancer families, including 1 family with male breast cancer. *Am J Hum Genet* 1995;57: 1–7.

18. Gayther SA, Warren W, Mazoyer S, et al. Germline mutations of the BRCA1 gene in breast and ovarian cancer families provide evidence for a genotype-phenotype correlation. *Nat Genet* 1995;11:428–433.

19. Matsushima M, Kobayashi K, Emi M, et al. Mutation analysis of the BRCA1 gene in 76 Japanese ovarian cancer patients: four germline mutations, but no evidence of somatic mutation. *Hum Mol Genet* 1995;4:1953–1956.

20. Plummer SJ, Anton-Culver H, Webster L, et al. Detection of BRCA1 mutations by the protein truncation test. *Hum Mol Genet* 1995;4:1989–1991.

21. Rodabaugh KJ, Biggs RB, Qureshi JA, et al. Detailed deletion mapping of chromosome 9p and p16 gene alterations in human borderline and invasive epithelial ovarian tumors. *Oncogene* 1995;11:1249–1254.

22. Serova O, Montagna M, Torchard D, et al. A high incidence of BRCA1 mutations in 20 breast-ovarian cancer families. *Am J Hum Genet* 1996; 58:42–51.

23. Bowcock AM, Anderson LA, Friedman LS, et al. THRA1 and D17S183 flank an interval of <4 cM for the breast-ovarian cancer gene (BRCA1) on chromosome 17q21. *Am J Hum Genet* 1993;52: 718–722.

24. Kacinski BM, Chambers SK. Molecular biology of ovarian cancer. *Curr Opin Oncol* 1991;3: 889–900. Review.

25. Kainu T, Kononen J, Johansson O, et al. Detection of germline BRCA1 mutations in breast cancer patients by quantitative messenger RNA in situ hybridization. *Cancer Res* 1996;56: 2912–2915.

26. Rodenhiser D, Chakraborty P, Andrews J, et al. Heterogeneous point mutations in the BRCA1 breast cancer susceptibility gene occur in high frequency at the site of homonucleotide tracts, short repeats and methylatable CpG/CpNpG motifs. *Oncogene* 1996;12:2623–2629.

27. Johannsson O, Ostermeyer EA, Hakansson S, et al. Founding BRCA1 mutations in hereditary breast and ovarian cancer in southern Sweden. *Am J Hum Genet* 1996;58:441–450.

28. Jandrig B, Grade K, Seitz S, et al. BRCA1 mutations in German breast-cancer families. *Int J Cancer* 1996;68:188–192.

29. Caligo MA, Ghimenti C, Cipollini G, et al. BRCA1 germline mutational spectrum in Italian families from Tuscany: a high frequency of novel mutations. *Oncogene* 1996;13:1483–1488.

30. Montagna M, Santacatterina M, Corneo B, et al. Identification of seven new BRCA1 germline mutations in Italian breast and breast/ovarian cancer families. *Cancer Res* 1996;56:5466–5469.

31. Couch FJ, Garber J, Kiousis S, et al. Genetic analysis of eight breast-ovarian cancer families with suspected BRCA1 mutations. *Monogr Natl Cancer Inst* 1995;17:9–14.

32. Tonin P, Serova O, Lenoir G, et al. BRCA1 mutations in Ashkenazi Jewish women. *Am J Hum Genet* 1995;57:189.

33. Struewing JP, Abeliovich D, Peretz T, et al. The carrier frequency of the BRCA1 185delAG mutation is approximately 1 percent in Ashkenazi Jewish individuals. *Nat Genet* 1995;11:198–200.

34. Roa BB, Boyd AA, Volcik K, Richards CS. Ashkenazi Jewish population frequencies for common mutations in BRCA1 and BRCA2. *Nat Genet* 1996;14:185–187.

35. Neuhausen SL, Mazoyer S, Friedman L, et al. Haplotype and phenotype analysis of six recurrent BRCA1 mutations in 61 families: results of an international study. *Am J Hum Genet* 1996;58: 271–280.

36. Tonin P, Weber B, Offit K, et al. Frequency of recurrent BRCA1 and BRCA2 mutations in Ashkenazi Jewish breast cancer families. *Nat Med* 1996;2:1179–1183.

37. Steichen-Gersdorf E, Gallion HH, Ford D, et al. Familial site-specific ovarian cancer is linked to BRCA1 on 17q12-21. *Am J Hum Genet* 1994;55: 870–875.

38. Miki Y, Swensen J, Shattuck-Eidens D, et al. A strong candidate for the breast and ovarian cancer susceptibility gene BRCA1. *Science* 1994; 266:66–71.

39. Tonin P, Moslehi R, Green R, et al. Linkage analysis of 26 Canadian breast and breast-ovarian cancer families. *Hum Genet* 1995;95: 545–550.

40. Stratton JF, Gayther SA, Russell P, et al. Contribution of *BRCA1* mutations to ovarian cancer. *N Engl J Med* 1997;336:1125–1130.

41. Whittemore AS, Gong G, Itnyre J. Prevalence and contribution of BRCA1 mutations in breast cancer and ovarian cancer: results from three U.S. population-based case-control studies of ovarian cancer. *Am J Hum Genet* 1997;60: 496–504.

42. Brown MA, Nicolai H, Xu CF, et al. Regulation of BRCA1. *Nature* 1994;372:733.

43. Brown MA, Xu C, Nicolai H, et al. The 5′ end of the BRCA1 gene lies within a duplicated region of human chromosome 17q21. *Oncogene* 1996;2507–2513.

44. Campbell IG, Nicolai HM, Foulkes WD, et al. A novel gene encoding a B-box protein within the BRCA1 region at 17q21.1. *Hum Mol Genet* 1994; 3:589–594.

45. Berman DB, Wagner-Costalas J, Schultz DC, et al. Two distinct origins of a common BRCA1 mutation in breast-ovarian cancer families: a genetic study of 15 185delAG-mutation kindreds. *Am J Hum Genet* 1996;58:1166–1176.

46. Rubin SC, Benjamin I, Behbakht K, et al. Clinical and pathological features of ovarian cancer in women with germ-line mutations of BRCA1. *N Engl J Med* 1996;335:1413–1416.

47. Wooster R, Bignell G, Lancaster J, et al. Identification of the breast cancer susceptibility gene BRCA2. *Nature* 1995;378:789–792.

48. Wooster R, Neuhausen SL, Mangion J, et al. Localization of a breast cancer susceptibility

gene, BRCA2, to chromosome 13q12-13. *Science* 1994;265:2088–2090.

49. Lancaster JM, Wooster R, Mangion J, et al. BRCA2 mutations in primary breast and ovarian cancers. *Nat Genet* 1996;13:238–240.

50. Neuhausen S, Gilewski T, Norton L, et al. Recurrent BRCA2 6174delT mutations in Ashkenazi Jewish women affected by breast cancer. *Nat Genet* 1996;13:126–128.

51. Couch FJ, Farid LM, Deshano ML, et al. BRCA2 germline mutations in male breast cancer cases and breast cancer families. *Nat Genet* 1996; 13:123–125.

52. Friedman LS, Gayther SA, Kurosaki T, et al. Mutation analysis of BRCA1 and BRCA2 in a male breast cancer population. *Am J Hum Genet* 1997;60:313–319.

53. Goggins M, Schutte M, Lu J, et al. Germline BRCA2 gene mutations in patients with apparently sporadic pancreatic carcinomas. *Cancer Res* 1996;56:5360–5364.

54. Phelan CM, Lancaster JM, Tonin P, et al. Mutation analysis of the BRCA2 gene in 49 site-specific breast cancer families. *Nat Genet* 1996;13:120–122.

55. Modrich P. Mismatch repair, genetic stability, and cancer. *Science* 1994;266:1959–1960.

56. Karran P. Appropriate partners make good matches. *Science* 1995;268:1857–1858.

57. Nystrom-Lahti M, Parsons R, Sistonen P, et al. Mismatch repair genes on chromosome 2p and 3p account for a major share of hereditary nonpolyposis colorectal cancer families evaluable by linkage. *Am J Hum Genet* 1994; 55:659–665.

58. Lynch HT, Lanspa S, Smyrk T, et al. Hereditary nonpolyposis colorectal cancer (Lynch syndromes I & II): genetics, pathology, natural history, and cancer control, part I. *Cancer Genet Cytogenet* 1991;53:143–160.

59. Lynch HT, Cavalieri RJ, Lynch JF, Casey MJ. Gynecologic cancer clues to Lynch syndrome II diagnosis: a family report. *Gynecol Oncol* 1992; 44:198–203.

60. Aarnio M, Mecklin J, Aaltonen LA, et al. Lifetime risk of different cancers in hereditary nonpolyposis colorectal cancer (HNPCC) syndrome. *Int J Cancer* 1995;64:430–433.

61. Malkin D. Germline p53 gene mutations and cancer—Pandora's box or open sesame? *J Natl Cancer Inst* 1994;86:326–328.

62. Milner BJ, Allan LA, Eccles DM, et al. p53 Mutation is a common genetic event in ovarian carcinoma. *Cancer Res* 1993;53:2128–2132.

63. Kohler MF, Kerns BJ, Humphrey PA, et al. Mutation and overexpression of p53 in early-stage epithelial ovarian cancer. *Obstet Gynecol* 1993; 81:643–650.

64. Runnebaum IB, Tong XW, Moebus V, et al. Multiplex PCR screening detects small p53 deletions and insertions in human ovarian cancer cell lines. *Hum Genet* 1994;93:620–624.

65. Skilling JS, Sood A, Niemann T, et al. An abundance of p53 null mutations in ovarian carcinoma. *Oncogene* 1996;13:117–123.

66. Kim JW, Cho YH, Kwon DJ, et al. Aberrations of the p53 tumor suppressor gene in human epithelial ovarian carcinoma. *Gynecol Oncol* 1995;57:199–204.

67. Buller RE, Anderson B, Connor JP, Robinson R. Familial ovarian cancer. *Gynecol Oncol* 1993; 51:160–166.

68. Jolly KW, Malkin D, Douglass EC, et al. Splice-site mutation of the p53 gene in a family with hereditary breast-ovarian cancer. *Oncogene* 1994;9:97–102.

69. Buller RE, Skilling JS, Kaliszewski S, et al. Absence of significant germ line p53 mutations in ovarian cancer patients. *Gynecol Oncol* 1995; 58:368–374.

70. Lamovec J, Bracko M, Cerar O. Familial occurrence of small-cell carcinoma of the ovary. *Arch Pathol Lab Med* 1995;119:523–527.

71. Young RH, Oliva E, Scully RE. Small cell carcinoma of the ovary, hypercalcemic type: a clinicopathological analysis of 150 cases. *Am J Surg Pathol* 1994;18:1102–1116.

72. Cole DEC, Gallinger S, McCready DR, et al. Genetic counseling and testing for susceptibility to breast, ovarian and colon cancer: where are we today? *Can Med Assoc J* 1996;154:149–155.

73. Biesecker BB, Boehnke M, Calzone K, et al. Genetic counseling for families with inherited susceptibility to breast and ovarian cancer. *JAMA* 1993;269:1970–1974.

74. Bombard AT, Fields AL, Auffox S, Ben-Yishay M. The genetics of ovarian cancer: an assessment of current screening protocols and recommendations for counseling families at risk. *Clin Obstet Gynecol* 1996;39:860–872.

75. Robinson GE, Rosen BP, Bradley LN, et al. Psychological impact of screening for familial

ovarian cancer: reactions to initial assessment. *Gynecol Oncol* 1997;65:197–205.

76. Narod SA. Should a family history be taken from every woman with ovarian cancer? *Arch Intern Med* 1995;155:893–894. Editorial.

77. Eng C, Stratton M, Ponder B, et al. Familial cancer syndromes. *Lancet* 1994;343:709–713.

78. Hartenbach EM, Schink JC. The genetics of ovarian cancer: concepts in testing and counseling. *Curr Opin Obstet Gynecol* 1996;8:339–342.

79. Bourne TH, Campbell S, Reynolds KM, et al. Screening for early familial ovarian cancer with transvaginal ultrasonography and colour blood flow imaging. *BMJ* 1993;306:1025–1029.

80. Carter JR, Lau M, Fowler JM, et al. Blood flow characteristics of ovarian tumors: implications for ovarian cancer screening. *Am J Obstet Gynecol* 1995;172:901–907.

81. Guidozzi F. Screening for ovarian cancer. *Obstet Gynecol Surv* 1996;51:696–701.

82. American College of Physicians. Screening for ovarian cancer: recommendations and rationale. *Ann Intern Med* 1994;121:141–142.

83. Dorum A, Kristensen GB, Abeler VM, et al. Early detection of familial ovarian cancer. *Eur J Cancer* 1996;32A:1645–1651.

84. Karlan BY, Platt LD. Ovarian cancer screening: the role of ultrasound in early detection. *Cancer* 1995;76:2011–2015.

85. Tobacman JK, Tucker MA, Kase R, et al. Intra-abdominal carcinomatosis after prophylactic oophorectomy in ovarian-cancer–prone families. *Lancet* 1982;2:795–797.

86. Struewing JP, Watson P, Easton DF, et al. Effectiveness of prophylactic oophorectomy in inherited breast/ovarian cancer families. *Am J Hum Genet Suppl* 1994;55:A70.

87. Kerlikowske K, Brown JS, Grady DG. Should women with familial ovarian cancer undergo prophylactic oophorectomy? *Obstet Gynecol* 1992;80:700–707.

88. Kontoravdis A, Kalogirou D, Antoniou G, et al. Prophylactic oophorectomy in ovarian cancer prevention. *Int J Gynecol Obstet* 1996;54:257–262.

89. Ford D, Easton DF, Peto J. Estimates of the gene frequency of BRCA1 and its contribution to breast and ovarian cancer incidence. *Am J Hum Genet* 1995;57:1457–1462.

90. Early Breast Cancer Trialists Collaborative Group. Ovarian ablation in early breast cancer: overview of the randomised trials. *Lancet* 1996; 348:1189–1196.

91. Claus EB, Schwartz PE. Familial ovarian cancer: update and clinical applications. *Cancer* 1995; 76:1998–2003.

92. Offit K, Bowles B, Burt RW, et al. Statement of the American Society of Clinical Oncology: genetic testing for cancer susceptibility. *J Clin Oncol* 1996;14:1730–1736.

93. Narod S. Hereditary breast-ovarian cancer: how can we use the new DNA markers to improve patient management? *Clin Invest Med* 1993;16: 314–317.

94. Rosenblatt DS, Narod SA. Genetic screening for breast cancer. *N Engl J Med* 1996;334:1200–1201.

95. Olopade OI. Genetics in clinical cancer care––the future is now. *N Engl J Med* 1996;335: 1455–1456.

96. Struewing JP, Lerman C, Kase RG, et al. Anticipated uptake and impact of genetic testing in hereditary breast and ovarian cancer families. *Cancer Epidemiol Biomarkers Prev* 1995;4: 169–173.

97. Sox HCJ. Preventive health services in adults. *N Engl J Med* 1994;330:1589–1595.

98. Schrag D, Kuntz KM, Garber JE, Weeks JC. Decision analysis––effects of prophylactic mastectomy and oophorectomy on life expectancy among women with *BRCA1* or *BRCA2* mutations. *N Engl J Med* 1997;336:1465–1471.

99. Botkin JR, Croyle RT, Smith KR, et al. A model protocol for evaluating the behavioral and psychosocial effects of BRCA1 testing. *J Nat Cancer Inst* 1996;88:872–882.

100. Lerman C, Narod S, Schuman K, et al. BRCA1 testing in families with hereditary breast-ovarian cancer: a prospective study of patient decision making and outcome. *JAMA* 1996;275:1885–1892.

101. ACOG Committee. Breast-ovarian cancer screening. *Am Coll Obstet Gynecol* 1996;176:1–2.

102. Berchuck A, Cirisano F, Lancaster JM, et al. Role of BRCA1 mutation screening in the management of familial ovarian cancer. *Am J Obstet Gynecol* 1996;175:738–746.

103. Petty EM, Killeen AA. BRCA1 mutation testing: controversies and challenges. *Clin Chem* 1997; 43:6–8.

104. Stoppa-Lyonnet D, Fricker JP, Essioux L, et al. Segregation of two BRCA1 mutations in a single family. *Am J Hum Genet* 1996;59:479–481.

105. Ramus SJ, Friedman LS, Gayther SA, et al. A breast/ovarian cancer patient with germline mutations in both BRCA1 and BRCA2. *Nat Genet* 1997;15:14–15.

106. Cole DEC. Familial ovarian cancer. *Clin Lab News* 1995;21:18–19.

107. Durocher F, Shattuck-Eidens D, McClure M, et al. Comparison of BRCA1 polymorphisms, rare sequence variants and/or missense mutations in unaffected and breast/ovarian cancer populations. *Hum Mol Genet* 1996;5:835–842.

108. Lynch HT, Severin MJ, Mooney MJ, Lynch J. Insurance adjudication favoring prophylactic surgery in hereditary breast-ovarian cancer syndrome. *Gynecol Oncol* 1995;57:23–26.

109. Rowley PT, Loader S. Attitudes of obstetrician-gynecologists toward DNA testing for a genetic susceptibility to breast cancer. *Obstet Gynecol* 1996;88:611–615.

110. Spurdle AB, Jenkins T. The origins of the Lemba "black Jews" of southern Africa: evidence from p12F2 and other Y-chromosome markers. *Am J Hum Genet* 1996;59:1126–1133.

111. Feunteun J, Lenoir GM. BRCA1, a gene involved in inherited predisposition to breast and ovarian cancer. *Biochim Biophys Acta* 1996; 1242:177–180.

112. Ford D, Easton DF, Bishop DT, et al. Risks of cancer in BRCA1-mutation carriers. *Lancet* 1994; 343:692–695.

113. Fishel R, Lescoe MK, Rao MRS, et al. The human mutator gene homolog MSH2 and its association with hereditary nonpolyposis colon cancer. *Cell* 1993;75:1027–1038.

114. Papadopoulos N, Nicolaides NC, Wei YF, et al. Mutation of a mutL homolog in hereditary colon cancer. *Science* 1994;263:1625–1629.

115. Nicolaides NC, Papadopoulos N, Liu B, et al. Mutations of two PMS homologues in hereditary nonpolyposis colon cancer. *Nature* 1994;371: 75–80.

116. Vasen HF, Wijnen JT, Menko FH, et al. Cancer risk in families with hereditary nonpolyposis colorectal cancer diagnosed by mutation analysis. *Gastroenterology* 1996;110:1020–1027.

117. Xu C, Brown MA, Chambers JA, et al. Distinct transcription start sites generate two forms of BRCA1 mRNA. *Hum Mol Genet* 1995;4:2259–2264.

118. Berg JM, Shi Y. The galvanization of biology: a growing appreciation for the roles of zinc. *Science* 1996;271:1081–1085.

119. Bienstock RJ, Darden T, Wiseman R, et al. Molecular modeling of the amino-terminal zinc ring domain of BRCA1. *Cancer Res* 1996;56:2539–2545.

120. Wu LC, Wang ZW, Tsan JT, et al. Identification of a RING protein that can interact in vivo with the BRCA1 gene product. *Nat Genet* 1996;14: 430–440.

121. Chapman MS, Verma IM. Transcriptional activation by BRCA1. *Nature* 1996;382:678–679.

122. Monteiro ANA, August A, Hanafusa H. Evidence for a transcriptional activation function of BRCA1 C-terminal region. *Proc Natl Acad Sci USA* 1996;93:13595–13599.

123. Lu M, Conzen SD, Cole CN, Arrick BA. Characterization of functional messenger RNA splice variants of BRCA1 expressed in nonmalignant and tumor-derived breast cells. *Cancer Res* 1996; 56:4578–4581.

124. Wilson CA, Payton MN, Pekar SK, et al. BRCA1 protein products: antibody specificity. *Nat Genet* 1996;13:264–265.

125. Thomas JE, Smith M, Rubinfeld B, et al. Subcellular localization and analysis of apparent 180-kDa and 220-kDa proteins of the breast cancer susceptibility gene, BRCA1. *J Biol Chem* 1996;271:28630–28635.

126. Chen Y, Farmer AA, Chen C, et al. BRCA1 is a 220-kDa nuclear phosphoprotein that is expressed and phosphorylated in a cell cycle–dependent manner. *Cancer Res* 1996;56: 3168–3172.

127. Steeg PS. Granin expectations in breast cancer? *Nat Genet* 1996;12:223–225.

128. Jensen RA, Thompson ME, Jetton TL, et al. BRCA1 is secreted and exhibits properties of a granin. *Nat Genet* 1996;12:303–308.

129. Koonin EV, Altschul SF, Bork P. Functional motifs. *Nat Genet* 1996;13:266–268.

130. Scully RE, Anderson SF, Chao DM, et al. BRCA1 is a component of the RNA polymerase II holoenzyme. *Proc Nat Acad Sci USA* 1997;94: 5605–5610.

131. Holt JT, Thompson ME, Szabo C, et al. Growth retardation and tumour inhibition by BRCA1. *Nat Genet* 1996;12:298–302.

132. Lane TF, Deng C, Elson A, et al. Expression of BRCA1 is associated with terminal differentiation of ectodermally and mesodermally derived tissues in mice. *Genes Dev* 1995;9: 2712–2722.

133. Scully RE, Ganesan S, Brown M, et al. Location of BRCA1 in human breast and ovarian cancer cells. *Science* 1996;272:123–126.

134. Chen Y, Chen C, Riley DJ, et al. Aberrant subcellular localization of BRCA1 in breast cancer. *Science* 1995;270:789–791.

135. Merajver SD, Pham TM, Caduff RF, et al. Somatic mutations in the BRCA1 gene in sporadic ovarian tumours. *Nat Genet* 1995;9: 439–443.

136. Smith SA, Easton DF, Evans DG, Ponder BA. Allele losses in the region 17q12-21 in familial breast and ovarian cancer involve the wild-type chromosome. *Nat Genet* 1992;2:128–131.

137. Zelada-Hedman M, Torroella M, Mesquita R, et al. Loss of heterozygosity studies in tumors from families with breast-ovarian cancer syndrome. *Hum Genet* 1994;94:231–234.

138. Neuhausen SL, Marshall CJ. Loss of heterozygosity in familial tumors from three BRCA1-linked kindreds. *Cancer Res* 1994;54:6069–6072.

139. Futreal PA, Liu Q, Shattuck-Eidens D, et al. BRCA1 mutations in primary breast and ovarian carcinomas. *Science* 1994;266:120–122.

140. Takahashi H, Behbakht K, McGovern PE, et al. Mutation analysis of the BRCA1 gene in ovarian cancers. *Cancer Res* 1995;55:2998–3002.

141. Schildkraut JM, Collins NK, Dent GA, et al. Loss of heterozygosity on chromosome 17q11-21 in cancers of women who have both breast and ovarian cancer. *Am J Obstet Gynecol* 1995;172: 908–913.

142. Tangir J, Muto MG, Berkowitz RS, et al. A 400 kb novel deletion unit centromeric to the BRCA1 gene in sporadic epithelial ovarian cancer. *Oncogene* 1996;12:735–740.

143. Goldgar DE, Reilly PR. A common BRCA1 mutation in the Ashkenazim. *Nat Genet* 1995; 11:113–114.

144. Modan B, Gak E, Sade-Bruchim RB, et al. High frequency of BRCA1 185delAG mutation in ovarian cancer in Israel. *JAMA* 1996;276: 1823–1825.

145. Muto MG, Cramer DW, Tangir J, et al. Frequency of the BRCA1 185delAG mutation among Jewish women with ovarian cancer and matched population controls. *Cancer Res* 1996;56: 1250–1252.

146. Andersen TI, Borresen AL, Moller P. A common BRCA1 mutation in Norwegian breast and ovarian cancer families? *Am J Hum Genet* 1996;59:486–487.

147. Wagner TMU, Moslinger R, Zielinski C, et al. New Austrian mutation in BRCA1 gene detected in three unrelated families. *Lancet* 1996;347: 1263.

148. Cornelis RS, Vasen HFA, Meijers-Heijboer H, et al. Age at diagnosis as an indicator of eligibility for BRCA1 DNA testing in familial breast cancer. *Hum Genet* 1995;95:539–544.

149. Piver MS, Goldberg JM, Tsukada Y, et al. Characteristics of familial ovarian cancer: a report of the first 1000 families in the Gilda Radner familial ovarian cancer registry. *Eur J Gynecol Oncol* 1996;3:169–176.

150. Salazar H, Godwin AK, Daly MB, et al. Microscopic benign and invasive malignant neoplasms and a cancer-prone phenotype in prophylactic oophorectomies. *J Natl Cancer Inst* 1996;88: 1810–1820.

151. Shushan A, Paltiel O, Gordon L, Schenker JG. Ovarian cancer of low malignant potential is not associated with positive familial history. *Am J Obstet Gynecol* 1996;175:507–508.

152. Narod S, Tonin P, Lynch H, et al. Histology of BRCA1-associated ovarian tumours. *Lancet* 1994; 343:236.

153. Narod SA, Goldgar D, Cannon-Albright L, et al. Risk modifiers in carriers of BRCA1 mutations. *Int J Cancer* 1995;64:394–398.

154. Phelan CM, Rebbeck TR, Weber BL, et al. Ovarian cancer risk in BRCA1 carriers is modified by the HRAS1 variable number of tandem repeat (VNTR) locus. *Nat Genet* 1996; 12:309–311.

155. Gayther SA, Mangion J, Russell P, et al. Variation of risks of breast and ovarian cancer associated with different germline mutations of the BRCA2 gene. *Nat Genet* 1997;15:103–105.

156. Tavtigian SV, Simard J, Rommens J, et al. The complete BRCA2 gene and mutations in chromosome 13q-linked kindreds. *Nat Genet* 1996; 12:333–337.

157. Sharan SK, Morimatsu M, Albrecht U, et al. Embryonic lethality and radiation hypersensitivity mediated by Rad51 in mice lacking *Brca2*. *Nature* 1997;386:804–810.

158. Berman DB, Costalas J, Schultz DC, et al. A common mutation in BRCA2 that predisposes to a variety of cancers is found in both Jewish Ashkenazi and non-Jewish individuals. *Cancer Res* 1996;56:3409–3414.

159. Gudmundsson J, Johannesdottir G, Arason A, et al. Frequent occurrence of BRCA2 linkage in

Icelandic breast cancer families and segregation of a common BRCA2 haplotype. *Am J Hum Genet* 1996;58:749–756.

160. Teng DH-F, Bogden R, Mitchell J, et al. Low incidence of BRCA2 mutations in breast carcinoma and other cancers. *Nat Genet* 1996;13:241–244.

161. Takahashi H, Chiu H, Bandera CA, et al. Mutations of the BRCA2 gene in ovarian carcinomas. *Cancer Res* 1996;56:2738–2741.

162. Rajan JV, Wang M, Marquis ST, Chodosh LA. BRCA2 is coordinately regulated with BRCA1 during proliferation and differentiation in mammary epithelial cells. *Proc Natl Acad Sci USA* 1996;93:13078–13083.

163. Friedman LS, Ostermeyer EA, Lynch ED, et al. The search for BRCA1. *Cancer Res* 1994;54:6374–6382.

164. Hacia JG, Brody LC, Chee MS, et al. Detection of heterozygous mutations in BRCA1 using high density oligonucleotide arrays and two-colour fluorescence analysis. *Nat Genet* 1996;14:441–447.

165. Hogervorst FBL, Cornelis RS, Bout M, et al. Rapid detection of BRCA1 mutations by the protein truncation test. *Nat Genet* 1995;10:208–212.

166. Lancaster JM, Cochran CJ, Brownlee HA, et al. Detection of BRCA1 mutations in women with early-onset ovarian cancer by use of the protein truncation test. *J Natl Cancer Inst* 1996;88:552–554.

167. Ozcelik H, Antebi YJ, Cole DEC. Heteroduplex and protein truncation analysis of the BRCA1 185delAG mutation. *Hum Genet* 1996;98:310–312.

168. Gayther SA, Harrington P, Russell P, et al. Rapid detection of regionally clustered germ-line BRCA1 mutations by multiplex heteroduplex analysis. *Am J Hum Genet* 1996;58:451–456.

169. Kozlowski P, Sobczak K, Napierala M, et al. PCR-SSCP-HDX analysis of pooled DNA for more rapid detection of germline mutations in large genes. The BRCA1 example. *Nucleic Acids Res* 1996;24:1177–1178.

170. Rohlfs EM, Learning WG, Friedman KJ, et al. Direct detection of mutations in the breast and ovarian cancer susceptibility gene BRCA1 by PCR-mediated site-directed mutagenesis. *Clin Chem* 1997;43:24–29.

171. Mok SC, Bell DA, Knapp RC, et al. Mutation of K-ras protooncogene in human ovarian epithelial tumors of borderline malignancy. *Cancer Res* 1993;53:1489–1492.

172. Gallion HH, Pieretti M, DePriest PD, van Nagell JR Jr. The molecular basis of ovarian cancer. *Cancer* 1995;76:1992–1997.

173. Zheng J, Benedict WF, Xu H, et al. Genetic disparity between morphologically benign cysts contiguous to ovarian carcinomas and solitary cystadenomas. *J Natl Cancer Inst* 1995;87:1146–1153.

174. Liu E, Nuzum C. Molecular sleuthing: tracking ovarian cancer progression. *J Natl Cancer Inst* 1995;87:1099–1101. Editorial.

175. Hoskins WJ. Histologic changes in the ovaries of cancer-prone women: an indication of premalignant change? *J Natl Cancer Inst* 1996;88:1790–1793.

176. Shelling AN, Cooke IE, Ganesan TS. The genetic analysis of ovarian cancer. *Br J Cancer* 1995;72:521–527.

177. Naber SP. Molecular pathology—detection of neoplasia. *N Engl J Med* 1994;331:1508–1510.

CHAPTER *40*

Women at Risk for Heritable Cancers: Social and Psychological Considerations

BRIAN D. DOAN

The identification of geneic mutations associated with heritable breast and ovarian cancers has progressed with exceptional speed. It is now possible, in a limited way, to identify women who are susceptible to such cancers prior to disease onset. On the surface, the potential benefit of this new genetic technology is compelling: the early identification of mutation carriers allows, at least in principle, for the de-velopment of targeted surveillance and management strategies that would enhance prevention and early detection, and ultimately prolong survival, of women at increased risk.

However promising, the application of genetic testing to cancer susceptibility is far from straightforward. A woman's needs and attitudes related to familial cancer extend beyond the question of her eligibility or non-eligibility for genetic testing, to her understanding of cancer risk information and its implications for her own and her family's future well-being and peace of mind. Genetic testing and counseling is of benefit to women concerned about their cancer risk only if it yields reassuring information or prompts action that will help prevent cancer or facilitate its early detection (1). If information about heritable risk has the potential to cause psychological harm, it is crucial that such hazards be identified and ways found to minimize or eliminate them (2,3).

This chapter examines a range of social and psychological issues raised by the development of genetic testing and counseling services related to cancer-predisposing mutations. In the first section, I consider the current literature on the demand for genetic testing for cancer susceptibility: Why women presumed to be at risk might want to know their mutation status, and how they might decide to participate in or decline predictive testing. In the second section, I examine the psychological benefits and hazards of testing and counseling for susceptibility to heritable female cancers. In the third and final section, I consider the latest findings suggesting that ethnicity can be a primary heritable risk category, regardless of family history, and examine the ethical, legal, and sociobehavioral implications of using ethnicity rather than family history to identify a population as being at increased risk for breast and ovarian cancer.

Demand for Genetic Testing for Cancer Predisposition

North Americans are understandably intrigued by developments in genetics. Media reports almost every week are raising public awareness of new discoveries in molecular genetics and their potential to predict the occurrence of disease (4). Despite heightened media attention, however, the scientific literacy of the general public regarding human genetics remains limited (5,6). For example, a study of educated laypeople tested on their understanding of a selection of media reports on health research found an error rate near 40% (7). Many people are uncertain about probability principles, which can impede their comprehension of risk estimates (8–10). In general, the public is more familiar with genetic defects that result in developmental disability than with those that are associated with disease susceptibility (11,12).

These limitations of public awareness and comprehension make it all the more difficult to predict the public's interest in and response to the availability of new genetic tests for susceptibility to particular diseases. Croyle and Lerman (13) reported that the majority of the general population, including those at increased risk, hold favorable attitudes toward genetic testing and screening. However, expressed interest in genetic testing may not be a strong predictor of subsequent participation in genetic testing. The fact is, public attitudes toward genetic testing for susceptibility to disease have not yet been widely investigated. The few available insights come mainly from studies of the attitudes towards presymptomatic testing of people at risk for Huntington disease (HD). Evidently, the number of people who actually pursue predictive testing for HD is not as high as expected based on their prior expressed interest (14). There are several reasons why many at-risk individuals choose not to avail themselves of predictive testing for HD: 1) HD is incurable, 2) they are concerned about losing their health insurability, 3) they are concerned about the impact of positive results on their children, 4) they are concerned about financial costs, and 5) they are concerned about their inability to undo the knowledge.

It remains unclear whether the pattern of participation in genetic testing for HD is generalizable to the setting of cancer susceptibility. Participants in a study on attitudes towards testing for susceptibility to colon cancer had a high level of interest, especially if they also considered themselves to be at risk due to a strong family history (15). In contrast to HD, colon cancer is understood to be treatable, especially with early intervention.

The situation appears to be similar with regard to receptivity to testing for genetic susceptibility for breast cancer. Chaliki et al (16) recently reported that 90% of women undergoing mammograms or visiting their gynecologist indicated that they would take a test for *BRCA1*, and would recommend it to their relatives. Roughly one fourth of these women had at least one first or second degree relative with breast or ovarian cancer. Their main reasons for wanting to be tested: 1) they believed that early breast cancer is curable, 2) they wanted to pursue active surveillance, and 3) they worried about developing breast cancer.

Lerman et al (17) found that three fourths of first degree female relatives of ovarian cancer patients indicated they would definitely want to be tested for *BRCA1*, and another 20% said they probably would. Their most commonly cited reasons for pursuing testing were: 1) to learn about their children's risk, 2) to ensure an appropriate level of surveillance, and 3) to be reassured. Interestingly, many of these women did not expect testing to reduce their cancer anxiety and still intended to pursue *BRCA1* testing when available (17,18). Colleagues and I have also obtained comparable levels of interest in a Canadian sample of 100 women attending a Diagnostic Breast Clinic (unpublished data; Doan, Chart, Warner & Eakin, 1996). Other studies have also estimated interest in pursuing genetic testing for cancer susceptibility as being considerably higher (40%–60%) than has been the case for HD (19,20).

At the present time, little more than this is known about the potential demand for genetic testing for breast and ovarian cancers: It appears that a moderately high enrollment in testing can be anticipated. Beyond that, there are a number of social and psychological factors that influence a given woman's pursuit of information regarding cancer risk about which we know comparatively little. Clinical reports suggest that a woman is more likely to seek information about her risk when she is supported by affected family members (e.g., a mother or sister with breast cancer) or by her family physician (21).

A woman's perception of her vulnerability to cancer, her anxiety about it, and her typical style of coping with threat may also influence how interested she will be in knowing more about her risk status (15,17,22). Some women are prone to coping with a health threat by scanning for and attending to threatening cues;

others are more inclined to avoidance or distraction in dealing with threat-relevant information. The former, "high monitors," are information seekers, tend to worry more, and may be inclined to overuse cancer screening tests, genetic tests, or prophylactic surgery (23). In other words, women who seek risk information likely constitute a more psychologically vulnerable group. In contrast, "low monitors" who are at high risk for cancer and who cope by avoiding information may represent a more physically vulnerable group. They may also present the greater clinical challenge. After all, steps can be taken to provide emotional support to anxious risk information seekers as part of a comprehensive genetic testing service. But what would be the best clinical approach for high risk women who prefer not to know? The matter warrants close attention by investigators.

Preexisting communication patterns within a given family may also be potentially powerful mediators of demand for genetic testing (24). A woman's current eligibility for testing frequently depends on her ability to contact and inform affected and nonaffected relatives about the need for all of them to take part in a cancer risk assessment and, possibly, predictive testing. In some cases, disrupted communication among relatives due to distance, illness, or conflict may impede participation in a predictive testing and cancer surveillance program (25,26). Here again, too little of the research conducted so far has considered the impact of the familial context on demand for genetic testing and counseling.

To summarize: At the present, early stage in the development of genetic tests for cancer susceptibility, demand for hereditary cancer risk information—including predictive testing—appears to be substantial. The limited research reported to date indicates that against a background of generally favorable public attitudes towards genetics, seeking cancer risk information is influenced significantly by a woman's perceptions of her susceptibility to breast and ovarian cancers, by her distress about it, and by her typical style of coping with health threats. Family experiences with cancer and family communication patterns can also serve to support or restrict cancer risk information seeking. Further elaboration is needed of how family experiences with cancer and individual family members' worries about cancer risk influence their decisions about pursuing genetic

testing and related familial risk information. Indeed, a better understanding of how these psychological factors influence test participation is crucial to the success of any effort to educate and empower high risk women to access surveillance and intervention programs that could ultimately enhance their and their family's survival.

Of course, all of this rests on the assumption that the putative benefits of participation in predictive testing will outweigh any possible hazards incurred either by the provision of risk information itself or by subsequent actions designed to reduce a woman's risk of breast and ovarian cancer. Accordingly, I now turn to the probable psychological impact of genetic testing for cancer susceptibility in high risk women.

Psychological Costs and Benefits of Genetic Testing and Cancer Risk Counseling

Given the very early stage of development of the field, it should come as no surprise that there are presently very few empirical data about the psychological impact of testing for cancer susceptibility per se, although the literature on the subject is growing. Indirect evidence for the psychological benefits and risks of testing for heritable breast and ovarian cancer comes from three sources: studies of the impact of testing for other genetic disorders such as HD and cystic fibrosis (27,28), studies of the impact of cancer screening and surveillance programs (29–31), and studies of women at high risk for familial breast or ovarian cancers attending surveillance programs (17,32).

Benefits of Predictive Testing

Studies of the demand for genetic tests—be they prenatal screens (33), carrier screens (34,35), or predictive tests (36–38)—have noted the main reasons for wanting to be tested. People in high risk groups typically are seeking reassurance and want to reduce anxiety about their own and their children's health risks.

Recent studies indicate that a majority of women with a family history of breast cancer overestimate their personal risk for the disease (39,40). Such inflated perceptions of their risk contribute to their higher levels of distress and hence their interest in seeking reassuring information. In one study (7), a majority of the women surveyed who were interested in genetic testing anticipated that a negative test result would improve their quality of life (83%), make them feel less anxious (83%), make them feel less depressed (68%), and allow them to feel more in control (82%). On the surface, predictive testing for susceptibility to breast and ovarian cancer has a high likelihood of yielding good news for the majority of women who are worried about their risk of carrying a cancer-predisposing gene mutation.

The reassuring value of any test for breast and ovarian cancers depends crucially on its actual predictive power. Test accuracy is crucial to prevent adverse psychological effects from either false positive or false negative results. Moreover, given that the penetrance of cancer-related genes is lower than it is for other hereditary diseases, test results may not provide a level of certainty that is decisive or reassuring. In the case of familial breast cancer, for example, a positive test result does not necessarily mean that a breast cancer phenotype will be expressed and cancer will develop. Nor, for that matter, does a negative test result reduce a woman's risk of developing sporadic breast cancer. To illustrate: Lerman et al (17) found that 72% of women with strong family histories of breast or ovarian cancer thought they would continue to worry about developing the disease even if they tested negative for a mutation on the *BRCA1* gene.

In short, while there appears to be widespread agreement that predictive testing for breast and ovarian cancer susceptibility might reassure those who are most worried about their cancer risk, the overall psychological impact of such testing remains unclear. For example, a recent controlled study of risk perception and distress among women enrolled in genetic counseling (41) found that despite genetic counseling, many high risk women remained more vulnerable to cancer-specific distress, and continued to perceive their risk of breast cancer inaccurately. In contrast, in the only randomized trial of breast cancer risk counseling reported to date (32), Lerman et al found the counseling to be effective: Women who received it had significantly less cancer-specific distress at 3-month follow-up than did matched control subjects, and the benefits were greatest for women with less formal education. While this new evidence of the benefits of cancer risk counseling is heartening, careful

evaluation of the actual psychological outcomes of predictive testing and counseling for breast and ovarian cancer risk must remain a continuing research priority.

Psychological Costs of Predictive Testing

A woman's desire for reassurance and "good news" can conflict with her desire for definitive information about her risk status (42). Consequently, some women may have adverse emotional responses to genetic risk information if the test results are uncertain or positive. The experience with predictive testing for HD provides some telling insights into the reactions of people tested who either did or did not receive their test results (43,44).

Whether or not they received their test results, participants in HD testing experienced mild anxiety before being offered their results. Those who tested positive exhibited immediate and acute distress, as well as depression, increased anxiety, anger, intrusive thinking, and sleep disturbance for several weeks. After six months, the acute distress had subsided but the scores of those tested for well-being remained low. Distress continued to decline over the year. A negative test result for HD was reassuring to most participants, but approximately 10% of the group at decreased risk also suffered adverse effects of being tested for several months afterward (45). Having lived for years with the expectation of eventually developing HD, they were unprepared for the good news that they were unlikely to get HD. As well, those participants who refused to be tested, or whose test results were indeterminate, remained more distressed through to the 12-month follow-up than did those who did participate.

Although the penetrance for cancer susceptibility is lower than that for HD, predictive testing for breast and ovarian cancer will also identify a proportion of women who really are at increased risk. It seems reasonable to predict that being informed definitively of increased cancer risk will be devastating to them. Being told of a positive result after tests to detect cancer (e.g., mammography) is known to have a major psychological impact (29). And most women anticipating a genetic test for breast or ovarian cancer susceptibility expect that upon receiving a positive test result they too would become depressed (80%), become anxious (77%), and have an impaired quality of life (32%) (33). Case reports from genetic linkage studies of families with a high risk of cancer tend to corroborate the likelihood of adverse emotional reactions to positive test results (38,46) and have also reported negative sequelae—notably guilt and shame—among some family members who are notified that they are not likely to have an altered *BRCA1* gene (26). A study by Lynch et al (47) noted that many of the women who tested negative still worried, expressed disbelief that they were not gene carriers, and still wanted intense surveillance. Some negative carriers said they might still consider prophylactic surgical intervention, and those negatives who had previously undergone such surgeries reported that in retrospect they did not regret their decision.

To summarize the evidence so far: 1) seeing oneself at high risk of breast or ovarian cancer is distressing to the majority of women from families with a high incidence of cancer; 2) genetic testing and counseling for breast and ovarian cancer susceptibility may in fact be reassuring the majority of high risk women about their vulnerability; but 3) it appears that testing and counseling can also adversely affect women—for example, when test results are positive or uncertain, or in some cases, even when they are negative; and 4) cancer risk counseling is not always effective either in helping women to understand their actual risk status or in helping to reduce their anxiety and distress about developing cancer.

In addition, increased worry about breast or ovarian cancer among high risk women may deter them from adhering to breast surveillance programs, including breast self-examination (BSE), biannual clinical breast examination (CBE), and yearly mammograms (48,49). Such findings highlight a difficult predicament for genetic counselors: Giving notification to a healthy woman of a positive genetic test result could deter her from potentially life-prolonging surveillance.

There are broader, troubling social issues to consider as well. Problems of self-image and stigmatization follow carrier testing for sickle cell and Tay-Sachs disease (TSD) genes (50–52). One study of health perceptions before and after TSD carrier testing reported that those who tested positive had a diminished view of their future health even though they would never get the disease (53). It remains unclear whether this lowered self-esteem is specific to certain diseases or disorders, or stems from the recognition that one is a "carrier" of some defect. In

the latter case, it would seem probable that a positive predictive test result for susceptibility to breast or ovarian cancer would also diminish self-esteem. Beyond that, could having an identifiable vulnerability to breast or ovarian cancer also lead to negative perceptions by society of women at increased risk? It seems possible. Could this ability to determine who is at increased risk for cancer lead to the creation of what Nelkin (54) referred to as a new "genetic underclass," the "presymptomatic ill"? We have yet to find out.

Psychological Issues Associated with Prevention and Surveillance

One of the putative benefits of genetic testing and counseling is that they offer opportunities for cancer prevention or early detection. Our evaluation of the psychological impact of predictive testing for breast or ovarian cancer susceptibility must therefore take into account the possible impact of strategies aimed at reducing a high risk woman's susceptibility.

Surveillance

There are well-established protocols for increased surveillance of women at risk of developing breast or ovarian cancer, including transvaginal ultrasound screening, CBE, mammography, and regular BSE. The efficacy of such surveillance activities remains unclear for mutation carriers, nor is it certain that cancer mortality among high-risk groups is at all reduced with increased surveillance (46,55,56). Some research has shown that recommended surveillance strategies are underutilized by the majority of women who have a positive family history of breast cancer (57). Participation in predictive testing could potentially increase adherence to surveillance strategies, as was found in a recent controlled study of genetic counseling in the United Kingdom (41). It has been noted, however, that risk notification itself can engender psychological distress (58), and increased cancer anxiety can reduce adherence to mammography, CBE, and BSE (29,59).

In view of these contradictory findings, there is a need for careful intervention studies focused on barriers to surveillance and on strategies that promote adherence to surveillance among high-risk women. Among the strategies that bear further investigation are those that address known facilitators of adherence in the general oncological setting: physician support, patient education to reduce anxieties about radiation, and clinical service models that promote a secure, emotionally supportive setting for surveillance with minimal embarrassment and anxiety.

Prophylactic Oophorectomy

Among the preventive options, prophylactic oophorectomy has been recommended for women genetically predisposed (i.e., having as high as a 50% lifetime risk) to ovarian cancer (60). Although the protective effects of oophorectomy have been questioned due to reports of postsurgical intra-abdominal carcinomatosis (61), it appears that this risk may have been overestimated (62). There are medical risks owing to early menopause following oophorectomy, and possibly also with long-term hormone replacement. In addition, there are psychological costs to oophorectomy, especially among younger women of reproductive age (63). It remains unclear, however, how women at risk for ovarian cancer weigh these potential costs of surgery against the relief from the risk of ovarian cancer (64).

Prophylactic Mastectomy

Prophylactic mastectomy is another preventive option for women at risk for familial breast cancer, but it too raises complex psychological, social, and ethical concerns (46,55). The psychological impact of mastectomy is relatively well understood for women who have already been diagnosed with cancer (65) but the effect of mastectomy on younger, asymptomatic women is unknown. For some women, the psychological impact may be less given that the women choose mastectomy as a preventive measure (66). The psychological benefits of that choice include reduced cancer worry and reduced need for upsetting surveillance and its attendant risks such as false positive findings on mammograms. Other women may find that the negative impact of mastectomy on their sense of their femininity and maternality overrides its reassuring value. Our own data suggest that the majority of high risk women contemplating genetic testing for cancer susceptibility consider a prophylactic mastectomy to be more radical than is warranted despite their elevated risk (unpublished data; Doan, Chart, Warner, &

Eakin, 1996). There are no findings to date to indicate whether or not the high risk woman's view of prophylactic mastectomy would be different in the face of a positive, negative, or uncertain genetic test result.

Chemoprevention

Women at high risk for ovarian cancer are advised to consider oral contraceptive therapy to decrease the risks, and this is generally viewed as a safe and non-distressing preventive strategy by health care professionals and consumers (60). High risk women can also elect to enroll in the Tamoxifen Chemoprevention Trial (46). However, widely publicized reports of increased risks of uterine cancer from tamoxifen may add an additional burden to women already worried about their cancer risk. Clinical experience suggests that there are some adverse psychological responses associated with tamoxifen therapy for a proportion of women with breast cancer, but at present no systematic studies that have specifically addressed the psychological costs or benefits of chemoprevention. Indeed, it is unclear to what extent healthy women may be predisposed to avoid any but the most benign forms of chemoprevention, such as dietary modification (67). Clearly, the impact on high risk women's psychological adjustment of a range of interventions, from chemoprevention trials to dietary and other lifestyle changes, requires continuing investigation.

Implications for the Family

All of the psychological benefits and hazards considered so far pertain to individual women at risk. What is the psychological and social impact of predictive testing and genetic counseling on families (27,68)? Family-related issues are paramount for the women who participate in predictive testing (43). The ability to make an early diagnosis of hereditary cancer will have far-reaching implications for both affected and unaffected family members. Until now, families might be aware that they had a high incidence of cancer, and family members, believing themselves to be all at equal, elevated risk, would support one another through mutual concern. Now that individual family members can learn with some degree of certainty who in the family is at high risk, family dynamics will inevitably change (69).

It is at the level of family relationships where further research is most needed to improve our understanding of the psychological costs and benefits of genetic testing for cancer susceptibility. For example, how does notification of increased cancer susceptibility affect the spouse of a high-risk woman? Does it alter the couple's marital and sexual relationship, reproductive choices, and future plans? How best can a genetic counselor assess the family dynamics involved in risk notification? What are the most pressing family issues for those living at high risk? How do we assess and deal with them? What is the impact of risk notification on the parent-offspring relationship? What are the anxieties of "at risk" mothers or fathers of children? When—and how—should offspring be informed of their risk status? What are the psychological risks of parents being told of their children's cancer susceptibility? How might cancer risk information about either the parent or child affect the child's psychosocial development? What are the effects on relationships between high risk siblings when some elect to be tested and others do not? Does having genetic cancer risk information alter family members' responses when cancer is subsequently diagnosed, or when a death occurs among them? Does having that information alter the family's socioeconomic status (i.e., their employability or insurability)? Answers to any and all of these questions will go a long way towards clarifying the hazards and the benefits to families of predictive testing for breast and ovarian cancers.

Primary Heritable Risk Categories: Ethnicity and Family History

Until 1995, heritable breast cancer was linked to persons with a strong family history of the disease. In late 1995, a mutation of *BRCA1* 185delAG was found to be eight times more common among people of Ashkenazi Jewish descent, than those who were not, regardless of family history of breast cancer (70). It was inferred that 1% of Ashkenazi women carry this genetic mutation. Then, a second *BRCA1* mutation—5382insC—was found to be most prevalent among Ashkenazi women (71). By October 1996, a third mutation, 6174delT on *BRCA2*, was announced as common to Ashkenazi women and unrelated to family history of breast or ovarian cancer (72). The discovery of these three mutations doubled the projected number of Ashkenazi women carrying a cancer predisposing mutation from 1 in 100 to 1 in 50 (73).

The findings regarding these mutations fall within a tradition of ethnically identified genetic predisposition to disease. Race has long been linked to predisposition to sickle cell anemia, and the correlation between geographic location (Asia, Middle East, the Mediterranean) and genetic predisposition to thalassemia is widely cited (74,75). Being Jewish has also been reported as the strongest predisposing factor to TSD (76). However, the incidence of breast cancer and the number of Ashkenazi women now identified as being at increased risk makes genetic susceptibility to breast cancer the most common predisposition to a potentially lethal, late-onset disease (77).

The clinical, informational, and psychosocial needs of this newly defined at risk population required immediate attention. In early 1996, a population-based trial was initiated in the Washington, DC, area. Volunteers were recruited to donate blood from a finger-prick for genomic DNA blood analysis and to complete a brief family history. The purpose of the trial was to determine whether 185delAG is associated with an increased risk of breast cancer. Within 2 months more than 5000 persons identifying themselves as Ashkenazi Jews had come forward to be anonymously tested for this *BRCA1* mutation, and entry to the trial was closed half-way into the projected accrual period because the number of participants required had been reached (78–81).

Heated debate ensued regarding the ethical and legal ramifications of conducting a community based trial in this manner (82). Some speculated that the guarantee of anonymity prompted many Ashkenazim to enter the trial, while others argued that the women may have assumed that the identification of this particular *BRCA1* mutation indicated an increased incidence of breast cancer among the Ashkenazim, and were therefore motivated to participate in the trial by fear of a potential epidemic. The fact is, decisions had been made to offer testing for the mutations to a community rather than to individuals, without important baseline information regarding the potential community response, and with little consideration of the possible consequences of identifying *any* given ethnic community as being at increased risk for heritable cancer (83).

The use of ethnic origin as a predictor of genetic susceptibility to a disease has generally been associated with some positive, but many negative, consequences (84–87). Even so, it is difficult to anticipate the precise positive and negative effects of using ethnic origin as a predictor of susceptibility to heritable breast or ovarian cancer. Information about Jewish reaction to other genetic conditions such as TSD and cystic fibrosis does not lend itself to extrapolation, because of the differences between these diseases and breast cancer, including differences in penetrance and the late onset of breast cancer. Other ethnic experiences such as Afro-American sickle cell disease also are not directly applicable to the problem of Ashkenazi susceptibility to cancer, and what little is known about the effects of breast or ovarian cancer risk information on *families* is not easily generalizable to an entire ethnic community (88). Consequently, there remains a pressing need for information about: 1) who in the Ashkenazi community perceives themselves to be at increased risk for breast cancer, and how they arrive at their estimates; 2) who is best suited to serve as the community's translators and disseminators of genetic risk information; 3) who will be likely to request genetic testing and what they will do with test results; and 4) what, if any, psychological and social support will be required by those who are identified as mutation carriers.

The discovery of three Ashkenazi-specific mutations was unexpected, but will not be the last. Other mutations have recently been reported to be associated with different ethnic communities. For all such communities, it is essential to know: 1) What genetic risk information they require and who should provide it? 2) What genetic services and what other support services should be provided? 3) How can such community based genetic services be evaluated? In particular, evaluative efforts must attend to the risk of discriminatory practices towards segments of the population who are identified as genetically susceptible to cancer, especially when such practices are also, *de facto,* discriminatory along ethnic lines.

Summary and Conclusions

In this chapter, I examined a range of social and psychological issues raised by the development of genetic testing and counseling services related to cancer-predisposing mutations. First, I considered the demand for genetic testing for cancer susceptibility: why women presumed to be at risk might want to know their mutation status, and how they might decide to participate in or decline predictive testing. So far, interest and demand for genetic testing for cancer susceptibility appears to be quite high, especially among the more worried, vigilant monitors. I then examined the psychological benefits and hazards of testing and counseling for susceptibility to heritable female cancers. The benefits include reassurance and an opportunity for planned surveillance and early detection. The hazards include increased worry about cancer, and a host of other potential risks associated with 1) the provision of risk information, 2) the delivery of a genetic test result, and 3) subsequent preventive options (e.g., intense surveillance, prophylactic surgery, or a chemoprevention trial). The findings to date reinforce the need for caution in the development of genetic testing and counseling services, and careful attention to the provision of safeguards and supports to mitigate any adverse psychological consequences of participation in genetic counseling, testing, and related cancer surveillance and preventive services.

Finally, I considered the latest findings suggesting that ethnicity can be a primary heritable risk category, regardless of family history. I drew attention to some of the ethical and psychosocial implications of using ethnicity to identify a population at increased risk for breast and ovarian cancer. These recent discoveries highlight the need for immediate, ongoing, and careful evaluations of the genetic services that are developing. In particular, such evaluations must attend to the possible adverse and distressing social consequences of predictive testing that could arise, such as employment and insurance discrimination against healthy women carriers, their relatives, or their ethnic community.

Knowledge of the role that heredity plays in relation to breast and ovarian cancer has increased dramatically in the past few years. Unfortunately, the negative consequences of providing familial cancer risk information to individual women, families and communities are only beginning to be understood. The greatest uncertainties lie in the arena of social, psychological, and ethical issues. As we have seen, the critical concerns are the possibilities that risk information might cause already vulnerable women undue worry and distress, that it might be used to their disadvantage, and might lead to the creation of a genetic "underclass" of women, and/or ethnic communities.

We must add to this list of concerns the problem of demand on an already overtaxed health care system. All that we know so far about the impact of familial cancer risk information has been acquired from research programs that have had the resources to offer comprehensive, multi-disciplinary services. The extent to which this experience can be generalized to community-based health care programs that have to compete for scarce resources remains unclear. There is every indication that demand for cancer risk information and predictive testing will continue to grow. Instead of simply responding to this demand on an emergent basis, researchers, policy makers, and clinicians have both an opportunity and an obligation to proceed with caution and foresight to ensure that cancer risk information programs continue to meet the social and psychological needs of women.

REFERENCES

1. MacDonald KG, Doan B, Kelner M, Taylor KM. A sociobehavioural perspective on genetic testing and counseling for heritable breast, ovarian and colon cancer. *Can Med Assoc J* 1996;154:457–464.

2. Croyle RT, Lerman C. Psychological impact of genetic testing. In: Croyle RT, ed. *Psychosocial effects of screening for disease prevention and detection.* New York: Oxford University Press, 1995:11–38.

3. Croyle RT, Jemmott JB. Psychological reactions to risk factor testing. In: Skelton JA, Croyle RT, eds. *Mental representation in health and illness.* New York: Springer, 1991:86–107.

4. Elmer-Dewitt P. The genetic revolution. *Time,* January 17, 1994:46–53.

5. Halliwell JE, chairman: *Genetics in canadian health care* Report 42. Ottawa: Science Council of Canada, 1991:1–14, 53–90.

6. Miller JD. *The public understanding of science and technology in the United States, 1990: A report to the National Science Foundation.* Washington, DC: National Science Foundation, 1991:4–22.

7. Yeaton WH, Smith D, Rogers K. Evaluating understanding of popular press reports of health research. *Health Educ Q* 1990;17:223–234.

8. Palmer CGS, Sainfort F. Toward a new conceptualization and operationalization of risk perception within the genetic counseling domain. *J Genet Counsel* 1993;2:275–294.

9. Robinson A. Genetic diagnosis: present and prospects. *Can Med Assoc J* 1994;150:49–52.

10. Shiloh S, Saxe L. Perception of risk in genetic counseling. *Psychol Health* 1989;3:45–61.

11. Singer E. Public attitudes toward genetic testing. *Popul Res Policy Rev* 1991;10:235–255.

12. Singer E. Public attitudes toward fetal diagnosis and the termination of life. *Soc Indic Res* 1993;28:117–136.

13. Croyle RT, Lerman C. Psychological impact of genetic testing. In: RT Croyle, ed. *Psychosocial effects of screening for disease prevention and detection.* New York: Oxford University Press, 1995:11–38.

14. Quaid K, Morris M. Reluctance to undergo predictive testing: the case of Huntington disease. *Am J Med Genet* 1993;45:41–45.

15. Croyle RT, Lerman C. Interest in genetic testing for colon cancer susceptibility: cognitive and emotional correlates. *Prev Med* 1993;22:284–292.

16. Chaliki H, Loader S, Levenkron JC, et al. Women's receptivity to testing for a genetic susceptibility to breast cancer. *Am J Public Health* 1995;85:1133–1135.

17. Lerman C, Daly M, Masny A, Balshem A. Attitudes about genetic testing for breast-ovarian cancer susceptibility. *J Clin Oncol* 1994;12:843–850.

18. Mohammed S, Barnes C, Watts S, et al. Attitudes to predictive testing for *BRCA1. J Med Genet* 1995;32:140.

19. Watson M, Murday V, Lloyd S, et al. Genetic testing in breast/ovarian cancer (*BRCA1*) families. *Lancet* 1995;346:583.

20. Evans DG. Genetic testing for cancer predisposition: Need and demand. *J Med Genet* 1995; 32:161.

21. Mahon SM, Casperson DS. Hereditary cancer syndrome: part 2—psychosocial issues, concerns and screening: results of a qualitative study. *Oncol Nurs Forum* 1995;22:775–782.

22. Miller SM. Monitoring versus blunting styles of coping with cancer influence the information patients want and need about their disease:

Implications for cancer screening and management. *Cancer* 1995;76(2):167–177.

23. Schwartz MD, Lerman C, Miller SM, et al. Coping disposition, perceived risk, and psychological distress among women at increased risk for ovarian cancer. *Health Psychol* 1995;14:232–235.

24. Chalmers MA, Thompson K, Degner LF. Information, support and communication needs of women with a family history of breast cancer. *Cancer Nurs* 1996;19:204–213.

25. Kelly PT. Information needs of individuals and families with hereditary cancers. *Semin Oncol Nurs* 1992;5:65–79.

26. Ayme S, Macquart-Moulin G, Julian-Reynier C, et al. Diffusion of information about genetic risk within families. *Neuromusc Disord* 1993;3: 571–574.

27. Decruyenaere M, Evers-Kiebooms G, Van de Berghe H. Perception of predictive testing for Huntington's disease by young women: Preferring uncertainty to certainty? *J Med Genet* 1993; 30:557–561.

28. Wertz DC, Janes SR, Rosenfield JM, Erbe RW. Attitudes toward the prenatal diagnosis of cystic fibrosis: Factors in decision making among affected families. *Am J Hum Genet* 1992;50: 1077–1085.

29. Wardle J, Pope R. The psychological costs of screening for cancer. *J Psychosom Res* 1992; 36:609–624.

30. Lerman C, Trock B, Rimer BK, et al. Psychological side effects of breast cancer screening. *Health Psychol* 1991;10:259–267.

31. Vernon SW, Laville EA, Jackson GL. Participation in breast screening programs: A review. *Soc Sci Med* 1990;30:1107–1118.

32. Lerman C, Schwartz MD, Miller SM, et al. A randomized trial of breast cancer risk counseling: Interacting effects of counseling, educational level, and coping style. *Health Psychol* 1996; 15:75–83.

33. Lippman A. Research studies in applied human genetics: A quantitative analysis and critical review of recent literature. *Am J Med Genet* 1991;41:105–111.

34. Watson EK, Mayall GS, Lamb J, et al. Psychological and social consequences of community carrier screening programme for cystic fibrosis. *Lancet* 1992;340:619–621.

35. Becker MH, Kaback MM, Rosenstock IM, Ruth MV. Some influences on public participation in a genetic screening program. *J Commun Health* 1975;1:3–14.

36. Bloch M, Fahy M, Fox S, Hayden MR. Predictive testing for Huntington disease: II. Demographic characteristics, life-style patterns, attitudes and psychosocial assessments of the first fifty-one test candidates. *Am J Med Genet* 1989;32:217–224.

37. Bloch M, Adam S, Wiggins S, et al. Predictive testing for Huntington disease in Canada: The experience of those receiving an increased risk. *Am J Med Genet* 1992;42:499–507.

38. Biesecker BB, Moehnke M, Calzone K, et al. Genetic counseling for families with inherited susceptibility to breast and ovarian cancer. *JAMA* 1993;269:1970–1974.

39. Evans DG, Burnell LD, Hopwood P, Howell A. Perception of risk in women with a family history of breast cancer. *Br J Cancer* 1993;67: 612–634.

40. Lerman C, Lustbaer E, Riber B, et al. Effect of individualized breast cancer risk counseling: A randomized trial. *J Nat Cancer Inst* 1995;87: 286–292.

41. Lloyd S, Watson M, Waites B, Meyer L, Eeles R, Ebbs S, Tylee A. Familial breast cancer: a controlled study of risk perception, psychological morbidity and health beliefs in women attending for genetic counseling. *Br J Cancer* 1996; 74:482–487.

42. Croyle RT, Lerman C. Psychological impact of genetic testing. In: Croyle RT, ed. *Psychosocial effects of screening for disease prevention and detection*. New York: Oxford University Press, 1995:11–38.

43. Wiggins S, Whyte P, Huggins M, et al. The psychological consequences of predictive testing for Huntington's Disease. *N Engl J Med* 1992;327: 1401–1405.

44. Huggins M, Bloch M, Kanani S, et al. Ethical and legal dilemmas arising during predictive testing for adult-onset disease: The experience of Huntington disease. *Am J Med Genet* 1990;47: 4–12.

45. Huggins M, Bloch M, Wiggins S, et al. Predictive testing for Huntington Disease in Canada: Adverse effects and unexpected results in those receiving a decreased risk. *Am J Med Genet* 1992;42:508–515.

46. King M, Rowell S, Love SM. Inherited breast and ovarian cancer: What are the risks? What are the choices? *JAMA* 1993;269:1975–1980.

47. Lynch HT, Watson P, Conway TA, et al. DNA screening for breast/ovarian cancer susceptibility based on linked markers: A family study. *Arch Intern Med* 1993;153:1979–1987.

48. Kash KM, Holland JC, Halper MS, et al. Psychological distress and surveillance behaviours of women with a family history of breast cancer. *J Nat Cancer Inst* 1992;84:24–30.

49. Lerman C, Trock B, Rimer BK, Boyce A, et al. Psychological and behavioral implications of abnormal mammograms. *Ann Intern Med* 1991; 114:657–661.

50. Charo RA. Legal and regulatory issues surrounding carrier testing. *Clin Obstet Gynecol* 1993;36:568–597.

51. Childs B, Gordis L, Kaback MM, Kazazian HH Jr. Tay-Sachs screening: Motives for participating and knowledge of genetics and probability. *Am J Hum Genet* 1976;28:537–549.

52. Antley RM. The genetic counselor as facilitator of the counselee's decision process. In: Capron A, Lappe M, Murray RF Jr, et al, eds. *Genetic counseling: facts, values and norms.* New York: Arliss, 1979:51–84.

53. Marteau TM, van Duijn M, Ellis I. Effects of genetic screening on perceptions of health: A pilot study. *J Med Genet* 1992;29:24–26.

54. Nelkin K. The social power of genetic information. In: Kevles DJ, Hood L, eds. *The Code of codes.* Cambridge, MA: Harvard University Press, 1992:177–190.

55. Lerman C, Croyle R. Psychological issues in genetic screening for breast cancer susceptibility. *Ann Intern Med* 1994;154:609–616.

56. Moens F. Familial ovarian cancer: Screening and prevention. *Can J Cont Med Educ* 1994;6:33–44.

57. Vogel VG, Graves DS, Vernon SW, et al. Mammographic screening of women with increased risk of breast cancer. *Cancer* 1990;66: 1613–1620.

58. Lerman C, Rimer BK, Engstrom PF. Cancer risk notification: Psychological and ethical implications. *J Clin Oncol* 1991;9:1275–1282.

59. Rimer BK. Understanding the acceptance of mammography by women. *Ann Behav Med* 1992;7:69–74.

60. Kerlikowske K, Brown JS, Grady DG. Should women with familial ovarian cancer undergo prophylactic oophorectomy? *Obstet Gynecol* 1992;80:700–707.

61. Schlesselman JJ. Cancer of the breast and reproductive tract in relation to use of oral contraceptives. *Contraception* 1989;40:1–27.

62. Evans DGR, Ribiero G, Warrell D, Donnai D. Ovarian cancer family and prophylactic choices. *J Med Genet* 1992;29:416–418.

63. Green J, Murton F, Statham H. Psychological issues raised by a familial ovarian cancer register. *J Med Genet* 1993;30:575–579.

64. Daly MB, Lerman C. Ovarian cancer risk counseling: A guide for the practitioner. *Oncology* 1993;7:27–41.

65. Ganz PA, Schag AG, Lee JJ, et al. Breast conservation versus mastectomy: Is there a difference in psychological adjustment on quality of life in the year after surgery? *Cancer* 1992;69: 1727–1738.

66. Breo DL. Altered fates—Counseling families with inherited breast cancer. *JAMA* 1993;269: 2017–2022.

67. Henderson M. Current approaches to breast cancer prevention. *Science* 1993;259:630–632.

68. Houlston RS, Lemoine L, McCarter E, et al. Screening and genetic counseling for relatives of patients with breast cancer in a family cancer clinic. *J Med Genet* 1992;29:691–694.

69. Slattery ML, Kerber RA. A comprehensive evaluation of family history and breast cancer risk. *JAMA* 1993;270:1563–1568.

70. FitzGerald MG, MacDonald DJ, Krainer M, et al. Germ-line *BRCA1* mutations in Jewish and non-Jewish women with early-onset breast cancer. *N Engl J Med* 1996;334:143–149.

71. Kuska B. BRCA1 alteration found in eastern European Jews. *J Nat Cancer Inst* 1995;87:1505.

72. Neuhausen S, Gilewski T, Norton L. Recurrent *BRCA2* 6174delT mutations in Ashkenazi Jewish women affected by breast cancer. *Nat Genet* 1996;13:126–128.

73. Easton DF, Ford D, Bishop DT, the Breast Cancer Linkage Consortium. Breast and ovarian cancer incidence in *BRCA1* mutation carriers. *Am J Hum Genet* 1995;56:265–271.

74. Offit K. Breast cancer and *BRCA1* mutations. *N Engl J Med* 1996;334:1197–1198.

75. Rund D, Cohen T, Filon D, et al. Evolution of a genetic disease in a genetic ethnic isolate: B-Thalassemia in the Jews of Kurdistan. *Proc Nat Acad Sci USA* 1991;88:310–314.

76. Triggs-Raine BI, Feigenbaum ASJ, Natowicz M, et al. Screening for carriers of Tay-Sachs disease

among Ashkenazi Jews: A comparison of DNA based and enzyme based tests. *N Engl J Med* 1990;323:6–12.

77. Shattuck-Eidens D, McClure M, Simard J, et al. A collaborative survey of 80 mutations in the *BRCA1* breast/ovarian cancer susceptibility gene. *JAMA* 1995;273:535–541.

78. NIH Studies specific breast cancer gene alteration in Ashkenazi Jews. NCI Press Office, February 26, 1996.

79. Struewing JP, Abeliovich D, Peretz T, et al. The carrier frequency of the *BRCA1* 185delAG mutation is approximately 1 percent in Ashkenazi Jewish individuals. *Nat Genet* 1995;11:198–200.

80. Nelson N. Caution guides genetic testing for cancer susceptibility genes. *J Nat Cancer Inst* 1995;88:70–72.

81. Recruitment effort for *BRCA1* Ashkenazi study is complete: National Institutes of Health. NCI Press Office, June 4, 1996.

82. Collins FS. *BRCA1*—Lots of mutations, lots of dilemmas. *N Engl J Med* 1996;334:186–188.

83. Scrimgeour D. Ethics are local: Engaging cross-cultural variation in the ethics for clinical research. *Soc Sci Med* 1993;37:957–958.

84. Fost N. Ethical implications of screening asymptomatic individuals. *FASEB J* 1992;6:2813–2817.

85. Robertson JA. Legal and ethical issues arising from the new genetics. *J Reprod Med* 1992;37:521–524.

86. Caplan AL. Twenty years after, the legacy of the Tuskegee Syphilis Study: When evil intrudes. *Hastings Cent Rep* 1992;22:29–32.

87. Macaulay AC. Ethics of research in Native communities. *Can Fam Phys* 1994;40:1888–1890.

88. Lerman C, Narod S, Schulman K, et al. *BRCA1* testing in families with hereditary breast-ovarian cancer. *JAMA* 1996;275:1885–1892.

CHAPTER *41*

The Evolving Role of the Physician in Heritable Female Cancer

KATHRYN M. TAYLOR
LOUISE MURPHY
INGRID AMBUS

Background

Many diseases have a heritable component. Specialist physicians such as geneticists and pediatricians were the ones usually responsible for the complex and sensitive process of conveying specific genetic information to a relatively small number of people who had comparatively rare conditions such as Huntington's disease, Gaucher's disease, or Tay-Sachs disease. Information provision for some heritable cancers has, for example, been primarily on the identification of genetic predisposition, and rarely on specific recommendations for treatment. Before 1990 the provision of this information was usually the responsibility of few members of the health care system, and genetic counseling had been an important but modest portion of any health care budget. These singular services were most often provided in highly specialized clinics, most often within research centers.

However, the search for the genetic mutation of breast and ovarian cancer expanded the number of persons predisposed to a late-onset, potentially lethal disease. The cloning of *BRCA1* in 1993 (1), followed by the development of a blood test for heritable breast/ovarian cancer in 1994 (1), escalated the possibility of widespread genetic testing. The availability of a simple test for *BRCA1* and *-2* signified that general physicians or medical oncologists no longer had to rely solely on a strong family history or link-age analysis to suggest to their patients that they *may* be at increased risk of breast and/or ovarian cancer. Physicians could be more precise about who among their patients may be actually at increased risk of developing the disease sometime over their lifetimes.

As a result of these findings and the identification of the breast and ovarian cancer mutation, the number of persons who could be confirmed as being predisposed to a relatively frequent disease (breast and/or ovarian cancer) has increased exponentially. Over the years, it had been assumed that breast and ovarian cancer account for approximately 45% of all cancer deaths in North America. Of these, approximately 5% to 10% may be genetically linked (2,3).

Testing for heritable female cancers has become a reality, and is generally accessible in a wide range of health care settings. Specifically, testing for breast and ovarian cancer genes and their mutations is currently available in broad research experiments that purport to ensure confidentiality (4), as a public health care service, and from commercial sources (Myrid, Inc., Philadelphia, PA, 1966; Oncormed, Inc., Gaithersburg, MD, 1966). The availability of the test has preceded the development of definitive therapies (5,6).

The identification and cloning of several breast and ovarian cancer genes, the commercial availability of genetic tests, and an increasing public awareness of genetic technologies are factors that, together, have dramatically changed the process of genetic testing in North America. A key transformation has been the dramatic increase in persons seeking this information, and the escalating number of physicians (not necessarily geneticists) who wish to provide this service for their patients. Patients are no longer restricted to asking questions of the limited number of geneticists in research labs. More and more women are asking questions of surgeons, family physicians, medical oncologists, and other physicians who had not previously provided genetic information on a regular basis.

A wider range of specialists are now being asked to provide genetic risk information. At the same time, they often have a limited comprehension of the complexity of this new information (7). Many physicians can easily provide access to a blood test and report the results to the patients. However, many are becoming aware that they have insufficient information or experience with 1) the psychological implications of providing this information and who should be responsible for potential distress; 2) physicians' responsibilities of privacy and confidentiality, and to whom are they primarily responsible; and 3) what should be said to persons identified as being at high risk with regard to follow-up, surveillance, or any medical intervention.

Scientific advances in the genetic identification of breast and ovarian cancer are being noted almost daily in the professional and popular press. They continue to raise the pace of the compelling questions physicians can, should, or may want to respond to. The traditional role of physician as diagnostician, treatment decision maker, and supervisor of treatment for individual patients has not usually included the role of heritable cancer risk information provider (8). The discrepancy between the increasing ability to predict genetic predisposition to female cancers and the comparatively slow evolution of effective interventions raises questions about the role and responsibility of physicians. How will physicians respond to the continuing explosion of scientific information generated in the lab? What do they see as their role and how do others perceive it? This

is one of the most critical questions for physicians in the 1990s.

Physicians have often undertaken responsibilities that have not necessarily received unanimous approval of their peers, or of those outside the profession. For example, such endeavors as promoting cancer prevention, advising on public health problems, or discussing abortion continue to be a topic of heated debate. What role do physicians and society believe doctors could, should, or want to play?

Some contend that physicians are in an ideal position to provide leadership in this area and should be encouraged to do so (9). Yet some researchers strongly disagree, citing the potential "geneticization" of medicine, maintaining that much of the responsibility in cancer genetics should be given to others (e.g., genetic counselors, trained nurse specialists, lay persons, sociologists, psychologists) rather than left exclusively in the medical domain (10). In another example, the related ethical, legal, and social implications of cancer genetic testing are complex, intense, and often inadequately appreciated; physicians are expected to provide leadership in each of these areas. They are asked to consider multiple and often conflicting perspectives simultaneously and integrate them into routine clinical practice. The acquisition and use of information gained through cancer genomic testing are obliging many physicians to make decisions in areas where there is a limited precedent, exceptional controversy, and debate.

The availability to acquire detailed information regarding predisposition to female cancers raises serious questions for the medical profession, while offering few concrete solutions. These decisions are not unique products of cancer genome research; they reflect issues relevant to progress in many biomedical fields. However, the genetic underpinnings of health problems often have stigmatizing connotations, and physicians have traditionally seen themselves as gatekeepers of this information, working with individual patients and families on exceptionally complex, emotional, genetic-related decisions (11).

This has been true in many diseases other than cancer; Tay-Sachs disease, cystic fibrosis, thalassemia, and Huntington's disease are but a few examples. However, predisposition to female cancer affects larger numbers of individuals. The risk is also possible for both those with a strong family history of the disease and those with an ethnically defined risk, regardless of family history (12). The sheer volume of persons that can now be identified as being at increased risk for heritable breast and ovarian cancer from a single blood test changes the task from a narrowly focused dilemma for a few patients who are cared for by a limited number of physicians specialized in these diseases, to a challenge faced by entire populations cared for by physicians from a wide range of specialties, not all of whom have experience, skills, or specific interest in this area. This significant distinction will require immediate attention; addressing this issue is no longer optional, it is essential. The potential for misuse of this once medically dominated information obliges the profession to act quickly to define its role and responsibilities in an era in which the basic science data are changing at a rapid pace.

As well, many physicians face these choices with potentially contentious political implications. Moreover, the choices are made against the backdrop of past experiences—the relatively recent misfortune with sickle cell screening (13) and the possible emergence of a modern eugenics movement (14). This backdrop evokes intense and directive responses regarding what physicians should or should not do; this in the face of limited data on what physicians *are* currently doing, and what role they expect to play. The majority of discussions are currently based on anecdotal evidence, and the stronger arguments come from those already committed to a definite position, some of whom stand to gain from remaining "controllers of the information" (15). While the perspective of consumers who seek cancer genetic risk information is increasingly being investigated, there is limited information published regarding what physicians are actually doing or feeling (16).

For example, in recent days, there has been wide publication of study results suggesting that prophylactic mastectomy and oophorectomy may indeed reduce the lifetime risk by 91%, for those identified as being carriers of *BRCA1* or *BRCA2* and its mutations (17). Does this clarify or obscure the role of the physician? Are these early data to be accepted without question, or do they fly in the face of the lumpectomy issue, which showed that less surgery was as equally effective as more radical surgery? How will physicians answer the questions of young women identified as carriers of *BRCA1* or *-2* mutations, but are still in child-bearing

years and reluctant to have their ovaries removed?

It appears that the role of the physician is unfolding, primarily driven by the rapid evolution of discoveries in the laboratory. How the role will unfold is not yet known, but it is clear that there are key issues to be researched. There are fundamental questions, the answers to which in part determine what position the physician will play as information from the human genome continues to unfold at its rapid pace.

Currently, there is much uncertainty and confusion regarding the role and responsibility of physicians in this rapidly evolving field of breast and ovarian cancer genetics. Time is of the essence, unfortunately, since laboratory science is evolving at an unprecedented rate, and physicians are obliged to act, whether or not they feel they are fully prepared.

What Is the Current Role of Physicians in Cancer Genetics and How Will It Unfold?

The current role of the physician in cancer genetics is evolving alongside the growing number of discoveries made in the lab. Physicians are increasingly screening patients they believe may be at potentially increased risk. This may include relatives of affected persons, especially when a family history reveals many close relatives with breast and/or ovarian and other cancers, especially at a young age. This screening is becoming more and more a part of routine history-taking by family physicians, medical oncologists, and surgeons (18). Often patients are notified that further investigation may be warranted, and if they agree, other members of their family are contacted. It is important to note that unlike the traditional individual doctor–individual patient relationship, the shift is to an entire family, a concept often unfamiliar to the physician and not a part of routine medical education. Even more complex is the physicians' screening of patients ethnically identified as being at potentially increased risk, regardless of family history. Dealing with patients who are not necessarily affected, and whose risk is in fact ethnically determined, is often a unique situation for many clinicians. In these cases, they have little precedent for their actions.

These patients, who may or may not be

affected by the disease, require information to provide them details of their *actual* risk (high, medium, or low) and whether testing is warranted. This process is often unfamiliar to clinicians. Those who work in centers where they can call on or refer to genetic counselors have an opportunity to do so easily. On the other hand, the vast majority of clinicians must choose to provide, or not provide, the information themselves. This is among the most arduous tasks for physicians: how to elicit accurate information and how to handle families in which some members choose to obtain this information while others do not. In addition, it is not always clear how much information to give and to whom, as the information has the potential of disrupting previously cohesive families. This has been particularly noted as a concern among families and cultures that may unconsciously wish to lay blame on the carrier of the genetic mutation. There is little in the literature that addresses the concerns of the information providers (7).

For those patients the clinician believes should be tested, to confirm or repudiate the existence of a genetic mutation, the explanation of the implications of these tests is a long, complex, emotional undertaking. Unlike many other tests for routine medical conditions, the act of testing itself comes with major cautions. Unlike most other tests, genetic testing impacts directly on other members of the family. A positive test has been known to result in denial of health insurance and life insurance and in overt or covert employability discrimination. These potential harms must be carefully explained to each patient, and the clinicians' inability to ensure *absolute* confidentiality of her record adds to the dilemma. In addition, the need to explain the relative accuracy of the test, and the potential for a false positive or false negative, adds to the emotional burden of the discussion. Many of these tasks are relatively unfamiliar to clinicians.

If and when the decision is made to test, and the test results (whether positive or negative) are available, the follow-up is usually equivocal. For those identified as not carrying the specific genetic mutation that was tested for, it does not mean that 1) they do not carry other mutations that simply were not tested for or found due to the less than perfect accuracy of the test or 2) that they will not get the breast or ovarian cancer even if it is not genetically linked. How to follow these low-risk (geneti-

cally speaking) patients is controversial (2). Even more questionable is what to do with patients who prove to be at high risk. Recent data suggest that prophylactic mastectomy/ oophorectomy can reduce the incidence by 91%, but these data remain controversial (17). Increased surveillance is also recommended by many clinicians. However, the effectiveness of increased surveillance apart from possibly helping to reduce patient anxiety is not clear (17). Cancer specialists must be fully informed of the range of issues involved in genetic testing (4). Health care professionals may often feel a compelling responsibility to examine and assess the validity of new genetic tests, but in an era of a constant influx of new information, it is becoming extremely difficult for researchers and clinicians to keep constantly abreast of the implications of the new genetic findings (18). Physicians, in general, are currently unsure as to how to provide the necessary information given the often minimal training and experience in counseling of cancer genetics provided in most medical education (7).

How Do We Study the Evolving Physician Role?

The complexity and uncertainty of the clinician's role and obligation make the researching of physicians who provide cancer risk information of great importance and, at the same time, a major challenge. The initial requirement is to develop a novel framework within which scientists can explore physician attitudes and behavior toward cancer genetic predisposition. Such a framework requires in-depth examination and understanding of the issues face practitioners. The existing literature pro limited guidance. In addition, it is not suff....... to rely on anecdotal or outdated accounts of physician behavior in other types of genetic testing. What is needed is a solid foundation constructed from immediate experiences. Data collection must be comprehensive and responsive to rapid changes in medical genetics; omitting this step could have negative consequences.

An example from other physician behavior research illustrates this point. The lack of sufficient numbers of cancer patients being entered into randomized trials comparing removal of the breast with removal of the lump, with or without radiation to the breast, was initially attributed to patient reluctance to participate (19). It was generally assumed that physician-investigators approached almost all of their eligible patients, asking them to take part in the study. An in-depth investigation of a small group of cancer physicians, however, revealed that many of them had a fundamental discomfort with the entire concept of randomization, and it was the physicians' discomfort, not the patients', that accounted for the majority of the refusals to join the protocol (20). Randomized trials oblige physicians to integrate competing allegiances—on the one hand the needs of their patients and on the other hand the collection of data that may benefit future patients. Many physicians find this a virtually insurmountable obstacle, curtailing the number of patients they might put on any randomized study. Subsequent research on 1800 physician members of a cancer cooperative group confirmed the generalizability of the preliminary findings (21). Such findings challenged existing assumptions about randomized clinical trial participation. Now, interventions to increase patient accrual are most often directed at physicians as well as patients. Without a genuine understanding of accrual to trials, the focus would likely have remained on patients' attitudes and behavior, rather than on those of the physicians.

Appropriate research on physicians and cancer genetics must carefully examine and often attempt to challenge predetermined concepts extracted from apparently similar, but essentially dissimilar, situations. For example, genetic research on disorders such as Huntington's disease and cystic fibrosis has been done with excellent multidisciplinary collaboration by investigative groups in high-risk research clinics of academic centers. These programs have not generally focused on the treating physician outside an academic environment. In contrast with past experience, the cost and burden on the health care system make it unlikely that such highly regarded interdisciplinary efforts can be easily replicated, especially for common diseases such as heritable breast, ovarian, and colon cancer (22). In addition, there are inherent dangers in extrapolating conclusions regarding the role of physicians and cancer genetic testing from their role in other less common heritable disease risks. The Huntington's disease and cystic fibrosis experiences provide important clues to understanding physician response to genetic cancer testing, and their experiences cannot be entirely discounted; the challenge is

to extract what is useful and disregard experiences that will not be helpful.

Another critical issue is the parameters of physician role and responsibility in medicine. Most physicians are accustomed to a "do-something" approach to medicine, and screening and prevention are only recently becoming part of the activities of some physician subspecialties (7). Although geneticists practicing in specialized clinics have been trained in this new area, many family physicians or surgeons have not. The pressure for practicing physicians to conduct new tasks, quite unlike most of their treatment-based work, is increasing. Their response is likely to be one of uncertainty and a feeling that they need more information and education on an ongoing basis. Some physicians may be less than comfortable in this role and accommodation than others. Research can provide significant data from which evidence-based educational interventions can be established and evaluated.

The current role of physicians in cancer genetics is evolving alongside the growing number of discoveries made in genetics research (23). Attempts are being made to integrate genetic testing into routine clinical management of cancer patients and their families, and oncologists and family physicians are being asked to take on new tasks (16). Women in all risk categories are seeking information on their heritable cancer risk status, and therefore the primary care physicians are being asked to assess familial risk factors, to provide individual risk information, and to offer surveillance recommendations (2). The public demand for testing seems to depend on the perception of the potential for a cure (18), and the improved prognosis offered through technological advances in treatment ensures that the number of individuals seeking testing will increase.

To date, genetics have not played a key role in general medical diagnosis or treatment (23). The increasing prominence of genetics in medicine is shifting the medical treatment paradigm and is redefining the physician–patient relationship. Increasingly, the primary care giver not only treats the individual patient, but now must deal with other relatives who may also be concerned about their heritable cancer risk.

Cancer specialists must be fully informed of the range of issues involved in genetic testing (4). Until recently, genetics were not a prominent part of medical education. Furthermore, there are few clear guidelines for heritable cancer genetic information provision, and there is no single consensual framework for physicians to refer to when dealing with these patients and their families. Most health professionals are not well prepared to integrate genetics into their clinical practice at this time (7).

It is increasingly recognized that the approach used to counsel individuals with non-cancer genetic conditions such as Huntington's disease is not necessarily applicable to heritable cancer risk assessment (24). For example, a positive test for Huntington's disease almost guarantees onset of this disease, whereas there may be some potential measures for disease prevention with identification of a cancer-predisposing mutation: the ambiguity presented by the multifactorial (e.g., environmental and heritable factors) etiology of cancer makes genetic counseling for this disease extremely challenging.

The increase in the number of genetic tests means that there is a greater need for heritable cancer risk information provision, which is time consuming and often not cost recoverable (18). The greater number of tests available, the fewer the number of professionals available to deal with the demand. While more specialist personnel will be needed (e.g., genetic counselors, medical geneticists) to attend to the increasing demands for heritable cancer risk information (9), it is suggested that other specialists (e.g., family physicians, medical oncology surgeons) may ultimately be responsible for a large part of heritable cancer risk information provision. They may be well suited for this role because of their existing close relationships with the families.

Physicians must have considerable training in the basic science of genetics and a working knowledge of the implications of having a predisposition to cancer (7). Not all practitioners may be sufficiently prepared for or interested in becoming heritable cancer information providers. One study found that most primary care physicians could answer less than 75% of questions related to genetic concepts and facts required to offer genetic testing and counseling.

The traditional role has been to reduce uncertainty for patients by explaining the meaning of sometimes contradictory evidence, but the purpose of providing heritable cancer risk information is not to reduce uncertainty (11). The goal is usually to educate patients, to facilitate informed decisions, and to promote long-term changes in risk-related health behaviors and surveillance patterns (16).

The enhanced role of physicians in heritable cancer risk information has led to calls for unified recommendations by some medical professional associations. The American Society of Clinical Oncologists, for example, has proposed guidelines for the role of the clinician in this capacity. They proposed that medical oncologist tasks include documenting the family history of cancer in their patients, providing counseling regarding familial cancer risk, and presenting options for prevention and early detection of disease.

Typically, a patient seeking heritable cancer risk information interfaces with the medical oncologist as follows. At the initial physician–patient meeting in clinic, a medical history is obtained, and a family medical history is sought. While practitioners strive to acquire information on as many family members as possible, it is recognized that the accuracy of information on relatives beyond immediate family (e.g., first-degree relatives) can be inaccurate and sketchy. From this information a pedigree or detailed family history is created. A pedigree identifies familial and hereditary tendencies toward heritable cancer (25). Through this activity, high-risk individuals in the family can be identified and perhaps screened (26). Traditionally, detailed pedigrees have been taken by clinical geneticists and genetic counselors, but with the increased demand for genetic information, many types of physician are now expected to have current genetic knowledge and perform these duties. A more complex issue is the physician's screening of patients ethnically identified as being at potentially increased risk, regardless of family history, as is the case with the Ashkenazi Jewish population (27).

Physicians have often served as gatekeepers of information, by helping families make informed decisions about extremely complex and emotional issues. In genetic predisposition doctors must remain sensitive to the sometimes conflicting view points of those seeking testing (11). Many physicians cannot or do not wish to deal with patient anxiety when undergoing genetic testing. Physicians do not always agree on the value of so-called nondirective counseling (18). This method attempts to provide information, explain procedures, and answer questions, without offering the patient specific recommendations. In nondirective counseling, the physician must allow the patients to come to their decisions on their own, without answering typical patient questions such as "what would you do if you were me?" and "what do you think I should do?" Rather, the physician is instructed to present complex information, explain probabilities of disease penetrance, and respond obliquely to questions of "what should I do?" while at the same time providing empathy and support (28). However, recent studies have shown that information given to some women at risk is often fragmented, sometimes inaccurate, occasionally inappropriate, and often unsatisfying (29). Patients believe that information may preserve hope and promote adaptation of relatives to cancer illness. The method assumes that the patients have accurate risk perception and is intended to minimize anxiety and hopelessness, while increasing personal control and predictability (29). However, new evidence suggests that this is not always the case (29).

The physician is viewed as the entry point for patient information, "lump detector," controller of the mammography, reassurer, teacher of breast self-examination, and referrer for other health care providers. Although many believe that family physicians can take on the role of "provider of information on genetic testing" to the growing numbers of women seeking information, advances in medical education must be initiated as quickly as possible (29).

In recognition of the special needs of patients seeking heritable cancer risk information, it appears that physicians who work in multidisciplinary clinics where physicians can consult genetic counselors often do so (30). A multidisciplinary genetics (high-risk) clinic team typically comprises geneticists, medical and surgical oncologists, genetic counselors, oncology nurses, and others (2,31). Each patient is seen by a team of at least three people. The team, which usually includes a physician, strives to provide elaborate education, explanation, implications, intervention, and counseling. The emphasis on comprehensive care arises from the recognition that the heritable disease information screening, testing, and counseling process may have economic and social implications that the individual physician may not feel comfortable providing. Information is provided to ensure the patient knows that positive test results may lead to loss of health and life insurance, employment discrimination, anxiety, depression, and even suicide (32).

As physician involvement in the heritable cancer risk information process becomes more routine, however, and not only restricted to those people at high risk for predisposition to cancer, providing cancer risk information for patients may well become standard health care and not occur in specialized clinics (32). In families that appear to have only a low risk of heritable cancer, genetic testing will likely not proceed. In other families, the pedigree may indicate that the family has a moderate to high risk of heritable cancer. The physician must then begin to advise the patient and her family as to what the options are. Further investigation may be warranted and, if the patient agrees, other family members may be contacted. The patient must be given sufficient information to make adequately informed decisions (28) regarding the risks and benefits of having (or not having) genetic testing done. Even well-adjusted families may suffer terrible strains in their relationships when going through this process (33). Physicians must also outline the issues of confidentiality and the physician's obligation to disclose information in some circumstances, and, in the instance of a positive test, further options. Time constraints, financial limitations, concerns about liability, and low tolerance for diagnostic ambiguity may all impede physicians from giving optimal genetic information.

Providing excellent heritable cancer risk information is a complicated procedure. Genetic screening may help determine heritable cancer risk, but it may also bring with it adverse psychological and social outcomes for the patient (12). With few strong data from which to work, clinicians are beginning to make recommendations regarding cancer screening and, in some cases, prophylactic oophorectomy or mastectomy to women with gene mutations. Physicians may assume that women from high-risk families may be more inclined to want prophylactic surgical procedures (mastectomy, oophorectomy). Tumors may still develop in residual tissues, and the psychological ramifications of this type of radical surgery may be extremely damaging. The option of the increased surveillance is also recommended by many clinicians; however, the effectiveness of increased surveillance apart from possibly helping to reduce patient anxiety has not been confirmed (33).

Research into the evolving role of the physician in cancer genetics is needed urgently to provide data. Evidence from a multitude of effective interventions must be established and evaluated as soon as possible if physicians are to play a key role in enhancing the promise of the Human Genome Project.

REFERENCES

1. Cannon-Albright LA, Skolnick MH. The genetics of familial breast cancer. *Semin Oncol* 1996; 23(suppl 2):1–5.

2. Hoskins KF, Stopfer JE, Calzone A, et al. Assessment and counseling for women with a history of breast cancer: a guide for clinicians. *JAMA* 1995;273:577–585.

3. Goulet RJ. Breast cancer genetics: family history, heterogeneity, molecular genetic diagnosis, and genetic counselling. *Curr Probl Cancer* 1996; Nov/Dec: 331–362.

4. Baron RH, Borgen PI. Genetic susceptibility for breast cancer: testing and primary prevention options. *Oncol Nursing Forum* 1997;24(3):461–468.

5. Parker SL, Tong T, Bolden S, Wingo PW. Cancer Statistics, 1997. *CA-A Cancer J Clinicians* 1997;47:5–27.

6. National Cancer Institute of Canada. Canadian cancer statistics, 1997. Toronto: Statistics Canada, 1997.

7. Pyeritz RE. Family history and genetic risk factors. *JAMA* 1997;278:1284–1285.

8. Whittaker LA. The implications of the Human Genome Project for family practice. *J Fam Pract* 1992;35:294–301.

9. Collins FS. Preparing health professionals for the genetic revolution. *JAMA* 1997;278:1285–1286.

10. Lippman A. Led (astray) by genetic maps: the cartography of the human genome and health care. *Soc Sci Med* 1992;35:1469-1476.

11. Taylor KM, Kelner MJ. The emerging role of the physician in genetic counselling and testing for heritable breast, ovarian, and colon cancer. *Can Med Assoc J* 1996;154:1155–1277.

12. Struewing JP, Lerman C, Kase RG, et al. Anticipated uptake and impact of genetic testing in hereditary breast and ovarian cancer families. *Cancer Epidemiol Biomarkers Prevent* 1995;4: 169–173.

13. Markel H. The stigma of disease: implications of genetic screening. *Am J Med Genet* 1992;93: 209–215.

14. Annas GJ, Elias S, eds. *Gene mapping: using law and ethics as guides.* New York: Oxford University Press, 1992.

15. Garver KL, Garver B. Eugenics: past, present, and the future. *Am J Hum Genet* 1991;49:1109–1118.

16. Lerman C, Croyle RT. Emotional and behavioral responses to genetic testing for susceptibility to cancer. *Oncology* 1996;10:191–199.

17. Schrag D, Kuntz KM, Garber JE, Weeks JC. Decision analysis—effects of prophylactic mastectomy and oophorectomy on life expectancy among women with *BRCA1* or *BRCA2* mutations. *N Engl J Med* 1997;336:1465–1471.

18. Macdonald KG, Doan B, Kelner M, Taylor KM. A sociobehavioural perspective on genetic testing and counselling for heritable breast, ovarian, and colon cancer. *Can Med Assoc J* 1996;154:457–464.

19. Spodick DH. Randomized controlled clinical trials: the behavioural case. *JAMA* 1982;247: 2258–2260.

20. Taylor KM. Decision difficult: breast cancer physicians [doctoral thesis]. McGill University, Montreal, 1986.

21. Taylor KM, Feldstein M, Skeel R, et al. Fundamental dilemmas with physician participation in randomized clinical trials. *J Clin Oncol* 1994; 12:1796–1806.

22. Biesecker BB, Boehnke M, Calzone K, et al. Genetic counseling for families with inherited susceptibility to breast and ovarian cancer. *JAMA* 1993;269:1970–1974.

23. Palmer SE, Stephens K. From the clinic to the research laboratory: the role of the clinician in molecular genetic studies. *Arch Dermatol* 1993; 129:1424–1429.

24. Julian-Reynier C, Lisinger R, Vennin P, et al: Attitudes towards cancer predictive testing and transmission of information to the family. *J Med Genet* 1996;33:731–736.

25. Narod SA, Madlensky L, Bradley L, et al. Hereditary and familial ovarian cancer in southern Ontario. *Cancer* 1994;74:2341–2346.

26. Lancaster JM, Wiseman RW, Berchuck A. An inevitable dilemma: prenatal testing for mutations in the *BRCA1* breast-ovarian cancer susceptibility gene. *Obstet Gynecol* 1996;87:306–309.

27. Berman DB, Costalas J, Schultz DC, et al. A common mutation in *BRCA2* that predisposes to a variety of cancers is found in both Jewish Ashkenazi and non-Jewish individuals. *Cancer Res* 1996;56:3409–3414.

28. Dickens BM, Pei N, Taylor KM. Legal and ethical issues in genetic testing and counselling for susceptibility to breast, ovarian, and colon cancer. *Can Med Assoc J* 1996;154:813–818.

29. Chalmers K, Thomson K, Degner LF. Information, support, and communication needs of women with a family history of breast cancer. *Cancer Nursing* 1996;19(3):204–213.

30. Bombard AT, Fields AL, Aufox S, Ben-Yishay M. The genetics of ovarian cancer: an assessment of current screening protocols and recommen-dations for counseling families at risk. *Clin Obstet Gynecol* 1996;39:860–872.

31. Peters JA, Biesecker BB. Genetic counseling and hereditary cancer. *Am Cancer Soc* 1997;80: 576–586.

32. Nelson C. Must doctors become genetic coun-sellors? *J Nat Cancer Inst* 1994;86:1574–1576.

33. Croyle RT, Achilles JS, Lerman C. Psychologic aspects of cancer genetic testing. *Cancer* 1997; 80(suppl):569–575.

CHAPTER 42

Sexual Rehabilitation in Gynecologic Oncology

A. DENNY DEPETRILLO
LESLEE J. THOMPSON

*S*exual dysfunction is not a rare occurrence in the gynecologic patient. According to the literature, 75% of all women experience sexual difficulties during their lifetime, with sexual dysfunction affecting 50% of all couples in a stable relationship (1,2). These sexual problems go unrecognized and untreated because the patient is reluctant to discuss the pertinent issues or the health-care team has constraints in terms of time or knowledge. Although a woman's view of her sexuality is shaped from her past experience, cultural attitudes, and identity of herself, gynecologic cancer increases the number of women who become sexually inactive, compared to the number of women without cancer (3). Unfortunately, when a gynecologic cancer is added to the problem, up to 90% of women will report some form of sexual dysfunction (2,4). Although sexuality should invoke images of life, love, pleasure, and energy, and cancer invokes images of pain, suffering, darkness, and death, there are numerous misconceptions around linking the concept of punishment and pain to etiologic aspects of sexual problems and cancer. In fact, "sex is one of the very few human issues clouded with as much ignorance and taboo as cancer" (5). Myths regarding cancer and sexuality should be addressed and appropriate information conveyed to the patient and her partner, to lessen the impact of adverse sexual consequences.

When women are diagnosed with gynecologic cancer, their reported decrease in sexual activity and satisfaction may be due in part to misconceptions held about the relationship of past sexual activity and the onset of cancer.

Some patients fear they will transmit the cancer to their partner (6); others claim that they received little or no information to help them prepare or adjust to these problems (7). Much is known about the physiologic and psychological impact of gynecologic cancer on sexuality and sexual function; however, application of that knowledge into clinical practice is limited. Our challenge is to balance the attention to the disease and its treatment with the ever-changing complex needs of the person who is living with that disease and the effects of its treatment.

Quality of life issues for the gynecologic cancer patient have been the subject of increasing research in the past few years. However, the overall impact of cancer needs to be assessed not only in terms of the magnitude of emotional, physical, social, and sexual changes, but also in terms of the patient's perceived and actual ability to compensate for and cope with these changes. The outcome of cancer treatment cannot be viewed simply as the presence or absence of disease and 5-year survival statistics. To date, the focus of research and clinical practice has been on the extension of disease-free intervals, manifestation of disease response, and shifting the survival curve "to the right" (8). Survival is typically measured in terms of the number of years added to a patient's life, although the quality of that life, regardless of the number of years involved, is rarely addressed. It is our belief that the treatment goals of cancer care need to be redefined to integrate the concept of survival in terms of "life to years," not just "years to life." The driving force of cancer care is rehabilitation—the rebuilding of life, hope, and sense of survival. Rehabilitation must be given the same priority in the planning of care, allocation of resources, and treatment of people with cancer, as the more traditional aspects of medical therapy. To achieve sexual rehabilitation, the entire spectrum of human sexuality must be addressed. That means viewing the patient as a vital being worthy of love and affection, despite the devastations perceived such as barriers of age, marital status, type of disease, prognosis, or religion. Sexual health goes beyond the intercourse of penis and vagina; it encompasses the needs for physical comfort, tenderness, affection, and love that are within each of us from birth to death. The assessment of the unique needs and desires of each patient requires sensitivity and skill on the part of the health-care team. Interventions must be tailored to these individual needs and integrated into the overall plan of care.

The Research on Assessment of Sexual Function and the Impact of Gynecologic Cancer

It is difficult to evaluate the reported studies on the assessment of sexual function in cancer patients. There are differences in the logical design, outcome variability, and end results. In her excellent review of different multidimensional scales of assessment, Cull (9) concluded that there is no brief, well-researched, self-reported measure on sexual function that can be recommended for use in its entirety in cancer clinical trials. However, with the various available scales and quality of life questionnaires it is possible to construct a measure appropriate to both sexes by incorporating a small number of questions concerning specific dysfunctions that are gender, disease, or treatment specific.

Nevertheless, several reports in the literature tend to address the psychosocial/psychosexual impact of gynecologic cancer. Roberts et al (10) found that patients treated for gynecologic cancer with surgery reported a good quality of life. Their scores reflected moderately elevated levels of psychological distress that were comparable to levels in breast cancer patients who had participated in an earlier study. However, the authors found a strong negative correlation between age and psycho-

logical distress; younger patients appeared to be more at risk for problems than did older patients after radical gynecologic surgery. On the contrary, Corney et al (11) reported that 66% of patients who had radical surgery for gynecologic cancer had problems more than 6 months later and 15% never resumed intercourse. Eighty-two percent of those younger than 50 years who had radiotherapy had sexual dysfunction. Lack of desire was the most common problem and half of the women felt that their sexual relationship had deteriorated (11). Krumm and Lamberti (12) found that women who undergo radiation therapy for cervical cancer experience a deterioration in their sexual interest and activity. There was a high degree of noncompliance that was not necessarily attributable to radiation alone, but to underlying psychosexual concerns that antedated the diagnosis of disease (12). These authors designed a sexual behavior questionnaire for patients undergoing radiation therapy with a formalized patient education program. The reader is also referred to the review by Dobkin and Bradley (13) on the assessment of sexual dysfunction in oncology patients and their proposed test battery and interview.

Issues Related to Evaluation and Management

The rest of this chapter provides an overview of the existing issues regarding sexuality and sexual function for the patient with gynecologic malignancy and offers practical suggestions around effective assessment, communication, and intervention when dealing with sexual issues and concerns of cancer patients.

The earliest concerns for sexual problems of cancer patients were expressed in articles written in 1952 focusing on adaptation to radical mastectomy and colostomy (14,15). Issues relating to the emotional response in body changes, changes in sexual response patterns, and disruptions to sexual activity in marital relations were all discussed. However, research in this area was severely flawed, particularly in the areas of design and interpretation of study results. It is through the efforts of Andersen et al (16), Schover (17), and Auchincloss (18) that the evaluation and management of sexual dysfunction after treatment of gynecologic cancer and other cancer types have been emphasized.

In order to assess the dimension of the problem completely, the health-care professional must be aware that these problems do not differ in principle from the sexual difficulties of many healthy women. Therefore, an understanding of both the normal aspects of female sexuality and sexual problems, as well as of the physical and psychological dimensions of the cancer experience, is necessary. One must also be aware of the biases regarding sexuality that are present in our society. The "body beautiful" concept bombards each of us through the media every day. Through heightened attention to fabulous breasts, hair, smell, and other body parts, we are led to believe that the achievement, possession, and use of a beautiful body is the key to success, happiness, and life itself. This provides a benchmark not only from which some women come to measure themselves and their self-worth, but also for those who believe that the image is what women truly want. Surgeons involved with neovaginal reconstruction are sometimes enthralled more with the surgical technique rather than the true assessment of the quality of life following that surgery. The assumption that intercourse is essential for sexual rehabilitation is another bias. A review of the literature on vaginal reconstruction revealed that the majority of the papers deemed the mere presence of a vaginal "receptacle" and the fact that the patient had intercourse following surgery were indeed indicative of sexual rehabilitation (19,20). Patient satisfaction, pleasure, and self-image were not addressed.

There is a growing body of research examining the relationship between cancer and self-concept. A widely accepted definition of self-concept is "the sum total of all that a person feels about himself/herself" (21). Sexuality, body image, and femininity are all dimensions of this global sense of self, and therefore cannot be separated out from it. There is increasing recognition that the definition of one's self and how that is projected to others will vary over time, depending on the circumstances at hand. For women with cancer, we have observed that the patient's attention to sexuality issues changes over time, depending on the phase of their illness experience.

Through the diagnosis and treatment of the disease, the patient is concerned with mortality issues as well as issues in self-perception. She will rely on members of the health-care team for advice, support, and information that should be available. There is sufficient information available to implement programs focused on the prevention and resolution of sexual problems that surface within the cancer experience. However, educational programs have not kept pace with this information and new practitioners are ill-prepared to deal with this. Because of a gap in attention to such issues, few role models exist for students and seasoned practitioners.

When polled about their reasons why sexual concerns were not dealt with as part of their daily practice, members of health-care teams identified a variety of responses, as outlined in Table 42-1. Personal discomfort in dealing with the issues was exemplified through comments such as "none of our business," "too embarrassed," "afraid I won't have the right answer," and "uncomfortable with non-scientific language." With these types of personal barriers set up, it is easy to rationalize further that if the patient does not bring up the topic of sex or sexuality, then the caregiver needs not assume any responsibility for assessing this issue further. Research has shown, however, that patients do expect physicians, or another health-care team member, to bring up the subject first, thus giving permission to discuss these concerns (7,22). In one study (7), 56% of

T A B L E   **42-1**

Psychosexual Concerns—Why Clinicians' Hesitancy?

Issue is too private, none of our business
Too embarrassed
Afraid to be misinterpreted, or give wrong information
Patient will be angry for bringing up this topic when she is sick
Afraid won't have the right answer to her "nonmedical" questions
Patient too old, not sexually active right now, or doesn't have a partner
Afraid to deal with potential that patient is not heterosexual, or prefers "different" way of getting sexual pleasure
Nowhere to refer patient if problem surfaces
No time
Uncomfortable with nonscientific language
Not enough privacy
Not enough formal "how to" preparation for talking about these issues, no role models
Uncomfortable personally with these issues
Not a priority in light of "everything else"

the patients surveyed wanted more information than was given to them, and 79% of those people said that they would not ask the physician for more information themselves. Further analysis of this situation would probably reveal that education about dealing with sexual issues and concerns needs to happen at the consumer level as well as the health-care provider level.

Annon (23) proposed a model of dealing with sexual issues and concerns that outlines four levels of intervention. Each level requires more skill and experience on the part of the practitioner, and reflects more in-depth work with the patient. The model recognizes that very few people actually require intensive sexual therapy. In fact, the needs of patients can almost always be met by providing an atmosphere of comfort and permission to talk about issues regarding sexuality. Then, by providing some basic information, problems can be prevented, or be made easier to cope with. It is essential that in a multidisciplinary approach model such as this, a member of the team be identified as the person responsible for discussing sexual issues. This need not be a physician, and in fact our program involves a nurse who specializes in talking to patients about such concerns. Communication among team members around who has talked to the patient, what was said, and what the patient's response was is also important in enhancing overall continuity of care.

The role and contribution of the patient's partner in successful sexual rehabilitation has been under discussion for some time. Many people believe that an informed and supportive partner is critical (24). Involving both the patient and her partner in the discussions about upcoming treatment and its impact helps prepare both people at the same time so that they are at a similar level of understanding right from the start.

Anticipatory Guidance

The more patients understand and know prior to their treatment, the more in control they will feel of their responses after treatment. There are eight steps that can be easily followed in helping to prepare for coping with gynecologic cancer and its treatment (Table 42-2). First, determine the patient's perception about the current situation. What do they understand about their illness and what meaning have they

TABLE 42-2

Anticipatory Guidance

1. Patient's perception of the situation.
2. Biggest concern? Fear?
3. Myths and misconceptions.
4. What to expect before, during, and after.
5. Provide ongoing opportunities for open, honest communication.
6. Facilitate reality-based expectations, and a philosophy of hope.
7. Keep avenues of support open with different members of the health-care team.
8. Referral as needed.

attributed to it? Finding out that a patient feels the cancer is a punishment for promiscuous sexual behavior will be important in the planning of supportive care for that patient.

The second step is determining the patient's biggest concern or fear right now. The patient who is thinking about the possibility of dying as a result of her surgery will not be ready to talk about resuming sexual activity 6 weeks later.

Concerns and fears of the person with cancer may change over time, depending on the surrounding circumstances. No one has tracked the changing perceptions of the sexual needs of women with gynecologic cancer over time as they relate to their physical and psychosocial needs, although this would be a very fruitful area for research. Clinicians often ask when the "best" time to talk about sexual concerns is, given the fact that their patient is also coping with a diagnosis of cancer and its treatment. It is important to address these issues prior to treatment, for although attention may not be focused on this right away, dealing with sexual issues and concerns becomes more meaningful to the patient once the uncertainty about the effects of immediate treatment is reduced. By setting the stage for discussion of sexual issues before treatment, the patient will feel more comfortable talking with the clinician about them afterward.

Clarifying myths and misconceptions about cancer, its treatment, and the effects of both on the body is also critical to helping enhance the patient's ability to cope. Many people are afraid to even acknowledge how they think things might be for fear of being seen as silly or misinformed, and worse yet, the person may not even question some of the things he or she has heard under the assumption that this was indeed the truth. Two approaches may be helpful in this situation. One is to ask the patient whether she or her family has heard anything about the illness or its treatment from others that she would like to clarify with the clinician. This allows the patient some comfort in her ability to make the "others" who might have told her something responsible for the issue being brought forward, and take the onus of thinking about it off of herself. Secondly, if the clinician suspects that the patient may be harboring some questions that have not been brought out, the clinician could use third person to say, for example, "Some people think that having sexual relations while on radiation therapy is dangerous to her partner; however, we know that the effects of radiation cannot be transmitted from one person to the next, through general or intimate contact." With this approach, the patient does not need to even ask the question, which in certain situations may be a big relief for the patient.

Describing for the patient what she can expect before, during, and after treatment or a procedure is also useful in helping her feel more in control of her situation. Research has shown that by providing information that not only outlines the sequence of events, but also explains how the person may feel, best facilitates retention of that information.

Identifying both structural and functional changes that can be expected after treatment and letting patients know what they can do to manage these changes can also help enhance sexual rehabilitation. Diagrams, three-dimensional models, and simple analogies can help clarify the meaning of "before" and "after" effects of treatment. Often a former patient can provide a personal perspective of the treatment experience and rehabilitative process.

Keeping the avenues of support open with different members of the health-care team is also an important strategy in helping patients prepare for and cope with their cancer experience. Fostering dependency on one individual can have negative ramifications for the patient. No one person can meet all of the complex needs of people with cancer, and each member of the health team, by virtue of their own professional perspective and personal style, has something unique to offer. Often treatment involves different modalities, and maintaining good communication among all team members is critical. We have found that multidisciplinary

patient rounds are a good forum for talking and learning from each other ways of communicating more effectively with patients about sexuality, body image, and general self-esteem.

Tricks of the Trade

When talking to patients and their partners about sexuality before or after treatment, we have found the following principles useful in guiding the discussion. These are outlined in Table 42-3. An atmosphere of comfort is paramount in obtaining the patient's confidence. Initial discussions should be held together with the patient and her partner in a room that ensures privacy and confidentiality. Asking the patient if she has any sexual concerns when the clinician and five others are standing at the foot of the bed during morning rounds is obviously not an appropriate strategy. Sitting down, talking or listening to the patient even for a short period of time can be highly effective, to clearly demonstrate concern for her and her situation.

If a sexual history is required, beginning with the least sensitive questions is important in helping to reduce anxiety and to maximize comfort in talking about a highly personal and private matter. Letting the patient know why detailed questions need to be asked helps the patient feel comfortable in providing the information needed. For example, the following statement might be used: "I would like to ask you some more specific questions about how you and your body are feeling before, during, and after intercourse, to get a clearer picture of

T A B L E 42-3
Tricks of the Trade

1. Create an atmosphere of comfort for self and patient.
2. Begin with least sensitive questions.
3. Pair questions with rationale.
4. Move from general to specific.
5. Move from past to present.
6. Ask when and how often, instead of "do you."
7. Use third person to introduce questions, e.g., "most people."
8. Prepare question with a statement that validates a range of normalcy.
9. Refer to how often an experience occurs in others.
10. Listen, observe, and maintain a sensitive, nonjudgmental attitude.

why the symptoms you have are occurring." Phrasing questions in a way that moves from the more general to the specific is also helpful. For example: "Radiation affects your body in a variety of different ways. Have you noticed any changes in your ability to enjoy sexual relations?"

Recognizing that the present time is highly stressful for the patient, moving the discussion from the past to the present can ease the person into discussions about sexual problems. "Tell me about how you were feeling before the cancer, and how that has changed over time." Other principles that underlie effective communication with patients about sexuality are captured in the following questions. "Many women undergoing this type of surgery have questions or concerns about what it feels like sexually afterwards. Is this an area of concern to you?" Using the third person to introduce questions lets the patient know that she is not alone and that the health-care team appreciates the fact that this is an area that might be of concern to her too. This establishes not only a sense of normalcy for the patient, but also an ability for the patient to talk about these issues with the health-care team. Finally, listening, observing, and maintaining a sensitive, nonjudgmental attitude is absolutely essential. Noting changes over time, and dealing with them in an open and honest way can significantly enhance the overall sexual rehabilitation of the patient.

Sexual Adjustment

When considering sexual rehabilitation, it is important to be aware of the sexual relationship of the patient before treatment. Andersen et al (16) hypothesized, however, that because some people have never had to cope with any type of sexually related problem, they may in fact be more at risk for difficulties because they may have fewer coping skills to draw on, especially if the problems are severe and persistent. The onset of sexual difficulties for women with cancer is typically acute, appearing in the immediate posttreatment phase. The woman may anticipate how such difficulties will make her or her partner feel and actually avoid any sexual encounters, or the problem (e.g., dyspareunia) may be experienced once intercourse or other activity is resumed. Some people will have long-term underlying problems that become exacerbated throughout the cancer experience. If the

relationship was problematic before cancer, the same pattern is likely to continue afterward. The emergence of a highly dysfunctional relationship as a result of the cancer itself is unlikely. Some people actually experience a strengthening of the existing relationship, and others have the confidence to develop a new one.

In working with gynecologic cancer patients, we have learned that despite radical treatment and the experience of distressing symptoms, a positive sexual rehabilitation is possible for the majority of women. Rehabilitation does not always mean a resumption of pretreatment sexual activity, but may involve a heightened awareness of one's capacity for intimacy through alternative expressions of sexuality. A motivated and informed patient or couple can overcome the challenges imposed by this disease and its treatment. A knowledgeable and sensitive health-care team can help ease the transition from diagnosis, through treatment, and afterward, so that a healthy sense of sexuality and self-confidence is maintained by the patient. In this way, the overall quality of life for women with gynecologic cancer may be enhanced.

REFERENCES

1. Halvorsen J. Sexual dysfunction—diagnosis, management and prognosis. *J Am Board Fam Pract* 1992;5:117–192.
2. Andersen BL, Turnquist DC. Psychological issues. In: Berek JS, Hacker NF, eds. *Practical gynecologic oncology.* Baltimore: Williams & Wilkins, 1989:631–660.
3. Bachmann G, Ayers C. Psychosexual gynecology. *Med Clin North Am* 1995;79:1299–1317.
4. Mooradian A, Greiff V. Sexuality in older women. *Cancer* 1990;150:1033–1038.
5. van Eschenbach AC, Schover LR. Sexual rehabilitation of cancer patients. In: Gunn AE, ed. *Cancer rehabilitation.* New York: Raven, 1984: 155–173.
6. Andersen BL. Yes there are sexual problems; now what can we do about them? *Gynecol Oncol* 1994;52:10–19.
7. Vincent CE, Vincent B, Greiss FG, Linton EB. Some marital-sexual concomitants of carcinoma of the cervix. *South Med J* 1975;68:552–558.
8. DePetrillo AD, Thompson LJ. Care of the patient with ovarian cancer: a quality of life per-

spective. In: Sharp F, Mason WP, Leake RE, eds. *Ovarian cancer: biological and therapeutic challenges.* London: Chapman and Hall Medical, 1989:315–322.

9. Cull A. The assessment of sexual function in cancer patients. *Eur J Cancer* 1992;28:1680–1686.

10. Roberts C, Rossetti K, Cine D, Cavanagh D. Psychosocial impact of gynecologic cancer. A descriptive study. *J Psychosoc Oncol* 1992;10:99–109.

11. Corney RH, Crowther ME, Everett H, et al. Psychosexual dysfunction in women with gynecological cancer following radical pelvic surgery. *Br J Obstet Gynaecol* 1993;100:73–78.

12. Krumm S, Lamberti J. Changes in sexual behavior following radiation therapy for cervical cancer. *J Psychosom Obstet Gynaecol* 1993;14:51–63.

13. Dobkin PL, Bradley I. Assessment of sexual function in oncology patients: review critique and suggestions. *J Psychosoc Oncol* 1991;9:43–74.

14. Bard M, Sutherland AM. Adaptation to radical mastectomy. *Cancer* 1952;8:656.

15. Sutherland AM, Orbach CF, Dyk RB, Bard M. The psychological impact of cancer and cancer surgery. I: adaptation to the drug colostomy. *Cancer* 1952;5:857.

16. Andersen BL, VanderDoes J, Anderson B. Sexual morbidity following gynecologic cancer. Conceptualization, description and prevention.

In: Coppleson M, Monaghan J, Morrow P, Tattersall M, eds. *Gynecologic oncology.* Edinburgh: Churchill Livingstone, 1992.

17. Schover LR. The impact of breast cancer on sexuality, body image and intimate relationships. *CA Cancer J Clin* 1991;41:112–120.

18. Auchincloss S. Psychosocial issues in gynecologic cancer survivorship. *Cancer* 1995; 76(suppl):2117–2124.

19. DePetrillo AD, Thompson LJ. Use of the amnion graft for vaginal reconstruction in gynecologic oncology. Abstract presented at the annual meeting of the Western Association of Gynecologic Oncologists, 1989.

20. Chamberlain G, Parker Y, Dewhurst DJ. Sexual activity after treatment of carcinoma of the cervix. *J Obstet Gynecol* 1986;6:281–283.

21. Curbow B, Somerfield M, Legro M, Sonnega J. Self concept and cancer in adults: theoretical and methodological issues. *Soc Sci Med* 1990;31:115–128.

22. Bullard D, Causey G, Newman A, et al. Sexual health care and cancer: a needs assessment. *Front Radiat Ther Oncol* 1980;14:51–54.

23. Annon J. *Behaviorial treatment of sexual problems: brief therapy.* Hagerstown, MD: Harper and Row, 1976.

24. Lamont J, DePetrillo AD, Sargeant EJ. Psychosexual rehabilitation and exenterative surgery. *Gynecol Oncol* 1978;6:236–242.

CHAPTER *43*

Quality of Life in Women with Cancer

ANDREA BEZJAK

Quality of life (QOL) is a term that is gaining increasing prominence in the field of oncology. It is frequently used in the context of clinical trials (1), in clinical decision making (2), as well as by the patients and cancer survivors (3). Although the 1990s have witnessed an exponentially increasing bibliography on QOL (4), it is by no means a new term or concept. In 1948 Karnofsky and Burchenal (5) described assessment of functional status of cancer patients treated with palliative chemotherapy (nitrogen mustard). Around the same time, the World Health Organization issued its definition of health, as "...a state of complete physical and mental wellbeing, and not just absence of disease and infirmity..." (6). This definition does not confine health to its biomedical model, rooted in anatomy, pathology, and physiology, but takes into account psychological and functional well-being in addition to physical well-being.

There are several reasons why interest and research in QOL in oncology have increased since the early 1980s. Firstly, treatment of cancer has become more aggressive, and cancer patients live longer. In many instances, cancer has become a chronic disease, with several treatment options available, all of which impact significantly on patients' physical, emotional, and functional well-being. Secondly, behavioral research and tools have become recognized as useful, and have gained a place in medicine, bridging the gap between social sciences (psychology, sociology) and medicine. Thirdly, at least in the Western world, patients are getting more involved in treatment decisions about their health, necessitating a patient-based approach, emphasizing functional ability and overall impact on the person, rather than the traditional organ-based or even the more modern problem-based approach to medicine.

Definition of Quality of Life

Quality of life is a term that is familiar and intuitively understood by most people, but may mean different things to many people. Philosophers and ethicists may never reach agreement on the full spectrum and meaning of this broad term. For research purposes, a number of operational (working) definitions have been formulated. These operational definitions describe what those researchers mean by the term; implicit is an understanding that QOL may be a broader concept than what they have included in their definition. Calman (7), for example, defined QOL as "the extent to which a person's hopes and ambitions are matched and fulfilled by experience." Ferrans (8) described it as referring to "a person's sense of wellbeing that stems from satisfaction or dissatisfaction with areas of life that are important to him/her." de Haes (9) stated that "QOL is the subjective evaluation of life as a whole."

Because of the broad scope of these definitions, and many factors other than health that can influence QOL, within the field of medicine the concept of QOL is commonly restricted to refer to health-related quality of life. One report (10) defined this as "including psychologic and social functioning as well as physical functioning and incorporating positive

610

aspects of wellbeing as well as negative aspects of disease and infirmity." Other operational definitions in the literature are similar but may emphasize different aspects, such as ". . . patients' appraisal of and satisfaction with their current level of functioning compared to what they perceive to be possible or ideal . . ." (11). The term *health-related quality of life* thus more accurately describes the majority of QOL research in oncology, which centers on the effect of cancer and cancer treatment on a patient. Despite that, most of the medical literature has not yet adopted the term; the remainder of the chapter therefore uses the generic *QOL* in its restricted meaning of health-related QOL.

What most definitions of QOL agree on is the multidimensional nature of QOL. It is more than just the person's performance status, or physical well-being, or psychological well-being—it is a combination of all those and many other dimensions, such as social functioning, role functioning, spirituality, sexuality, body image, and other aspects that contribute to their QOL. It is this multidimensional aspect of QOL that sets QOL apart from measures of performance status or emotional well-being.

Is Quality of Life Measurable?

One of the major perceived barriers to widespread acceptance of QOL assessment in medicine is the misconception that QOL is a vague subjective concept that cannot be measured (12). This view is voiced frequently, although studies do not universally document it. A survey of 621 oncology nurses in the United States (13) revealed that 42% of nurses felt that there was no way to objectively quantify QOL. In contrast, 78% of U.S. physicians who responded to another survey (14) thought it was possible to measure QOL. Similarly, in each of several phases of a project to describe oncologists' views on QOL, colleagues and I (15–17) documented the belief of Canadian, U.S., and international oncologists that QOL can be defined, quantified, and measured. This research is ongoing to determine whether these findings are generalizable beyond the selected sample of physicians included in these studies (18).

A number of arguments can be given to illustrate the scientific validity of quantifying and measuring QOL. The main argument is the vast experience gained by social scientists in measuring other "vague subjective concepts" such as intelligence and attitude. Who of us does not remember being subjected to at least one of such tests during our years of education? Decades of research have accumulated a lot of evidence of the ability to measure such concepts. Another argument derives from comparison of such "soft subjective" data to "objective and accurate" measures, such as tumor size and response rate. Although we tend to rely on the latter measures, and often base major decisions on them, there is convincing evidence for their inaccuracy, in view of great interobserver and intraobserver variations in clinical or radiologic measurement of tumor size (19). These inaccuracies translate into uncertainties in recording response rates in studies. Even survival data are not immune from errors in measurement; cause-specific survival is especially prone to bias as the diagnosis of cancer at some point in one's life almost inevitably leads to it assuming a prominent position on the death certificate of that patient. Finally, the subjective nature of QOL is its strength rather than weakness—it reflects the experiences that only a patient with cancer can know about and judge. Rather than relying on "objective" toxicity scales that may record the level of hematologic parameters as a measure of treatment toxicity (a measure that is only indirectly relevant to patients, by causing a reduction in treatment intensity and thus minimizing the risk of significant complications), a QOL scale directly reflects the relevant experience of a patient. Besides, for many important effects of cancer and its treatment, there are no good and easily quantifiable proxy measures. An excellent example is pain; a subjective assessment of the patient experiencing pain is the gold standard of measuring pain.

In summary, QOL is a concept that is quantifiable and measurable, but it is important that researchers and clinicians specify what they mean by the term QOL. It is no more prone to inaccurate measurement than many other end points used in oncology, and may be of greater relevance to patients.

Methodology of Assessment

Considerable progress has been made in the last 15 years in measuring QOL. A number of methodologic issues have been clarified, including how, who, and when to measure QOL; how to develop QOL questionnaires and what properties they should possess; and how to validate QOL questionnaires.

How to Measure Quality of Life

QOL can be evaluated through interviews with patients, or through administration of questionnaires. Interviews provide in-depth information but require considerable time. They need to be structured (i.e., to follow a script or list of questions) and need to be administered by trained personnel in a neutral setting, if they are to accurately assess a subject's QOL. Following the interview the information needs to be transcribed and recorded in a written form, which adds to the time and work needed. Because of these requirements, questionnaires are more commonly utilized; they are usually self-administered. Their advantage is that the subject directly records the answers, that the questions are uniformly posed to all subjects, that the subjects may be more comfortable answering questions of a personal or sensitive nature without the presence of an interviewer, and that the personnel time and therefore cost are reduced. The disadvantage of questionnaires is that they usually only exist in a few languages, which limits the spectrum of subjects and therefore the generalizability of study findings. This is currently a problem in QOL studies; efforts are underway to translate and culturally validate QOL questionnaires (20).

Who Should Measure Quality of Life?

There are several possible sources of information regarding a patient's QOL: the health-care professional (physician or nurse) who is looking after the patient, the patient's family or caregiver, or the patient herself. In medicine we are most accustomed to health-care providers supplying the information, but this information is second-hand (i.e., they need to question the patient if they are to give us an assessment of the patient's experiences); otherwise we have obtained their impression of patients' QOL, which may be biased and inaccurate. Similarly, the assessment obtained from family or caregivers is influenced by how they perceive patient actions and experiences, and thus also are prone to bias. A number of studies have indeed documented discrepancies between observer assessment of a patient's QOL and that patient's own assessment of QOL. To illustrate, Sprangers and Aaronson (21) studied the role

of proxy raters and found that both health-care providers and family members underestimate patients' QOL to a similar degree, including underestimating patients' pain. Similarly, Fossa et al (22) documented that physicians underestimated subjective morbidity (pain, decreased performance status) in 30% to 50% of patients with metastatic prostatic cancer. Moreover, Starr et al (23) showed that physicians' inferior rating of QOL for elderly patients influences their resuscitation orders.

Therefore, the patient's perspective has been accepted as the gold standard of QOL assessment, as it is the individual perception of her QOL that is being assessed. However, this methodology is not without its drawbacks: Some patients may be unable to provide QOL information because of confusion, delirium, or generalized debility. This may be especially common in preterminal stages of the illness. Despite that, successful QOL assessment is possible in the palliative-care setting (24), especially if simple instruments are used, and supplemented by nursing and family observations of patients' mental status changes (25).

When to Measure Quality of Life

In prospective longitudinal QOL studies, QOL should be assessed at baseline, and at time intervals that correspond to significant points in the illness trajectory. For example, when the impact of surgery on a cancer patient's QOL is being assessed, measurements may be done at the following time points: baseline (prior to surgery), soon after surgery (to assess the acute morbidity), a few weeks or months after surgery (to assess possible difficulties recuperating), and at a time when the patient is expected to reach her new baseline. In radiotherapy studies, QOL is usually assessed prior to the start of radiation, at the time of greatest radiation toxicity (e.g., last week of radiation), a few months following radiation (to document extent of recovery from acute side effects), and at one or more time points in the future, when late effects, disease control, or cancer relapse are expected to occur. Depending on the schedule and intent of radiation, these time points will differ. For example, in patients with cervical cancer treated with curative pelvic radiation, the time points chosen may be at baseline, the last week of radiation, the end of brachytherapy, and then 1, 3, 6, 12, 24, 48, and 60 months after radiation. In breast cancer patients who undergo palliative radiation for bone metastases, the appropriate time points may be at baseline, the week following radiation (when toxicity may be maximal), and 1, 3, and 6 months after radiation.

In the instructions to patients that precede most QOL questionnaires, there is often a specified time frame that the patient should consider when giving answers. It may be "during the last day" (e.g., linear analogue scales), "during the last week" [e.g., European Organization for Research and Treatment of Cancer (EORTC), Functional Living Index–Cancer (FLIC)], "during the last month" [e.g., Medical Outcomes Study (MOS) Short Form 36 (SF-36)], or some other time frame. This time frame of a particular QOL instrument may have an impact on the timing of QOL assessment, especially in chemotherapy studies. It is customary to administer the QOL questionnaire just prior to the next cycle of chemotherapy, but if the time frame is "last week," and in an every-3-week cycle of chemotherapy the greatest impact on QOL is in week 2, QOL may not be represented by the measurement that pertains to week 3. However, one should not deal with this problem by arbitrarily changing the time frame of the questionnaire, as studies point out that longer time frames (e.g., "last month") may bring out the tendency of a person to complain or minimize problems, whereas a shorter time frame may more accurately reflect the actual experience of that person (26). A study of antiemetics performed by the National Cancer Institute of Canada (NCIC) Clinical Trials Group (27) demonstrated that patients accurately distinguish between a 4-day and 7-day time frame—patients reported more nausea when asked 1 week after chemotherapy how they felt during the last 7 days, than when asked how they felt during the last 4 days.

Types and Examples of Questionnaires

Numerous questionnaires have been developed for assessment of QOL in cancer patients. They are broadly categorized as generic or disease specific. Table 43-1 lists the advantages and disadvantages of these two categories of QOL instruments. Generic questionnaires measure concepts that are relevant to everyone, regardless of age, disease, or treatment groups. The most generic questionnaires have been developed for healthy populations. Examples include MOS SF-36 (28), Nottingham Health Profile (29),

T A B L E   43-1

Characteristics of Generic and Disease-Specific Quality of Life (QOL) Instruments

Generic QOL Instruments	Disease-Specific QOL Instruments
Advantages	
Readily available	Tailor made
Extensively tested for reliability/validity	Focus on question of interest
Applicable to any situation	May be more likely to detect change
Allow comparisons across studies	
Disadvantages	
May not focus on area of interest	Time and effort to design instrument
All questions may not be relevant	Reliability and validity testing neccessary
May not be sensitive to change	Instrument may not be comprehensive
	May not be applicable/ acceptable to others
	Cannot compare across studies

and Sickness Impact Profile (SIP) (30). Disease-specific measures, on the other hand, have been developed for a specific disease, and are intended to capture the specific effects of the disease on QOL, in addition to some general issues of health-related QOL. They range from cancer-specific questionnaires, such as Cancer Rehabilitation Evaluation System (CARES) (31), FLIC (32), Functional Assessment of Can-cer Therapy–General (FACT-G) (33), EORTC Quality of Life Questionnaire (QLQ)-C30 (QOL questionnaire core) (34); to site-specific questionnaires such as the Breast Cancer Questionnaire (BCQ) (35); to treatment-specific and trial-specific questionnaires. A common approach is to use a core questionnaire that applies to all types of cancer, followed by a trial-specific or site-specific module, such as QLQ-C30 with a breast cancer module (36) or FACT questionnaire with a breast, ovary, or bone marrow transplant module (37).

Table 43-2 lists some of the more commonly used QOL questionnaires in oncology, including the structure and domains (areas) covered, as well as the reference that provides a description of their development or evidence for their validity. The reader who wishes to see the actual questionnaires in this list is referred to the *Oncology* issue edited by Tchekmedyian

TABLE 43-2

Some of the Quality of Life Instruments Used in Oncology

Instrument	References	Population	Dimensions	Items/Format
Cancer Rehabilitation Evaluation System (CARES)	Heinrich et al, 1984 (121); Ganz et al, 1992 (31)	General ca	Phy, Fnc, Fam, Emo, Tre, Sex, Soc, Occ, Tot	139 Likert plus box to check asking for help Self-report
European Organization for Research and Treatment of Cancer Quality of Life Questionnaire (EORTC-QLQ)	Aaronson et al, 1993 (34)	General ca	Phy, Fnc, Fam, Emo, Tre, Soc, Occ, Tot	40+ Likert/yes-no (30 general; 10 or more in disease-specific modules) Self-report
Functional Assessment of Cancer Therapy (FACT)	Cella et al, 1993 (33)	Lung ca, Breast ca, colon ca, general ca, head and neck ca	Phy, Fnc, Fam, Emo, Spi, Tre, Fut, Sex	42+ Likert (33 general; 9 or more disease-specific) Self-report
Functional Living Index–Cancer (FLIC)	Schipper et al, 1984 (32)	General ca	Phy, Fnc, Fam, Emo, Tre, Soc, Occ, Tot	22 Likert/analogue Self-report
Linear analogue self-assessment (LASA)	Priestman and Baum, 1976 (70)	Breast ca, General ca	Phy, Fnc, Fam, Emo, Tre, Soc	25 Analogue Self-report
Linear analogue self-assessment (LASA)	Coates et al, 1983 (122)	General ca	Phy, Emo	5 Analogue Self-report
Linear analogue self-assessment (LASA)	Selby et al, 1984 (72)	Breast ca	Phy, Fnc, Fam, Emo, Sex, Soc, Occ	31 Analogue (18 general; 13 specific) Self-report Observer rated
Medical Outcome Study (MOS) Short-Form General Health Survey	Ware and Sherboburne, 1992 (28)	General illness	Phy, Fnc, Emo, Soc	20 Likert/categorical (MOS) Self-report
Nottingham Health Profile	Hunt et al, 1981 (29)	General illness	Phy, Fnc, Emo, Sex, Soc, Occ	38 Yes-no Self-report
Psychological Adjustment to Illness Scale (PAIS)	Derogatis, 1983 (123)	General illness	Fnc, Fam, Emo, Tre, Fut, Sex, Soc, Occ, Tot	46 Ordered choices Self-report and interview versions
Quality of Life Index (QLI)	Ferrans and Powers, 1985 (124)	General ca	Phy, Fnc, Fam Spi, Fut, Sex Soc, Occ, Tot	64 Likert Self-report
Quality of Life Index (QLI)	Padilla et al, 1983 (125)	General ca	Phy, Fnc, Tre, Sex, Occ, Tot	14 Analogue Self-report
Quality of Life Index (QL-index)	Spitzer et al, 1981 (126)	General ca	Phy, Fnc, Fut, Soc, Tot	5 Ordered choices 1 Confidence rating Observer-rated
Rotterdam Symptom Checklist (RSCL)	de Haes et al, 1990 (40)	Breast ca, Ovarian ca	Phy, Fnc, Emo, Fut, Sex, Tot	30 Symptom items, 8 activity items Likert scale Self-report
Sickness Impact Profile (SIP)	Bergner et al, 1981 (30)	General illness	Phy, Fnc, Fam, Emo, Tre, Sex, Soc, Occ, Tot	136 Yes-no Self-report

Ca = cancer; Phy = physical concerns (e.g., symptoms, pain); Emo = emotional well-being; Sex = sexuality/intimacy (includes body image); Fnc = functional ability (e.g., mobility); Spi = spirituality; Soc = social functioning; Fam = family well-being; Tre = treatment satisfaction (includes financial concerns); Occ = occupational functioning; Fut = future orientation (planning; hope); Tot = total score (i.e., whether items are summed or a global rating is made).

Source: Adapted with permission from Cella DF, Tulsky DS, Measuring quality of life today: methodological aspects. *Oncology* 1990;4:29–38.

and Cella (38), which includes a number of questionnaires in the appendix. Most of these questionnaires can be obtained by requesting permission from the authors; updated versions of the questionnaires as well as instructions for scoring are provided, and a user's agreement usually needs to be signed.

There is no consensus as to which QOL questionnaire in oncology is best. Maguire and Selby (39), in their review of QOL assessment, suggested using the Rotterdam Symptom Checklist (40) and Hospital Anxiety and Depression Scale (HADS) (41), which at the time of that review (1989) were considered valid and suitable for clinical trials. Since that time a number of other questionnaires have been validated. Currently, the most widely used generic QOL questionnaire seems to be MOS SF-36, and the most commonly used cancer-specific questionnaires are probably EORTC QLQ-C30, FLIC, and FACT. Some questionnaires are widely advertised (usually by their authors) as being useful, although little has been published about their properties, so that caution is needed when choosing a QOL instrument. Therefore, the reader needs to be familiar with the essential attributes of QOL measures.

Properties of Questionnaires—Reliability, Validity, Responsiveness

QOL questionnaires need to have a few essential features before one can use them to indeed measure QOL. The most important properties are reliability, validity, and responsiveness. *Reliability* is the measure of the amount of random error associated with a measurement. In the case of QOL questionnaires, repeated measures of QOL when patients are stable should yield very similar or identical results; this is termed *test-retest reliability*. *Validity* is a term that describes whether a measurement method indeed measures what it intends to measure. Proving validity is a complex process, outlined in the next section. *Responsiveness* or *sensitivity to change* means that QOL questionnaires detect changes that occur in individuals or groups over time. Some authors stress responsiveness as a particularly important property (42) whereas others view it as an integral part of validity (43).

How Are Questionnaires Validated?

There are several types of validity, and a number of standard approaches to assessing it.

Content validity describes the extent to which the content of a questionnaire appears logical and complete. This can be performed by critically reviewing the items in a questionnaire, preferably by patients as well as health-care personnel.

Criterion validity is the extent to which a questionnaire compares to the gold standard. This type of validity is difficult to prove because in the QOL arena there is no definite gold standard. However, comparison to an existing well-validated QOL questionnaire would be a reasonable approximation of a gold standard.

Construct validity is the extent to which a questionnaire confirms hypotheses about the concepts (constructs) it is measuring. It is tested by designing experiments to test if the instrument behaves as the theory predicts it should. For example, hypotheses are generated about the relationship between QOL and some measurable events, and experiments are designed to test those hypotheses. The following are descriptions of a few different subtypes of construct validity.

Concurrent validity is the extent to which a questionnaire is correlated with other external measures of what it is measuring. For example, the physical domain of QOL would be correlated with observed physical activity, psychological domain would be correlated with other measures of psychological distress, and so on.

Convergent validity is the extent to which two or more questionnaires agree with each other, if they are supposed to measure the same thing. To test convergent validity, one can apply several instruments; the QOL instrument should correlate more closely with similar tests (e.g., measures of performance status), and less closely with more different tests (e.g., measures of depression).

Discriminant validity is the extent to which a questionnaire reflects differences in individuals (or populations) that we would expect to be different, such as patients with early-stage versus those with metastatic disease, or patients with excellent versus those with poor performance status.

Predictive validity is the extent to which an instrument can predict future developments. If a study shows that patients with a poorer baseline QOL have a shorter median survival time than do those with a better QOL, this would illustrate the predictive validity of that QOL instrument, and add to the evidence for its validity.

It should be noted that validation of QOL questionnaires is an ongoing process. The more types of validity that are tested and confirmed, the more confidence one can have in that questionnaire as being truly valid. Each new study that uses the questionnaire adds evidence for its validity, or perhaps challenges some assumptions regarding its validity. It is primarily for this reason that authors of questionnaires request that data obtained using the questionnaire be available to them, so that more evidence for their validity is accumulated. Many of the QOL questionnaires listed in Table 43-2 have published evidence pointing to their validity. A major argument for using one of those questionnaires rather than an "ad hoc" developed list of questions is the greater confidence that the former questionnaires really measure QOL.

Other Methodologic Issues

Response Format

QOL instruments differ in their format of responses. A common response format is the linear analogue self-assessment scale (LASA), also known as *visual analogue scale* (VAS), which is a 10-cm line with descriptors at each end of the line, called *anchors*, which represent extremes (e.g., not at all and extremely severe). Patients are instructed to place a slash mark at the point on the line that most closely represents how they feel or at what level their pain is. Another common response format is categorical, in which the respondent is asked to circle a category; the number of categories varies from four (e.g., QLQ-C30) up to seven or 10 (e.g., BCQ). These are usually *Likert scales*, meaning that each category is greater than the one before (e.g., not at all, a little bit, quite a bit, very much). There is evidence for validity of both of these response formats; studies comparing the performance of VAS and category scales (44) provide no evidence of superiority of one response format to another, although VASs may require more instructions to patients.

Feasibility

Feasibility refers to practical aspects of instrument administration, namely, the length of administration (10–15 minutes seems reasonable, anything longer requires a motivated patient population); ease of administration (how much instruction do patients need, can they complete VASs); timing and frequency of administration (should the questionnaire be given before or after seeing a physician, will the timing of a scheduled QOL assessment require an extra clinic visit); acceptability to patients (content of items, domains); acceptability to clinicians (barriers may at times be greater among clinicians than patients); and setting and personnel (will the patient be undisturbed to complete the questionnaire, are the personnel administering the questionnaire well trained and familiar with the procedure).

Statistical Issues

Several statistical issues need to be considered when analyzing QOL data. One is the way in which a specific questionnaire or instrument can be summarized (i.e., does it have a total score or not). FLIC, for example, has a total score which is a summary of the individual 27 item scores. However, many other questionnaires have subscale scores; for example, the EORTC QLQ-C30 questionnaire has a physical functioning score, emotional functioning score, role functioning score, and so on. They may also have one or more questions that yield a global QOL score that is not obtained by summing up individual subscores.

Another important statistical issue is longitudinal analysis of QOL when some data are missing, especially as missing data are not random but are due to patients deteriorating and dying. If one analyzes only the available data (i.e., from patients who are doing well), the findings will be quite misleading. The optimal way in which missing data can be incorporated is still being resolved.

Integrating Quality of Life and Other End Points

Although QOL is an extremely relevant end point, and at times is the primary end point of a study, it is usually assessed in parallel with other outcomes such as survival and remission duration. There are several ways in which results of such studies can then be presented. One is to present each end point separately. For example, a randomized study may reveal that patients in one study arm had a median survival prolongation of 2 months, but worsened global QOL and physical-domain QOL in comparison to patients in the other study arm. The reader is then left to judge the overall survival benefit at the expense of QOL, present this information to the patient, and make or help arrive at a treatment decision on the basis of these disparate results.

Alternatively, the researchers can present QOL data in such a way that they are already integrated with other outcomes. There are several ways of achieving this. One is to adjust ("correct") the length of survival by quality, that is, to express survival in terms of quality-adjusted life years (QALYs). The usual QOL measures may not be suitable for this, as they do not provide a value by which to adjust for a certain level of QOL. This concept, that is, a person's preference for a certain level of health state (i.e., certain QOL), is termed her *utility* for that state. The two main methods for deriving utilities are standard gamble and time trade-off techniques (45). In the standard gamble technique, a person is asked to choose between the certainty of a particular health state (described to the person or actually experienced by them) and a varying probability (X) of perfect health (and a converse risk of 1 minus the probability X of immediate death). As the probability X is varied from 1 (i.e., 100% probability of perfect health) toward zero (zero probability of perfect health), the responder will reach a point at which she is indifferent to the choice; that is, the particular health state is equally desirable as X probability of perfect health. The higher the number X (e.g., 0.8) is, the more desirable that particular health state is, and the less the respondent is willing to risk to achieve perfect health (or lose it all).

In the time trade-off technique the subjects are asked to choose between the rest of their life in a particular health state and a variable (but shorter) length of time in perfect health. How much time are they willing to trade off for perfect health? The less time they will trade off, the more they value that particular health state, that is, the higher their utility. Once a utility value is obtained, that number is used to weigh survival by multiplying the length of survival in years, and thus obtaining QALYs.

Gelber and Goldhirsch (46) developed another way of integrating QOL with other outcomes, termed *TWiST* (time without symptoms and toxicity). With this concept, study results can be depicted by a survival curve that is partitioned into time on treatment (i.e., time with toxicity), time in remission (presumed to be good quality, i.e., without symptoms or toxic-

ity), and time after relapse (i.e., time with symptoms of disease). The study arms can then be compared not just by length of overall survival, but also by length of time without symptoms and toxicity. If utilities of these time intervals are known or measured, they can be used to adjust the TWiST and result in Q-TWiST, providing further information about the patient's perception of the quality and length of the various health states of relevance to cancer patients throughout their disease trajectory.

Purposes of Assessment

There are several possible purposes of QOL assessment in oncology. Firstly, QOL instruments are commonly used to evaluate the change in QOL in groups over time, and to compare QOL between different treatments. This is the common use of QOL in clinical trials. Secondly, baseline QOL of patients is an important prognostic factor in a number of different cancers including lung cancer (47,48), breast cancer (49), and melanoma (50). It is likely that QOL may become a stratifying variable to be used in studies. Cella and Tulsky (51) described three general purposes of QOL assessment: to assess rehabilitation needs, to use as an end point in evaluating treatment outcome, and to use as a predictor of response to future treatment. Osoba et al (52) referred to additional purposes of measuring QOL: screening, such as finding high-risk individuals; describing health profiles (describing the QOL of a cohort of patients, using QOL profiles for comparing two groups of patients or a single cohort over time) or stratifying patients according to their QOL parameters; using QOL for assessment of preferences, such as measuring utilities (see above); and using QOL measurements in clinical decision making (see below).

Role in Clinical Trials

A number of clinical trial groups have issued statements regarding guidelines for QOL assessment. For example, the National Cancer Institute (NCI) in the United States, in its report from a workshop on QOL assessment in cancer clinical trials, organized in 1990 (53), identified the various QOL issues of relevance in particular disease sites and treatment comparisons; they also made recommendations regarding assessment, implementation, and analysis of QOL data. The NCIC Clinical Trials Group has a policy that each phase III clinical trial needs to have a statement about the impact of that trial on patients' QOL, and whether QOL will be assessed (54). The Southwest Oncology Group (SWOG) guidelines regarding QOL assessment (55) lists the following recommendations: to measure physical and emotional functioning, symptoms, and global QOL using separate validated QOL measures; to consider measuring social functioning and other trial-specific issues if resources are available; and to use patient-based brief questionnaires with categorical scales, rather than VASs. The Radiation Therapy Oncology Group (RTOG) published their experience with QOL assessment design, analysis, and data management (56); their decision was to focus on the long-term impact of treatment on QOL, and not on the acute side effects of treatment. The EORTC formulated the following criteria for including QOL assessment in phase III clinical trials: if the other end points of interest are expected to be similar, but QOL differences are anticipated; if a treatment arm is expected to produce superior survival but at the expense of toxicity; if a treatment is very burdensome, new, or invasive; or if the patient population has a poor prognosis (57). A recent monograph of the NCI (1) on QOL in clinical cancer trials provided an updated perspective and experience with QOL assessment from these and other cooperative groups.

Role of Quality of Life in Clinical Practice

At the present time, QOL research has developed a solid foundation and methodology for measuring QOL in clinical trials, but the clinical relevance of the findings and whether or not QOL information will ever be useful in daily practice is still being questioned (58–60). One of the most serious challenges to QOL research is the assurance that published QOL information will be appropriately utilized, rather than remain in the domain of academic interest (61,62). Whether or not QOL assessment is useful in individual patients and whether it should be incorporated in routine clinical practice are controversial issues that are currently subjects of several studies (Aaronson N, personal communication, 1996) (63). We need to wait for data to support or refute the clinical applicability of QOL questionnaires to individual patients. At the broader level of clinical application of the results of QOL research to

patient populations, there is more convincing evidence of usefulness of QOL information to clinical practice, that is, new knowledge gained from QOL research that can (and has) influence(d) practice (64,65). At the Third Conference on Advances in Health Status Assessment (61), strategies for implementing health status assessment in the clinical setting were discussed (66). Panelists believed that health status measurements are ready for clinical implementation, but noted a number of potential barriers, including suspicion on the part of the clinician as to why outcomes of patients are being assessed, a belief that physicians already do outcome assessment in traditional ways, a lack of knowledge on how to collect and interpret new health status information from formal questionnaires, and a lack of time and resources in busy practices (67,68).

Physicians have traditionally been rewarded for prolonging survival, and have been trained using a traditional biomedical model that considers disease response rather than overall patient functioning and well-being. Recently, however, the Health Services Research Committee of the American Society of Clinical Oncology (ASCO) declared patient outcomes such as survival and QOL as higher priorities than cancer outcomes such as response rates (69), paving the way perhaps to a broader perspective of oncologists on cancer care, and broader incorporation of QOL in clinical practice.

The following sections review some of the research on QOL in breast cancer and gynecologic malignancies.

Quality of Life in Breast Cancer

The field of breast cancer has seen the greatest proliferation of QOL research in comparison to cancer at other sites. Some of the published studies will be used to illustrate areas of QOL research as well as specific findings related to breast cancer. Table 43-3 (pp. 622–623) lists some of the current cooperative group trials in breast and gynecologic cancers that have a QOL endpoint.

Quality of Life Questionnaires Specific for Breast Cancer

Published studies use a variety of QOL questionnaires—some generic, some cancer specific, and some developed specifically for breast cancer. Priestman and Baum (70) were among the first to evaluate the effect of treatment in women with metastatic breast cancer using the LASA scale to assess pain, nausea, appetite, mood, anxiety, level of activity, ability to perform housework, social activities, feelings of well-being, and opinion on whether treatment is helping. They documented an improvement in symptoms and QOL in patients who had a response to treatment. This correlation is, however, not always seen. For example, Tannock (71), in a study of 117 patients with metastatic breast cancer treated with chemotherapy, recorded tumor response and change in symptomatic complaints. The tumor size was decreased in 29 patients, only a third of whom (10/29) had an associated improvement in symptoms. A similar number of patients (28) had symptomatic improvement, but almost two thirds (18/28) showed no corresponding decrease in tumor size.

In a randomized study of chemotherapy, Bell at al (72) used an expanded version of the LASA scales, developed by Selby et al (73) and consisting of 31 items on functional status and disease or treatment-related symptoms.

Some of the core questionnaires have had modules developed specifically for breast cancer. For example, the EORTC QLQ-C30 core questionnaire has been supplemented with a breast cancer–specific module, BCM-23, which is undergoing final validity testing after a few years of development (36). Similarly, the FACT questionnaire has a module specific for breast cancer patients, FACT-B, which differs from FACT-G, the general form of the questionnaire, by having 10 additional items specific to breast cancer (74).

The BCQ (35) was developed and psychometrically tested in a trial of a short versus a prolonged course of adjuvant chemotherapy for early-stage breast cancer. It is sensitive to changes in QOL related to treatment, and documented a decrease in QOL during treatment but then a recovery to baseline levels following treatment. Interested readers are referred to the description of the development of this questionnaire, which adheres to the published guidelines with a description of various steps in developing a questionnaire (75).

A group in the United Kingdom (76) developed a daily diary card to measure QOL specifically in patients with advanced breast cancer. This diary card contains questions per-taining to four domains—symptoms and side effects, psychological aspects, relationships, and physical functioning. Patients are asked to choose among 23 items from the domains that are most important to them, and to evaluate daily how severe each of the resulting four to six items is for them. It has been validated by comparing it with LASA scores and the Nottingham health profile, a validated generic QOL measure.

Other questionnaires that were not specifically developed for breast cancer were nevertheless tested in breast cancer populations and used in trials, and will be mentioned in examples below. The specific items and areas addressed by the questionnaire should be taken into consideration when various studies are reviewed, to ascertain that those aspects of QOL that are indeed important to patients were addressed. Sutherland et al (77) asked patients with metastatic breast cancer to rate the relative importance of 28 items using two methods, Q sort (ranking of cards listing different items) and a linear analogue rating. General health items, specifically self-care, mobility, physical activity, appetite, sleep, and family relationship, were ranked significantly higher than common side effects of chemotherapy. This would suggest that including mostly items related to the side effects of chemotherapy would not address the health-related QOL of patients with metastatic breast cancer.

Effect of Surgery on Quality of Life

A number of studies documented the impact of surgery on QOL. The two main areas that appear affected by surgery are body image (78) and sexual functioning (79). Ganz et al (80) studied 109 patients with breast cancer who had either mastectomy or lumpectomy. Although their QOL was comparable, there were differences in body image and sexual functioning, with the mastectomy group having worse impairment. Similarly, de Haes et al (78) found the same in a randomized trial of mastectomy versus lumpectomy; both the younger and older women in the mastectomy group had more severely impaired body image. Interestingly, fear of recurrence was not related to the type of treatment in that study.

Kiebert et al (81) confirmed these results in their review of 18 studies investigating the impact of breast cancer treatment on QOL, and concluded that there is no definite proof of better psychological adjustment to breast-conserving surgery and no substantial differences on the major domains of QOL except for body image and sexual functioning.

Effect of Radiation on Quality of Life

A number of studies described QOL during radiation therapy. For example, Wallace et al (82) examined 63 patients, participants in a randomized clinical trial of two different radiotherapy regimens and tamoxifen for early breast cancer. Overall, there was little deterioration of QOL but the longer radiotherapy regimen did have slightly more impact, with disruption of private life and transient weight change. McArdle et al (83) studied patients in a randomized trial of adjuvant radiation with or without adjuvant chemotherapy; they found the same levels of anxiety but less psychological morbidity, in addition to the expected lower levels of side effects in patients treated with radiation alone.

Similarly, studies of palliative radiotherapy in breast cancer are starting to measure QOL in addition to other end points. As part of a larger randomized study of chest wall radiation with or without hyperthermia in recurrent breast cancer, colleagues and I (84) used the guidelines for assessment of QOL in hyperthermia trials (85), and administered a nine-item LASA scale, Rotterdam Symptom Checklist, and a questionnaire about patient perception of the inconvenience of treatment. Despite the premature closure of the trial, and a resultant small sample size, this study demonstrated the feasibility and clinical relevance of those guidelines.

Other studies on palliative radiotherapy currently include measuring QOL and pain relief after palliative radiotherapy for bone metastases; subjective assessment of pain relief is considered necessary, in addition to recording analgesic intake, to assess the degree of palliative response to radiation.

Effect of Chemotherapy on Quality of Life

A number of studies of adjuvant chemotherapy documented increased psychological morbidity but a return to baseline after the chemotherapy was completed. Similar to the Levine trial (35), the Eastern Co-operative Group (ECOG) conducted a randomized trial of CAF versus a 16-week chemotherapy regimen in an adjuvant setting in breast cancer patients (86). They doc-

umented a greater decrease in QOL in the aggressive treatment arm but recovery after 4 months following treatment. Hurny et al (87) used a four-item LASA scale to measure QOL in International Breast Cancer Study Group trials VI and VII on more than 2000 patients. They documented a measurable adverse affect of adjuvant chemotherapy on QOL but the effect was transient and was noted with subsequent courses of chemotherapy.

QOL research not only has confirmed what we already know but also on occasions has given new insight into the patients' experience. In a widely quoted study, Coates et al (88) measured QOL using LASA in patients receiving chemotherapy for metastatic breast cancer. Patients were randomized to receive continuous chemotherapy (i.e., continuing the chemotherapy regime if their cancer was responding) or intermittent chemotherapy (i.e., stopping chemotherapy when response was achieved, and restarting it when disease progresses). The expectation was that patients with intermittent chemotherapy will have a better QOL as they will be spared chemotherapy toxicity. However, the finding was the opposite, in that patients in the continuous chemotherapy arm had a better QOL. The explanation was found when specific items in the LASA questionnaire were examined: In the patients receiving intermittent chemotherapy the effects of cancer were worse, which led to impaired QOL.

Other studies confirmed the finding that at times aggressive chemotherapy can lead to a better QOL. For example, Fraser et al (89) evaluated 40 patients randomized to receive either the combination cyclophosphamide, methotrexate, and fluorouracil (CMF) or a weekly low dose of epirubicin. The response rates were superior in the CMF treatment arm although the survival rates were similar in both groups. Patients who responded to chemotherapy improved their QOL. Despite the greater toxicity of CMF, there was no difference in the overall global scores of QOL. As a group patients on single-agent chemotherapy had a low response rate, and despite low toxicity had no improvement in QOL.

Assessment of QOL is also essential in the process of evaluating newer agents, and has been accepted by the U.S. Food and Drug Administration and other agencies as a requirement and criterion for approving chemotherapeutic medications in certain settings. For example, a recent review of QOL analysis in trials using vinorelbine (90) described QOL assessment using items from MOS SF-20 and MOS SF-36 (28) to measure physical and role functioning, symptom assessment using the Symptom Distress Scale (91), and LASA uniscale to measure global QOL. In the patients treated with vinorelbine, they documented better physical functioning and otherwise comparable QOL to patients receiving intravenous melphalan. QOL assessment in vinorelbine studies was performed at baseline, every 2 weeks for the first 8 weeks of treatment, and then monthly. QOL questionnaires were administered before examination by the physician and before treatment, as they are in most clinical studies. In these as in many other studies, there were problems collecting information because patients get progressively sicker. Patients with better baseline scores tend to stay in studies longer. Therefore, analysis of time trend can result in a false overestimation of QOL in the patient population. If the attrition rate in the two groups is not comparable, this can bias the results.

Similarly, a number of studies utilizing taxol measured QOL as a secondary end point. In one study (92), several validated instruments, including the Memorial Symptom Assessment Scale (93), FLIC, Brief Pain Inventory, and Memorial Pain Assessment Card, were completed prior to treatment and at regular intervals during chemotherapy. QOL assessment correlated with clinical response, in that patients with progressive disease experienced deterioration of QOL whereas others had improved or unchanged QOL scores. Important information about specific symptoms and their impact on patient functioning was revealed through QOL assessment. In addition, baseline QOL predicted survival more accurately than did a number of other standard prognostic variables.

Clinical Usefulness of Quality of Life Data from Breast Cancer Studies

As discussed earlier in this chapter, there are a number of potential clinical applications of QOL data that become available through studies on breast cancer patients. In addition to descriptive information, as in the examples already listed on the effects of various therapies, they include the comparison of treatment alternatives, evaluation of programs or interventions, prognostic value of QOL scores, and facilitation of communication with patients, among others. Examples of each follow.

In a few studies QOL was used as a primary end point. Kornblith et al (94) assessed QOL in patients receiving three different doses of megestrol acetate, by using FLIC, the Rand Mental Health Inventory, the Rand Functional Limitation Scale, and the Body Image Subscale. The lowest dose of megestrol, 160 mg/day, was associated with the least severe side effects, best functioning, and an improvement in overall QOL. On the basis of this finding and in view of no survival advantage documented for higher doses, the lowest dose was recommended as optimal.

QOL has also been an important end point in prevention trials and screening trials. It has also been used to assess various interventions. For example, the Italian group GIVIO (Interdisciplinary Group for Cancer Care Evaluation) (95) performed a randomized trial of intensive surveillance for patients with primary breast cancer versus clinic visits with additional diagnostic tests performed when clinically indicated. The primary end points were overall survival and health-related QOL assessed by a self-administered questionnaire at 6, 12, 24, and 60 months. With a median follow-up time of 71 months and 1320 patients available for analysis, there were no differences in overall survival, percentage of asymptomatic patients in whom metastases were detected, and time to diagnosis of metastatic disease. Health-related QOL including overall health and QOL, emotional well-being, and satisfaction with care was the same in the two groups, suggesting that a policy of clinical assessment and tests guided by clinical findings does not adversely affect patient outcome and QOL. Argument for close clinical follow-up and surveillance is that it reassures patients; that is, there is a beneficial psychological effect of frequent testing, reassuring patients that the disease is in remission. An alternative hypothesis would be that frequent testing increases stress and anxiety, at least until negative results are communicated. Interestingly, Liberati's large study (95) did not lend support to either of these hypotheses, showing instead that QOL was the same in these two large patient groups. The QOL questionnaire used in this study was not described in detail, although it was specifically developed for the study and had good internal reliability and documented content, convergent, and discriminative validity. These results are intriguing and challenge our clinical practice.

Several studies confirmed the prognostic importance of QOL scores in breast cancer (49).

T A B L E   **43-3**

Active Cooperative Group Therapy Trials With Quality of Life (QOL)
Components—Breast and Gynecologic Cancers

Cooperative Group/ Protocol Number	Title/Description of Trial	Phase	QOL Instrument
Breast			
CALGB-9342	Study of paclitaxel (Taxol) at three dose levels in the treatment of patients with metastatic breast cancer	III	Functional Living Index–Cancer, Symptom Distress Scale
E 1193	Trial of doxorubicin versus paclitaxel versus paclitaxel plus doxorubicin plus G-CSF in metastatic breast cancer	III	Functional Assessment of Cancer Therapy–(FACT) Breast
INT-0121/EST-2190	Study of conventional adjuvant chemotherapy versus high-dose chemotherapy and ABMT as adjuvant intensification therapy following conventional adjuvant chemotherapy in patients with stage II or III breast cancer at high risk of recurrence	III	Breast Chemotherapy Questionnaire (BCQ)
INT-0142/E-3193	Comparison of tamoxifen versus tamoxifen with ovarian ablation in premenopausal women with axillary node-negative receptor-positive breast cancer <2 cm	III	FACT–Breast, ECOG Menopausal Symptom Form
T90-0180/PBT-1	Randomized comparison of maintenance chemotherapy with CTX, MTX, and 5-FU versus high-dose chemotherapy with CTX, thiotepa, and carboplatinium + ABMT support for women with metastatic breast cancer responding to conventional induction chemotherapy	III	Medical Outcomes Study Short-Form (SF)-20, Symptom Distress Scale, Profile of Mood States, Mental Adjustment
NCIC MA.10	Dose-intensive chemotherapy for locally advanced/inflammatory cancer	III	QLQ-C30 + trial-specific checklist
NCIC MA.11	Escalating FEC with G-CSF support	I/II	BCQ
NCIC MA.14	Octreotide + tamoxifen vs tamoxifen alone for stage I/II postmenopausal breast cancer	III	QLQ-C30 + trial-specific checklist
NCIC MA.16	High-dose chemotherapy/ABMT vs standard chemotherapy for metastatic breast cancer	III	QLQ-C30, trial-specific checklist, FACT-BMT subscale
NCIC MA.17	Vorozole vs placebo after 5 yr of tamoxifen for ER-, PR-positive postmenopausal breast cancer	III	SF-36, menopausal checklist
EORTC	Preoperative vs postoperative chemotherapy for early-stage breast cancer	III	QLQ-C30
	Dose-intensive chemotherapy for inflammatory breast cancer	III	QLQ-C30
	Taxol vs doxorubicin as first-line chemotherapy for advanced breast cancer	III	QLQ-C30
	Oral pamidronate vs placebo in patients with breast cancer and newly diagnosed bone metastases	III	QLQ-C30

T A B L E   **43-3**

Continued

Cooperative Group/ Protocol Number	Title/Description of Trial	Phase	QOL Instrument
Gynecologic			
E2E93	Clinical trial of an outpatient paclitaxel and carboplatin regimen in the treatment of suboptimally debulked epithelial carcinoma of the ovary	II	FACT–Ovarian
GOG-145	Randomized study of surgery vs surgery plus vulvar radiation in the management of poor-prognosis primary vulvar cancer and of radiation vs radiation and chemotherapy for positive inguinal nodes	III	FACT–General, GOG Symptom Inventory, Groningen Arousability Scale, Groningen Body Image Scale
GOG-152	Randomized study of cisplatin and paclitaxel with interval secondary cytoreduction vs cisplatin and paclitaxel in patients with suboptimal stage III or IV epithelial ovarian carcinoma	III	FACT–Ovarian
GOG-9102	Effect of alopecia on cancer patients' body image and the role of audiovisual information on body image	Other	Secourd and Jourard Body Cathexis Index
GOG-LAP1	Orientation and evaluation study of surgeon proficiency in performing a GOG-standardized procedure for laparoscopic staging in adenocarcinoma of the endometrium	Other	FACT–General, Medical Outcomes Survey–Physical
SWOG-9324	Trial of vinorelbine tartrate (Navelbine) for patients with relapsed ovarian cancer	II	Medical Outcomes Study SF-36
NCIC CX.2	Radiation ± cisplatin for locally advanced squamous cell cancer of the cervix	III	QLQ-C30 + trial-specific checklist
NCIC OV.10	Platinum and paclitaxel versus platinum and cyclophosphamide for advanced ovarian cancer	III	QLQ-C30 + trial-specific checklist
NCIC EN.5	Surgery ± pelvic radiation for stage I carcinoma of the endometrium	III	QLQ-C30 + trial-specific checklist, Sexual Adjustment Questionnaire
EORTC	Taxol/platinum vs cyclophosphamide/platinum for advanced ovarian cancer	III	QLQ-C30
	Cyclophosphamide/platinum vs abdominal pelvic radiation for high risk ovarian cancer	III	QLQ-C30

CALGB = Cancer and Leukemia Group B; E = Eastern Co-operative Group; INT = Intergroup study; NCIC = National Cancer Institute of Canada; EORTC = European Organization for Research and Treatment in Cancer; GOG = Gynecologic Oncology Group; SWOG = Southwest Oncology Group; CTX = Cytoxan (cyclophosphamide); MTX = methotrexate; 5-FU = 5-fluorouracil; ABMT = autologous bone marrow transplantation; G-CSF = granulocyte colony-stimulating factor; FEC = fluorouracil, epirubicin, cyclophosphamide; ER = estrogen receptor; PR = progestin receptor.

Source: Adapted with permission from McCabe M. Quality of life in clinical cancer trials. *J Natl Cancer Inst Monogr* 1996;20.

Patients with poor QOL at baseline have a worse prognosis even when controlling for other known prognostic factors (including performance status). On the other hand, it is not possible to accurately predict variations and deterioration of QOL in patients. For example, Ganz et al (80) found no significant correlation between important clinical variables such as type of surgery and administration of chemotherapy, and patient-rated QOL.

In other studies, it may be necessary to integrate survival and QOL results for comparisons of treatment groups. One well-described methodology is Q-TWiST—quality-adjusted time without symptoms or toxicity—developed by adaptation of the TWiST methodology of Gelber and Goldhirsch (46), and detailed earlier in this chapter.

Quality of Life in Gynecologic Malignancies

The literature on QOL in gynecologic malignancies is considerably smaller than that in breast cancer. A number of recent reviews summarized the current state of knowledge (96–103).

Quality of Life Questionnaires Used in Gynecologic Cancer

Numerous QOL questionnaires have been used in studies of QOL of patients with gynecologic cancers. Two well-known and validated QOL questionnaires that have been developed in patients with ovarian cancer are the Rotterdam Symptom Checklist and the EORTC QLQ-C30 questionnaire. The Rotterdam Symptom Checklist (40) consists of 34 physical and psychological symptoms and eight items referring to the patient's functional status; it takes 8 to 10 minutes to complete and yields scores for physical distress and psychological distress as well as data about specific symptoms.

The EORTC QLQ-C30 core questionnaire was validated in a large study of 535 patients with varying cancer diagnoses, including 111 patients with ovarian cancer (104). Patients with ovarian cancer had advanced disease and were treated with platinum chemotherapy. In comparison to patients with breast cancer, some of whom had adjuvant chemotherapy and some chemotherapy for metastatic disease, ovarian

cancer patients had lower scores on domains of physical functioning, role functioning, and social function; had more fatigue and pain; and had lower QOL global scores. They had especially low scores on role functioning. Following chemotherapy, nausea, vomiting, and fatigue scores had worsened; however, role functioning, social function, and global QOL scores changed less than in other patients treated with chemotherapy. In this group pain improved with the aid of chemotherapy, in comparison to baseline levels prior to chemotherapy.

Psychological Adjustment to Gynecologic Cancer

A large proportion of QOL studies in patients with gynecologic cancers dealt with psychological adjustment to cancer, its treatment, and the resulting sequelae. A related area of impact of gynecologic cancer and its treatment on sexuality is covered in another chapter of this book. The following examples illustrate some types of studies that describe the psychosocial domain of QOL.

Zacharias et al (105) studied QOL and coping in 40 patients with gynecologic malignancies and their spouses. QOL was measured using the Ferrans QOL Index–Cancer Version (QLI-CV) (8), which assesses satisfaction with and importance of 34 items within the health/functioning domain, socioeconomic domain, psychological/spiritual domain, and family domain. Coping was measured with a 51-item coping scale, which describes six different ways of coping with the illness experience. QOL overall was fairly high. Patients and spouses expressed an importance of the same domains of QOL, rating family life as most important and giving them greatest satisfaction. The health/functioning domain was not rated as important to patients and spouses but health care was perceived as important. The area of lowest satisfaction and importance for both patients and spouses was sex life. Patients also reported dissatisfaction with their lack of energy. Differences in coping strategies were found between patients and their spouses. Interestingly, different coping strategies correlated with different QOL domains. Patients who had poor QOL used more wish-fulfilling fantasy as a coping mechanism (wishing the cancer to go away).

This study illustrates that when using a

general QOL questionnaire rather than a health-related QOL questionnaire, the QOL of cancer patients and their spouses is similar to that of the general population. Family interactions and family life are two of the most important domains of all QOL factors, and effective medical and nursing intervention aimed at the entire family may best bring about improved QOL in patients with gynecologic malignancies.

Padilla et al (106) evaluated the effect of several factors in the adaptation process related to uncertainty of values on health-related QOL, using 100 women with newly diagnosed gynecologic cancer. Interestingly, coping strategy did not predict health-related QOL. The theory of uncertainty and illness explained some of the adaptation process and resultant QOL. The key variables of health-related QOL were mood states, ambiguity about illness or wellness, danger-focused appraisal, and mastery.

Cain et al (107) reported on psychological reactions to cancer and treatment in a study of 60 newly diagnosed patients with cancer of the cervix, uterus, or ovary. Depression, anxiety, and impairment in work, domestic, and sexual functioning were common. Depression was especially pronounced in patients with ovarian cancer, those on chemotherapy, and those with poorly differentiated tumors of the ovary and endometrium. This last finding led the authors to conclude that patients who perceive their prognosis as poor are especially prone to depression. As there is evidence that psychotherapy and support groups can improve psychological distress, QOL, and possibly survival, identifying patients who are at risk and would benefit from such interventions is important.

Andersen (108) studied emotional distress in newly diagnosed gynecologic cancer patients and compared it to women with benign gynecologic disorders. Depressed mood and confusion were significantly high in cancer patients. Interestingly, anxiety and fatigue were similar in women with cancer as in those with benign disease.

Other studies (101) reported increasing levels of depression and anxiety during and after radiotherapy. Increased anxiety and agitation were particularly pronounced just before patients underwent intracavitary irradiation for gynecologic cancer. Anxiety was not decreased in patients who required a second intracavitary treatment, suggesting that knowledge about the procedure does not necessarily reduce the anxiety level (109).

Quality of Life with Ovarian Cancer

QOL in patients with ovarian cancer is particularly relevant because of the high mortality rates of patients with this cancer, relatively prolonged time to death, and significant toxicity of treatment. As with breast cancer, there are a number of clinical applications of QOL data from these studies—descriptive information, assessment or comparison of treatment alternatives, evaluation of programs or interventions, and facilitation of communication with patients. Examples of each follow.

The group from Memorial Sloan-Kettering reported on QOL in 151 ovarian cancer patients, most with advanced-stage disease (110). QOL was assessed at 3-month intervals using FLIC, Memorial Pain Assessment Card, Memorial Symptom Assessment Scale, Mental Health Inventory, and Karnofsky Performance Status. Assessment at baseline was done through a questionnaire or by interview, but most of the follow-up assessments were largely done through mailed questionnaires. At 12-month follow-up, only 42% of the patients were available for assessment, mostly because many had died or were debilitated. The attrition rate of that degree over a 12-month study period presents methodologic problems in generalizing results to all patients. This patient group exhibited on average nine physical and psychological symptoms, with pain being most common. It often interfered with functioning and well-being to a moderate or great degree. One third or more of patients reported symptoms of anxiety or depression at moderate to very severe intensity. Patients who scored high in the psychological distress categories also had significant physical symptoms. Patients in high distress were more likely to have advanced-stage disease and to be inpatients. Patients who survived the longest showed significant improvement in their physical symptom scores over time, suggesting that both their quality and length of survival were superior. Patients who died within 120 days of their last assessment had documented steep worsening in all of their QOL dimensions.

QOL in ovarian cancer patients at baseline in this study was compared to QOL in a mixed group of cancer patients and a group of breast cancer patients, for whom the FLIC was also utilized. The mean FLIC score in women with ovarian cancer was 108.2, comparable to hospitalized cancer patients and breast cancer patients who were identified as being at high risk for psychosocial distress. The ovarian cancer patients whose Karnofsky performance status score was 80 or lower had worse FLIC mean scores than did either of the comparison groups. They also had significantly more psychological distress, more physical symptoms, and worse social functioning than did patients with a Karnofsky score of 90 to 100.

This and other studies identified factors that predict greater stress and poorer QOL in patients with ovarian cancer: advanced-stage disease, disease recurrence, treatment failure, diminished physical functioning, limited financial resources, poor social support, and prior psychiatric history.

Blythe and Wahl (111) reported that debulking surgery in ovarian cancer patients can improve QOL. Although other authors reported the same conclusions, this is one of a minority of studies using a QOL instrument. Rather, in many studies (112) performance status measurement was used as a proxy for QOL.

Payne et al (113) performed an intervention study that had a QOL end point. They compared hospital-based versus home-based palliative chemotherapy; the group that had delivery of chemotherapy at home had a better QOL (other outcomes were equivalent in the two groups). In another intervention study, Ovesen et al (114) assessed the relationship between nutritional counseling, dietary intake, and QOL in patients with ovarian, breast, or lung cancer. Patients with weight loss at study entry (i.e., due to cancer) had a worse outlook and social interactions than did those without weight loss.

In communicating the expected effect of treatment to patients, it is useful to be able to combine the survival results and QOL data. To that extent, Willemse et al (115) from the Netherlands applied the TWiST methodology (time without symptoms and toxicity) to a cohort of 68 patients with stage III or IV ovarian cancer treated with CAP chemotherapy for six cycles and second-look laparotomy. There was no formal QOL evaluation. TWiST was calculated by subtracting from the number of days of progression-free survival the following: All time spent in hospital was subtracted day per day. Any day that patients had side effects of treatment was subtracted as a half day. Peripheral neuropathy was graded, and grade II or III neuropathy was subtracted from survival, arbitrarily choosing 50% of the duration of the symptomatic period (in days) to subtract from progression-free survival. In this way, in addition to the traditional end points of response rate, median survival time, progression-free survival time, and incidence of toxicity, time without symptoms and toxicity, and presumably with good quality, can be calculated as well. In this study, the median progression-free survival time was 18 months; median overall survival time, 22 months; and median duration of TWiST, 10 months. In 24 of 68 patients, the ratio of TWiST to progression-free survival was less than 50%, indicating that any symptom-free time gained by the patient did not exceed time consumed with treatment and its symptoms. As expected, clinical variables such as extent of residual disease after initial laparotomy predicted the likelihood of response. Therefore, patients with microscopic disease prior to chemotherapy had improved progression-free survival, and the proportion of their survival time spent with symptoms or toxicity was significantly less. The weakness of this study is that patients' own weighing of toxicity was not used in assessing the burden of toxicity and symptoms. Patients did provide information on duration of their symptoms, although it was not clear what amount of time should be discounted for duration of symptoms, hospital admissions, and so on. Patients' perspective is especially important in treatments that impact on their well-being in more than one sphere, such as chemotherapy and debulking surgery.

Simes (116) described the application of a statistical decision tree to help in the decision making with respect to treatment selection for advanced ovarian cancer. The treatment alternatives and their consequences are listed, probabilities of these various outcomes are assigned from the literature, and utilities of these outcomes are obtained or assigned. A sensitivity analysis, done by varying the probabilities and utility values, revealed that the treatment decision is most sensitive to the variation in survival data and to whether patients place more importance on the immediate or the long-term future.

Other Studies in Gynecologic Cancers

Bye et al (117) reported on QOL during pelvic radiotherapy in a randomized trial of a low-fat, low-lactose diet to prevent acute radiation-induced diarrhea. One hundred forty-three women with gynecologic malignancies receiving radiotherapy were evaluated using the EORTC QLQ-C30 questionnaire and a diary. The diary recording of diarrhea appeared more accurate than did the diarrhea question on the EORTC questionnaire. Patients with diarrhea had more fatigue and malaise and poor physical functioning. The authors speculated that the patients' ability to cope with diarrhea may have been favorably influenced by the dietary intervention.

King et al (118) studied home parenteral nutrition in patients with gynecologic malignancies and used QOL as an end point. QOL was assessed through evaluation of physical and social well-being, social interactions, and symptom assessment retrospectively from the chart or interview with a health-care provider. Home parenteral nutrition was believed to have improved QOL as judged by improvement in gastrointestinal symptoms, morale, and social interactions.

QOL issues may be particularly germane in elderly patients, for whom treatment decisions are more likely under the influence of external factors such as age, comorbidity, toxicity of treatment, patients' functional status, and the weighing of benefit versus risk. In his review on ovarian cancer in the elderly patient, Moore (119) suggested that patients' own values and QOL assessment be used to guide the decision making. He pointed out that elderly patients have been documented to rate their own QOL higher than their physicians do. Assumptions should therefore not be made about patients' values and the benefit that they place on QOL versus improvement in survival. Patients should be allowed to state their own preferences regarding treatment, utilizing their own assessments of their QOL, and provided with information about expected impairment in functioning related to treatment and disease.

QOL concerns are also of relevance when considering the issue of hormone replacement therapy in patients with gynecologic malignancies, especially endometrial cancer. Despite concern that endometrial and ovarian cancers are hormone-sensitive tumors, it is not clear whether estrogen replacement therapy increases the recurrence rate of these cancers. Proponents of replacement therapy point to improvement in menopausal symptoms and the expected improvement in cardiac morbidity as well as osteoporosis. In this setting, survival and QOL are relevant end points, both in clinical studies and in treatment decisions for individual patients (120).

Conclusions

As our research and treatment efforts strive to improve survival rates from various types of cancer in women, QOL remains an important issue both to women who will be cured of their disease and to the ones who will eventually die from their malignancy. QOL is a multidimensional concept that can be operationally defined, measured, and evaluated. Considerable progress has been achieved over the last two decades in assessing health-related QOL in patients with cancer. Numerous questionnaires and instruments are available, and have been shown to reliably and validly measure health-related QOL. They can be used in clinical trials to assess the impact of cancer and its treatment on patients' well-being. They may also have a role to play in everyday clinical practice. We need to continue with research to evaluate and improve the QOL of patients with cancer.

REFERENCES

1. Anonymous. Quality of life in clinical cancer trials. *J Natl Cancer Inst Monogr* 1996;20:1–116.

2. Sutherland HJ, Till JE. Quality of life assessments and levels of decision making; differentiating objectives. *Qual Life Res* 1993;2:297–303.

3. Leigh S. Influencing social change: the cancer survivorship movement. *Proceedings of the 8th International Symposium Support Care Cancer* 1996;51–52.

4. Spilker B, Simpson RL, Tilson HH. Quality of life bibliography and indexes; 1991 update. *J Clin Res Pharmacoepidemiol* 1992;6:205–266.

5. Karnofsky D, Burchenal J. The clinical evaluation of chemotherapeutic agents in cancer. In: Macleod C, ed. *Evaluation of chemotherapeutic agents.* New York: Columbia University Press, 1949:191.

6. World Health Organization. *The first ten years of the World Health Organization.* Geneva: World Health Organization, 1958.

7. Calman K. The quality of life in cancer patients—an hypothesis. *J Med Ethics* 1984; 10:124.

8. Ferrans C. Development of a quality of life index for patients with cancer. *Oncol Nurs Forum* 1990;17:15–19.

9. de Haes J, van Knippenberg F. Quality of life of cancer patients. *Soc Sci Med* 1985;20:809–817.

10. Till JE, McNeil BJ, Bush RS. Measurement of multiple components of quality of life. *Cancer Treat Symp* 1984;1:177–181.

11. Cella D, Cherin E. Quality of life during and after cancer treatment. *Compr Ther* 1988;14:69–75.

12. Osoba D. Measuring the effect of cancer in quality of life. In: Osoba D, ed. *Effect of cancer on quality of life.* Boca Raton: CRC Press, 1991:25–40.

13. Lindley C, Hirsch J. Oncology nurses' attitudes, perceptions, and knowledge of quality-of-life assessment in patients with cancer. *Oncol Nurs Forum* 1994;21:108–110.

14. Walsh D, Emrich L. Measuring cancer patients' quality of life—a look at physician attitudes. *NY State J Med* 1988;88:354–357.

15. Taylor K, Macdonald K, Bezjak A, et al. Physician's perspectives on quality of life: an exploratory study of oncologists. *Qual Life Res* 1996;5:5–14.

16. Bezjak A, Ng P, Macdonald K, et al. A preliminary survey of oncologists' perceptions of quality of life information. *Psychooncology* 1997;6:107–113.

17. Bezjak A, Taylor K, Ng P, et al. Physician willingness to use quality of life information—development of a predictive model. *Qual Life Res* 1995;4:374.

18. Taylor K, Ng P, Bezjak A, et al. Predicting oncologists' use of quality-of-life (QOL) data; results of a survey of Eastern Co-operative Group (ECOG) physicians. *Proc Am Soc Clin Oncol* 1997;16:54a.

19. Warr D, McKinney S, Tannock I. Influence of measurement error on assessment of response to anticancer chemotherapy: proposal for new criteria of tumor response. *J Clin Oncol* 1984;2:1040–1046.

20. Bullinger M, Anderson R, Cella D, Aaronson N. Developing and evaluating cross-cultural instruments—from minimum requirements to optimal models. *Qual Life Res* 1993;2:451–459.

21. Sprangers M, Aaronson N. The role of health care providers and significant others in evaluating the quality of life of patients with chronic disease: a review. *J Clin Epidemiol* 1992;45:743–760.

22. Fossa S, Aaronson N, Newling D, et al. Quality of life and treatment of hormone resistant metastatic prostatic cancer. *Cancer* 1990;26:1133–1136.

23. Starr T, Pearlman R, Uhlmann R. Quality of life and resuscitation decisions in elderly patients. *J Gen Intern Med* 1986;1:373–379.

24. Cohen S, Mount B, Strobel M, Bim F. The McGill Quality of Life Questionnaire—a measure of quality of life appropriate for people with advanced disease. A preliminary study of validity and acceptability. *Palliat Med* 1995;9:207–219.

25. Bruera J, Kuehn N, Miller M, et al. The Edmonton Symptom Assessment System (ESAS); a simple method for the assessment of palliative care patients. *J Palliat Care* 1991;7(2):6–9.

26. Huisman SJ, Van Dam FSAM, Aaronson NK, Hanewald GJFP. On measuring complaints of cancer patients; some remarks on the time span of the question. In: Aaronson NK, Beckmann J, eds. *The quality of life of cancer patients.* New York: Raven, 1987:101–109.

27. Pater J, Palmer M, Zee B, et al. Day of assessment (DA) and question time frame (TF) affect reported quality of life (QOL) after moderately emetogenic chemotherapy (MEC). *Support Care Cancer* 1995;3:375.

28. Ware JE, Sherbourne CD. The MOS 36-item short-form health survey (SF-36). *Med Care* 1992;30:473–483.

29. Hunt S, McKenna S, McEwen J, et al. The Nottingham health profile; subjective health status and medical consultations. *Soc Sci Med* 1981;15A:221–229.

30. Bergner M, Bobbitt R, Carter W, Gilson B. The Sickness Impact Profile: development and final revision of a health status measure. *Med Care* 1981;19:787–805.

31. Ganz PA, Schag CAC, Lee JJ, Sim MS. The CARES: a generic measure of health-oriented quality of life for patients. *Qual Life Res* 1992;1:19–29.

32. Schipper H, Clinch J, McMurray A, Levitt M. Measuring the quality of life of cancer patients: the Functional Living Index–Cancer: development and validation. *J Clin Oncol* 1984;2:472–483.

33. Cella DF, Tulsky DS, Gray G, et al. The Functional Assessment of Cancer Therapy scale:

development and validation of the general measure. *J Clin Oncol* 1993;11:570–579.

34. Aaronson NK, Ahmedzai S, Bergman B, et al. The European Organization for Research and Treatment of Cancer QLQ-C30: a quality-of-life instrument for use in international trials in oncology. *J Natl Cancer Inst* 1993;85:365–376.

35. Levine M, Guyatt G, Gent M. Quality of life in stage II breast cancer; an instrument for clinical trials. *J Clin Oncol* 1988;6:1798–1810.

36. Sprangers M, Groenvold M, Arraras J, et al. The European Organization for Research and Treatment of Cancer Breast Cancer-Specific Quality-of-Life Questionnaire module: first results from a three-country field study. *J Clin Oncol* 1996;14:2756–2768.

37. McQuellon R, Russell G, Cella D, et al. Quality of life measurement in bone marrow transplantation: development of the Functional Assessment of Cancer Therapy-Bone Marrow Transplant (FACT-BMT) scale. *Bone Marrow Transplant* 1997;19:357–368.

38. Tchekmedyian NS, Cella DF. Quality of life in current oncology practice and research. *Oncology* 1990;4.

39. Maguire P, Selby P. Assessing quality of life in cancer patients. *Br J Cancer* 1989;60:437–440.

40. de Haes JCJM, van Knippenberg FCE, Neijt JP. Measuring psychological and physical distress in cancer patients: structure and application on the Rotterdam Symptom Checklist. *Br J Cancer* 1990;62:1034–1038.

41. Zigmond A, Snaith R. The Hospital Anxiety and Depression Scale. *Acta Psychiatr Scand* 1983;67:361.

42. Guyatt GH, Kirschner B, Jaeschke R. Measuring health status; what are the necessary measurement properties? *J Clin Epidemiol* 1992;45:1341–1345.

43. Hays RD, Hadorn D. Responsiveness to change: an aspect of validity, not a separate dimension. *Qual Life Res* 1992;1:73–75.

44. Jaeschke R, Singer J, Guyatt GH. A comparison of seven-point and visual analogue scales; data from a randomized trial. *Control Clin Trials* 1990;11:43–51.

45. Torrance G. Utility approach to measuring health-related quality of life. *J Chron Dis* 1987;40:593–600.

46. Gelber RD, Goldhirsch A. A new endpoint for the assessment of adjuvant therapy in post-menopausal women with operable breast cancer. *J Clin Oncol* 1986;4:1772–1779.

47. Ruckdeschel J, Piantadosi S. Assessment of quality of life (QL) by the Functional Living Index–Cancer (FLIC) is superior to performance status for prediction of survival in patients with lung cancer. *Proc Am Soc Clin Oncol* 1989;8:311.

48. Ganz PA, Lee JJ, Siau J. Quality of life assessment: an independent prognostic variable for survival in lung cancer. *Cancer* 1991;67:3131–3135.

49. Coates A, Gebski V, Signorini D, et al. Prognostic value of quality-of-life scores during chemotherapy for advanced breast cancer. *J Clin Oncol* 1992;10:1833–1838.

50. Coates A, Thompson D, McLeod GRM, et al. Prognostic value of quality of life scores in a trial of chemotherapy with or without interferon in patients with metastatic malignant melanoma. *Eur J Cancer* 1993;29A:1731–1734.

51. Cella DF, Tulsky DS. Quality of life in cancer: definition, purpose, and method of measurement. *Cancer Invest* 1993;11:327–336.

52. Osoba D, Aaronson N, Till J. A practical guide for selecting quality-of-life measures in clinical trials and practice. In: Osoba D, ed. *Effect of cancer on quality of life*. Boca Raton: CRC Press, 1991:90–104.

53. Nayfield SG, Ganz PA, Moinpour CM, et al. Report from a National Cancer Institute (USA) workshop on quality of life assessment in cancer clinical trials. *Qual Life Res* 1992;1:203–210.

54. Osoba D. The Quality of Life Committee of the Clinical Trials Group of the National Cancer Institute of Canada: organization and functions. *Qual Life Res* 1992;1:203–211.

55. Moinpour CM, Hayden KA, Thompson IM, et al. Quality of life assessment in Southwest Oncology Group trials. *Oncology* 1990;4(5):79–89.

56. Scott CB, Stetz J, Bruner DW, Wasserman TH. Radiation Therapy Oncology Group quality of life assessment; design, analysis and data management issues. *Qual Life Res* 1994;3:199–206.

57. Kiebert G, Kaasa S. Quality of life in clinical cancer trials: experience and perspective of the European Organization for Research and Treatment of Cancer. *J Natl Cancer Inst Monogr* 1996;20:91–95.

58. Till JE, Osoba D, Pater JL, Young JR. Research on health-related quality of life: dissemination into practical applications. *Qual Life Res* 1994; 3:279–283.

59. Greenfield S, Nelson E. Recent developments and future issues in the use of health status assessment measures in clinical settings. *Med Care* 1992;30:MS23–MS41. Review.

60. Selby P. The value of quality of life scores in clinical cancer research. *Eur J Cancer* 1993; 29A:1656–1657.

61. Lohr K. Applications of health status assessment measures in clinical practice. *Med Care* 1992; 30:MS1–MS14.

62. Schipper H. Guidelines and caveats for quality of life measurement in clinical practice and research. *Oncology* 1990;4:51–57.

63. Bezjak A. Assessing the clinical application of a symptom assessment and a quality of life instruments in oncology. Master's thesis, McMaster University, Hamilton, Ontario, Canada, 1995.

64. Meyerowitz BE. Quality of life in breast cancer patients: the contribution of data to the care of patients. *Eur J Cancer* 1993;29A(suppl 1): S59–S62.

65. Osoba D. Lessons learned from measuring health-related quality of life in oncology. *J Clin Oncol* 1994;12:608–616.

66. Ware JE. Comments on the use of health status assessment in clinical settings. *Med Care* 1992; 30(5, suppl):MS205–MS209.

67. Wasson J, Keller A, Rubenstein L, et al. Benefits and obstacles of health status assessment in ambulatory settings: the clinician's point of view. *Med Care* 1992;30(5, suppl):MS42–MS49.

68. Deyo RA, Patrick DL. Barriers to the use of health status measures in clinical investigation, patient care and policy research. *Med Care* 1989;27:S254–S268.

69. Anonymous. Outcomes of cancer treatment for technology assessment and cancer treatment guidelines. *J Clin Oncol* 1996;14:671–679.

70. Priestman T, Baum M. Evaluation of quality of life in patients receiving treatment for advanced breast cancer. *Lancet* 1976;1:1899.

71. Tannock IF. Treating the patient, not just the cancer. *N Engl J Med* 1987;317:1534–1535.

72. Bell DR, Tannock IF, Boyd NF. Quality of life measurement in breast cancer patients. *Br J Cancer* 1985;51:577–580.

73. Selby P, Chapman J, Etazadi-Amoli J, et al. The development of a method for assessing the quality of life of cancer patients. *Br J Cancer* 1984;50:13.

74. Cella D. Manual for the Functional Assessment of Cancer Therapy (FACT) scales. Chicago: Rush-Presbyterian-St. Luke's Medical Center, 1994.

75. Kirshner B, Guyatt G. A methodologic framework for assessing health indices. *J Chron Dis* 1985;38:27–36.

76. Fraser S, Ramirez A, Ebbs S, et al. A daily diary for quality of life measurement in advanced breast cancer trials. *Br J Cancer* 1993;67:341–346.

77. Sutherland H, Lockwood G, Boyd N. Ratings of the importance of quality of life variables: therapeutic implications for patients with metastatic breast cancer. *J Clin Epidemiol* 1990;43:661–666.

78. de Haes J, van Oostrom M, Welvaart K. The effect of radical and conserving surgery on the quality of life of early breast cancer patients. *Eur J Surg Oncol* 1986;12:337–342.

79. Wolberg W, Romsaas E, Tanner M, Malec J. Psychosexual adaptation to breast cancer surgery. *Cancer* 1989;63:1645–1656.

80. Ganz P, Schag C, Cheng H-L. Assessing the quality of life—a study in newly-diagnosed breast cancer patients. *J Clin Epidemiol* 1990; 43:75–86.

81. Kiebert G, de Haes J, van de Velde C. The impact of breast-conserving treatment and mastectomy on the quality of life of early-stage breast cancer patients: a review. *J Clin Oncol* 1991;9:1059–1070.

82. Wallace L, Priestman S, Dunn J, Priestman T. The quality of life of early breast cancer patients treated by two different radiotherapy regimens. *Clin Oncol* 1993;5:228–233.

83. McArdle C, Calman K, Cooper A, et al. The social, emotional and financial implications of adjuvant chemotherapy in breast cancer. *Br J Surg* 1981;68:261–264.

84. Liu F, Bezjak A, Levin W, et al. Assessment of palliation in women with recurrent breast cancer. *Int J Hyperthermia* 1996;12:825–826.

85. Nielsen OS, Munro AJ, Warde PR. Assessment of palliative response in hyperthermia. *Int J Hyperthermia* 1992;8:1–10.

86. Fairclough D, Fetting J, Cella D, et al. Quality of life (QL) on a breast cancer adjuvant trial com-

paring CAF with a 16 week multidrug regimen. *Proc Am Soc Clin Oncol* 1995;14:890.

87. Hurny C, Bernhard J, Coates A, et al. Impact of adjuvant therapy on quality of life in women with node-positive operable breast cancer. *Lancet* 1996;347:1279–1284.

88. Coates A, Gebski V, Bishop JF, et al. Improving the quality of life during chemotherapy for advanced breast cancer; a comparison of intermittent and continuous treatment strategies. *N Engl J Med* 1987;317:1490–1495.

89. Fraser S, Dobbs H, Ebbs S, et al. Combination or mild single agent chemotherapy for advanced breast cancer? CMF vs epirubicin measuring quality of life. *Br J Cancer* 1993;67: 402–406.

90. Bertsch L, Donaldson G. Quality of life analyses from vinorelbine (Navelbine) clinical trials of women with metastatic breast cancer. *Semin Oncol* 1995;22:45–54.

91. McCorkle R, Young K. Development of a symptom distress scale. *Cancer Nurs* 1978;(Oct 1978):373–378.

92. Seidman AD, Portenoy R, Yao TJ, et al. Quality of life in phase II trials; a study of methodology and predictive value in patients with advanced breast cancer treated with paclitaxel plus granulocyte colony-stimulating factor. *J Natl Cancer Inst* 1995;87:1316–1322.

93. Portenoy R, Thaler H, Kornblith A, et al. The Memorial Symptom Assessment Scale: an instrument for the evaluation of symptom prevalence, characteristics and distress. *Eur J Cancer* 1994;30A:1326–1336.

94. Kornblith A, Hollis D, Zuckerman E, et al. Effect of megestrol acetate on quality of life in a dose-response trial in women with advanced breast cancer. *J Clin Oncol* 1993;11:2081–2089.

95. Liberati A. The GIVIO trial on the impact of follow-up care on survival and quality of life in breast cancer patients. *Ann Oncol* 1995;6: S41–S46.

96. Andersen B. Quality of life for women with gynecologic cancer. *Curr Opin Obstet Gynecol* 1995;7:69–76.

97. Andersen B. Predicting sexual and psychologic morbidity and improving the quality of life for women with gynecologic cancer. *Cancer* 1992; 71(4 suppl):1678–1690.

98. Anderson B. Quality of life in progressive ovarian cancer. *Gynecol Oncol* 1994;55:S151–S155.

99. Makar A, Trope C. Gynecologic malignancy and surgery: from quantity to quality of life. *Curr Opin Obstet Gynecol* 1992;4:419–429.

100. Romagnolo C. Quality of life in gynaecological oncology. *Clin Exp Obstet Gynecol* 1991;18: 203–205.

101. McCartney C, Larson D. Quality of life in patients with gynecologic cancer. *Cancer* 1987; 60:2129–2136.

102. Audet-Lapointe P. Quality of life in gynaecological cancer. *Eur J Gynaecol Oncol* 1987; 8:569–574.

103. Montazeri A, McEwen J, Gillis C. Quality of life in patients with ovarian cancer: current state of research. *Support Care Cancer* 1996;4:169–179.

104. Osoba D, Zee B, Pater J, et al. Psychometric properties and responsiveness of the EORTC quality of life questionnaire (QLQ-C30) in patients with breast, ovarian and lung cancer. *Qual Life Res* 1994;3:353–364.

105. Zacharias D, Gilg C, Foxall M. Quality of life and coping in patients with gynecologic cancer and their spouses. *Oncol Nurs Forum* 1994; 21:1699–1706.

106. Padilla G, Grant M, Ferrell B. Nursing research into quality of life. *Qual Life Res* 1992;1:341–348.

107. Cain E, Kohorn E, Quinlan D, et al. Psychosocial reactions to the diagnosis of gynecologic cancer. *Obstet Gynecol* 1983;62:635–641.

108. Andersen B. Psychological responses and sexual outcomes of gynecologic cancer. In: Sciarra J, ed. *Gynecology and obstetrics*, vol. 4. Philadelphia: Harper and Row, 1987:1–15.

109. Andersen B, Karlsson J, Anderson B, Tewfik H. Anxiety and cancer treatment: response to stressful radiotherapy. *Health Psychol* 1984;3: 535–551.

110. Kornblith A, Thaler H, Wong G, et al. Quality of life of women with ovarian cancer. *Gynecol Oncol* 1995;59:231–242.

111. Blythe J, Wahl T. Debulking surgery: does it increase the quality of survival? *Gynecol Oncol* 1982;14:396–408.

112. Janicke F, Holscher M, Kuhn W, et al. Radical surgical procedure improves survival time in patients with recurrent ovarian cancer. *Cancer* 1992;70:2129–2136.

113. Payne S. A study of quality of life in cancer patients receiving palliative chemotherapy. *Soc Sci Med* 1992;35:1505–1509.

114. Ovesen L, Hannibal J, Mortensen E. The inter-relationship of weight loss, dietary intake, and quality of life in ambulatory patients with cancer of the lung, breast, and ovary. *Nutr Cancer* 1993;19:159–167.

115. Willemse P, Van Lith J, Mulder N, et al. Risks and benefits of cisplatin in ovarian cancer. A quality-adjusted survival analysis. *Eur J Cancer* 1990;26:345–352.

116. Simes R. Treatment selection for cancer patients: application of statistical decision theory to the treatment of advanced ovarian cancer. *J Chron Dis* 1985;38:171–186.

117. Bye A, Ose T, Kaasa S. Quality of life during pelvic radiotherapy. *Acta Obstet Gynecol Scand* 1995;74:147–152.

118. King L, Carson L, Konstantinides N, et al. Outcome assessment of home parenteral nutrition in patients with gynecological malignancies; what have we learned in a decade of experience. *Gynecol Oncol* 1993;51:377–382.

119. Moore D. Ovarian cancer in the elderly patient. *Oncology* 1994;8(12):21–30.

120. Roberts W. Gynecologic cancer: screening, treatment options, and quality-of-life considerations. *Cancer Control* 1996;3:94–95.

121. Heinrich RL, Schag CC, Ganz P. Living with cancer: the cancer inventory of problem situations. *J Clin Psychol* 1984;40:972–980.

122. Coates A, Fischer Dillenbeck C, McNeil DR, et al. On the receiving end—II. Linear analogue self-assessment (LASA) in evaluation of aspects of the quality of life of cancer patients receiving therapy. *Eur J Cancer Clin Oncol* 1983;19:1633–1637.

123. Derogatis L. The brief symptom inventory—an introductory report. *Psychol Med* 1983;13:595–605.

124. Ferrans CE, Powers MJ. Quality of life index: development and psychometric properties. *Adv Nurs Sci* 1985;8:15–24.

125. Padilla GV, Presant C, Grant MM, et al. Quality of life index for patients with cancer. *Res Nurs Health* 1983;6:117–126.

126. Spitzer WO, Dobson AJ, Hall J, et al. Measuring the quality of life of cancer patients: a concise QL-Index for use by physicians. *J Chronic Dis* 1981;34:585–597.

CHAPTER *44*

Symptom Management and Supportive Care in Women with Advanced Cancer

JANE POULSON

The Nature of Palliative Care

Many patients and their families undergo the cancer experience without the benefit and support of a palliative-care service. This is due to misunderstanding on behalf of the general population and many clinicians about the scope of services palliative care can offer. There exists a general belief that enlisting the support of a palliative-care service is akin to admitting defeat to the illness. The transition to palliative care is viewed as the end of "active" treatment, that the patient is no longer of interest to the oncology team. Modern palliative care has developed far beyond this limited perspective. Palliative-care providers currently play an important role on the oncology team, working in conjunction with oncologists to provide symptom management, care, and support to families and patients with advanced-stage disease.

The World Health Organization (WHO) (1) defined palliative care as follows:

The active total care of patients whose disease is not responsive to curative treatment. Control of pain of other symptoms, and of psychological, social and spiritual problems, is paramount. The goal of palliative care is achievement of the best quality of life for patients and their families. Many aspects of palliative care are also applicable earlier in the course of the illness in conjunction with anti-cancer treatment.

To further clarify the meaning and goals of palliative care, the WHO (1) further stated:

Palliative care: affirms life and regards dying as a normal process, . . . neither hastens nor postpones death, . . . provides relief from pain and other distressing symptoms, . . . integrates the psychological and the spiritual aspects of care, . . . offers a support system to help patients live as actively as possible until death, . . . offers a support system to help the family cope during the patient's illness and their own bereavement.

Palliative care, then, is centered on ensuring the patient lives as comfortably as possible until death occurs. Palliative care is an interdisciplinary specialty, utilizing the talents of physicians, nurses, pharmacists, rehabilitation professionals, chaplains, and social workers. Treatment revolves around the needs of the patient and her family. The patient is guided in reclaiming control of her life. As each woman is unique, each woman's goals differ. These professionals function synergistically in assisting the patient in realizing her goals. Volunteers are also an important component of a palliative-care program, providing services and support that exhausted families desperately need.

Many oncology teams attempt to offer the

633

services and supports mentioned above. The transition from striving for cure to focusing on quality of life issues is often difficult for care teams and patients alike. Women have many concerns about leaving their children and preparing for possible death in the coming months. Many patients experience guilt when asking their oncologist about family problems or expressing concern about dying. The patients are reluctant to raise these issues with the team, which is still striving to control the disease or prolong life. Although always sad, the period of time preceding death can be one of profound growth for individuals and families. Unfortunately, when patients and families are not encouraged to address end-of-life issues, this interval is often foreshortened or missed altogether. Palliative-care services are not preoccupied with death, grief, and mourning. Neither is death romanticized. Rather, the essence of palliative care is the affirmation of life in its fullest until the conclusion of the journey.

Many patients and clinicians are reluctant to request intervention from a palliative-care service because the concept of palliative care is confused with terminal care (2). This is an unfortunate misunderstanding. As Doyle et al (3) stated, the term *terminal care* is ambiguous and confusing. When does terminal care begin? Is it hours, days, or weeks before death occurs? Could it begin at the time when it becomes clear that the goal of care has changed from cure to quality of life? Patients often sense death will be the ultimate outcome long before the physician or care team is prepared to acknowledge this fact. Does terminal care begin at this point? The term *terminal care* implies great "negativity and passivity" (3). Many people perceive it as the end to active treatment. As a result, the whole concept of a palliative-care consultation is rejected. Education underscoring the falseness of these suppositions is needed, both to health-care providers and to the population at large.

Good palliative care is based on providing good medical care. Symptom management is primary. It is unrealistic to attempt to help a woman deal with the psychological and social issues involved in the preparation for death when she is experiencing pain, severe shortness of breath, or uncontrolled nausea and vomiting. Palliative-care physicians receive training specific to managing these symptoms. Once symptoms are controlled, the team embarks on addressing psychosocial issues, helping the patient identify and achieve her goals.

Another function of a palliative-care service is to ensure the patient receives care in the setting of her choice. Palliative care for the woman who prefers to die at home is arranged by the palliative-care team. If care at home becomes too onerous, transfer to a palliative-care unit is often appropriate. Once physical care is facilitated, the patient and family are encouraged to continue focusing on accomplishing their personal and family goals.

Symptom Management in Advanced Cancer

Patients with advanced and terminal malignant disease experience a wide variety of symptoms posing a diversity of problems. The most commonly reported symptoms include pain, dyspnea, weakness, fatigue, nausea and vomiting, anorexia, and weight loss (4–10). There are also a variety of psychological and psychiatric disorders, such as anxiety, depression, and alterations of cognitive function (6,10–14). Many patients also complain of sleep disorders, ranging from nightmares to hypersomnia and insomnia (11–13). Careful management of these various symptoms can make a tremendous difference to the quality of life of both the patient and the family. The bereavement process of the family is much affected by the condition of the patient in the last days of life (15). The mourning period is eased if recollection of the patient is one of relative comfort and peace. Three clinical problems—pain, dyspnea, and bowel obstruction—are discussed in detail. Pain and dyspnea are frequent findings in both breast and gynecologic tumors and are the two symptoms most feared by cancer patients (11). Bowel obstruction is a very common terminal event in women with gynecologic tumors but may also result from widespread peritoneal metastases from tumors at other sites (16).

Management of Cancer Pain

Pain is the most persistent and debilitating symptom of metastatic cancer (11). Moderate and severe pain has been identified as a significant health problem globally (1,11,17–19). When poorly managed, it leads to a limitation of function and impairment of quality of life (20).

It is well recognized that despite validated practice guidelines from the WHO (21,22), the

American Pain Society (23), the American Medical Association (24), and the U.S. Department of Health and Human Resources (25), cancer pain continues to be poorly managed (11,17,26,27). One third of patients in active treatment experience significant function-limiting pain (20,26). This number rises to greater than 50% in patients with more advanced illness and to 70% in patients with advanced and terminal disease (28). In contrast, in a palliative-care program, satisfactory pain control is achieved with the vast majority of patients (29–31). Most patients will develop their symptoms months and even years before becoming terminally ill. It is essential, then, that health-care workers caring for cancer patients in all disciplines become familiar with techniques of good cancer pain management (4).

Three major barriers to good pain management have been identified:

1. *The health-care delivery system* contributes by not recognizing the time required for good pain assessment and management. Physicians are not appropriately remunerated for their services. This discourages proper investigation (25). Regulation of the prescription of opioids discourages appropriate utilization of these medications (25,32). Medical and postgraduate education focuses on cure and does not underline the importance of symptom management.

2. *Patients and families* contribute to poor pain management by failing to report significant discomfort (32,33). Many people believe that pain is simply part of the cancer experience and do not report function-limiting symptoms to their physician (33). Patients do not wish to "bother" the physician, "wasting" precious time talking about non-life-threatening issues with the physician (33). Worsening pain is often viewed as advance of the disease; patients do not want to admit this or fear being ineligible for treatment protocols (32). Finally, there is much misunderstanding about drug dependence, addiction, and tolerance to opioids (32,33). Patients and families believe the cost of good pain management is potential drug dependence or intolerable side effects (32). Much patient education is required (32).

3. *Health-care professionals* also have knowledge gaps regarding the use, abuse, and side effect profile of opioids (25,32,34). Many physicians feed into the myth that early opioid use will lead to poor pain control in advanced disease, or will produce patients addicted to opioid medications (35). Many are reluctant to prescribe opioids due to federal regulations on controlled drugs. Most significant, many physicians are lacking the skills of cancer pain assessment and investigation (27,32,36,37). Because pain is an interdisciplinary symptom, proper pain management skills are often not taught in medical and postgraduate training programs (37–40).

Cancer pain is a complex phenomenon, combining physical, psychological, social, and spiritual components. Patients often define their pain in terms of loss of function (e.g., "I used to jog five miles daily, now I can scarcely walk fifty feet") or in terms of threat to the future (e.g., "What will happen if the pain gets so bad I can't walk to the bathroom?"). The experience of pain is heightened if patients believe their disease is punishment for past real or imagined misdemeanors. The management of pain is greatly influenced by 1) surrounding caregivers, 2) past experience with illness, and 3) attitudes or fears about pain medications. Cultural background plays a significant role in the expression of pain. People from diverse cultural backgrounds who are experiencing similar pain will have varying expressions of their discomfort, depending on cultural expectations or the meaning and value of pain. Suffering is not proportional to or equivalent with pain. Patients fearing disease recurrence or experiencing guilt may suffer more distress from smaller amounts of pain. We cannot measure nociception, pain, or suffering (11). One can only observe pain behavior. Many factors other than nociceptive input can impact on this behavior. Figure 44-1 illustrates how a multitude of factors, none of which can be quantified, may overlie the original nociceptive stimuli. The first observable outcome is pain behavior, which is the result of a combination of personal, social, and cultural influences. A patient who is quietly enduring pain does not necessarily have better pain control than a very demonstrative patient. A corollary conclusion is that pharmacologic intervention alone is often insufficient to relieve the suffering in cancer pain. A multidisciplinary approach, addressing social,

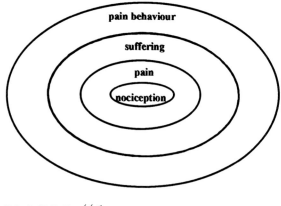

F I G U R E **44-1**

A conceptual model of pain.

psychological, and spiritual concerns, is essential for complete symptom management.

Assessment of Cancer Pain

The key to good cancer pain management is a careful initial assessment of the patient and repeat reassessments after therapy has begun. It is important to note that the pain picture will change as the disease progresses; management strategies will change accordingly.

A good pain history includes a detailed description of the site and nature of the pain: 1) What factors trigger the pain or make it worse? 2) What factors relieve the pain? 3) How long does it take for analgesics to alleviate the pain? 4) How complete is the alleviation? 5) How long does pain relief last? A psychological assessment is also included in the initial interview. The examiner is looking for indications of emotional factors that will affect the patient's symptoms (11).

The physical examination is targeted toward a general assessment of the patient with particular focus on the neurologic examination. It is important to note how well the patient is able to move and her functional capacity. Patients with chronic severe pain present differently from patients with acute severe pain (11). Acute pain is often accompanied by overt distress, restlessness, tachycardia, and tachypnea. Patients may be diaphoretic and hypertensive. In contrast, patients with chronic pain rarely demonstrate such findings. They are often quiet and have no hemodynamic alterations or tachypnea. A common mistake is to underestimate the distress of these patients because

they are not presenting the signs associated with acute pain syndromes.

Classification of Cancer Pain

A careful description of the pain along with a neurologic assessment is required to assist with classification of the pain syndrome. This is important as the appropriate treatment modalities depend on the pathophysiology of the pain (11).

Cancer pain is generally divided into two broad categories: nociceptive and neuropathic. Nociceptive pain is further subclassified into somatic and visceral categories. *Nociceptive pain* refers to a pathophysiology whereby pain is precipitated by activation of peripheral nociceptive receptors and transmitted centrally by large A fibers and smaller unmyelinated C fibers. The impulses ascend the spinothalamic tract via the dorsal root ganglion and thalamus, and eventually reach the cerebral cortex. The pain is described by patients in usual pain terms such as sharp, dull, or aching. The patient clearly recognizes the sensation as pain. Somatic pain results from involvement of the musculoskeletal system such as bony metastases or soft tissue tumors. The pain is usually sharp, well localized, and nonradiating. It is often made worse by movement and the patient prefers to find and maintain a comfortable posture. Visceral pain results from involvement of abdominal viscera such as pancreas or liver or obstruction of hollow viscera such as the bowel or bladder. This pain is poorly localized and is often diffuse. It is frequently associated with nausea or diaphoresis. With obstruction, the pain is colicky in nature. Patients often have difficulty finding a comfortable position and may demonstrate restlessness.

Neuropathic pain results from spontaneous discharge of damaged nerve fibers. Damage may result from tumor invasion, compression, or therapies such as chemotherapy or radiation. The anatomic connections of neuropathic pain are not well known. Patients describe the pain as burning, itching, lancinating, tingling, numb, or cold (41). Most patients will relate that they have not experienced this type of feeling before. When a limb is involved, there may be a corresponding motor deficit.

Systemic Analgesic Therapy

As pain is so debilitating, it is appropriate to begin therapy with systemic analgesics even prior to making a definitive pain diagnosis. It is important to note, however, that systemic analgesic therapy only treats symptoms and does not remedy the underlying cause of the pain. Even if the patient has advanced disease, definitive interventions should be considered for pain control (e.g., surgery, chemotherapy, or radiation). For example, the best management of bone pain due to a pathologic fracture is stabilization of the fractured bone. This usually requires surgical intervention. Even minor shrinking of a tumor may relieve neuropathic pain due to nerve compression.

Often, there is no definitive therapy or the patient is too debilitated to undergo rigorous interventions and aggressive pharmacologic management is required. The WHO has issued practice guidelines for the appropriate use of analgesic medications (22). These guidelines are summarized in the WHO ladder (Fig. 44-2). For mild pain, initial therapy consists of nonopioid medications such as salicylates, nonsteroidal anti-inflammatory medications (NSAIDs), or acetaminophen, either singly or in combination. For moderately severe pain, the initial drug of choice should be a weak opioid such as codeine or oxycodone in combination with salicylates or acetaminophen. More severe pain is managed by strong opioids in combination with adjuvant analgesics. Adjuvants may be used at any stage in the therapeutic process. Other nonpharmacologic interventions such as physiotherapy, massage, relaxation therapies, and mental imaging should be encouraged at all stages (11).

Nonopioid Analgesics

The most commonly used medications are salicylates, NSAIDs, and acetaminophen. These are appropriate for use in patients with mild to moderate pain and as adjunctive therapy in those with moderate to severe pain. There is a ceiling to their analgesic effect.

Although usually well tolerated, these medications have significant side effect profiles and patients should be selected with caution. Salicylates and NSAIDs can cause significant bleeding via their antiplatelet actions and propensity to produce gastric duodenal ulceration. Patients with a history of gastrointestinal bleeding should receive concurrent therapy with cytoprotective agents. Renal failure can be precipitated, particularly in patients who are volume depleted.

No clinical trials have demonstrated clear superiority of any single NSAID in managing cancer pain. There is considerable interpatient variability in response to therapy. If a patient fails to respond to one medication, after 1 week, switching to an NSAID medication in a different class is recommended (Table 44-1).

Opioid Analgesics

Opioid analgesics are traditionally classified into weak or strong opioids (Table 44-2). This distinction is based on clinical criteria rather than differences in pharmacology. All opioid actions are mediated via interaction with opioid receptors. Opioid receptors are widely distributed throughout the body including the central nervous system and respiratory and gastrointestinal tracts. Opioid actions can be reversed by administration of specific opioid antagonists (e.g., naloxone) (see Table 44-2). The most commonly used weak opioids are codeine and oxycodone. They are most efficacious when used in combination with aspirin or acetaminophen. Weak opioids not recommended for use in cancer pain include propoxyphene and pentazocine.

There are a number of strong opioids available for clinical use. The most commonly used

F I G U R E **44-2**

The WHO three-step analgesic step ladder.

T A B L E **44-1**

Recommended Dosages of Some Common Nonsteroidal Anti-inflammatory Drugs

Trade Name	Generic Name	Route	Recommended Dosage	Frequency	Caution
Naprosyn E[a]	Naproxen	PO	375 mg	bid	GI bleeding, renal failure, platelet dysfunction
Naprosyn	Naproxen	Suppository	100 mg	Daily	Same
Voltaren SR	Diclofenac sodium	PO	100 mg	Daily	Same
Voltaren	Diclofenac sodium	Suppository	100 mg	Daily	Same
Toradol	Ketorolac tromethamine	PO	10 mg	Daily, q6h prn	Same
Toradol	Ketorolac tromethamine	IM	30 mg	q6h prn	[b]
Indocid	Indomethacin	PO	25 mg	tid	GI bleeding, etc. (see above)
Indocid	Indomethacin	Suppository	50 mg	Once a day	Same
Motrin	Ibuprofen	PO	400 mg	tid	Same

[a] Naprosyn E reflects enteric coated formulation.

[b] Recommended for short course only (e.g., 5–7 days). May precipitate serious GI bleeding.

include morphine, hydromorphone, levorphanol, heroin, and methadone. The widest clinical experience is with morphine which should be considered the strong opioid of choice for therapy of moderate to severe pain. Opioids are versatile medications. They are well absorbed orally but are also available for parenteral epidural and intrathecal administration. They are widely distributed throughout the central nervous system and peripheral tissues. They are metabolized in the liver and excreted in the urine. Doses must be reduced for elderly patients or those with hepatic or renal failure (Table 44-3). Morphine has two known metabolites: morphine-3-glucuronide and morphine-6-glucuronide. The half-life of these metabolites is longer than the half-life of the active drug and may be responsible for some of the observed side effects. Meperidine also has an active metabolite: normeperidine. Its half-life is considerably longer than that of active meperidine and it is seizurogenic. Meperidine is not recommended for use in chronic cancer pain management. Hydromorphone is not currently known to have any metabolites. For patients who are not experiencing desired analgesia, or who have intolerable side effects with one opioid agent, other opioids should be tried sequentially, as ineffectiveness or side effects

with one agent does not predict similar problems with other drugs in this class (Tables 44-4 and 44-5).

The oral route is the preferred method of administration. It is generally recommended that therapy be initiated with short-acting preparations for rapid achievement of analgesia. Once the required dose has been determined, patients may be switched to a sustained-release preparation, administered every 8 to 12 hours. Analgesics should be administered around the clock and not on an "as required" basis. Provision must always be made for a breakthrough or rescue dose. This is generally 50% of the regular dose administered every 2 hours as required. If patients require frequent rescue doses, the regular dose of opioid should be increased accordingly.

Managing Opioid Side Effects

Patients who are experiencing poor analgesia or intolerable side effects with one opioid should be switched to a series of different opioids before one concludes that therapy is ineffective or intolerable. On occasion, changing the route of administration may also provide improved pain management.

There are multiple side effects associated

TABLE **44-2**

Guidelines for the Utilization of Opioids and Opioid Antagonists

Drug	Recommended Starting Dose	Route	Frequency (hr)	Peak Effect (hr)	Duration (hr)	Side Effect
Weak Opioids						
Codeine 15–30 mg/ acetaminophen	1–2 tablets	PO	q4	1–2	4–6	Constipation, nausea and vomiting
Codeine	30–60 mg	SC	q4	0.5	4–6	Same
Codeine contin.	50–100 mg	PO	q12	N/A	12	Same
Oxycodone 5 mg/ acetaminophen	1–2 tablets	PO	q4	1–2	4–6	Same
Strong Opioids						
Morphine elixir	5–10 mg	PO	q4	1–2	4–6	Sweet taste may precipitate nausea
Morphine tablet	5–10 mg	PO	q4	1–2	4–6	See Table 44-6
Morphine sustained release	15–30 mg	PO	8–12	N/A	8–12	See Table 44-6
Morphine parenteral[a]	5–10 mg (see Table 44-5)	SC	q4	0.25–0.50	4–6	See Table 44-6
Hydromorphone	1–2 mg	PO	q4	1–2	4–6	See Table 44-6
Hydromorphone parenteral	0.5–1.0 mg	SC	q4	0.5	4–6	See Table 44-6
Demerol[b]	100–150 mg	PO	4	1–2	3–4	Generally less effective given orally
Demerol parenteral[b]	75 mg	IM	4	0.5–1.0	3–4	Repeated administrations are seizurogenic
Fentanyl patch	[c]	Dermal patch[d]	Change patch q3d	N/A	N/A	[e]
Naloxone (Narcan)	0.2–0.4 mg	IV	q5min prn	Immediate	Variable[f]	Acute abstinence syndrome[g]

N/A = not applicable.

[a] Subcutaneous and intravenous doses are equivalent. The onset of action and side effects is more rapid with intravenous injection. If given intravenously, recommend low initial dose with gradual dose augmentation.

[b] Not recommended for cancer pain.

[c] Based on previous response to short-acting opioids (e.g., morphine or hydromorphone).

[d] Oral preparation currently not available.

[e] Prolonged duration of both effects and side effects due to subdermal pooling of medication. No oral preparation available for breakthroughs.

[f] Action is via competitive antagonism at the opioid receptor. Competition between agonist and antagonist may persist for 3–4 hours. Patients must be carefully monitored as repeated naloxone injections may be required.

[g] Precipitation of acute abstinence syndrome: attempt to administer minimum required dose to reverse life-threatening respiratory depression without reversing all desirable opioid effects (e.g., analgesia).

with opioid therapy (Table 44-6). Many of these can be prevented with good prophylactic medical management. All patients will experience constipation, which can be serious enough to result in bowel obstruction. Tolerance to this effect does not develop and all patients receiving opioids should receive concurrent stool softeners and bowel stimulants. Nausea and vomiting are frequently seen with early opioid therapy. Tolerance usually develops over 3 to 5 days but all patients should be provided with concurrent antiemetic therapy as required. Tol-

TABLE 44-3
Factors Influencing Dose

Factor	Influence
Age	Elderly patients very susceptible to opioid effects. Halve doses in geriatric patients.
Renal and hepatic failure	All opioids are metabolized by liver and excreted in urine. Reduce dose and/or lengthen interval of administration in patients with renal/hepatic failure or reduced PO intake and dehydration.
Prior exposure	Patients who are opioid naive will have greater effect from initial opioid therapy. Doses should be lowered.

TABLE 44-4
Equianalgesic Doses

Drug	SC	PO
Morphine	10	20–30
Hydromorphone	1.5	3–5
Codeine	120	120

TABLE 44-5
Dose Conversion from Oral Morphine to Transdermal Fentanyl

Oral Morphine (mg/day)	Initial TTS Fentanyl Dose (μg/h)
45–134	25
135–224	50
225–314	75
315–404	100

TABLE 44-6
Opioid Side Effects

Side Effect	Frequency	Management
Constipation	Universal	All patients receiving opioids should receive concurrent stool softeners and laxatives.
Nausea	Frequent	Antiemetics should be available, particularly in early phases of opioid therapy.
Respiratory depression (RD)	Variable and dose dependent	Can be fatal. If RD significant, naloxone, a competitive antagonist, should be administered. RD may reoccur following antagonist: observe patient closely for 4 hr following event. Repeated naloxone administration may be required.
Sedation	Variable, tolerance quickly develops	Dose reduction. If remains problematic, switch opioids. Occasionally addition of methylphenidate (Ritalin) 5 mg bid allows analgesia without sedation.
Cognitive impairment	Variable	Switch opioids if cognitive state does not improve within 48 hr.
Dry mouth	Frequent	Mouth irrigation and chewing gum/sour candies to stimulate saliva.
Urinary retention	Infrequent	Always consider other possible etiology (e.g., cord compression).
Pruritus	Infrequent Does not represent allergy	Opioids release histamine from mast cells. Concurrent treatment with antihistamines sometimes required. True allergy to opioids is extremely rare.

erance usually develops to the sedative effects of opioids and patients should be encouraged to persist with therapy for at least 72 hours. Respiratory depression is the most serious side effect and can be life-threatening. This is rare if initial doses are appropriate and gradually escalated. Reversal of respiratory depression is rapidly achieved with the administration of the specific antagonist (naloxone). It is important to note that the half-life of naloxone is very short relative to morphine and patients may require repeat administration of this agent to prevent return of respiratory depression.

Adjuvant Analgesic Therapies

Adjuvant analgesics are medications that are not primarily analgesic in nature, but which act syn-

Adjuvant Analgesics for Neuropathic Pain

Adjuvant Analgesic	Dose	Mechanism of Action	Caution
Tricyclic antidepressants (amitriptyline, nortriptyline)	Initial dose: 10–25 mg qhs with gradual increase to 150–200 mg	Enhanced catecholamine neurotransmitters for analgesic pathways	May produce anticholinergic side effects
Anticonvulsants			
A. Carbamazepine	100 mg tid increase to 800 mg daily	Neuromembrane stabilization	Drowsiness, rash, bone marrow suppression
B. Valproic acid	250 mg bid increase to 1 g daily	Same	Monitor liver function tests for hepatotoxicity
Antiarrhythmics (mexiletine)	100 mg bid to maximum 600–800 mg daily	Same	Severe nausea, not responsive to antiemetics, arrhythmias if underlying cardiac disease
Steroids (dexamethasone)	2–4 mg qid	Not well defined	Peptic ulcer disease, long-term use has many complications
NMDA receptor blockers (ketamine)	Continuous SC infusion with anesthesia supervision	NMDA receptor blockade interrupts aberrant pain pathways at level of central nervous system	Hypotension, confusion, disorientation, aggression

T A B L E   **44-8**

Adjuvant Analgesics for Bone Pain

Adjuvant Analgesic	Dose	Mechanism of Action	Caution
Nonsteroidal anti-inflammatories	See Table 44-1	Interrupted prostaglandin synthesis	See Table 44-1
Bisphosphonates (pamidronate)	60 mg IV over 6 hr	Decreased osteoclastic activity	Monitor serum calcium and phosphate; may require repeated administration to control pain
Steroids (dexamethasone)	2–4 mg bid to qid	In part anti-inflammatory but incompletely understood	Peptic ulcer disease and long-term complications

ergistically with analgesic medications to enhance pain relief. There is wide interpatient variability in responses to adjuvant analgesic therapy. It is important to identify neuropathic components of pain syndromes as adjuvant analgesics are almost always required to manage neuropathic pain (Tables 44-7 and 44-8).

Invasive Analgesic Approaches

Unfortunately, there remains a small but significant proportion of cancer patients who will not achieve adequate pain management with systemic opioid administration or who develop unacceptable side effect profiles at doses required to control their pain. A number of different approaches are available for this patient population. The dose of opioids required to achieve analgesia is significantly reduced when the medication is administered centrally (e.g., epidural or intraventricular administration). Administration of opioids via these routes preserves motor and sensory functions. Once analgesia has been achieved, patients may resume normal activities. Morphine or hydromorphone can be administered, but many anesthetists select fentanyl due to its short duration of action and lipophilicity, which reduces central redistribution. Analgesia may be enhanced by the addition of low-dose anesthetic agents (e.g., bupivacaine). Postural hypotension is the major significant limitation of this approach.

Consultation with an anesthetist with a special interest in pain management is recommended for consideration of blocks or neurolytic procedures.

Neurosurgical Techniques

Similarly, in a small proportion of patients, consultation with a neurosurgeon is appropriate for consideration of surgical interruption of anatomic pathways (e.g., cordotomy or thalamotomy). The complications of these procedures are significant and the success rate variable and these approaches are generally reserved for intractable pain that has not responded to all other approaches.

Myths About Morphine: Tolerance, Addiction, and Dependence

There is broad misunderstanding by health-care providers, patients, and families about the risk of developing opioid dependence. This is an extremely rare phenomenon. There is an important clinical distinction between physical and psychological dependence. All patients receiving regular opioid therapy will develop physical dependence. This is defined as the development of the abstinence or withdrawal syndrome upon cessation of therapy. Patients exhibit salivation, lacrimation, piloerection, pain, and diarrhea. Abrupt cessation of opioid therapy should always be avoided. Patients who have been receiving regular opioid therapy should have their dose tapered before discontinuation. In this way, the withdrawal syndrome is avoided. Psychological dependence implies drug-seeking behavior and inappropriate use of medication. This is rare in cancer patients and has no relation to physical dependence.

Tolerance is a pharmacologic concept referring to the need for an increased dosage to achieve a similar outcome. Tolerance develops to many of the opioid side effects, but is rarely seen to analgesia. Patients who develop increasing pain following a period of stable opioid usage should be investigated for advancing underlying disease. Opioid therapy should never be withheld at an earlier stage of illness in order to reserve strong medication until the end.

Addiction is a pattern of compulsive drug use characterized by a continued craving for an opioid, the need to use the opioid for effects other than pain relief. Addiction is extremely rare in cancer patients. It is, however, a major cause of concern for patients and families, who must be repeatedly reassured.

Specific Pain Syndromes

Postmastectomy Pain

Up to 10% of women will develop this syndrome following partial or total mastectomy (42). The pain is neuropathic in nature and described as constricting, bandlike, or burning (41). It is often aggravated by movement of the arm (41–43). Some women will develop a frozen shoulder from holding the arm immobile and flexed to prevent pain (41). This syndrome follows neuroma or damage of the intercostobrachial nerve during surgery (28,41,42,44,45). The anatomic distribution of this nerve is highly variable, which accounts for the wide variability in clinical presentation. This symptom may present in the immediate postoperative period or up to 6 months postoperatively (43,44). Treatment is difficult and consists of a topical application of capsaicin, local anesthetics (e.g., lidocaine or lidocaine-prilocaine) (42,44), medications directed to neuropathic pain (e.g., carbamazepine), and adjuvant analgesics (41). Occasionally injection of a neurolytic agent into an identified neuroma may be helpful.

Postherpetic Neuralgia

Acute herpetic cutaneous eruptions are extremely painful and may be complicated by the development of postherpetic neuralgia, a chronic pain syndrome. Patients with cancer are five times as likely to develop zoster compared with the general population (46). Patients with gynecologic tumors are more likely to develop zoster in the lumbosacral region. Women with breast tumors are more likely to have thoracic zoster whereas patients with hematologic malignancies most often present with cervical zoster. Cancer patients are five times more likely to develop postherpetic neuralgia following acute herpetic eruptions (46). This pain is neuropathic in nature, described as burning, itching, or lancinating. Patients will also demonstrate hyperesthesia and allodynia (47). Pain from this syndrome can be debilitating and treatment is difficult. Different management approaches have been suggested, including systemic opioids, carbamazepine, and topical application of capsaicin (3,47).

Management of Dyspnea

Dyspnea is an unpleasant sensation of an increased awareness of breathing (48,49). It is seen in 29% to 74% of patients with terminal cancer (48–52) and may occur in the absence of pulmonary involvement (49). It is a significant cause of distress for both patient and family (4,51). Dyspnea is a frequent complication of advanced breast carcinoma. It is important to note that dyspnea is an entirely subjective sensation (48,49,53). There are no objective measures of dyspnea. The best single objective criterion is respiratory rate. Significant to the experience of dyspnea is the patient's prior history of respiratory disease (49). Patients with chronic obstructive pulmonary diseases have a life history of respiratory compromise and may be less symptomatic with more disease than a patient who has never experienced any shortness of breath (49).

The etiology of dyspnea is multifactorial (Table 44-9); there are usually several major synergistic factors contributing to any single patient's symptoms (6,49). Tumor-related factors may include invasion or compression of the bronchial tree, superior vena caval compression, pleural or pericardial effusion, lymphangitic involvement, and vocal cord paralysis (6,49). Associated conditions such as pneumonia (aspiration or postobstructive), pulmonary embolism, cardiac disease, ascites, anemia, hepatomegaly, and generalized muscle weakness may contribute to dyspnea (6,49,50). Treatment-related causes include pulmonary fibrosis (from either chemotherapy or radiation) and surgical resection of pulmonary tissues. Anxiety, a frequent companion to dyspnea, can significantly contribute to patient discomfort (6,49). One must also consider preexisting cardiac or respiratory diseases such as asthma, chronic obstructive pulmonary disease, and congestive heart failure (49,54).

Behavioral, Environmental, and Psychological Management

Effective management of shortness of breath requires a multifactorial approach (6,51). These approaches can be summarized as behavioral, environmental, psychological, and pharmacologic. Most patients benefit from interventions in all four categories; the first three are discussed in this section (Table 44-10).

Behavioral approaches are largely based on the concept of energy conservation. Typically taught by occupational and physiotherapy specialists, these techniques educate the patient on methods of energy conservation and minimizing respiratory demands. Examples of energy-conserving techniques include helping patients reorganize activities. Tasks such as bathing and dressing are difficult for patients with dyspnea. Patients are instructed to rest between these activities and during scheduled periods, especially prior to an expected activity. There are many effective aids that assist in dressing, reaching, and bending. Various postures are explored to identify those most comfortable.

Environmental interventions include arranging the patient's environment to minimize the need for mobilization. Again, these interventions are best managed by occupational and physiotherapy therapists. Patients are advised to move to a bedroom situated near the bathroom.

T A B L E   **44-9**

Etiology of Dyspnea

Airway obstruction by tumor
Pleural effusion
Lymphangitis carcinomatosa
Lung metastases
Tracheoesophageal fistula
Embolism (tumor or venous)
Anxiety
Pneumonia (aspiration or obstructive)
Vocal cord paralysis
Pericardial effusion
Ascites
Hepatomegaly

T A B L E   **44-10**

Strategies for the Management of Dyspnea

Behavioral
   A. Postural adjustment
   B. Energy conservation
Environmental
   Arrangement of environment to minimize need
      for mobilization
Psychological
   A. Stress management
   B. Relaxation
   C. Imaging

Alternatively, bedside commodes are provided to obviate the need for patients to walk to the bathroom. Other aids may be provided in the home or hospital (such as wheelchairs) to conserve the patient's energy and breathing capacity for other activities.

Psychological interventions include relaxation therapy to manage anxiety and stress which can precipitate or exacerbate dyspnea. Family counseling may be helpful as caregivers can transfer anxiety to the patient.

Pharmacologic Management

Appropriate management of contributing medical conditions (e.g., infection or pleural effusion) should be undertaken (Table 44-11). Moderate to severe dyspnea usually requires treatment with a combination of medications (Table 44-12). Opioids are thought to be effective by decreasing the sensation of breathlessness: a decrease in ventilatory drive in response to stimuli such as hypoxia and hypercapnia, and a decrease in oxygen consumption at any given level of exercise. These effects are achieved without altering arterial oxygen saturation, carbon dioxide pressure, or respiratory rate (52). Opioids may be administered subcutaneously or intravenously if rapid effects are required. In opioid-naive patients, small doses (5 mg) are recommended initially (52). Alterna-

TABLE 44-11

Medical Management of Dyspnea

Chemotherapy or radiation to shrink obstructing
   lesion
Thoracentesis with or without pleurodesis
Treatment of pneumonia
Pericardiocentesis
Paracentesis
Blood transfusion
Re-expansion of pneumothorax
Oxygen therapy

TABLE 44-12

Pharmacologic Management of Dyspnea

Morphine (nebulized or parenteral)
Benzodiazepines
Corticosteroids
Bronchodilators
Local anesthetics
Anticholinergics

tively, morphine may be administered orally if the clinical situation is less acute. Trials of nebulized opioids are currently ongoing. No clear advantage over nebulized saline solution has been demonstrated, but some subgroups of patients appear to benefit significantly from this approach (53). Further studies are required to identify which patients are most likely to benefit from this route of administration. Benzodiazepines (e.g., lorazepam 1–2 mg sublingually every 2–4 hours as required) will reduce the associated anxiety (6,49). Many patients, particularly those with lymphangitic involvement, will benefit significantly from corticosteroid therapy (49,53) [e.g., dexamethasone (Decadron) 2–4 mg orally or intravenously every 6 hours]. This effect is not apparent until 4 to 6 hours following initial administration. Phenothiazines (e.g., chlorpromazine 10–25 mg orally every 6 hours) may contribute to relief (55). Secretions in the large airways contribute to congestion and terminal "death rattle." This can be significantly relieved by the administration of scopolamine (e.g., Hyoscine 0.4–0.6 mg subcutaneously every 2 hours as required or glycopyrrolate 200 µg orally or subcutaneously every 6 hours). Patients with a history of chronic obstructive pulmonary disease or with audible wheezing may benefit from bronchodilator therapy (54) (e.g., methylxanthines or nebulized salbutamol). There are anecdotal reports that patients with persistent cough may benefit from inhaled local anesthetic agents.

Management of Malignant Bowel Obstruction in Advanced Cancer

Malignant bowel obstruction (MBO) presents difficult management issues in patients with advanced cancer. The exact prevalence of this condition is not known, but MBO is seen in 25% to 42% of patients with ovarian carcinoma (16,56). Obstruction can be complete or partial. Patients present with abdominal pain, colic, nausea, and vomiting (7,8,56–58). The symptoms are a cause of major distress for the patient and family, and usually require admission to a hospital for management.

Traditional management of MBO has been surgical intervention aimed at relieving the obstruction and restoring bowel patency. When the patient is not deemed to be a suitable surgical candidate, alternative therapies have included nasogastric (NG) suction with aggressive volume repletion (8). Poor prognostic factors for surgical intervention include diffuse carcinomatosis causing intestinal motility problems, severe preoperative malnutrition, recurrent ascites, previous abdominal or pelvic radiation, preceding combination chemotherapy, palpable masses or liver involvement, extensive distant metastatic disease or pleural effusion, multiple sites of partial obstruction, and prolonged hospital admissions. Traditional outcome measures to assess the results of surgical interventions are generally expressed as length of survival postoperatively. These measures do not include assessment of quality of life. These patients often experience recurrent intermittent partial bowel obstruction, poor wound healing, infection, venous thrombosis, and other surgical complications. Repeat institution of NG suction is often required. NG suction is uncomfortable and restricts the patient to bed.

An alternative approach for patients with MBO who are poor surgical candidates has been developed by the hospice movement. This approach involves aggressive pharmacologic management of symptoms and obviates the need for NG suction. This approach was first introduced by Baines at St. Christopher's Hospice in London (8), and has been further developed by various hospice programs (7,56, 59). The approach is still largely confined to a palliative-care or hospice program but should be introduced to more general usage.

The principal symptoms of bowel obstruction include pain, nausea, and vomiting. The pain is both continuous from tumor involvement of the bowel and pelvic organs and colicky from obstruction of the bowel lumen (7,57,60). Nausea and vomiting are universally present but their incidence and severity vary depending on the location of the obstruction. Higher levels of obstruction are associated with increased nausea and vomiting (16). The key features of this approach include the following.

Pain Management

Pain is controlled via the use of intermittent or continuous subcutaneous administration of opioids. Various techniques are available for simple subcutaneous administration of medications (e.g., syringe drivers or infusers). These devices are small, lightweight, and portable, allowing for patient mobility. Colicky pain may require the use of antispasmodic medications such as scopolamine (Hyoscine), dicyclomine (Bentyl), or loperamide (Imodium).

Relief of Constipation

Constipation is a major contributor to the symptoms of MBO, particularly when the obstruction is partial. Aggressive use of stool softeners, enemas, and suppositories is required. Oral laxatives are not indicated when obstruction is complete.

Relief of Nausea and Vomiting

The symptom of nausea is a major cause of morbidity in MBO (Table 44-13). Aggressive management includes intermittent or continuous subcutaneous administration of different antiemetics, often used in combination (e.g., metoclopramide, dimenhydrinate, haloperidol, scopolamine, prochlorperazine). Corticosteroids can also be useful in this setting, both as antiemetics and possibly by reducing bowel wall edema, thus relieving some obstruction. Different studies report using dexamethasone, methylprednisolone, and prednisone (61–63). These medications can be administered via continuous subcutaneous infusion. In some instances, reducing the volume of bowel fluids relieves nausea and vomiting. Medications used in this setting include scopolamine and somatostatin. Again, these medications can be administered intermittently or via continuous subcutaneous infusion. When nausea and vomiting are not adequately controlled by pharmacologic methods alone, a percutaneous venting gastrostomy may be helpful. This is far more acceptable to patients than NG suction and permits patient mobility. Infusion of combination antiemetics provides good relief of nausea. Patients may continue to vomit intermittently, but if nausea is well controlled, this is not objectionable to most patients.

Advantages of the Symptom Management Approach

Site of Care

Using the symptom management approach, patients with MBO can be managed at home with the supervision of a physician and nurse familiar with this approach. Patients are not confined to bed and are able to dress and move

T A B L E **44-13**

Nausea and Vomiting

Source of Stimulus	Stimulus	Site of Action*	Antiemetics
Brain	Increased intracranial pressure	TVC	Corticosteroids
Cerebral cortex	Fear, anxiety, offensive smell, offensive sight	TVC	Antihistamines, corticosteroids, cannabinoids, benzodiazepines
Vestibular apparatus	Motion sickness (narcotics), brain tumors	TVC	Antihistamines
GI tract: vagal stimulation	Gastric stasis, GI obstruction, pharyngeal stimulation, gastric irritants (blood, iron, acetylsalicylic acid, NSAID)	TVC	Metoclopramide, domperidone
GI tract: sympathetic afferents	Same as above	CTZ	Phenothiazine, butyrophenones, (haloperidol), metoclopramide
Circulatory factors	Drugs: chemotherapy, opioids, digitalis, estrogens; metabolic: uremia, hypercalcemia, infection, radiotherapy	CTZ	Phenothiazines, butyrophenones, metoclopramide

GI = gastrointestinal.

*TVC: True vomiting center. Lateral reticular formation of medulla, close to respiratory and salivary centers. Several different kinds of receptors, activated by different neuronal transmitters. Common pathway of all stimuli leading to emesis. CTZ: Chemoreceptor trigger zone. Floor of fourth ventricle outside blood-brain barrier, linked to the TVC.

about as they wish. If the patient or family find care at home too difficult, patients can be cared for at a palliative-care unit or other nonacute care settings.

Patient Comfort

NG suction is physically uncomfortable and distasteful to many patients and families. Studies indicate good control of pain and nausea without excessive medical interventions (7,56, 57,59,61,64). Dignity is restored as patients are relieved of tubes, are able to dress, and in most instances, remain at home until or shortly before death.

Nutrition

Patients are encouraged to satisfy their wish for oral intake. It is explained to patients that increasing oral intake is likely to increase the incidence or volume of vomiting. Most patients receive considerable satisfaction from ingesting foods or beverages that appeal to them. Apart from anything else, this restores to the patient a sense of control (i.e., they can decide whether they wish to eat or drink, depending on their desires and tolerance for symptoms). It is emotionally devastating for patients to be told they can never eat or drink again.

There is considerable debate in the litera-

ture regarding hydrating patients with advanced disease (6,21). Volume repletion may cause an increased volume of gastrointestinal secretions, ascites, or pleural effusions. This may cause increased volume of vomiting or other symptoms, such as dyspnea or abdominal pain. Proponents of volume repletion report improved mental status and physical strength (64). Many patients and families have emotional difficulty with the concept of dehydration. In instances where volume replacement becomes a critical issue, this can be achieved in the home setting via hypodermoclysis—the subcutaneous administration of fluids (5). Again, this permits care at home and patient mobility without excessive medical intervention.

Infusion Devices

There are different lightweight infusion devices available. A variety of medications can be mixed and administered together without inactivating any of the components. These devices are portable and can be concealed beneath the patient's clothing.

Conclusions

Pain, dyspnea, nausea, and vomiting are frequent and distressing symptoms of advanced malignant disease. There are, however, a multitude of other symptoms experienced by patients with terminal illness, ranging from headache and blurred vision to dry skin and ulceration. These symptoms can be a source of profound despair to both patients and caregivers. Currently, insufficient attention is devoted to the management of these problems. However, the quality of life for patients can be considerably improved by interventions to control these symptoms. There are effective management strategies for many of these complaints. Readers are referred to comprehensive textbooks on the management of patients with advanced disease (3,62,65). It will be important to consolidate active palliative care into current treatment regimens to ensure comprehensive care for women with neoplastic disease.

Appendix: Definitions

Adjuvant analgesics: Medications that are not primarily analgesics but that act synergistically when used with analgesics.

Breakthrough analgesic: Analgesic made available to the patient as a rescue dose if a regular analgesic provides insufficient relief. If a breakthrough dose is required frequently, it is no longer considered a breakthrough dose and regular medications should be increased. Breakthrough analgesia is also useful to administer prophylactically if a painful event is anticipated (e.g., physiotherapy, physical care, or procedure).

Equianalgesic dose: An important clinical concept that facilitates switching from one medicine to another (e.g., morphine to hydromorphone) or switching from one route to another (oral to subcutaneous). Equianalgesic dose charts do not provide information about usual doses or recommended starting doses.

Neuropathic pain: Pain resulting from activation of damaged nerves. It is an "abnormal" pain consisting of burning, lancinating, or altered sensation (e.g., light touch is perceived as painful) or dysesthesia. Classically neuropathic pain is less responsive to opioid therapy.

Nociceptive pain: Pain resulting from activation of peripheral pain receptors, transmitted via A fibers and smaller un-

myelinated C fibers via the ascending spinothalamic tracts. Two subcategories include somatic and visceral.

Total pain: A concept whereby the patient expresses global despair (spiritual, psychological, emotional, and existential), using the word "pain." It is important to recognize this concept, as the use of analgesic medications alone is unlikely to improve the patient's suffering. A multidisciplinary approach is required to manage a total pain picture. It should be noted that a patient's suffering is not proportional to physical pain.

REFERENCES

1. Cancer pain relief and palliative care. *World Health Organ Tech Rep Ser* 1990;804.

2. Doyle D, Hanks GWC, MacDonald N. Introduction. In: *Oxford textbook of palliative medicine.* Oxford: Oxford University Press, 1993;3–8.

3. Foley KM, Doyle D, Hanks GWC, MacDonald N. Pain syndromes associated with cancer treatment. In: *Oxford textbook of palliative medicine.* Oxford: Oxford University Press, 1993:148–165.

4. Coyle N, Adelhardt J, Foley KM. Character of terminal illness in the advanced cancer patient: pain and other symptoms during the last four weeks of life. *J Pain Symptom Manage* 1990;5:83–93.

5. Bruera E, Legris MA, Kuehn N, Miller MJ. Hypodermoclysis for the administration of fluids and narcotic analgesics in patients with advanced cancer. *J Pain Symptom Manage* 1990;5:218–220.

6. Storey P. Symptom control in advanced cancer. *Semin Oncol* 1994;21:748–753.

7. Fainsinger RL, Spachynski K, Hanson J, Bruera E. Symptom control in terminally ill patients with malignant bowel obstruction (MBO). *J Pain Symptom Manage* 1994;9:12–18.

8. Baines M, Oliver DJ, Carter RL. Medical management of intestinal obstruction in patients with advanced malignant disease. *Lancet* 1985;2:990–993.

9. Bruera E, MacDonald RN. Nutrition in cancer patients: an update and review of our experience. *J Pain Symptom Manage* 1988;3:133–140.

10. Fainsinger R, Miller MJ, Bruera E. Symptom control during the last week of life on a palliative care unit. *J Palliat Med* 1991;7:5–11.

11. Foley KM. The treatment of cancer pain. *N Engl J Med* 1985;313:84–95.

12. Bottomley DM, Hanks G. Subcutaneous midazolam infusion in palliative care. *J Pain Symptom Manage* 1990;5:259–261.

13. Holland JC, Morrow GR, Schmale A, et al. A randomized clinical trial of alprazolam versus progressive muscle relaxation in cancer patients with anxiety and depressive symptoms. *J Clin Oncol* 1991;9:1004–1011.

14. Breitbart W, Bruera E, Chochinov H, Lynch M. Neuropsychiatric syndromes and psychological symptoms in patients with advanced cancer. *J Pain Symptom Manage* 1995;10:131–141.

15. Linn MW, Linn BS, Harris R. Effects of counseling for late stage cancer patients. *Cancer* 1982;49:1048–1055.

16. Tang E, Davis J, Silberman H. Bowel obstruction in cancer patients. *Arch Surg* 1995; 130:832–837.

17. Cleeland CS, Gonin R, Hatfield AK, et al. Pain and its treatment in outpatients with metastatic cancer. *N Engl J Med* 1994;330:592–596.

18. Greenwald HP, Bonica JJ, Bergner M. The prevalence of pain in four cancers. *Cancer* 1987; 60:2563–2569.

19. Twycross RG, Fairfield S. Pain in far-advanced cancer. *Pain* 1982;14:303–310.

20. Cleeland CS. Impact of pain on the patient with cancer. *Cancer* 1984;54:2635–2641.

21. Ventafridda V, Oliveri E, Caraceni A, et al. A retrospective study on the use of oral morphine in cancer pain. *J Pain Symptom Manage* 1987;2:77–82.

22. World Health Organization. *Cancer pain relief.* Geneva: World Health Organization, 1986:1–74.

23. Committee on Quality Assurance Standards, American Pain Society. American Pain Society quality assurance standards for relief of acute pain and cancer pain. In: Bond MR, Charlton JE, Woolf CJ, eds. *Proceedings of the VIth World Congress on Pain*, vol. 6. New York: Elsevier Science, 1991:185–189.

24. McGivney WT, Crooks GM. The care of patients with severe chronic pain in terminal illness. *JAMA* 1984;251:1182–1188.

25. Jacox A, Carr DB, Payne R. New clinical-practice guidelines for the management of pain in patients with cancer. *N Engl J Med* 1994; 330:651–655.

26. Bonica JJ. Cancer pain. In: Bonica JJ, ed. *Pain.* New York: Raven, 1980:335–362.

27. Marks RM, Sacher EJ. Undertreatment of medical inpatients with narcotic analgesics. *Ann Intern Med* 1973;38:173–181.

28. Portenoy RK. Cancer pain: epidemiology and syndromes. *Cancer* 1989;63:2298–2307.

29. Grond S, Zech S, Schug SA, et al. Validation of the World Health Organization guidelines for cancer pain relief during the last days and hours of life. *J Pain Symptom Manage* 1991;6:411–422.

30. Melzack R, Ofiesh JG, Mount BM. The Brompton mixture: effects on pain in cancer patients. *Can Med Assoc J* 1976;115:125–129.

31. Saunders C. Current views of pain relief and terminal care. In: Swerdlow M, ed. *The therapy of pain.* Lancaster: MTP Press, 1981:215.

32. Wilder-Smith CH, Schuler L. Postoperative analgesia: pain by choice? The influence of patient attitudes and patient education. *Pain* 1992;50:257–262.

33. Francke AL, Theeuwen I. Inhibition in expressing pain: a qualitative study among Dutch surgical breast cancer patients. *Cancer Nurs* 1994; 17:193–199.

34. Clarke EB, French B, Bilodeau ML, et al. Pain management knowledge, attitudes and clinical practice: the impact of nurses' characteristics and education. *J Pain Symptom Manage* 1996;1:18–31.

35. Cleeland CS, Cleeland LM, Dar R, Rinehardt LC. Factors influencing physician management of cancer pain. *Cancer* 1986;58:796–800.

36. Cleeland C. Research in cancer pain: what we know and what we need to know. *Cancer* 1991; 67:823–827.

37. Cooper S, Bean G, Alpery R, Baum JH. Medical students' attitudes toward cancer. *J Med Educ* 1980;55:434–439.

38. Margolies R, Wachtel AB, Sutherland KR, Blum RH. Medical students' attitudes toward cancer: concepts of professional distance. *J Psychosoc Oncol* 1983;1:35–49.

39. Kaye H, Appel M, Joseph R. Attitudes of medical students and residents toward cancer. *J Psychol* 1981;107:87–96.

40. Love RR, Hayward J, Stone HL. Attitudes about cancer medicine among primary care residents and their teachers. *J Med Educ* 1980;55:211–212.

41. Stevens PE, Dibble SL, Miaskowski C. Prevalence, characteristics, and impact of postmastectomy pain syndrome: an investigation of women's experiences. *Pain* 1995;61:61–68.

42. Dini D, Bertelli G, Gozza A, Forno GG. Treatment of the post-mastectomy pain syndrome with topical capsaicin. *Pain* 1993;54:223–226.

43. Maunsell E, Brisson J, Deschenes L. Arm problems and psychological distress after surgery for breast cancer. *Can J Surg* 1993;36:315–320.

44. Watson CPN, Evans RJ. The postmastectomy pain syndrome and topical capsaicin: a randomized trial. *Pain* 1992;51:375–379.

45. Foley K. Cancer pain syndromes. *J Pain Symptom Manage* 1987;2:S13–S17.

46. Rusthoven JJ, Ahlgren P, Elhakim T, et al. Risk factors for varicella zoster disseminated infection among adult cancer patients with localized zoster. *Cancer* 1988;62:1641–1646.

47. Bowsher D. Postherpetic neuralgia and its treatment: a retrospective survey of 191 patients. *J Pain Symptom Manage* 1996;12:290–299.

48. Gift AG. Dyspnea. *Nurs Clin North Am* 1990; 25:955–965.

49. Horn LW. Terminal dyspnea: a hospice approach. *Am J Hospice Palliat Care* 1992; (March/April):24–32.

50. Shepard KV. Dyspnea in cancer patients. *PCL Rev* 1990;2(6): insert 1.

51. Bruera E, De Stoutz N, Velasco-Leiva A, et al. Effects of oxygen on dyspnoea in hypoxaemic terminal-cancer patients. *Lancet* 1993;342:13–14.

52. Bruera E, Macmillan K, Pither J, et al. Effects of morphine on the dyspnea of terminal cancer patients. *J Pain Symptom Manage* 1990;5: 341–344.

53. Cowcher K, Hanks GW. Long-term management of respiratory symptoms in advanced cancer. *J Pain Symptom Manage* 1990;5:320–330.

54. Manning HL, Schwartzstein RM. Pathophysiology of dyspnea. *N Engl J Med* 1995;333:1547–1553.

55. O'Neill PA, Morton PB, Stark RD. Chlorpromazine—a specific effect on breathlessness? *Br J Pharmacol* 1985;19:793–797.

56. Ventafridda V, Ripamonti C, Caraceni A, et al. The management of inoperable gastrointestinal obstruction in terminal cancer patients. *Tumori* 1990;76:389–393.

57. Baines M. Medical management of intestinal obstruction. *Baillieres Clin Oncol* 1987;1:357–371.

58. Phillips RKS, Hittinger R, Fry JS, Fielding LP. Malignant large bowel obstruction. *Br J Surg* 1985;72:296–302.

59. Isbister WH, Elder P, Symons L. Non-operative management of malignant intestinal obstruction. *J R Coll Surg Edinb* 1990;35:369–372.

60. De Conno R, Caraceni A, Zecca E. Continuous subcutaneous infusion of hyoscine butylbromide reduces secretions in patients with gastrointestinal obstruction. *J Pain Symptom Manage* 1991; 6:484–486.

61. Reid DB. Palliative management of bowel obstruction. *Med J Aust* 1988;148–154.

62. Twycross RG, Lack SA. *Therapeutics in terminal cancer.* 2nd ed. New York: Churchill Livingstone, 1990.

63. Bruera E, Roca E, Cedaro L, et al. Action of oral methylprednisolone in terminal cancer patients: a prospective randomized double-blind study. *Cancer Treat Rep* 1985;69:751–754.

64. Gemlo B, Rayner AA, Lewis B, et al. Home support of patients with end-stage malignant bowel obstruction using hydration and venting gastrostomy. *Am J Surg* 1986;152:100–104.

65. McGuire DB, Yarbro CH, Ferrell BR. *Cancer pain management.* 2nd ed. Boston: Jones and Bartlett, 1995.

Index